T0362420

Third Edition

Electrical Power Transmission System Engineering

Analysis and Design

Third Edition

Electrical Power Transmission System Engineering

Analysis and Design

Turan Gönen
California State University, Sacramento, USA

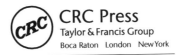

CRC Press
Taylor & Francis Group
Boca Raton   London   New York

CRC Press is an imprint of the
Taylor & Francis Group, an **informa** business

MATLAB® is a trademark of The MathWorks, Inc. and is used with permission. The MathWorks does not warrant the accuracy of the text or exercises in this book. This book's use or discussion of MATLAB® software or related products does not constitute endorsement or sponsorship by The MathWorks of a particular pedagogical approach or particular use of the MATLAB® software.

CRC Press
Taylor & Francis Group
6000 Broken Sound Parkway NW, Suite 300
Boca Raton, FL 33487-2742

© 2014 by Taylor & Francis Group, LLC
CRC Press is an imprint of Taylor & Francis Group, an Informa business

No claim to original U.S. Government works

Printed by CPI Group (UK) Ltd, Croydon, CR0 4YY on sustainably sourced paper
Version Date: 20140210

International Standard Book Number-13: 978-1-4822-3222-6 (Hardback)

Library of Congress Cataloging-in-Publication Data

Gonen, Turan.
  [Electric power distribution system engineering]
  Electric Power Transmission Engineering : Aanalysis and design / author, Turan Gonen. -- Third edition.
      pages cm
  Revised edition of: Electric power distribution system engineering / Turan Gonen. 2008.
  Includes bibliographical references and index.
    ISBN 978-1-4822-0700-2 (hardcover : alk. paper) 1. Electric power distribution. I. Title.

TK3001.G58 2014
621.319--dc23
                                                                          2013047009

**Visit the Taylor & Francis Web site at
http://www.taylorandfrancis.com**

**and the CRC Press Web site at
http://www.crcpress.com**

It is with great sadness that we learn of Turan's passing. Such a vibrant, funny, brilliant man, and a true professional. Thank you for all of the knowledge you have passed on to us with your words—your books have taught many great things to many great engineers.

On behalf of all of us at CRC Press, you will be greatly missed, Turan!

Nora Konopka, Publisher of Engineering

Turan's editor, friend, and one of his biggest fans.

OBITUARY

Dr. Turan Gönen, a leading expert and popular professor of electrical engineering at California State University, Sacramento, died Feb. 24 of a stroke, his family said. He was 72.

Dr. Gönen was widely respected in academia and industry for his scholarship in electrical and electronic engineering. Specializing in the area of electric power transmission, he authored numerous books and papers and traveled to many countries as a technical consultant to utilities, trade groups and government agencies.

He belonged to major professional and scientific organizations in the United States and his native Turkey. His 2013 textbook, "Electric Power Distribution System Engineering," is taught in college classrooms worldwide.

"I was meeting with someone the other day from the electric power industry and shared the sad news about Turan, and asked if he knew him," Tom Matthews, CSUS chair of electrical and electronic engineering. "He said, 'Only by reputation.' He was pretty well known."

Besides his impressive research, Dr. Gönen earned a reputation as a caring teacher and mentor. He supervised more than 100 graduate students over the years and helped many find jobs in industry and teaching. He was recognized by CSUS with outstanding teacher awards in 1997 and 2009.

Raised in a home that stressed education, Dr. Gönen was born Sept. 2, 1941, in Bursa, Turkey, to a family that included professional engineers in various fields. With a bachelor's and master's degree in electrical engineering from Istanbul Technical University, he determined at 27 to leave home for new opportunities.

"He didn't know any English, but he said, 'I'm going to go to the United States and make something of my life,'" his daughter Sevil said. "He got on a plane with an English dictionary and studied it all the way to Florida. He got off the plane and could speak a few words, enough to get around."

Dr. Gönen earned advanced degrees – including two doctorates in engineering – at Iowa State University and University of Oklahoma. He taught for three years at University of Missouri before joining CSUS in 1986.

Dr. Gönen had been active in the Sacramento chapter of the Turkish American Association of California. He lived in Sacramento and enjoyed gardening, visiting art museums and vacationing in Carmel.

"He was a serious person, but he loved to laugh and to make people laugh," his daughter said.

In addition to his daughter, Dr. Gönen is survived by his fiancée, Diane Kelly-Abrams.

We are all ignorant, just
about different things.

Mark Twain

There is so much good in the worst of us,
And so much bad in the best of us,
That it little behooves any of us,
To talk about the rest of us.

J. M.

For everything you have missed,
You have gained something else;
And for everything you gain,
You lose something else.

R. W. Emerson

Dedicated to my late brother,
Zaim Suat Gönen,
for giving me the motivation

Contents

Preface

The structure of the electric power system is very large and complex. Nevertheless, its main components (or subsystems) can be identified as the generation system, transmission system, and distribution system. These three systems are the basis of the electric power industry. Today, there are various textbooks dealing with a broad range of topics in the power system area of electrical engineering. Some of them are considered to be classics. However, they do not particularly concentrate on the topics dealing with electric power transmission. Therefore, this text is unique in that it is written specifically for an in-depth study of modern power transmission engineering.

This book has evolved from the content of courses given by the author at California State University, Sacramento, the University of Missouri at Columbia, the University of Oklahoma, and Florida International University. It has been written for senior-level undergraduate and beginning-level graduate students, as well as practicing engineers in the electric power utility industry. It can serve as a text for a two-semester course, or by judicious selection, the material in the text can also be condensed to suit a one-semester course.

This book has been particularly written for a student or practicing engineer who may want to teach himself or herself. Basic material has been explained carefully, clearly, and in detail with numerous examples. Each new term is clearly defined when it is first introduced. The special features of the book include ample numerical examples and problems designed to apply the information presented in each chapter. An effort has been made to familiarize the reader with the vocabulary and symbols used in the industry.

The addition of the numerous impedance tables for overhead lines, transformers, and underground cables makes the text self-contained.

The text is primarily divided into two parts: Section I—Electrical Design and Analysis and Section II—Mechanical Design and Analysis. Section I includes topics such as transmission system planning; basic concepts; environmental impact of transmission lines; transmission line parameters and the steady-state performance of transmission lines; flexible ac transmission systems (FACTS); supervisory control and data acquisition (SCADA); disturbance of the normal operating conditions and other problems; symmetrical components and sequence impedances; in-depth analysis of balanced and unbalanced faults; extensive review of transmission system protection; detailed study of transient overvoltages and insulation coordination; underground cables; and limiting factors for extra-high- and ultrahigh-voltage transmission in terms of corona, radio noise, and audible noise.

Section II includes topics such as construction of overhead lines, factors affecting transmission line route selection, right of way, insulator types, conductor vibration, sag and tension analysis, profile and plan of right of way, and templates for locating structures. Also included is a review of the methods for allocating transmission line fixed charges among joint users, new trends and regulations in transmission line construction, a guide to FERC: electric transmission facilities permit process, order number 1000 of FERC Federal Energy Regulatory Commission, and a glossary for transmission system engineering terminology.

Turan Gönen

MATLAB® is a registered trademark of The MathWorks, Inc. For product information, please contact:

The MathWorks, Inc.
3 Apple Hill Drive
Natick, MA 01760-2098 USA
Tel: 508-647-7000
Fax: 508-647-7001
E-mail: info@mathworks.com
Web: www.mathworks.com

Acknowledgments

I would like to express my sincere appreciation to Dr. Dave D. Robb of D. D. Robb and Associates for his encouragement and invaluable suggestions and friendship over the years.

I am indebted to numerous students who studied portions of the book, at California State University, Sacramento, the University of Missouri at Columbia, and the University of Oklahoma, and made countless contributions and valuable suggestions for improvements. I am also indebted to my past graduate students Mira Lopez; Joel Irvine of Pacific Gas & Electric Inc. and Tom Lyons of the Sacramento Municipal Utility District; Alex Takahashi, president of West Power Inc.; R.K. Ravuri of California State University, Sacramento; and Trevor Martin Oneal of Lawrence Livermore National Laboratory for their kind help.

Author

Turan Gönen is professor of electrical engineering at California State University, Sacramento (CSUS). He received his BS and MS in electrical engineering from Istanbul Technical College (1964 and 1966, respectively) and his PhD in electrical engineering from Iowa State University (1975). Dr. Gönen also received an MS in industrial engineering (1973) and a PhD comajor in industrial engineering (1978) from Iowa State University, as well as an MBA from the University of Oklahoma (1980).

Professor Gönen is the director of the Electrical Power Educational Institute at CSUS. Prior to this, he was professor of electrical engineering and director of the Energy Systems and Resources Program at the University of Missouri–Columbia. Professor Gönen also held teaching positions at the University of Missouri–Rolla, the University of Oklahoma, Iowa State University, Florida International University, and Ankara Technical College. He has taught electrical electric power engineering for over 40 years.

Professor Gönen also has a strong background in the power industry. He worked as a design engineer in numerous companies both in the United States and abroad for eight years. He has also served as a consultant for the United Nations Industrial Development Organization, Aramco, Black & Veatch Consultant Engineers, and the public utility industry. Recently, he was a consultant/senior engineer at the San Diego Gas and Electric company. Professor Gönen has written over 100 technical papers as well as four other books: *Modern Power System Analysis, Electric Power Distribution System Engineering, Electrical Machines*, and *Engineering Economy for Engineering Managers*.

Professor Gönen is a fellow of the Institute of Electrical and Electronics Engineers and a senior member of the Institute of Industrial Engineers. He served on several committees and working groups of the IEEE Power Engineering Society and is a member of numerous honor societies, including Sigma Xi, Phi Kappa Phi, Eta Kappa Nu, and Tau Alpha Pi. Professor Gönen received the Outstanding Teacher Award at CSUS in 1997 and 2009.

Section I

Electrical Design and Analysis

1 Transmission System Planning

It is curious that physical courage should be
so common in the world and moral courage so rare.

Mark Twain

1.1 INTRODUCTION

An *electrical power system* can be considered to consist of a *generation system*, a *transmission system*, a *subtransmission system*, and a *distribution system*. In general, the generation and transmission systems are referred to as the *bulk power supply*, and the subtransmission and distribution systems are considered to be the final means to transfer the electric power to the ultimate customer.

In the United States, the alternating current (ac) transmission system was developed from a necessity to transfer large blocks of energy from remote generation facilities to load centers. As the system developed, transmission additions were made to improve reliability, to achieve economic generation utilization through interconnections, and to strengthen the transmission backbone with higher-voltage overlays. *Bulk power transmission* is made up of a high-voltage network, generally 138–765 kV ac, designed to interconnect power plants and electric utility systems and to transmit power from the plants to major load centers.

Table 1.1 gives the standard transmission voltages up to 700 kV as dictated by ANSI Standard C-84 of the American National Standards Institute (ANSI). In the United States and Canada, 138, 230, 345, 500, and 765 kV are the most common transmission grid voltages. In Europe, voltages of 130, 275, and 400 kV are commonly used for the bulk power grid infrastructures.

The *subtransmission* refers to a lower-voltage network, normally 34.5–115 kV, interconnecting bulk power and distribution substations. The voltages that are in the range of 345–765 kV are classified as *extrahigh voltages* (EHVs). The EHV systems dictate a very thorough system design. While, on the contrary, high-voltage transmission systems up to 230 kV can be built in relatively simple and well-standardized designs, voltages above 765 kV are considered as the *ultrahigh voltages* (UHVs). Currently, the UHV systems, at 1000, 1100, 1500, and 2250 kV voltage levels, are in the R&D stages [34].

Figures 1.1 and 1.2 show three-phase double-circuit transmission lines made of steel towers. Figure 1.3 shows the installation of a 345 kV double-circuit transmission tower made of steel cage. Figure 1.4 shows a transmission line is being upgraded.

Figure 1.5 shows the trends in technology and cost of electrical energy (based on 1968 constant dollars). Historically, the decreasing cost of electrical energy has been due to the technological advances reflected in terms of economies of scale and operating efficiencies.

1.2 AGING TRANSMISSION SYSTEM

In the United States, the transmission network was built primarily in the 1950s or so to reliably serve local demands for power and interconnect neighboring utilities. By and large, it has done these without any significant problems. However, for the past 20 years, the growth of electricity demand has far outpaced the growth in transmission capacity. With limited new transmission capacity available, the loading of existing transmission lines has extremely increased. Since 1980, for example, the country's electricity use has increased by 75%. Based on the recent predictions, the demand will grow by another 30% within the next 10 years.

TABLE 1.1
Standard System Voltages

Rating	
Nominal (kV)	Maximum (kV)
34.5	36.5
46	48.3
69	72.5
115	121
138	145
161	169
230	242
345	362
500	550
700	765

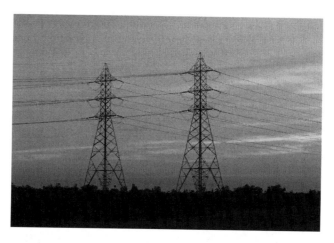

FIGURE 1.1 A three-phase double-circuit transmission line made of steel towers.

Nowadays, the transmission grid is also carrying a growing number of wholesale electricity transactions. Just in the last 5 years, the amount of these deals has grown by 300%. At times, this has left the transmission grid facing more requests for transmission than it can handle. This means that generation from distant sources, which can often be more economical, cannot get through.

According to Fama [37], after recognizing the growing demand being placed on the transmission grid, today the utility industry is beginning to spend more money on new transmission lines and/or upgrading existing transmission lines. As it is indicated in Table 1.2, both integrated and stand-alone transmission companies are investing heavily to expand transmission capacity. During 1999–2003, for example, privately owned utilities increased their annual transmission investment by 12% annually, for a total of US $17 billion. Through year 2008, preliminary data indicated that utilities invested, or planned to invest, US $28 billion more. This is a 60% increase over the previous 5 years.

However, even with this new spending, the continually increasing demand for electricity, together with the expanding number of wholesale market transactions, means that more investment will be necessary.

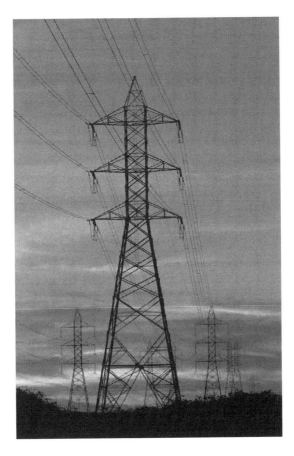

FIGURE 1.2 A three-phase double-circuit transmission line made of steel towers.

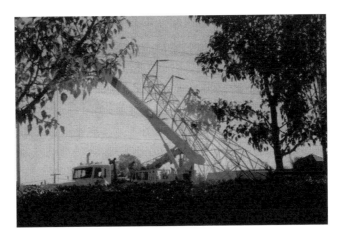

FIGURE 1.3 Installation of a 345 kV double-circuit transmission tower made of steel cage.

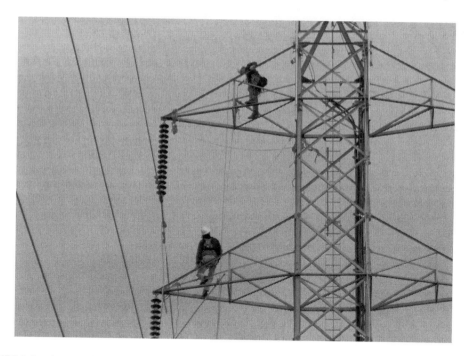

FIGURE 1.4   A transmission line is being upgraded.

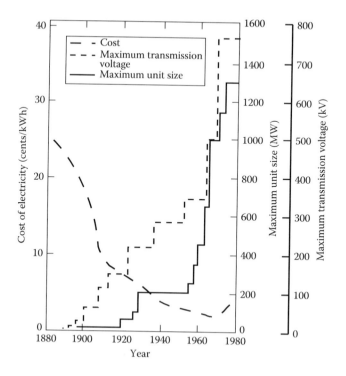

FIGURE 1.5   Historical trends in technology and cost of electrical energy of the past until year 1980. (From Electric Power Research Institute, *Transmission Line Reference Book: 345 kV and Above*, EPRI, Palo Alto, CA, 1979. © 1979 Electric Power Research Institute. Used by permission.)

TABLE 1.2
Actual and Planned Transmission Investment
by Privately Owned Integrated and Stand-Alone
Transmission Companies

Year	Actual Transmission Investment (in Million US $)	Planned Transmission Investment (in Million US $)
1999	2585	—
2000	3614	—
2001	3704	—
2002	3785	—
2003	4107	—
2004	—	4567
2005	—	5678
2006	—	6041
2007	—	6141
2008	—	6111

1.3 BENEFITS OF TRANSMISSION

The primary function of transmission is to transmit bulk power from sources of desirable generation to bulk power delivery points. Benefits have traditionally included lower electrical energy costs, access to renewable energy such as wind and hydro, locating power plants away from large population centers, and access to alternative generation sources when primary sources are not available.

In the past, transmission planning and its construction have been done by individual utilities with a focus on local benefits. However, today proponents of nationwide transmission policies now consider the transmission system as an *enabler* of energy policy objectives at even the national level. According to Morrow and Brown [36], this view is reasonable since a well-planned transmission grid has the potential to provide for the following:

1. *Hedge against generation outages.* The transmission system should typically permit access to alternative economic energy sources to replace lost sources.
2. *Efficient bulk power markets.* Bulk power needs should be met by the lowest-cost generation, instead of by higher-cost electricity purchases to prevent violation of transmission loading constraints. (The difference between the actual price of electricity at the point of usage and the lowest price on the grid is called the *congestion cost.*)
3. *Operational flexibility.* The transmission system should permit for the economic scheduling of maintenance outages and for the economic reconfiguration of the grid when unforeseen events take place.
4. *Hedge against fuel price changes.* The transmission system should permit purchases to economically access generation from diversified fuel resources as a hedge against fuel disruptions due to various causes.
5. *Low-cost access to renewable energy.* The transmission system should usually permit developers to build renewable energy sources without the need for expensive transmission upgrades.

The aforementioned benefits are not fully achieved on a regional or national level, since planning has traditionally been focused on providing these benefits at the local level [36].

TABLE 1.3

1980 Regional Transmission Lines in Miles

	Voltage (kV)						
	HVAC				HVDC		
Region	230	345	500	765	250	400/450	800
ECAR	934	9.850	796	1.387	0	0	0
ERCOT	0	4.110	0	0	0	0	0
MAAC	4.400	160	1.263	0	0	0	0
MAIN	258	4.852	0	90	0	0	0
MARCA (United States)	6.477	3.504	138	0	465	436	0
NPCC (United States)	1.557	3.614	5	251	0	0	0
SERC	16.434	2	4.363	0	0	0	0
SPP	3.057	2.843	1.432	0	0	0	0
WSCC (United States)	27.892	5.923	7.551	0	0	0	844
NERC (United States)	61.009	34.858	15.548	1.728	465	436	844

Source: National Electric Reliability Council, *10th Annual Review of Overall Reliability and Adequacy of the North American Bulk Power Systems*, NERC, Princeton, NJ, 1980.

1.4 POWER POOLS

Interchange of power between neighboring utilities using interconnecting transmission lines was economically advantageous in the past. But, when a system is interconnected with many neighbors, the process of setting up one transaction at a time with each neighbor can become very time consuming and would have rarely resulted in the best economic interchange. In order to solve this problem, several utilities may have formed a power pool that incorporates a central dispatch office.

Hence, the power pool was administered from a central location that had responsibility for setting up interchanges between members as well as other administrative tasks. For example, if one member's transmission system was heavily loaded with power flows that mainly benefited that member's neighbors, then that system was entitled to a reimbursement for the use of the transmission lines.

In the United States, there are also regional reliability councils that coordinate the reliability aspects of the transmission operations. Table 1.3 gives the lengths of the high-voltage ac (HVAC) and high-voltage dc (HVDC) transmission lines installed in the service areas of the regional reliability councils up to the year 1980.

1.5 TRANSMISSION PLANNING

Transmission planning is closely related to generation planning. The objectives of transmission planning are to develop year-to-year plans for the transmission system based on existing systems, future load and generation scenarios, right-of-way (ROW) constraints, cost of construction, line capabilities, and reliability criteria.

In general, transmission lines have two primary objectives: (1) to transmit electrical energy* from the generators to the load centers within a single utility and (2) to provide paths for electrical energy to flow between utilities. These latter lines are called *tie lines* and enable the utility companies to operate as a team to gain benefits that would otherwise not be obtainable. Interconnections,

---

* The term *energy* is being increasingly used in the electric power industry to replace the conventional term *power*. Here, they are used interchangeably.

or the installation of transmission circuits across utility boundaries, influence both generation and transmission planning of each utility involved.

When power systems are electrically connected by transmission lines, they must operate at the same frequency, that is, the same number of cycles per second, and the pulse of the ac must be coordinated. As a corollary, generator speeds, which determine frequency, must also be coordinated. The various generators are said to be *stable*.

A sharp or sudden change in loading at a generator will affect the frequency, but if the generator is strongly interconnected with other generators, they will normally help to absorb the effect on the changed loading so that the change in frequency will be negligible and system stability unaffected. Hence, the installation of an interconnection affects generation planning substantially in terms of the amount of generation capacity required, the reserve generation capacity, and the type of generation capacity required for operation.

Also, interconnections may affect the generation planning through the installation of apparatus owned jointly by neighboring utilities and the planning of generating units with greater capacity than would be otherwise feasible for a single utility without interconnections. Furthermore, interconnection planning affects transmission planning by moving required bulk power deliveries away from or to interconnection substations, that is, bulk power substations, and often the addition of circuits on a given utility's own network [32].

Subtransmission planning includes planning activities for the major supply of bulk stations, subtransmission lines from the stations to distribution substations, and the high-voltage portion of the distribution substations.

Furthermore, distribution planning must take into consideration not only substation siting, sizing, number of feeders to be served, voltage levels, and type and size of the service area but also the coordination of overall subtransmission, and even transmission planning efforts, in order to ensure the most reliable and cost-effective system design [40].

1.6 TRADITIONAL TRANSMISSION SYSTEM PLANNING TECHNIQUES

The purpose of *transmission system planning* is to determine the timing and type of new transmission facilities required in order to provide adequate transmission network capability to cope with the future generating capacity additions and load-flow requirements.

Figure 1.6 shows a functional block diagram of a typical transmission system planning process. This process may be repeated, with diminishing detail, for each year of a long-range (15–20-year) planning horizon. The key objective is to minimize the long-range capital and operating costs involved in providing an adequate level of system reliability, with due consideration of environmental and other relevant issues.

Transmission planning may include not only existing but also new service areas. The starting point of the planning procedure is to develop load forecasts in terms of annual peak demand for the entire system, as well as for each region and each major present and future substation, and then finding specific alternatives that satisfy the new load conditions. The system performance is tested under *steady-state* and *contingency* conditions.

The logic diagram for transmission expansion study is shown in Figure 1.7. The main objective is to identify the potential problems, in terms of unacceptable voltage conditions, overloading of facilities, decreasing reliability, or any failure of the transmission system to meet performance criteria. After this analysis stage, the planner develops *alternative plans* or *scenarios* that not only will prevent the foreseen problems but also will best meet the long-term objectives of system reliability and economy. The effectiveness of the alternative plans is determined by *load-flow*, or *power-flow*, *studies under both normal and emergency operations*.

The load-flow programs now in use by the utilities allow the calculation of currents, voltages, and real and reactive power flows, taking into account the voltage-regulating capability of generators, transformers, synchronous condensers, specified generation schedules, as well as net interchange among

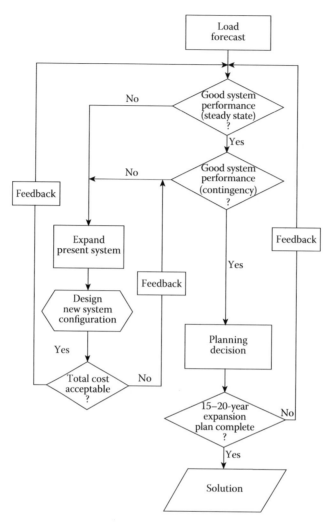

FIGURE 1.6 Block diagram of typical transmission system planning process.

interconnected systems, automatically. By changing the location, size, and number of transmission lines, the planner can achieve to design an economical system that meets the operating and design criteria.

After determining the best system configuration from load-flow studies, the planner studies the system behavior under fault conditions. The main objectives of short-circuit studies can be expressed as follows: (1) to determine the current-interrupting capacity of the circuit breaker so that the faulted equipment can be disconnected successfully, therefore clearing the fault from the system, and (2) to establish the relay requirements and settings to detect the fault and cause the circuit breaker to operate when the current flowing through it exceeds the maximum allowable current.

The short-circuit studies can also be used to (1) calculate voltages during faulted conditions that affect insulation coordination and lightning arrester applications, (2) design the grounding systems, and (3) determine the electromechanical forces affecting the facilities of the system.

Finally, the planner performs stability studies in order to be sure that the system will remain stable following a severe fault or disturbance. Here, the *stability analysis* is defined as the transient behavior of the power system following a disturbance. It can be classified as transient stability analysis. The *transient stability* is defined as the ability of the system to maintain synchronous operation following a disturbance, usually a fault condition.

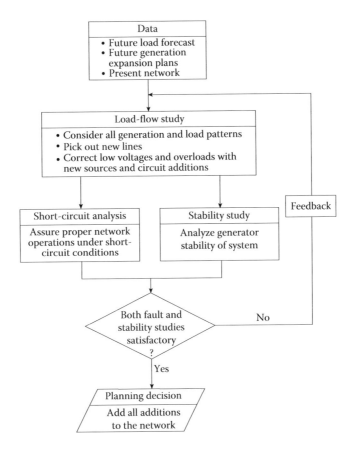

FIGURE 1.7   Logic diagram for transmission expansion study.

Unless the fault condition is cleared rapidly by circuit breakers, the generators, which are connected to each other through a transmission network, will get out with respect to one another, that is, they will *not run in synchronism*.

This situation, in turn, will cause large currents to flow through the network, transferring power from one generator to another in an oscillating way and causing the power system to become *unstable*. Consequently, the protective relays will detect these excessive amounts of currents and activate circuit breakers all over the network to open, causing a complete loss of power supply.

Usually, the first swing of rotor angles is considered to be an adequate indicator of whether or not the power system remains stable. Therefore, the simulation of the first few seconds following a disturbance is sufficient for transient stability. Whereas steady-state stability analysis is defined as long-term fluctuations in system frequency and power transfers resulting in *total blackouts*,* in this case, the system is simulated from a few seconds to several minutes.

There are various computer programs available for the planner to study the transient and steady-state stabilities of the system. In general, a *transient stability program* employs the data, in terms of initial voltages and power flows, provided by a load-flow program as the input and transforms the system to that needed for the transient stability analysis.

---

* The IEEE (Institute of Electrical and Electronics Engineers) has redefined *steady-state stability* to include the manifestation formerly included in both *steady-state* and *dynamic stabilities*. The purpose of this change is to bring American practice into agreement with international practice. Therefore, dynamic stability is no longer found in the IEEE publications unless the reviewers happened to overlook the old usage.

Usually, the *critical switching time*, that is, the time during which a faulted system component must be tripped to assure stability, is used as an indicator of *stability margin*. The critical switching times are calculated for various fault types and locations. The resultant *minimum required clearing time* is compared to actual relay and circuit breaker operating time.

If the relays and circuit breakers cannot operate rapidly enough to maintain stable operation, the planner may consider a change in the network design or a change in the turbine-generator characteristics or perhaps control apparatus.

1.7 MODELS USED IN TRANSMISSION SYSTEM PLANNING

In the past, the transmission system planning and design were rather intuitive and based substantially on the planner's past experience. Today, the planner has numerous analysis and synthesis tools at his disposal. These tools can be used for design and planning activities, such as (1) transmission route identification and selection, (2) transmission network expansion planning, (3) network analysis, and (4) reliability analysis. The first two of these will be discussed in this chapter.

1.8 TRANSMISSION ROUTE IDENTIFICATION AND SELECTION

Figure 1.8 shows a typical *transmission route (corridor)* selection procedure. The restricting factors affecting the process are safety, engineering and technology, system planning, institutional, economics, environmental, and aesthetics. Today, the planner selects the appropriate transmission route based on his knowledge of the system, results of the system analysis, and available ROWs.

However, recently, two computer programs, Power and Transthetics, have been developed to aid the planner in transmission route identification and selection [1–3]. The Power computer program can be used to locate not only transmission line corridors but also other types of corridors. In contrast, the Transthetics computer program is specifically designed for electrical utilities for the purpose of identifying and selecting potential transmission line corridors and purchasing the necessary ROWs.

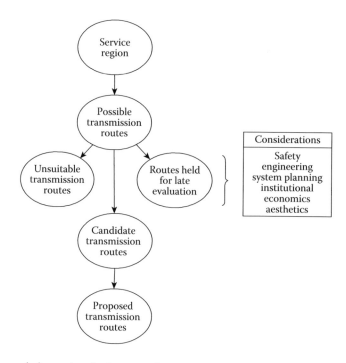

FIGURE 1.8   Transmission route selection procedure.

1.9 TRADITIONAL TRANSMISSION SYSTEM EXPANSION PLANNING

In the past, the system planner mostly used to use tools such as load-flow, stability, and short-circuit programs in analyzing the performance of specific transmission system alternatives. However, some utilities also employed the use of so-called automatic expansion models to determine the optimum system.

Here, the optimality claim is in the mathematical sense; that is, the optimum system is the one that minimizes an objective function (performance function) subject to restrictions. In general, the automatic expansion models can be classified into three basic groups:

1. Heuristic models
2. Single-stage optimization models
3. Time-phased optimization models

1.9.1 HEURISTIC MODELS

The primary advantage of the *heuristic models* was interactive planning. The system planner can observe the *expansion process* and direct its direction as it is desired. According to Meckiff et al. [4], the characteristics of the heuristic models are (1) simple model and logic, (2) user interaction, and (3) families of *feasible*, *near-optimal* plans.

In contrast, the characteristics of the mathematical programming models are (1) no user interaction, (2) fixed model by program formulation, (3) detailed logic or restriction set definition, and (4) single *global* solution.

The heuristic models can be considered to be custom-made, contrary to mathematical models. Some help to simulate the way a system planner uses analytical tools such as load-flow programs [5,6] and reliability analysis [6] involving simulations of the planning process through automated design logic. The classical paper by Garver [7] describes a method that unites heuristic logic for circuit selection with optimization techniques. The proposed method is to determine the most direct route transmission network from the generation to load without causing any circuit overloads. In heuristic approach, the best circuit addition or exchange is given to the planner by the computer program automatically at each stage of the synthesis process. The planner may select to accept it or modify it as he desires. Further information on heuristic models is given in Baldwin et al. [8–11].

1.9.2 SINGLE-STAGE OPTIMIZATION MODELS

The *single-stage* or *single-state* (or so-called *static*) optimization models can be used for determining the *optimum network expansion* from one stage to the next. But *they do not give the timing of the expansion*. Therefore, even though they provide an optimum solution for year-by-year expansion, they may not give the optimum solution for overall expansion pattern over a time horizon. The mathematical programming techniques used in single-state optimization models include (1) linear programming (LP), (2) integer programming, and (3) gradient search method.

1.9.2.1 Linear Programming

LP is a mathematical technique that can be used to minimize or maximize a given linear function, called the *objective function* in which the variables are subject to linear constraints. The objective function takes the linear form

$$Z = \sum_{i=1}^{n} c_i x_i \qquad (1.1)$$

where Z is the value to be optimized. (In expansion studies, Z is the total cost that is to be minimized.) The x_i represents n unknown quantities, and the c_i are the costs associated with one unit of x_i. The c_i may be positive or negative, whereas the x_i must be defined in a manner as to assume only positive values. The constraints, or restrictions, are limitations on the values that the unknowns may assume and must be a linear combination of the unknowns. The constraints assume the form

$$\sum a_{ji} =, \geq, \leq b_j \quad x_i \geq 0 \tag{1.2}$$

or

$$a_{11}x_1 + a_{12}x_2 + \cdots + a_{1n}x_n =, \geq, \leq b_1$$

$$a_{21}x_1 + a_{22}x_2 + \cdots + a_{2n}x_n =, \geq, \leq b_2$$

$$\cdots\cdots\cdots\cdots\cdots\cdots\cdots\cdots\cdots\cdots\cdots\cdots\cdots\cdots$$

$$a_{m1}x_1 + a_{m2}x_2 + \cdots + a_{mn}x_n =, \geq, \leq b_m$$

$$x_1 \geq 0, x_2 \geq 0, \ldots, x_n \geq 0$$

where

$$j = 1, 2, \ldots, m \quad \text{and} \quad j = 1, 2, \ldots, n$$

where there are m constraints of which any number may be equalities or inequalities. Also, the number of constraints, m, may be greater than, less than, or equal to the number of unknowns, n. The coefficients of the unknowns, a_{ij}, may be positive, negative, or zero but must be constants. The b_j are also constants, which may be positive, negative, or zero. The constraints define a region of solution feasibility in n-dimensional space. The optimum solution is the point within this space whose x_i values minimize or maximize the objective function Z. In general, the solutions obtained are real and positive.

In 1970, Garver [7] developed a method that uses LP and linear flow estimation models in the formulation of an *automated transmission-system-planning algorithm*. The method helps to determine where capacity shortages exist and where to add new circuits to alleviate overloads. The objective function is the sum of the circuit lengths (guide numbers) times the magnitude of power that they transport.

Here, the power flows are calculated using *a linear loss function network model* that is similar to a transportation model. This model uses Kirchhoff's current law (i.e., at each bus, the sum of all flows in and out must sum to zero) but not Kirchhoff's voltage law to specify flows. Instead, the model uses *guide potentials* to assure that conventional circuits are not overloaded. However, the flow model also uses *overload paths*, in which power can flow if required, to determine where circuit additions are to be added. The network is expanded one circuit at a time to eliminate the path with the largest overload until no overload paths exist. After the completion of the network expansion, the system is usually tested, employing an ac load-flow program. As mentioned, the method is also heuristic partly due to the fact that assigning the guide numbers involves a great deal of judgment [12,13]. A similar method has been suggested by Kaltenbach et al. [14]. However, it treats the problem more rigidly as an optimization problem.

1.9.2.2 Integer Programming

The term *integer programming* refers to the class of LP problems in which some or all of the decision variables are restricted to be integers. For example, in order to formulate the LP given in

Equations 1.1 and 1.2 as an integer program, a binary variable can be introduced for each line to denote whether it is selected or not:

$$x_i = 1 \quad \text{if line } i \text{ is selected}$$

$$x_i = 0 \quad \text{if line } i \text{ is } not \text{ selected}$$

Therefore,

$$\text{minimize } Z = \sum_{i=1}^{n} c_i x_i \tag{1.3}$$

subject to

$$\sum_{i=1}^{n} a_{ji} x_i \le b_j \quad x_i = 0,1 \tag{1.4}$$

where $j = 1, 2,…, m$ and $i = 1, 2,…, n$.

In general, integer programming is *more suitable* for the transmission expansion problem than LP because it takes into account the discrete nature of the problem; that is, a line component is either added or not added to the network. The integer program wherein all variables are restricted to be (0–1) integer valued is called a *pure integer program*. Conversely, if the program restricts some of the variables to be integers while others can take continuous (fractional) values, it is called a *mixed-integer program*.

In 1960, Knight [15,16] applied integer programming to the transmission expansion problem. Adams and Laughton [17] used mixed-integer programming for optimal planning of power networks. Lee et al. [18] and Sjelvgren and Bubenko [19] proposed methods that employ a combination of sensitivity and screening procedures to restrict the search on a limited number of new additions that are most likely to meet all restrictions.

The method proposed by Lee et al. [18] starts with a direct current (dc) load-flow solution to distinguish the overloaded lines as well as to compute the line-flow sensitivities to changes in admittances in all transmission corridors. In order to reduce the dimension of the integer programming problem in terms of number of variables and therefore the computer time, it employs a screening process to eliminate ineffective corridors.

The resulting problem is then solved by a branch-and-bound technique. It adds capacity only in discrete increments as defined by the optimal capacity cost curves. The process is repeated as many times as necessary until all restrictions are satisfied. Further information on integer programming models is given in Gönen et al. [21,22].

1.9.2.3 Gradient Search Method

The gradient search method is a nonlinear mathematical programming applicable to the so-called automated transmission system planning. Here, the objective function that is to be minimized is a performance index of the given transmission network.

The method starts with a *dc load-flow solution* for the initial transmission network and future load and generation forecasts. The system performance index is calculated, and the necessary circuit modifications are made using the partial derivatives of the performance index with respect to circuit admittances. Again, a dc load-flow solution is obtained, and the procedure is repeated as many times as necessary until a network state is achieved for which no further decrease in the performance index can be obtained.

The method proposed by Fischl and Puntel [23] applies Tellegen's theorem. The gradient information necessary to update the susceptances associated with effective line additions as aforementioned was implemented. More detailed information can also be found in Puntel et al. [24,25].

1.9.3 TIME-PHASED OPTIMIZATION MODELS

The single-stage transmission network expansion models do not take into account the timing of new installations through a given time horizon. Therefore, as Garver [26] points out, there is a need for *a method of finding a sequence of yearly transmission plans which result in the lowest revenue requirements through time but which may be higher in cost than really needed in any one particular year.*

A *time-phased* (*through-time*, or *multistate*, or the so-called *dynamic*) optimization model can include inflation, interest rates, as well as yearly operating cost in the comparison of various network expansion plans.

Both integer programming and dynamic programming optimization methods have been used to solve the time-phased network expansion models [27]. The *integer programming* has been applied by dividing a given time horizon into numerous annual subperiods. Consequently, the objective function in terms of present worth of a cost function is minimized in order to determine the capacity, location, and timing of new facilities subject to defined constraints [17,22,28].

The *dynamic programming* [24] has been applied to network expansion problems by developing a set of network configurations for each year (stage). Only those feasible plans (states) that satisfy the defined restrictions are accepted. However, as Garver [26] points out, *the dynamic programming method has organized the search so that a minimum number of evaluations were necessary to find the lowest cost expansion. However, the dynamic programming method by itself cannot introduce new plans (states), it only links given states together in an optimal manner.*

Dusonchet and El-Abiad [29] applied discrete dynamic optimization employing a combination of dynamic programming, a random search, and a heuristic stopping criterion. Henault et al. [28] studied the problem in the presence of uncertainty. Mamandur and Berg [30] applied the *k-shortest paths* method to replace dynamic programming for transmission network expansion. The k-shortest paths technique [31] is employed to determine the expansion plans with the minimum costs.

1.10 TRADITIONAL CONCERNS FOR TRANSMISSION SYSTEM PLANNING*

In the previous sections, some of the techniques used by the system planning engineers of the utility industry performing transmission system planning have been discussed. Also, the factors affecting the transmission system planning have been reviewed. The purpose of this section is to examine what today's trends are likely to bring for the future of the planning process.

There are several traditional economic factors that will still have significant effects on the transmission system planning of the future. The first of these is inflation; fueled by energy shortages, energy source conversion costs, environmental concerns, and large government deficits, it will continue to play a major role.

The second important economic factor will still be the increasing expense of acquiring capital. As long as inflation continues to decrease the real value of the dollar, attempts will be made by the government to reduce the money supply. This, in turn, will increase the competition for attracting the capital necessary for expansions in power systems.

---

* This section is based on Gönen [32]. Included with permission of CRC Press.

The third factor, which must be considered, is increasing difficulty in increasing customer rates. This rate increase *inertia* also stems in part from inflation as well as from the results of customers being made more sensitive to rate increases by consumer activist groups.

Predictions about the future methods for transmission system planning must necessarily be extrapolations of present methods. Basic algorithms for network analysis have been known for years and are not likely to be improved upon in the near future. However, the superstructure that supports these algorithms and the problem-solving environment used by the system designer is expected to change significantly to take advantage of new methods technology has made possible. Before giving a detailed discussion of these expected changes, the changing role of transmission system planning needs to be examined.

For the economic reasons listed earlier, transmission systems will become more expensive to build, expand, and modify. Thus, it is particularly important that each transmission system design be as cost-effective as possible. This means that the system must be optimal from many points of view over the time period from the first day of operation to the planning time horizon. In addition to the accurate load growth estimates, components must be phased in and out of the system so as to minimize capital expenditure, meet performance goals, and minimize losses [20].

In the utility industry, the most powerful force shaping the future is that of economics. Therefore, any new innovations are not likely to be adopted for their own sake. These innovations will be adopted only if they reduce the cost of some activity or provide something of economic value that previously had been unavailable for comparable costs. In predicting that certain practices or tools will replace current ones, it is necessary that one judge their acceptance on this basis.

The expected innovations that satisfy these criteria are planning tools implemented on a digital computer that deals with transmission systems in network terms. One might be tempted to conclude that these planning tools would be adequate for industry use throughout the future.

1.10.1 PLANNING TOOLS

Tools to be considered fall into two categories: network design tools and network analysis tools. Analysis tools may become more efficient but are not expected to undergo any major changes, although the environment in which they are used will change significantly. This environment will be discussed in the next section.

Design tools, however, are expected to show the greatest development since better planning could have a significant impact on the utility industry. The results of this development will show the following characteristics:

1. Network design will be optimized with respect to many criteria using programming methods of operations research.
2. Network design will be only one facet of transmission system management directed by human engineers using a computer system designed for such management functions.
3. So-called network editors [33] will be available for designing trial networks; these designs in digital form will be passed to extensive simulation programs that will determine if the proposed network satisfies performance and load growth criteria.

1.10.2 SYSTEMS APPROACH

A collection of computer programs to solve the analysis problems of a designer does not necessarily constitute an efficient problem-solving system nor even does such a collection when the output of one can be used as the input of another.

The systems approach to the design of a useful tool for the designer begins by examining the types of information required and its sources. The view taken is that this information generates decisions and additional information that pass from one stage of the design process to

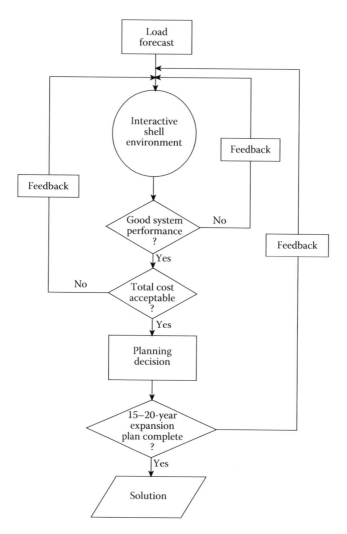

FIGURE 1.9   Schematic view of transmission planning system.

another. At certain points, it is noted that the human engineer must evaluate the information generated and add his inputs. Finally, the results must be displayed for use and stored for later reference.

With this conception of the planning process, the systems approach seeks to automate as much of the process as possible, ensuring in the process that the various transformations of information are made as efficiently as possible. One representation of this information flow is shown in Figures 1.9 and 1.10. Here, the outer circle represents the interface between the engineer and the system. Analysis programs forming part of the system are supported by a database management system (DBMS) that stores, retrieves, and modifies various data on transmission systems.

1.10.3 DATABASE CONCEPT

As suggested in Figure 1.10, the database plays a central role in the operation of such a system. It is in this area that technology has made some significant strides in the past 5 years so that not only is it possible to store vast quantities of data economically, but it is also possible to retrieve desired data with access times on the order of seconds.

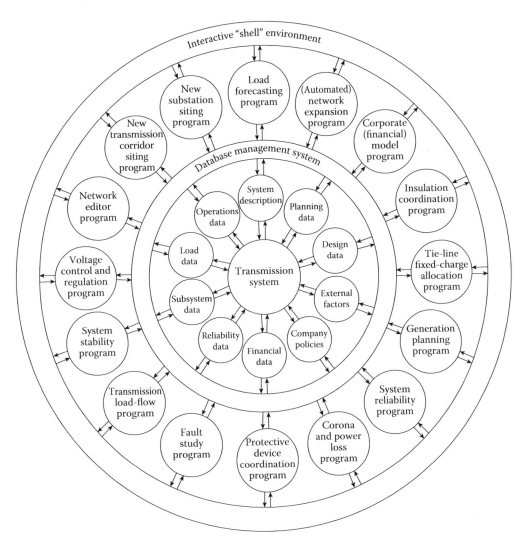

FIGURE 1.10 Block diagram of future transmission-system-planning process.

The DBMS provides the interface between the process, which requires access to the data, and the data itself. The particular organization likely to emerge as the dominant one in the near future is based on the idea of a relation. Operations on the database are performed by the DBMS.

In addition to the database management program and the network analysis programs, it is expected that some new tools will emerge to assist the designer in arriving at the optimal design. One such new tool that has appeared in the literature is known as a network editor [41].

Future transmission systems will be more complex than those of today. This means that the distribution system planner's task will be more complex. If the systems being planned are to be optimal with respect to construction cost, capitalization, performance, and operating efficiency, better planning tools are required. While it is impossible to foresee all of the effects that technology will have on the way in which transmission system planning will be done, it is possible to identify the major forces beginning to institute a change in the methodology and extrapolate.

The most important single influence is that of the computer, which will permit the automating of more and more of the planning activity. The automation will proceed along two major avenues.

First, increased application of operations research techniques will be made to meet performance requirements in the most economical way.

Second, improvements in database technology will permit the planner to utilize far more information in an automatic way than has been possible in the recent past. Interactive computer systems will display network configurations, cost information, device ratings, etc., at the whim of the planner. Moreover, this information will be available to sophisticated planning programs that will modify the database as new systems are designed and old ones are modified.

1.11 NEW TECHNICAL CHALLENGES

With authority over the rates, terms, and conditions of wholesale electric sales and transmission in interstate commerce, the Federal Energy Regulatory Commission (FERC) plays an important role in stimulating investment in the grid.

Today, the primary technical challenges for the transmission planning are reliability and congestion. Here, reliability relates to unexpected transmission contingencies, including faults, and the ability of the system to respond to these contingencies without interrupting load. Congestion takes place when transmission reliability limitations dictate to use higher-cost generation than would be the case without any reliability constraints.

In the United States, transmission reliability is tracked and managed by National Electric Reliability Council (NERC) that now serves as the federal electric reliability organization (ERO) under the jurisdiction of the FERC since 2006.

In the past, the main reliability consideration used by the NERC for transmission planning has been known as $N - 1$. This concept can be explained as follows. For a system that has N main components, the $N - 1$ criterion is satisfied if the system can perform satisfactorily with only $N - 1$ components in service. A given $N - 1$ analysis consists of a steady-state and a dynamic part.

The purpose of the steady-state analysis is to find out if the transmission system can withstand the loss of any single major piece of apparatus, such as a large transformer or a transmission line, without sacrificing voltage or equipment loading limits. On the other hand, the purpose of the dynamic analysis is to find out if the system can retain synchronism after all potential faults.

Up to now, $N - 1$ has served the power industry well. But it has several challenges when applied to transmission planning today. The first one is its *deterministic nature*. That is, $N - 1$ treats all contingencies as equal regardless of how likely such contingencies are to take place or the severity of consequences. The second one is the inability of $N - 1$, and $N - 2$, to take into account for the increased risk associated with a more heavily interconnected system and a more heavily loaded system.

When a system is able to withstand any single major contingency, it is called $N - 1$ *secure*. A moderately loaded $N - 1$ secure system can handle most single contingencies more or less fairly. However, a single contingency can significantly stress the system when many components of the transmission system are operated close to their thermal or stability limits. This situation can be prevented if all protection systems operate perfectly and preventive actions are taken properly and promptly. Heavily loaded systems can carry the risk of widespread outages in the event of a protection system failure. The $N - 1$ and $N - 3$ secure systems are not secure enough for wide-area events since blackouts involve multiple contingencies and/or cascading events. In the event that transmission failure rates double due to aging and greater loading, the possibility of a third-order event increases by a factor of eight or more.

According to Morrow and Brown [36], transmission system planners also face the problem of congestion. The basic congestion planning steps are as follows:

1. Hourly loads for an entire year are assigned to each bulk power delivery point.
2. A power flow is performed for each hour, taking into account scheduled generation and transmission maintenance.
3. If transmission reliability criteria are violated, the necessary corrective actions are taken. For example, generation redispatch is done until the restrictions are removed.
4. The additional energy costs due to these corrective actions are assigned to congestion cost.

In general, there are numerous ways to solve existing congestion problems. However, it is difficult to combine congestion planning with reliability planning. Hence, a congestion simulation that takes into account for unplanned contingencies is required.

In the past, a transmission planner was mainly concerned with the transmission of bulk power to load centers without violating any local restrictions. Today, a transmission planner has to have a wide-area perspective, being aware of aging infrastructure, having an economic mindset, willing to coordinate extensively, and having an ability for effectively integrating the new technologies with traditional methods.

Today, the North American power grid faces many challenges that it was not designed and built for properly handling them. On the one hand, congestion and atypical power flows threaten to overwhelm the transmission grid system of the country, while on the other hand, demand increases for higher reliability and improved security and protection. Because of the fact that modern infrastructure systems are so highly interconnected, a change in conditions at any one location can have immediate impact over a wide area. Hence, the effect of a local disturbance even can be magnified as it propagates through a network. The vulnerability of the US transmission grid to cascading effects has been demonstrated by the wide-area outages of the late 1990s and summer of 2003. The increased risks due to interdependencies have been compounded by the following additional reasons:

1. Deregulation and the growth of competition among the electricity providers have eroded spare transmission capacity that served as a useful shock absorber.
2. Mergers among infrastructure providers have led to further pressures to reduce spare capacity as companies have sought to eliminate excess costs.
3. The issue of interdependent and cascading effects among infrastructures has received very minimum attention.

Today, practical methods, tools, and technologies (based on advances in the fields of engineering, computation, control, and communications) are allowing power grids and other infrastructures to locally self-regulate, including automatic reconfiguration in the event of failures or disturbances [39].

According to Amin and Wollenberg [39], power transmission systems in the United States also suffer from the fact that intelligence is only applied locally by protection systems and by central control through the supervisory control and data acquisition (SCADA) system. In some cases, the central control system is too slow. Also, the protection systems by design are only limited to the protection of specific components.

Amin and Wollenberg [39] suggest providing intelligence to an electric power transmission system by adding independent processors into each component and at each substation and power plant. They must be able to act as *independent agents* that can communicate and cooperate with others, establishing a large distributed computed platform. Hence, each agent must be connected to sensors related to its own component or its own substation so that it can assess its own operating conditions and report them to its neighboring agents via the communications paths. For example, a processor associated with a circuit breaker would have the ability to communicate with sensors built into the breaker and communicate the sensor values using high-bandwidth fiber communications connected to other such processor agents.

At the present time, there are two kinds of intelligent systems that are used to protect and operate transmission systems in the United States. These are the protection systems and the SCADA/EMS/ independent system operator (ISO) systems.

According to Amin and Wollenberg [39], based on the modern computer and communication technologies, the transmission system planners must think beyond existing protection systems and the central control systems (i.e., the SCADA/EMS/ISO systems) to a fully distributed system that places intelligent devices at each component, substation, and power plant. Such distributed system will finally enable the utility industry to build a *truly smart transmission grid*.

1.12   TRANSMISSION PLANNING AFTER OPEN ACCESS

In 1996, the FERC Order 888 has created the *Open Access Tariff* in the United States. It requires functional separation of generation and transmission within a vertically integrated utility. For example, a generation queue process is now required to be sure that generation interconnection requests are processed in a nondiscriminatory way and in the order of FIFO, that is, first-in first-out or served order.

Also, the FERC Order 889 (the companion of Order 888) has established an Open Access Same-time Information System (OASIS) process that requires transmission service request, both external and internal, to be publicly posted and processed in the order in which they are entered.

Similarly, Order 889 requires each utility to ensure nonpreferential treatment of its own generation plan. Effectively, generation and transmission planning, even within the same utility, are not permitted to be coordinated and integrated. This has been done to protect nondiscriminatory, open access to the electric system for all parts.

Also, these landmark orders have removed barriers to market participation by entities such as independent power producers (IPPs) and power marketers. They force utilities to follow standardized protocols to address their needs and permit for addition of new generation capacity. These orders also complicate the planning process, since information flow within planning departments becomes unidirectional. Transmission planners know all the details of proposed generation plans through the queue process, but not vice versa.

A good transmission plan is now supposed to address the economic objectives of all users of the transmission grid by designing plans to accommodate generation entered into the generation queue and to ensure the viability of long-term firm transmission service requests entered through OASIS. However, utility transmission planners continue to design their transmission system basically to satisfy their own company's reliability objectives.

Furthermore, the FERC Order 2000 has established the concept of the *regional transmission operator* (RTO) and requires transmission operators to make provisions to form and participate in these organizations. Accordingly, RTOs have the authority to perform regional planning and have the ultimate responsibility for planning within its region. Thus, the US electric system now has the potential for a coordinated, comprehensive regional planning process.

1.13   POSSIBLE FUTURE ACTIONS BY THE FERC

The FERC has the authority over the rates, terms, and conditions of wholesale electric sales and transmission in interstate commerce. Hence, it plays an important role in stimulating investment in the grid. According to Fama of the Edison Electric Institute [37], the utility industry is expecting the FERC to have the following regulatory policies:

1. Establish a lasting regulatory framework that assures those who are willing to invest in the grid will be able to fully recover their investment, along with their cost of capital, through electricity rates.
2. Encourage a variety of corporate structures and business models for building transmission. It is clear that many different structures and business models can coexist in a competitive wholesale marketplace, provided there are fair rules in place for all market participants.
3. Permit alternative transmission pricing and cost recovery approaches for states with renewable resources goals so that their renewable resources that lack siting flexibility can be developed.
4. Permit utilities to recover construction work-in-process costs under customer rates to improve cash flow and rate stability.
5. Grant accelerated depreciation in ratemaking to improve financial flexibility and promote additional transmission investment.

6. Work closely with state policy makers
   a. To allow full recovery of all prudently incurred costs to design, study, precertify, and permit transmission facilities, as well as amend its own rules to allow full recovery of the prudently incurred costs of transmission projects that are later abandoned
   b. To allow that the appropriate regulatory mechanisms are in place to allow for full cost recovery and the avoidance of unrecoverable or trapped costs, which arise when federal and state regulatory policies diverge

In addition to the FERC, the US Congress also has the opportunity to stimulate wholesale competition by making investment in the grid more attractive.

In North America, NERC is composed of 10 regional reliability councils (RRCs), which cover the continental United States, Canada, and parts of Mexico. The councils oversee compliance with NERC reliability standards, by which the grid is operated, as well as those standards that must be followed to ensure that the grid is operated securely.

According to Fama [37], the role of the regional state committees (RSCs) should be based on the following principles:

1. RSCs should consider individual state needs but act in the best interest of its region.
2. RSCs should facilitate the necessary state regulatory approvals for parties seeking to build new transmission facilities that cross state boundaries.
3. RSCs should minimize regulatory uncertainty and assist in a timely transition to regional wholesale electricity markets but not create another level of regulation.
4. RSCs should support recovery of costs associated with forming and operating RTOs and ISOs.
5. RSCs should support timely recovery of costs associated with forming and operating RTOs and ISOs.

It is clear that developing a stronger and more flexible transmission grid will not be easy or fast. However, as suggested by the Edison Electric Institute, by creating a financial environment that encourages investment and by achieving greater cooperation among the regulatory groups, it can be accomplished.

REFERENCES

1. Power: A computer system for corridor location, NTIS Rep. No. PB-261 960. U.S. Department of Commerce, Washington, DC, 1976.
2. Hulett, J. P. and Denbrock, F. A. *Transthetics—Environmental Treatment for Utilities*, Southeastern Electric Exchange, Atlanta, GA, 1973.
3. Hulett, J. P. Transthetics, *J. Power Div.* (*Am. Soc. Civ. Eng.*) 98, 1971, Pap. No. 8989, 901.
4. Meckiff, C., Boardman, J. T., Richards, I., and Green, J. R. Comparative analysis of heuristic synthesis methods for electricity transmission networks, *IEEE Power Engineering Society Winter Power Meeting*, 1978, Pap. No. F78 259-4.
5. DeSalvo, C. A. and Smith, H. L. Automated transmission planning with AC load flow and incremental transmission loss evaluation, *IEEE Trans. Power Appar. Syst.* PAS-84, 1965, 156–163.
6. Bhavaraju, M. P. and Billington, R. Transmission planning using a quantitative reliability criterion, *Proceedings of the Sixth Power Industry Computer Applications Conference*, Denver, CO, 1969, pp. 115–124.
7. Garver, L. L. Transmission network estimation using linear programming, *IEEE Trans. Power Appar. Syst.* PAS-89, 1970, 1088–1097.
8. Baldwin, C. J., DeSalvo, C. A., Hoffman, C. H., and Ku, W. S. A model for transmission planning by logic, *AIEE Trans. Power Appar. Syst.*, part 3, 78, 1960, 1638–1645.
9. Burstall, R. M. Computer design of electricity supply networks by a heuristic method, *Comput. J.* 9, 1966, 253–274.

10. Baldwin, C. J., Montwest, F. E., Shortley, P. B., and Benson, R. U. Techniques for simulation of sub-transmission and distribution system expansion, *Proceedings of the Sixth Power Industry Computer Applications Conference*, Denver, CO, 1969, pp. 71–80.

11. Whysong, J. L., Uram, R., Brown, H. E., King, C. W., and DeSalvo, C. A. Computer program for automatic transmission planning, *Trans. Am. Inst. Electr. Eng.* part 3, 81, 1963, 774–781.

12. Platts, J. E., Sigley, R. B., and Garver, L. L. A method for horizon-year transmission planning, *IEEE Power Engineering Symposium on Winter Power Meeting*, 1972, Pap. No. C72 166-2.

13. Quiroga, L. F., Parrondo, M., Rosales, J. I., and Tamarit, J. Long term transmission expansion (1974–1993) within a system with a nuclear generation alternative, CIGRE 32-07, 1976.

14. Kaltenbach, J. C., Peschon, J., and Gehrig, E. H. A mathematical optimization technique for the expansion of electric power transmission systems, *IEEE Trans. Power Appar. Syst.* PAS-90(1), 1970, 113–119.

15. Knight, U. G. The logical design of electrical networks using linear programming methods, *Proc. Inst. Electr. Eng.*, Part A 107, 1960, 306–314.

16. Knight, U. G. *Power Systems Engineering and Mathematics*, Pergamon Press, New York, 1972.

17. Adams, R. N. and Laughton, M. A. Optimal planning of power networks using mixed-integer programming, part I. Static and time-phased network synthesis, *Proc. Inst. Electr. Eng.* 121(2), 1974, 139–147.

18. Lee, S. T. Y., Hicks, K. L., and Hnyilicza, E. Transmission expansion by branch-and bound integer programming with optimal cost, capacity curves, *IEEE Trans. Power Appar. Syst.* PAS-96(2), 1977, 657–666.

19. Sjelvgren, D. V. and Bubenko, J. A. Nonlinear integer programming for transmission expansion planning, *IEEE Power Engineering Society Winter Meeting*, 1977, Pap. No. A 77 150-6, 1977.

20. Sarvey, R. M. and Zinn, C. D. A mathematical model for long range expansion planning of generation and transmission in electric utility systems, *IEEE Trans.* PAS-96(2), 1977, 657–666.

21. Gönen, T. and Foote, B. L. Distribution system planning using mixed-integer programming, *Proc. Inst. Electr. Eng.* 128(2), 1981, 70–79.

22. Gönen, T. and Foote, B. L. Mathematical dynamic optimization model for electrical distribution system planning, *Electr. Power Energy Syst.* 4(2), 1982, 129–136.

23. Fischl, J. and Puntel, W. R. Computer-aided design of electric power transmission networks, *IEEE Power Engineering Society Winter Power Meeting*, 1972, Pap. No. C 72 168-8, 1972.

24. Puntel, W. R. et al. An automated method for long-range planning of transmission networks, *Proceedings of the 10th Power Industry Computer Applications Conference*, Toronto, Ontario, Canada, 1973, pp. 38–46.

25. Fischl, R. and Puntel, W. R. Efficient method for computing electric power transmission network sensitivities, *IEEE Power Engineering Society Winter Power Meeting*, 1972, Pap. C 72 167-0, 1972.

26. *Application of Optimization Methods in Power System Engineering*, IEEE Tutorial Course, IEEE Publishing No. 76 CH1107-2-PWR, IEEE, New York, 1976.

27. Baleriaux, H., Jamoulle, E., Doulliez, P., and Van Kelecom, J. Optimal investment policy for a growing electrical network by a sequential decision method, CIGRE 32-08, 1970.

28. Henault, P. H., Eastvedt, R. B., Peschon, J., and Hadju, L. P. Power system long-term planning in the presence of uncertainty, *IEEE Trans. Power Appar. Syst.* PAS-89(1), 1970, 156–163.

29. Dusonchet, Y. P. and El-Abiad, A. H. Transmission planning using discrete dynamic optimizing, *IEEE Trans. Power Appar. Syst.* PAS-92(4), 1973, 1358–1371.

30. Mamandur, K. R. C. and Berg, G. J. Alternative long-range expansion plans for transmission systems, *IEEE Power Eng. Soc. Winter Power Meet.*, 1978, paper no. A 78 042-4, 1978.

31. Yen, J. Y. Finding the K-shortest loopless paths in a network, *Manage. Sci.* 17, 1971, 712–716.

32. Gönen, T. *Modern Power System Analysis*, John Wiley & Sons, New York, 1988.

33. National Electric Reliability Council. *10th Annual Review of Overall Reliability and Adequacy of the North American Bulk Power Systems*, NERC, Princeton, NJ, 1980.

34. Electric Power Research Institute. *Transmission Line Reference Book: 345 kV and Above*, EPRI, Palo Alto, CA, 1979.

35. Dunlop, R. D., Gutman, R., and Marchenko, P. P. Analytical development of loadability characteristics of EHV and UHV transmission lines, *IEEE Trans. PAS*, PAS-98, March–April 1979, 606–617.

36. Morrow, D. J. and Brown, R. E. Future vision: The challenge of effective transmission planning, *IEEE Power Energy Mag.* 5(5), September–October 2007, 36–104.

37. Fama, J. Reenergizing the grid, *IEEE Power Energy Mag.* 3(5), September–October 2005, 30–33.

38. IEEE Task Force on Terms and Definitions. Proposed terms and definition for power system stability, *IEEE Trans. PAS* PAS-101(7), July 1982, 1894–1898.

39. Amin, S. M. and Wollenberg, B. F. Toward a smart grid, *IEEE Power Energy Mag.* 3 (5), September–October, 2005, 34–41.
40. Gönen, T., *Electrical Power Distribution System Engineering*, 2nd edn., CRC Press, Boca Raton, FL, 2008.
41. Gönen, T., Foote, B. L., and Thompson, J. C. Development of advanced methods for planning electric energy distribution systems, Report No. C00-4830-3, U.S. Department of Energy, Washington, DC, 1979.

GENERAL REFERENCES

Dougherty, J. J. Higher efficiency for transmission and distribution, *EPRI J.* 8 (3), 1983, 18–21.

Edison Electric Institute. *EHV Transmission Line Reference Book*, EEI, New York, 1968.

Electric Power Research Institute. *Transmission Line Reference Book: 115–138 kV Compact Line Design*, EPRI, Palo Alto, CA, 1978a.

Electric Power Research Institute. *Transmission Line Reference Book: HVDC to ±600 kV*, EPRI, Palo Alto, CA, 1978b.

Electric Power Research Institute. *Transmission Line Reference Book: 345 kV and Above*, EPRI, Palo Alto, CA, 1979.

Fink, D. G. and Beaty, H. W. *Standard Handbook for Electrical Engineers*, 11th edn., McGraw-Hill, New York, 1978.

Fink, L. H. and Carlsen, K. Systems engineering for power: Status and prospects, *Proceedings of an Engineering Foundation Conference*, CONF-750867, U.S. Energy Research and Development Administration, Washington, DC, 1975.

Gönen, T., *Engineering Economy for Engineering Managers: With Computer Applications*, Wiley, New York, 1990.

Gönen, T. and Anderson, P. M. The impact of advanced technology on the future electric energy supply problem, *Proceedings of IEEE Energy Conference*, Tulsa, OK, 1978, pp. 117–121.

Gönen, T., Anderson, P. M., and Bowen, D. W. Energy and the future, *Proceedings of the First World Hydrogen Energy Conference*, Miami Beach, FL, 1976, vol. 3 (2c), pp. 55–78.

Gönen, T. and Bekiroglu, H. Some views on inflation and a Phillips curve for the U.S. economy, *Proceedings of the American Institute for Decision Sciences Conference*, Albany, NY, 1977, pp. 328–331.

Haden, R. et al. Regional power systems planning: A state of the art assessment, Final Rep. U.S. Department of Energy, University of Oklahoma, Norman, OK, 1978.

IEEE Committee Report. The significance of assumptions implied in long-range electric utility planning studies, *IEEE Trans. Power Appar. Syst.* PAS-99, 1980, 1047–1056.

Merrill, H. M., Schweppe, F. C., and White, D. C. Energy strategy planning for electric utilities, part I. Smarte methodology, *IEEE Trans. Power Appar. Syst.* PAS-101(2), 1982, 340–346.

Serna, C., Duran, J., and Camargo, A. A model for expansion planning of transmission systems: A practical application example, *IEEE Trans. Power Appl. Syst.* PAS-97(2), 1978, 610–615.

U.S. Department of the Interior. *Environmental Criteria for Electrical Transmission Systems*. U.S. Government Printing Office, Superintendent of Documents, Washington, DC, 1970.

2 Transmission Line Structures and Equipment

I would have my ignorance rather than another man's knowledge,
because I have so much of it.

Mark Twain

2.1 INTRODUCTION

The function of the overhead (OH) three-phase electric power transmission line is to transmit bulk power to load centers and large industrial users beyond the primary distribution lines. A given transmission system comprises all land, conversion structures, and equipment (such as step-down transformers) at a primary source of supply, including interconnecting transmission lines, switching, and conversion stations, between a generating or receiving point and a load center or wholesale point. It includes all lines and equipment whose main function is to increase, integrate, or tie together power supply sources.

2.2 DECISION PROCESS TO BUILD A TRANSMISSION LINE

The decision to build a transmission line results from system planning studies to determine how best to meet the system requirements. At this stage, the following factors need to be considered and established:

1. Voltage level
2. Conductor type and size
3. Line regulation and voltage control
4. Corona and losses
5. Proper load flow and system stability
6. System protection
7. Grounding
8. Insulation coordination
9. Mechanical design:
    a. Sag and stress calculations
    b. Conductor composition
    c. Conductor spacing
    d. Insulation and conductor hardware selection
10. Structural design:
    a. Structure types
    b. Stress calculations

Once the decision to build a particular transmission line has been reached, after considering all the previously mentioned factors, there is a critical path that needs to be followed in its design.

According to the Electric Power Research Institute (EPRI) [1], the critical path steps in an EHV line design are as follows:

1. Define needs and list alternative system layouts.
2. Acquisition of ROW.
3. Load flow (i.e., power flow) and stability study.
4. Determine overvoltage.
5. Set performance criteria and formulate weather conditions.
6. Preliminary line design.
7. Specification of apparatus.
8. Purchase of apparatus.
9. Installation of station.
10. Economic conductor solution.
11. Electrical design of towers.
12. Lightning performance design.
13. Audible and radio noise (RN) analysis.
14. Addressing special design problems.
15. Insulation planning.
16. Final tower design.
17. Optimization of tower locations.
18. Line construction.
19. Fulfillment of power needs.

Figure 2.1 shows the order of these critical path steps in EHV line design. Further, the levels of various types of line compensation and other system impedances affect load flow, stability, voltage drop, and other transmission system performances. Accordingly, the most accurate transmission line performance computation must take all of these considerations into account and must be performed by using a digital computer program. The obtained results must be reflected in the transmission line design effectively.

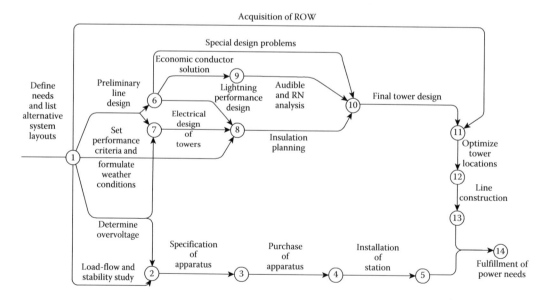

FIGURE 2.1 Critical path steps in an EHV line design. (From Electric Power Research Institute, 1979. Used by permission. © 1979 Electric Power Research Institute.)

TABLE 2.1
Line Design Characteristics Affecting Cost

Line voltage
Loading (MW)
Number of conductors
Number of circuits
Phase bundle configuration
Phase spacing
Insulation characteristics
Span length range
GWs: diameter, weight
Number, type, and cost of insulator units
Tower type
Wind pressure on conductors
Ice thickness
Unloaded loaded tension
Broken conductors and broken conductors' tension
Allowable conductor temperature
Ground clearances
Grounding
Transpositions
Tower and foundation weight factors
Tower and foundation steel excavation and backfill costs
Tower setup and assembly costs
Pulling, sagging, and clipping costs

The optimum line design is the design that meets all the technical specifications and the other requirements at the lowest cost. The process of finding such line design with the lowest cost can be accomplished by using a computerized design. The transmission line design engineer can then quickly examine thousands of different combinations of line parameters by using such computer design program to achieve the best solution. Table 2.1 gives some of the line design characteristics that affect the transmission line cost.

2.3 DESIGN TRADE-OFFS

There are also various design trade-offs that need to be considered in the areas of insulation, corona performance, and environment. For example, with respect to insulation, a tower with legs of small cross section inhibits switching-surge flashover in the gap between conductor and tower leg. Small tower legs increase tower inductance. Hence, the lightning performance is negatively affected.

In EHV and UHV design, increasing line height or adding auxiliary conductors for field control can reduce the maximum field under the line at the ground level and the field at the edge of the ROW. However, such design would be expensive and suffer in appearance. Minimizing insulation clearances would decrease line cost but increase corona, especially at UHV. Since the corona effects are small, line compaction is most easily done at 69–110 kV voltage range designs.

In double-circuit line designs, there are trade-offs in the areas of corona and electric field for various phasing arrangements. For example, to improve the corona performance of a line, the tower-top configuration must have the nearby phases in the following order:

$$
\begin{array}{cc}
\mathbf{A} & \mathbf{A} \\
\mathbf{B} & \mathbf{B} \\
\mathbf{C} & \mathbf{C}
\end{array}
$$

However, in such order while conductor surface gradients improve, the ground-level electric field increases. On the other hand, the following phase order is best for ground field and worse for corona performance [1]:

$$
\begin{array}{cc}
\mathbf{A} & \mathbf{C} \\
\mathbf{B} & \mathbf{B} \\
\mathbf{C} & \mathbf{A}
\end{array}
$$

Note that the use of underbuilt auxiliary conductors and circuits with or without applied voltage would separate the relationship between the conductor surface electric field and the ground-level electric field. Also, in a single-circuit horizontal arrangement, the conductor surface gradient and the electric field at the edge of the ROW are affected by phase spacing. Hence, decreasing the phase spacing in a design would help its electric field but would affect negatively on its conductor surface gradient. But the use of a vertical design arrangement would change or tend to decouple this relationship [1].

2.4 TRADITIONAL LINE DESIGN PRACTICE

In the present practice, each support structure (i.e., pole or tower) supports a half-span of conductors and OH lines on either side of the structure. For a given line voltage, the conductors and the overhead ground wires (OHGWs) are arranged to provide, at least, the minimum clearance mandated by the National Electric Safety Code (NESC) in addition to other applicable codes. The resultant configuration is designed to control the following:

1. The separation of energized parts from other energized parts
2. The separation of energized parts from the support structures of other objects (located along the ROW)
3. The separation of energized parts above ground

The NESC divides the United States into three loading zones: heavy, medium, and light, as explained in Section 12.5.3. It specifies the minimum load levels that must be employed within each loading zone. Furthermore, the NESC uses the concept of an *overload capacity factor* (OCF) to take into account uncertainties resulting from the following factors:

1. Likelihood of occurrence of the specified load
2. Grade of construction
3. Dispersion of structure strength
4. Structure function, for example, suspension, dead end, and angle
5. Determination of strength during service life
6. Other line support components, for example, guys and foundations

In general, the following *steps are used for the design of a transmission line*:

1. A list of loading events is prepared by the utility company that would own the transmission lines. This list includes the following:
   a. Mandatory regulations from the NESC and other codes
   b. Possible climatic events that are expected in the loading zone in which the line is located
   c. Specific contingency loading events such as broken conductors
   d. Expectations and special requirements
   Note that each of these loading events is multiplied by its own OCF to take care of uncertainties involved to come up with an agenda of final ultimate design loads.
2. A ruling span is determined according to sag/tension requirements of the preselected conductor.
3. A structure type is selected based on past experience or on possible suppliers' recommendations.
4. Ultimate design loads due to the ruling span are applied statistically as components in the longitudinal, transverse, and vertical directions and the structure deterministically designed.
5. Ground line reactions are calculated and used to design the foundation by using the loads and structure configuration.
6. The ruling span line configuration is adjusted to fit the actual ROW profile.
7. To adjust for variations in actual span lengths and changes in elevation and running angles the structure/foundation designs are modified.
8. Since the tangent structures are the weakest link in the line, accordingly, hardware, insulators, and other accessory components are selected to be stronger than the structure.

2.4.1 Factors Affecting Structure-Type Selection

According to Pohlman [4], there are usually many factors that affect the determination of the structure type to be used in a given OH transmission line design. Some of them are listed as follows:

1. *Public concerns.* In order to take into account of the general public, living, working, or coming in proximity to the line, it is customary to have hearings as part of the approval process for a new transmission line. To hold such public meetings that are satisfactory is a prerequisite for the required permit.
2. *Erection technique.* In general, different structure types dictate different erection techniques. For example, a tapered steel pole is probably to be manufactured in a single piece and erected directly on its previously installed foundation in one hoist. Steel lattice towers have hundreds of individual parts that must be bolted together, assembled, and erected onto the four previously installed foundations.
3. *Inspection, assessment, and maintenance.* The structures are inspected by human inspectors who may use diagnostic technologies in addition to their personal inspection techniques. Some of the techniques may involve observations from ground or fly by patrol. Climbing, bucket trucks, or the use of helicopters. The necessary line maintenance activities are also needed to be considered.
4. *Possible future upgrading or uprating.* It is difficult to get the necessary ROWs and required permits to build new transmission lines. Because of these considerations, some utilities select structure types for the new transmission lines in a manner that would allow easy upgrading and/or uprating, if it is needed in the future.

2.4.2 IMPROVED DESIGN APPROACHES

Today, there are many techniques to assess the true capability of an OH transmission line that was designed by using the conventional practice of specifying ultimate static loads and designing a structure that would properly support them.

So far, the best technique was developed by Ostendorp [5] and is presently under development by CIGRE Study Committee 22: *Recommendations for Overhead Lines* [6]. This technique is known as "improved design criteria of overhead transmission lines based on reliability concepts." It is based on the concept that loads and strengths are statistical variables and the combined reliability is computable if the statistical functions of loads and strengths are known. The flow diagram of the methodology of this technique is shown in Figure 2.2. The steps of this recommended methodology for designing transmission line components are as follows:

1. Collect preliminary line design data and available climatic data.
2. Do the following in this step:
   a. Select the reliability level in terms of return period of design loads.
   b. Select the security requirements (failure containment).
   c. List safety requirements imposed by mandatory regulations and construction and maintenance loads.

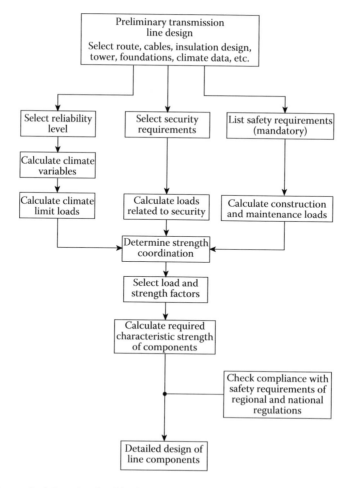

FIGURE 2.2 The methodology involved in developing improved design criteria of OH transmission lines based on reliability concepts.

3. Calculate climatic variables corresponding to the selected return period of design loads.
4. Do the following in this step:
    a. Calculate climatic limit loadings on components.
    b. Calculate loads corresponding to security requirements.
    c. Calculate loads related to safety requirements during construction and maintenance.
5. Determine the suitable strength coordination between line components.
6. Select appropriate load and strength equations.
7. Calculate the characteristic strengths required for components.
8. Design line components for the strength requirements.

2.5 TRANSMISSION LINE STRUCTURES

In order to put it into a historical perspective, it should be mentioned that it was in the late 1887 when Tesla filed for several patents in the field of polyphase ac systems. Among them was a patent on power transmission. Among polyphase systems, Tesla strongly preferred two-phase configurations. In 1893, George Westinghouse and his Niagara Falls Power Company decided on the adoption of polyphase (two phases) ac. Later in August 1895, the power system went into operation, including a higher-voltage transmission line in Buffalo, New York, about 20 mi away. In 1903, when the next Niagara plant extension took place, the new ac generators were built with three phases, as were all the following plant additions. However, the birth of first long-distance three-phase power transmission was achieved by Swiss engineers in 1891. This 30 kV transmission line was connected between Lauffen and Frankfurt by means of Tesla's system.

As displayed in Table 1.1, the standard transmission voltages are continuously creeping up historically. In the design of a system, the voltage selected should be the one best suited for the particular service on the basis of economic considerations. The ac transmission system in the United States developed from a necessity to transfer large blocks of energy from remote generation facilities to load centers. As the system grew, transmission additions were made to improve reliability, to achieve economic generation utilization through interconnections, and to strengthen the transmission backbone with higher-voltage overlays.

Numerous transmission lines with 115–230 kV are used as primary transmission or become underlay to higher-voltage lines. At the end of 1974, about 85% (i.e., 208,000 mi) of transmission lines in service in the United States were in the range of 115–230 kV. Today, it is estimated that this class of transmission lines are about more than half of the total transmission lines of all classes.

In general, the basic structure configuration selected depends on many interrelated factors, including aesthetic considerations, economics, performance criteria, company policies and practice, line profile, ROW restrictions, preferred materials, and construction techniques.

2.5.1 COMPACT TRANSMISSION LINES

For a long time (about 30 years), the transmission lines in the 115–230 kV class saw very little change in design practices than the previous ones. But, in 1960s, this voltage class has seen major changes due to two reasons: (1) the induction of prefabricated steel poles, laminated structures, and armless structures and (2) the increasing difficulties in obtaining new ROWs due to increasing environmental pressures that, in turn, forced the utilities to uprate the existing 69 kV circuits to 138 kV circuits and 138 kV circuits to 230 kV circuits. This trend has demonstrated the applicability of EHV technology to lower voltage circuits.

Later, the practicality of using vertical postinsulators and 3 ft phase-to-phase spacing on a wood pole line was demonstrated on a 138 kV transmission line at Saratoga, New York, in 1973. Other applications verified that compact 138 kV constructions were feasible in 1974. Figure 2.3 shows typical compact configurations for horizontal unshielded, horizontal shielded, vertical, delta, and vertical delta.

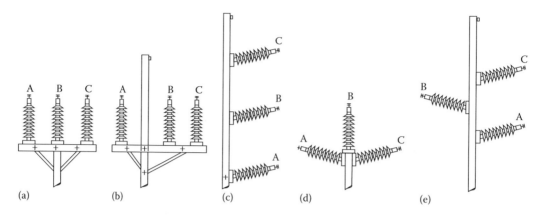

FIGURE 2.3 Typical compact configurations (not to scale): (a) horizontal unshielded, (b) horizontal shielded, (c) vertical, (d) delta, and (e) vertical delta. (From Electric Power Research Institute, *Transmission Line Reference Book: 115–138 kV Compact Line Design*, 2nd edn., EPRI, Palo Alto, CA, 1978. Used by permission. © 1978 Electric Power Research Institute.)

The double-circuit 138 kV lines that are shown in Figures 2.4 and 2.5 were built by using steel poles, having two 138 kV top circuits and a 34.5 kV single circuit underbuilt. Figure 2.6 also shows a double-circuit 138 kV line that was built by using steel poles, having two 34.5 kV double circuits underbuilt.

The studies on such compact line design have verified that the insulation and clearance requirements with respect to electrical strength of air gaps and insulators were adequate. The compact

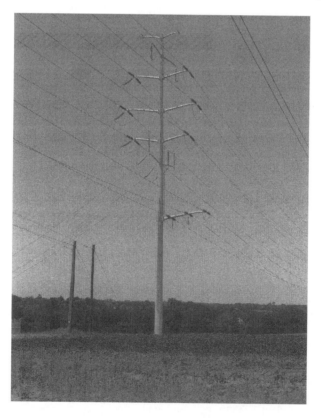

FIGURE 2.4 A double-circuit 138 kV line built by using steel poles, having two 138 kV top circuits and a 34.5 kV single circuit underbuilt. (Courtesy of Union Electric Company.)

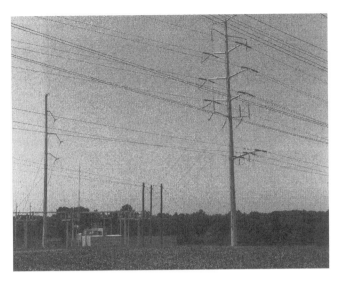

FIGURE 2.5   A double-circuit 138 kV line built by using steel poles, having two 138 kV top circuits and a 34.5 kV single circuit underbuilt. (Union Electric Company.)

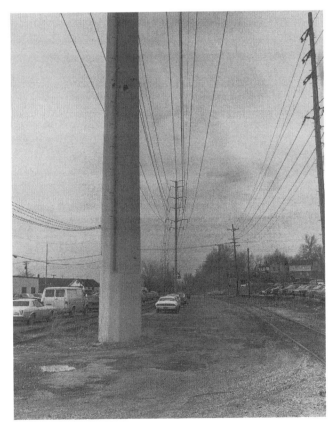

FIGURE 2.6   A double-circuit 138 kV line built by using steel poles, having two 138 kV circuits underbuilt. (Union Electric Company.)

designs were further tested for motion caused by wind, ice shedding from conductors, and fault currents. However, such lines were not tested for switching surges and lightning responses since neither criterion poses any serious problem to compaction. Also, studies have shown that for most compact line and conductor dimensions, RN and other manifestation of corona were well below levels normally acceptable at EHV. But, special attention must be given to line hardware, since most 138 kV hardware is not designed to operate at electric field gradients comparable to those of EHV lines.

Several provisions of the NESC are directly applicable to 138 kV compact lines especially in the areas of phase-to-phase spacing and maintenance clearances. Compact lines, due to reduced design margins, dictate more rigorous analysis of insulation and mechanical parameters to ensure adequate reliability than is needed for conventional lines.

2.5.2 Conventional Transmission Lines

Higher-voltage lines with higher loading capabilities continue to experience higher growth rates. As loads grow, 765 kV is a logical voltage for the overlay of 345 kV having a previous underlay of 138 kV. Similarly, 500 kV will continue to find its place as an overlay of 230 and 161 kV. Here, higher voltages mean higher power transfer capability, as can be observed from the surge imped-ance loading (SIL) capabilities of typical EHV transmission lines. Some power systems rate their transmission voltages by the nominal voltages; others may use the maximum voltage. Typically, 345, 500, 700, and 765 kV and their corresponding maximums are classified as EHV. They are used extensively and commercially in the United States and are gaining popularity in other parts of the world. In addition, 380 or 400 kV EHV transmission is used mainly in Europe.

EHV systems require an entirely new concept of system design. Contrarily, voltages 230 kV and below are relatively simple and well standardized in design and construction practices. EHV dictates complete and thorough reconsideration of all normally standardized design features, such as necessity for bundled conductors and switching surges that control the insulation, corona, radio interference (RI), lightning protection, line-charging current, clearances, and construction practices.

The 345 kV system established the practice of using bundle conductors, the V-configuration of insulator strings (to restrain conductor swinging), and the use of aluminum in line structures. The first 500 kV transmission line was built in 1964 to tie a mine-mouth power plant in West Virginia to load centers in the eastern part of the state. The main reason for preferring to use 500 kV over the 345 kV voltage level was that upgrading from 230 to 345 kV provided a gain of only 140% increase in the amount of power that can be transmitted in comparison to a 400% gain that can be obtained by using the 500 kV level.

Also in 1964, Hydro-Quebec inaugurated its 735 kV 375 mi line. A line voltage of 765 kV was introduced into service by AEP in 1969. The 1980s witnessed the Bonneville Power Administration's (BPA) 1100 kV transmission line.

The trend toward higher voltages is basically motivated by the resulting increased line capacity while reducing line losses. The reduction in power losses is substantial. Also, the better use of land is a side benefit as the voltage level increases. For example, for building a transmission line with a capacity of 10,000 MW, a ROW width of 76 m is required for a 500 kV line having a double circuit, whereas the required ROW width for a 1,100 kV line is only 56 m.

The power transmission voltages above 765 kV, generally in the range of 1100 and 1500 kV, are known as the UHVs. They are subject to intensive research and development before they can be included in practical line designs and apparatus for commercial service. The problems associated with UHV transmission include audible noise (AN), RN, electrostatic field effects, contamina-tion, and switching overvoltages. However, research into higher-voltage transmission will help utilities to transmit up to six times the electric power possible with the lines in use in the 1970s. But, it is well known that engineering and physical problems become more complex at operating voltages above 765 kV.

2.5.3 DESIGN OF LINE SUPPORT STRUCTURES

After the proper considerations of voltage drop, power loss, thermal overloading, and other considerations, the design of a transmission line has simply become of the adaptation of available standard designs to best fit the requirements of a particular job at hand. Otherwise, designing a complete transmission line from scratch is a complex and tedious process.

However, once a good design is developed, it can be used repeatedly or it can be adapted to the situation at hand easily. Using computers and standard line designs, a new line can be designed rather quickly. In general, companies only change a standard structure after much consideration and after the proper testing and production of the necessary materials. In the United States, originally, three engineering companies were responsible for all of the design work for 80% of the transmission lines. Eventually, the best of all available designs was adopted and used in all designs in the country.

Also, conductors, fittings, and hardware were standardized by the IEEE and the National Electrical Manufacturing Association (NEMAS). Towers were standardized by major steel tower manufacturers.

Furthermore, the federal government is also in electric power business with the Tennessee Valley Authority (TVA), BPA, and Bureau of Water Power and the Rural Electrification Association (REA). The use of the design guides prepared by the REA is mandatory for all borrowers of federal funds through the REA program.

Figure 2.7 shows a typical 345 kV transmission line with single circuit and a wood H-frame. Figure 2.8 shows a typical 345 kV transmission line with bundled conductors and double circuit on steel towers. Figure 2.9 shows a typical 345 kV transmission line with bundled conductors and

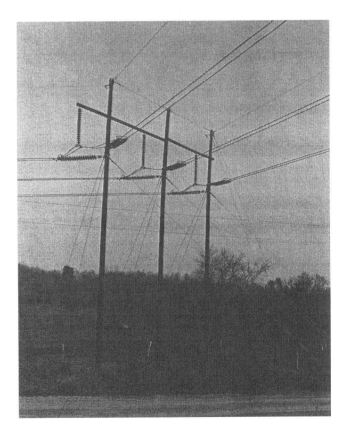

FIGURE 2.7 A typical 345 kV transmission line with single-circuit and wood H-frame. (Union Electric Company.)

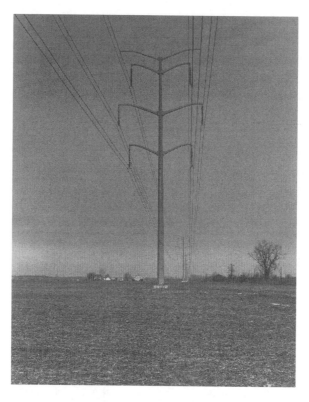

FIGURE 2.8   A typical 345 kV transmission line with bundled conductors and double circuit on steel towers. (Union Electric Company.)

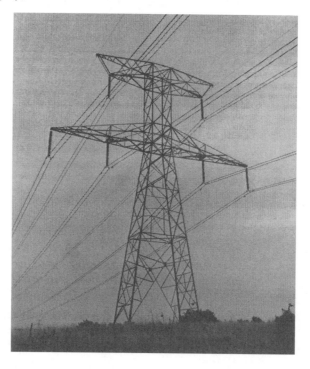

FIGURE 2.9   A typical 345 kV transmission line with bundled conductors and double circuit on steel towers. (Union Electric Company.)

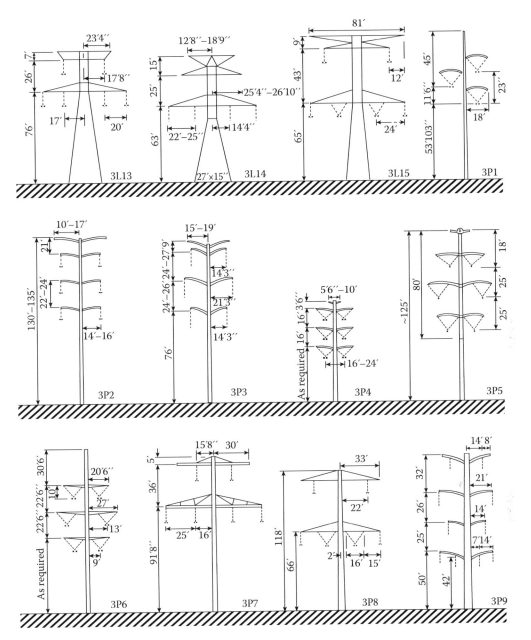

FIGURE 2.10 Typical pole- and lattice-type structures for 345 kV transmission systems. (From Electric Power Research Institute, *Transmission Line Reference Book: 345 kV and Above*, 2nd edn., EPRI, Palo Alto, CA, 1982. Used with permission. © 1979 Electric Power Research Institute.)

double circuit on steel pole. Figure 2.10 shows typical pole- and lattice-type structures for 345 kV transmission systems. The construction of OH lines is discussed further in Chapter 12. Figure 2.11 shows typical wood H-frame-type structures for 345 kV transmission systems. Figure 2.12 shows typical pole- and lattice-type structures for 500 kV transmission systems. Figure 2.13 shows typical pole- and lattice-type structures for 735–800 kV transmission systems. Figure 2.14 shows a typical 230 kV transmission line steel tower with bundled conductors and double circuit. Figure 2.15 shows a lineman working from a helicopter platform.

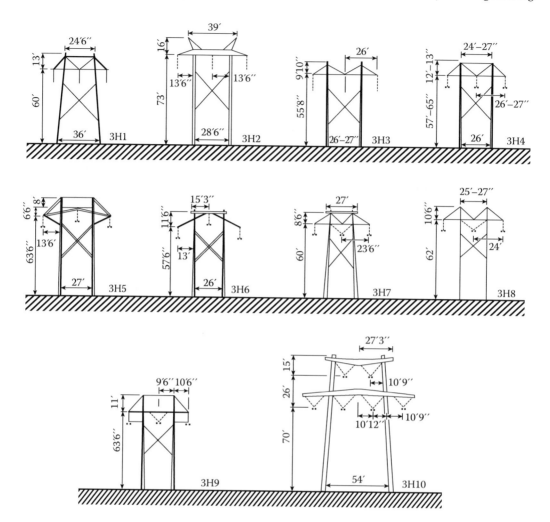

FIGURE 2.11 Typical wood H-frame-type structures for 345 kV transmission systems. (From Electric Power Research Institute, *Transmission Line Reference Book: 345 kV and Above*, 2nd edn., EPRI, Palo Alto, CA, 1982. Used by permission. © 1979 Electric Power Research Institute.)

2.6 SUBTRANSMISSION LINES

The subtransmission system is that part of the electric utility system that delivers power from the bulk power sources, such as large transmission substations. The subtransmission circuits may be made of OH open-wire construction or wood poles with post-type insulators. Steel tube or concrete towers are also used. The line has a single conductor in each phase. Postinsulators hold the conductor without metal crossarms.

One grounded shield conductor located on the top of the tower provides the necessary shielding for the phase conductors against lightning. The shield conductor is grounded at each tower or pole. Plate or vertical tube electrodes, also known as *ground rods*, are used for grounding. Occasionally, the subtransmission lines are also built using underground cables.

The voltage of these circuits varies from 12.47 to 230 kV, with the majority at 69, 115, and 138 kV voltage levels. There is a continuous trend in usage of the higher voltage as a result of the increasing use of higher primary voltages. Typically, the maximum length of subtransmission lines is in the range of 50–60 mi. In cities, most subtransmission lines are located along streets and alleys.

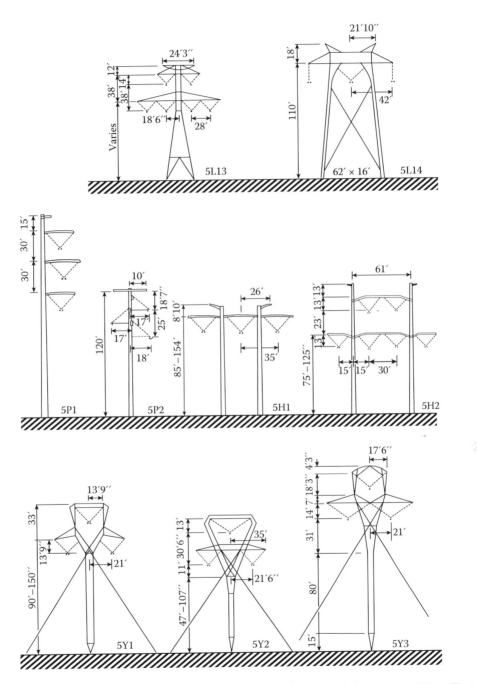

FIGURE 2.12 Typical pole- and lattice-type structures for 500 kV transmission systems. (From Electric Power Research Institute, *Transmission Line Reference Book*: *345 kV and Above*, 2nd edn., EPRI, Palo Alto, CA, 1982. Used by permission. © 1979 Electric Power Research Institute.)

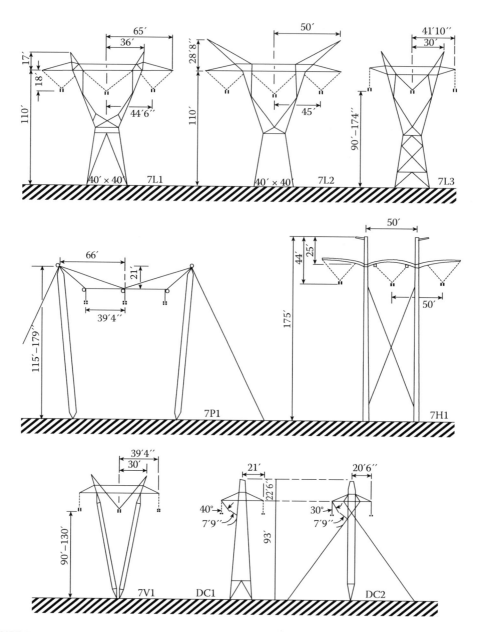

FIGURE 2.13 Typical pole- and lattice-type structures for 735–800 kV transmission systems. (From Electric Power Research Institute, *Transmission Line Reference Book: 345 kV and Above*, 2nd edn., EPRI, Palo Alto, CA, 1982. Used by permission. © 1979 Electric Power Research Institute.)

The subtransmission system designs vary from simple radial systems to a subtransmission network. The major considerations affecting the design are cost and reliability. Figure 2.28 shows a radial subtransmission system. It is a simple system and has a low first cost but also has low service continuity. Because of this, the radial system is not generally used. Instead, an improved form of radial-type subtransmission design is preferred, as shown in Figure 2.29. It allows relatively faster service restoration when a fault occurs on one of the subtransmission circuits.

In general, due to higher service reliability, the subtransmission system is designed as loop circuits or multiple circuits, forming a form of subtransmission grid or network. Figure 2.30 shows a

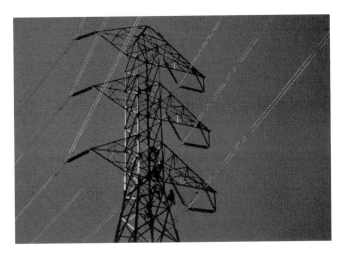

FIGURE 2.14 A typical 230 kV transmission line steel tower with bundled conductors and double circuit.

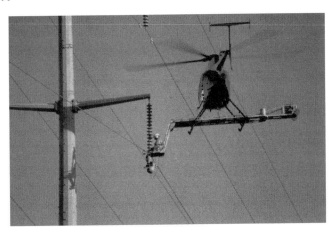

FIGURE 2.15 A lineman working from a helicopter platform.

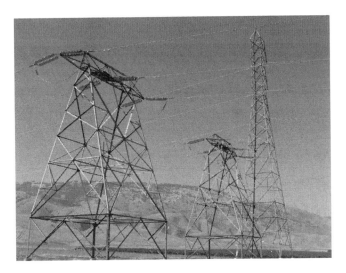

FIGURE 2.16 Two 345 and 230 kV transmission lines side by side. (Courtesy of West Power Inc.)

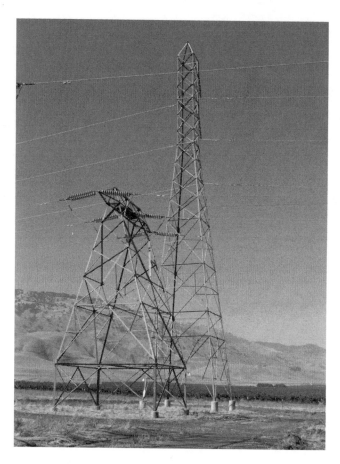

FIGURE 2.17   A 345 kV transmission line and a 230 kV transmission line side by side. (Courtesy of West Power Inc.)

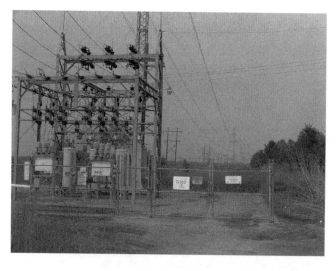

FIGURE 2.18   A 230/161 kV substation with a 230 kV transmission line passing by. (Courtesy of West Power Inc.)

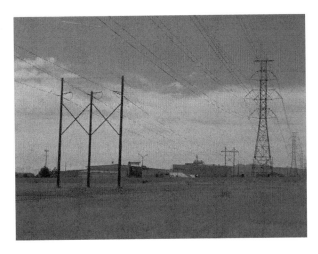

FIGURE 2.19 A 115 kV transmission line and a 230 kV transmission line side by side. (Courtesy of West Power Inc.)

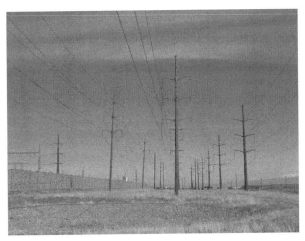

FIGURE 2.20 A cluster of four transmission lines side by side. (Courtesy of West Power Inc.)

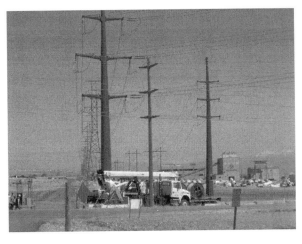

FIGURE 2.21 A 115 kV transmission line and a 345 kV transmission line with corner towers. (Courtesy of West Power Inc.)

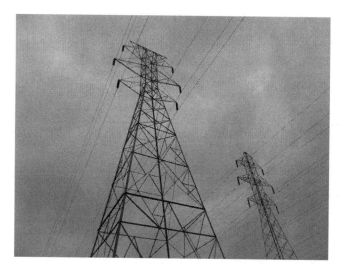

FIGURE 2.22   A 345 kV transmission line and a 115 kV transmission line side by side. (Courtesy of West Power Inc.)

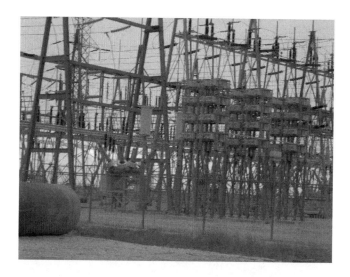

FIGURE 2.23   A 230 kV switchyard. (Courtesy of West Power Inc.)

loop-type subtransmission system. In this design, a single circuit originating from a bulk power bus runs through a number of substations and returns to the same bus.

Figure 2.31 shows a grid-type subtransmission that has multiple circuits. Here, the distribution substations are interconnected, and also the design may have more than one bulk power source. Therefore, it has the greatest service reliability, but it requires costly control of power flow and relaying. It is the most commonly used form of subtransmission.

Occasionally, a subtransmission line has a double circuit, having a wooden pole and post-type insulators. Steel tube or concrete towers are also used. The line may have a single conductor or bundled conductors in each phase. Postinsulators carry the conductors without metal crossarms. One grounded shield conductor (or OHGW) on the top of the tower shields the phase conductors from lightning. The shield conductor is grounded at each tower. Plate or vertical tube electrodes (ground rod) are used for grounding.

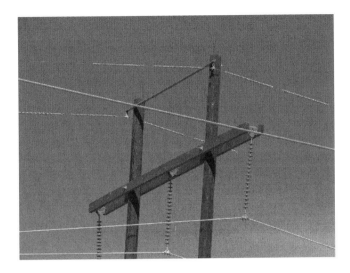

FIGURE 2.24 A pole-top view. (Courtesy of West Power Inc.)

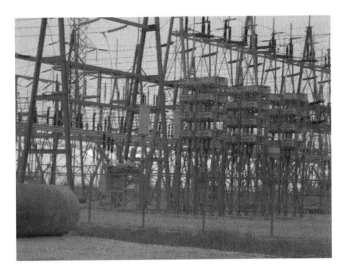

FIGURE 2.25 A 230/34.5 kV switchyard. (Courtesy of West Power Inc.)

Figure 2.32 shows a 34.5 kV line with a double circuit and wood poles. (It has a newer style pole-top configuration.) Figure 2.33 shows a 34.5 kV line with a single circuit and wood poles. It has a 12.47 kV underbuilt line and 34.5 kV switch. (It has an old style pole-top configuration.) Figure 2.34 shows a typical 34.5 kV line with a double circuit and wood poles. It has a 4.16 kV underbuilt line and a 34.5 kV switch. Figure 2.35 shows a typical 12.47 kV line with a single circuit and wood pole. It has a newer type pole-top construction.

2.6.1 Subtransmission Line Costs

Subtransmission line costs at the end of the line are associated with the substation at which it is terminated. According to the *ABB Guidebook* [5], based on 1994 prices, costs can run from as low as $50,000 per mile for a 46 kV wooden pole subtransmission line with perhaps 50 MVA capacity ($1 per kVA-mile) to over $1,000,000 per mile for a 500 kV double-circuit construction with 2000 MVA capacity ($0.5 per kVA-mile).

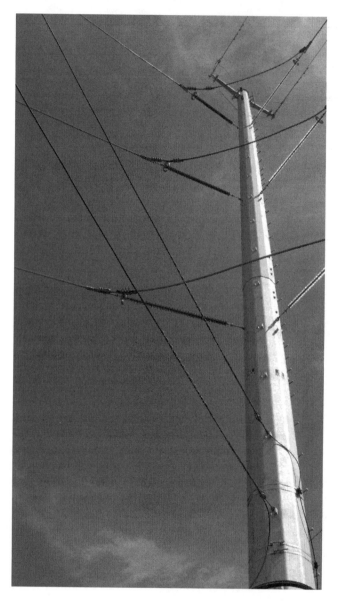

FIGURE 2.26 A galvanized dead-end corner pole of a 230 kV transmission line. (Courtesy of West Power Inc.)

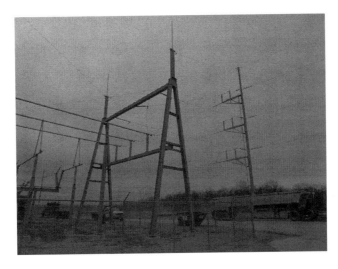

FIGURE 2.27 A substation connection of transmission lines. (Courtesy of West Power Inc.)

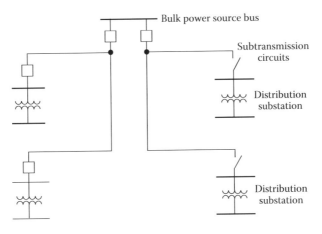

FIGURE 2.28 A radial-type subtransmission. (Courtesy of West Power Inc.)

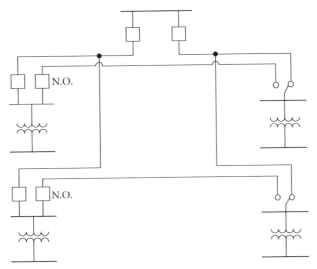

FIGURE 2.29 An improved form of radial-type subtransmission. (Courtesy of West Power Inc.)

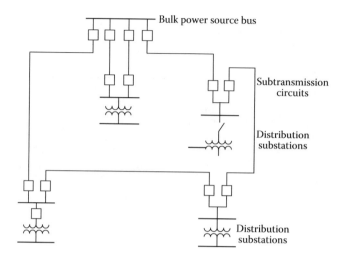

FIGURE 2.30   A loop-type subtransmission.

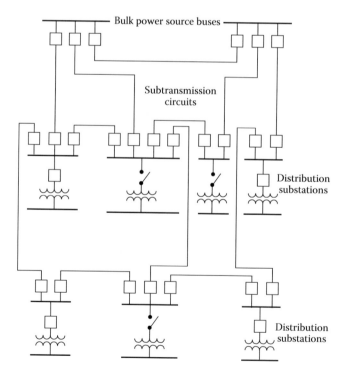

FIGURE 2.31   A grid- or network-type subtransmission.

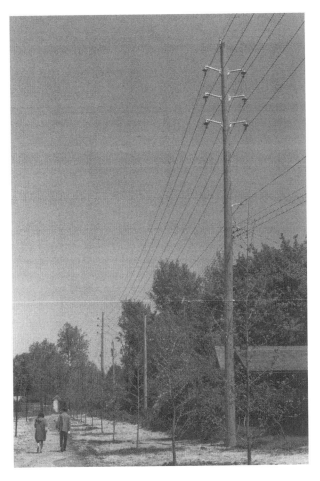

FIGURE 2.32 A typical 34.5 kV line with a double circuit and wood poles. It has a newer style construction. (Union Electric Company.)

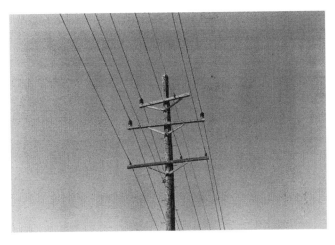

FIGURE 2.33 A 34.5 kV line with a single circuit and wood poles. It also has a 12.47 kV underbuilt line and 34.5 kV switch. It has an old style construction. (Union Electric Company.)

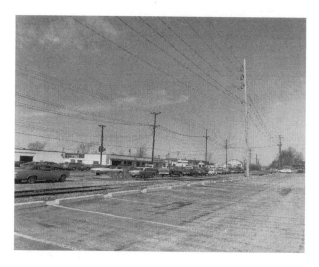

FIGURE 2.34   A typical 34.5 kV line with a double circuit and wood poles. It also has a 4.16 kV underbuilt line and a 34.5 kV switch. (Union Electric Company.)

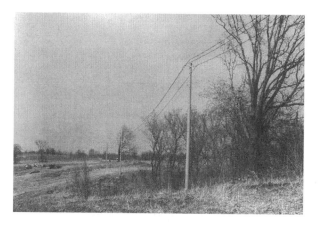

FIGURE 2.35   A typical 12.47 kV line with a single circuit and wood pole. It has a newer type of pole-top construction. (Union Electric Company.)

2.7 TRANSMISSION SUBSTATIONS

In general, there are four main types of electric substations in the ac power systems, namely, the following:

1. Switchyard
2. Customer substation
3. Transmission substation
4. Distribution substation

The switchyard is located at a generating plant (or station). They are used to connect the generators to the transmission grid and also provide off-site power to the plant. Such generator switchyards are usually very large installations covering large areas.

The customer substation functions as the primary source of electric power for one specific industrial/business customer. Its type depends on the customer's requirements. Transmission substations are also known as *bulk power substations*. They are large substations and are located at the ends of the transmission lines emanating from generating switchyards. They provide power to distribution switchyards and distribution substations, often over subtransmission lines. They are *enablers* of sending large amount of power from the power plants to the load centers. These substations are usually very large and very expensive to build.

Distribution substations provide power to the customers over primary and secondary lines, using distribution transformers. They are most common facilities and are typically located close to the load centers [8]. However, the purpose of this chapter is to discuss the transmission substations. Whether it is a large distribution substation or a transmission substation, establishment of a new substation is a long and tedious process, as shown in Figure 2.36.

The objective of a transmission substation design is to provide maximum reliability, flexibility, and continuity of service and to meet objectives with the lowest investment costs that satisfy the system requirements. Thus, a substation performs one or more of the following functions:

1. *Voltage transformation*: Power transformers are used to raise or lower the voltages as necessary.
2. *Switching functions*: Connecting or disconnecting parts of the system from each other.
3. *Reactive power compensation*: Shunt capacitors, shunt reactors, synchronous condensers, and static var systems are used to control voltage. Series capacitors (SCs) are used to reduce line impedance.

Transmission substations serving bulk power sources operate at voltages from usually 69 to 765 kV or more. As an integral part of the transmission system, the substation or switching station functions as a connection and switching point for transmission lines, subtransmission lines, generating circuits, and step-up and step-down transformers. A transmission substation changes voltages to or from transmission level voltages and operates CBs in response to transmission line or substation faults. It also has the following functions: controlling power to an area, housing protective relays and instrument transformers, and housing switching arrangements that allow maintenance of any substation equipment without disrupting the power to any area served by the substation.

Essentially, a transmission substation performs all of the functions of an important distribution substation at much higher voltage and power levels. Most of the apparatus is the same and operates the same as the equipment at a distribution substation, except that it is larger and has some larger capacity functions.

In addition, there are other differences between transmission and distribution substations. For example, spacing between conductors is greater, autotransformers are often used, reactors are sometimes housed, and also grounding is more critical in bulk power substations. Figure 2.37 shows a bulk power substation operating at 138/34.5 kV voltage level. On the other hand, Figure 2.38 shows a distribution substation operating at 34.5/12.47 kV voltage level. Similarly, Figure 2.39 shows another distribution substation operating at 34.5/4.16 kV voltage level.

2.7.1 Additional Substation Design Considerations

The design of an HV substation includes basic station configuration and physical system layout, grounding, transformer selection, CB selection, bus designs, switches, lightning protection, lightning shielding, and protective relaying systems. The essential information that is needed, in determining the selection of a basic substation configuration, includes the following:

1. The estimation of initial and future loads to be served by the substation
2. A careful study of the transmission facilities and operating voltages
3. The study of service reliability requirements
4. Determination of space availability for station facilities and transmission line access

In general, the need for improved reliability dictates for additional apparatus that, in turn, requires more space. For a given substation design, the size of the bays depends on the voltages used. For example, they vary from about 24 ft^2 at 34.5 kV to about 52 ft^2 at 138 kV voltage level.

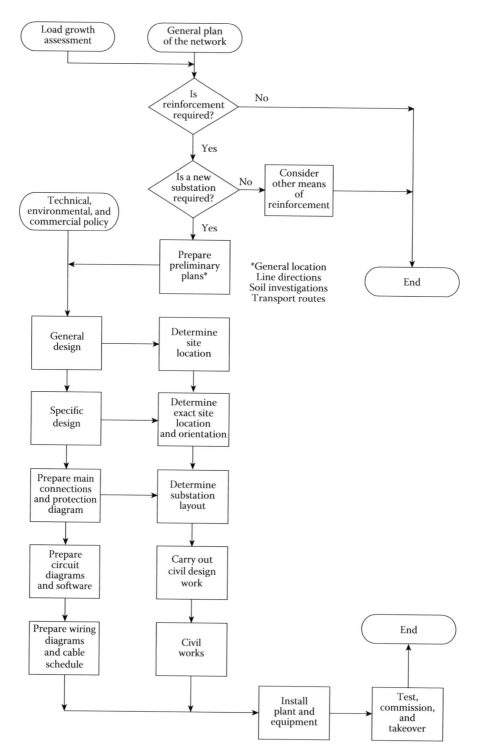

FIGURE 2.36 Establishment of a new substation. (From Burke, J. and Shazizian, M., How a substation happens?, in *Electric Power Substation Engineering*, J. D. McDonald, ed., CRC Press, Boca Raton, FL, 2007.)

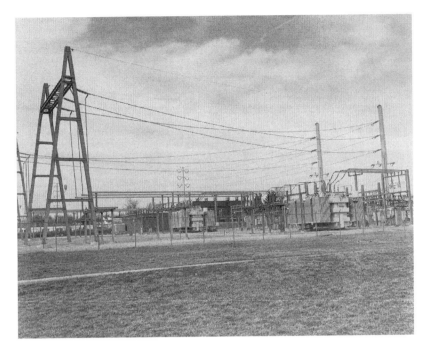

FIGURE 2.37   A bulk power substation operating at 138/34.5 kV voltage level. (Union Electric Company.)

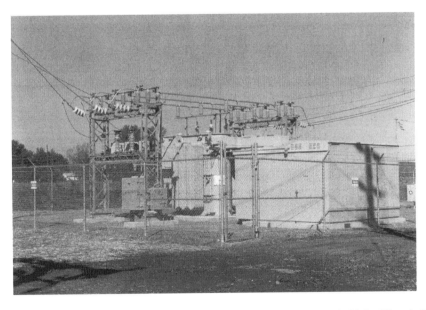

FIGURE 2.38   A distribution substation operating at 34.5/12.47 kV voltage level. (Union Electric Company.)

In order to improve the substation reliability, it is usual that more substation area is needed. This, in turn, increases the cost of the substation. The determination of reliability dictates the knowledge of the frequency of each piece of equipment and the cost of the outage. Failure rates for substations vary, depending on substation size, degree of contamination, and the definition of what is a failure.

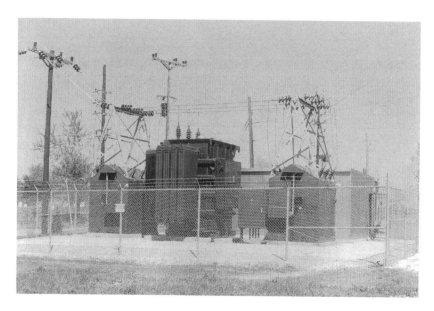

FIGURE 2.39 A distribution substation operating at 34.5/4.16 kV voltage level. (Union Electric Company.)

2.7.2 SUBSTATION COMPONENTS

A typical substation may include the following equipments: (1) power transformers, (2) CBs, (3) disconnecting switches, (4) substation buses and insulators, (5) current-limiting reactors, (6) shunt reactors, (7) current transformers (CTs), (8) potential transformers, (9) capacitor VTs, (10) coupling capacitors, (11) SCs, (12) shunt capacitors, (13) grounding system, (14) lightning arresters and/or gaps, (15) line traps, (16) protective relays, (17) station batteries, and (18) other apparatus.

2.7.3 BUS AND SWITCHING CONFIGURATIONS

In general, the substation switchyard scheme (or configuration) selected dictates the electrical and physical arrangement of the switching equipment. It is affected by the emphasis put on reliability, economy, safety, and simplicity as warranted by the function and importance of the substation. Additional factors that need to be considered are maintenance, operational flexibility, relay protection cost, and also line connections to the facility. The following are the most commonly used bus schemes:

1. Single-bus scheme
2. Double-bus–double-breaker scheme
3. Main-and-transfer bus scheme
4. Double-bus–single-breaker scheme
5. Ring bus scheme
6. Breaker-and-a half scheme

Figure 2.40a shows a typical single-bus scheme, Figure 2.40b presents a typical double-bus–double-breaker scheme, Figure 2.40c illustrates a typical main-and-transfer bus scheme, Figure 2.41a shows a typical double-bus–single-breaker scheme, Figure 2.41b presents a typical ring bus scheme, and Figure 2.41c illustrates a typical breaker-and-a-half scheme.

Each scheme has some advantages and disadvantages depending upon economical justification of a specific degree of reliability. Table 2.2 gives a summary of switching schemes' advantages and disadvantages.

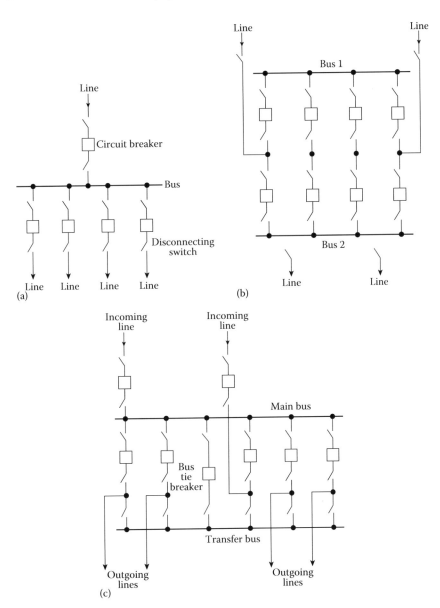

FIGURE 2.40 Most commonly used substation bus schemes: (a) single-bus scheme, (b) double-bus–double-breaker scheme, and (c) main-and-transfer bus scheme.

2.7.4 SUBSTATION BUSES

The substation buses, in HV substations or EHV substations, are a most important part of the substation structure due to the fact that they carry a large amount of energy in a confined space. The design of substation buses is a function of a number of elements. For example, it includes current-carrying capacity, short-circuit stresses, and establishing maximum electrical clearances.

They are designed and built in a manner so that the bus construction is strong enough to withstand the maximum stresses imposed on the conductors, and on the structure, by heavy currents under short-circuit conditions. In the past, the HV substations usually had the strain buses. The strain bus is similar to a transmission line and was merely a conductor such as aluminum conductor, steel reinforced (ACSR) that was strung between substation structures.

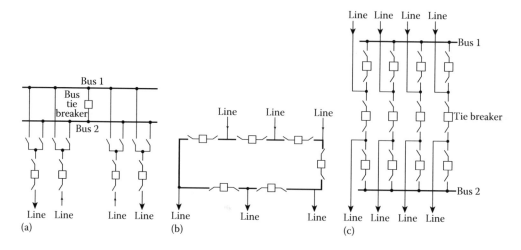

FIGURE 2.41 Most commonly used substation bus schemes: (a) double-bus–single-breaker scheme, (b) ring bus scheme, and (c) breaker-and-a-half scheme.

On the other hand, EHV substations use the rigid-bus technique. The use of rigid buses has the advantages of low substation profile and ease of maintenance and operation. In a conventional substation arrangement, it is normally a combination of mixing of rigid-and strain-bus construction. For example, the 765 kV EHV substation design has both rigid- and strain-bus arrangements. According to [7], the advantages of using the rigid-bus design are as follows:

- Less steel is used and structures are simple.
- The rigid bus is lower in height.
- Low profile with the rigid bus provides good visibility of conductors and equipment. Hence, it gives a good appearance to the substation.
- Rigid conductors are not under constant strain.
- Individual pedestal-mounted insulators are more accessible for cleaning.

The disadvantages of using the rigid bus are as follows:

- Rigid-bus designs are more expensive.
- Rigid-bus designs require more land.
- It requires more insulators and supports. (Hence, it has more insulators to clean.)
- This design is more sensitive to structural deflections that results in misalignment problems and possible bus damages.

On the other hand, the advantages of using strain bus are as follows:

- Fewer structures are required.
- It needs lesser land to occupy.
- It has a lesser cost.

The disadvantages of using strain bus are as follows:

- It requires larger structures and foundations.
- Painting of high steel structures is costly and hazardous.
- Its insulators are not conveniently accessible for cleaning.
- Conductor repairs are more difficult in emergency.

TABLE 2.2

Summary of Comparison of Switching Schemes

Switching Scheme	Advantages	Disadvantages
1. Single bus	1. Lowest cost.	1. Failure of bus or any CB results in shutdown of the entire substation. 2. Difficult to do any maintenance. 3. Bus cannot be extended without completely deenergizing substation. 4. Can be used only where loads can be interrupted or have other supply arrangements.
2. Double bus–double breaker	1. Each circuit has two dedicated breakers. 2. Has flexibility in permitting feeder circuits to be connected to either bus. 3. Any breaker can be taken out of service for maintenance. 4. High reliability.	1. Most expensive. 2. Would lose half the circuits for breaker failure if circuits are not connected to both buses.
3. Main and transfer	1. Low initial and ultimate cost. 2. Any breaker can be taken out of service for maintenance. 3. Potential devices may be used on the main bus for relaying.	1. Requires one extra breaker for the bus tie. 2. Switching is somewhat complicated when maintaining a breaker. 3. Failure of bus or any CB results in shutdown of the entire substation.
4. Double bus–single breaker	1. Permits some flexibility with two operating buses. 2. Either main bus may be isolated for maintenance. 3. Circuit can be transferred readily from one bus to the other by the use of bus-tie breaker and bus selector disconnect switches.	1. One extra breaker is required for the bus tie. 2. Four switches are required per circuit. 3. Bus protection scheme may cause loss of substation when it operates if all circuits are connected to that bus. 4. High exposure to bus faults. 5. Line breaker failure takes all circuits connected to that bus out of service. 6. Bus-tie breaker failure takes entire substation out of service.

(*continued*)

TABLE 2.2 (continued)
Summary of Comparison of Switching Schemes

Switching Scheme	Advantages	Disadvantages
5. Ring bus	1. Low initial and ultimate cost. 2. Flexible operation for breaker maintenance. 3. Any breaker can be removed for maintenance without interrupting load. 4. Requires only one breaker per circuit. 5. Does not use main bus. 6. Each circuit is fed by two breakers. 7. All switching is done with breakers.	1. If a fault occurs during a breaker maintenance period, the ring can be separated into two sections. 2. Automatic reclosing and protective relaying circuitry rather complex. 3. If a single set of relays is used, the circuit must be taken out of service to maintain the relays. (Common on all schemes.) 4. Requires potential devices on all circuits since there is no definite potential reference point. These devices may be required in all cases for synchronizing, live line, or voltage indication. 5. Breaker failure during a fault on one of the circuits causes loss of one additional circuit owing to operation of breaker failure relaying.
6. Breaker and a half	1. Most flexible operation. 2. High reliability. 3. Breaker failure of bus side breakers removes only one circuit from service. 4. All switching is done with breakers. 5. Simple operation; no disconnect switching required for normal operation. 6. Either main bus can be taken out of service at any time for maintenance. 7. Bus failure does not remove any feeder circuits from service.	1. One and a half breakers per circuit. 2. Relaying and automatic reclosing are somewhat involved since the middle breaker must be responsive to either of its associated circuits.

The current-carrying capacity of a bus is restricted by the heating effects generated by the current. Buses are rated according to the temperature rise that can be allowed without heating equipment terminals, bus connections, and joints. According to IEEE, NEMA, and ANSI standards, the permissible temperature rise for plain copper and aluminum buses is restricted to 30°C above an ambient temperature of 40°C. EHV substation bus phase spacing is based on the clearance required for switching-surge impulse values plus an allowance for energized equipment projections and corona rings.

2.7.4.1 Open-Bus Scheme

A typical conventional open-bus substation scheme has basically open-bus construction that has either only rigid- or strain-buses design or combinations of rigid and strain buses.

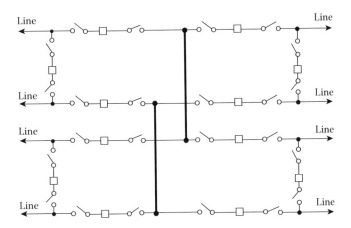

FIGURE 2.42   A low-profile EHV substation using inverted breaker-and-a-half scheme.

In arrangements employing double-bus schemes (e.g., the breaker-and-a half scheme), the buses are arranged to run the length of the substation. They are usually located toward the outside of the station.

The transmission line exists usually crossover the main bus and is dead-ended on takeoff tower structures. The line drops into one of the bays of the substation and connects to the disconnecting switches and CBs. In such arrangement, three distinct bus levels are required to make the necessary crossovers and connections to each substation bay. The open-bus scheme has the advantage of requiring a minimum of land area per bay and relative ease of maintenance [7].

2.7.4.2   Inverted-Bus Scheme

In designing EHV substations, this scheme is usually preferred. Figure 2.42 shows a one-line diagram of a substation illustrating many variations of the inverted-bus scheme. In this scheme, all of the outgoing circuit takeoff towers are located on the outer perimeter of the substation. This eliminates the line crossovers and exit facilities. Main buses are located in the middle of the substation, with all disconnecting switches, CBs, and all bay equipment located outboard of the main buses. Such inverted-bus scheme provides a very low-profile substation. It has the advantages of beauty and aesthetics, resulting in better public relations.

2.8   SF$_6$-INSULATED SUBSTATIONS

Today, there are various types of sulfur hexafluoride (SF$_6$) substations ranging from 69 kV up to 765 kV, up to 4000 A continuous current, and up to 80 kA symmetric interrupting rating.

In such substation, the buses, CBs, isolators, instrument transformers, cable sealing ends, and connections are contained in metal enclosures filled with SF$_6$. The advantages of SF$_6$ substations are little space requirement, short installation time, positive protection against contact, low noise, very little maintenance, protection against pollution, and modular design for all components, which can be installed horizontal or vertical.

Basically, an SF$_6$ substation has the same components as a conventional substation, including CBs, buses, bushings, isolators and grounding switches, and instrument transformers. The metal enclosure, made up of tubular elements, totally covers all live parts. In addition, SF$_6$-insulated cables are also being used in the following applications: (1) line crossings, (2) connections of EHV OH lines, (3) HV and/or high-current links in underground power stations, (4) HV links from offshore power plants, (5) HV cable links in city networks and substation areas, (6) power transmission in road tunnels, and (7) power transmission to airports.

2.9 TRANSMISSION LINE CONDUCTORS

In transmission line design, the determination of conductor type and size is very important. This is done due to the fact that the selection of conductor affects the cost of construction of the line but it affects perhaps more crucially the cost of transmitting power through the transmission line throughout its life.

2.9.1 CONDUCTOR CONSIDERATIONS

When selecting transmission line conductors, the following factors have to be taken into account:

1. The maximum amount of allowed current in the conductor
2. The maximum amount of power loss allowed on the line
3. The maximum amount of voltage loss allowed
4. The required spa and sag between spans
5. The tension on the conductor
6. The climate conditions at the line location (the possibility of wind and ice loading)
7. The possibility of conductor vibration
8. The possibility of having corrosive atmospheric conductors

The selected conductor should be suitable to overcome these conditions.

2.9.2 CONDUCTOR TYPES

The most commonly used transmission types are the following:

- ACSR (aluminum conductor, steel reinforced)
- ACSR/AW (aluminum conductor, aluminum-clad steel reinforced)
- ACSR-SD (aluminum conductor, steel reinforced/self-damping)
- ACAR (aluminum conductor, allow reinforced)
- AAC-1350 (aluminum alloy conductor composed of 1350 aluminum alloy)
- AAAC-201 (all aluminum alloy conductor composed of 6201 alloy)

ACSR consists of a central core of steel strands surrounded by layers of aluminum strands. Thus, an ACSR conductor with a designation of 26/7 means that it has 7 strands of galvanized steel wires in its core and 26 strands of aluminum wires surrounding its core. The galvanizing is a zinc coating placed on each of the steel wire strand. The thickness of the coating is listed as *class A* for normal thickness, *class B* for medium, and *class C* for heavy duty. The degree of conductor and atmospheric contamination dictates the class of galvanization for the core.

ACSR/AW conductor is similar to ACSR with the exception that its core is made up of high-strength steel clad in an aluminum coating. It is more expensive than ACSR. However, it can be used in worse corrosive atmospheric conditions than is the ACSR with class *C* galvanizing.

ACSR-SD conductor has two layers of trapezoidal-shaped strands or two layers of trapezoidal strands and one of round strands around a conventional steel core. They are built to have a self-damping against aeolian vibration. They can be used at very high tensions without having any auxiliary dampers.

ACAR conductors have high-strength aluminum core. It is lighter than the ACSR and is just as strong, but higher in cost. They are used in long spans in a corrosive atmosphere.

AAC-1350 is used for any construction that needs good conductivity and has short spans.

AAAC-6201 has high-strength aluminum alloy strands. It is as strong as ACSR but is much lighter and more expensive. It is used in long spans in a corrosive atmosphere.

2.9.3 CONDUCTOR SIZE

When subjected to motions such as wind gust and ice droppings, large conductors are more mechanically stable than small conductors, mainly due to their higher inertia. However, the choice of conductor size is often largely based on electrical (power loss and voltage drop considerations), thermal capacity (ampacity), and economic requirements rather than on motion considerations. Other factors include the required tensions for span and sag considerations and the breakdown voltage of the air. The voltage per unit surface area is a function of the voltage and the circumference of the chosen conductor.

Conductor sizes are based on the circular mil. A *circular mil* is the area of a circle that has a diameter of 1 mil. A mil is equal to 1×10^{-3} in. The cross-sectional area of a wire in square inches equals its area in circular mils multiplied by 0.7854×10^{-6}.

For smaller conductors, up to 211,600 circular mils, the size is usually given by a gauge number according to the American Wire Gauge (AWG) standard, formerly known as the Brown and Sharpe (B&S) wire gauge. Gauge sizes decrease as the wire increases in size. The larger the gauge size, the smaller the wire. These numbers start at 40, the smallest, which is assigned to a wire with a diameter of 3.145 mils. The largest size is number 0000, written as 4/0 and read as four odds. Above 4/0, the size is determined by cross-sectional area in circular mils. In summary,

$$1 \text{ linear mil} = 0.001 \text{ in.}$$

$$= 0.0254 \text{ mm}$$

$$1 \text{ circular mil} = \text{area of circle 1 linear mil in diameter}$$

$$= \frac{\pi}{4} \text{ square mils}$$

$$= \frac{\pi}{4} \times 10^{-6} = 0.7854 \times 10^{-6} \text{ square in.}$$

One thousand circular mils is often used as a unit, for example, a size given as 250 kcmil (or MCM) refers to 250,000 circular mils or 250,000 cmil.

A given conductor may consist of a single strand or several strands. If of a single strand, it is solid; if of more than one strand, it is stranded. A solid conductor is often called a *wire*, whereas a stranded conductor is called a *cable*. A general formula for the total number of strands in concentrically stranded cables is

$$\text{Number of strands} = 3n^2 - 3n + 1$$

where n is the number of layers, including the single center strand.

In general, distribution conductors larger than 2 AWG are stranded. Insulated conductors for underground distribution or aerial cable lines are classified as cables and usually are stranded. Table 2.3 gives standard conductor sizes.

2.9.3.1 Voltage Drop Considerations

Also, voltage drop considerations dictate that not only must the given conductor meet the minimum size requirements but must transmit power at an acceptable loss. Common minimum size conductors that are typically used for the given voltages are as follows:

For 69 kV	4/0
For 138 kV	336.4 MCM (or kcmil)
For 230 kV	795 MCM (or kcmil) single conductor
For 345 kV	795 MCM (or kcmil) bundle of two conductors
For 500 kV	795 MCM (or kcmil) bundle of three conductors
For 750 KV	795 MCM (or kcmil) bundle of four conductors

Note that Europeans have adopted a standard of 556 mm bundle of four for 500 kV.

TABLE 2.3
Standard Conductor Sizes

Size (AWG or kcmil)	(Circular mils)	Number of Wires	Solid or Stranded
18	1,620	1	Solid
16	2,580	1	Solid
14	4,110	1	Solid
12	6,530	1	Solid
10	10,380	1	Solid
8	16,510	1	Solid
7	20,820	1	Solid
6	26,250	1	Solid
6	26,250	3	Stranded
5	33,100	3	Stranded
5	33,100	1	Solid
4	41,740	1	Solid
4	41,740	3	Stranded
3	52,630	3	Stranded
3	52,630	7	Stranded
3	52,630	1	Solid
2	66,370	1	Solid
2	66,370	3	Stranded
2	66,370	7	Stranded
1	83,690	3	Stranded
1	83,690	7	Stranded
0 (or 1/0)	105,500	7	Stranded
00 (or 2/0)	133,100	7	Stranded
000 (or 3/0)	167,800	7	Stranded
000 (or 3/0)	167,800	12	Stranded
0000 (or 4/0)	211,600	7	Stranded
0000 (or 4/0)	211,600	12	Stranded
0000 (or 4/0)	211,600	19	Stranded
250	250,000	12	Stranded
250	250,000	19	Stranded
300	300,000	12	Stranded
300	300,000	19	Stranded
350	350,000	12	Stranded
350	350,000	19	Stranded
400	400,000	19	Stranded
450	450,000	19	Stranded
500	500,000	19	Stranded
500	500,000	37	Stranded
600	600,000	37	Stranded
700	700,000	37	Stranded
750	750,000	37	Stranded
800	800,000	37	Stranded
900	900,000	37	Stranded
1,000	1,000,000	37	Stranded

This requirement is often expressed as a maximum voltage drop of 5% across the transmission line for a particular system. The total series impedance of the line is equal to the maximum allowable voltage drop divided by the maximum load current. Hence,

$$Z_L = |R + jX_L| = \frac{VD_{max}}{I_{max}} \tag{2.1}$$

where
Z_L is the magnitude of the total impedance of the line
R is the total resistance of the line
X_L is the total inductive reactance of the line
VD_{max} is the maximum allowable voltage drop for the line
I_{max} is the maximum load current

Note that R is inversely proportional to the area of the conductor size.

2.9.3.2 Thermal Capacity Considerations

When a phase conductor is sized, the thermal capacity of the conductor (ampacity) has to be taken into account. In another words, *the conductor should be able to carry the maximum expressed long-term load current without experiencing any overheating.* Typically, a conductor must be able to withstand a temperature of 75°C (167°F) without a decrease in the strength. Above that temperature, the strength of the conductor decreases as a function of the amount and duration of the excessive heat.

In general, the ampacity of a conductor is a function of the generated heat by the current itself, the heat from the sun, and the cooling of the winds. Conductor heating is expressed as ambient temperature plus load temperature, less cooling effects of the wind.

2.9.3.3 Economic Considerations

Economic considerations are very important in the determination of conductor size of a transmission line. Usually, the conductor that meets the minimum aforementioned factors is not the most economical one.

The present worth of the savings that result from the lower power losses during the entire useful life of a conductor has to be taken into account. Hence, a larger conductor, than the one that just barely meets the minimum requirements, is often more justifiable. In other words, the marginal additional cost involved will be more than offset by the cost savings of the future.

To make any meaningful conductor size selection, the transmission planning engineer should make a cost study associated with the line. The cost analysis for the proper conductor size should include the following: (1) investment cost of installed line with the particular conductor being considered, (2) cost of energy loss due to total I^2R losses in the line conductors, and (3) cost of demand lost, that is, the cost of useful system capacity lost (including generation, transmission, and distribution systems), in order to resupply the line losses. Hence, the total present worth of line cost (TPWL) at a given conductor size is

$$\text{TPWL} = \text{PWIC} + \text{PWEC} + \text{PWDC} \ \$/\text{mi} \tag{2.2}$$

where
TPWL is the total present worth cost of the line in dollar per mile
PWEC is the present worth of the investment cost of the installed feeder in dollar per mile
PWEC is the present worth of energy cost due to I^2R losses in the line conductors in dollar per mile
PWDC is the present worth of the demand cost incurred to maintain adequate system capacity to resupply I^2R losses in the line conductors in order to compensate for the line losses in dollar per mile

In addition to these considerations, the future load growth is also needed to be considered.

2.9.4 Overhead Ground Wires

OHGWs are also called the shield wires. They are the wires that are installed above the phase conductors (or wires). They are used to protect the line from lightning and to even out the ground potential and are sometimes even used for low-voltage (LV) communication. The OHGWs do not conduct the load current, but they very rapidly conduct the very heavy current of a lightning strike to the ground, through their many grounded connections. Every transmission structure is all grounded and the OHGW is grounded at every structure (whether it is a pole or tower).

High-strength or extra-strength galvanized steel wires are used. The allowable sizes for the high-strength wires are 3/8 and 7/16 in., while the allowable sizes for the extra-strength wires are 5/26, 3/8, and 7/16 in. The sags of the OHGWs must be the same as the sags of the phase conductors.

2.9.5 Conductor Tension

The conductor tension of a transmission line may vary between 10% and 60% or even more of its rated conductor strength. This is due to change in line loading and temperature. Normal tensions may be more important for determination of the life of the conductor of a line than higher tensions that do not occur frequently. The proper conductor tensions are given in the NESC based on ice and wind loadings in the loading districts of heavy, medium, and light loading.

2.10 INSULATORS

2.10.1 Types of Insulators

An *insulator* is a material that prevents the flow of an electric current and can be used to support electrical conductors. The function of an insulator is to provide for the necessary clearances between the line conductors, between conductors and ground, and between conductors and the pole or tower. Insulators are made of porcelain, glass, and fiberglass treated with epoxy resins. However, porcelain is still the most common material used for insulators.

The basic types of insulators include *pin-type insulators*, *suspension insulators*, and *strain insulators*. The pin insulator gets its name from the fact that it is supported on a pin. The pin holds the insulator, and the insulator has the conductor tied to it. They may be made in one piece for voltages below 23 kV, in two pieces for voltages from 23 to 46 kV, in three pieces for voltages from 46 to 69 kV, and in four pieces for voltages from 69 to 88 kV. Pin insulators are seldom used on transmission lines having voltages above 44 kV, although some 88 kV lines using pin insulators are in operation. The glass pin insulator is mainly used on LV circuits. The porcelain pin insulator is used on secondary mains and services, as well as on primary mains, feeders, and transmission lines.

A modified version of the pin-type insulator is known as the *post-type insulator*. The post-type insulators are used on distribution, subtransmission, and transmission lines and are installed on wood, concrete, and steel poles. The line postinsulators are constructed for vertical or horizontal mountings. The line postinsulators are usually made as one-piece solid porcelain units. Figure 2.43 shows a typical post-type porcelain insulator. Suspension insulators consist of a string of interlinking separate disks made of porcelain. A string may consist of many disks depending on the line voltage.* For example, as an average, for 115 kV lines, usually 7 disks are used and for 345 kV lines, usually 18 disks are used.

---

* In average practice, the number of units used in an insulator string is approximately proportional to the line voltage, with a slight increase for the highest voltages and with some allowances for the length of insulator unit. For example, 4 or 5 units have generally been used at 69 kV, 7 or 8 at 115 kV, 8–10 at 138 kV, 9–11 at 161 kV, 14–20 at 230 kV, 15–18 at 345 kV, 24–35 at 500 kV (with the 35 unit insulator strings used at high altitudes), 33–35 at 735 kV (Hydro-Quebec), and 30–35 at 765 kV.

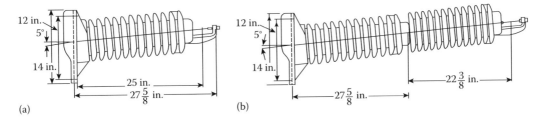

FIGURE 2.43 Typical (side) post-type insulators used in (a) 69 kV and (b) 138 kV.

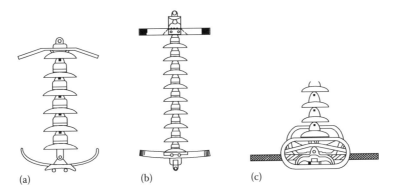

FIGURE 2.44 Devices used to protect insulator strings: (a) suspension string with arcing horns, (b) suspension string with grading shields (or *arcing rings*), and (c) suspension string with control ring. (Courtesy of The Ohio Brass Company.)

The *suspension insulator*, as its name implies, is suspended from the crossarm (or pole or tower) and has the line conductor fastened to lower end. When there is a dead end of the line, or there is corner or a sharp curve, or the line crosses a river, etc., then the line will withstand great strain. The assembly of suspension units arranged to dead-end the conductor of a structure is called a *dead-end*, or *strain*, insulator.

In such an arrangement, suspension insulators are used as strain insulators. The dead-end string is usually protected against damage from arcs by using one to three additional units and installing arcing horns or rings, as shown in Figure 2.44. Such devices are designed to ensure that an arc (e.g., due to lightning impulses) will hold free of insulator string.

The arcing horns protect the insulator string by providing a shorter path for the arc, as shown in Figure 2.44a. Contrarily, the effectiveness of the arcing ring (or grading shield), shown in Figure 2.44b, is due to its tendency to equalize the voltage gradient over the insulator, causing a more uniform field.

Thus, the protection of the insulator is not dependent on simply providing a shorter arcing path, as is the case with horns. Figure 2.44c shows a control ring developed by The Ohio Brass Company that can be used to *control* the voltage stress at the line end of the insulator strings.

It has been shown that their use can also reduce the corona formation on the line hardware. Control rings are used on single-conductor HV transmission lines operating above 250 kV. Transmission lines with bundled conductors do not require the use of arcing horns and rings nor control rings, provided that the bundle is not made of two conductors one above the other.

2.10.2 TESTING OF INSULATORS

The operating performance of a transmission line depends largely on the insulation. Experience has shown that for a satisfactory operation, the dry flashover operating voltage of the assembled insulator must be equal to three to five times the nominal operating voltage and its leakage path must be about twice the shortest air gap distance. Insulators used on OH lines are subject to tests that can generally be classified as (1) design tests, (2) performance tests, and (3) routine tests. The *design tests* include dry flashover test, pollution flashover test, wet flashover test, and impulse test.

The *flashover voltage* is defined as the voltage at which the insulator surface breaks down (by ionization of the air surrounding the insulator), allowing current to flow on the outside of the insulator between the conductor and the crossarm. Whether or not an insulator breaks down depends not only on the magnitude of the applied voltage but also on the rate at which the voltage increases.

Since insulations have to withstand steep-fronted lightning and switching surges when they are in use, their design must provide the flashover voltage* on a steep-fronted impulse waveform that is greater than that on a normal system waveform. The ratio of these voltages is defined as the *impulse ratio*. Hence,

$$\text{Impulse ratio} = \frac{\text{impulse flashover voltage}}{\text{power frequency flashover voltage}} \tag{2.3}$$

Table 2.4 gives flashover characteristics of suspension insulator strings and air gaps [10]. The performance tests include puncture tests, mechanical test, temperature test, porosity test, and electromechanical test (for suspension insulators only). The event that takes place, when the dielectric of the insulator breaks down and allows current to flow inside the insulator between the conductor and the crossarm, is called the *puncture*.

Therefore, the design must facilitate the occurrence of flashover at a voltage that is lower than the voltage for puncture. An insulator may survive flashover without damage but must be replaced when punctured. The test of the glaze on porcelain insulators is called the *porosity test*. The routine tests include proof test, corrosion test, and HV test (for pin insulators only).†

2.10.3 Voltage Distribution over a String of Suspension Insulators

Figure 2.45 shows the voltage distribution along the surface of a single clean insulator disk (known as the *cap-and-pin insulator unit*) used in suspension insulators. Note that the highest voltage gradient takes place close to the cap and pin (which are made of metal), whereas much lower voltage gradients take place along most of the remaining surfaces. The underside (i.e., the inner skirt) of the insulator has been given the shape, as shown in Figure 2.45, to minimize the effects of moisture and contamination and to provide the longest path possible for the leakage currents that might flow on the surface of the insulator.

In the figure, the voltage drop between the cap and the pin has been taken as 100% of the total voltage. Approximately, 24% of this voltage is distributed along the surface of the insulator from the cap to point 1 and only 6% from point 1 to point 9. The remaining 70% of this voltage is distributed between point 9 and the pin.

The main problem with suspension insulators having a string of identical insulator disks is the nonuniform distribution voltage over the string. Each insulator disk with its hardware (i.e., cap and pin) constitutes a capacitor, the hardware acting as the plates or electrodes, and the porcelain as the

---

* This phenomenon is studied in the laboratory by subjecting insulators to voltage impulses by means of a *lightning generator*.
† For further information, see the ANSI standard C29.1–C29.9.

TABLE 2.4

Flashover Characteristics of Suspension Insulator Strings and Air Gaps

Impulse Air Gap		Impulse Flashover (Positive Critical), kV	Number of Insulator Units[a]	Wet 60 Hz Flashover, kV	Wet 60 Hz Air Gap	
in.	mm				mm	in.
8	203	150	1	50	254	10
14	356	255	2	90	305	12
21	533	355	3	130	406	16
26	660	440	4	170	508	20
32	813	525	5	215	660	26
38	965	610	6	255	762	30
43	1092	695	7	295	889	35
49	1245	780	8	335	991	39
55	1397	860	9	375	111	44
60	1524	945	10	415	1245	49
66	1676	1025	11	455	1346	53
71	1803	1105	12	490	1473	58
77	1956	1185	13	525	1575	62
82	2083	1265	14	565	1676	66
88	2235	1345	15	600	1778	70
93	2362	1425	16	630	1880	74
99	2515	1505	17	660	1981	78
104	2642	1585	18	690	2083	82
110	2794	1665	19	720	2183	86
115	2921	1745	20	750	2286	90
121	3073	1825	21	780	2388	94
126	3200	1905	22	810	2464	97
132	3353	1985	23	840	2565	101
137	3480	2065	24	870	2692	106
143	3632	2145	25	900	2794	110
148	3759	2225	26	930	2921	115
154	3912	2305	27	960	3023	119
159	4039	2385	28	990	3124	123
165	4191	2465	29	1020	3251	128
171	4343	2550	30	1050	3353	132

Source: Edison Electric Institute, *EHV Transmission Line Reference Book*, EEI, New York, 1968.

[a] Insulator units are 146 × 254 mm (5¾ × 10 in.) or 146 × 267 mm (5¾ ×10½ in.).

dielectric. Figure 2.46 shows the typical voltage distribution on the surfaces of three clean cap-and-pin insulator units connected in series [10]. The figure clearly illustrates that when several units are connected in series, (1) the voltage on each insulator over the string is not the same, (2) the location of the unit within the insulator string dictates the voltage distribution, and (3) the maximum voltage gradient takes place at the (pin of the) insulator unit nearest to the line conductor.

As shown in Figure 2.47, when several insulator units are placed in series, two sets of capacitances take place: the series capacitances C_i (i.e., the capacitance of each insulator unit) and the shunt capacitances to ground, C_2. Note that all the charging current I for the series and shunt capacitances flows through the first (with respect to the conductor) of the series capacitances C_1. The I_1 portion of this current flows through the first shunt capacitance C_2, leaving the remaining I_1

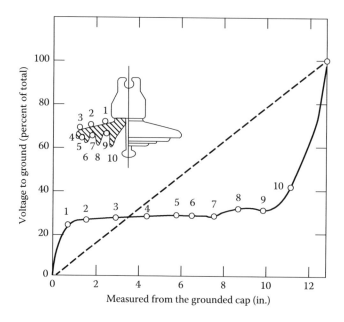

FIGURE 2.45 Voltage distribution along the surface of single clean cap-and-pin suspension insulator.

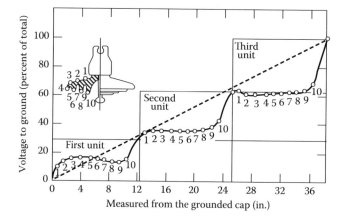

FIGURE 2.46 A typical voltage distribution on surfaces of three clean cap-and-pin suspension insulator units in series.

portion of the current to flow through the second series capacitance, and so on. The diminishing current flow through the series capacitances C_1 results in a diminishing voltage (drop) distribution through them from conductor end to ground end (i.e., crossarm), as illustrated in Figure 2.47. Thus,

$$V_5 > V_4 > V_3 > V_2 > V_1$$

In summary, the voltage distribution over a string of identical suspension insulator units is not uniform due to the capacitances formed in the air between each cap/pin junction and the grounded (metal) tower.

However, other air capacitances exist between metal parts at different potentials. For example, there are air capacitances between the cap/pin junction of each unit and the line conductor.

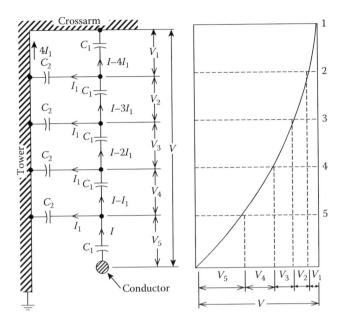

FIGURE 2.47 Voltage distribution among suspension insulator units.

Figure 2.48 shows the resulting equivalent circuit for the voltage distribution along a clean eight-unit insulator string. The voltage distribution on such a string can be expressed as

$$V_k = \frac{V_n}{\beta^2 \sinh \beta n} \left[\frac{C_2}{C_1} \sinh \beta k + \frac{C_3}{C_1} \sinh \beta (k-n) + \frac{C_3}{C_1} \sinh \beta n \right] \quad (2.4)$$

where
V_k is the voltage across k units from ground end
V_n is the voltage across n units (i.e., applied line-to-ground voltage in volts)

$$\beta = \text{a constant} = \left(\frac{C_2 + C_3}{2} \right)^{1/2} \quad (2.5)$$

C_1 is the capacitance between cap and pin of each unit
C_2 is the capacitance of one unit to ground
C_3 is the capacitance of one unit to line conductor

The capacitance C_3 is usually very small, and therefore, its effect to the voltage distribution can be neglected. Hence, Equation 2.4 can be expressed as

$$V_k = V_n \left(\frac{\sinh \alpha k}{\sinh \alpha n} \right) \quad (2.6)$$

where

$$\alpha = \text{a constant} = \left(\frac{C_2}{C_1} \right)^{1/2} \quad (2.7)$$

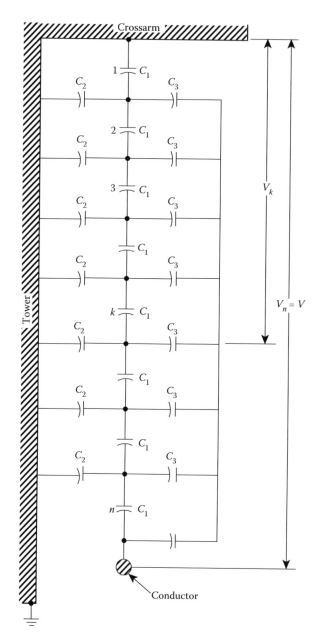

FIGURE 2.48 An equivalent circuit for voltage distribution along clean eight-unit insulator string. (Adopted from Edison Electric Institute, *EHV Transmission Line Reference Book*, EEI, New York, 1968.)

Figure 2.49 shows how the voltage changes along the eight-unit string of insulators when the ratio C_2/C_1 is about 1/12 and the ratio C_3/C_1 is about zero (i.e., $C_3 = 0$). However, a calculation based on Equation 2.33 gives almost the same result. The ratio C_2/C_1 is usually somewhere between 0.1 and 0.2.

Furthermore, there is also the air capacitance that exists between the conductor and the tower. But it has no effect on the voltage distribution over the insulator string, and therefore, it can be neglected. This method of calculating the voltage distribution across the string is based on the assumption that the insulator units involved are clean and dry, and thus, they act as a purely capacitive voltage divider. In reality, however, the insulator units may not be clean or dry.

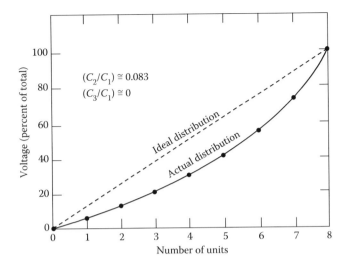

FIGURE 2.49   Voltage distribution along a clean eight-unit cap-and-pin insulator string.

Thus, in the equivalent circuit of the insulator string, each capacitance C_1 should be shunted by a resistance R representing the leakage resistance. Such resistance depends on the presence of contamination (i.e., pollution) on the insulator surfaces and is considerably modified by rain and fog. If, however, the units are badly contaminated, the surface leakage (resistance) currents could be greater than the capacitance currents, and the extent of the contamination could vary from unit to unit, causing an unpredictable voltage distribution.

It is also interesting to note that if the insulator unit nearest to the line conductor is electrically stressed to its safe operating value, then all the other units are electrically understressed, and consequently, the insulation string as a whole is being inefficiently used. The string efficiency (in per units) for an insulator string made of n series units can be defined as

$$\text{String efficiency} = \frac{\text{voltage across string}}{n\left(\text{voltage across unit adjacent to line conductor}\right)} \tag{2.8}$$

If the unit adjacent to the line conductor is about to flashover, then the whole string is about to flashover. Here, the string efficiency can be reexpressed as

$$\text{String efficiency} = \frac{\text{flashover voltage of string}}{n\left(\text{flashover voltage across of one unit}\right)} \tag{2.9}$$

Note that the string efficiency decreases as the number of units increases.

The methods to improve the string efficiency (grading) include the following:

1. By grading the insulators so that the top unit has the minimum series capacitances C_1 whereas the bottom unit has the maximum capacitance. This may be done by using different sizes of disks and hardware or by putting metal caps on the disks or by a combination of both methods.* But this is a rarely used method since it would involve stocking spares of different types of units, which is contrary to the present practice of the utilities to standardize on as few types as possible.

---

* Proposed by Peek [11,12].

2. By installing a large circular or oval grading shield ring (i.e., an arcing ring) at the line end of the insulator string [10]. This method introduces a capacitance C_3, as shown in Figure 2.48, from the ring to the insulator hardware to neutralize the capacitance C_2 from the hardware to the tower. This method substantially improves the string efficiency. However, it is not usually possible in practice to achieve completely uniform voltage distribution by using the gradient shield, especially if the string has a large number of units.

3. By reducing the air (shunt) capacitances C_3, between each unit and the tower (i.e., the *ground*), and by increasing the length of the crossarms. However, this method is restricted in practice due to the reduction on crossarm rigidity and the increase in tower cost.

4. By using a semiconducting (or stabilizing) high-resistance glaze on the insulator units to achieve a resistor voltage divider effect. This method is based on the fact that the string efficiency increases due to the increase in surface leakage resistance when the units are wet. Thus, the leakage resistance current becomes the same for all the units, and the voltage distribution improves since it does not depend on the capacitance currents only. This method is restricted by the risk of thermal instability.

2.10.4 Insulator Flashover due to Contamination

An insulator must be capable of enduring extreme sudden temperature changes such as ice, sleet, and rain as well as environmental contaminants such as smoke, dust, salt, fogs, saltwater sprays, and chemical fumes without deterioration from chemical action, breakage from mechanical stresses, or electric failure. Further, the insulating material must be thick enough to resist puncture by the combined working voltage of the line, and any probable transient whose time lag to spark over is great. If this thickness is greater than the desirable amount, then two or more pieces are used to achieve the proper thickness.

The thickness of a porcelain part must be so related to the distance around it that it will flashover before it will puncture. The ratio of puncture strength to flashover voltage is called the *safety factor* of the part or of the insulator against puncture. This ratio should be high enough to provide sufficient protection for the insulator from puncture by the transients.

The insulating materials mainly used for the line insulators are (1) wet-process porcelain, (2) dry-process porcelain, and (3) glass. The wet-process porcelain is used much more than dry porcelain. One of the reasons for this is that wet porcelain has greater resistance to impact and is practically incapable of being penetrated by moisture without glazing, whereas dry porcelain is not.

However, in general, dry-process porcelain has somewhat higher crushing strength. Dry-process porcelain is only used for the lowest voltage lines. As a result of recent development in the technology of glass manufacturing, the glass insulators that can be very tough and have a low internal resistance can be produced. Because of this, the usage of glass insulators is increasing.

In order to select insulators properly for a given OH line design, not only the aforementioned factors but also the geographic location of the line needs to be considered. For example, the OH lines that will be built along the seashore, especially in California, will be subjected to winds blowing in from the ocean, which carry a fine salt vapor that deposits salt crystals on the windward side of the insulator.

On the other hand, if the line is built in areas where rain is seasonal, the insulator surface leakage resistance may become so low during the dry seasons that insulators flashover without warning. Another example is that if the OH line is going to be built near gravel pits, cement mills, and refineries, its insulators may become so contaminated that extra insulation is required.

Contamination flashover on transmission systems is initiated by airborne particles deposited on the insulators. These particles may be of natural origin or they may be generated by pollution that is mostly a result of industrial, agricultural, or construction activities. When line insulators are contaminated, many insulator flashovers occur during light fogs unless arcing rings protect the insulators or special fog-type insulators are used.

TABLE 2.5
Numbers of Flashovers Caused by Various Contaminant, Weather, and Atmospheric Conditions

Type of Contaminant	Weather and Atmospheric Conditions								
	Fog	Dew	Drizzle, Mist	Ice	Rain	No Wind	High Wind	Wet Snow	Fair
Sea salt	14	11	22	1	12	3	12	3	—
Cement	12	10	16	2	11	3	1	4	—
Fertilizer	7	5	8	—	1	1	—	4	—
Fly ash	11	6	19	1	6	3	1	3	1
Road salt	8	2	6	—	4	2	—	6	—
Potash	3	3	—	—	—	—	—	—	
Cooling tower	2	2	2	—	2	—	—	—	—
Chemicals	9	5	7	1	1	—	—	1	1
Gypsum	2	1	2	—	2	—	—	2	—
Mixed contamination	32	19	37	—	13	1	—	1	—
Limestone	2	1	2	—	4	—	2	2	—
Phosphate and sulfate	4	1	4	—	3	—	—	—	
Paint	1	1	—	—	1	—	—	—	
Paper mill	2	2	4	—	2	—	—	1	—
Acid exhaust	2	3	—	—	—	—	1	—	
Bird droppings	2	2	3	—	1	2	—	—	2
Zinc industry	2	1	2	—	1	—	—	1	—
Carbon	5	4	5	—	—	4	3	3	—
Soap	2	2	1	—	—	1	—	—	—
Steel works	6	5	3	2	2	—	—	1	—
Carbide residue	2	1	1	1	—	—	—	1	—
Sulfur	3	2	2	—	—	1	—	1	—
Copper and nickel salt	2	2	2	—	—	2	—	1	—
Wood fiber	1	1	1	—	1	—	—	1	—
Bulldozing dust	2	1	1	—	—	—	—	—	
Aluminum plant	2	2	1	—	1	—	—	—	
Sodium plant	1	1	—	—	—	—	—	—	
Active pump	1	1	1	—	—	—	—	—	
Rock crusher	3	3	5	—	1	—	—	—	
Total flashover	146	93	166	8	68	26	19	38	4
Percent weather	25.75	16.4	29.3	1.4	12	4.58	3.36	6.52	0.71

Table 2.5 lists the types of contaminants causing contamination flashover [1]. The mixed contamination condition is the most common caused by the combination of industrial pollution and sea salt or by the combination of several industrial pollutions. Table 2.5 also presents the prevailing weather conditions at the time of flashover. Fog, dew, drizzle, and mist are common weather conditions, accounting for 72% of the total. In general, a combination of dew and fog is considered as the most severe wetting condition, even though fog is not necessary for the wetting process.

The surface leakage resistance of an insulator is unaffected by the dry deposits of dirt. However, when these contamination deposits become moist or wet, they constitute continuous conducting layers. Leakage current starts to flow in these layers along the surface of the insulators. This leakage

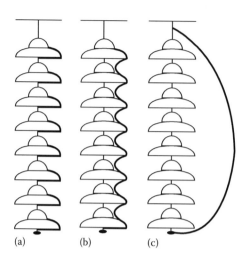

(a)   (b)   (c)

FIGURE 2.50 Changes in channel position of contaminated flashover.

current heats the wet contamination, and the water starts to evaporate from those areas where the product of current density and surface resistivity is greater, causing the surface resistivity further to increase.

This, in turn, produces more heat, which evaporates the moisture in the surrounding regions, causing the formation of circular patterns known as *dry bands* until the leakage currents decreased to a value insufficient to sustain further evaporation and the voltage builds up across the dry bands.

Further wetting results in further reduction of the resistance, and small flashovers taking place on the insulator are in the same condition; the arcs extend rapidly over the whole surface, forcing all the dry bands to discharge in a rapid cascade known as the *flashover* of the insulator. Figure 2.50 illustrates the phenomenon of insulator flashover due to contamination.

Severe contamination may reduce the 60 Hz flashover voltage from approximately 50 kV root-mean-square (rms) per unit to as low as 6–9 kV rms per unit. The condition of such flashover may be developed during the melting of contaminated ice on the insulator by leakage currents.

An insulator flashover due to contamination is easily distinguished from other types of flashover due to the fact that the arc always begins close to the surface of the insulator unit, as shown in Figure 2.50a. As shown in Figure 2.50c, only in the final stage does the flashover resemble an air strike. Furthermore, since the insulator unit at the conductor end has the greatest voltage, the flashover phenomenon usually starts at that insulator unit.

To prevent insulator flashovers, the insulators of an OH transmission line may be cleaned simply by washing them, a process that can be done basically either by the conventional techniques or by the new technique. In the conventional techniques, the line is deenergized, and its conductors are grounded at each pole or tower where the members of an insulator cleaning crew wash and wipe the insulators by hand.

In the new technique, the line is kept energized, while the insulators may be cleaned by high-pressure water jets produced by a truck-mounted high-pressure pump that forces water through a nozzle at 500–850 psi, developing a round solid stream. The water jets strike the insulator with a high velocity, literally tearing the dirt and other contaminants from the insulator surface. The cost of insulator cleaning per unit is very low by this technique. Certain lines may need insulator cleaning as often as three times a year.

To overcome the problem of surface contamination, some insulators may be covered with a thin film of silicone grease that absorbs the dirt and makes the surface water form into droplets rather than a thin film. This technique is especially effective for spot contamination where maintenance is possible, and it is also used against sea salt contamination. Finally, specially built semiconducting glazed insulators having arc-resistive coating are used. The heat produced by the resistive coating keeps the surface dry and provides for relatively linear potential distribution.

2.10.5 INSULATOR FLASHOVER ON OVERHEAD HVDC LINES

Even though mechanical considerations are similar for both ac and dc lines, electrical characteristics of insulators on dc lines are significantly different from those on dc lines, and flashover takes place much more frequently than on an ac line of equivalent voltage. This is caused partly by the electrostatic forces of the steady dc field, which increases the deposit of pollution on the insulator surface. Further, arcs tend to develop into flashovers more readily in the absence of voltage zero.

To improve the operating performance and reduce the construction cost of OH HVDC lines by using new insulating materials and new insulator configurations particularly suited to dc voltages' stress, more compact line design can be produced, therefore, saving money on towers and ROWs.

For example, to improve the operating performance and reduce the construction cost of OH HVDC lines, EPRI has sponsored the development of a new insulator. One of the more popular designs, the composite insulator, uses a fiberglass rod for mechanical and electrical strength and flexibility skirts made of organic materials for improved flashover performance. The composite insulator appears to be especially attractive for use on HVDC lines because it is better able to withstand flashover in all types of contaminated environments, particularly in areas of light and medium contamination.

Furthermore, there are various measures that may be taken into account to prevent contamination flashovers, for example, overinsulation, installment of v-string insulators, and installment of horizontal string insulators. Overinsulation may be applicable in the areas of heavy contamination. Up to 345 kV, the overinsulation is often achieved by increasing the number of insulators. However, several contaminations may dictate the use of very large leakage distances that may be as large as double the minimal requirements. Thus, electrical, mechanical, and economic restrictions may limit the use of this design measure. The use of the v-string insulators can prevent the insulation contamination substantially. They self-clean more effectively in rain than vertical insulators since both sides of each insulator disk are somewhat exposed to rain. They can be used in heavy contamination areas very effectively. The installment of horizontal insulator strings is the most effective design measure that can be used to prevent contamination flashovers in the very heavy contamination areas. The contaminants are most effectively washed away on such strings. However, they may require a strain tower support depending on the tower type.

Other techniques used include the installation of specially designed and built insulators. For example, the use of fog-type insulators has shown that the contamination flashover can be effectively reduced since most of the flashovers occur in conditions where there is mist, dew, and fog.

2.11 SUBSTATION GROUNDING

2.11.1 ELECTRICAL SHOCK AND ITS EFFECTS ON HUMANS

To properly design a grounding (called *equipment grounding*) for the HV lines and/or substations, it is important to understand the electrical characteristics of the most important part of the circuit, the human body. In general, shock currents are classified based on the degree of severity of the shock they cause. For example, currents that produce direct physiological harm are called primary shock currents.

Whereas currents that cannot produce direct physiological harm but may cause involuntary muscular reactions are called *secondary shock currents*. These shock currents can be either steady state or transient in nature. In ac power systems, steady-state currents are sustained currents of 60 Hz or its harmonics. The transient currents, on the other hand, are capacitive discharge currents whose magnitudes diminish rapidly with time.

TABLE 2.6

Effect of Electric Current (in mA) on Men and Women

	DC		AC (60 Hz)	
Effects	Men	Women	Men	Women
1. No sensation on hand	1	0.6	0.4	0.3
2. Slight tingling; per caption threshold	5.2	3.5	1.1	0.7
3. Shock not painful and muscular control not lost	9	6	1.8	1.2
4. Painful shock painful but muscular control not lost	62	41	9	6
5. Painful shock—let-go threshold[a]	76	51	16	10.5
6. Painful and severe shock, muscular contractions, breathing difficult	90	60	23	15
7. Possible ventricular fibrillation from short shocks:				
(a) Shock duration 0.03 s	1300	1300	1000	1000
(b) Shock duration 3.0 s	500	500	100	100
(c) Almost certain ventricular fibrillation (if shock duration over one heartbeat interval)	1375	1375	275	275

[a] Threshold for 50% of the males and female tested.

Table 2.6 gives the possible effects of electrical shock currents on humans. Note that the threshold value for a normally healthy person to be able to feel a current is about 1 mA. (Experiments have long ago established the well-known fact that *electrical shock effects are due to current, not voltage* [11].) This is the value of current at which a person is just able to detect a slight tingling sensation on the hands or fingers due to current flow. Currents of approximately 10–30 mA can cause lack of muscular control. In most humans, a current of 100 mA will cause ventricular fibrillation. Currents of higher magnitudes can stop the heart completely or cause severe electrical burns. The ventricular fibrillation is a condition where the heart beats in an abnormal and ineffective manner, with fatal results. Therefore, its threshold is the main concern in grounding design.

Currents of 1 mA or more but less than 6 mA are often defined as the secondary shock currents (*let-go currents*). The let-go current is the maximum current level at which a human holding an energized conductor can control his muscles enough to release it. The 60 Hz minimum required body current leading to possible fatality through ventricular fibrillation can be expressed as

$$I = \frac{0.116}{\sqrt{t}} \text{ A} \qquad (2.10)$$

Equipment protection is only part of the reason that substations are so well grounded. Personnel protection is a major consideration. A continuous current of 0.15 A flowing through the trunk part of the body is almost always fatal. To properly design a grounding (called *equipment grounding*) for the HV lines and/or substations, it is important to understand the electrical characteristics of the most important part of the circuit, the human body.

In general, shock currents are classified based on the degree of severity of the shock they cause. For example, currents that produce direct physiological harm are called *primary shock currents*. However, currents that cannot produce direct physiological harm but may cause involuntary muscular reactions are called *secondary shock currents*. These shock currents can be either steady state or transient in nature. In ac power systems, steady-state currents are sustained currents of 60 Hz or its harmonics. The transient currents, on the other hand, are capacitive currents of whose magnitudes diminish rapidly with time.

The threshold value for a normally healthy person to be able to feel a current is about 1 mA. (Experiments have long ago established the well-known fact that *electrical shock effects are due to current, not voltage.*) This is the value of current at which a person is just able to detect a slight tingling sensation on the hands or fingers due to current flow.

Currents of 1 mA or more but less than 6 mA are often defined as the *secondary shock currents* (*let-go currents*). The let-go current is the maximum current level at which a human holding an energized conductor can control his muscles enough to release it. Currents of approximately 10–30 mA can cause lack of muscular control. In most humans, a current of 100 mA will cause ventricular fibrillation. Currents of higher magnitudes can stop the heart completely or cause severe electrical burns.

The *ventricular fibrillation* is a condition where the heart beats in an abnormal and inefficient manner, with fatal results. Therefore, its threshold is the main concern in grounding design. IEEE Std. 80-2000 gives the following equation to find that the nonfibrillating current of magnitude I_B at durations ranging from 0.03 to 3.0 s is related to the energy absorbed by the body as

$$S_B = (I_B)^2 \times t_s \tag{2.11}$$

where
  I_B is the rms magnitude of the current through the body in amperes
  t_s is the duration of the current exposure in seconds
  S_B is the empirical constant related to the electrical shock energy tolerated by a certain percent of a given population

The effects of an electric current passing through the vital parts of a human body depend on the duration, magnitude, and frequency of this current. The body resistance considered is usually between two extremities, either from one hand to both feet or from one foot to the other one.

Experiments have shown that the body can tolerate much more current flowing from one leg to the other than it can when current flows from one hand to the legs. Treating the foot as a circular plate electrode gives an approximate resistance of $3\rho_s$, where ρ_s is the soil resistivity. The resistance used for the body itself is usually about 2300 Ω hand to hand or 1100 Ω hand to foot [12]. However, IEEE Std. 80-2000 [14] recommends the use of 1000 Ω as a reasonable approximation for body resistance. Figure 2.51a shows a touch contact with current flowing from hand to feet. On the other hand, Figure 2.51b shows a step contact where current flows from one foot to the other. Note that in each case, the body current I_b is driven by the potential difference points *A* and *B*.

Currents of 1 mA or more but less than 6 mA are often defined as the secondary shock currents (*let-go currents*). The let-go current is the maximum current level at which a human holding an energized conductor can control his muscles enough to release it. For 99.5% of population, the 60 Hz minimum required body current, I_B, leading to *possible fatality through ventricular fibrillation* can be expressed as

$$I_B = \frac{0.116}{\sqrt{t_s}} \text{ A} \quad \text{for 50 kg body weight} \tag{2.12a}$$

or

$$I_B = \frac{0.157}{\sqrt{t_s}} \text{ A} \quad \text{for 70 kg body weight} \tag{2.12b}$$

where *t* is in seconds in the range from approximately 8.3 ms to 5 s.

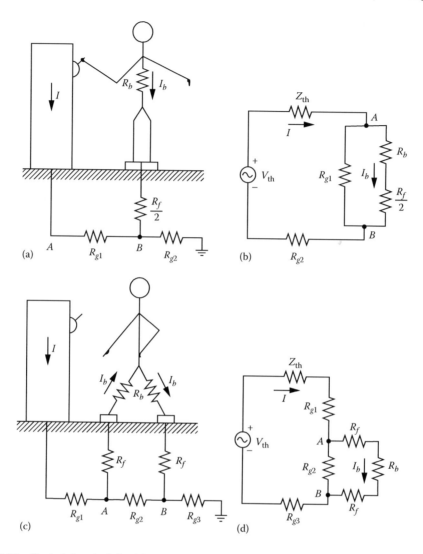

FIGURE 2.51 Typical electrical shock hazard situations: (a) touch potential, (b) its equivalent circuit, (c) step potential, and (d) its equivalent circuit.

The effects of an electric current passing through the vital parts of a human body depend on the duration, magnitude, and frequency of this current. The body resistance considered is usually between two extremities, either from one hand to both feet or from one foot to the other one. Figure 2.52 shows five basic situations involving a person and grounded facilities during fault.

On the other hand, the *touch voltage* represents the potential difference between the ground potential rise (GPR) and the surface potential at the point where a person is standing while at the same time having a hand in contact with a grounded structure. The *transferred voltage* is a special case of the touch voltage where a voltage is transferred into or out of the substation from or to a remote point external to the substation site [14].

Finally, GPR is the maximum electrical potential that a substation grounding grid may have relative to a distant grounding point assumed to be at the potential of remote earth. This voltage, GPR, is equal to the maximum grid current times the grid resistance. Under normal conditions, the grounded electrical equipment operates at near-zero ground potential. That is, the potential of a grounded neutral conductor is nearly identical to the potential of remote earth. During a

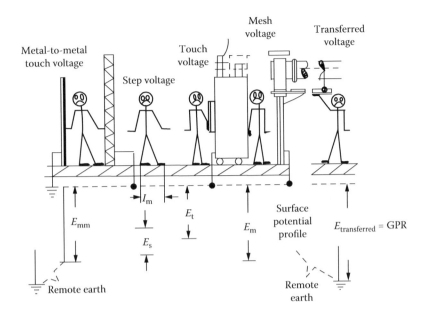

FIGURE 2.52 Possible basic shock situations. (From Keil, R.P., Substation grounding, in *Electric Power Substation Engineering*, Chapter 11, Figure 11.6, CRC Press, Boca Raton, FL, 2003, pp. 11-7. With permission.)

ground fault, the portion of fault current that is conducted by substation grounding grid into the earth causes the rise of the grid potential with respect to remote earth.

Exposure to touch potential normally poses a greater danger than exposure to step potential. The step potentials are usually smaller in magnitude (due to the greater corresponding body resistance), and the allowable body current is higher than the touch contacts. In either case, the value of the body resistance is difficult to establish.

As said before, experiments have shown that the body can tolerate much more current flowing from one leg to the other than it can when current flows from one hand to the legs. Treating the foot as a circular plate electrode gives an approximate resistance of $3\rho_s$, where ρ_s is the soil resistivity. The resistance of the body itself is usually used as about 2300 Ω hand to hand or 1100 Ω hand to foot.

However, IEEE Std. 80-2000 [14] recommends the use of 1000 Ω as a reasonable approximation for body resistance. Therefore, the total branch resistance, *for hand-to-foot currents*, can be expressed as

$$R_B = 1000 + 1.5\rho_s \ \Omega \quad \text{for touch voltage} \tag{2.13a}$$

and, *for foot-to-foot currents*,

$$R_B = 1000 + 6\rho_s \ \Omega \quad \text{for step voltage} \tag{2.13b}$$

where ρ_s is the soil resistivity in ohmmeters. If the surface of the soil is covered with a layer of crushed rock or some other high-resistivity material, its resistivity should be used in Equations 2.13a and b.

The *touch voltage limit* can also be determined from

$$V_{touch} = \left(R_B + \frac{R_f}{2} \right) I_B$$

and the *step voltage limit* can also be determined from

$$V_{step} = \left(R_B + 2R_f\right)I_B$$

where

$$R_f = 3C_s\rho_s$$

where

R_B is the resistance of human body, typically $1000\ \Omega$ for 50 and 60 Hz

R_B is the ground resistance of one foot

I_B is the rms magnitude of the current going through the body in A, per Equations 2.12a and b

C_s is the surface layer derating factor based on the thickness of the protective surface layer spread above the earth grade at the substation (per IEEE Std. 80-2000, if no protective layer is used, then $C_s = 1$)

$$R_B = 1000 + 1.5\rho_s\ \Omega \quad \text{for touch voltage}$$

and, for foot-to-foot currents,

$$R_B = 1000 + 6\rho_s\ \Omega \quad \text{for step voltage}$$

where ρ_s is the soil resistivity in ohmmeters. If the surface of the soil is covered with a layer of crushed rock or some other high-resistivity material, its resistivity should be used in Equations 2.13 and 2.17.

Since it is much easier to calculate and measure potential than current, the fibrillation thresholds, given by Equations 2.12a and b, are usually given in terms of voltage.

If no protective surface layer is used, the maximum allowable (or tolerable) touch voltages, for a person with a body weight of 50 or 70 kg, respectively, can be expressed as

$$V_{touch\ 50} = \frac{0.116\left(1000 + 1.5\rho_s\right)}{\sqrt{t_s}}\ V \quad \text{for 50 kg body weight} \tag{2.14a}$$

and

$$V_{touch\ 70} = \frac{0.157\left(1000 + 1.5\rho_s\right)}{\sqrt{t_s}}\ V \quad \text{for 70 kg body weight} \tag{2.14b}$$

If no protective surface layer is used, the maximum allowable (or tolerable) step voltages, for a person with a body weight of 50 or 70 kg, respectively, can be expressed as

$$V_{step\ 50} = \frac{0.116\left(1000 + 6\rho_s\right)}{\sqrt{t_s}}\ V \quad \text{for 50 kg body weight} \tag{2.15a}$$

and

$$V_{step\ 70} = \frac{0.157\left(1000 + 6\rho_s\right)}{\sqrt{t_s}}\ V \quad \text{for 70 kg body weight} \tag{2.15b}$$

If no protective surface layer is used, for the metal-to-metal touch in V, since $\rho_s = 0$, the aforementioned equations become

$$V_{\text{mm-touch } 50} = \frac{116}{\sqrt{t_s}} \text{ V} \quad \text{for 50 kg body weight} \tag{2.16a}$$

and

$$V_{\text{mm-touch } 70} = \frac{157}{\sqrt{t_s}} \text{ V} \quad \text{for 70 kg body weight} \tag{2.16b}$$

If a protective layer does exist, then the *maximum allowable (or tolerable) step voltages,* for a person with a body weight of 50 or 70 kg, are given, respectively, as

$$V_{\text{step } 50} = \frac{116(1000 + 6C_s\rho_s)}{\sqrt{t_s}} \text{ V} \quad \text{for 50 kg body weight} \tag{2.17a}$$

and

$$V_{\text{step } 70} = \frac{0.157(1000 + 6C_s\rho_s)}{\sqrt{t_s}} \text{ V} \quad \text{for 70 kg body weight} \tag{2.17b}$$

If a protective layer does exist, then the *maximum allowable (or tolerable) touch voltages,* for a person with a body weight of 50 or 70 kg, are given, respectively, as

$$V_{\text{step } 50} = \frac{116(1000 + 6C_s\rho_s)}{\sqrt{t_s}} \text{ V} \quad \text{for 50 kg body weight} \tag{2.18a}$$

$$V_{\text{step } 70} = \frac{0.157(1000 + 6C_s\rho_s)}{\sqrt{t_s}} \text{ V} \quad \text{for 70 kg body weight} \tag{2.18b}$$

Again, these equations are applicable only in the event that a protection surface layer is used. For metal-to-metal contacts, use $\rho_s = 0$ and $C_s = 1$. For more detailed applications, see IEEE Std. 2000 [12]. Also, it is important to note that in using these equations, it is assumed that they are applicable to 99.5% of the population. There are always exceptions.

Furthermore, the *touch voltage limit* can also be expressed as

$$V_{\text{touch}} = \left(R_B + \frac{R_f}{2}\right)I_B \tag{2.19}$$

Similarly, the *step voltage limit* can also be expressed as

$$V_{\text{step}} = \left(R_B + 2R_f \right) I_B \tag{2.20}$$

where

$$R_f = 3C_s \rho_s \tag{2.21}$$

where

R_B is the resistance of human body, typically 1000 Ω for 50 and 60 Hz
R_f is the ground resistance of one foot
I_B is the rms magnitude of the current going through the body in A, per Equations 2.12 and 2.13
C_s is the surface layer derating factor based on the thickness of the protective surface layer spread above the earth grade at the substation. (per IEEE Std. 80-2000, if no protective layer is used, then $C_s = 1.0$.)

Since it is much easier to calculate and measure potential than current, the fibrillation thresholds, given by Equations 2.12 and 2.13, are usually given in terms of voltage.

2.11.2 REDUCTION OF FACTOR C_s

Note that according to IEEE Std. 80-2000, a *thin layer of highly resistive protective surface material* such as gravel spread across the earth at a substation greatly reduced the possibly shock current at a substation. IEEE Std. 80-2000 gives the required equations to determine the ground resistance of one foot on a thin layer of surface material as

$$C_s = 1 + \frac{1.6b}{\rho_s} \sum_{n=1}^{\infty} K^n R_{m(2nh_s)} \tag{2.22}$$

and

$$C_s = 1 - \frac{0.09 \left(1 - \left(\rho / \rho_s \right) \right)}{2h_s + 0.09} \tag{2.23}$$

where

$$K = \frac{\rho - \rho_s}{\rho + \rho_s} \tag{2.24}$$

where

C_s is the surface layer derating factor (it can be considered as a corrective factor to compute the effective foot resistance in the presence of a finite thickness of surface material) (see Figure 2.53)
ρ_s is the surface material resistivity in ohmmeters
K is the reflection factor between different material resistivities
ρ is the resistivity of earth beneath the substation in ohmmeters
h_s is the thickness of the surface material in meters
b is the radius of circular metallic disk representing the foot in meters
$R_{m(2nh_s)}$ is the mutual ground resistance between two similar, parallel, coaxial plates that are separated by a distance of $(2nh_s)$ in ohmmeters

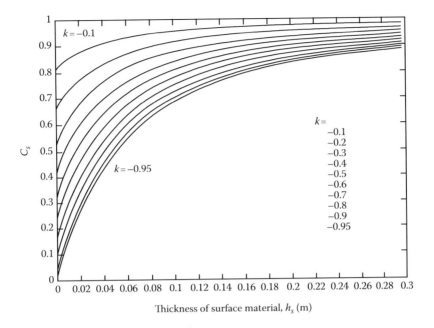

FIGURE 2.53 Surface layer derating factor C_s versus thickness of surface material in meters. (From From Keil, R.P., Substation grounding, in *Electric Power Substation Engineering*, Chapter 11, CRC Press, Boca Raton, FL, 2003. With permission.)

Again, note that Figure 2.53 gives the exact value of C_s instead of using the empirical equation (2.22) for it. The empirical equation gives approximate values that are within 5% of the values that can be found in the equation.

Example 2.1

Assume that a human body is part of a 60 Hz electric power circuit for about 0.25 s and that the soil type is average earth. Based on the IEEE Std. 80-2000, determine the following:

(a) Tolerable touch potential for 50 kg body weight
(b) Tolerable step potential for 50 kg body weight

Solution

(a) Using Equation 2.18a, for 50 kg body weight,

$$V_{touch} = \frac{0.116(1000 + 1.5\rho_s)}{\sqrt{t}} = \frac{0.116(1000 + 1.5 \times 100)}{\sqrt{0.25}} \cong 267 \text{ V}$$

(b) Using Equation 2.19b, for 50 kg body weight,

$$V_{step} = \frac{0.116(1000 + 6\rho_s)}{\sqrt{t}} = \frac{0.116(1000 + 6 \times 100)}{\sqrt{0.25}} \cong 371 \text{V}$$

Example 2.2

Assume that a human body is part of a 60 Hz electric power circuit for about 0.49 s and that the soil type is average earth. Based on the IEEE Std. 80-2000, determine the following:

(a) Tolerable touch potential for 50 kg body weight
(b) Tolerable step potential for 50 kg body weight
(c) Tolerable touch voltage limit for metal-to-metal contact if the person is 50 kg
(d) Tolerable touch voltage limit for metal-to-metal contact if the person is 70 kg

Solution

(a) Using Equation 2.18a, for 50 kg body weight,

$$V_{\text{touch }50} = \frac{0.116(1000 + 1.5\rho_s)}{\sqrt{t_s}}$$

$$= \frac{0.116(1000 + 1.5 \times 100)}{\sqrt{0.49}}$$

$$\cong 191\,\text{V}$$

(b) Using Equation 2.18c,

$$V_{\text{touch }50} = \frac{0.116(1000 + 6\rho_s)}{\sqrt{t_s}}$$

$$= \frac{0.116(1000 + 6 \times 100)}{\sqrt{0.49}}$$

$$\cong 265\,\text{V}$$

(c) Since $\rho_s = 0$,

$$V_{\text{mm-touch }50} = \frac{116}{\sqrt{t_s}} = \frac{116}{\sqrt{0.49}} = 165.7\,\text{V} \quad \text{for 50 kg body weight}$$

(d) Since $\rho_s = 0$,

$$V_{\text{mm-touch }70} = \frac{157}{\sqrt{t_s}} = \frac{157}{\sqrt{0.49}} = 224.3\,\text{V} \quad \text{for 70 kg body weight}$$

Table 2.7 gives typical values for various ground types. However, the resistivity of ground also changes as a function of temperature, moisture, and chemical content. Therefore, in practical applications, the only way to determine the resistivity of soil is by measuring it.

TABLE 2.7

Resistivity of Different Soils

Ground Type	Resistivity, ρ_s
Seawater	0.01–1.0
Wet organic soil	10
Moist soil (average earth)	100
Dry soil	1000
Bedrock	10^4
Pure slate	10^7
Sandstone	10^9
Crushed rock	1.5×10^8

2.11.3 Ground Resistance

Ground is defined as a conducting connection, either intentional or accidental, by which an electric circuit or equipment becomes grounded. Therefore, *grounded* means that a given electric system, circuit, or device is connected to the earth serving in the place of the former with the purpose of establishing and maintaining the potential of conductors connected to it approximately at the potential of the earth and allowing for conducting electric currents from and to the earth of its equivalent. A *safe grounding design* should provide the following:

1. A means to carry and dissipate electric currents into ground under normal and fault conditions without exceeding any operating and equipment limits or adversely affecting continuity of service
2. Assurance for such a degree of human safety so that a person working or walking in the vicinity of grounded facilities is not subjected to the danger of critic electrical shock

However, a low ground resistance is not, in itself, a guarantee of safety. For example, about three or four decades ago, a great many people assumed that any object grounded, however crudely, could be safely touched. This misconception probably contributed to many tragic accidents in the past. Since there is no simple relation between the resistance of the ground system as a whole and the maximum shock current to which a person might be exposed, a system or system component (e.g., substation or tower) of relatively low ground resistance may be dangerous under some conditions, whereas another system component with very high ground resistance may still be safe or can be made safe by careful design.

GPR is a function of fault current magnitude, system voltage, and ground (system) resistance. The current through the ground system multiplied by its resistance measured from a point remote from the substation determines the GPR with respect to remote ground.

The ground resistance can be reduced by using electrodes buried in the ground. For example, metal rods or *counterpoise* (i.e., buried conductors) is used for the lines of the grid system made of copper-stranded copper cable, and rods are used for the substations.

The grounding resistance of a buried electrode is a function of (1) the resistance of the electrode itself and connections to it, (2) contact resistance between the electrode and the surrounding soil, and (3) resistance of the surrounding soil, from the electrode surface outward. The first two resistances are very small with respect to soil resistance and therefore may be neglected in some applications. However, the third one is usually very large depending on the type of soil, chemical ingredients, moisture level, and temperature of the soil surrounding the electrode.

Table 2.8 presents data indicating the effect of moisture contents on the soil resistivity. The resistance of the soil can be measured by using the three-electrode method or by using self-contained instruments such as the Biddle Megger ground resistance tester.

TABLE 2.8
Effect of Moisture Content on Soil Resistivity

	Resistivity (Ω-cm)	
Moisture Content (wt.%)	Topsoil	Sandy Loam
0	$>10^9$	$>10^9$
2.5	250,000	150,000
5	165,000	43,000
10	53,000	18,500
15	19,000	10,500
20	12,000	6,300
30	6,400	4,200

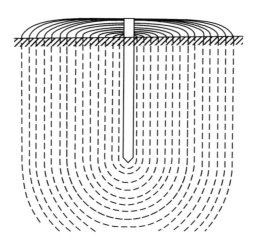

FIGURE 2.54 Resistance of earth surrounding an electrode.

If the surface of the soil is covered with a layer of crushed rock or some other high-resistivity material, its resistivity should be used in the previous equations. Table 2.6 gives typical values for various ground types. However, the resistivity of ground also changes as a function of temperature, moisture, and chemical content. Thus, in practical applications, the only way to determine the resistivity of soil is by measuring it.

In general, soil resistivity investigations are required to determine the soil structure. Table 2.7 gives only very rough estimates. The soil resistivity can vary substantially with changes in temperature, moisture, and chemical content. To determine the soil resistivity of a specific site, soil resistivity measurements are required to be taken. Since soil resistivity can change both horizontally and vertically, it is necessary to take more than one set of measurements. IEEE Std. 81-1983 [19] describes various measuring techniques in detail. There are commercially available computer programs that use the soil data and calculate the soil resistivity and provide a confidence level based on the test. There is also a graphical method that was developed by Sunde [20] to interpret the test results.

Figure 2.54 shows a ground rod driven into the soil and conducting current in all directions. Resistance of the soil has been illustrated in terms of successive shells of the soil of equal thickness. With increased distance from the electrode, the soil shells have greater area and therefore lower resistance. Thus, the shell nearest the rod has the smallest cross section of the soil and therefore the highest resistance. Measurements have shown that 90% of the total resistance surrounding an electrode is usually with a radius of 6–10 ft.

The assumptions that have been made in deriving these formulas are that the soil is perfectly homogeneous and the resistivity is of the same known value throughout the soil surrounding the electrode. Of course, these assumptions are seldom true. The only way one can be sure of the resistivity of the soil is by actually measuring it at the actual location of the electrode and at the actual depth.

Figure 2.55 shows the variation of soil resistivity with depth for a soil having uniform moisture content at all depths [25a]. In reality, however, deeper soils have greater moisture content, and the advantage of depth is more visible. Some nonhomogeneous soils can also be modeled by using the two-layer method [26–29].

The resistance of the soil can be measured by using the three-electrode method or by using self-contained instruments such as the Biddle Megger ground resistance tester. Figure 2.56 shows the approximate ground resistivity distribution in the United States.

If the surface of the soil is covered with a layer of crushed rock or some other high-resistivity material, its resistivity should be used in the previous equations. Table 2.9 gives typical values for various ground types. However, the resistivity of ground also changes as a function of temperature,

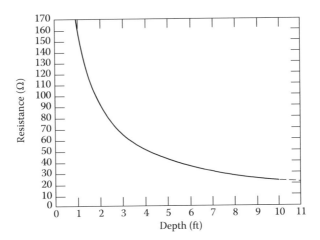

FIGURE 2.55 Variation of soil resistivity with depth for soil having uniform moisture content at all depths. (From National Bureau of Standards Technical Report 108.)

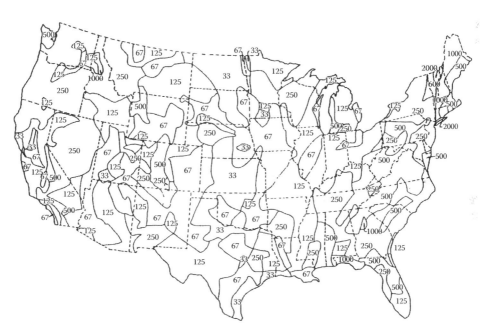

FIGURE 2.56 Approximate ground resistivity distribution in the United States. *Notes:* All figures on this map indicate ground resistivity (Rho) in ohm-meters. These data are taken from FCC figure M3, February 1954. The FCC data indicate ground conductivity in milliohms per meter. Resistivities of special note from Transmission Line Reference Book by EPRI in ohmmeters: Swampy ground (10–100), pure slate (10,000,000), and sandstone (100,000,000). (From Keil, R.P., Substation grounding, in *Electric Power Substation Engineering*, Chapter 11, CRC Press, Boca Raton, FL, 2003.)

moisture, and chemical content. Thus, in practical applications, the only way to determine the resistivity of soil is by measuring it.

In general, soil resistivity investigations are required to determine the soil structure. Table 2.9 gives only very rough estimates. The soil resistivity can vary substantially with changes in temperature, moisture, and chemical content. To determine the soil resistivity of a specific site, soil resistivity

TABLE 2.9

Material Constants of the Typical Grounding Material Used

Description	K_f	T_m (°C)	α_r Factor at 20°C (1/°C)	ρ_r, 20°C ($\mu\Omega \cdot$ cm)	K_0 at 0°C (0°C)	Fusing Temperature T_m (0°C)	Material Conducting (%)	TCAP Thermal Capacity [J/cm³·°C]
Copper annealed, soft drawn	7	1083	0.0393	1.72	234	1083	100	3.42
Copper annealed, hard drawn	1084	1084	0.00381	1.78	242	1084	97	3.42
Copper-clad steel wire	1084	12.06	0.00378	5.86	245	1084	30	3.85
Stainless steel 304	1510	14.72	0.00130	15.86	749	1400	2.4	3.28
Zinc-coated steel rod	28.96	28.96	0.0030	72	293	419	8.6	4.03

measurements are required to be taken. Since soil resistivity can change both horizontally and vertically, it is necessary to take more than one set of measurements. IEEE Std. 80-2000 [12] describes various measuring techniques in detail. There are commercially available computer programs that use the soil data and calculate the soil resistivity and provide a confidence level based on the test. There is also a graphical method that was developed by Sunde [20] to interpret the test results.

2.11.4 SOIL RESISTIVITY MEASUREMENTS

Table 2.9 gives estimates on soil classification that are only an approximation of the actual resistivity of a given site. Actual resistivity tests therefore are crucial. They should be made at a number of places within the site. In general, substation sites where the soil has uniform resistivity throughout the entire area and to a considerable depth are seldom found.

2.11.4.1 Wenner Four-Pin Method

More often than not, there are several layers, each having a different resistivity. Furthermore, lateral changes also take place, however with respect to the vertical changes; these changes usually are more gradual. Hence, soil resistivity tests should be made to find out if there are any substantial changes in resistivity with depth. If the resistivity varies considerably with depth, it is often desirable to use an increased range of probe spacing in order to get an estimate of the resistivity of deeper layers.

IEEE Std. 81-1983 describes a number of measuring techniques. The Wenner four-pin method is the most commonly used technique. Figure 2.57 illustrates this method. In this method, four probes

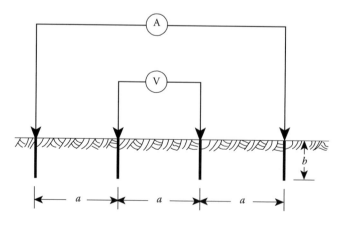

FIGURE 2.57   Wenner four-pin method.

(or pins) are driven into the earth along a straight line, at equal distances apart, driven to a depth b. The voltage between the two inner (i.e., potential) electrodes is then measured and divided by the current between the two outer (i.e., current) electrodes to give a value of resistance R. The apparent resistivity of soil is determined from

$$\rho_a = \frac{4\pi a R}{1 + 2a / \left(\sqrt{a^2 + 4b^2} \right) - \dfrac{a}{\sqrt{a^2 + 4b^2}}} \qquad (2.25)$$

where
ρ_a is the apparent resistivity of the soil in ohmmeters
R is the measured resistivity in ohms
a is the distance between adjacent electrodes in meters
b is the depth of the electrodes in meters

In the event that b is small in comparison to a, then

$$\rho_a = 2\pi a R \qquad (2.26)$$

The current tends to flow near the surface for the small probe spacing, whereas more of the current penetrates deeper soils for large spacing. Because of this fact, the previous two equations can be used to determine the apparent resistivity ρ_a at a depth a.

The Wenner four-pin method obtains the soil resistivity data for deeper layers without driving the test pins to those layers. No heavy equipment is needed to do the four-pin test. The results are not greatly affected by the resistance of the test pins or the holes created in driving the test pins into the soil. Because of these advantages, the Wenner method is the most popular method.

2.11.4.2 Three-Pin or Driven-Ground Rod Method

IEEE Std. 81-1983 describes *a second method of measuring soil resistivity.* It is illustrated in Figure 2.58. In this method, the depth (L_r) of the driven rod located in the soil to be tested is varied.

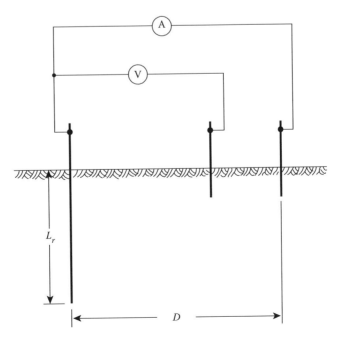

FIGURE 2.58 Circuit diagram for three-pin or driven-ground rod method.

The other two rods are known as *reference rods*. They are driven to a shallow depth in a straight line. The location of the voltage rod is varied between the test rod and the current rod. Alternatively, the voltage rod can be placed on the other side of the driven rod. The apparent resistivity is found from

$$\rho_a = \frac{2\pi L_r R}{\ln(8L_r/d) - 1} \qquad (2.27)$$

where

    L_r is the length of the driven rod in meters
    d is the diameter of the rod in meters
    R is the measured resistivity in ohms

A plot of the measured resistivity value ρ_a versus the rod length (L_r) provides a visual aid for finding out earth resistivity variations with depth. An advantage of the driven-rod method, even though not related necessarily to the measurements, is the ability to determine to what depth the ground rods can be driven. This knowledge can save the need to redesign the ground grid. Because of hard layers in the soil such as rock and hard clay, it becomes practically impossible to drive the test rod any further resulting in insufficient data.

A *disadvantage of the driven-rod method* is that when the test rod is driven deep in the ground, it usually losses contact with the soil due to the vibration and the larger diameter couplers resulting in higher measured resistance values. A ground grid designed with these higher soil resistivity values may be unnecessarily conservative. Thus, this method presents an uncertainty in the resistance value.

2.12 SUBSTATION GROUNDING

Grounding at substation has paramount importance. Again, the purpose of such a grounding system includes the following:

1. To provide the ground connection for the grounded neutral for transformers, reactors, and capacitors
2. To provide the discharge path for lightning rods, arresters, gaps, and similar devices
3. To ensure safety to operating personnel by limiting potential differences that can exist in a substation
4. To provide a means of discharging and deenergizing equipment in order to proceed with the maintenance of the equipment
5. To provide a sufficiently low-resistance path to ground to minimize rise in ground potential with respect to remote ground

A multigrounded, common neutral conductor used for a primary distribution line is always connected to the substation grounding system where the circuit originates and to all grounds along the length of the circuit. If separate primary and secondary neutral conductors are used, the conductors have to be connected together provided the primary neutral conductor is effectively grounded.

The substation grounding system is connected to every individual equipment, structure, and installation so that it can provide the means by which grounding currents are connected to remote areas. It is extremely important that the substation ground has a low ground resistance, adequate current-carrying capacity, and safety features for personnel. It is crucial to have the substation ground resistance very low so that the total rise of the ground system potential will not reach values that are unsafe for human contact.*

The substation grounding system normally is made of buried horizontal conductors and driven-ground rods interconnected (by clamping, welding, or brazing) to form a continuous grid

---

* *Mesh voltage* is the worst possible value of a touch voltage to be found within a mesh of a ground grid if standing at or near the center of the mesh.

(also called mat) network. A continuous cable (usually it is 4/0 bare copper cable buried 12–18 in. below the surface) surrounds the grid perimeter to enclose as much ground as possible and to prevent current concentration and thus high gradients at the ground cable terminals. Inside the grid, cables are buried in parallel lines and with uniform spacing (e.g., about 10 × 20 ft).

All substation equipment and structures are connected to the ground grid with large conductors to minimize the grounding resistance and limit the potential between equipment and the ground surface to a safe value under all conditions. All substation fences are built inside the ground grid and attached to the grid in short intervals to protect the public and personnel. The surface of the substation is usually covered with crushed rock or concrete to reduce the potential gradient when large currents are discharged to ground and to increase the contact resistance to the feet of personnel in the substation.

IEEE Std. 80-1976 [13] provides a formula for a quick simple calculation of the grid resistance to ground after a minimum design has been completed. It is expressed as

$$R_{grid} = \frac{\rho_s}{4r} + \frac{\rho_s}{L_T} \qquad (2.28)$$

where
   ρ_s is the soil resistivity in ohmmeters
   L_T is the total length of grid conductors in m
   R is the radius of circle with an area equal to that of grid in m

IEEE Std. 80-2000 [19] provides the following equation to determine the grid resistance after a minimum design has been completed:

$$R_{grid} = \frac{\rho_s}{4r} \sqrt{\frac{\pi}{A}} \qquad (2.29)$$

Also, IEEE Std. 80-2000 provides the following equation to determine *the upper limit for grid resistance to ground after a minimum design has been completed*:

$$R_{grid} = \frac{\rho_s}{4r} \sqrt{\frac{\pi}{A}} + \frac{\rho_s}{L_T} \qquad (2.30)$$

where
   R_{grid} is the grid resistance in ohms
   ρ is the soil resistance in ohmmeters
   A is the area of the ground in square meters
   L_T is the total buried length of conductors in meters

But Equation 2.30 requires a uniform soil resistivity. Hence, a substantial engineering judgment is necessary for reviewing the soil resistivity measurements to decide the value of soil resistivity. However, it does provide a guideline for the uniform soil resistivity to be used in the ground grid design. Alternatively, Sverak [19] provides the following formula for the grid resistance:

$$R_{grid} = \rho_s \left[\frac{1}{L_T} + \frac{1}{\sqrt{20A}} \left(1 + \frac{1}{1 + h\sqrt{20/A}} \right) \right] \qquad (2.31)$$

where
   R_{grid} is the substation ground resistance in ohms
   ρ_s is the soil resistivity in ohmmeters
   A is the area occupied by the ground grid in square meters
   H is the depth of the grid in meters
   L_T is the total buried length of conductors in meters

IEEE Std. 80-1976 also provides formulas to determine the effects of the grid geometry on the step and mesh voltage (which is the worst possible value of the touch voltage) in volts. *Mesh voltage* is the worst possible value of a touch voltage to be found within a mesh of a ground grid if standing at or near the center of the mesh. They can be expressed as

$$E_{\text{step}} = \frac{\rho_s \times K_s \times K_i \times I_G}{L_s} \qquad (2.32)$$

and

$$E_{\text{mesh}} = \frac{\rho_s \times K_m \times K_i \times I_G}{L_m} \qquad (2.33)$$

where

ρ_s is the average soil resistivity in ohmmeters
K_s is the step coefficient
K_m is the mesh coefficient
K_i is the irregularity coefficient
I_G is the maximum rms current flowing between ground grid and earth in amperes
L_s is the total length of buried conductors, including cross connections and (optionally) the total effective length of ground rods in meters
L_m is the total length of buried conductors, including cross connections and (optionally) the combined length of ground rods in meters

Many utilities have computer programs for performing grounding grid studies. The number of tedious calculations that must be performed to develop an accurate and sophisticated model of a system is no longer a problem.

In general, in the event of a fault, OHGWs, neutral conductors, and directly buried metal pipes and cables conduct a portion of the ground fault current away from the substation ground grid and have to be taken into account when calculating the maximum value of the grid current. Based on the associated equivalent circuit and resultant current division, one can determine what portion of the total current flows into the earth and through other ground paths. It can be used to determine the approximate amount of current that did not use the ground as flow path. The fault current division factor (also known as the *split factor*) can be expressed as

$$S_{\text{split}} = \frac{I_{\text{grid}}}{3I_{ao}} \qquad (2.34)$$

where

S_{split} is the fault current division factor
I_{grid} is the rms symmetrical grid current in amperes
I_{ao} is the zero-sequence fault current in amperes

The *split factor* is used to determine the approximate amount of current that did not use the ground flow path. Computer programs can determine the split factor easily, but it is also possible to determine the split factor through graphs. With the Y ordinate representing the split factor and the X axis representing the grid resistance, it is obvious that the grid resistance has to be known to determine the split factor.

As previously said, the split factor determines the approximate amount of current that does use the earth as return path. The amount of current that does enter the earth is found from the following equation. Hence, the design value of the maximum grid current can be found from

$$I_G = D_f \times I_{\text{grid}} \tag{2.35}$$

where
I_G is the maximum grid current in amperes
D_f is the decrement factor for the entire fault duration of t_f, given in seconds
I_{grid} is the rms symmetrical grid current in amperes

Here, Figure 2.59 illustrates the relationship between asymmetrical fault current, dc decaying component, and symmetrical fault current and the relationship between variables I_F, I_f, and D_f for the fault duration t_f.

The *decrement factor* is an adjustment factor that is used in conjunction with the symmetrical ground fault current parameter in safety-oriented grounding calculations. It determines the rms

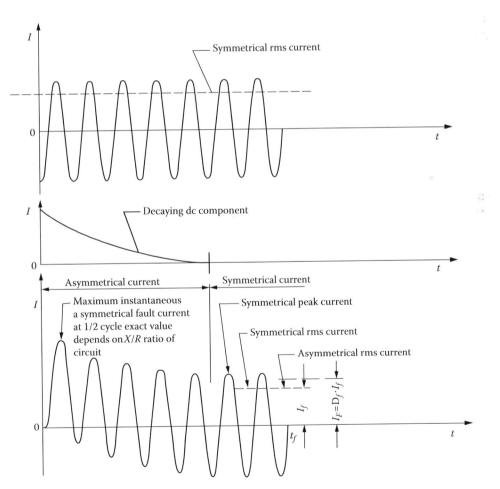

FIGURE 2.59 The relationship between asymmetrical fault current, dc decaying component, and symmetrical fault current.

equivalent of the asymmetrical current wave for a given fault duration, accounting for the effect of initial dc offset and its attenuation during the fault. The decrement factor can be calculated from

$$D_f = \sqrt{1 + \frac{T_a}{I_f}\left(1 - e^{2t_f/T_a}\right)} \tag{2.36}$$

where t_f is the time duration of fault in seconds.

$$T_a = \frac{X}{\omega R} = \text{dc offset time constant in seconds}$$

Here, t_f should be chosen as the fastest clearing time. The fastest clearing time includes breaker and relay time for transmission substations. It is assumed here that the ac components do not decay with time.

The *symmetrical grid current* is defined as that portion of the symmetrical ground fault current that flows between the grounding grid and surrounding earth. It can be expressed as

$$I_{\text{grid}} = S_f \times I_f \tag{2.37}$$

where

I_f is the rms value of symmetrical ground fault current in amperes
S_f is the fault current division factor

IEEE Std. 80-2000 provides a series of current based on computer simulations for various values of ground grid resistance and system conditions to determine the grid current. Based on those split-current curves, one can determine the maximum grid current.

2.13 GROUND CONDUCTOR SIZING FACTORS

The flow of excessive currents will be very dangerous if the right equipment is not used to help dissipate the excessive currents. Ground conductors are means of providing a path for excessive currents from the substation to ground grid. Hence, the ground grid then can spread the current into the ground, creating a zero potential between the substation and the ground. Table 2.9 gives the list of possible conductors that can be used for such conductors.

In the United States, there are only two types of conductors that are used, namely, copper and/ or copper-clad steel conductors that are used for this purpose. The copper one is mainly used due to its high conductivity and the high resistance to corrosion. The next step is to determine the size of ground conductor that needs to be buried underground.

Thus, based on the *symmetrical conductor current*, the required conductor size can be found from

$$I_f = A_{\text{mm}^2}\left[\left(\frac{\text{TCAP} \times 10^{-4}}{t_c \times \alpha_r \times \rho_r}\right)\ln\left(\frac{K_0 + T_{\max}}{K_0 + T_{\text{amb}}}\right)\right]^{1/2} \tag{2.38}$$

If the conductor size needs to be found in mm², the conductor size can be found from

$$A_{\text{mm}^2} = \frac{I_f}{\left[\left(\dfrac{\text{TCAP} \times 10^{-4}}{t_c \times \alpha_r \times \rho_r}\right)\ln\left(\dfrac{K_0 + T_{\max}}{K_0 + T_{\text{amb}}}\right)\right]^{1/2}} \tag{2.39}$$

Alternatively, in the event that the conductor size needs to be found in kcmil, since

$$A_{\text{kcmil}} = 1.974 \times A_{\text{mm}^2} \tag{2.40}$$

then, Equation 2.31 can be expressed as

$$I_f = 5.07 \times 10^{-3} A_{\text{kcmil}} \left[\left(\frac{\text{TCAP} \times 10^{-4}}{t_c \times \alpha_r \times \rho_r} \right) \ln \left(\frac{K_0 + T_{\text{max}}}{K_0 + T_{\text{amb}}} \right) \right]^{1/2} \tag{2.41}$$

Note that both α_r and ρ_r can be found at the same reference temperature of T_r °C. Also, note that Equations 2.38 and 2.39 can also be used to determine the short-time temperature rise in a ground conductor. Thus, taking other required conversions into account, the conductor size in kcmil can be found from

$$A_{\text{kcmil}} = \frac{197.4 \times I_f}{\left[\left(\frac{\text{TCAP} \times 10^{-4}}{t_c \times \alpha_r \times \rho_r} \right) \ln \left(\frac{K_0 + T_{\text{max}}}{K_0 + T_{\text{amb}}} \right) \right]^{1/2}} \tag{2.42}$$

where
I_f is the rms current (without dc offset) in kiloamperes
A_{mm^2} is the conductor cross section in square millimeters
A_{kcmil} is the conductor cross section in kilocircular mils
TCAP is the thermal capacity per unit volume, J/(cm³ · °C) (it is found from Table 2.9, per IEEE Std. 80-2000)
t_c is the duration of current in seconds
α_r is the thermal coefficient of resistivity at reference temperature T_r, 1/°C (it is found from Table 2.9, per IEEE Std. 80-2000 for 20°C)
ρ_r is the resistivity of the ground conductor at reference temperature T_r, microohm centimeters (it is found from Table 2.9, per IEEE Std. 80-2000 for 20°C)
$K_0 = 1/\alpha_0$ or $(1/\alpha_r) - T_r$ in degree Celsius
T_{max} is the maximum allowable temperature in degree Celsius
T_{amb} is the ambient temperature in degree Celsius
I_f is the rms current (without dc offset) in kiloamperes

For a given conductor material, the TCAP is found from Table 2.9 or calculated from

$$\text{TCAP} \left[\frac{\text{J}}{\left(\text{cm}^3 \cdot °\text{C} \right)} \right] = 4.184 \left(\frac{\text{J}}{\text{cal}} \right) \times \text{SH} \left[\frac{\text{cal}}{\left(\text{g} \cdot °\text{C} \right)} \right] \times \text{SW} \left(\frac{\text{g}}{\text{cm}^3} \right) \tag{2.43}$$

where SH is the specific heat, in cal/(g · °C), and is related to the thermal capacity per unit volume in

$$\frac{\text{J}}{\left(\text{cm}^3 \cdot °\text{C} \right)}$$

SW is the specific weight, in g/cm³, and is related to the thermal capacity per unit volume in

$$\frac{J}{\left(cm^3 \cdot °C\right)}$$

Thus, TCAP is defined by

$$TCAP\left[\frac{J}{\left(cm^3 \cdot °C\right)}\right] = 4.184\left(\frac{J}{cal}\right) \times SH\left[\frac{cal}{\left(g \cdot °C\right)}\right] \times SW\left(\frac{g}{cm^3}\right) \qquad (2.44)$$

Asymmetrical fault currents consist of subtransient, transient, and steady-state ac components and the dc offset current component. To find the *asymmetrical fault current* (i.e., if the effect of the dc offset is needed to be included in the fault current), the equivalent value of the asymmetrical current I_F is found from

$$I_F = D_f \times I_f \qquad (2.45)$$

where I_F is representing the rms value of an asymmetrical current integrated over the entire fault duration, t_c, which can be found as a function of X/R by using D_f, before using Equations 2.36 or 2.39 and where D_f is the decrement factor and is found from

$$D_f = \left[1 + \frac{T_a}{t_f}\left(1 - e^{-2t_f/T_a}\right)\right]^{1/2} \qquad (2.46)$$

where
  t_f is the time duration of fault in seconds
  T_a is the dc offset time constant in seconds

Note that

$$T_a = \frac{X}{\omega R} \qquad (2.47)$$

and for 60 Hz,

$$T_a = \frac{X}{120\pi R} \qquad (2.48)$$

The resulting I_F is always greater than I_f. However, if the X/R ratio is less than 5 and the fault duration is greater than 1 s, the effects of the dc offset are negligible.

2.14 MESH VOLTAGE DESIGN CALCULATIONS

If the GPR value exceeds the tolerable touch and step voltages, it is necessary to perform the mesh voltage design calculations to determine whether the design of a substation is safe. If the design is again unsafe, conductors in the form of ground rods are added to the design until the design is considered safe. The mesh voltage is the maximum touch voltage and it is found from

$$E_{\text{mesh}} = \frac{\rho \times K_m \times K_i \times I_G}{L_M} \tag{2.49}$$

where

ρ is the soil resistivity in ohmmeters
K_m is the mesh coefficient
K_i is the correction factor for grid geometry
I_G is the maximum grid current that flows between ground grid and surrounding earth in amperes
L_m is the length of $L_c + L_R$ for mesh voltage in meters
L_c is the total length of grid conductor in meters
L_R is the total length of ground rods in meters

The mesh coefficient K_m is determined from

$$K_m = \frac{1}{2\pi}\left[\ln\left(\frac{D^2}{16 \times h \times d} + \frac{(D + 2 \times h)^2}{8 \times D \times d} - \frac{h}{4 \times D}\right) + \frac{K_{ii}}{K_h}\ln\left(\frac{8}{\pi(2 \times 14 - 1)}\right)\right] \tag{2.50}$$

where

d is the diameter of grid conductors in meters
D is the spacing between parallel conductors in meters
K_{ii} is the irregularity factor (*corrective weighting factor* that adjusts for the effects of inner conductors on the corner mesh)
K_h is the corrective weighting factor that highlights for the effects of grid depth
n is the geometric factor
h is the depth of ground grid conductors in meters

As it can be observed from Equation 2.50, the geometric factor K_m has the following variables: D_s, the spacing between the conductors; n_s, the number of conductors; d, the diameter of the conductors used; and h, the depth of the grid. The effect of each variable on the K_m is different. Figure 2.60 shows the effect of the spacing (D) between conductors on K_m. Figure 2.61 shows the effect of the number of conductors (n) on the K_m. Figure 2.62 show the relationship between the diameter of the conductor (d) and the K_m. Figure 2.63 shows the relationship between the depth of the conductor (h) and K_m [17].

Note that the value of K_{ii} depends on the following circumstances:

1. For the grids with ground rods existing in grid corners as well as perimeter,

$$K_{ii} = 1 \tag{2.51}$$

2. For the grids with no or few ground rods with none existing in corners or perimeter,

$$K_{ii} = \frac{1}{(2n)^{2/n}} \tag{2.52}$$

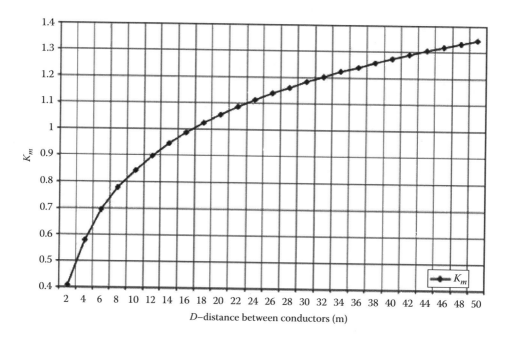

FIGURE 2.60 The effect of the spacing (D) between conductors on K_m. (From Keil, R.P., Substation grounding, in *Electric Power Substation Engineering*, Chapter 11, CRC Press, Boca Raton, FL, 2003. With permission.)

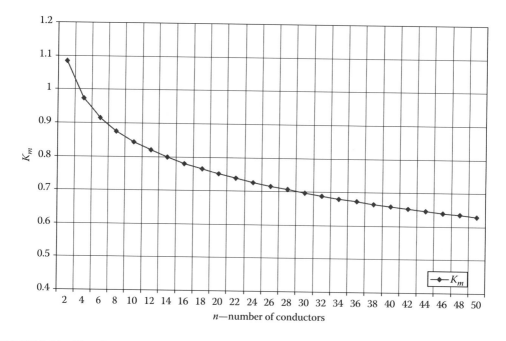

FIGURE 2.61 The effect of the number of conductors (n) on the K_m. (From Keil, R.P., Substation grounding, in *Electric Power Substation Engineering*, Chapter 11, CRC Press, Boca Raton, FL, 2003. With permission.)

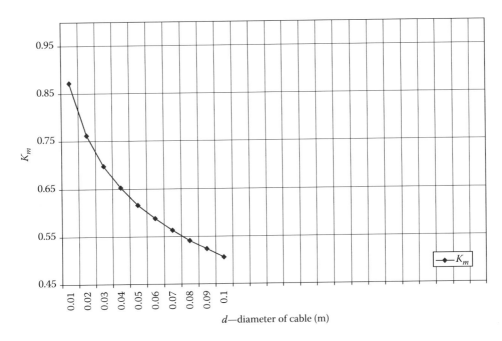

FIGURE 2.62 The relationship between the diameter of the conductor (d) and the K_m. (From Keil, R.P., Substation grounding, in *Electric Power Substation Engineering*, Chapter 11, CRC Press, Boca Raton, FL, 2003. With permission.)

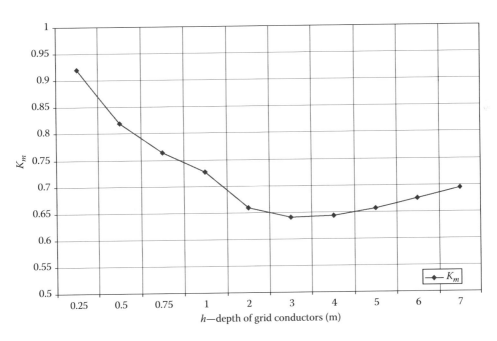

FIGURE 2.63 The relationship between the depth of the conductor (h) and K_m. (From Keil, R.P., Substation grounding, in *Electric Power Substation Engineering*, Chapter 11, CRC Press, Boca Raton, FL, 2003. With permission.)

and

$$K_h = \sqrt{1 + \frac{h}{h_0}} \tag{2.53}$$

where h_0 is the grid reference depth = 1 m.

The effective number of parallel conductors (n) given in a given grid is found from

$$n = n_a \times n_b \times n_c \times n_d \tag{2.54}$$

where
$n_a = 2L_c/L_p$
$n_b = 1$, for square grids
$n_c = 1$, for square and rectangular grids
$n_d = 1$, for square, rectangular, and L-shaped grids

Otherwise, the following equations are used to determine the n_b, n_c, and n_d so that

$$n_b = \sqrt{\frac{L_p}{4\sqrt{A}}} \tag{2.55}$$

$$n_c = \left[\frac{L_X \times L_Y}{A}\right]^{0.7A/L_X \times L_Y} \tag{2.56}$$

$$n_d = \frac{D_m}{\sqrt{L_X^2 + L_Y^2}} \tag{2.57}$$

where
L_p is the peripheral length of the grid in meters
L_C is the total length of the conductor in the horizontal grid in meters
A is the area of the grid in square meters
L_X is the maximum length of the grid in the x direction in meters
L_Y is the maximum length of the grid in the y direction in meters
d is the diameter of grid conductors in meters
D is the spacing between parallel conductors in meters
D_m is the maximum distance between any two points on the grid in meters
h is the depth of ground grid conductors in meters

Note that the irregularity factor is determined from

$$K_{ii} = 0.644 + 0.148n \tag{2.58}$$

The effective buried length (L_M) for grids:

1. With little or no ground rods but not located in the corners or along the perimeter of the grid,

$$L_M = L_C + L_R \tag{2.59}$$

where
L_R is the total length of all ground rods in meters
L_C is the total length of the conductor in the horizontal grid in meters

2. With ground rods in corners and along the perimeter and throughout the grid,

$$L_M = L_C + \left[1.55 + 1.22 \left(\frac{L_g}{\sqrt{L_X^2 + L_Y^2}} \right) \right] L_R \tag{2.60}$$

where L_R is the length of each ground rod in meters.

2.15 STEP VOLTAGE DESIGN CALCULATIONS

According to IEEE Std. 80-2000, in order for the ground system to be safe, step voltage has to be less than the tolerable step voltage. Furthermore, step voltages within the grid system designed for safe mesh voltages will be well within the tolerable limits; the reason for this is both feet and legs are in series rather than in parallel and the current takes the path from one leg to the other rather than through vital organs. The step voltage is determined from

$$E_{\text{step}} = \frac{\rho \times K_s \times K_i \times I_G}{L_S} \tag{2.61}$$

where
K_s is the step coefficient
L_S is the buried conductor length in meters

Again, for grids with or without ground rods,

$$L_S = 0.75 L_C + 0.85 L_R \tag{2.62}$$

so that the step coefficient can be found from

$$K_S = \frac{1}{\pi} \left[\frac{1}{2h} + \frac{2}{D+h} + \frac{1}{D} \left(1 - 0.5^{n-2} \right) \right] \tag{2.63}$$

where h is the depth of ground grid conductors in meters, usually between $0.25\ \text{m} < h < 2.5\ \text{m}$.

As in Equation 2.63, the geometric factor K_s is a function of D, n, d, π, and h. Figure 2.64 shows the relationship between the distance (D) between the conductors and the geometric factor K_s.

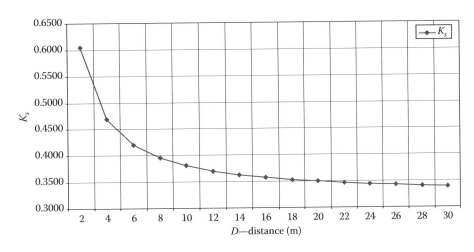

FIGURE 2.64 The relationship between the distance (D) between the conductors and the geometric factor K_s. (From Keil, R.P., Substation grounding, in *Electric Power Substation Engineering*, Chapter 11, CRC Press, Boca Raton, FL, 2003. With permission.)

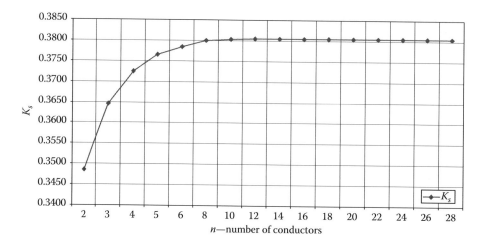

FIGURE 2.65 The relationship between the number of conductors (n) and the geometric factor K_s. (From Keil, R.P., Substation grounding, in *Electric Power Substation Engineering*, Chapter 11, CRC Press, Boca Raton, FL, 2003. With permission.)

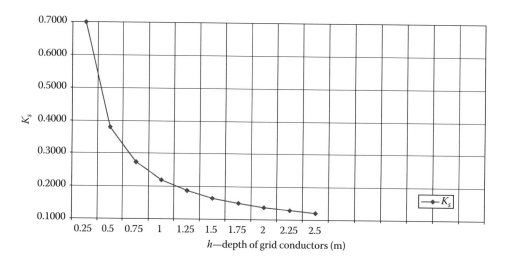

FIGURE 2.66 The relationship between the depth of grid conductors (h) in meter and the geometric factor K_s. (From Keil, R.P., Substation grounding, in *Electric Power Substation Engineering*, Chapter 11, CRC Press, Boca Raton, FL, 2003. With permission.)

Figure 2.65 shows the relationship between the number of conductors (n) and the geometric factor K_s. Figure 2.66 shows the relationship between the depth of grid conductors (D) in meters and the geometric factor K_s.

2.16 TYPES OF GROUND FAULTS

In general, it is difficult to determine which fault type and location will result in the greatest flow of current between the ground grid and surrounding earth because no simple rule applies. IEEE Std. 80-2000 recommends not to consider multiple simultaneous faults since their probability of occurrence is negligibly small. Instead, it recommends investigating single line-to-ground (SLG) and line-to-line-to-ground faults.

2.16.1 Line-to-Line-to-Ground Fault

For a line-to-line-to-ground (i.e., double line-to-ground [DLG]) fault, IEEE Std. 80-2000 gives the following equation to calculate the zero-sequence fault current:

$$I_{a0} = \frac{E\left(R_2 + jX_2\right)}{\left(R_1 + jX_1\right)\left[R_0 + R_2 + 3R_f + j\left(X_0 + X_2\right) + \left(R_2 + jX_2\right)\left(R_0 + 3R_f + jX_0\right)\right]} \tag{2.64}$$

where

I_{a0} is the symmetrical rms value of zero-sequence fault current in amperes
E is the phase-to-neutral voltage in volts
R_f is the estimated resistance of the fault in Ω (normally it is assumed R_f is 0)
R_1 is the positive-sequence system resistance in ohms
R_2 is the negative-sequence system resistance in ohms
R_0 is the zero-sequence system resistance in ohms
X_1 is the positive-sequence system reactance (subtransient) in ohms
X_2 is the negative-sequence system reactance in ohms
X_0 is the zero-sequence system reactance in ohms

The values of R_0, R_1, R_2, and X_0, X_1, X_2 are determined by looking into the system from the point of fault. In other words, they are determined from the Thévenin equivalent impedance at the fault point for each sequence.* Often, however, the resistance quantities given in the previous equation are negligibly small. Hence,

$$I_{a0} = \frac{E \times X_2}{X_1\left(X_0 + X_2\right)\left(X_0 + X_2\right)} \tag{2.65}$$

2.16.2 Single Line-to-Ground Fault

For an SLG fault, IEEE Std. 80-2000 gives the following equation to calculate the zero-sequence fault current:

$$I_{a0} = \frac{E}{3R_f + R_0 + R_1 + R_2 + j\left(X_0 + X_1 + X_2\right)} \tag{2.66}$$

Often, however, the resistance quantities in the previous equation are negligibly small. Hence,

$$I_{a0} = \frac{E}{X_0 + X_1 + X_2} \tag{2.67}$$

2.17 GROUND POTENTIAL RISE

The GPR is a function of fault current magnitude, system voltage, and ground system resistance. The GPR with respect to remote ground is determined by multiplying the current flowing through the ground system by its resistance measured from a point remote from the substation. Here, the current flowing through the grid is usually taken as the maximum available line-to-ground fault current.

---

* It is often acceptable to use $X_1 = X_2$, especially if an appreciable percentage of the positive-sequence reactance to the point of fault is that of static equipment and transmission lines.

GPR is a function of fault current magnitude, system voltage, and ground (system) resistance. The current through the ground system multiplied by its resistance measured from a point remote from the substation determines the GPR with respect to remote ground. Hence, GPR can be found from

$$V_{GPR} = I_G \times R_g \tag{2.68}$$

where
V_{GPR} is the GPR in volts
R_g is the ground grid resistance in ohms

For example, if a ground fault current of 20,000 A is flowing into a substation ground grid due to a line-to-ground fault and the ground grid system has a 0.5 Ω resistance to the earth, the resultant IR voltage drop would be 10,000 V. It is clear that such 10,000 V IR voltage drop could cause serious problems to communication lines in and around the substation in the event that the communication equipment and facilities are not properly insulated and/or neutralized. The ground grid resistance can be found from

$$R_g = \rho \left[\frac{1}{L_T} + \frac{1}{\sqrt{20A}} \left(1 + \frac{1}{1 + h\sqrt{20/A}} \right) \right] \tag{2.69}$$

where
L_T is the total buried length of conductors in meters
h is the depth of the grid in meters
A is the area of substation ground surface in square meters

Figure 2.67 shows the effects of number of grid conductors (n), without ground rods, on the ground grid resistance. It shows that area (A) has a substantial influence on the grid resistance. Figure 2.68 shows the relationship between the burial depth of the grid (h), in meter, and the grid resistance. Here, the depth is varied from 0.5 to 2.5 m and the number of conductors from 4 to 10 [17].

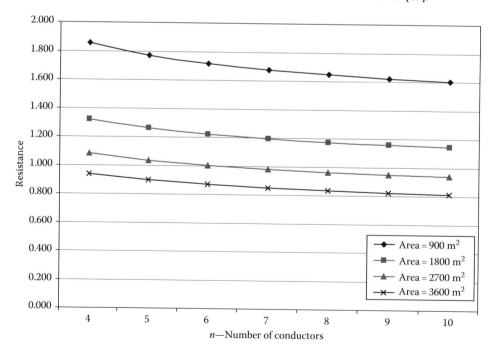

FIGURE 2.67 The effects of number of grid conductors (n), without ground rods, on the ground grid resistance.

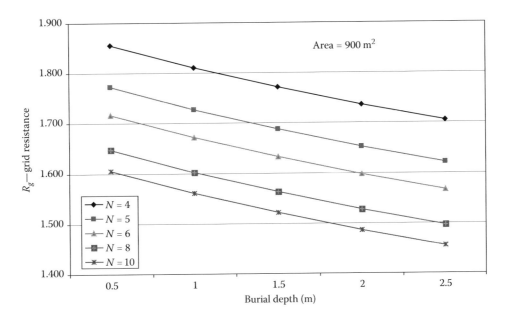

FIGURE 2.68 The effects of varying the depth of burial of the grid (*h*) from 0.5 to 2.5 m and the number of conductors from 4 to 10. (From Keil, R.P., Substation grounding, in *Electric Power Substation Engineering*, Chapter 11, CRC Press, Boca Raton, FL, 2003; Electric Power Research Institute, *Transmission Line Reference Book: 345 kV and Above*, 2nd edn., EPRI, Palo Alto, CA, 1982. With permission.)

In order to aid the substation grounding design engineer, the IEEE Std. 80-2000 includes a design procedure that has a 12-step process, as shown in Figure 2.69, in terms of substation grounding design procedure block diagram, based on a preliminary of a somewhat arbitrary area, that is, the standard suggests the grid be approximately the size of the distribution substation. But, some references state a common practice that is to extend the grid 3 m beyond the perimeter of the substation fence.

Example 2.3

Let the starting grid be an 84.5 m by 49.6 m ground grid. Design a proper substation grounding to provide safety measures for anyone going near or working on a substation. Hence, use the IEEE 12-step process shown in Figure 2.69 and then build a grid large enough to dissipate the ground fault current into the earth. (A large grounding grid extending far beyond the substation fence and made of a single copper plate would have the most desirable effect for dispersing fault currents to remote earth and thereby ensure the safety of personnel at the surface. Unfortunately, a copper plate of such size is not economically viable option.)

A grounding system is considered for this three-phase 230 kV system that feeds two step-down transformers that step down the voltage from 230 to 69 kV. The two transformers are connected in parallel with respect to each other. One of the transformers feeds a switchyard. The other one is connected to a transformer bank (which has three single-phase 4 MVA transformers) that steps down the 69 to 13.8 kV and feeds an industrial facility.

One alternative is to design a grid by using a series of horizontal conductors and vertical ground rods. Of course, the application of conductors and rods depends on the resistivity of the substation ground.) Change the variables as necessary in order to meet specifications for grounding of the substation.

The variables include the size of the grid, the size of the conductors used, the amount of conductors used, and the spacing of each grounding rod. Use 17,000 A, as the maximum value fault current, a maximum clearing time of 1 s, and a conductor diameter of 210.5 kcmil, based on the given information. The soil resistivity is 50 Ω-m and the crushed rock resistivity on the surface of the substation is 2500 Ω-m.

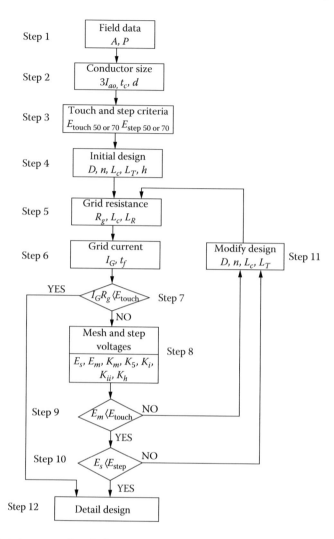

FIGURE 2.69   Substation grounding design procedure block diagram.

Assume that the incoming transmission line into the substation has no shield wires, but there are four distribution neutrals. Design a grounding grid system by using a series of horizontal conductors and vertical ground rods, based on the resistivity of the soil.

Solution

Step 1: Field Data

Assume a uniform average soil resistivity of the substation ground is measured to be 50 Ω-m. Initial design parameters are given in Table 2.10.

Step 2: Conductor Size

The analysis of the grounding grid should be based on the most conservative fault conditions. For example, the fault current $3I_{ao}$ is assumed maximum value, with all current dispersed through the grid (i.e., there is no alternative path for ground other than through the grid to remote earth). As said before, the maximum value of the fault current is given as 17,000 A; thus, the conductor size is selected based on this current and the duration of the fault. Thus, use 17,000 A as the maximum

TABLE 2.10

Initial Design Parameters

ρ	A	L_T	L_C	L_R	L_T	h	L_X	L_Y	D
50 Ω-m	4204.6 m²	3.048 m	1825	76	1901	1.524 m	84.6 m	49.6 m	4.97 m

t_c	h_s	d	$3I_{a0}$	ρ_s	D_f	L_p	n_c	n_d	t_f
1 s	0.11 m	0.018 m (for 500 kcmil)	17,000 A	2500 Ω-m	1.026	75 m	1	1	0.5 s

value fault current, and a maximum clearing time of 0.5 s. A conductor diameter of 210.5 kcmil is determined from the following calculation:

$$
\begin{aligned}
A_{kcmil} &= I \times K \times \sqrt{t_c} \\
&= 17 \times 10.45 \times \sqrt{1} \\
&= 210.5 \text{ kcmil}
\end{aligned}
\tag{2.70}
$$

However, the conductor selected is 500 kcmil. This is based on the given guidelines so that the size is more than enough to handle the fault current. The diameter of the conductor can be found from Table A.1. Based on the selected conductor, the diameter (d) of the conductor is 0.018 m. The crushed rock resistivity is 2500 Ω-m. Surface derating factor is 0.714.

Step 3: Touch and Step Voltage Criteria

In order to move to the third step in the design process, it is first needed to determine the surface layer derating factor

$$
\begin{aligned}
C_s &= 1 - \frac{0.09\left(1 - \left(\rho/\rho_s\right)\right)}{2h_s + 0.09} \\
&= 1 - \frac{0.09\left(1 - \left(50/2500\right)\right)}{2 \times 0.1524 + 0.09} \\
&= 0.78
\end{aligned}
$$

According to the federal law, all known hazards must be eliminated when the GPR takes place for the safety of workers at a work site. In order to remove the hazards associated with GPR, a grounding grid is designed to reduce the hazardous potentials at the surface. First, it is necessary to determine what was not hazardous to the body. For two body types, the potential safe touch and step voltages a human could withstand before the fault is cleared need to be determined from Equations 2.14b and 2.18b, respectively, as

$$
\begin{aligned}
V_{touch\ 70} &= \left(1000 + 1.5C_s \times \rho_s\right)\frac{0.157}{\sqrt{t_s}} \\
&= \left(1000 + 1.5 \times 0.78 \times 2500\right)\frac{0.157}{\sqrt{0.5}} \\
&= 871.5 \text{ V}
\end{aligned}
$$

and

$$V_{step\ 70} = \left(1000 + 6C_s \times \rho_s\right)\frac{0.157}{\sqrt{t_s}}$$

$$= \left(1000 + 1.6 \times 0.78 \times 2500\right)\frac{0.157}{\sqrt{0.5}}$$

$$= 2819.5\ V$$

Step 4: Initial Design

Step 4 deals with the layout of the grounding conductors and the amount of conductors being used for the design. The initial design consists of factors obtained from the general knowledge of the substation. The preliminary size of the grounding grid system is largely based on the size of the substation to include all dimensions within the perimeter of the fence. To establish economic viability, the maximum area is considered and formed the shape of a square with an area of 4204.6 m². The spacing of conductors (D) is selected as 4.97 m.

Therefore, an alternative grid size is developed as shown in Figure 2.70. The maximum lengths (L_x) of the conductor in the x direction and the y direction (L_y) are determined to be 84.6 and 49.6 m, respectively. Based on the information given in this section, the total length of the grounding conductor is 1825 m. The length of the ground rods (L_r) is 3.048 m. A total of 25 ground

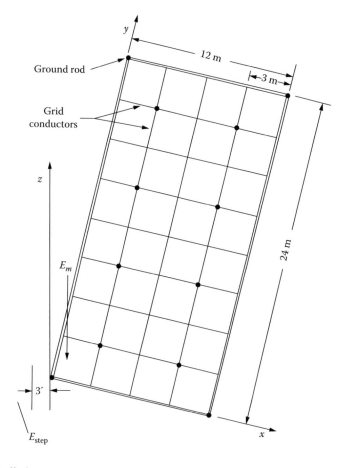

FIGURE 2.70   Preliminary design.

rods are used, which gives the total length of the ground rods (L_R) to be approximately 76 m. Thus, the total conductor length that includes the conductor plus the ground rods is 1901 m.

The depth of the ground grid (h) is determined as 1.525 m below the surface. The next step is to take into account the geometry of the ground grid. Given the length of each side of the grounding grid, it is determined that the shape of the grid design will be a rectangle. The geometric factor can be calculated by determining n_a, n_b, n_c, and n_d as

$$n_a = \frac{2 \times L_c}{L_p}$$
$$= \frac{2 \times 1825}{268}$$
$$= 14$$

and

$$n_b = \sqrt{\frac{L_p}{4 \times \sqrt{A}}}$$
$$= \sqrt{\frac{268}{4 \times \sqrt{4204.6}}}$$
$$= 1.03$$

and

$$n_c = \left[\frac{L_x \times L_y}{A}\right]^{0.7 \times A / L_x \times L_y}$$
$$= \left[\frac{84.6 \times 49.6}{4204.6}\right]^{0.7 \times 4204.6 / 84.6 \times 49.6}$$
$$= 1.00$$

and

$$n_d = \frac{D_m}{\sqrt{L_x^2 + L_y^2}}$$
$$= \frac{98.1}{\sqrt{84.6^2 + 49.6^2}}$$
$$= 1.00$$

The geometric factor is then calculated to be

$$n = n_a \times n_b \times n_c \times n_d$$
$$= 14 \times 1.03 \times 1 \times 1$$
$$= 14$$

Thus, they are approximately equal to 1 due to the shape of the grid.

Step 5: Grid Resistance

A good grounding system provides a low resistance to remote earth in order to minimize the GPR. The next step is to evaluate the grid resistance by using Equation 2.71. All design parameters can be found in Table 2.10. Table 2.11 gives approximate equivalent impedance of transmission line

TABLE 2.11

Approximate Equivalent Impedance of Transmission Line OH Shield Wires and Distribution Feeder Neutrals

Number of Transmission Lines	Number of Distribution Neutrals	$R_{tg} = 15$ and $R_{d\phi} = 25\ R + jX\Omega$	$R_{tg} = 15$ and $R_{d\phi} = 25\ R + jX\Omega$
1	1	$0.91 + j0.485\ \Omega$	$3.27 + j0.652\ \Omega$
1	2	$0.54 + j0.33\ \Omega$	$2.18 + j0.412\ \Omega$
1	4	$0.295 + j0.20\ \Omega$	$1.32 + j0.244\ \Omega$
4	4	$0.23 + j0.12\ \Omega$	$0.817 + j0.16\ \Omega$
0	4	$0.322 + j0.242\ \Omega$	$1.65 + j0.291\ \Omega$

OH shield wires and distribution feeder neutrals, according to their numbers. From Equation 2.168 for $L_T = 1901$ m, a grid area of $A = 4205$ m^2, $\rho = 50$ Ω-m, and $h = 1.524$ m, the grid resistance is

$$R_g = \rho\left[\frac{1}{L_T} + \frac{1}{\sqrt{20 \times A}}\left(1 + \frac{1}{1 + h \times \sqrt{20 \times A}}\right)\right]$$

$$= 50\left[\frac{1}{1901} + \frac{1}{\sqrt{20 \times 4205}}\left(1 + \frac{1}{1 + 1.524 \times \sqrt{20 \times 4205}}\right)\right]$$

$$= 0.35\ \Omega$$

Step 6: Grid Current

In Step 6 of the logic flow diagram of the IEEE Std. 80-2000, the amount of current that flows within the designed grid (I_G) is determined. The GPR is determined as

$$V_{GPR} = I_G \times R_g$$

Determining the GPR and comparing it to the tolerable touch voltage is the first step to find out whether the grid design is a safe design for the people in and around the substation. The next step is to find the grid current I_G. But, it is first needed to determine the split factor from the following equation:

$$S_f = \left|\frac{Z_{eq}}{Z_{eq} + R_g}\right| \tag{2.71}$$

Since the substation has no impedance line shield wires and four distribution neutrals, from Table 2.11, the equivalent impedance can be found as $Z_{eq} = 0.322 + j0.242$ Ω. Thus, $R_g = 1.0043$ Ω with a total fault current of $3I_{a0} = 17,000$ A and a decrement factor of $D_f = 1.026$. Thus, the current division factor (or the split factor) can be found as

$$S_f = \left|\frac{Z_{eq}}{Z_{eq} + R_g}\right|$$

$$= \left|\frac{(0.322 + j0.242)}{(0.322 + j0.242) + 1.0043}\right|$$

$$\cong 0.2548$$

since

$$I_g = S_f \times 3I_{a0}$$
$$= 0.2548 \times 17,000$$
$$= 4,331.6 \text{ A}$$

thus,

$$I_G = D_f \times I_g$$
$$= 1.026 \times 4331.6$$
$$= 4444.2 \text{ A}$$

Step 7: Determination of GPR

As said before, the product of I_G and R_g is the GPR. It is necessary to compare the GPR to the tolerable touch voltage, $V_{\text{touch } 70}$. If the GPR is larger than the $V_{\text{touch } 70}$, further design evaluations are necessary and the tolerable touch and step voltages should be compared to the maximum mesh and step voltages. Hence, first determine the GPR as

$$\text{GPR} = I_G \times R_g$$
$$= 4444.2 \times 0.35$$
$$= 1555.48 \text{ V}$$

Check to see whether

$$\text{GPR} > V_{\text{touch } 70}$$

Indeed,

$$1555.2 \text{ V} > 871.5 \text{ V}$$

As it can be observed from the results, the GPR is much larger than the step voltage. Therefore, further design considerations are necessary, and thus, the step and mesh voltages must be calculated and compared to the tolerable touch and step voltage as follows.

Step 8: Mesh and Step Voltage Calculations

1. Determination of the Mesh Voltage

In order to calculate the mesh voltage by using Equation 2.49, it is necessary first to calculate the variables K_h, K_m, and K_{ii}. Here, the correction factor that accounts for the depth of the grid (K_{ii}) can be determined from Equation 2.53 as

$$K_h = \sqrt{1 + \frac{h}{h_0}}$$
$$= \sqrt{1 + \frac{1.524}{1}}$$
$$= 1.59$$

The corrective factor for grid geometry (K_{ii}) can be calculated from Equation 2.57 as

$$K_{ii} = 0.644 + 0.148 \times n$$
$$= 0.644 + 0.148 \times 4$$
$$= 2.716$$

2. Comparison of Mesh Voltage and Allowable Touch Voltage

Using K_h and K_{ii}, the spacing factor for mesh voltage (K_m) can be calculated. Here, the corrective weighting factor that can be used to adjust conductors on the corner mesh (K_{ii}) is considered to be 1.0 due to the shape of the grid being rectangular. Hence,

$$K_m = \frac{1}{2\pi}\left[\ln\left(\frac{D^2}{16\times h\times d}+\frac{(D+2\times h)^2}{8\times D\times d}-\frac{h}{4\times d}\right)+\frac{K_{ii}}{K_h}\ln\left(\frac{8}{\pi(2\times 14-1)}\right)\right]$$

$$=\frac{1}{2\pi}\left[\ln\left(\frac{4.97^2}{16\times 1.524\times 0.018}+\frac{(4.97+2\times 1.524)^2}{8\times 4.97\times 0.018}-\frac{1.524}{4\times 0.018}\right)+\frac{1}{1.589}\ln\left(\frac{8}{\pi(2\times 14-1)}\right)\right]$$

$$=0.53$$

Thus, the mesh voltage can now be calculated as

$$E_m = \frac{\rho\times I_G\times K_m\times K_{ii}}{L_C+\left[1.55+1.22\left(L_r/\sqrt{(L_x^2+L_y^2)}\right)\right]L_R}$$

$$=\frac{50\times 4444.2\times 0.53\times 2.716}{1825+\left[1.55+1.22\left(3.048/\sqrt{(84.6^2+49.6^2)}\right)\right]76.2}$$

$$=164.39\,\text{V}$$

3. Determination of the Step Voltage

In order for the ground to be safe, step voltage has to be less than the tolerable step voltages. Also, step voltages within a grid system designed for mesh voltages will be well within the tolerable limits. To determine the step voltage (E_{step}), unknown variables of K_s and L_s are to be calculated. Thus, the spacing factor for step voltage (K_s) can be found from

$$K_s = \frac{1}{\pi}\left[\frac{1}{2\times h}+\frac{1}{D+h}+\frac{1}{D}\left(1-0.5^{n-2}\right)\right]$$

$$=\frac{1}{\pi}\left[\frac{1}{2\times 1.524}+\frac{1}{3.97+1.524}+\frac{1}{4.97}\left(1-0.5^{14-2}\right)\right]$$

$$=0.22$$

The effective length (L_s) for the step voltage is

$$L_s = 0.75\times L_c+0.85\times L_R$$

$$=0.75\times 1825+0.85\times 76$$

$$=1433.5\,\text{m}$$

Thus, the step voltage (E_{step}) is determined as

$$E_{step} = \frac{\rho\times I_G\times K_s\times K_{ii}}{L_s}$$

$$=\frac{50\times 4444.2\times 0.22\times 2.716}{1433.5}$$

$$=92.62\,\text{V}$$

Step 9: Comparison of E_{mesh} versus V_{touch}

Here, the mesh voltage that is calculated in Step 8 is compared with the tolerable touch voltages calculated in Step 4. If the calculated mesh voltage E_{mesh} is greater than the tolerable $V_{touch\,70}$, further design evaluations are necessary. If the mesh voltage E_{mesh} is smaller than the $V_{touch\,70}$, then it can be moved to the next step and E_{step} can be compared with $V_{step\,70}$. Accordingly,

$$E_{mesh} < V_{touch70}\,(?)$$

$$164.39\text{ V} < 871.5\text{ V}$$

Here, the original grid design passes the second critical criteria in step 9. Hence, it can be moved to step 10 to find out whether the final criterion is met.

Step 10: Comparison of E_{step} versus $V_{step\,70}$

This is the final step that the design has to meet before the grounding system is considered safe. At this step, E_{step} is compared with the calculated tolerable step voltage $V_{step\,70}$. If

$$E_{step} > V_{step\,70}\,(?)$$

A refinement of the preliminary design is necessary and can be accomplished by decreasing the total grid resistance, closer grid spacing, adding more ground grid rods, if possible, and/or limiting the total fault current.

On the other hand, if

$$E_{step} < V_{step\,70}\,(?)$$

then the designed grounding grid is considerably safe. Since here,

$$92.62\text{ V} < 2819.8\text{ V}$$

then for the design,

$$E_{step} < V_{step\,70}$$

In summary, according to the calculations, the calculated mesh and step voltages are smaller than the tolerable touch and step voltages; therefore, in a typical shock situation, humans (weighting 70 kg) that become part of the circuit during a fault will have only what is considered a safe amount of current passing through their bodies.

There are many variables that can be changed in order to meet specifications for grounding a substation. Some variables include the size of the grid, the size of the conductors used, the amount of conductors used, and the spacing of each ground rod. After many processes an engineer has to go through, the project would then be put into construction if it is approved. Designing safe substation grounding is obviously not an easy task, but there are certain procedures that an engineer can follow to make the designing substation grounding easier.

2.18   TRANSMISSION LINE GROUNDS

HV transmission lines are designed and built to withstand the effects of lightning with a minimum damage and interruption of operation. If the lightning strikes an OHGW (also called *static wire*) on a transmission line, the lightning current is conducted to ground through the ground wire (GW) installed along the pole or through the metal tower. The top of the line structure is raised in potential to a value determined by the magnitude of the lightning current and the surge impedance of the ground connection.

In the event that the impulse resistance of the ground connection is large, this potential can be in the magnitude of thousands of volts. If the potential is greater than the insulation level of the apparatus, a flashover will take place, causing an arc. The arc, in turn, will start the operation of protective relays, causing the line to be taken out of service. In the event that the transmission structure is well grounded and there is a sufficient coordination between the conductor insulation and the ground resistance, flashover can generally be avoided.

The transmission line grounds can be in various ways to achieve a low ground resistance. For example, a pole butt grounding plate or butt coil can be employed on wood poles. A butt coil is a spiral coil of bare copper wire installed at the bottom of a pole. The wire of the coil is extended up the pole as the GW lead. In practice, usually one or more ground rods are employed instead to achieve the required low ground resistance.

The sizes of the rods used are usually 5/8 or 3/4 in. in diameter and 10 ft in length. The thickness of the rod does not play a major role in reducing the ground resistance as does the length of the rod. Multiple rods are usually used to provide the low ground resistance required by the high-capacity structures. But, if the rods are moderately close to each other, the overall resistance will be more than if the same number of rods were spaced far apart. In other words, adding a second rod does not provide a total resistance of half that of a single rod unless the two are several rod lengths apart (actually infinite distance). Lewis [22] has shown that at 2 ft apart, the resistance of two pipes (used as ground rods) in parallel is about 61% of the resistance of one of them, and at 6 ft apart, it is about 55% of the resistance of one pipe.

Where there is bedrock near the surface or where sand is encountered, the soil is usually very dry and therefore has high resistivity. Such situations may require a grounding system known as the *counterpoise*, made of buried metal (usually galvanized steel wire) strips, wires, or cables. The counterpoise for an OH transmission line consists of a special grounding terminal that reduces the surge impedance of the ground connection and increases the coupling between the GW and the conductors.

The basic types of counterpoises used for transmission lines located in areas with sandy soil or rock close to the surface are the continuous type (also called the *parallel type*) and the radial (also called the *crowfoot type*), as shown in Figure 2.71. The continuous counterpoise is made of one or more conductors buried under the transmission line for its entire length.

The counterpoise wires are connected to the OH ground (or *static*) wire at all towers or poles. But, the radial-type counterpoise is made of a number of wires and extends radially (in some fashion) from the tower legs. The number and length of the wires are determined by the tower location and the soil conditions. The counterpoise wires are usually installed with a cable plow at a length of 18 in. or more so that they will not be disturbed by cultivation of the land.

A multigrounded, common neutral conductor used for a primary distribution line is always connected to the substation grounding system where the circuit originates and to all grounds along the length of the circuit. If separate primary and secondary neutral conductors are used, the conductors have to be con-

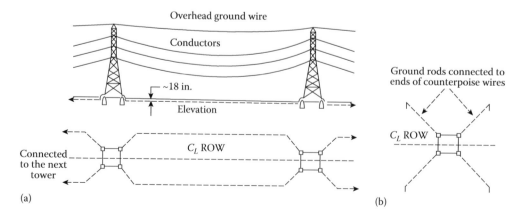

(a)　　　　　　　　　　　　　　　　　　　　　　(b)

FIGURE 2.71　Two basic types of counterpoises: (a) continuous (parallel) and (b) radial.

nected together provided that the primary neutral conductor is effectively grounded. The resistance of a single buried horizontal wire, when it is used as radial counterpoise, can be expressed as [16]

$$R = \frac{\rho}{\pi\ell}\left(\ln\frac{2\ell}{2(ad)^{1/2}} - 1\right) \quad \text{when } d \ll \ell \tag{2.72}$$

where
  ρ is the ground resistivity in ohmmeters
  ℓ is the length of wire in meters
  a is the radius of wire in meters
  d is the burial depth in meters

It is assumed that the potential is uniform over the entire length of the wire. This is only true when the wire has ideal conductivity. If the wire is very long, such as with the radial counterpoise, the potential is not uniform over the entire length of the wire. Hence, Equation 2.39 cannot be used. Instead, the resistance of such a continuous counterpoise when $\ell(r/\rho)^{1/2}$ is large can be expressed as

$$R = (r\rho)^{1/2}\coth\left[\left(\ell\left(\frac{r}{\rho}\right)^{1/2}\right)\right] \tag{2.73}$$

where r is the resistance of wire in ohmmeters.

If the lightning current flows through a counterpoise, the effective resistance is equal to the surge impedance of the wire. The wire resistance decreases as the surge propagates along the wire. For a given length counterpoise, the transient resistance will diminish to the steady-state resistance if the same wire is used in several shorter radial counterpoises rather than as a continuous counterpoise. Thus, the first 250 ft of counterpoise is most effective when it comes to grounding of lightning currents.

2.19 TYPES OF GROUNDING

In general, transmission and subtransmission systems are solidly grounded. Transmission systems are usually connected grounded wye, but subtransmission systems are often connected in delta. Delta systems may also be grounded through grounding transformers. In most HV systems, the neutrals are solidly grounded, that is, connected directly to the ground. The advantages of such grounding are as follows:

1. Voltages to ground are limited to the phase voltage.
2. Intermittent ground faults and HVs due to arcing faults are eliminated.
3. Sensitive protective relays operated by ground fault currents clear these faults at an early stage.

The grounding transformers used are normally either small distribution transformers (which are connected normally in wye–delta, having their secondaries in delta) or small grounding autotransformers with interconnected wye or *zigzag* windings, as shown in Figure 2.72. The three-phase autotransformer has a single winding. If there is a ground fault on any line, the ground current flows equally in the three legs of the autotransformer. The interconnection offers the minimum impedance to the flow of the single-phase fault current.

The transformers are only used for grounding and carry little current except during a ground fault. Because of that, they can be fairly small. Their ratings are based on the stipulation that they carry current for no more than 5 min since the relays normally operate long before that. The grounding transformers are connected to the substation ground.

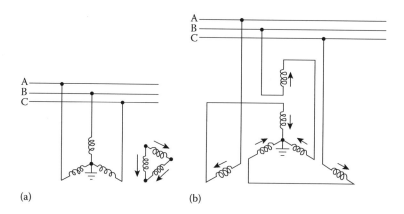

FIGURE 2.72 Grounding transformers used in delta-connected systems: (a) using wye–delta-connected small distribution transformers or (b) using grounding autotransformers with interconnected wye or *zigzag* windings.

All substation equipment and structures are connected to the ground grid with large conductors to minimize the grounding resistance and limit the potential between equipment and the ground surface to a safe value under all conditions. All substation fences are built inside the ground grid and attached to the grid at short intervals to protect the public and personnel. Furthermore, the surface of the substation is usually covered with crushed rock or concrete to reduce the potential gradient when large currents are discharged to ground and to increase the contact resistance to the feet of personnel in the substation.

As said before, the substation grounding system is connected to every individual equipment, structure, and installation in order to provide the means by which grounding currents are conducted to remote areas. Thus, it is extremely important that the substation ground has a low ground resistance, adequate current-carrying capacity, and safety features for personnel.

It is crucial to have the substation ground resistance very low so that the total rise of the grounding system potential will not reach values that are unsafe for human contact. Therefore, the substation grounding system normally is made up of buried horizontal conductors and driven-ground rods interconnected (by clamping, welding, or brazing) to form a *continuous grid* (also called *mat*) network.

Notice that a continuous cable (usually it is 4/0 bare stranded copper cable buried 12–18 in. below the surface) surrounds the grid perimeter to enclose as much ground as possible and to prevent current concentration and thus high gradients at the ground cable terminals. Inside the grid, cables are buried in parallel lines and with uniform spacing (e.g., about 10 × 20 ft).

Today, many utilities have computer programs for performing grounding grid studies. Thus, the number of tedious calculations that must be performed to develop an accurate and sophisticated model of a system is no longer a problem.

The GPR depends on grid burial depth, diameter and length of conductors used, spacing between each conductor, fault current magnitude, system voltage, ground system resistance, soil resistivity, distribution of current throughout the grid, proximity of the fault electrodes, and the system grounding electrodes to the conductors. IEEE Std. 80-1976 [14] provides a formula for a quick simple calculation of the grid resistance to ground after a minimum design has been completed. It is expressed as

$$R = \frac{\rho}{4r} + \frac{\rho}{L} \ \Omega \tag{2.74}$$

where
ρ is the soil resistivity in ohmmeters
L is the total length of grid conductors in meters
R is the radius of circle with area equal to that of grid in meters

IEEE Std. 80-1976 also provides formulas to determine the effects of the grid geometry on the step and mesh voltage (which is the worst possible value of the touch voltage) in volts. They can be expressed as

$$V_{\text{step}} = \frac{K_s K_i \rho I_G}{L} \tag{2.75}$$

and

$$V_{\text{mesh}} = \frac{K_m K_i \rho I_G}{L} \tag{2.76}$$

where

K_s is the step coefficient
K_m is the mesh coefficient
K_i is the irregularity coefficient

Many utilities have computer programs for performing grounding grid studies. The number of tedious calculations that must be performed to develop an accurate and sophisticated model of a system is no longer a problem.

2.20 TRANSFORMER CLASSIFICATIONS

In power system applications, the single- or three-phase transformers with ratings up to 500 kVA and 34.5 kV are defined as *distribution transformers*, whereas those transformers with ratings over 500 kVA at voltage levels above 34.5 kV are defined *as power transformers*. Most distribution and power transformers are immersed in a tank of oil for better insulation and cooling purposes.

Today, for reasons of efficiency and economy, most electric energy is generated, transmitted, and distributed using a three-phase system rather than a single-phase system. Three-phase power may be transformed by the use of either a single three-phase transformer or three single-phase trans- formers, which are properly connected with each other for a three-phase operation. A three-phase transformer, in comparison to a bank of three single-phase transformers, weighs less, costs less, needs less floor space, and has a slightly higher efficiency. In the event of failure, however, the entire three-phase transformer must be replaced.

On the other hand, if three separate single-phase units (i.e., *a three-phase transformer bank*) are used, only one of them needs to be replaced.* Also, a standby three-phase transformer is more expensive than a single-phase spare transformer. There are the two versions of three-phase core construction that are normally used: core type and shell type.

In the *core-type* design, both the primary and secondary windings of each phase are placed only on one leg of each transformer. For balanced, three-phase sinusoidal voltages, the sum of the three-core fluxes at any given time must be zero. This is a requirement that does not have to be met in the *shell-type* construction. In the *core-type construction,* the magnetic reluctance of the flux path of the center phase is less than that of the outer two phases.

A *shell-type transformer* is quite different in character from a core-type transformer. In such design, the flux in the outside paths of the core is reduced by 42% since in *a shell-type construction,* the center phase windings are wound in the opposite direction of the other two phases.

Since all yoke cross sections are equal, not only is the amount of core requirement reduced, but also the manufacturing process involved is simplified. Furthermore, in a shell-type transformer, the no-load losses are less than those in a core-type transformer.

Figure 2.73 shows a 40 MVA, 110 kV ± 16%/21 kV three-phase core-type transformer. Notice that its primary-side voltage can be adjusted by ±16%. Figure 2.74 shows a 850/950/1100 MVA,

---

* However, it is not possible to use transformers to convert a single-phase system to a three-phase system for a large amount of power. Relatively very small amounts of power can be developed from a single-phase system using $R-C$ phase shift networks (or an induction phase converter) to produce two-phase power, which in turn can be transformed into three-phase power.

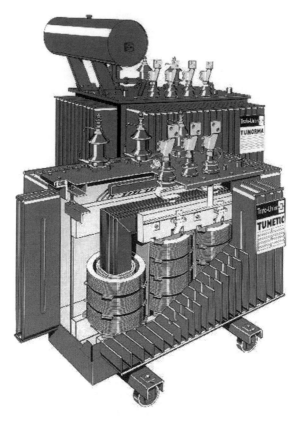

FIGURE 2.73   A 40 MVA, 110 kV ± 16%/21 kV, three-phase, core-type transformer, 5.2 m high, 9.4 m long, 3 m wide, weighing 80 tons. (Courtesy of Siemens AG.)

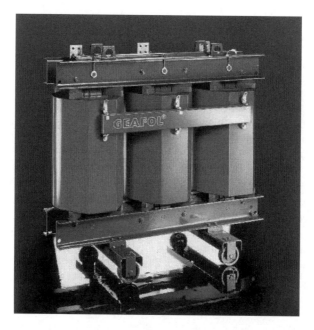

FIGURE 2.74   A 850/950/1100 MVA, 415 kV ± 11%/27 kV, three-phase, shell-type transformer, 11.3 high, 14 long, 5.7 wide, weighing (without cooling oil) 552 tons. (Courtesy of Siemens AG.)

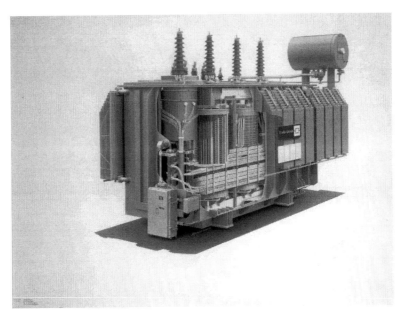

FIGURE 2.75   The 10 MVA and 50 kVA, core-type three-phase transformers with GEAFOL solid dielectric cores. (Courtesy of Siemens AG.)

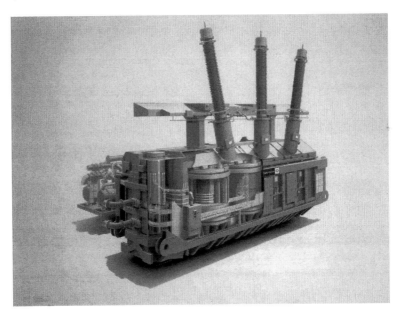

FIGURE 2.76   A typical core and coil assembly of a three-phase, core-type, power transformer. (Courtesy of Siemens AG.)

415 kV ± 11%/27 kV, three-phase shell-type transformer. Figure 2.75 shows a 10 MVA and a 40 WA core-type three-phase transformer with *GEAFOL solid dielectric core*. Finally, Figure 2.76 shows a typical core and coil assembly of a three-phase core-type power transformer. Notice that its core and coil assembly are rigidly supported and clamped by heavy, fabricated clamping structures. The windings are concentrically placed on the core legs and laterally braced by inserting kiln-dried, maple wood dowels between the windings and the core. The complete assembly is rigidly braced to withstand the mechanical forces experienced under fault conditions and to resist vibration

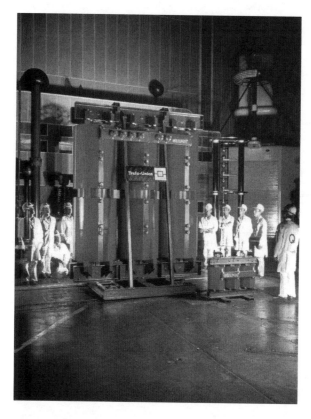

FIGURE 2.77 The 10MVA and 50 kVA, core-type three-phase transformers with GEAFOL solid dielectric cores. (Courtesy of Siemens AG.)

and shock forces encountered during shipment and installation. All HV leads are brought to tap changers, terminal blocks, or bushings. Figure 2.77 shows 10 MVA and 50 kVA, core-type three-phase transformers with GEAFOL solid dielectric cores. Figure 2.78 shows a core-type three-phase transformer with GEAFOL solid dielectric core.

Today, various methods are in use in power transformers to get the heat pot of the tank more effectively. Historically, as the transformer sizes increased, the losses outgrew any means of self-cooling that was available at the time, thus a water-cooling method was put into practice. This was done by placing metal coil tubing in the top oil, around the inside of the tank. Water was pumped through this cooling coil to get rid of the heat from oil.

Another method was circulating the hot oil through an external oil-to-water heat exchanger. This method is called *forced-oil-to-water* (FOW) *cooling* . Today, the most common of these forced-oil-cooled power transformers uses an external bank of oil-to-air heat exchangers through which the oil is continuously pumped. It is known as type FOA.

In present practice, fans are automatically used for the first stage and pumps for the second, in triple-rated transformers that are designated as type OA/FA/FOA. These transformers carry up to about 60% of maximum nameplate rating (i.e., FOA rating) by natural circulation of the oil (OA) and 80% of maximum nameplate rating by forced cooling that consists of fans on the radiators (FA). Finally, at maximum nameplate rating (FOA), not only is oil forced to circulate through external radiators, but fans are also kept on to blow air onto the radiators as well as into the tank itself. In summary, the power transformer classes are

OA: Oil-immersed, self-cooled
OW: Oil-immersed, water-cooled

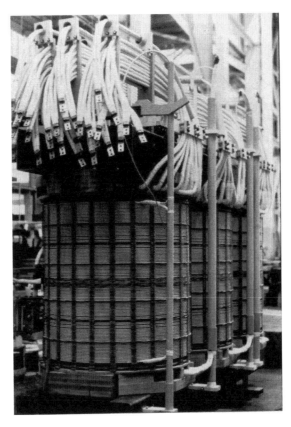

FIGURE 2.78 A core-type three-phase transformer with GEAFOL solid dielectric core. (Courtesy of Siemens AG.)

OA/FA: Oil-immersed, self-cooled/forced-air-cooled
OA/FA/FOA: Oil-immersed, self-cooled/forced-air-cooled/forced-oil-cooled
FOA: Oil-immersed, forced-oil-cooled with forced-air cooler
FOW: Oil-immersed, forced-oil-cooled with water cooler

In a distribution substation, power transformers are used to provide the conversion from subtransmission circuits to the distribution level. Most are connected in delta–wye grounded to provide ground source for the distribution neutral and to isolate the distribution grounding system from the subtransmission system.

Substation transformers can range from 5 MVA in smaller rural substations to over 80 MVA at urban stations (in terms of base ratings). As mentioned earlier, power transformers have multiple ratings, depending on cooling methods. The base rating is the self-cooled rating, just due to the natural flow to the surrounding air through radiators. The transformer can supply more load with extra cooling turned on, as explained before.

However, the ANSI ratings were revised in the year 2000 to make them more consistent with IEC designations. This system has a four-letter code that indicates the cooling (IEEE C57.12.00-2000):

First letter—internal cooling medium in contact with the windings

O: Mineral oil or synthetic insulating liquid with fire point = 300°C
K: Insulating liquid with fire point >300°C
L: Insulating liquid with no measurable fire point

TABLE 2.12
Equivalent Cooling Classes

Year 2000 Designations	Designation Prior to Year 2000
ONAN	OA
ONAF	FA
ONAN/ONAF/ONAF	OA/FA/FA
ONAN/ONAF/OFAF	OA/FA/FOA
OFAF	FOA
OFWF	FOW

Source: IEEE Std. C57.12.00-2000.

Second letter—circulation mechanism for internal cooling medium

N: Natural convection flow through cooling equipment and in windings

F: Forced circulation through cooling equipment (i.e., *coolant pumps*); natural convection flow in windings (also called *nondirected flow*)

D: Forced circulation through cooling equipment, directed from the cooling equipment into at least the main windings

Third letter—external cooling medium

A: Air

W: Water

Fourth letter—circulation mechanism for external cooling medium

N: Natural convection

F: Forced circulation, fans (*air cooling*), pumps (*water cooing*)

   Therefore, *OA/FA/FOA* is equivalent to *ONAN/ONAF/OFAF*. Each cooling level typically provides an extra one-third capability: 21/28/35 MVA. Table 2.12 shows equivalent cooling classes in old and new naming schemes.

   Utilities do not overload substation transformers as much as distribution transformers, but they do not run them hot at times. As with distribution transformers, the trade-off is loss of life versus the immediate replacement cost of the transformer. Ambient conditions also affect loading. Summer peaks are much worse than winter peaks. IEEE Std. C57.91-1995 provides detailed loading guidelines and also suggests an approximate adjustment of 1% of the maximum nameplate rating for every degree C above or below 30°C.

   The hottest-spot-conductor temperature is the critical point where insulation degrades. Above the hot-spot-conductor temperature of 110°C, life expectancy of a transformer decreases exponentially. *The life of a transformer halves for every* 8°C *increase in operating temperature.* Most of the time, the hottest temperatures are nowhere near this. The impedance of substation transformers is normally about 7%–10%. This is the impedance on the base rating, the self-cooled rating (OA or ONAN).

2.20.1 Transformer Connections

Figure 2.79 shows various three-phase transformer connections, including wye–wye, delta–delta, wye–delta, and delta–wye connections. The complete windings have to be insulated for full line-to-line voltages. Because of this, wye-connected transformers with graded insulation are used for transmission voltages above 73 kV due to the costs involved. Additionally, the delta–delta

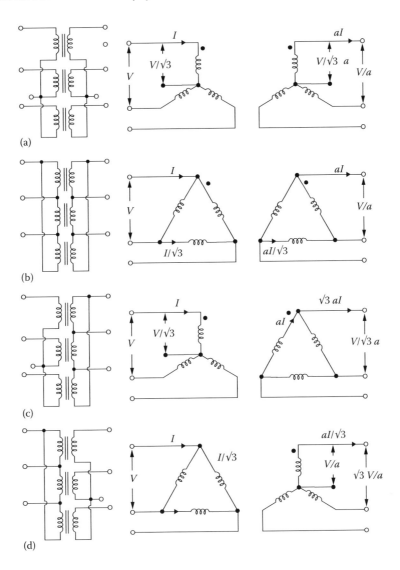

(a)

(b)

(c)

(d)

FIGURE 2.79 Possible three-phase transformer connections.

transformers can be operated as open delta, if the need arises. In that case, the transformer bank capacity becomes 86.6% of the capacity of the remaining transformers.

The delta–wye connection is in common use for both step-up and step-down operations. The HV winding is wye-connected when used for voltage step-down. On the other hand, the LV winding is usually wye-connected when used in order to provide a grounded neutral for secondary transmission. Delta-connected HV windings are rarely used for transmission voltages of 138 kV and above. The delta–wye transformer connection almost completely suppresses the triple harmonics (i.e., the third harmonic and its odd multiples) with the neutral solidly grounded.

Wye–wye connected transformers are seldom used on HV transmission systems. When used with both neutrals grounded, if the transformers have three phases with shell-type core, they have been used with wye-connected generator(s). In that event, there must be solid neutral connecting the generator(s) and the low-VT neutral to minimize triple harmonic problems. Wye–wye connected transformers with delta-connected tertiary windings solve the problems that are associated with simple wye–wye connections.

2.20.2 Transformer Selection

The selection of the proper transformer can have a major impact on the cost of a substation, since the transformer represents the major cost item. Nameplate rating is only a preliminary guide to the transformer application.

The transformer is applicable as a self-cooled unit, or it can be purchased with additional steps of forced cooling that use fan or sets of fans and oil pumps, as explained in the previous section. Transformer ratings can be increased from 25% to 66% by the addition of fans and pumps.

The nameplate rating is based on a continuous load that is producing a 55°C conductor temperature rise over ambient. Since many transformers do not carry continuous loads, advantages can be obtained from the thermal time lag to carry higher peak loads without being over the temperature limits.

Transformer ratings are based on the assumption that only an extremely small amount of insulation deterioration takes place due to aging process under normal operation. A considerable increase in rating can be obtained at the expense of the loss of insulation life. This increase in rating might be close to 200% for an hour or two and about 20% for 24 h.

The additional factors that affect the transformer selection are as follows:

1. Transformer impedances should be chosen after taking into account their effects on short-circuit duties and low-side breaker ratings, both the initial and future stations' developments.
2. When applicable, the transformer impedance should be selected to achieve a proper load division in the parallel operation of transformers.
3. It may be necessary to provide bus regulation if the HV side and LV side voltages vary over a wide range during the load cycle of the transformer.
4. If the bus regulation is needed, determine the actual regulation by using the system and load characteristics. The bus regulation may also be provided in the transformer itself by using load tap-changing (LTC) equipment.
5. If there is no need for such bus regulation at the present time, consider the possibility of such requirement in the future. If so, it may be economical. For the time being, just to leave space in the substation for future regulations, and bus transformers without LTC equipment.

It is important to note that autotransformers are employed almost universally in EHV stations. This is true even for transformations from EHV directly to subtransmission voltage levels. For such applications, low impedance is desirable.

2.21 ENVIRONMENTAL IMPACT OF TRANSMISSION LINES

2.21.1 Environmental Effects

Designing a transmission line with minimum environmental effects dictates a study of three key factors, namely, the effects of electric fields, the visual effects of the design, and the effects of physical location.

In addition to the transmission lines, substations also generate electric and magnetic fields (EMFs). In substations, typical sources of EMFs include the following: both transmission and distribution lines entering or exiting the substation, bus work, switchgear, cabling, CBs, transformers, air core reactors, line traps, grounding grid, capacitors, computers, and battery charges.

The HV gradients of EHV lines near the phase conductors can cause breakdowns of the air around the conductors. Such breakdowns may in turn cause corona loss, electromagnetic interference (EMI), RN, television interference (TVI), AN, and ozone generation. The transmission line designer is guided by the established acceptable levels of each of the previous concerns.

The RN is an undesirable electromagnetic radiation in the radio-frequency (RF) band and interferes with the existing radio signals. It can be caused by corona on EHV transmission lines. Hence, the designer must take into account the electric fields near the conductors.

AN is also produced by high-field gradients like the RN. It generates pressure waves in the air that fall within the audible frequency range. The AN manifests itself as a cracking sound or hum and is audible especially at night. The environmental effects mentioned earlier are even more since corona activity is usually greater during heavy rain.

Also, ungrounded equipment located near HV lines will develop an oscillating electric field. Because of this, the line designer has to be sure that the line height is sufficient to keep the discharge current below the proper levels for all apparatus that are located within the ROW.

2.21.2 BIOLOGICAL EFFECTS OF ELECTRIC FIELDS

Electric fields are present whenever voltage exists on a line conductor. Electric fields are not dependent on the current but voltage. Electric substations produce EMFs. In a substation, the strongest fields are located around the perimeter fence and come from transmission and distribution lines entering and leaving the substation. The strength of fields from apparatus that is located inside the fence decreases rapidly with the distance, reaching very low levels at relatively short distances beyond substation fences.

Electric fields are not dependent on the current. The magnitude of the electric field is a function of the operating voltage and decreases with square of the distance from the source. The strength of electric fields is measured in volts per meter or kilovolts per meter. The electric field can be easily shielded (i.e., its strength can be reduced) by any conducting surface, such as trees, fences, walls, building, and most other structures. Furthermore, in substations, the electric field is extremely variable because of the effects of existing grounded steel structures that are used for bus and equipment support.*

Due to the public concerns with respect to EMFs levels and government regulations, the substation designer has to consider design measures to lower EMF levels. The electric field levels, especially near-HV equipment, can reach to very high levels, but the level decreases significantly toward

---

* (The source for the following information is Electric Power Research Institute (EPRI) [26]: "Concerns have been expressed since the advent of EHV transmission above the possible effects of chronic exposure to ac electric fields. (W.B. Kouwenhoven et al., "Medical evaluation of man working in AC electric fields," *IEEE Transactions on Power Apparatus and Systems*, pp. 506–511, 1967.) Recently, these concerns have increased because of the expansion of EHV transmission systems and because of USSR reports of health complaints by personnel working in EHV substations. (V.P. Korobkova et al., "Influence of the electric fields in 500 kV and 750 kV switchyards on maintenance staff and means for its protection," CIGRE, Institute of Electrical and Electronics Engineers, 1972 Session Report 23-06) (Study in the USSR of medical effects of electric fields on electric power systems, 1978 special publication No. 10, IEEE-PES, 78 CHO 1020-7-PWR.)

"The body of research literature on effects of electric fields on test animals and plants has been reviewed and commented upon by many organizations." [(J.W. Bankoske et al., "Some biological effects of high intensity, low frequency (60 Hz) electric fields on small birds and animals," Electric Power Research Institute, EPRI Research Project RP 129, Final Report, December 1977.) ("Research on the biological effects of electric and magnetic fields," *Revue Generale D. L'electricite Numero Special,* July 1976.) (IIT Research Institute, "Biological effects of high-voltage electric fields: an update," EPRI EA-1123, Vol. 1 & 2, Project 857-1, Final Report, July 1979.) (J.E. Bridges, "Environmental effects of power frequency (50 or 60 Hz) electrical fields," *IEEE Transactions on Power Apparatus and Systems,* Vol. PAS-97, Jan/Feb 1978.) (G. E. Atoian, "Are there biological and psychological effects due to extra high voltage installations?" *IEEE Transactions on Power Apparatus and Systems,* Vol. PAS-97, No. 1, Jan/Feb 1978.)"]

"Even though it is not presently possible to draw definite conclusions, it is, nevertheless, necessary for systems planners, line designers, and public service commissions to make recommendations and to make decisions on the design, construction, and operation of transmission lines. Some effects have been found in several instances on test animals, but in no case have they been confirmed by independent research."

"Although health complaints by substation workers in the USSR were reported [(V.P. Korobkova et al., "Influence of the electric fields in 500 kV and 750 kV switchyards on maintenance staff and means for its protection," CIGRE, Institute of Electrical and Electronics Engineers, 1972 Session Report 23-06) and (Study in the USSR of medical effects of electric fields on electric power systems, 1978 special publication No. 10, IEEE-PES, 78 CHO 1020-7-PWR.)] medical examinations of linemen in the USA, in Sweden, and in Canada, failed to find health problems ascribable to ac electric fields. As a result of unclear findings and of research in progress, no rules for electric-field intensity and outside the transmission corridor have been established to allow construction of EHV transmission lines to precede with the maximum possible guaranteed protection of people from possible health risks."

TABLE 2.13
Russian Rules for Duration of Work in Live Substations

Field Intensity (kV/m)	Permissible Duration (Min/Day)
>5	No restrictions
5–10	180
10–15	90
15–20	10
20–25	5

the fence line. For example, the level of electric field may be 13 kV/m in the vicinity of a 500 kV CB, but the fence line, which has to be located according to NESC at least 6.4 m (21 ft) away from the nearest 500 kV conductor, becomes almost zero.

In general, the electric field produced by a transmission line has been considered having no harmful health effects. Nevertheless, design rules have been established to allow construction of EHV transmission lines to be built with the maximum possible guaranteed protection of people from possible health risks. In Russia [9], the rules for the EHV substations and EHV transmission lines have been established long ago. For example, the limits for the duration of daily work in live substation, which is subject to various electric fields, have been limited, as indicated in Table 2.13.

For transmission lines, taking into account the frequency and nonsystematic exposure, higher values of the accepted field intensities are as follows:

10–12 kV	For road crossings
15–20 kV/m	For unpopulated regions
20 kV/m	For difficult terrains

2.21.3 BIOLOGICAL EFFECTS OF MAGNETIC FIELDS

Magnetic fields are present whenever current flows in a conductor, and they are not voltage dependent. The factors that affect the level of a magnetic field are magnitude of the current, spacing among the phases, bus height, phase configurations, distance from the source, and the amount of phase unbalance in terms of magnitude and angle. The level of such magnetic fields also decreases with distance from the source. Also, magnetic fields cannot easily be shielded. Contrary to electric fields, conducting materials have little shielding effects on magnetic fields. The magnetic flux density B, instead of the magnetic field strength ($H = B/\mu$), is used to describe the magnetic field generated by currents in the conductors of transmission lines.

According to Deno and Zaffanela [1], the magnetic induction near the ground level appears to be of less concern for power transmission lines than electric induction for the following reasons:

1. The induced current densities in the human body are less than one-tenth of those caused by electric field induction.
2. Magnetic induced current density is greatest in the human body periphery, where electric current is thought to be of least concern.
3. Magnetic fields do not cause transient currents of high peak value and current density such as those caused by electric field-induced spark discharges.

However, there have been increasing reports in recent years indicating that the exposure to magnetic fields increases the cancer occurrence. Also, several studies linked the childhood leukemia to transmission line-generated magnetic field exposure. Furthermore, magnetic fields have been reported to affect blood composition, growth, behavior, immune systems, and neural functions. At the present time, there is a worldwide research on the health effects of magnetic fields. The studies are conducted in the following three major groups: epidemiological studies, laboratory studies, and exposure assessment studies.

2.21.4 MAGNETIC FIELD CALCULATION

It is well known that an electric current in a cylindrical transmission line conductor produces magnetic field surrounding the conductor. Such magnetic field lines are represented by concentric circles. At any given point around the conductor, the strength of the magnetic field (or intensity) is defined by a field vector that is perpendicular to the radius. Figure 2.80 illustrates such current-carrying conductor, its circular magnetic field lines, and its magnetic field vector H at a given point of observation. Note that the field vector H is divided into its horizontal and vertical components. The point of observation and the conductor are indicated by (X, Y) and (x, y) coordinates, respectively. The magnetic field intensity is determined by using the ampere's law so that

$$H = \frac{I}{2\pi r} = \frac{I}{2\pi \left[\left(x_1 - X\right)^2 + \left(y_1 - Y\right)^2 \right]^{1/2}} \tag{2.77}$$

where
H is the field intensity in ampere per meter
I is the current in the conductor
r is the distance from the conductor

In a three-phase system, each current generates a magnetic field. The phase currents are apart with respect to each other by 120°. Thus,

$$\mathbf{I}_a = I_a \angle 0°, \quad \mathbf{I}_b = \angle 120°, \quad \text{and} \quad \mathbf{I}_c = \angle 240°$$

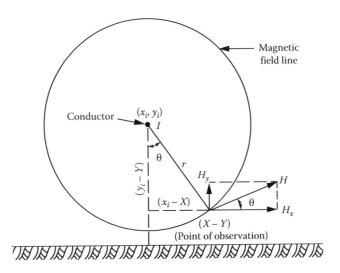

FIGURE 2.80 Magnetic field generation by a current-carrying conductor.

Similarly, their corresponding field vectors are also apart with respect to each other by 120°. The field intensity of three-phase line is determined by using the conductor currents and coordinates in the equations describing the horizontal and vertical field components in order to obtain horizontal and vertical three-field vectors. For a three-phase line, the total magnetic field can be defined in terms of horizontal and vertical components, respectively, as

$$\sum H_x = H_{x,a} + H_{x,b} + H_{x,c} \tag{2.78}$$

and

$$\sum H_x = H_{x,a} + H_{x,b} + H_{x,c} \tag{2.79}$$

Hence, the total magnetic field intensity can be described as

$$H_{3\phi \; line} = \left[\left(\sum H_x \right)^2 + \left(\sum H_x \right)^2 \right]^{1/2} \tag{2.80}$$

Hence, the magnetic field density of the three-phase line is determined from

$$B_{3\phi \; line} = \mu_0 \times H_{3\phi \; line} \tag{2.81}$$

where

$$\mu_0 = 4\pi \times 10^{-7} \tag{2.82}$$

Figure 2.81 shows the magnetic flux density distribution under the transmission line at a location that is 1 m above the ground. As it is expected, the maximum flux density is under the middle of the ROW and decreases rapidly with distance. Even though the acceptable level of magnetic field density is not given by national or international standards, utility companies in the United States try to maintain less than 100 mG (10 μT) at the edge of the ROW and less than 10 mG (1 μT) at the neighboring residential areas [25]. Note that 1 Tesla $= 1 \times 10^4$ Gauss.

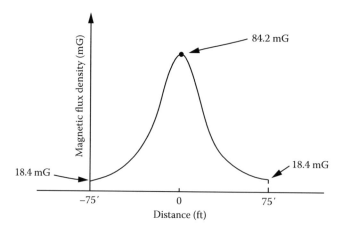

FIGURE 2.81 Magnetic field density distribution.

Example 2.4

Assume a three-phase 400 MVA, 230 kV double-circuit transmission line operating at 0.85 lagging power factor (PF) using 500 kcmil ACSR conductors. Each circuit carries 200 MVA using such conductors that has an ampacity of 690 A. Assume that the width of ROW of the line is 150 ft and that the height of the towers used is 150 ft. Other specifics of the towers used have been represented in Figure 2.82. Consider the magnetic field effects of the line and determine the following:

(a) The magnetic field intensity of the line at 1 m above the ground at the edge of its ROW.
(b) The magnetic field density of the line at 1 m above the ground at the edge of its ROW.
(c) The magnetic field intensity of the line at 1 m above the ground in the middle of its ROW.
(d) The magnetic field density of the line at 1 m above the ground in the middle of its ROW.

Solution

The current in each conductor is

$$I_R = \frac{S_{3\phi}}{\sqrt{3} \times kV_{L\text{-}L}}$$

$$= \frac{200 \times 10^6}{\sqrt{3}\left(230 \times 10^3\right)}$$

$$\cong 502 \text{ A}$$

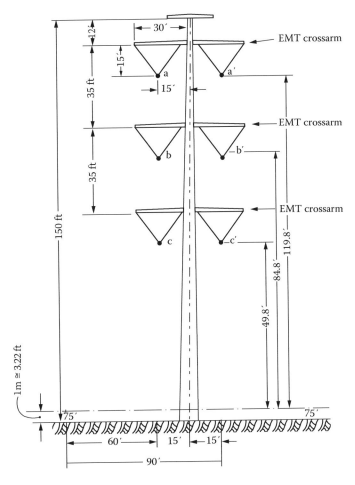

FIGURE 2.82 A typical tower used in Example 2.4.

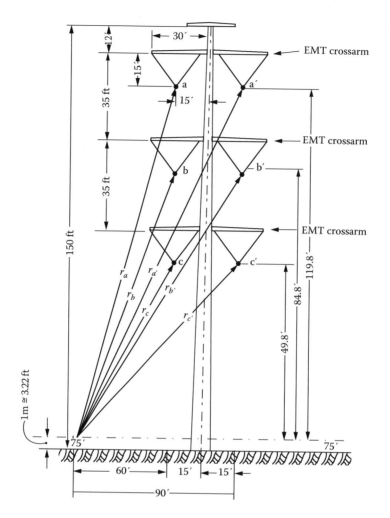

FIGURE 2.83   The radiuses in question in terms of the geometry involved with respect to the edge of the ROW.

Consider the illustration of a typical tower of the line in Figure 2.82, and determine the radiuses (the distances from the conductor of each phase) of circular magnetic field lines with respect to the edge of the ROW, as shown in Figure 2.83. After taking into account the geometry that is involved, the radiuses can be determined for each phase of the left circuit as

$$r_a^{\text{left}} = \left(60^2 + 119.8^2\right)^{1/2}$$
$$= \left(133.99 \text{ ft}\right)\left(0.3048 \text{ m/ft}\right)$$
$$= 40.84 \text{ m}$$

$$r_b^{\text{left}} = \left(60^2 + 84.8^2\right)^{1/2}$$
$$= \left(103.88 \text{ ft}\right)\left(0.3048 \text{ m/ft}\right)$$
$$= 31.66 \text{ m}$$

$$r_c^{\text{left}} = \left(60^2 + 49.8^2\right)^{1/2}$$
$$= \left(77.97 \text{ ft}\right)\left(0.3048 \text{ m/ft}\right)$$
$$= 23.77 \text{ m}$$

Similarly, radiuses for the right three-phase circuit are

$$r_a^{right} = \left(90^2 + 119.8^2\right)^{1/2}$$
$$= (149.84 \ ft)(0.3048 \ m/ft)$$
$$= 45.67 \ m$$

$$r_b^{right} = \left(90^2 + 84.8^2\right)^{1/2}$$
$$= (123.66 \ ft)(0.3048 \ m/ft)$$
$$= 37.69 \ m$$

$$r_c^{right} = \left(90^2 + 49.8^2\right)^{1/2}$$
$$= (102.86 \ ft)(0.3048 \ m/ft)$$
$$= 31.35 \ m$$

(a) The magnetic field intensity of the conductors of the *first circuit* of the line at 1 m above the ground at the edge of its ROW for each phase conductor is determined so that the following applies:

For phase a,

$$\mathbf{H}_a^{left} = \frac{\mathbf{I}_a}{2\pi r_a^{left}} = \frac{502\angle 0°}{2\pi (40.84 m)} \cong 1.956\angle 0° \ A/m$$

In terms of its horizontal and vertical components,

$$H_x^a = 1.956 \ A/m \quad and \quad H_y^a = 0$$

For phase b,

$$\mathbf{H}_b^{left} = \frac{\mathbf{I}_b}{2\pi r_b^{left}} = \frac{502\angle 0°}{2\pi (31.66 \ m)} \cong 2.528\angle -120° \ A/m$$

In terms of its horizontal and vertical components,

$$H_x^b = -1.264 \ A/m \quad and \quad H_y^b = -2.1893 \ A/m$$

For phase c,

$$\mathbf{H}_c^{left} = \frac{\mathbf{I}_c}{2\pi r_c^{left}} = \frac{502\angle -240°}{2\pi (23.77 \ m)} \cong 3.361\angle -240° \ A/m$$

In terms of its horizontal and vertical components,

$$H_x^c = -1.6905 \ A/m \quad and \quad H_y^c = 2.9107 \ A/m$$

The magnetic field intensity of the conductors of the *second circuit* of the line at 1 m above the ground at the edge of its ROW for each phase conductor is determined so that

For phase a',

$$\mathbf{H}_{a'}^{right} = \frac{\mathbf{I}_{a'}}{2\pi r_{a'}^{left}} = \frac{502\angle 0°}{2\pi (45.67 \ m)} \cong 1.7494\angle 0° \ A/m$$

In terms of its horizontal and vertical components,

$$H_x^{a'} = 1.7494 \ A/m \quad and \quad H_y^{a'} = 0$$

For phase b',

$$\mathbf{H}_{b'}^{\text{left}} = \frac{\mathbf{I}_{b'}}{2\pi r_{b'}^{\text{left}}} = \frac{502\angle 0°}{2\pi (37.69\,\text{m})} \cong 2.1198\angle -120°\,\text{A/m}$$

In terms of its horizontal and vertical components,

$$H_x^b = -1.0599\,\text{A/m} \quad \text{and} \quad H_y^b = -1.8358\,\text{A/m}$$

For phase c,

$$\mathbf{H}_{c'}^{\text{left}} = \frac{\mathbf{I}_{c'}}{2\pi r_{c'}^{\text{left}}} = \frac{502\angle -240°}{2\pi (31.35\,\text{m})} \cong 2.5485\angle -240°\,\text{A/m}$$

In terms of its horizontal and vertical components,

$$H_x^c = -1.27425\,\text{A/m} \quad \text{and} \quad H_y^c = 2.20707\,\text{A/m}$$

At a given point on the ground, 1 m above the ground, at the edge of ROW, the resulting magnetic field intensity is the sum of all six conductor's magnetic intensities at that point. Thus, their sums on the X and Y coordinates are

$$H_x = \sum_{n=1}^{6} H_x = H_x^a + H_x^b + H_x^c + H_x^{a'} + H_x^{b'} + H_x^{c'}$$

$$= 1.956 + 1.264 - 1.6805 + 1.7494 - 1.0599 + 1.2743$$

$$= 0.9753\,\text{A/m}$$

and

$$H_y = \sum_{n=1}^{6} H_y = H_y^a + H_y^b + H_y^c + H_y^{a'} + H_y^{b'} + H_y^{c'}$$

$$= 0 - 2.1893 + 2.9107 + 0 - 1.8358 + 2.20707$$

$$= 1.09267\,\text{A/m}$$

Hence, magnetic field intensity for the double-circuit line is

$$H_{\substack{\text{double} \\ \text{circuit}}} = \left(H_x^2 + H_y^2\right)^{1/2}$$

$$= \left(0.9753^2 + 1.09267^2\right)^{1/2}$$

$$\cong 1.46463\,\text{A/m}$$

(b) Thus, the flux density on the ground at the edge of ROW is

$$B_{\substack{\text{double} \\ \text{circuit}}} = \mu_0 \times H_{\substack{\text{double} \\ \text{circuit}}}\,\text{T}$$

$$= \left(4\pi \times 10^{-7}\right)(1.46493\,\text{A/m})$$

$$\cong 1.8409\,\mu\text{T}$$

$$\cong 18.41\,\text{mG} < 100\,\text{mG}$$

which is less than 100 mG. Note that $1\,\text{T} = 1\times 10^4$ G. Also note that per industry standards, the point on the ground is considered to be 1 m high from the ground, at the point of consideration. The calculations are done accordingly.

(c) Before determining the magnetic field intensity of the line, at 1 m above the ground, in the middle of its ROW, as illustrated in Figure 2.84, the associated radiuses need to be found as

$$r_a^{\text{left}} = r_{a'}^{\text{right}} = \left(15^2 + 119.8^2\right)^{1/2}$$

$$\cong \left(120.73 \text{ ft}\right)\left(0.3048 \text{ m/ft}\right)$$

$$\cong 36.8 \text{ m}$$

$$r_b^{\text{left}} = r_{b'}^{\text{right}} = \left(15^2 + 84.8^2\right)^{1/2}$$

$$\cong \left(86.12 \text{ ft}\right)\left(0.3048 \text{ m/ft}\right)$$

$$\cong 26.25 \text{ m}$$

$$r_c^{\text{left}} = r_{c'}^{\text{right}} = \left(15^2 + 49.8^2\right)^{1/2}$$

$$\cong \left(52 \text{ ft}\right)\left(0.3048 \text{ m/ft}\right)$$

$$\cong 15.85 \text{ m}$$

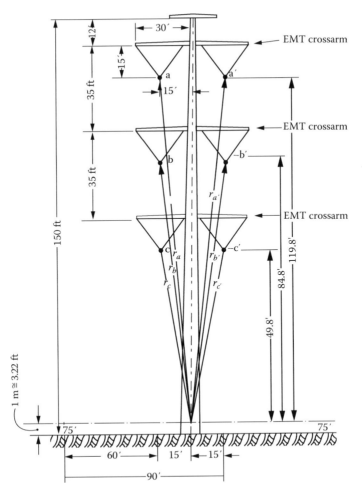

FIGURE 2.84 The radiuses in question in terms of the geometry involved with respect to the center of the ROW.

so that the magnetic field intensity of the conductors of the *first circuit* of the line at 1 m above the ground at the edge of its ROW for each phase conductor is determined as follows:

For phase *a*,

$$\mathbf{H}_a^{\text{left}} = \frac{\mathbf{I}_a}{2\pi r_a^{\text{left}}} = \frac{1004\angle 0°}{2\pi(36.8\,\text{m})} \cong 4.342\angle 0°\,\text{A/m}$$

In terms of its horizontal and vertical components,

$$H_x^a = 2342.956\,\text{A/m} \quad \text{and} \quad H_y^a = 0$$

For phase *b*,

$$\mathbf{H}_b^{\text{left}} = \frac{\mathbf{I}_b}{2\pi r_b^{\text{left}}} = \frac{1004\angle 0°}{2\pi(26.25\,\text{m})} \cong 6.0873\angle -120°\,\text{A/m}$$

In terms of its horizontal and vertical components,

$$H_x^b = -3.04364\,\text{A/m} \quad \text{and} \quad H_y^b = -5.27176\,\text{A/m}$$

For phase *c*,

$$\mathbf{H}_c^{\text{left}} = \frac{\mathbf{I}_c}{2\pi r_c^{\text{left}}} = \frac{1004\angle -240°}{2\pi 15(23.85\,\text{m})} \cong 10.0814\angle -240°\,\text{A/m}$$

In terms of its horizontal and vertical components,

$$H_x^c = -5.04\,\text{A/m} \quad \text{and} \quad H_y^c = 8.7308\,\text{A/m}$$

The magnetic field intensity of the conductors of the *second circuit* of the line at 1 m above the ground in the middle of its ROW for each phase conductor is the same so that

For phase *a'*,

$$\mathbf{H}_{a'}^{\text{right}} = \frac{\mathbf{I}_{a'}}{2\pi r_{a'}^{\text{right}}} = \frac{1004\angle 0°}{2\pi(36.8\,\text{m})} \cong 4.342\angle 0°\,\text{A/m}$$

In terms of its horizontal and vertical components,

$$H_x^{a'} = 2.342\,\text{A/m} \quad \text{and} \quad H_y^{a'} = 0$$

For phase *b'*,

$$\mathbf{H}_{b'}^{\text{right}} = \frac{\mathbf{I}_{b'}}{2\pi r_{b'}^{\text{right}}} = \frac{1004\angle 0°}{2\pi(26.25\,\text{m})} \cong 6.0873\angle -120°\,\text{A/m}$$

In terms of its horizontal and vertical components,

$$H_x^b = -3.04364 \text{ A/m} \quad \text{and} \quad H_y^b = -5.27176 \text{ A/m}$$

For phase c,

$$\mathbf{H}_{c'}^{\text{right}} = \frac{\mathbf{I}_{c'}}{2\pi r_{c'}^{\text{right}}} = \frac{100\angle -240°}{2\pi (15.85 \text{ m})} \cong 10.0814 \angle -240° \text{ A/m}$$

In terms of its horizontal and vertical components,

$$H_x^c = 5.04 \text{ A/m} \quad \text{and} \quad H_y^c = 8.7308 \text{ A/m}$$

At a given point on the ground, 1 m above the ground, in the middle of the ROW, the resulting magnetic field intensity is the sum of all six conductor's magnetic intensities at that point. Thus, their sums on the X and Y coordinates are

$$H_x = \sum_{n=1}^{6} H_x = H_x^a + H_x^b + H_x^c + H_x^{a'} + H_x^{b'} + H_x^{c'}$$

$$= 1171 - 1.52182 - 2.520 + 1.171 - 1.52182 - 2.520$$

$$= -5.74164 \text{ A/m}$$

and

$$H_y = \sum_{n=1}^{6} H_y = H_y^a + H_y^b + H_y^c + H_y^{a'} + H_y^{b'} + H_y^{c'}$$

$$= 0 - 2.63588 + 4.3654 + 0 - 2.63588 + 4.3654$$

$$= 3.45904 \text{ A/m}$$

Hence, magnetic field intensity for the double-circuit line is

$$H_{\substack{\text{double} \\ \text{circuit}}} = \left(H_x^2 + H_y^2 \right)^{1/2}$$

$$= \left(-5.74164^2 + 3.45904^2 \right)^{1/2}$$

$$\cong 6.703 \text{ A/m}$$

(d) Thus, the flux density on the ground is

$$B_{\substack{\text{double} \\ \text{circuit}}} = \mu_0 \times H_{\substack{\text{double} \\ \text{circuit}}} \text{ T}$$

$$= \left(4\pi \times 10^{-7} \right) \left(6.703 \text{ A/m} \right)$$

$$\cong 8.8232 \text{ μT}$$

$$\cong 84.232 \text{ mG}$$

The associated magnetic flux density distribution is indicated in Figure 2.80.

2.22 HIGH-VOLTAGE BUSHINGS WITH DRAW LEADS AND THEIR FAILURES

Typically, power transformers of about 50 MVA are usually built with draw-lead bushings if the current rating is less than about 800 A. Using such bushing permits, without lowering the oil levels involved, makes the replacement of the bushings much easier, as a result saving time and money. However, numerous failures of 230 kV bushings have occurred at various utility companies since 2001. The bushings involved were manufactured by various manufacturers. All these failures involve damage to the draw leads. All the resultant arching is located between the draw-lead cable and the central tube at one or more locations along the length of the bushings. All failed bushings do so violently with explosion and usually with subsequent fire. Due to the explosion, several parts of the bushing fly over several hundred feet, covering large areas.

Typically, one can make some common observations that include the following: It happens mostly to bushings of 230 kV rated 750 and 900 kV BIL. They all have draw-lead bushings and arching occurred from lead to tube at one or more random locations above and below flange. Condenser bushings were destroyed in all failures. Failures took place early morning, mostly between midnight and 6:00 AM. In all locations, SF6 breakers and/or SF6 circuit switches were employed. There was a 50 ft separation between transformer and breaker. The power ratings were ranged from 15 to 132 MVA, but mostly about 50 MVA. Failures took place within 4–13 years of installation but main tank gassing was reported within 2 years of installation. In all, power distribution systems were rarely switched; most of them were lightly loaded. An IEEE committee has reported that the arching within bushing tube is most likely initiated by a high-frequency transient (HFT) or fast front transients and then sustained by the power frequency voltage.

The committee chaired by Hopkinson et al. [27] believes that the failure progression evolves over a period of months or years in the fallowing fashion:

1. At first, a frequency transient enters the top of the bushing, causing traveling waves to flow down the cable lead and the tube at slightly different speeds.
2. The wave in the lead is somewhat faster due to the larger impedance of transformer winding, causing a reflected wave of the same polarity as the original. This, in turn, results in a magnitude that is between 1.0 and 2.0 pu of the original wave.
3. Further, the wave in the aluminum tube is reflected when it comes across the open end of the tube, causing a reflected wave of the same magnitude and polarity as the original wave. The magnitude of the resulting wave is twice that of the original wave.
4. Here, the distance that the lead wave has to travel is longer than the tube wave due to the additional distance between the bottom of the bushing and the bottom of the winding. As a result, the tube wave starts its return before the lead wave returns to the bottom of the bushing.
5. When the voltage difference exceeds the withstand capability of the insulation and oil film surrounding the lead, an arcing is initiated between the cable lead and tube. Such flashovers result in numerous discharge marks between the lead and tube interior.
6. Gases from the degradation of oil film are produced by the arcing, and arcing is eventually sustained by the power frequency current. In time, erosion takes place between the lead and tube, additional gassing occurs.
7. The rising gas level in the tube may push the oil level down until it is below the region of arcing. This in turn reduces the heat of the system.
8. When discharge deposits enough carbon and/or ionized gases in the region to effectively place the lead in contact with the tube, then the power frequency current is able to flow, with as much as 50% of the load current flowing through the tube.

9. The tube heats up to the degree that it begins to degrade the adjacent paper insulation in the bushing condenser outside the tube.

10. The entire condenser eventually fails radially, pressure builds up within the bushing due to gases produced by degradation of oil and insulation, and the bushing explodes, often resulting in fire.

11. In some cases, a small hole is burned in the aluminum tube. This may happen due to either the heat produced by the arcing or the resultant flashover in the condenser [2009] [27].

REFERENCES

1. Deno and Zaffanda. Electric Power Research Institute. *Transmission Line Reference Book: 345 kV and Above*, 2nd edn., EPRI, Palo Alto, CA, 1982.

2. Electric Power Research Institute. *Transmission Line Reference Book: 115–138 kV Compact Line Design*, 2nd edn., EPRI, Palo Alto, CA, 1978.

3. Rural Electrification Administration. *Transmission Line Manual*, REA Bull. No. 62-1, U.S. Dept. of Agriculture, U.S. Govt. Printing Office, Washington, DC, 1972.

4. Pholman, J. C. Transmission line structures, in *Electric Power Generation, Transmission, and Distribution*, L. L. Grigsby, ed., CRC Press, Boca Raton, FL, 2007.

5. Ostendorp, M. Longitudinal loading and cascading failure assessment for transmission line upgrades, *ESMO Conference*, Orlando, FL, April 26–30, 1998.

6. CIGRE. Improved design criteria of overhead transmission lines based on reliability concepts, CIGRE SC-22 Report, October 1995.

7. Basilesco, J. Substation design, in *Standard Handbook for Electrical Engineers*, D. G. Fink and H. W. Beaty, eds., 11th edn., McGraw-Hill, New York, 1978.

8. Burke, J. and Shazizian, M. How a substation happens?, in *Electric Power Substation Engineering*, J. D. McDonald, ed., CRC Press, Boca Raton, FL, 2007.

9. Lyskov, Y. I., Emma, Y. S., and Stolarov, M. D. Electrical field as a parameter considered in designing electric power transmission of 750–1150 kV, in *USS-USSR Symposium on Ultra-high Voltage Transmission*, Washington, DC, 1976.

10. Edison Electric Institute. *EHV Transmission Line Reference Book*, EEI, New York, 1968.

11. Peek, F. W. Jr. Electric characteristics of the suspension insulator, Part I, *Trans. Am. Inst. Electr. Eng.* 319, 1912, 907–930.

12. Peek, F. W. Jr. Electric characteristics of the suspension insulator, Part II, *Trans. Am. Inst. Electr. Eng.* 39, 1920, 1685–1705.

13. Gönen, T. *Modern Power System Analysis*, Wiley, New York, 1988.

14. IEEE Standard 2000. *IEEE Guide for Safety in AC Substation Grounding*, IEEE Std. 80-2000.

15. Sciaca, S. C. and Block, W. R. Advanced SCADA concepts, *IEEE Comput. Appl. Power* 8 (1), January 1995, 23–28.

16. Sunde, E. D. *Earth Conduction Effect in Transmission System*, Macmillan, New York, 1968.

17. Keil, R. P. Substation grounding, in *Electric Power Substation Engineering*, Chapter 11, CRC Press, Boca Raton, FL, 2003.

18. Gönen, T. and Haj-mohamadi, M. S. Electromagnetic unbalance of untransposed and transposed transmission lines with "N" overhead ground wires, *Int. J. Comput. Math. Electr. Electron. Eng. (COMPEL)* 7 (3), 1988, 107–122.

19. IEEE Standard. *IEEE Guide for Measuring Earth Resistivity, Ground Impedance, and Earth Surface Potentials of a Ground System*, IEEE Std. 81-1983.

20. Sunde, E. D. *Earth Conduction Effect in Transmission System*, Macmillan, New York, 1968.

21. Sverak, J. G. Simplified analysis of electrical gradients above a ground grid. Part 1: How good is the present IEEE method? *IEEE Trans. Power Apparatus Syst.* 103, 1984, 7–25.

22. Lewis, W. W. *The Protection of Transmission Systems against Lightning*, Dover, New York, 1965.

23. Farr, H. H. *Transmission Line Design Manual*, U.S. Dept. of Interior, Water and Power Resources Service, Denver, CO, 1980.

24. Karady, G. G. Environmental impact of transmission lines, in *Electric Power Generator, Transmission and Generation*, Chapter 19, 2nd edn., CRC Press, Boca Raton, FL, 2007.

25. Bricker, S., Rubin, L., and Gönen, T. Substation automation techniques and advantages, *IEEE Comput. Appl. Power* 14 (3), July 2001, 31–37.
26. Electric Power Research Institute. *Transmission Line Reference Book: 345 kV and Above*, Revised Second Edition, Palo Alto, CA, 1982, pp. 379–380.
27. Hopkinson, P. et al. Progress report on failures of high voltage bushings with draw leads, presented at *2009 IEEE/PES Power Systems Conference and Exposition*, Seattle, WA, April 2009.

3 Flexible AC Transmission System (FACTS) and Other Concepts

A diplomat is a person who tells you to go to hell in such a way that you actually look forward to the trip.

Anonymous

3.1 INTRODUCTION

As previously said, the main function of a transmission system is to transmit electric energy in bulk from generating plants that are located at various distances from the load centers. Such transmission systems carry economically dispatched power not only during normal conditions but also during emergency conditions. In addition to sharing the lowest-cost generated power, the transmission system facilitates large reductions in the required reserve capacities among the utilities.

3.2 FACTORS AFFECTING TRANSMISSION GROWTH

The factors affecting transmission growth especially at EHV–UHV voltage levels are

1. Load growth
2. Generation siting
3. Fuel cost and availability
4. Reliability
5. Ecology
6. Government
7. Energy centers

The main influence on transmission growth in the past has been the increase in electrical load. Increasingly, the growth in loads is being met by building transmission lines that operate at EHV and/or UHV levels in order to make the transmission process economical. In urban areas, new generating sites are almost impossible to have due to environmental concerns and unavailability of suitable land. Hence, the electric power is increasingly being transmitted from remote areas, some of them being several hundred miles from load centers.

The rising cost of fuel and increasing dependency on foreign oil have already influenced the use of transmission systems to supply electric energy from remote coal, hydro, and nuclear plants. Even without considering load growth, new transmission systems can be justified to improve reliability during emergency conditions and to supply less expensive base loading from remote generating sites.

The growth in transmission beyond that demanded by load growth requires greater reliability as the margin between peak load and generating capability decreases especially in interties between adjacent companies and regions. It is often more economical to add the needed reliability by strengthening interties at EHV and UHV levels. Also, increased interregional power transfer without added transmission reduces stability margins and leaves subtransmission lines vulnerable to overload. But if the required reliability is to be maintained, new transmission with stronger interties is required.

The environmental impacts of transmission lines are mainly visual impact, land usage, biological interaction, and communications interference. Minimization of the biological and visual impact dictates a thorough study of the compatibility of alternative transmission routes with the various tower types, vegetation, and terrain types. Occasionally, a considerable number of proposed lines are delayed or rerouted due to legal intervention by the public.

The electrical load growth for some good number of years in the future will be strongly influenced by government regulations, the cost of funds, and the establishment of a sustainable national energy policy, and perhaps government-financed projects are needed. The reduced availability of unacceptable generating sites near load centers will increasingly be forcing the development of energy centers with ever-increasing power-generating capacities.

3.3   STABILITY CONSIDERATIONS

Power system stability can be defined as that ability of the system that enables the synchronous machines of the system to respond to a disturbance from a normal operating condition so as to return to a condition where their operation is again normal. In other words, the state of operating equilibrium, after being subject to a physical disturbance such as a transmission fault, sudden load changes, loss of generating units, or line switching, is kept intact, and hence, the system integrity is preserved. Integrity of the system is preserved when practically the entire power system remains intact with no tripping of generators and loads, with the exception of those disconnected by isolation of the faulted elements or intentionally tripped elements to preserve the continuity of operation of the rest of the system.

In a broad definition, stability is a condition of equilibrium between opposing forces. By the same token, instability can be defined as a disturbance that leads to a sustained imbalance between the opposing forces. In the event that the system is unstable, it will result in a runaway situation. As a result, there will be a progressive increase in angular separation of generator rotors or a progressive decrease in bus voltages.

However, the loss of synchronism is not the only cause of an unstable operation. For example, an alternator that supplies power to an induction motor may become unstable due to collapse of load voltage. Here, the problem is the stability and control of voltage instead of the issue of synchronism.

In general, stability problems, for the sake of convenience of analysis, are divided into two major problems by the IEEE [5]. These are steady-state instability and transient instability:

1. *Steady-state instability* occurs when the power system is forced into a condition for which there is an equilibrium condition. For example, the power output of an alternator may be slowly increased until maximum power is transferred. At this point, either an increase or a decrease in alternator angle will result in a reduction in power transferred. Any further increase in alternator output will cause a steady-state instability and a loss of synchronism between that alternator and the rest of the system. *Dynamic instability*, another form of steady-state instability, is characterized by hunting or steadily growing oscillations, ultimately leading to a loss of synchronism.

2. *Transient instability* applies to a system's inability to survive a major disturbance. Hence, it causes an abrupt and large transient change in the electric power supplied by the synchronous machines. For example, the occurrence of a fault or the sudden outage of a transmission line carrying heavy load from an alternator will cause a severe momentary unbalance between the input power and the electrical load on one or more generators. If the input/output power unbalance is large enough or lasts long enough, the result will be a transient instability [5].

In some sense, a transmission system is designed so that all generators remain in synchronism under steady-state and transient operating conditions. The power that is sent over a transmission line is inversely proportional to the inductive reactance of the system. In that sense, reactance sets a limit on the maximum power that can be transmitted by a line for a given transmission voltage. For example, consider a system in which a transmission line connects a generator to a remote system. The amount of power transferred over the line is expected as

$$P = \left(\frac{E_{gen} \times E_{sys}}{X_L} \right) \sin \delta \qquad (3.1)$$

where
  P is the power transferred
  E_{gen} is the generator (or source) voltage
  E_{sys} is the system voltage
  X_L is the total inductive reactance between E_{gen} and E_{sys}, including the reactance of the transmission line and terminal connections
  δ is the angle between the source voltage E_{gen} and the remote system voltage E_{sys}

In most systems, $\mathbf{Z}_L (= R + jX_L)$ is predominantly inductive reactance and R can be neglected with little error. For a given system operating at a constant voltage, the power transmitted is proportional to the sine of the power angle δ. The maximum power that can be transferred under stable steady-state conditions takes place at an angular displacement of 90° and is

$$P_{max} = \frac{E_{gen} \times E_{sys}}{X_L} \qquad (3.2)$$

A transmission system with its connected synchronous machines must also be able to withstand, without loss of stability, sudden changes in generation, loads, and faults. All of these disturbances cause transients on the system voltage and power angle. In the United States, reliability coordinating council of each region dictates the stability requirements that have to be met under such transient conditions, forcing the power angle to be limited to an angle that is much less than 90° for the maximum power transfer. Typically, it is usually somewhere between 30° and 45°. The speed of the circuit breakers and the operation time of the backup relay, in the event of primary circuit-breaker failure, are crucial to transient stability.

Consider that a three-phase line fault has taken place so that there is no power that is being sent from the alternator to the system during the fault interval. This causes the whole turbine output to accelerate the generator rotor during this time period.

If the fault is cleared, the system tries to return to normal state. But the speed of the rotor is now above the synchronous speed. This, in turn, causes the electric output power to be greater than the mechanical input power. This difference will now decelerate the rotor, but not before the power angle has increased still further. However, the power angle starts to decrease after the rotor speed reaches the synchronous speed. The electric output power of the alternator will continue to oscillate around the mechanical input power until damping stabilizes the system.

If the fault exists in the long run, the swing may be greater than the point where the power angle will continue to increase even with the electric power output less than the mechanical input power. If this happens, the system will become unstable and the alternator has to be shut down.

Thus, the more rapidly the fault is removed by the circuit-breaker operation, the more stable the system becomes. In a sense, circuit breakers with independent pole operation improve transient stability by guaranteeing that a three-phase fault is reduced to a single-phase fault when there is a stuck pole because of a circuit-breaker tripping failure.

In general, the ability of the power to adjust to its previous steady state or to a new stable operating condition, without loss of synchronism, is a function of the inertias of the connected machines, the response of their exciters and turbine governors, and the system voltage and reactance. It is also important to point out that the transient stability criterion usually dictates that the transmission line loading and therefore the power angle be restricted to a value that is considerably below the steady-state limit [3].

It is well known that the power system stability can be improved by reducing the inductive reactance between the generators and the rest of the system. The use of additional lines, conductor bundling, and SCs can produce such a result.

3.4 POWER TRANSMISSION CAPABILITY OF A TRANSMISSION LINE

It can be observed that the higher-voltage transmission lines with higher loading capabilities continue to experience a higher growth rate. Higher voltages mean higher power transfer capability, as illustrated by the SIL capabilities of typical EHV transmission lines in Table 3.1.

3.5 SURGE IMPEDANCE AND SURGE IMPEDANCE LOADING OF A TRANSMISSION LINE

For a single-phase lossless line, the *surge impedance* (also called *characteristic impedance*) is expressed as

$$Z_S = \sqrt{\frac{X_L}{Y_C}}, \; \Omega \tag{3.3}$$

where X_L and Y_C are the series impedance and the shunt admittance per unit length of line, respectively. Where line losses are ignored, Z_S is dimensionally a pure resistance. For a three-phase lossless line, the SIL is expressed as

$$SIL = \frac{\left| kV_{R(L\text{-}L)} \right|^2}{Z_S} \; MW \tag{3.4}$$

TABLE 3.1
SIL Capability

Nominal System Voltage (kV)	Maximum System Voltage (kV)	Line (or Tower Top) Type	Phase Conductor Diameter (in.)	Conductor per Phase	Phase Spacing (ft)	Surge Impedance (Ω)	SIL Capability (MVA)
345	362	Horizontal	1.76	1	24.6	366	325
345	362	Horizontal	1.11	2	24.6	285	418
345	362	Delta	1.11	2	29.5	283	421
500	550	Horizontal	1.76	2	32.8	287	871
500	550	Vertical	1.17	4	29.5	235	1,064
500	550	Delta	1.60	3	32.8	247	1,012
765	800	Horizontal	1.38	4	45.9	258	2,268
765	800	Delta	1.38	4	55.1	257	2,277
1100	1200	Horizontal	1.60	8	60.7	232	5,216
1100	1200	Delta	1.60	8	72.2	231	5,238
1500	—	Horizontal	1.60	12	73.8	225	10,000

A loaded transmission line or its SIL has no net reactive power flow into or out of the line and will have approximately a flat voltage profile along its length. SILs are given in Table 3.1 for a variety of typical and proposed EHV and UHV transmission lines.

Example 3.1

A 345 kV three-phase transmission line with a horizontal tower top configuration has a 24.6 ft phase spacing between the adjacent conductors. Each phase conductor has a diameter of 1.76 in. Its surge impedance is 366 Ω. Determine the SIL of the line.

Solution

The SIL of the line is

$$\text{SIL} = \frac{\left|kV_{R(L-L)}\right|^2}{Z_S}$$

$$= \frac{345^2}{366} \cong 325 \text{ MW}$$

3.6 LOADABILITY CURVES

The line loadability is defined simply as that degree of line loading, in terms of percent of surge impedance load, as a function of surge impedance load, and as a function of line length that is allowable considering thermal limits, voltage drop, or stability limits. Also, the voltage drop and the stability limits have to be considered for both steady-state and transient conditions. Dunlop et al. [4] developed a set of curves that represent loadability characteristics and practical limits on line loading of EHV and UHV transmission lines.

Consider the system model shown in Figure 3.1 for developing the transmission line loadability curves. Assume that the terminal short-circuit capacities at each end of the line is 50 kA. Use the heavy loading criteria of having a maximum voltage drop of 5% along the transmission line and an

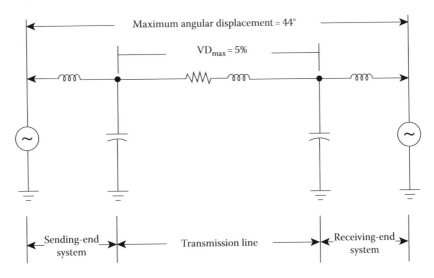

FIGURE 3.1 Illustration of the power system model used for the transmission line loadability curves.

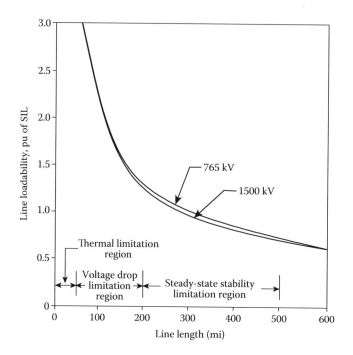

FIGURE 3.2   Transmission line loadability curves for EHV and UHV lines.

angular displacement of 44° across the system as shown in Figure 3.1. Here, the 44° corresponds to the steady-state stability margin of 30%. The percent stability margin is expressed as

$$\% \text{ Stability margin} = \frac{P_{\max} - P_{\text{rated}}}{P_{\max}} \times 100 \tag{3.5}$$

where

$P_{\max}$ is the maximum power transfer capability of the system
P_{rated} is the operating level

Note that the governing criteria of the loading of the transmission line are thermal limitations for its first 50 mi segment voltage drop limitations for its 50–200 mi segment and stability limitations for the segment that is beyond 200 mi. No series shunt compensation is considered in developing the curves that are shown in Figure 3.2. It shows the EHV and UHV transmission line loadability (in terms of per unit of SIL) curves as a function of the line length.

It is important for a good line design to study the cost sensitivity, in terms of both relative and absolute, with regard to line loading. In general, economic loadings are determined for a given transmission line using a conductor economics program. Figure 3.3 shows the cost of power in $/kW/year/mi versus the load in MW for the voltage levels of 230, 345, and 765 kV. It is clear that there is a considerable economic benefit for increasing line voltage. Also, it can be observed that as system voltage is increased, the U curves get to be flatter.

3.7   COMPENSATION

Figure 3.4 shows a power system that has lines with both series compensation and shunt compensation. Here, shunt compensation will be considered first. The general purpose of shunt compensation is to keep the voltage rises down during light- or no-load conditions. In general, shunt compensation can be implemented by the use of shunt reactors, shunt capacitors, static var control (SVC),

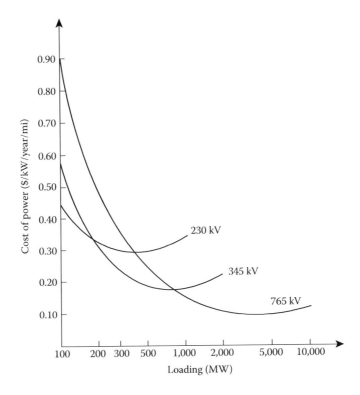

FIGURE 3.3   Cost of power versus loading of the line.

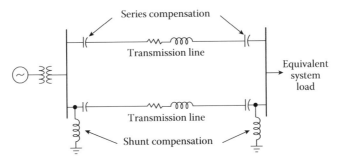

FIGURE 3.4   A transmission system with both series and shunt compensation.

and synchronous condensers. The most widely used shunt compensation is shunt capacitors. But with the arrival of higher-voltage lines, the need for and usage of shunt reactors have increased considerably. For example, today, shunt reactors are fundamental shunt compensation used on EHV lines. These reactors are implemented to compensate for the unwanted voltage effects due to the line capacitance.

The amount of shunt compensation provided by a reactor is based on a percentage of the positive-sequence susceptance of the transmission line. For EHV lines, this percentage is usually between 0% and 90%. It depends on various factors, including the line characteristics, the expected loading, and the system operating policy. A given transmission line's reactive power increases directly as the square of its voltage and is proportional to its line capacitance and length.

The line capacitance has two related voltage effects. The first one is known as the *Ferranti effect*. It is the rise in voltage along the line due to the capacitive current of the line flowing through the line inductance. The second one is the rise in voltage due to the capacitive current of the line flowing through the source impedance at the line terminations. Under no-load or particularly light-load conditions, these two effects may produce undesirably HVs. The application of shunt reactors can reduce these voltages.

3.8 SHUNT COMPENSATION

3.8.1 Effects of Shunt Compensation on Transmission Line Loadability

Consider the power system model shown in Figure 3.1 for the transmission line loadability. Still assume that the terminal short-circuit capacities at each end of the line are 50 kA. Use the *heavy loading criteria* of having a maximum voltage drop of 5% along the transmission line and angular displacement of 44° that corresponds to the steady-state stability margin of 30%.

Assume that a 765 kV three-phase transmission line has an SIL of 2250 MW and is made up of 4–1351 kcmil ACSR conductors. The shunt compensations of 0% and 100% are considered for two separate cases. For the first case, its short-circuit capacity (S/C) and its reactance are given as 50 kA and 0.151%, respectively. For the second case, the S/C and its reactance are given as 12.5 kA and 0.604%, respectively.

Figure 3.5 shows the effects of shunt reactance compensation on the line loadability. As it can be observed in the figure, for transmission lines with low source impedance, the effects of shunt compensation on the loadability are small. However, sources with high impedance can reduce the loadability of a given transmission line and increase the sensitivity of loadability to the changes in shunt compensation, as it can be observed in Figure 3.5.

On the other hand, when reactive power is supplied by using shunt compensation apparatus such as shunt capacitors, synchronous condensers, and SVC, the transmission line loadability can be increased.

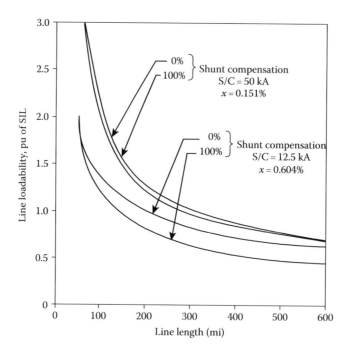

FIGURE 3.5 The effects of having only shunt reactor compensation on the line loadability.

3.8.2 SHUNT REACTORS AND SHUNT CAPACITOR BANKS

Shunt reactors may be either line connected or bus connected. It is often that they are connected on the tertiary windings of large-network transformers due to overvoltage concerns. Shunt capacitor banks are always bus, rather than line, connected. The main purpose of transmission system shunt compensation on the transmission system near load areas is load stabilization or voltage control. Mechanically switched shunt capacitor (MSC) banks are installed at major substations in load areas. The MSCs have several disadvantages. For example, the switching may not be fast enough for some applications. But compared to static var compensation, MSC banks have the advantage of much lower cost. However, capacitor bank energization allowing a transmission line outage should be adequately delayed to allow time for line reclosing. Current limiting reactors minimize switching transients. For voltage stability, shunt capacitor banks are very beneficial in allowing nearby generators to operate near-unity power factor.

3.9 SERIES COMPENSATION

Series compensation is the application of SCs to a transmission line. SCs improve the stability by canceling part of the inductive reactance. For example, a 50% compensation means canceling one-half of the transmission line reactance. This results in improved transient and steady-state stability, more economical loading, improved loading balance between parallel transmission lines, and minimum voltage dip on load buses. Studies [1] have shown that the addition of SCs on EHV transmission lines can more than double the *transient stability load limit* of having lines at a fraction of the cost of a transmission line.

However, despite all these aforementioned benefits, there has been a reluctance to use SCs in such applications. This is primarily due to the lack of a reliable high-speed protective device to limit the voltage across the capacitor bank during disturbances and to bypass the high currents during faults. The customary solution for this problem is to provide an automatic bypass during faults and then to reinsert the capacitors after the clearing of the fault.

3.9.1 EFFECTS OF SERIES COMPENSATION ON TRANSMISSION LINE LOADABILITY

The series compensation has a profound effect on the loadability of a transmission line. Also, the series compensation has a great impact on the criteria of voltage drop and stability. They, in turn, reduce the electrical length of the line.

Consider the same power system model that is shown in Figure 3.1. Assume that a 1100 kV three-phase transmission line has an SIL of 5185 MW and is made up of 8–1781 kcmil ACSR conductors. The series compensations of 0% and 75% are considered for two separate cases. Figure 3.6 shows the effects of series reactance compensation on the line loadability for both cases. For the first case of terminal system (given in solid lines in the figure), the S/C and its reactance are given as 50 kA and 0.105%, respectively. For the second case (given in dashed lines in the figure), the S/C and its reactance are given as 12.5 kA and 0.420%, respectively. The criteria for both cases are given as 5% for line voltage drop and 30% for steady-state stability margin.

The considerations of having series or shunt compensations are determined by the system impedance that is expressed in terms of terminal system S/C. Consider a 765 kcmil three-phase transmission system that has 4–1351 kcmil ACSR conductors per phase, having an SIL of 2250 MW. The angular stability limit of 44° and the voltage drop criterion of 5% are given for the transmission line. Figure 3.7 shows the effects of system impedance on the line loadability, without having any series or shunt compensation, for a range of S/C from 12.5 to 75 kA.

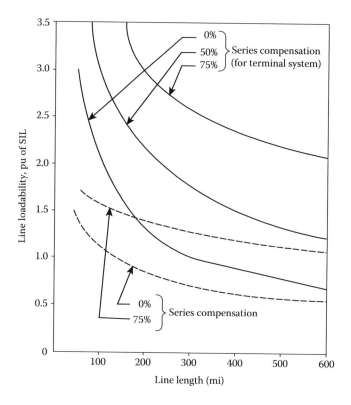

FIGURE 3.6 Effects of having only series compensation on the line loadability.

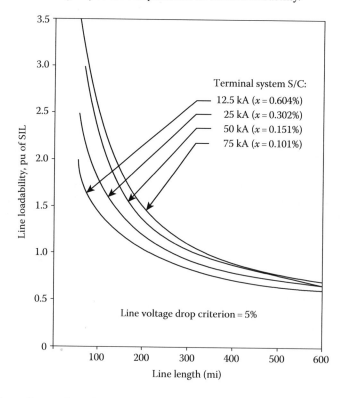

FIGURE 3.7 Effects of system impedance on line loadability without having any series or shunt compensation.

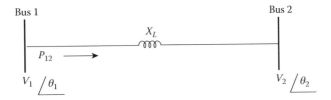

FIGURE 3.8   Power flow through a transmission line.

3.9.2 SERIES CAPACITORS

Consider the power flow through a transmission line, as shown in Figure 3.8. The amount of power that is transmitted from bus 1 (sending-end bus) to bus 2 (receiving-end bus) can be expressed as

$$P_{12} = \frac{V_1 \times V_2}{X_L} \sin \delta \tag{3.6}$$

where
   P_{12} is the power transmitted through the transmission system
   V_1 is the voltage at the sending end of the line
   V_2 is the voltage at the receiving end of the line
   X_L is the reactance of the transmission line
   δ is the phase angle between phasors $\mathbf{V}_1$ and $\mathbf{V}_2$, that is, $\delta = \theta_1 - \theta_2$

If the total reactance of a transmission system is reduced by installation of capacitors in series with the line, the power transmitted through the line can be increased. In that case, the amount of power that is transmitted can be expressed as

$$P_{12} = \frac{V_1 \times V_2}{X_L - X_C} \sin \delta \tag{3.7}$$

or

$$P_{12} = \frac{V_1 \times V_2}{X_L \left(1 - K\right)} \sin \delta \tag{3.8}$$

where $K = \left(X_C / X_L \right)$ is the *degree of compensation.*

The degree of compensation K is usually expressed in percent. For example, 60% compensation means that the value of the SC in ohms is equal to 60% of the line reactance.

As said earlier, SCs are used to compensate for the inductive reactance of the transmission line. They may be installed remote from the load, for example, at an intermediate point on a long transmission line. The benefits of SC compensation are

1. Improved line loadability
2. Improved system steady-state stability
3. Improved system transient-state stability
4. Better load division on parallel circuits
5. Reduced voltage drops in load areas during severe disturbance
6. Reduced transmission losses
7. Better adjustment of line loadings

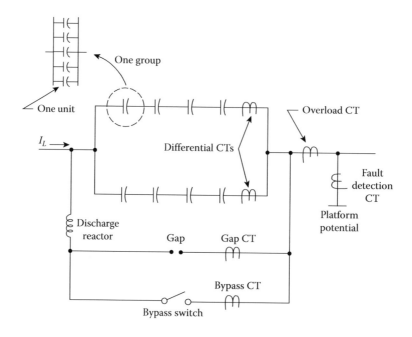

FIGURE 3.9   A simplified schematic diagram of an SC segment.

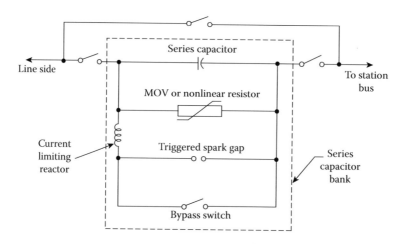

FIGURE 3.10   Schematic of typical SC compensation equipment.

Figure 3.9 shows a simplified schematic diagram of an SC segment. Figure 3.10 shows a schematic of typical SC compensation equipment. SCs are almost always in transmission lines, rather than within a substation bus arrangement.

SC compensation equipment is usually mounted on a platform at line potential and has the necessary amount of capacitors, spark gap protection, metal-oxide varistor (MOV), bypass switch (or breaker), and control and protection, as shown in Figure 3.9.

In three-phase applications, the capacitors are connected as a capacitor bank. Such capacitor banks are usually rated to withstand the line current for normal power flow considerations and power swing conditions. But it is not economical to design the capacitors to withstand the currents and voltages associated with faults. Under these conditions, capacitors are protected by MOV bank. The MOV has a highly nonlinear resistive characteristic and conducts ignorable amount of current until the voltage across it reaches the protective level.

In the event of internal faults, fault currents can be very high. Here, the internal faults are defined as the faults within the line section in which the SC bank is located. In such case, both the capacitor bank and MOV will be bypassed by the "triggered spark gap." The current limiting reactor (also called *dumping reactor*) will limit the capacitor discharge current and will damp the oscillations. Usually, such oscillations are caused by spark gap operations or when the bypass breaker is closed.

Here, the circuit parameters of C (of SC), L (of the current limiting reactor), and R (of the circuit) determine the amplitude, frequency of oscillations, and rate of damping of the SC discharge current. The energy discharge through the MOV is continually checked, and if it exceeds its rated value, the MOV will be protected by the firing of a triggered air gap, which will bypass the MOV. The triggered air gap provides a fast means of bypassing the SC bank and the MOV system when the triggered signal is issued under certain fault conditions (such as internal faults) or when the energy discharge passing through the MOV is greater than its rated value. In general, the bypass breaker is a standard line circuit breaker. It has a rated voltage that is suitable for the voltage across the capacitor bank.

As said earlier, series compensation reduces net inductive reactance of the transmission line. The reactive power generation of I^2X_C compensates for the reactive power consumption I^2X_L of the transmission line. As the load increases to the maximum value, the generation of reactive power by the capacitor also increases with the current squared. Hence, it provides reactive power when most needed. Here, the need of self-regulation becomes very obvious.

The application of series compensation increases the effective SIL of a transmission line. Contrarily, the application of shunt reactor compensation decreases the effective SIL.

In the event that the lumped compensation is approximated by the uniformly distributed compensation, the effective SIL for a compensated line can be determined from

$$SIL_{comp} = SIL_{uncomp}\sqrt{\frac{1-\Gamma_{shunt}}{1-\Gamma_{series}}} \qquad (3.9)$$

where
   SIL_{comp} is the surge impedance of a compensated line
   SIL_{uncomp} is the surge impedance of an uncompensated line
   Γ_{shunt} is the degree of shunt compensation using capacitors
   Γ_{series} is the degree of series compensation using capacitors

Consider two parallel transmission lines and assume that one of them is experiencing an outage. In such case, the current in the remaining line almost doubles. Also, the reactive power generated by SCs quadruples.

In the SC applications, the reactive power rating and the cost of series compensation are proportional to the current squared. Because of this, advantage is taken of short-time overload capability in such applications. For example, standards allow the current or voltage overload of 135% for 30 min or 150% for 5 min. This allows the dispatchers to reschedule generation, bring gas turbines on line, or shed load [7].

Example 3.2

Consider the 345 kV transmission line given in Example 3.1. In that example, the SIL was found to be 325 Ω. Investigate various compensation methods to improve the SIL of the transmission line. Determine the effective SIL for the following compensation choices:

   (a) A 50% shunt capacitive compensation and no series compensation
   (b) A 0% series capacitive compensation and 50% shunt compensation using shunt reactors
   (c) A 50% series capacitive compensation and no shunt compensation
   (d) A 50% series capacitive compensation and 20% shunt capacitive compensation

Solution

(a)

$$SIL_{comp} = SIL_{uncomp}\sqrt{\frac{1-\Gamma_{shunt}}{1-\Gamma_{series}}}$$

$$= (325 \ \Omega)\sqrt{\frac{1-0.50}{1-0.0}} = 230 \ \Omega$$

(b)

$$SIL_{comp} = SIL_{uncomp}\sqrt{\frac{1+\Gamma_{shunt}}{1-\Gamma_{series}}}$$

$$= (325 \ \Omega)\sqrt{\frac{1+0.50}{1-0.0}} = 398 \ \Omega$$

(c)

$$SIL_{comp} = SIL_{uncomp}\sqrt{\frac{1-\Gamma_{shunt}}{1-\Gamma_{series}}}$$

$$= (325 \ \Omega)\sqrt{\frac{1-0.0}{1-0.50}} = 460 \ \Omega$$

(d)

$$SIL_{comp} = SIL_{uncomp}\sqrt{\frac{1-\Gamma_{shunt}}{1-\Gamma_{series}}}$$

$$= (325 \ \Omega)\sqrt{\frac{1-0.20}{1-0.50}} = 411 \ \Omega$$

Note that the addition of shunt reactors in parallel will decrease the line capacitance. In turn, the propagation constant will be decreased, but the characteristic impedance will be increased, which is not desirable. The addition of capacitances in series with the line will decrease the line inductance. Hence, the characteristic impedance and the propagation constant will be reduced, which is desirable. Thus, the SC compensation of transmission lines is used to improve stability limits and voltage regulation, to provide a desired load division, and to maximize the load-carrying capability of the system.

Example 3.3

Consider two parallel transmission lines that are series compensated by using capacitor banks. Allow 150% voltage and current overload for a short period. The capacitor bank that is being considered to be employed must withstand twice the normal voltage and current. Determine the following:

(a) The rated current in terms of per unit of the normal load current.
(b) The amount of necessary increase in the bank's Mvar rating in per units.
(c) If the capacitor bank has a normal full-load current of 1000 A, find the rated current value.

Solution

(a) Since the capacitor bank must be able to withstand twice the normal voltage and current,

$$(1.5 \text{ pu}) \, I_{\text{rated}} = (2.0 \text{ pu}) \, I_{\text{normal}}$$

from which the rated current is

$$I_{\text{rated}} = (1.33 \text{ pu}) \, I_{\text{normal}}$$

(b) The increase in the bank's Mvar rating is

$$\text{Mvar rating increase} = (1.33 \text{ pu})^2 = 1.78 \text{ pu}$$

(c) The rated current value is

$$I_{\text{rated}} = (1.33) \, (1000 \text{ A}) = 1333 \text{ A}$$

3.10   FLEXIBLE AC TRANSMISSION SYSTEMS

A flexible ac transmission system (*FACTS*) is a power industry term for technologies that enhance the security, capacity, and flexibility of power transmission networks. IEEE defines FACTS as "a power electronic based system and other static equipment that provide control of one or more ac transmission system parameters to enhance controllability and increase power transfer capability."

FACTS solutions help power utility companies improve transmission capacity over existing ac power lines and its efficiency and enhance the security. It provides fast voltage regulation and active power control and power flow control in power networks. Succinctly put, its basic purpose is to minimize bottlenecks in existing transmission systems and improve the availability, reliability, stability, and quality of the power supply.

FACTS technology provides an alternative to building new power transmission lines or power generation facilities, which is an expensive and time-consuming process. Therefore, the use of FACTS technology is alternatively inexpensive and fast way to provide more power and control in existing networks, with minimum environmental impact.

In short, FACTS refers to a group of resources that are used to overcome certain limitations in the static and dynamic transmission capacity of electrical networks. These systems supply the power network as quickly as possible with inductive or capacitive reactive power that is adapted to its specific requirements while also improving transmission quality and efficiency of the electric power transmission system. Also, thanks to this technology, it is possible now to transmit power even over longer distances. The first FACTS installation was at the C.J. Slatt substation in Northern Oregon; it is a 500 kV, 60 Hz, three-phase substation and was developed by EPRI and the BPA. Transmission lines can be classified as

(I) Uncompensated transmission line
   Figure 3.11 shows an uncompensated transmission line and its voltage-phasor diagram.

(II) Transmission line with series compensation
   When FACTS is used for series compensation, it modifies line impedance. Thus, line impedance reactance X is decreased so as to increase the transmittable real power. However, this requires more reactive power. Here, the real and reactive powers, respectively, are

$$P = \frac{V^2}{X - X_c} \sin(\gamma) \tag{3.10}$$

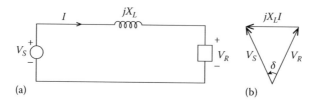

FIGURE 3.11   (a) An uncompensated transmission line and (b) its voltage-phasor diagram.

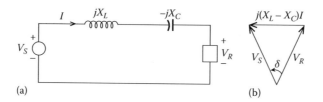

FIGURE 3.12   (a) A transmission line with series compensation and (b) its voltage-phasor diagram.

and

$$Q = \frac{V^2}{X - X_c}\left(1 - \cos\delta\right) \tag{3.11}$$

Series compensators provide an increase in transmission system stability and thus increase the capacity to transmit electric power on transmission lines. Applications of SCs include fixed series capacitors (FSC), thyristor-controlled series capacitors (TCSC), and thyristor-protected series capacitors (TPSC).

Figure 3.12a shows a transmission line with series compensation where the FACTS device is connected in series with the power system. In all ac transmission lines, a series inductance exists. On long transmission lines, when a current flows, it causes a large voltage drop. In order to compensate, SCs are connected in the line. They decrease the effect of the line reactance.

In the case of a no-loss line, voltage magnitude at the receiving end is the same as voltage magnitude at the sending end, that is,

$$V_S = V_R = V$$

Thus, the transmission results in a phase lag of δ that depends on line reactance X. It can be expressed that

$$\overline{V}_S = V \cos\left(\frac{\delta}{2}\right) + V \sin\left(\frac{\delta}{2}\right) \tag{3.12}$$

and

$$\overline{V}_S = V \cos\left(\frac{\delta}{2}\right) + V \sin\left(\frac{\delta}{2}\right) \tag{3.13}$$

and the current can be expressed as

$$I = \frac{\bar{V}_S - \bar{V}_R}{jX}$$

$$= \frac{2V \sin\left(\dfrac{\delta}{2}\right)}{X} \tag{3.14}$$

Since the line is a no-loss line, real power is the same at any point of the line. Hence,

$$P_S = P_R = P = V \cos\left(\frac{\delta}{2}\right)\left(\frac{2V \sin\left(\dfrac{\delta}{2}\right)}{X}\right) \tag{3.15}$$

or

$$P_S = P_R = P = \frac{V^2}{X} \sin(\delta) \tag{3.16}$$

Reactive power at the sending end is the opposite of reactive power at the receiving end. Thus,

$$Q_S = -Q_R = Q = V \sin\left(\frac{\delta}{2}\right)\left(\frac{2V \sin\left(\dfrac{\delta}{2}\right)}{X}\right) \tag{3.17}$$

and

$$Q_S = -Q_R = Q = \frac{V^2}{X}(1 - \cos\delta) \tag{3.18}$$

When FACTS is used for series compensation, it modifies line impedance. Thus, line reactance X is decreased so as to increase the transmittable real power. However, more reactive power must be provided. Here, the real and reactive powers, respectively, are

$$P = \frac{V^2}{X - X_C} \sin(\delta) \tag{3.19}$$

and

$$Q = \frac{V^2}{X - X_C}(1 - \cos\delta) \tag{3.20}$$

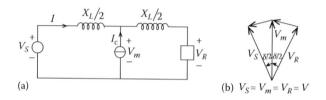

FIGURE 3.13   (a) A transmission line with shunt compensation and (b) its voltage-phasor diagram.

Examples of series compensation include the following:
1.   Static synchronous series compensation (SSSC).
2.   TCSC, that is, an SC bank that is shunted by a thyristor-controlled reactor.
3.   Thyristor-controlled series reactor (TCSR), that is, a series reactor bank that is shunted by a thyristor-controlled reactor.
4.   Thyristor-switched series capacitor (TSSR), that is, an SC bank that is shunted by a thyristor-switched reactor.
5.   Thyristor-switched series reactor (TSSR), that is, a series reactor bank that is shunted by a thyristor-switched reactor.

(III) Transmission lines with shunt compensation

Figure 3.13a shows a transmission line with shunt compensation. Here, the FACTS is connected in shunt (parallel) with the power system. The FACTS here operates as a controllable current source. The shunt compensation is of two types:

A.   Shunt capacitive compensation

This method is primarily used to improve power factor. Any time an inductive load is connected to the transmission line, power factor lags due to lagging current. In order to compensate for this, a shunt capacitor is connected, which draws current that leads the source voltage. As a result, there is an improvement in the power factor. Examples of shunt compensation include the following:

1.   Static synchronous compensator (STATCOM)

It is previously known as a static condenser (STATCON). It is connected in parallel with the line. It is a shunt-connected device injecting dynamically inductive or capacitive reactive power into the transmission grid. Its main functions are voltage stability and reactive power control of transmission systems and system buses. A different version of SVC is SVC Plus. It is a cost-efficient, space-saving, flexible solution to increase dynamic stability and power quality of transmission systems, based on multilevel voltage-source converter (VSC) technology.

2.   Static var compensators (SVCs)

They are a fast and reliable means of controlling voltage of lines and system's buses. The reactive power is changed by switchgear controlling reactive power elements connected to the secondary side of the transformer. Each capacitor bank is switched on or off by thyristor valve (thyristor-switched capacitor [TSC]).

Reactor can be either switched (thyristor-switched reactor [TSR]) or controlled (thyristor-controlled reactor [TCR]) by thyristor valves. When system voltage is low, the SVC supplies reactive power and raises the network voltage. When system voltage is high, the SVC generates inductive reactive power and reduces the system voltage. Most common SVCs are as follows:

(a)   *TCR*. This is a reactor that is connected in series with a bidirectional thyristor valve. The thyristor valve is phase controlled.
(b)   *TSR*. It is the same as TCR, but the thyristor is in either zero or full conduction. Here, the equivalent reactance is varied in stepwise manner.

(c) *TSC.* The capacitor is connected in series with a bidirectional thyristor valve. The thyristor is either in zero or full conduction. Equivalent reactance is varied in stepwise manner.

(d) *MSC/MSCDN.* The capacitor is switched mechanically by a circuit breaker. It compensates steady-state reactive power. It is only switched a few times a day. MSCs are a robust solution for voltage control and network stabilization under steady-state conditions.

The MSCDN is the advanced variation of MSC with a damping network to avoid resonance conditions in the electrical HV system.

B. Shunt inductive compensation

This method is employed either when charging the transmission line or when there is very low load at the receiving end. Due to very light load, or no load, a very small amount of current flows through the transmission line, and shunt capacitance in transmission line causes voltage increase. This is known as *Ferranti effect*. Occasionally, the receiving-end voltage may become double the sending-end voltage (usually in very long lines). In order to compensate, shunt inductors are connected across the transmission line. Therefore, the power transfer capability is increased as a result of the following equation:

$$P = \left(\frac{EV}{X}\right)\sin(\delta)$$

where δ is the power angle.

In such shunt compensation, reactive current is injected into the line to maintain voltage magnitude. This increases the transmittable real power, but more reactive power needs to be provided. Thus, the reactive power becomes

$$P = \frac{2V^2}{X}\sin\left(\frac{\delta}{2}\right)$$

and the reactive power becomes

$$Q = \frac{2V^2}{X}\left[1 - \cos\left(\frac{\delta}{2}\right)\right]$$

3.11 STATIC VAR CONTROL

In the past, shunt capacitor and SC (and synchronous condensers) have been used in many applications successfully. But in certain situations, it is crucial to have some form of compensation that will respond to rapid fluctuations in the system load with a minimum of delay of the order of a few milliseconds. The variable compensator (also known as *variable static compensator*) was a static device that could provide leading or lagging vars based on the requirements. The compensator also known as *static var supply* (SVC) device was made up of a reactor shunted across the supply and connected in parallel with a fixed or variable HV bank. The proportion of the lagging and leading vars to be supplied is totally dependent upon the individual requirements of a given transmission line or system.

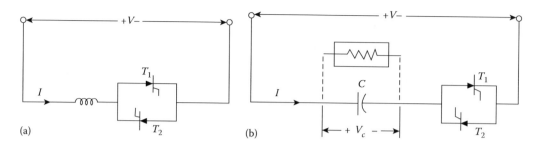

FIGURE 3.14 Principles of SVC compensation: (a) TCR and (b) TSC.

A thyristor valve, made up of two thyristors connected in antiparallel, will allow smooth regulation of the current flowing through a shunt reactor, as shown in Figure 3.12a. The current has high content of harmonics, and because of this, the device must have additional harmonic filters to help smooth the current waveform. Since such filters are very expansive, they share a large part of the compensator cost.

However, it is not possible to have smooth control of the current with capacitor because of the long time constant associated with the capacitor charge/discharge cycle. Hence, the thyristor valve can only switch the capacitor on or off, as shown in Figure 3.14b.

The thyristor firing circuits used in SVCs are usually controlled by a voltage regulator, which tries to keep bus voltage constant by controlling the amount and polarity of the reactive power injected into the bus. The regulator can also be employed to damp power swings in the system following a system disturbance.

Unfortunately, the cost of SVCs is typically several times that of an uncontrolled bank of shunt reactors or fixed capacitors (FCs). Hence, their use is somewhat restricted to those parts of a system where heavy fluctuations of real power take place and consequently compensation of both inductive and capacitive vars is needed.

Today's SVCs are shunt-connected power electronic devices. They vary the reactive power output by controlling (or switching) the reactive impedance components by means of power electronics. Typical SVC equipment classification includes the following:

1. TCRs with FCs
2. TCRs in combination with MSC or TSCs
3. TSCs

Typically, SVCs are used in the following applications:

1. Voltage regulation
2. Reduce temporary overvoltages
3. Reduce voltage flicker caused by varying loads such as arc furnaces
4. Increase power transfer capacity of transmission systems
5. Increase transient stability limits of a power system
6. Increase damping of power oscillations
7. Damp subsynchronous oscillations

The SVCs are generally cheaper than the synchronous condensers. The synchronous condensers have higher investment and operating and maintenance (O&M) costs. Their investment costs may be about 20%–30% higher than SVCs. However, the use of synchronous condensers has some advantages over SVC in voltage weak networks. The schematic representation of three types of SVCs, which include a TCR with FC bank, a TCR with switched capacitor banks, and a TSC compensator, is shown in Figure 3.15.

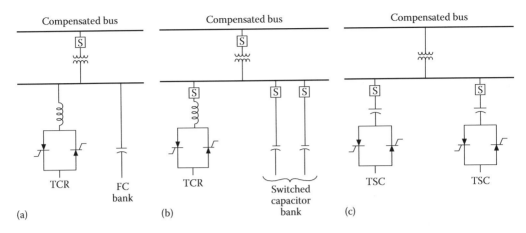

FIGURE 3.15 Schematic representation of three types of SVCs: (a) TCR with FC bank, (b) TCR with switched capacitor banks, and (c) TSC compensator.

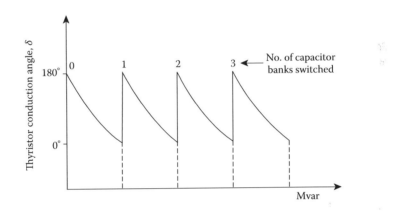

FIGURE 3.16 Reactive power variation of TCR with switched capacitor banks.

Note that a capacitor bank can be switched by mechanical breakers, if time delay, which is usually 5–10 cycles, is not an important factor, as shown in Figure 3.15b. Alternatively, they can be switched fast, in less than one cycle, by using thyristor switches, as shown in Figure 3.15c. Figure 3.16 illustrates the reactive power variation of a TCR with switched capacitor banks.

3.12 STATIC VAR SYSTEMS

CIGRÉ [15] distinguishes between SVCs and static var systems. A static var system is an SVC that can also control mechanical switching of shunt capacitor banks or reactors. Figure 3.17 shows a schematic diagram of a typical static var system. Its SVC includes TSCs, TCRs, and harmonic filters. The harmonic filters are used for the TCR-produced harmonics. The filters are capacitive at fundamental frequency and are 10%–30% of the TCRs' Mvar size. A static var system may also include FCs, TSRs, and a dedicated transformer.

3.13 THYRISTOR-CONTROLLED SERIES COMPENSATOR

It provides fast control and variation of the impedance of the SC bank. It is part of the FACTS. The FACTS, in turn, is an application of power electronics for control of the ac system to improve the power flow, operation, and control of the ac system. It has been shown that TCSC improves the

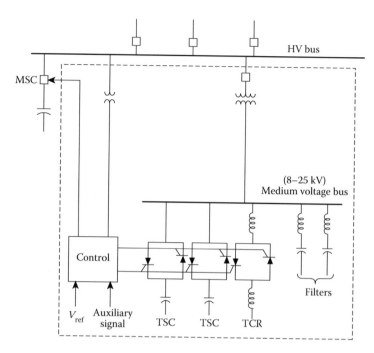

FIGURE 3.17   Schematic diagram of a typical static var system (as indicated by the dash signs).

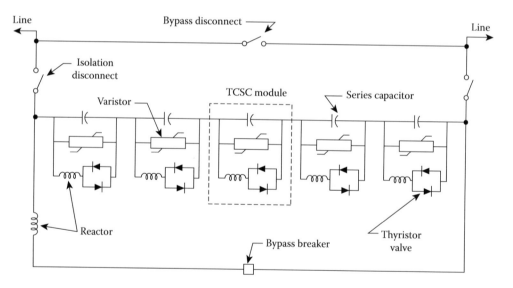

FIGURE 3.18   One-line diagram of a TCSC installed at a substation.

system performance for subsynchronous resonance (SSR) damping, power swing damping, transient stability, and power flow control. However, since it is relatively a new system, there have been only few applications. Figure 3.18 shows one-line diagram of a TCSC installed at a substation.

3.14   STATIC COMPENSATOR

A STATCOM is also called "gate turn-off (GTO) SVC" or "*advanced* SVC." It provides variable legging or leading reactive powers without using inductors or capacitors for the var generation. Reactive power generation is produced by regulating the terminal voltage of the converter.

The STATCOM is made up of a voltage-source inverter by using GTO thyristor that produces an ac voltage source, which is in phase with the transmission line voltage.

It is connected to the line through a series inductance. This reactance can be the transformer leakage inductance that is required to match the inverter voltage of the line voltage. When the terminal voltage of the voltage-source inverter is greater than the bus voltage, then STATCOM produces leading reactive power. On the other hand, when the terminal voltage is lower than the bus voltage, STATCOM produces lagging reactive power. In some sense, STATCOM is smaller to a synchronous condenser. In addition for being used for voltage control and var compensation, STATCOM can also be used to damp out electromechanical oscillations.

The operating principle of a STATCOM is illustrated in Figure 3.19. The GTO converter produces a fundamental frequency voltage V_2, which is in phase with the power system voltage V_1. As V_2 and V_1 are in phase, the difference between them results in a reactive current I, flowing through the transformer reactance X, which can be expressed as

$$I = \frac{V_1 - V_2}{jX} \tag{3.21}$$

When $V_2 > V_1$, then I leads V_1; thus, the reactive power is delivered to the bus that is connected to the line. Hence, the *converter behaves like a capacitor.*

On the other hand, if $V_2 < V_1$, then I lags V_1; thus, the reactive power is drawn from the bus and the *converter acts like a reactor.*

Note that for a transformer reactance of 0.1 pu, when there is a ±10% change on V_2, it produces ±1 pu change in the inserted reactive power.

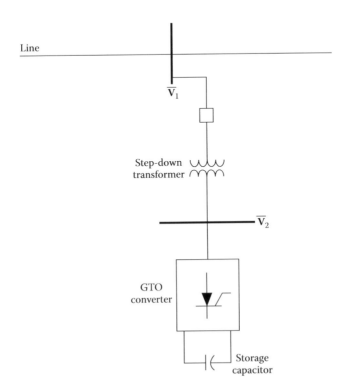

FIGURE 3.19 An illustration of the operation principle of STATCOM (or *advanced* SVC).

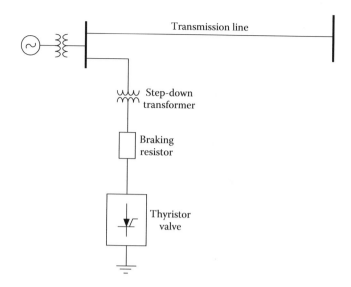

FIGURE 3.20   A thyristor-controlled braking resistor.

3.15   THYRISTOR-CONTROLLED BRAKING RESISTOR

In order to improve transient stability, a thyristor-controlled braking resistor can be used, as shown in Figure 3.20. It behaves as an additional resistive load capable of absorbing some of the generation in the event of a severe fault taking place near a generator. As a result of this, the loss of synchronism may be prevented.

3.16   SUPERCONDUCTING MAGNETIC ENERGY SYSTEMS

As a result of recent developments in the power electronics and superconductivity, the interest in using superconducting magnetic energy storage (SMES) units to store energy and/or damp power system oscillations has increased. In a sense, SMES can be seen as a controllable current source whose magnitude and phase can be changed within one cycle. The upper limit of this source is imposed by the dc current in the superconducting coil.

Figure 3.21 shows a typical configuration of an SMES unit with a double GTO thyristor bridge. In the configuration, the superconducting coil L is coupled to the transmission system via two converters and transformers. The converter firing angles α_1 and α_2 are determined by the PQI controller in order to control the real and reactive power outputs and the dc current I in the coil. The control strategy is determined by the modulation controller of SMES to damp out power swings in the network. The active and reactive power available from SMES depends on the type of ac/dc converter used. In essence, SMES is a powerful tool for transient stability enhancement and can be used to support primary frequency regulation.

3.17   SUBSYNCHRONOUS RESONANCE

As said earlier, the application of SCs is a very effective way of increasing the power transfer capability of a power system that has long transmission lines. SCs significantly increase transient and steady-state limits, in addition to being a near perfect means of var and voltage control. For a 500 kV transmission project with 1000 mi long lines, it was estimated that the application of SCs reduced the project cost by 25%. In the past, it was believed that up to 70% series compensation could be used in any transmission line with little or no concern.

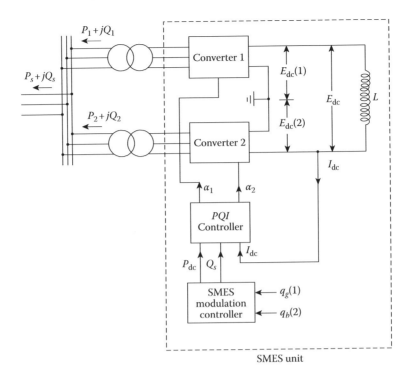

FIGURE 3.21 SMES unit with double GTO thyristor bridge.

However, there is an important problem with the use of series compensation. That is, series-compensated transmission systems and steam turbine generators can interact in a phenomenon that is known as SSR. This phenomenon may be described as the addition of SCs establishes a series-resonant circuit that can oscillate at a natural frequency below the normal synchronous frequency when stimulated by a disturbance. In certain EHV transmission circuit configurations with a high percentage of series compensation, the net resistance of the circuit can be negative, causing the oscillations to increase until they are limited by saturation effects. If the synchronous frequency minus the electrical resonant frequency approaches the frequency of one of the turbine-alternator natural torsional modes, substantial damage to the turbine-alternator shaft can occur. It may also cause insulation failure of the windings of the generator.

Also, some equipment damage may also take place due to switching series-compensated lines even though the steady-state net resistance for these oscillations is positive. The SSR problem can be corrected by modifying the alternator's excitation system, SC protective equipment, and the addition of special relaying and series blocking filters [3].

3.18   USE OF STATIC COMPENSATION TO PREVENT VOLTAGE COLLAPSE OR INSTABILITY

In general, *voltage collapse* and *voltage instability* are used interchangeably. A *voltage instability* can take place in the steady state, if the reactive demand of a load increases as the supply voltage decreases, which in turn causes a further decrease in voltage. Such voltage-collapse sequence can be triggered by a sudden disturbance. The end result is very costly, for example, in terms of loss of revenues to the utility company and loss of production to the manufacturing industry.

Some engineers view the *voltage stability* or *voltage collapse* as a steady-state problem that can be solved by using static analysis tools such as power flow. The ability to transfer reactive power from generators to loads during steady-state conditions is a main part of the voltage stability problem. Other engineers view the voltage instability or voltage collapse as a dynamic process. The word *dynamic* basically involves the loads and the methods for voltage control. It is often that voltage stability is also called as *load stability*.

It can be that a given power system has a *small-disturbance voltage stability*, if it can keep its load voltages at close or identical values (to the predisturbance values) after any small disturbance. Similarly, a power system can be said to have *voltage stability*, if it can keep its load voltages at postdisturbance equilibrium values following a disturbance. However, a power system can be said to have a voltage collapse, if it has postdisturbance equilibrium voltages that are below the acceptable limits following a disturbance. Voltage collapse may be total (i.e., *blackout*) or partial.

Voltage instability normally takes place after large disturbances in terms of rapid increases in load or power transfer. Often, the instability is an aperiodic but progressive decrease in voltage. However, oscillatory voltage instability may also be possible. In addition, control instabilities can also take place. For example, such control instabilities may result due to having a too high gain on an SVC or a too small deadband in a voltage relay that controls a shunt capacitor bank. The term *voltage security* defines the ability of a system for operating not only at a steady state but also remaining in a steady state following major contingencies or load increases [7].

The static shunt compensators can aid power system stability through rapid adjustment of its reactive power. The use of one or more compensators can complete with the alternative of additional transmission lines in meeting the need for greater power transfer capability. The controllability of TCR-based compensators allows the employment of supplementary damping signals to accelerate the settling of the power system following disturbance [6].

3.19 ENERGY MANAGEMENT SYSTEM

The main purpose of an electric power system is to efficiently generate, transmit, and distribute electric energy. The operations involved dictate geographically dispersed and functionally complex monitoring and control systems, as shown in Figure 3.22.

As illustrated in the figure, the *energy management system* (EMS) exercises overall control over the total system. The SCADA system involves generation and transmission systems. The *distribution automation and control* (DAC) system oversees the distribution system, including connected load. Automatic monitoring and control features have long been a part of the SCADA system.

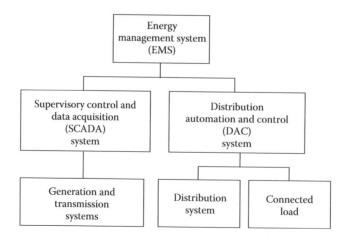

FIGURE 3.22 Monitoring and controlling an electric power system.

More recently, automation has become a part of the overall EMS, including the distribution system. Motivating objectives of the DAC system are

1. Improved overall system efficiency in the use of both capital and energy
2. Increased market penetration of coal, nuclear, and renewable domestic energy sources
3. Reduced reserve requirements in both transmission and generation
4. Increased reliability of service to essential load

Advances in digital technology have made the true EMS a reality. It is clear that future electric power systems will be more complex than those of today. If the systems being developed are to be operational with respect to construction costs, capitalization, performance reliability, and operating efficiency, better automation and controls are required.

3.20 SUPERVISORY CONTROL AND DATA ACQUISITION

SCADA is the equipment and procedures for controlling one or more remote stations from a master control station. It includes the digital control equipment, sensing and telemetry equipment, and two-way communications to and from the master stations and the remotely controlled stations.

The SCADA digital control equipment includes the control computers and terminals for data display and entry. The sensing and telemetry equipment includes the sensors, digital-to-analog and analog-to-digital converters, actuators, and relays used at the remote station to sense operating and alarm conditions and to remotely activate equipment such as circuit breakers. The communications equipment includes the modems (modulator/demodulator) for transmitting the digital data and the communications link (radio, phone line, microwave link, or power line).

Figure 3.23 shows a block diagram of a SCADA system. Typical functions that can be performed by SCADA are as follows:

1. Control and indication of the position of a two- or three-position device, for example, a motor-driven switch or a circuit breaker
2. State indication without control, for example, transformer fans on or off
3. Control without indication, for example, capacitors switched in or out
4. Set point control of remote control station, for example, nominal voltage for an automatic tap changer
5. Alarm sensing, for example, fire or the performance of a noncommanded function
6. Permit operators to initiate operations at remote stations from a central control station
7. Initiation and recognition of sequences of events, for example, routing power around a bad transformer by opening and closing circuit breakers or sectionalizing a bus with a fault on it
8. Data acquisition from metering equipment, usually via analog/digital converter and digital communication link

Today, in this country, all routine substation functions are remotely controlled. For example, a complete SCADA system can perform the following substation functions:

1. Automatic bus sectionalizing
2. Automatic reclosing after a fault
3. Synchronous check
4. Protection of equipment in a substation
5. Fault reporting
6. Transformer load balancing
7. Voltage and reactive power control

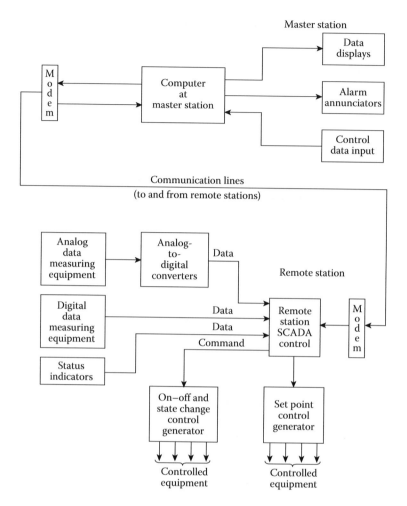

FIGURE 3.23   SCADA.

8. Equipment condition monitoring
9. Data acquisition
10. Status monitoring
11. Data logging

All SCADA systems have two-way data and voice communication between the master and the remote stations. Modems at the sending and receiving ends modulate, that is, put information on the carrier frequency, and demodulate, that is, remove information from the carrier, respectively. Here, digital codes are utilized for such information exchange with various error detection schemes to assure that all data are received correctly. The *remote terminal unit* (RTU) properly codes remote station information into the proper digital form for the modem to transmit and to convert the signals received from the master into the proper form for each piece of remote equipment.

When a SCADA system is in operation, it scans all routine alarm and monitoring functions periodically by sending the proper digital code to interrogate, or poll, each device. The polled device sends its data and status to the master station. The total scan time for a substation might be 30 s to several minutes subject to the speed of the SCADA system and the substation size. If an alarm condition takes place, it interrupts a normal scan. Upon an alarm, the computer polls the device at the substation that indicated the alarm. It is possible for an alarm to trigger a computer-initiated sequence of events, for example, breaker action to sectionalize a faulted bus. Each of the activated equipment has a code to activate it, that is, to make it listen, and another code to cause the controlled action to take place. Also, some alarm conditions may sound an alarm at the control station that indicates that an action is required by an operator. In that case, the operator initiates the action via a keyboard or a CRT. Of course, the computers used in SCADA systems must have considerable memory to store all the data, codes for the controlled devices, and the programs for automatic response to abnormal events.

3.21 ADVANCED SCADA CONCEPTS

The increasing competitive business environment of utilities, due to deregulation, is causing a reexamination of SCADA as a part of the process of utility operations, not as a process unto itself. The present business environment dictates the incorporation of hardware and software of the modern SCADA system into the corporation-wide, management information systems' strategy to maximize the benefits to the utility.

Today, the dedicated islands of automation gave way to the corporate information system. Tomorrow, in advanced systems, SCADA will be a function performed by workstation-based applications, interconnected through a *wide area network* (WAN) to create a virtual system, as shown in Figure 3.24.

This arrangement will provide the SCADA applications' access to a host of other applications, for example, substation controllers, automated mapping/facility management system, trouble call analysis, crew dispatching, and demand-side load management. The WAN will also provide the traditional link between the utility's EMS and SCADA processors. The workstation-based applications will also provide for flexible expansion and economic system reconfiguration.

Also, unlike the centralized database of most existing SCADA systems, the advanced SCADA system database will exist in dynamic pieces that are distributed throughout the network. Modifications to any of interconnected elements will be immediately available to all users, including the SCADA system. SCADA will have to become a more involved partner in the process of economic delivery and maintained quality of service to the end user.

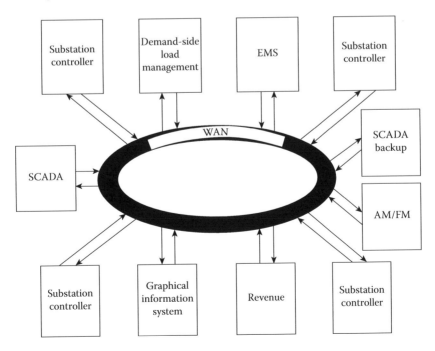

FIGURE 3.24 SCADA in virtual system established by WAN.

In most applications today, SCADA and the EMS operate only on the transmission and generation sides of the system. In the future, economic dispatch algorithms will include demand-side (load) management and voltage control/reduction solutions. The control and its hardware and software resources will cease to exist.

3.22 SUBSTATION CONTROLLERS

In the future, RTUs not only will provide station telemetry and control to the master station but also will provide other primary functions such as system protection, local operation, *graphical user interface* (GUI), and data gathering/concentration from other subsystems. Therefore, the future's RTUs will evolve into a class of devices that perform multiple substation control, protection, and operation functions. Besides these functions, the substation controller also develops and processes data required by the SCADA master, and it processes control commands and messages received from the SCADA master.

The substation controller will provide a gateway function to process and transmit data from the substation to the WAN. The substation controller is basically a computer system designed to operate in a substation environment. As shown in Figure 3.25, it has hardware modules and software in terms of the following:

1. *Data processing applications*: These software applications provide various users' access to the data of the substation controller in order to provide instructions and programming to the substation controller, collect data from the substation controller, and perform the necessary functions.
2. *Data collection applications*: These software applications provide the access to other systems and components that have data elements necessary for the substation controller to perform its functions.
3. *Control database*: All data reside in a single location, whether from a data processing application, data collection application, or derived from the substation controller itself.

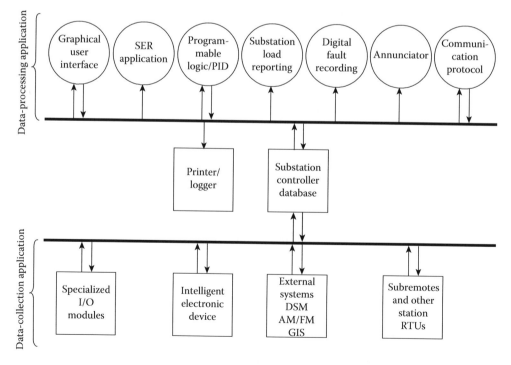

FIGURE 3.25 Substation controller.

Therefore, the substation controller is a system that is made up of many different types of hardware and software components and may not even be in a single location. Here, RTU may exist only as a software application within the substation controller system. Substation controllers will make all data available on WANs. They will eliminate separate stand-alone systems and thus provide greater cost savings to the utility company.

According to Sciacca and Block [29], the SCADA planner must look beyond the traditional roles of SCADA. For example, the planner must consider the following issues:

1. Reduction of substation design and construction costs
2. Reduction of substation operating costs
3. Overall lowering of power system operating costs
4. Development of information for non-SCADA functions
5. Utilization of existing resources and company standard for hardware, software, and database generation
6. Expansion of automated operations at the subtransmission and distribution levels
7. Improved customer relations

To accomplish these, the SCADA planner must join forces with the substation engineer to become an integrated team. Each must ask the other, "How can your requirements be met in a manner that provides positive benefits for my business?"

3.23 SIX-PHASE TRANSMISSION LINES

Recently, high-phase (i.e., 6-, 9-, and 12-phase) order transmission lines have been proposed to transmit more than three phases of electric power. Six-phase transmission lines are especially designed to increase power transfer over existing lines and reduce electrical environmental impacts [24–27]. The advantages of six-phase systems are as follows:

1. Increased thermal loading capacity of lines.
2. For a given conductor size and tower configuration, the stress on the conductor surface decreases with the number of phases, leading to reduced corona losses.
3. Their transmission efficiency is higher.
4. The double-circuit lines, with two three-phase circuits on each tower, can easily be converted to single-circuit six-phase lines.
5. The higher the number of phases, the smaller the line-to-line voltage becomes relative to the phase voltage. As a result, the existing rights of way can be better used since there is less need for phase-to-phase insulation requirement in the six-phase transmission.

In the three-phase ac systems, there are three phasors that are offset with respect to each other by 120°. Similarly, in the six-phase ac systems, there are six phasors that are offset with respect to each other by 60°. On the other hand, nine-phase ac systems have nine phasors that are offset by 40° and twelve-phase ac systems consist of twelve phasors offset by 30°.

However, three-phase transmission was accepted as the standard for ac transmission due to the following reasons:

1. Three phases are the least number required for power flow that is constant with time.
2. The power of electric machine does not increase as phases are increased more than three phases.

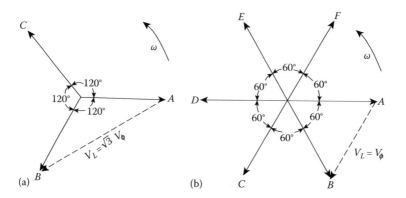

FIGURE 3.26 Polyphase phasor systems: (a) three-phase system and (b) six-phase system.

But electric power transmission with more than three phases has some advantages. For example, in six-phase transmission lines,* the conductor gradients are lower, which reduce both AN and electrostatic effects without requiring additional insulation. In multiphase transmission lines, if the line-to-ground voltage is fixed, then the line-to-line voltage decreases as the number of phases increases, thereby enabling the line-to-line insulation distance to be reduced. Figure 3.26 shows polyphase voltage phasors in three-phase phasor versus six-phase phasor systems. In the three-phase systems,

$$V_L = \sqrt{3}V_\phi$$

but in the six-phase systems,

$$V_L = V_\phi$$

that is, the line and phase voltages are the same. Hence, for example, for a given phase-to-ground voltage of 79.6 kV, the line-to-line voltage is 138 kV for three-phase systems. But it is 79.6 kV for six-phase systems. Similarly, for a phase-to-ground voltage of 199.2 kV, the line-to-line voltage is 345 kV for three-phase systems, but it is 199.2 kV for six-phase systems. The maximum complex power that six-phase transmission lines can carry is

$$\mathbf{S}_{6\phi} = 6\mathbf{V}_\phi\mathbf{I}_L^*$$ (3.22)

and the maximum complex power that a double-circuit three-phase line of the same phase voltage can carry is

$$\mathbf{S}_{3\phi} = 2\left(3\mathbf{V}_\phi\mathbf{I}_L^*\right)$$

$$= 6\mathbf{V}_\phi\mathbf{I}_L^* = \mathbf{S}_{6\phi}$$

which is the same as a six-phase transmission line. It is clear that the lower line-to-line voltage of the six-phase line permits the tower and other structures to be smaller than an equivalent double-circuit three-phase transmission line, as shown in Figure 3.27. As a result of this, the same amount

---

* A six-phase 93 kV transmission line was built between Goudey and Oakdale in New York by New York State Electric and Gas Company.

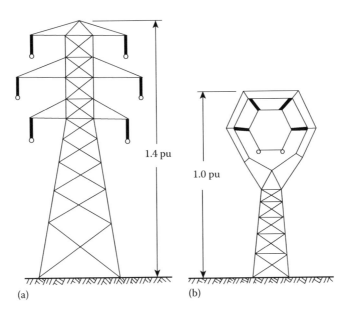

FIGURE 3.27 Comparative tower heights for a double-circuit (a) three-phase transmission line versus (b) a six-phase transmission line.

of complex power can be transmitted using smaller six-phase ROW for the same phase voltage and the same conductor current capacity.

Similarly, the power capacity of a six-phase transmission line with the same line voltage as an equivalent double-circuit three-phase transmission line is

$$\mathbf{S}_{6\phi} = 6\left(\sqrt{3}\mathbf{V}_{\phi}\mathbf{I}_{L}^{*}\right) \tag{3.23}$$

or

$$\mathbf{S}_{6\phi} = \sqrt{3}6\mathbf{V}_{\phi}\mathbf{I}_{L}^{*} \tag{3.24}$$

Therefore, for the same line voltage, the capacity of a six-phase line is 173% that of an equivalent double-circuit three-phase system. Also, the magnetic fields are three to four times lower in six-phase lines than an equivalent double-circuit three-phase line.

Since the electric field gradients on the conductors are lower in six-phase lines, its corona losses are also lower. Today, the need for six-phase transformers is met by using two regular three-phase transformers that are connected delta–wye and delta-inverted wye or wye–wye and wye-inverted wye, as illustrated in Figure 3.28.

The following types of protections are provided for the six-phase 93 kV transmission line that was built between Goudey and Oakdale in New York:

1. Current differential relaying employing pilot signal over a fiber-optic-based communication channel.
2. Phase-distance impedance relays with directional ground current relays.
3. Segregated phase comparison relays for backup. These relays can determine if an internal fault has taken place by comparing the phase at the ends of each conductor, using a fiber-optic communications system.

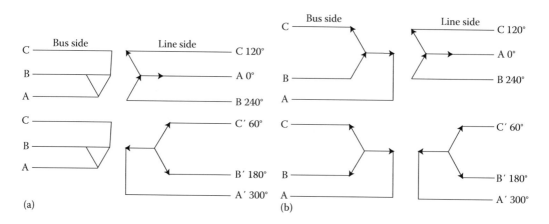

FIGURE 3.28 Six-phase transformer bank made up of two three-phase transformers connected as (a) delta–wye and delta-inverted wye and (b) wye–wye and wye-inverted wye.

In general, protection of a six-phase transmission line is more involved than for a double-circuit three-phase transmission line. There are more combinations of line-to-line and line-to-neutral faults that can take place.

REFERENCES

1. Electric Power Research Institute. *Transmission Line Reference Book: 345 kV and Above*, 2nd edn., EPRI, Palo Alto, CA, 1982.
2. Electric Power Research Institute. *Transmission Line Reference Book: 115–138 kV Compact Line Design*, 2nd edn., EPRI, Palo Alto, CA, 1978.
3. Rural Electrification Administration. Transmission line manual, REA Bulletin No. 62-1, U.S. Department of Agriculture, U.S. Government Printing Office, Washington, DC, 1972.
4. Dunlop, R. D., Gutman, R., and Morchenko, P. P. Analytical development of loadability characteristics for EHV and UHV transmission lines, *IEEE Trans. Power Appar. Syst.* PAS-98, March/April 1979, 606–617.
5. Kimbark, E. W. Improvement of system stability by series capacitors, *IEEE Trans. Power Appar. Syst.* PAS-85(2), February 1966, 180–188.
6. Miller, T. J. E. *Reactive Power Control in Electric Systems*, Wiley, New York, 1982.
7. Taylor, C. W. *Power System Voltage Stability*, McGraw-Hill, New York, 1994.
8. Hubacker, E. J., Meneatis, J. A., Rothenbuhler, W. N., and Sabath, J. 500-kV Series capacitor installations in California, *IEEE Trans. Power Appar. Syst.* PAS-90, May/June 1971, 1138–1149.
9. Crary, S. B. *Power System Stability*, vol. 1, Wiley, New York, 1948.
10. Benko, J. S., Bold, S. H., Rothenbuhler, W. N., Bock, L. E., Johnson, J. B., and Stevenson, J. R. Internal overvoltages and protective devices in EHV compensated systems-series capacitors and shunt reactors, CIGRÉ Paper 33-05, 1076.
11. Hanks, G. R. et al. Tennessee Valley Authority 500-kV shunt capacitor bank, *Proc. Am. Power Conf.* 36, April 1976, 15–21.
12. Concordia, C., Tice, J. B., and Bowler, E. E. J. Subsynchronous torques on generating units feeding series capacitor compensated lines, *Proc. Am. Power Conf.* 33, 1973, 1129–1136.
13. St. Clair, H. B. Practical concepts in capability and performance of transmission lines, *AIEE Trans. Power Appar. Syst.*, Paper 53-338, Presented at the *AIEE Pacific General Meeting*, Vancouver, British Columbia, Canada, September 1–4, 1953.
14. Hauth, R. L. and Moran, R. J. Basics of applying static var systems on HVAC power networks, *Proc. Trans. Static Var Systems Seminar*, Presented October 24, 1978, Minneapolis, MN, EPRI Report EL-1047-SR, 1979.
15. CIGRÉ Working Group Report, no. 38-01, Static var compensators, CIGRÉ, Paris, France, 1986.
16. Osborn, D. L. Factors for planning a static var system, *Elec. Power Syst. Res.* 17, 1989, 5–12.
17. Schander, C. et al. Development of a ±100 Mvar static condenser for voltage control of transmission systems, *IEEE Trans. Power Deliv.* 10(3), July 1995, 1486–1496.

18. Padiyar, K. R. *Analysis of Subsynchronous Resonance in Power Systems*, Kluwer Academic Publishers, Norwell, MA, 1999.
19. Anderson, P. M., Agrawal, B. L., and Van Ness, J. E. *Subsynchronous Resonance in Power Systems*, IEEE Press, New York, 1990.
20. Anderson, P. M. and Farmer, R. G. *Series Compensation on Power Systems*, PBLSH! Inc., Encinitas, CA, 1996.
21. Hammad, A. E. Analysis of power system stability enhancement by static var components, *IEEE Trans. Power Syst.* PAS-1(1), 1986, 222–227.
22. Gyugyi, L., Otto, R. A., and Putman, T. H. Principles and applications of thyristor-controlled shunt compensators, *IEEE Trans. Power Appar. Syst.* PAS-97, September/October 1978, 1935–1945.
23. Gyugyi, L. and Taylor, E. R., Jr. Characteristics of static thyristor-controlled shunt compensator for power transmission applications, *IEEE Trans. Power Appar. Syst.* PAS-99, September/October 1980, 1795–1804.
24. Barthold, L. O. and Barnes, H. C. High-phase order transmission, *Electra*, 24, 1972, 139–153.
25. Stewart, J. R., Kallaur, E., and Grant, I. S. Economics of EHV high phase order transmission, *IEEE Trans. Power Appar. Syst.* PAS-103, 1984, 3386–3392.
26. Stewart, J. R. and Wilson, D. D. High phase order transmission: Part A—Feasibility analysis, *IEEE Trans. Power Appar. Syst.* PAS-97, 1978, 2308–2317.
27. Gönen, T. and Haj-Mohamadi, M. S. Electromagnetic unbalances of six-phase transmission lines, *Electr. Power Energ. Syst.* 11(2), April 1989, 78–84.
28. Gönen, T. *Electric Power Distribution System Engineering*, 2nd edn., CRC Press, Boca Raton, FL, 2008.
29. Sciacca, S. C. and Block, W. R. Advanced SCADA concepts, *IEEE Comput. Appl. Power* 8(1), January 1995, 23–28.
30. Hingorani, N. G. and Gyugyi, L. *Understanding FACTS: Concepts and Technology of Flexible AC Transmission Systems*, Wiley–IEEE Press, New York, December 1999.
31. Edris, A. et al. Proposed term and definitions for flexible AC transmission system (FACTS), *IEEE Trans. Power Deliv.* 12(4), October 1997, 1848–1853.

4 Overhead Power Transmission

To see a world in a Grain of Sand and a Heaven in a Wild Flower.
Hold Infinity in the palm of your hand, and Eternity in an hour.

William Blake

4.1 INTRODUCTION

In this section, a brief review of fundamental concepts associated with steady-state ac circuits, especially with three-phase circuits, is presented. It is hoped that this brief review is sufficient to provide a common base, in terms of notation and references, that is necessary to be able to follow the forthcoming chapters.

Also, a brief review of transmission system modeling is presented in this chapter. Transmission lines are modeled and classified according to their lengths as

1. Short transmission lines
2. Medium-length transmission lines
3. Long transmission lines

The short transmission lines are those lines that have lengths up to 50 mi, or 80 km. The medium-length transmission lines are those lines that have lengths up to 150 mi, or 240 km. Similarly, the long transmission lines are those lines that have lengths above 150 mi or 240 km.

4.2 REVIEW OF BASICS

4.2.1 COMPLEX POWER IN BALANCED TRANSMISSION LINES

Figure 4.1a shows a per-phase representation (or one-line diagram) of a short three-phase balanced transmission line connecting buses i and j. Here, the term bus defines a specific nodal point of a transmission network. Assume that the bus voltages $\mathbf{V}_i$ and $\mathbf{V}_j$ are given in phase values (i.e., line-to-neutral values) and that the line impedance is $\mathbf{Z} = R + jX$ per phase. Since the transmission line is a short one, the line current 1 can be assumed to be approximately the same at any point in the line. However, because of the line losses, the complex powers $\mathbf{S}_{ij}$ and $\mathbf{S}_{ji}$ are not the same.

Therefore, the complex power per phase* that is being transmitted from bus i to bus j can be expressed as

$$\mathbf{S}_{ij} = P_{ij} + jQ_{ij} = \mathbf{V}_i\mathbf{I}^* \tag{4.1}$$

Similarly, the complex power per phase that is being transmitted from bus j to bus i can be expressed as

$$\mathbf{S}_{ji} = P_{ji} + jQ_{ji} = \mathbf{V}_j(-\mathbf{I})^* \tag{4.2}$$

---

* For an excellent treatment of the subject, see Elgerd [1].

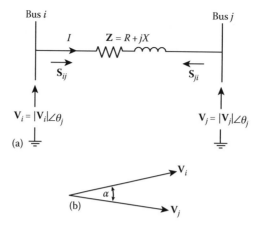

FIGURE 4.1 Per-phase representation of short transmission line: (a) a short transmission line and (b) voltage phasor diagram.

Since

$$\mathbf{I} = \frac{\mathbf{V}_j - \mathbf{V}_i}{\mathbf{Z}} \tag{4.3}$$

substituting Equation 4.3 into Equations 4.1 and 4.2,

$$\mathbf{S}_{ij} = \mathbf{V}_i \left(\frac{\mathbf{V}_i^* - \mathbf{V}_j^*}{\mathbf{Z}^*} \right)$$

$$= \frac{|\mathbf{V}_i|^2 - |\mathbf{V}_i||\mathbf{V}_j| \angle \theta_i - \theta_j}{R - jX} \tag{4.4}$$

and

$$\mathbf{S}_{ji} = \mathbf{V}_j \left(\frac{\mathbf{V}_j^* - \mathbf{V}_i^*}{\mathbf{Z}^*} \right)$$

$$= \frac{|\mathbf{V}_j|^2 - |\mathbf{V}_j||\mathbf{V}_i| \angle \theta_j - \theta_i}{R - jX} \tag{4.5}$$

However, as shown in Figure 4.1b, if the power angle (i.e., the phase angle between the two bus voltages) is defined as

$$\gamma = \theta_i - \theta_j \tag{4.6}$$

then the real and reactive power per phase values can be expressed, respectively, as

$$P_{ij} = \frac{1}{R^2 + X^2} \left(R|\mathbf{V}_i|^2 - R|\mathbf{V}_i||\mathbf{V}_j|\cos\gamma + X|\mathbf{V}_i||\mathbf{V}_j|\sin\gamma \right) \tag{4.7}$$

and

$$Q_{ij} = \frac{1}{R^2 + X^2}\left(X|\mathbf{V}_i|^2 - X|\mathbf{V}_i||\mathbf{V}_j|\cos\gamma - R|\mathbf{V}_i||\mathbf{V}_j|\sin\gamma\right) \tag{4.8}$$

Similarly,

$$P_{ji} = \frac{1}{R^2 + X^2}\left(R|\mathbf{V}_j|^2 - R|\mathbf{V}_i||\mathbf{V}_j|\cos\gamma - X|\mathbf{V}_i||\mathbf{V}_j|\sin\gamma\right) \tag{4.9}$$

and

$$Q_{ji} = \frac{1}{R^2 + X^2}\left(X|\mathbf{V}_j|^2 - X|\mathbf{V}_i||\mathbf{V}_j|\cos\gamma + R|\mathbf{V}_i||\mathbf{V}_j|\sin\gamma\right) \tag{4.10}$$

The three-phase real and reactive power can directly be found from Equations 4.7 through 4.10 if the phase values are replaced by the line values.

In general, the reactance of a transmission line is much greater than its resistance. Therefore, the line impedance value can be approximated as

$$\mathbf{Z} = jX \tag{4.11}$$

by setting $R = 0$. Therefore, Equations 4.7 through 4.10 can be expressed as

$$P_{ij} = \frac{|\mathbf{V}_i||\mathbf{V}_j|}{X}\sin\gamma \tag{4.12}$$

$$Q_{ij} = \frac{1}{X}\left(|\mathbf{V}_i|^2 - |\mathbf{V}_i||\mathbf{V}_j|\cos\gamma\right) \tag{4.13}$$

and

$$P_{ji} = \frac{|\mathbf{V}_j||\mathbf{V}_i|}{X}\sin\gamma = -P_{ij} \tag{4.14}$$

$$Q_{ji} = \frac{1}{X}\left(|\mathbf{V}_j|^2 - |\mathbf{V}_j||\mathbf{V}_i|\cos\gamma\right) \tag{4.15}$$

Example 4.1

Assume that the impedance of a transmission line connecting buses 1 and 2 is $100\angle60°\ \Omega$ and that the bus voltages are $73{,}034.8\angle30°$ and $66{,}395.3\angle20°$ V per phase, respectively. Determine the following:

(a) Complex power per phase that is being transmitted from bus 1 to bus 2
(b) Active power per phase that is being transmitted
(c) Reactive power per phase that is being transmitted

Solution

(a)

$$S_{12} = V_1 \left(\frac{V_1^* - V_2^*}{Z^*} \right)$$

$$= (73,034.8\angle 30°) \left(\frac{73,034.8\angle -30° - 66,395.3\angle -20°}{100\angle -60°} \right)$$

$$= 10,104,766.7\angle 3.56°$$

$$= 10,085,280.6 + j627,236.5 \text{ VA}$$

(b)

$$P_{12} = 10,085,280.6 \text{ W}$$

(c)

$$Q_{12} = 627,236.5 \text{ vars}$$

4.2.2 ONE-LINE DIAGRAM

In general, electric power systems are represented by a one-line diagram, as shown in Figure 4.2a. The one-line diagram is also referred to as the single-line diagram. Figure 4.2b shows the three-phase equivalent impedance diagram of the system given in Figure 4.2a. However, the need for the three-phase equivalent impedance diagram is almost nil in usual situations. This is due to the fact that a balanced three-phase system can always be represented by an equivalent impedance diagram per phase, as shown in Figure 4.2c. Furthermore, the per-phase equivalent impedance can also be simplified by neglecting the neutral line and representing the system components by standard symbols rather than by their equivalent circuits [1]. The result is the one-line diagram shown in Figure 4.2a. Table 4.1 gives some of the symbols that are used in one-line diagrams. Additional standard symbols can be found in Neuenswander [2].

At times, as a need arises, the one-line diagram may also show peripheral apparatus such as instrument transformers (i.e., CTs and VTs), protective relays, and lighting arrestors. Therefore, the details shown on a one-line diagram depend on its purpose. For example, the one-line diagrams that will be used in load flow studies do not show CBs or relays, contrary to the ones that will be used in stability studies. Furthermore, the ones that will be used in unsymmetrical fault studies may even show the positive-, negative-, and zero-sequence networks separately.

Note that the buses (i.e., the *nodal points* of the transmission network) that are shown in Figure 4.2a have been identified by their bus numbers. Also note that the neutral of generator 1 has been *solidly grounded*, that is, the neutral point has been directly connected to the earth, whereas the neutral of generator 2 has been *grounded through impedance* using a resistor. Sometimes, it is grounded using an inductance coil. In either case, they are used to limit the current flow to ground under fault conditions.

Usually, the neutrals of the transformers used in transmission lines are solidly grounded. In general, a proper generator grounding for generators is facilitated by burying a ground electrode system made of grids of buried horizontal wires. As the number of meshes in the grid is increased, its conductance becomes greater. Sometimes, a metal plate is buried instead of a mesh grid.

Transmission lines with OHGWs have a ground connection at each supporting structure to which the GW is connected. In some circumstances, a *counterpoise*, that is, a bare conductor, is buried under a transmission line to decrease the ground resistance, if the soil resistance is high. The best known

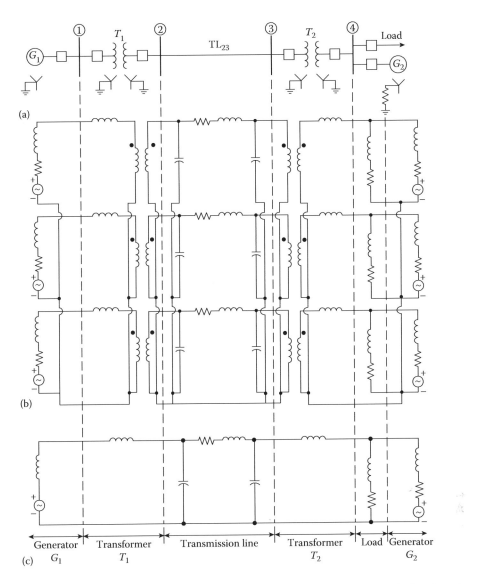

FIGURE 4.2 Power system representations: (a) one-line diagram, (b) three-phase equivalent impedance diagram, and (c) equivalent impedance diagram per phase.

example is the one that has been installed for the transmission line crossing the Mojave Desert. The counterpoise is buried alongside the line and connected directly to the towers and the OHGWs.

Note that the equivalent circuit of the transmission line shown in Figure 4.2c has been represented by a nominal π. The line impedance, in terms of the resistance and the series reactance of a single conductor for the length of the line, has been lumped. The line-to-neutral capacitance (or *shunt capacitive reactance*) for the length of the line has been calculated, and half of this value has been put at each end of the line.

The transformers have been represented by their equivalent reactances, neglecting their magnetizing currents and consequently their shunt admittances. Also neglected are the resistance values of the transformers and generators due to the fact that their inductive reactance values are much greater than their resistance values. Also not shown in Figure 4.2c is the ground resistor. This is due to no current flowing in the neutral under balanced conditions. The impedance diagram shown in Figure 4.2c is also referred to as the positive-sequence network or diagram. The reason is that the

TABLE 4.1

Symbols Used in One-Line Diagrams

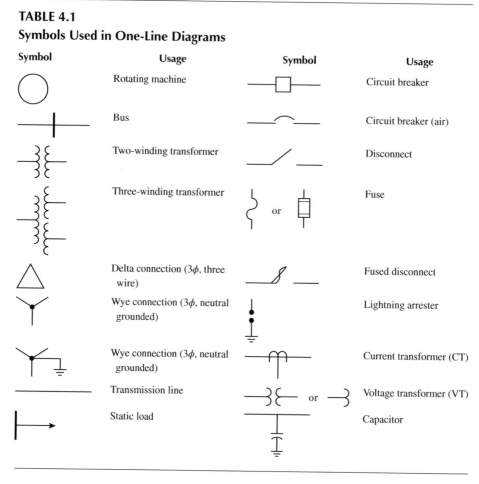

Symbol	Usage	Symbol	Usage
	Rotating machine		Circuit breaker
	Bus		Circuit breaker (air)
	Two-winding transformer		Disconnect
	Three-winding transformer	or	Fuse
	Delta connection (3ϕ, three wire)		Fused disconnect
	Wye connection (3ϕ, neutral grounded)		Lightning arrester
	Wye connection (3ϕ, neutral grounded)		Current transformer (CT)
	Transmission line	or	Voltage transformer (VT)
	Static load		Capacitor

phase order of the balanced voltages at any point in the system is the same as the phase order of the generated voltage, and they are positive. The per-phase impedance diagrams may represent a system given either in ohms or in per units.

4.2.3 PER-UNIT SYSTEM

Because of various advantages involved, it is customary in power system analysis calculations to use impedances, currents, voltages, and powers in per-unit values (which are scaled or normalized values) rather than in physical values of ohms, amperes, kilovolts, and megavolt-amperes (or megavars, or megawatts). A per-unit system is a means of expressing quantities for ease in comparing them. The per-unit value of any quantity is defined as the ratio of the quantity to an *arbitrarily* chosen base (i.e., *reference*) value having the same dimensions. Therefore, the per-unit value of any quantity can be defined as physical quantity:

$$\text{Quantity in per unit} = \frac{\text{Physical quantity}}{\text{Base value of quantity}} \tag{4.16}$$

where *physical quantity* refers to the given value in ohms, amperes, volts, etc. The *base value* is also called unit value since in the per-unit system, it has a value of 1, or unity. Therefore, a base current is also referred to as a unit current. Since both the physical quantity and base quantity have the same dimensions, the resulting per-unit value expressed as a decimal has no dimension and therefore is simply indicated by a subscript pu. The base quantity is indicated by a subscript B. The symbol for per unit is pu, or 0/1. The percent system is obtained by multiplying the per-unit value by 100. Therefore,

$$\text{Quantity in percent} = \frac{\text{Physical quantity}}{\text{Base value of quantity}} \times 100 \tag{4.17}$$

However, the percent system is somewhat more difficult to work with and more subject to possible error since it must always be remembered that the quantities have been multiplied by 100. Therefore, the factor 100 has to be continually inserted or removed for reasons that may not be obvious at the time. For example, 40% reactance times 100% current is equal to 4000% voltage, which, of course, must be corrected to 40% voltage. Thus, the per-unit system is preferred in power system calculations. The advantages of using the per unit include the following:

1. Network analysis is greatly simplified since all impedances of a given equivalent circuit can directly be added together regardless of the system voltages.
2. It eliminates the $\sqrt{3}$ multiplications and divisions that are required when balanced three-phase systems are represented by per-phase systems. Therefore, the factors $\sqrt{3}$ and 3 associated with delta and wye quantities in a balanced three-phase system are directly taken into account by the base quantities.
3. Usually, the impedance of an electrical apparatus is given in percent or per unit by its manufacturer based on its nameplate ratings (e.g., its rated volt-amperes and rated voltage).
4. Differences in operating characteristics of many electrical apparatus can be estimated by a comparison of their constants expressed in per units.
5. Average machine constants can easily be obtained since the parameters of similar equipment tend to fall in a relatively narrow range and therefore are comparable when expressed as per units based on rated capacity.
6. The use of per-unit quantities is more convenient in calculations involving digital computers.

4.2.3.1 Single-Phase System

In the event that any two of the four base quantities (i.e., base voltage, base current, base volt-amperes, and base impedance) are *arbitrarily* specified, the other two can be determined immediately. Here, the term arbitrarily is slightly misleading since in practice the base values are selected so as to force the results to fall into specified ranges. For example, the base voltage is selected such that the system voltage is normally close to unity.

Similarly, the base volt-ampere is usually selected as the kilovolt-ampere or megavolt-ampere rating of one of the machines or transformers in the system or a convenient round number such as 1, 10, 100, or 1000 MVA, depending on system size. As mentioned earlier, on determining the base volt-amperes and base voltages, the other base values are fixed. For example, current base can be determined as

$$I_B = \frac{S_B}{V_B} = \frac{\text{VA}_B}{V_B} \tag{4.18}$$

where
  I_B is the current base in amperes
  S_B is the selected volt-ampere base in volt-amperes
  V_B is the selected voltage base in volts

Note that

$$S_B = VA_B = P_B = Q_B = V_B I_B \tag{4.19}$$

Similarly, the impedance base* can be determined as

$$Z_B = \frac{V_B}{I_B} \tag{4.20}$$

where

$$Z_B = X_B = R_B \tag{4.21}$$

Similarly,

$$Y_B = B_B = G_B = \frac{I_B}{V_B} \tag{4.22}$$

Note that by substituting Equation 4.18 into Equation 4.20, the impedance base can be expressed as

$$Z_B = \frac{V_B}{VA_B/V_B} = \frac{V_B^2}{VA_B} \tag{4.23}$$

or

$$Z_B = \frac{(kV_B)^2}{MVA_B} \tag{4.24}$$

where
  kV_B is the voltage base in kilovolts
  MVA_B is the volt-ampere base in megavolt-amperes

The per-unit value of any quantity can be found by the *normalization process*, that is, by dividing the physical quantity by the base quantity of the same dimension. For example, the per-unit impedance can be expressed as

$$Z_{pu} = \frac{Z_{physical}}{Z_B} \tag{4.25}$$

or

$$Z_{pu} = \frac{Z_{physical}}{V_B^2/(kVA_B \times 1000)} \tag{4.26}$$

or

$$Z_{pu} = \frac{(Z_{physical})(kVA_B)(1000)}{V_B^2} \tag{4.27}$$

---

* It is defined as that impedance across which there is a voltage drop that is equal to the base voltage if the current through it is equal to the base current.

or

$$Z_{pu} = \frac{\left(Z_{physical}\right)\left(kVA_B\right)}{\left(kV_B\right)^2 \left(1000\right)} \tag{4.28}$$

or

$$Z_{pu} = \frac{\left(Z_{physical}\right)}{\left(kV_B\right)^2 / MVA_B} \tag{4.29}$$

or

$$Z_{pu} = \frac{\left(Z_{physical}\right)\left(MVA_B\right)}{\left(kV_B\right)^2} \tag{4.30}$$

Similarly, the others can be expressed as

$$I_{pu} = \frac{I_{physical}}{I_B} \tag{4.31}$$

or

$$V_{pu} = \frac{V_{physical}}{V_B} \tag{4.32}$$

or

$$kV_{pu} = \frac{kV_{physical}}{kV_B} \tag{4.33}$$

or

$$VA_{pu} = \frac{VA_{physical}}{VA_B} \tag{4.34}$$

or

$$kVA_{pu} = \frac{kVA_{physical}}{kVA_B} \tag{4.35}$$

or

$$MVA_{pu} = \frac{MVA_{physical}}{MVA_B} \tag{4.36}$$

Note that the base quantity is always a real number, whereas the physical quantity can be a complex number. For example, if the actual impedance quantity is given as $Z\angle\theta$ Ω, it can be expressed in the per-unit system as

$$\mathbf{Z}_{pu} = \frac{Z\angle\theta}{Z_B} = Z_{pu}\angle\theta \qquad (4.37)$$

that is, it is the magnitude expressed in per-unit terms. Alternatively, if the impedance has been given in rectangular form as

$$Z = R + jX \qquad (4.38)$$

then

$$\mathbf{Z}_{pu} = R_{pu} + jX_{pu} \qquad (4.39)$$

where

$$R_{pu} = \frac{R_{physical}}{Z_B} \qquad (4.40)$$

and

$$X_{pu} = \frac{X_{physical}}{Z_B} \qquad (4.41)$$

Similarly, if the complex power has been given as

$$S = P + jQ \qquad (4.42)$$

then

$$\mathbf{S}_{pu} = P_{pu} + jQ_{pu} \qquad (4.43)$$

where

$$P_{pu} = \frac{P_{physical}}{S_B} \qquad (4.44)$$

and

$$Q_{pu} = \frac{Q_{physical}}{S_B} \qquad (4.45)$$

If the actual voltage and current values are given as

$$\mathbf{V} = V\angle\theta_V \qquad (4.46)$$

and

$$\mathbf{I} = I \angle \theta_{\mathbf{I}} \tag{4.47}$$

the complex power can be expressed as

$$\mathbf{S} = \mathbf{VI}^* \tag{4.48}$$

or

$$S \angle \theta = \left(V \angle \theta_{\mathbf{V}} \right) \left(I \angle -\theta_{\mathbf{I}} \right) \tag{4.49}$$

Therefore, dividing through by S_B,

$$\frac{S \angle \theta}{S_B} = \frac{\left(V \angle \theta_{\mathbf{V}} \right) \left(I \angle -\theta_{\mathbf{I}} \right)}{S_B} \tag{4.50}$$

However,

$$S_B = V_B I_B \tag{4.51}$$

Thus,

$$\frac{S \angle \theta}{S_B} = \frac{\left(V \angle \theta_{\mathbf{V}} \right) \left(I \angle -\theta_{\mathbf{I}} \right)}{V_B I_B} \tag{4.52}$$

or

$$S_{\mathrm{pu}} \angle \theta = \left(V_{\mathrm{pu}} \angle \theta_{\mathbf{V}} \right) \left(I_{\mathrm{pu}} \angle -\theta_{\mathbf{I}} \right) \tag{4.53}$$

or

$$\mathbf{S}_{\mathrm{pu}} = \mathbf{V}_{\mathrm{pu}} \mathbf{I}_{\mathrm{pu}}^* \tag{4.54}$$

4.2.3.2 Converting from Per-Unit Values to Physical Values

The physical values (or system values) and per-unit values are related by the following relationships:

$$I = I_{\mathrm{pu}} \times I_B \tag{4.55}$$

$$V = V_{\mathrm{pu}} \times V_B \tag{4.56}$$

$$Z = Z_{\mathrm{pu}} \times Z_B \tag{4.57}$$

$$R = R_{\mathrm{pu}} \times Z_B \tag{4.58}$$

$$X = X_{pu} \times Z_B \tag{4.59}$$

$$S = VA = VA_{pu} \times VA_B \tag{4.60}$$

$$P = P_{pu} \times VA_B \tag{4.61}$$

$$Q = Q_{pu} \times VA_B \tag{4.62}$$

4.2.3.3 Change of Base

In general, the per-unit impedance of a power apparatus is given based on its own volt-ampere and voltage ratings and consequently based on its own impedance base. When such an apparatus is used in a system that has its own bases, it becomes necessary to refer all the given per-unit values to the system base values. Assume that the per-unit impedance of the apparatus is given based on its nameplate ratings as

$$Z_{pu(given)} = \left(Z_{physical}\right) \frac{MVA_{B(given)}}{\left[kV_{B(given)}\right]^2} \tag{4.63}$$

and that it is necessary to refer the very same physical impedance to a new set of voltage and volt-ampere bases such that

$$Z_{pu(new)} = \left(Z_{physical}\right) \frac{MVA_{B(new)}}{\left[kV_{B(new)}\right]^2} \tag{4.64}$$

By dividing Equation 4.63 by Equation 4.64 side by side,

$$Z_{pu(new)} = Z_{pu(given)} \left[\frac{MVA_{B(new)}}{MVA_{B(given)}}\right]\left[\frac{kV_{B(given)}}{kV_{B(new)}}\right]^2 \tag{4.65}$$

In certain situations, it is more convenient to use subscripts 1 and 2 instead of subscripts *given* and *new*, respectively. Equation 4.65 can be expressed as

$$Z_{pu(2)} = Z_{pu(1)} \left[\frac{MVA_{B(2)}}{MVA_{B(1)}}\right]\left[\frac{kV_{B(1)}}{kV_{B(2)}}\right]^2 \tag{4.66}$$

In the event that the kV bases are the same but the MVA bases are different, from Equation 4.65,

$$Z_{pu(new)} = Z_{pu(given)} \frac{MVA_{B(new)}}{MVA_{B(given)}} \tag{4.67}$$

Similarly, if the megavolt-ampere bases are the same but the kilovolt bases are different, from Equation 4.65,

$$Z_{\text{pu(new)}} = Z_{\text{pu(given)}} \left[\frac{kV_{B(\text{given})}}{kV_{B(\text{new})}} \right]^2 \tag{4.68}$$

Equations 4.65 through 4.68 must only be used to convert the given per-unit impedance from the base to another but not for referring the physical value of an impedance from one side of the transformer to another [3].

4.2.4 THREE-PHASE SYSTEMS

The three-phase problems involving balanced systems can be solved on a per-phase basis. In that case, the equations that are developed for single-phase systems can be used for three-phase systems as long as per-phase values are used consistently. Therefore,

$$I_B = \frac{S_{B(1\phi)}}{V_{B(\text{L-N})}} \tag{4.69}$$

or

$$I_B = \frac{VA_{B(1\phi)}}{V_{B(\text{L-N})}} \tag{4.70}$$

and

$$Z_B = \frac{V_{B(\text{L-N})}}{I_B} \tag{4.71}$$

or

$$Z_B = \frac{\left[kV_{B(\text{L-N})} \right]^2 (1000)}{kVA_{B(1\phi)}} \tag{4.72}$$

or

$$Z_B = \frac{\left[kV_{B(\text{L-N})} \right]^2}{MVA_{B(1\phi)}} \tag{4.73}$$

where the subscripts 1ϕ and L-N denote per phase and line to neutral, respectively. Note that, for a balanced system,

$$V_{B(\text{L-N})} = \frac{V_{B(\text{L-L})}}{\sqrt{3}} \tag{4.74}$$

and

$$S_{B(1\phi)} = \frac{S_{B(3\phi)}}{3} \qquad (4.75)$$

However, it has been customary in three-phase system analysis to use line-to-line voltage and three-phase volt-amperes as the base values. Therefore,

$$I_B = \frac{S_{B(3\phi)}}{\sqrt{3}V_{B(\text{L-L})}} \qquad (4.76)$$

or

$$I_B = \frac{kVA_{B(3\phi)}}{\sqrt{3}kV_{B(\text{L-L})}} \qquad (4.77)$$

and

$$Z_B = \frac{V_{B(\text{L-L})}}{\sqrt{3}I_B} \qquad (4.78)$$

$$Z_B = \frac{\left[kV_{B(\text{L-L})}\right]^2 (1000)}{kVA_{B(3\phi)}} \qquad (4.79)$$

or

$$Z_B = \frac{\left[kV_{B(\text{L-L})}\right]^2}{MVA_{B(3\phi)}} \qquad (4.80)$$

where the subscripts 3ϕ and L-L denote per three phase and line, respectively. Furthermore, base admittance can be expressed as

$$Y_B = \frac{1}{Z_B} \qquad (4.81)$$

or

$$Y_B = \frac{MVA_{B(3\phi)}}{\left[kV_{B(\text{L-L})}\right]^2} \qquad (4.82)$$

where

$$Y_B = B_B = G_B \qquad (4.83)$$

The data for transmission lines are usually given in terms of the line resistance R in ohms per mile at a given temperature, the line inductive reactance X_L in ohms per mile at 60 Hz, and the line shunt capacitive reactance X_c in megaohms per mile at 60 Hz. Therefore, the line impedance and shunt susceptance in per units for 1 mi of line can be expressed as*

$$\mathbf{Z}_{\text{pu}} = \left(\mathbf{Z}, \Omega/\text{mi} \right) \frac{\text{MVA}_{B(3\phi)}}{\left[kV_{B(\text{L-L})} \right]^2} \text{ pu} \tag{4.84}$$

where

$$\mathbf{Z} = R + jX_L = Z\angle\theta \ \Omega/\text{mi}$$

and

$$B_{\text{pu}} = \frac{\left[kV_{B(\text{L-L})} \right]^2 \times 10^{-6}}{\left[\text{MVA}_{B(3\phi)} \right]\left[X_c, \text{M}\Omega/\text{mi} \right]} \tag{4.85}$$

In the event that the admittance for a transmission line is given in microsiemens per mile, the per-unit admittance can be expressed as

$$Y_{\text{pu}} = \frac{\left[kV_{B(\text{L-L})} \right]^2 \left(Y, \mu S \right)}{\left[\text{MVA}_{B(3\phi)} \right] \times 10^6} \tag{4.86}$$

Similarly, if it is given as reciprocal admittance in megohms per mile, the per-unit admittance can be found as

$$Y_{\text{pu}} = \frac{\left[kV_{B(\text{L-L})} \right]^2 \times 10^{-6}}{\left[\text{MVA}_{B(3\phi)} \right]\left[Z, \text{M}\Omega/\text{mi} \right]} \tag{4.87}$$

Figure 4.3 shows conventional three-phase transformer connections and associated relationships between the HV- and LV-side voltages and currents. The given relationships are correct for a three-phase transformer as well as for a three-phase bank of single-phase transformers. Note that in the figure, n is the turns ratio, that is,

$$n = \frac{N_1}{N_2} = \frac{V_1}{V_2} = \frac{I_2}{I_1} \tag{4.88}$$

where the subscripts 1 and 2 are used for the primary and secondary sides. Therefore, an impedance Z_2 in the secondary circuit can be referred to the primary circuit provided that

$$Z_1 = n^2 Z_2 \tag{4.89}$$

---

* For further information, see Anderson [4].

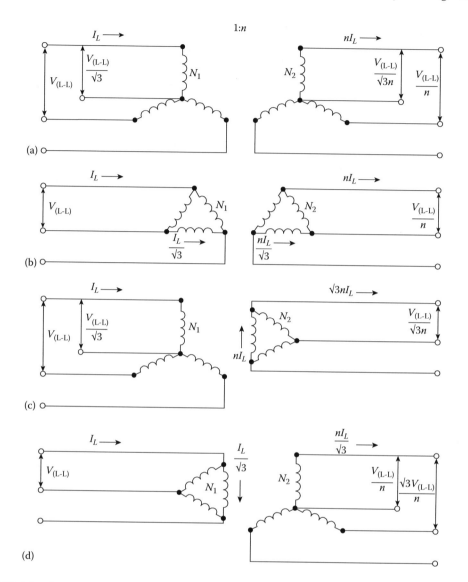

FIGURE 4.3 Conventional three-phase transformer connections: (a) wye–wye connection, (b) delta–delta connection, (c) wye–delta connection, and (d) delta–wye connection.

Thus, it can be observed from Figure 4.3 that in an ideal transformer, voltages are transformed in the direct ratio of turns, currents in the inverse ratio, and impedances in the direct ratio squared; and power and volt-amperes are, of course, unchanged. Note that a balanced delta-connected circuit of Z_Δ Ω/phase is equivalent to a balanced wye-connected circuit of Z_Y Ω/phase as long as

$$Z_Y = \frac{1}{3} Z_\Delta \tag{4.90}$$

The per-unit impedance of a transformer remains the same without taking into account whether it is converted from physical impedance values that are found by referring to the HV side or LV side of the transformer. This can be accomplished by choosing separate appropriate bases for each side of the transformer (whether or not the transformer is connected in wye–wye, delta–delta, delta–wye, or wye–delta since the transformation of voltages is the same as that made by wye–wye transformers as long as the same line-to-line voltage ratings are used).* In other words, the designated per-unit impedance values of transformers are based on the coil ratings.

Since the ratings of coils cannot alter by a simple change in connection (e.g., from wye–wye to delta–wye), the per-unit impedance remains the same regardless of the three-phase connection. The line-to-line voltage for the transformer will differ. Because of the method of choosing the base in various sections of the three-phase system, the per-unit impedances calculated in various sections can be put together on one impedance diagram without paying any attention to whether the transformers are connected in wye–wye or delta–wye.

Example 4.2

A three-phase transformer has a nameplate rating of 20 MVA, 345Y/34.5Y kV with a leakage reactance of 12% and the transformer connection is wye–wye. Select a base of 20 MVA and 345 kV on the HV side and determine the following:

(a) Reactance of transformer in per units
(b) HV-side base impedance
(c) LV-side base impedance
(d) Transformer reactance referred to the HV side in ohms
(e) Transformer reactance referred to the LV side in ohms

Solution

(a) The reactance of the transformer in per units is 12/100, or 0.12 pu. Note that it is the same whether it is referred to the HV or the LV sides.
(b) The HV-side base impedance is

$$Z_{B(HV)} = \frac{\left[kV_{B(HV)}\right]^2}{MVA_{B(3\phi)}}$$

$$= \frac{345^2}{20} = 5951.25\ \Omega$$

(c) The LV-side base impedance is

$$Z_{B(LV)} = \frac{\left[kV_{B(LV)}\right]^2}{MVA_{B(3\phi)}}$$

$$= \frac{34.5^2}{20} = 59.5125\ \Omega$$

(d) The reactance referred to the HV side is

$$X_{(HV)} = X_{pu} \times X_{B(HV)}$$
$$= (0.12)(5951.25) = 714.15\ \Omega$$

(e) The reactance referred to the LV side is

$$X_{(LV)} = X_{pu} \times X_{B(LV)}$$
$$= (0.12)(59.5125) = 7.1415\ \Omega$$

---

* This subject has been explained in greater depth in an excellent review by Stevenson [3].

or, from Equation 4.89,

$$X_{(LV)} = \frac{X_{(HV)}}{n^2}$$

$$= \frac{714.15 \, \Omega}{\left(\dfrac{345/\sqrt{3}}{34.5/\sqrt{3}}\right)^2} = 7.1415 \, \Omega$$

where n is defined as the turns ratio of the windings.

Example 4.3

A three-phase transformer has a nameplate rating of 20 MVA, and the voltage ratings of 345Y/34.5Δ kV with a leakage reactance of 12% and the transformer connection is wye–delta. Select a base of 20 MVA and 345 kV on the HV side and determine the following:

(a) Turns ratio of windings
(b) Transformer reactance referred to the LV side in ohms
(c) Transformer reactance referred to the LV side in per units

Solution

(a) The turns ratio of the windings is

$$n = \frac{345/\sqrt{3}}{34.5} = 5.7735$$

(b) Since the HV-side impedance base is

$$Z_{B(HV)} = \frac{\left[kV_{B(HV)}\right]^2}{MVA_{B(3\phi)}}$$

$$= \frac{345^2}{20} = 5951.25 \, \Omega$$

and

$$X_{(HV)} = X_{pu} \times X_{B(HV)}$$
$$= (0.12)(5951.25) = 714.15 \, \Omega$$

the transformer reactance referred to the delta-connected LV side is

$$X_{(LV)} = \frac{X_{(HV)}}{n^2}$$

$$= \frac{714.14 \, \Omega}{5.7735^2} = 21.4245 \, \Omega$$

(c) From Equation 4.90, the reactance of the equivalent wye connection is

$$Z_Y = \frac{Z_\Delta}{3}$$

$$= \frac{21.4245 \, \Omega}{3} = 7.1415 \, \Omega$$

Similarly,

$$Z_{B(LV)} = \frac{\left[kV_{B(LV)} \right]^2}{MVA_{B(3\phi)}}$$

$$= \frac{34.5^2}{20} = 59.5125 \ \Omega$$

Thus,

$$X_{pu} = \frac{7.1415 \ \Omega}{Z_{B(LV)}}$$

$$= \frac{7.1415 \ \Omega}{59.5125 \ \Omega} = 0.12 \ pu$$

Alternatively, if the line-to-line voltages are used,

$$X_{(LV)} = \frac{X_{(HV)}}{n^2}$$

$$= \frac{714.14 \ \Omega}{\left[345/\sqrt{3}(34.5) \right]^2} = 21.4245 \ \Omega$$

and therefore,

$$X_{pu} = \frac{X_{(LV)}}{Z_{B(LV)}}$$

$$= \frac{7.1415 \ \Omega}{59.5125 \ \Omega} = 0.12 \ pu$$

as before.

Example 4.4

Figure 4.4 shows a one-line diagram of a three-phase system. Assume that the line length between the two transformers is negligible and the three-phase generator is rated 4160 kVA, 2.4 kV, and 1000 A and that it supplies a purely inductive load of $I_{pu} = 2.08\angle{-90°}$ pu. The three-phase transformer T_1 is rated 6000 kVA, 2.4Y–24Y kV, with leakage reactance of 0.04 pu. Transformer T_2 is made up of three single-phase transformers and is rated 4000 kVA, 24Y–12Y kV, with leakage reactance of 0.04 pu. Determine the following for all three circuits, 2.4, 24, and 12 kV circuits:

(a) Base kilovolt-ampere values.
(b) Base line-to-line kilovolt values.
(c) Base impedance values.
(d) Base current values.
(e) Physical current values (neglect magnetizing currents in transformers and charging currents in lines).
(f) Per-unit current values.
(g) New transformer reactances based on their new bases.
(h) Per-unit voltage values at buses 1, 2, and 4.
(i) Per-unit apparent power values at buses 1, 2, and 4.
(j) Summarize results in a table.

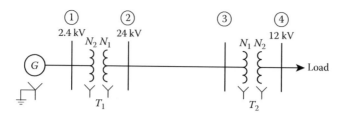

FIGURE 4.4 The one-line diagram for Example 4.4.

Solution

(a) The kilovolt-ampere base for all three circuits is arbitrarily selected as 2080 kVA.

(b) The base voltage for the 2.4 kV circuit is arbitrarily selected as 2.5 kV. Since the turns ratios for transformers T_1 and T_2 are

$$\frac{N_1}{N_2} = 10 \quad \text{or} \quad \frac{N_2}{N_1} = 0.10$$

and

$$\frac{N_1'}{N_2'} = 2$$

the base voltages for the 24 and 12 kV circuits are determined to be 25 and 12.5 kV, respectively.

(c) The base impedance values can be found as

$$Z_B = \frac{\left[kV_{B(L-L)}\right]^2 (1000)}{kVA_{B(3\phi)}}$$

$$= \frac{\left[2.5 \, kV\right]^2 1000}{2080 \, kVA} = 3.005 \, \Omega$$

and

$$Z_B = \frac{\left[25 \, kV\right]^2 1000}{2080 \, kVA} = 300.5 \, \Omega$$

and

$$Z_B = \frac{\left[12.5 \, kV\right]^2 1000}{2080 \, kVA} = 75.1 \, \Omega$$

(d) The base current values can be determined as

$$I_B = \frac{kVA_{B(3\phi)}}{\sqrt{3}kV_{B(L-L)}}$$

$$= \frac{2080 \, kVA}{\sqrt{3}\left(2.5 \, kV\right)} = 480 \, A$$

and

$$I_B = \frac{2080 \text{ kVA}}{\sqrt{3}\,(25 \text{ kV})} = 48 \text{ A}$$

and

$$I_B = \frac{2080 \text{ kVA}}{\sqrt{3}\,(12.5 \text{ kV})} = 96 \text{ A}$$

(e) The physical current values can be found based on the turns ratios as

$$I = 1000 \text{ A}$$

$$I = \left(\frac{N_2}{N_1}\right)(1000 \text{ A}) = 100 \text{ A}$$

$$I = \left(\frac{N'_1}{N'_2}\right)(100 \text{ A}) = 200 \text{ A}$$

(f) The per-unit current values are the same, 2.08 pu, for all three circuits.
(g) The given transformer reactances can be converted based on their new bases using

$$Z_{pu(new)} = Z_{pu(given)} \left[\frac{\text{kVA}_{B(new)}}{\text{kVA}_{B(given)}}\right] \left[\frac{\text{kV}_{B(given)}}{\text{kV}_{B(new)}}\right]^2$$

Therefore, the new reactances of the two transformers can be found as

$$Z_{pu(T_1)} = j0.04 \left[\frac{2080 \text{ kVA}}{6000 \text{ kVA}}\right] \left[\frac{2.4 \text{ kV}}{2.5 \text{ kV}}\right]^2 = j0.0128 \text{ pu}$$

and

$$Z_{pu(T_2)} = j0.04 \left[\frac{2080 \text{ kVA}}{4000 \text{ kVA}}\right] \left[\frac{12 \text{ kV}}{12.5 \text{ kV}}\right]^2 = j0.0192 \text{ pu}$$

(h) Therefore, the per-unit voltage values at buses 1, 2, and 4 can be calculated as

$$\mathbf{V}_1 = \frac{2.4 \text{ kV}\angle 0°}{2.5 \text{ kV}} = 0.96\angle 0° \text{ pu}$$

$$\mathbf{V}_2 = \mathbf{V}_1 - \mathbf{I}_{pu}\mathbf{Z}_{pu(T_1)}$$

$$= 0.96\angle 0° - (2.08\angle -90°)(0.0128\angle 90°) = 0.9334\angle 0° \text{ pu}$$

$$\mathbf{V}_4 = \mathbf{V}_2 - \mathbf{I}_{pu}\mathbf{Z}_{pu(T_2)}$$

$$= 0.9334\angle 0° - (2.08\angle -90°)(0.0192\angle 90°) = 0.8935\angle 0° \text{ pu}$$

TABLE 4.2
Results of Example 4.4

Quantity	2.4 kV Circuit	24 kV Circuit	12 kV Circuit
$kVA_{B(3\phi)}$	2080 kVA	2080 kVA	2080 kVA
$kV_{B(L-L)}$	2.5 kV	25 kV	12.5 kV
Z_B	3.005 Ω	300.5 Ω	75.1 Ω
I_B	480 A	48 A	96 A
$I_{physical}$	1000 A	100 A	200 A
I_{pu}	2.08 pu	2.08 pu	2.08 pu
V_{pu}	0.96 pu	0.9334 pu	0.8935 pu
S_{pu}	2.00 pu	1.9415 pu	1.8585 pu

(i) Thus, the per-unit apparent power values at buses 1, 2, and 4 are

$$S_1 = 2.00 \text{ pu}$$

$$S_2 = V_2 I_{pu} = (0.9334)(2.08) = 1.9415 \text{ pu}$$

$$S_4 = V_4 I_{pu} = (0.8935)(2.08) = 1.8585 \text{ pu}$$

(j) The results are summarized in Table 4.2.

4.2.5 CONSTANT-IMPEDANCE REPRESENTATION OF LOADS

Usually, the power system loads are represented by their real and reactive powers, as shown in Figure 4.5a. However, it is possible to represent the same load in terms of series or parallel combinations of its equivalent constant-load resistance and reactance values, as shown in Figure 4.5b and c, respectively [4].

In the event that the load is represented by the series connection, the equivalent constant impedance can be expressed as

$$\mathbf{Z}_s = R_s + jX_s \tag{4.91}$$

where

$$R_s = \frac{|\mathbf{V}|^2 \times P}{P^2 + Q^2} \tag{4.92}$$

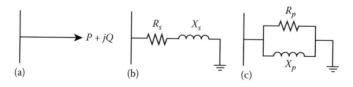

FIGURE 4.5 Load representations as (a) real and reactive powers, (b) constant impedance in terms of series combination, and (c) constant impedance in terms of parallel combination.

$$X_s = \frac{|\mathbf{V}|^2 \times Q}{P^2 + Q^2} \tag{4.93}$$

where
  R_s is the load resistance in series connection in ohms
  X_s is the load reactance in series connection in ohms
  $\mathbf{Z}_s$ is the constant-load impedance in ohms
  V is the load voltage in volts
  P is the real, or average, load power in watts
  Q is the reactive load power in vars

The constant impedance in per units can be expressed as

$$\mathbf{Z}_{\text{pu}(s)} = R_{\text{pu}(s)} + jX_{\text{pu}(s)} \text{ pu} \tag{4.94}$$

where

$$R_{\text{pu}(s)} = \left(P_{\text{physical}}\right) \frac{S_B \times \left(V_{\text{pu}}\right)^2}{P^2 + Q^2} \text{ pu} \tag{4.95}$$

$$X_{\text{pu}(s)} = \left(Q_{\text{physical}}\right) \frac{S_B \times \left(V_{\text{pu}}\right)^2}{P^2 + Q^2} \text{ pu} \tag{4.96}$$

If the load is represented by the parallel connection, the equivalent constant impedance can be expressed as

$$\mathbf{Z}_p = j\frac{R_p \times X_p}{R_p + X_p} \tag{4.97}$$

where

$$R_p = \frac{V^2}{P}$$

$$X_p = \frac{V^2}{Q}$$

where
  R_p is the load resistance in parallel connection in ohms
  X_p is the load reactance in parallel connection in ohms
  $\mathbf{Z}_p$ is the constant-load impedance in ohms

The constant impedance in per units can be expressed as

$$\mathbf{Z}_{\mathrm{pu}(p)} = j \frac{R_{\mathrm{pu}(p)} \times X_{\mathrm{pu}(p)}}{R_{\mathrm{pu}(p)} + X_{\mathrm{pu}(p)}} \ \mathrm{pu} \tag{4.98}$$

where

$$R_{\mathrm{pu}(p)} = \frac{S_B}{P} \left(\frac{V}{V_B} \right)^2 \ \mathrm{pu} \tag{4.99}$$

or

$$R_{\mathrm{pu}(p)} = \frac{V_{\mathrm{pu}}^2}{P_{\mathrm{pu}}} \ \mathrm{pu} \tag{4.100}$$

and

$$X_{\mathrm{pu}(p)} = \frac{S_B}{Q} \left(\frac{V}{V_B} \right)^2 \ \mathrm{pu} \tag{4.101}$$

or

$$X_{\mathrm{pu}(p)} = \frac{V_{\mathrm{pu}}^2}{Q_{\mathrm{pu}}} \ \mathrm{pu} \tag{4.102}$$

4.3 THREE-WINDING TRANSFORMERS

Figure 4.6a shows a single-phase three-winding transformer. They are usually used in the bulk power (transmission) substations to reduce the transmission voltage to the subtransmission voltage level. If excitation impedance is neglected, the equivalent circuit of a three-winding transformer can be represented by a wye of impedances, as shown in Figure 4.6b, where the primary, secondary, and tertiary windings are denoted by P, S, and T, respectively.

Note that the common point 0 is fictitious and is not related to the neutral of the system. The tertiary windings of a three-phase and three-winding transformer bank is usually connected in delta

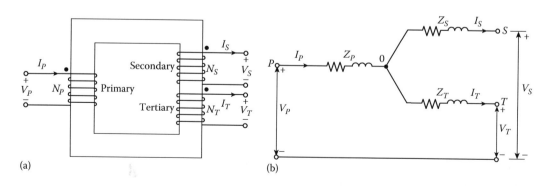

(a)   (b)

FIGURE 4.6 A single-phase three-winding transformer: (a) winding diagram and (b) equivalent circuit.

and may be used for (1) providing a path for zero-sequence currents, (2) in-plant power distribution, and (3) application of power-factor-correcting capacitors or reactors. The impedance of any of the branches shown in Figure 4.6b can be determined by considering the short-circuit impedance between pairs of windings with the third open. Therefore,

$$Z_{PS} = Z_P + Z_S \tag{4.103a}$$

$$Z_{TS} = Z_T + Z_S \tag{4.103b}$$

$$Z_{PT} = Z_P + Z_T \tag{4.103c}$$

$$Z_P = \frac{1}{2}\left(Z_{PS} + Z_{PT} - Z_{TS}\right) \tag{4.104a}$$

$$Z_S = \frac{1}{2}\left(Z_{PS} + Z_{TS} - Z_{PT}\right) \tag{4.104b}$$

$$Z_T = \frac{1}{2}\left(Z_{PT} + Z_{TS} - Z_{PS}\right) \tag{4.104c}$$

where
Z_{PS} is the leakage impedance measured in primary with secondary short circuited and tertiary open
Z_{PT} is the leakage impedance measured in primary with tertiary short circuited and secondary open
Z_{TS} is the leakage impedance measured in secondary with tertiary short circuited and primary open
Z_P is the impedance of primary winding
Z_S is the impedance of secondary winding
Z_T is the impedance of tertiary winding

In most large transformers, the value of Z_S is very small and can be negative. Contrary to the situation with a two-winding transformer, the kilovolt-ampere ratings of the three windings of a three-winding transformer bank are not usually equal. Therefore, all impedances, as defined earlier, should be expressed on the same kilovolt-ampere base. For three-winding three-phase transformer banks with delta- or wye-connected windings, the positive- and negative-sequence diagrams are always the same. The corresponding zero-sequence diagrams are shown in Figure 9.10.

4.4 AUTOTRANSFORMERS

Figure 4.7a shows a two-winding transformer. Viewed from the terminals, the same transformation of voltages, currents, and impedances can be obtained with the connection shown in Figure 4.7b. Therefore, in the autotransformer, only one winding is used per phase, the secondary voltage being tapped off the primary winding, as shown in Figure 4.7b. The *common winding* is the winding between the LV terminals, whereas the remainder of the winding, belonging exclusively to the HV circuit, is called the *series winding* and, combined with the common winding, forms the *series-common winding* between the HV terminals.

In a sense, an autotransformer is just a normal two-winding transformer connected in a special way. The only structural difference is that the series winding must have extra insulation. In a *variable autotransformer*, the tap is movable. Autotransformers are increasingly used to interconnect two HV transmission lines operating at different voltages. An autotransformer has two separate sets of ratios, namely, circuit ratios and winding ratios. For circuit ratios, consider the equivalent circuit

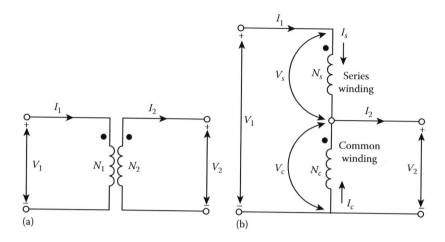

FIGURE 4.7   Schematic diagram of ideal (step-down) transformer connected as (a) two-winding transformer and (b) autotransformer.

of an ideal autotransformer (neglecting losses) shown in Figure 4.7b. Viewed from the terminals, the voltage and current ratios can be expressed as

$$a = \frac{V_1}{V_2} = \frac{N_1}{N_2} \tag{4.105a}$$

$$= \frac{N_c + N_s}{N_c} = \frac{N_1}{N_2} \tag{4.105b}$$

since

$$I_1 = \frac{I_2}{a} = \frac{N_2}{N_1} I_2$$

$$a = \frac{I_2}{I_1} = \frac{N_c + N_s}{N_c} \tag{4.105c}$$

and

$$a = \frac{I_2}{I_1} \tag{4.106}$$

From Equation 4.105c, it can be observed that the ratio a is always larger than 1.

For winding ratios, consider the voltages and currents of the series and common windings, as shown in Figure 4.7b. Therefore, the voltage and current ratios can be expressed as

$$\frac{V_s}{V_c} = \frac{N_s}{N_c} \tag{4.107}$$

and

$$\frac{I_c}{I_s} = \frac{I_2 - I_1}{I_1} \tag{4.108a}$$

$$= \frac{I_2}{I_1} - 1 \tag{4.108b}$$

From Equation 4.105c,

$$\frac{N_s}{N_c} = a - 1 \qquad (4.109)$$

Therefore, substituting Equation 4.109 into Equation 4.107 yields

$$\frac{V_s}{V_c} = a - 1 \qquad (4.110)$$

Similarly, substituting Equations 4.106 and (4.109) into Equation 4.108b simultaneously yields

$$\frac{I_c}{I_s} = a - 1 \qquad (4.111)$$

For an ideal autotransformer, the volt-ampere ratings of circuits and windings can be expressed, respectively, as

$$S_{\text{circuits}} = V_1 I_1 = V_2 I_2 \qquad (4.112)$$

and

$$S_{\text{windings}} = V_s I_s = V_c I_c \qquad (4.113)$$

The advantages of autotransformers are lower leakage reactances, lower losses, smaller exciting currents, and less cost than two-winding transformers when the voltage ratio does not vary too greatly from 1 to 1. For example, if the same core and coils are used as a two-winding transformer and as an autotransformer, the ratio of the capacity as an autotransformer to the capacity as a two-winding transformer can be expressed as

$$\frac{\text{Capacity as autotransformer}}{\text{Capacity as two-winding transformer}} = \frac{V_1 I_1}{V_s I_s} = \frac{V_1 I_1}{\left(V_1 - V_2\right) I_1} = \frac{a}{a - 1} \qquad (4.114)$$

Therefore, maximum advantage is obtained with relatively small difference between the voltages on the two sides (e.g., 161 kV/138 kV, 500 kV/700 kV, and 500 kV/345 kV). Therefore, a large saving in size, weight, the cost can be achieved over a two-windings-per-phase transformer. The disadvantages of an autotransformer are that there is no electrical isolation between the primary and secondary circuits and there is a greater short-circuit current than the one for the two-winding transformer.

Three-phase autotransformer banks generally have wye-connected main windings, the neutral of which is normally connected solidly to the earth. In addition, it is a common practice to include a third winding connected in delta, called the tertiary winding.

An autotransformer is never used as a distribution transformer because the lack of isolation can cause dangerously high voltages in a customer's location if the neutral opens. Autotransformers are generally used for transforming one transmission voltage to another when the ratio is 2:1 or less. They are used in a transmission substation to transform from one HV to another HV or from a transmission voltage to a substation voltage. They are normally connected in wye with the neutral solidly grounded, having a delta-connected tertiary for harmonic suppression.

The tertiary is also used to provide a supply of distribution voltage at the station. Autotransformers are better than two-winding transformers of the same MVA rating in terms of lower cost, smaller size and less weight, better regulation, and cooling requirements. Their main disadvantage is that their impedances are low. Because of this, in the event of a fault, the fault currents are higher than the faults would be for the equivalent two-winding transformers.

4.5 DELTA–WYE AND WYE–DELTA TRANSFORMATIONS

The three-terminal circuits encountered so often in networks are the delta and wye* configurations, as shown in Figure 4.8. In some problems, it is necessary to convert delta to wye or vice versa. If the impedances $\mathbf{Z}_{ab}$, $\mathbf{Z}_{bc}$, and $\mathbf{Z}_{ca}$ are connected in delta, the equivalent wye impedances $\mathbf{Z}_a$, $\mathbf{Z}_b$, and $\mathbf{Z}_c$ are

$$\mathbf{Z}_a = \frac{\mathbf{Z}_{ab}\mathbf{Z}_{ca}}{\mathbf{Z}_{ab} + \mathbf{Z}_{bc} + \mathbf{Z}_{ca}} \tag{4.115}$$

$$\mathbf{Z}_b = \frac{\mathbf{Z}_{ab}\mathbf{Z}_{bc}}{\mathbf{Z}_{ab} + \mathbf{Z}_{bc} + \mathbf{Z}_{ca}} \tag{4.116}$$

$$\mathbf{Z}_c = \frac{\mathbf{Z}_{bc}\mathbf{Z}_{ca}}{\mathbf{Z}_{ab} + \mathbf{Z}_{bc} + \mathbf{Z}_{ca}} \tag{4.117}$$

If $\mathbf{Z}_{ab} = \mathbf{Z}_{bc} = \mathbf{Z}_{ca} = \mathbf{Z}$,

$$\mathbf{Z}_a = \mathbf{Z}_b = \mathbf{Z}_c = \frac{\mathbf{Z}}{3} \tag{4.118}$$

On the other hand, if the impedances $\mathbf{Z}_a$, $\mathbf{Z}_b$, and $\mathbf{Z}_c$ are connected in wye, the equivalent delta impedances $\mathbf{Z}_{ab}$, $\mathbf{Z}_{bc}$, and $\mathbf{Z}_{ca}$ are

$$\mathbf{Z}_{ab} = \mathbf{Z}_a + \mathbf{Z}_b + \frac{\mathbf{Z}_a\mathbf{Z}_b}{\mathbf{Z}_c} \tag{4.119}$$

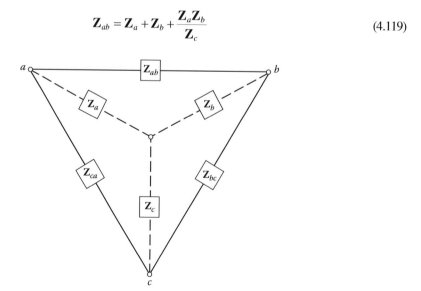

FIGURE 4.8   Delta-to-wye or wye-to-delta transformations.

---

* In Europe, it is called the *star configuration*.

$$\mathbf{Z}_{bc} = \mathbf{Z}_b + \mathbf{Z}_c + \frac{\mathbf{Z}_b\mathbf{Z}_c}{\mathbf{Z}_a} \tag{4.120}$$

$$\mathbf{Z}_{ca} = \mathbf{Z}_c + \mathbf{Z}_a + \frac{\mathbf{Z}_c\mathbf{Z}_a}{\mathbf{Z}_b} \tag{4.121}$$

If $\mathbf{Z}_a = \mathbf{Z}_b = \mathbf{Z}_c = \mathbf{Z}$,

$$\mathbf{Z}_{ab} = \mathbf{Z}_{bc} = \mathbf{Z}_{ca} = 3\mathbf{Z} \tag{4.122}$$

4.6 TRANSMISSION-LINE CONSTANTS

For the purpose of system analysis, a given transmission line can be represented by its resistance, inductance or inductive reactance, capacitance or capacitive reactance, and leakage resistance (which is usually negligible).

4.7 RESISTANCE

The dc resistance of a conductor is

$$R_{dc} = \frac{\rho l}{A} \ \Omega \tag{4.123}$$

where
  ρ is the conductor resistivity
  l is the conductor length
  A is the conductor cross-sectional area

In practice, several different sets of units are used in the calculation of the resistance. For example, in the International System of Units (SI units), l is in meters, A is in square meters, and ρ is in ohmmeters. However, in power systems in the United States, ρ is in ohm-circular-mils per foot, l is in feet, and A is in circular mils.

The resistance of a conductor at any temperature may be determined by

$$\frac{R_2}{R_1} = \frac{T_0 + t_2}{T_0 + t_1} \tag{4.124}$$

where
  R_1 is the conductor resistance at temperature t_1
  R_2 is the conductor resistance at temperature t_2
  t_1, t_2 is the conductor temperatures in degrees Celsius
  T_0 is the constant varying with conductor material
    = 234.5 for annealed copper
    = 241 for hard-drawn copper
    = 228 for hard-drawn aluminum

The phenomenon by which ac tends to flow in the outer layer of a conductor is called *skin effect*. Skin effect is a function of conductor size, frequency, and the relative resistance of the conductor material.

Tables given in Appendix A provide the dc and ac resistance values for various conductors. The resistances to be used in the positive- and negative-sequence networks are the ac resistances of the conductors.

4.8 INDUCTANCE AND INDUCTIVE REACTANCE

4.8.1 SINGLE-PHASE OVERHEAD LINES

Figure 4.9 shows a single-phase OH line. Assume that a current flows out in conductor a and returns in conductor b. These currents cause magnetic field lines that link between the conductors. A change in current causes a change in flux, which in turn results in an induced voltage in the circuit. In an ac circuit, this induced voltage is called the IX drop. In going around the loop, if R is the resistance of each conductor, the total loss in voltage due to resistance is $2IR$. Therefore, the voltage drop in the single-phase line due to loop impedance at 60 Hz is

$$\text{VD} = 2l\left(R + j0.2794\log_{10}\frac{D_m}{D_s}\right)I \tag{4.125}$$

where
  VD is the voltage drop due to line impedance in volts
  l is the line length in miles
  R is the resistance of each conductor in ohms per mile
  D_m is the equivalent or geometric mean distance (GMD) between conductor centers in inches
  D_s is the geometric mean radius (GMR) or self-GMD of one conductor in inches, $= 0.7788r$ for cylindrical conductor
  r is the radius of cylindrical conductor in inches (see Figure 4.9)
  I is the phase current in amperes

Therefore, the inductance of the conductor is expressed as

$$L = 2\times10^{-7}\ln\frac{D_m}{D_s}\ \text{H/m} \tag{4.126}$$

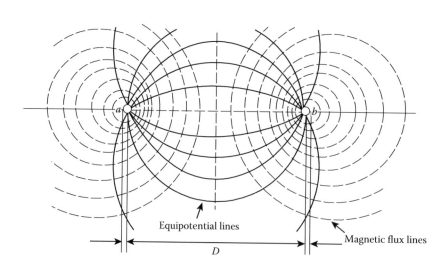

FIGURE 4.9   Magnetic field of single-phase line.

or

$$L = 0.7411 \log_{10} \frac{D_m}{D_s} \text{ mH/mi} \tag{4.127}$$

With the inductance known, the inductive reactance* can be found as

$$X_L = 2\pi f L = 2.02 \times 10^{-3} f \ln \frac{D_m}{D_s} \tag{4.128}$$

or

$$X_L = 4.657 \times 10^{-3} f \log_{10} \frac{D_m}{D_s} \tag{4.129}$$

or, at 60 Hz,

$$X_L = 0.2794 \log_{10} \frac{D_m}{D_s} \text{ } \Omega/\text{mi} \tag{4.130}$$

$$X_L = 0.1213 \ln \frac{D_m}{D_s} \text{ } \Omega/\text{mi} \tag{4.131}$$

By using the GMR of a conductor, D_s, the calculation of inductance and inductive reactance can be done easily. Tables give the GMR of various conductors readily.

4.8.2 THREE-PHASE OVERHEAD LINES

In general, the spacings D_{ab}, D_{bc}, and D_{ca} between the conductors of three-phase transmission lines are not equal. For any given conductor configuration, the average values of inductance and capacitance can be found by representing the system by one with equivalent equilateral spacing. The *equivalent spacing* is calculated as

$$D_{eq} \triangleq D_m = \left(D_{ab} \times D_{bc} \times D_{ca} \right)^{1/3} \tag{4.132}$$

In practice, the conductors of a transmission line are transposed, as shown in Figure 4.10. The transposition operation, that is, exchanging the conductor positions, is usually carried out at switching stations.

Therefore, the average inductance per phase is

$$L_a = 2 \times 10^{-7} \ln \frac{D_{eq}}{D_s} \text{ H/m} \tag{4.133}$$

or

$$L_a = 0.7411 \log_{10} \frac{D_{eq}}{D_s} \text{ mH/mi} \tag{4.134}$$

---

* It is also the same as the positive and negative sequence of a line.

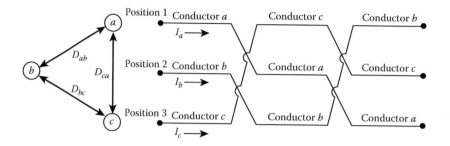

FIGURE 4.10   A complete transposition cycle of three-phase line.

and the inductive reactance is

$$X_L = 0.1213 \ln \frac{D_{eq}}{D_s} \ \Omega/\text{mi}$$

(4.135)

or

$$X_L = 0.2794 \log_{10} \frac{D_{eq}}{D_s} \ \Omega/\text{mi}$$

(4.136)

4.9 CAPACITANCE AND CAPACITIVE REACTANCE

4.9.1 Single-Phase Overhead Lines

Figure 4.11 shows a single-phase line with two identical parallel conductors a and b of radius r separated by a distance D, center to center, and with a potential difference of V_{ab} in volts. Let conductors a and b carry charges of $+q_a$ and $-q_b$ in farads per meter, respectively. The capacitance between conductors can be found as

$$C_{ab} = \frac{q_a}{V_{ab}}$$

$$= \frac{2\pi\varepsilon}{\ln\left(\dfrac{D^2}{r_a \times r_b}\right)} \ \text{F/m}$$

(4.137)

If $r_a = r_b = r$,

$$C_{ab} = \frac{2\pi\varepsilon}{2\ln\left(\dfrac{D}{r}\right)} \ \text{F/m}$$

(4.138)

Since

$$\varepsilon = \varepsilon_0 \times \varepsilon_r$$

where

$$\varepsilon_0 = \frac{1}{36\pi \times 10^9} = 8.85 \times 10^{-12} \ \text{F/m}$$

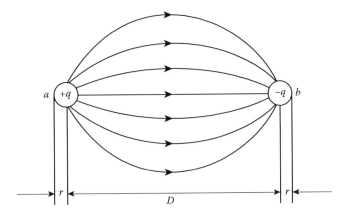

FIGURE 4.11 Capacitance of single-phase line.

and

$$\varepsilon_r \cong 1 \quad \text{for air,}$$

Equation 4.138 becomes

$$C_{ab} = \frac{0.0388}{2\log_{10}\left(\dfrac{D}{r}\right)} \ \mu\text{F/mi} \tag{4.139}$$

or

$$C_{ab} = \frac{0.0894}{2\ln\left(\dfrac{D}{r}\right)} \ \mu\text{F/mi} \tag{4.140}$$

or

$$C_{ab} = \frac{0.0241}{2\log_{10}\left(\dfrac{D}{r}\right)} \ \mu\text{F/km} \tag{4.141}$$

Stevenson [3] explains that the capacitance to neutral or capacitance to ground for the two-wire line is twice the line-to-line capacitance or capacitance between conductors, as shown in Figures 4.12 and 4.13. Therefore, the line-to-neutral capacitance is

$$C_N = C_{aN} = C_{bN} = \frac{0.0388}{\log_{10}\left(\dfrac{D}{r}\right)} \ \mu\text{F/mi} \ \text{ to neutral} \tag{4.142}$$

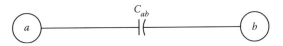

FIGURE 4.12 Line-to-line capacitance.

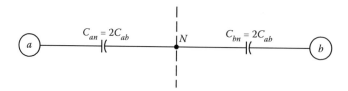

FIGURE 4.13 Line-to-neutral capacitance.

This can easily be verified since C_N must equal $2C_{ab}$ so that the capacitance between the conductors can be

$$C_{ab} = \frac{C_N \times C_N}{C_N + C_N}$$

$$= \frac{C_N}{2}$$

$$= C_{ab} \text{ as before}$$

(4.143)

With the capacitance known, the capacitive reactance between one conductor and neutral can be found as

$$X_c = \frac{1}{2\pi f C_N}$$

(4.144)

or, for 60 Hz,

$$X_c = 0.06836 \log_{10} \frac{D}{r} \text{ M}\Omega \text{ mi to neutral}$$

(4.145)

and the line-to-neutral susceptance is

$$b_c = \omega C_N$$

or

$$b_c = \frac{1}{X_c}$$

(4.146)

or

$$b_c = \frac{14.6272}{\log_{10}\left(\dfrac{D}{r}\right)} \text{ m}\Omega/\text{mi to neutral}$$

(4.147)

The charging current of the line is

$$\mathbf{I}_c = j\omega C_{ab} V_{ab} \text{ A/mi}$$

(4.148)

4.9.2 THREE-PHASE OVERHEAD LINES

Figure 4.14 shows the cross section of a three-phase line with equilateral spacing D. The line-to-neutral capacitance can be found as

$$C_N = \frac{0.0388}{\log_{10}\left(\dfrac{D}{r}\right)} \ \mu\text{F/mi to neutral} \tag{4.149}$$

which is identical to Equation 4.142.

On the other hand, if the spacings between the conductors of the three-phase line are not equal, the line-to-neutral capacitance is

$$C_N = \frac{0.0388}{\log_{10}\left(\dfrac{D_{eq}}{r}\right)} \ \mu\text{F/mi to neutral} \tag{4.150}$$

where

$$D_{eq} \triangleq D_m = \left(D_{ab} \times D_{bc} \times D_{ca}\right)^{1/3}$$

The charging current per phase is

$$\mathbf{I}_c = j\omega C_N V_{an} \ \text{A/mi} \tag{4.151}$$

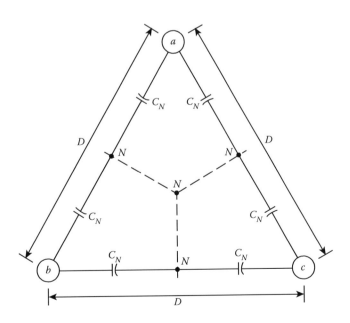

FIGURE 4.14 Three-phase line with equilateral spacing.

4.10 TABLES OF LINE CONSTANTS

Tables provide the line constants directly without using equations for calculation. This concept was suggested by W. A. Lewis [6]. According to this concept, Equation 4.131 for inductive reactance at 60 Hz, that is,

$$X_L = 0.1213 \ln \frac{D_m}{D_s} \ \Omega/\text{mi}$$

can be broken down to

$$X_L = 0.1213 \ln \frac{1}{D_s} + 0.1213 \ln D_m \ \Omega/\text{mi} \tag{4.152}$$

where
  D_s is the GMR, which can be found from the tables for a given conductor
  D_m is the GMD between conductor centers

Therefore, Equation 4.152 can be rewritten as

$$X_L = x_a + x_d \ \Omega/\text{mi} \tag{4.153}$$

where
  x_a is the inductive reactance at 1 ft spacing

$$= 0.1213 \ln \frac{1}{D_s} \ \Omega/\text{mi} \tag{4.154}$$

x_d is the inductive reactance spacing factor

$$= 0.1213 \ln D_m \ \Omega/\text{mi} \tag{4.155}$$

For a given frequency, the value of x_a depends only on the GMR, which is a function of the conductor type. But x_d depends only on the spacing D_m. If the spacing is greater than 1 ft, x_d has a positive value that is added to x_a. On the other hand, if the spacing is less than 1 ft, x_d has a negative value that is subtracted from x_a. Tables given in Appendix A give x_a and x_d directly.

Similarly, Equation 4.145 for shunt capacitive reactance at 60 Hz, that is,

$$x_c = 0.06836 \log_{10} \frac{D_m}{r} \ \text{M}\Omega \times \text{mi}$$

can be split into

$$x_c = 0.06836 \log_{10} \frac{1}{r} + 0.06836 \log_{10} D_m \ \text{M}\Omega \times \text{mi} \tag{4.156}$$

or

$$x_c = x_a' + x_d' \ \text{M}\Omega \times \text{mi} \tag{4.157}$$

where

x_a' is the capacitive reactance at 1 ft spacing

$$= 0.06836 \log_{10} \frac{1}{r} \ M\Omega \times mi \tag{4.158}$$

x_d' is the capacitive reactance spacing factor

$$= 0.06836 \log_{10} D_m \ M\Omega \times mi \tag{4.159}$$

Tables given in Appendix A provide x_a' and x_d' directly. The term x_d' is added or subtracted from x_a' depending on the magnitude of D_m.

Example 4.5

A three-phase, 60 Hz, transposed line has conductors that are made up of 4/0, 7-strand copper. At the pole top, the distances between conductors, center to center, are given as 6.8, 5.5, and 4 ft. The diameter of the conductor copper used is 0.1739 in. Determine the inductive reactances per mile per phase:

(a) By using Equation 4.135
(b) By using tables

Solution

(a) First calculating the equivalent spacing for the pole top,

$$D_{eq} = D_m = \left(D_{ab} \times D_{bc} \times D_{ca} \right)^{1/3}$$

$$= (6.8 \times 5.5 \times 4)^{1/3} = 5.3086 \ ft$$

From Table A.1, $D_s = 0.01579$ ft for the conductor. Hence, its inductive reactance is

$$X_L = 0.1213 \ln \frac{D_{eq}}{D_s}$$

$$= 0.1213 \ln \frac{5.3086 \ ft}{0.01579 \ ft}$$

$$= 0.705688 \ \Omega/mi \cong 0.7057 \ \Omega/mi$$

(b) From Table A.1, $X_a = 0.503$ Ω/mi, and from Table A.8, for $D_{eq} = 5.30086$ ft, by linear interpolation, $X_d = 0.2026$ Ω/mi. Thus, the inductive reactance is

$$X_L = X_a + X_d$$

$$= 0.503 + 0.2026$$

$$= 0.7056 \ \Omega/mi$$

Example 4.6

Consider the pole-top configuration given in Example 4.5. If the line length is 100 mi, determine the shunt capacitive reactance by using the following:

(a) Equation 4.156
(b) Tables

Solution

(a) By using the equation,

$$X_c = 0.06836 \log_{10} \frac{D_m}{r}$$

$$= 0.06836 \log_{10} \frac{5.3086 \text{ ft}}{\left(\dfrac{0.522}{2 \times 12}\right) \text{ft}}$$

$$= 0.06836 \log_{10} \frac{1}{\left(\dfrac{0.522}{2 \times 12}\right) \text{ft}} + 0.06836 \log_{10}(5.3086 \text{ ft})$$

$$= 0.113651284 + 0.49559632$$

$$\cong 0.163211 \ M\Omega \times mi$$

(b) From Table A.1, $X'_a = 0.1136 \ M\Omega \times mi$, and from Table A.9, $X'_d = 0.049543 \ M\Omega \times mi$. Hence,

$$X_c = X'_a + X'_d$$

$$= 0.1136 + 0.049543$$

$$= 0.163143 \ M\Omega \times mi$$

(c) The capacitive reactance of the 100 mi long line is

$$X_c = \frac{0.163143 \ M\Omega \times mi}{100 \ mi}$$

$$= 1.63143 \times 10^{-3} \ M\Omega$$

Example 4.7

A three-phase, 60 Hz, 100 mi long transposed line has conductors that are made up of 900 kcmil ACSR conductors, operating at 50°C. At a horizontal pole top, the distances between conductors, center to center, are given as 25, 25, and 50 ft. Determine the following:

(a) The resistance of the line per mile
(b) Self-inductive reactance of the conductor per mile
(c) Inductive reactance spacing factor per mile
(d) Inductive reactances per mile per phase
    1. By using Equation 4.135
    2. By using tables
(e) Total inductive reactance of the line
(f) Capacitive reactance spacing factor per mile
(g) Self-capacitive reactance per mile
(h) Capacitive reactance per mile
(i) Total capacitive reactance of the line
(j) Total line impedance

Solution

(a) From Table A.3, for 900 kcmil, the resistance of the line is $R_a = 0.1185$ Ω/mi.

(b) First calculating the equivalent spacing for the pole top,

$$D_{eq} = D_m = \left(D_{ab} \times D_{bc} \times D_{ca} \right)^{1/3}$$

$$= (25 \times 25 \times 50)^{1/3} = 31.498 \text{ ft}$$

From Table A.3, $D_s = 0.01579$ ft for the conductor.
The self-inductive reactance of the conductor per mile is

$$X_a = 0.1213 \ln \left(\frac{1}{D_s} \right)$$

$$= 0.1213 \ln \left(\frac{1}{0.0391} \right) = 0.39321 \text{ } \Omega/mi$$

(c) The inductive reactance spacing factor per mile is

$$X_d = 0.1213 \ln \left(D_m \right)$$

$$= 0.1213 \ln(31.498)$$

$$= 0.418476 \text{ } \Omega/mi$$

(d) The inductive reactance of the line is
   1. By using Equation 4.135,

$$X_L = 0.1213 \ln \frac{D_{eq}}{D_s}$$

$$= 0.1213 \ln \frac{31.498 \text{ ft}}{0.0391 \text{ ft}}$$

$$= 0.811686 \text{ } \Omega/mi \cong 0.8117 \text{ } \Omega/mi$$

   2. By using tables,
     From Table A.3,
     The self-inductive reactance is

$$X_a = 0.393 \text{ } \Omega/mi$$

The inductive reactance spacing factor is

$$X_d = 0.4186 \text{ } \Omega/mi$$

Thus, the inductive reactance of the line is

$$X_L = X_a + X_d$$

$$= 0.393 + 0.4186 = 0.8116 \text{ } \Omega/mi$$

(e) The total inductive reactance of the line is

$$\sum X_L = (X_a + X_d)\ell$$

$$= (0.8117 \ \Omega/\text{mi})(100 \ \text{mi})$$

$$= 81.17 \ \Omega$$

(f) The self-capacitive reactance per mile is

$$X'_a = 0.06836 \log_{10}\left(\frac{1}{r}\right)$$

$$= 0.06836 \log_{10}\left(\frac{1}{\dfrac{1.162}{2} \times \dfrac{1}{12}}\right)$$

$$= 0.089894 \ \text{M}\Omega \cdot \text{mi}$$

where the diameter of the conductor is 1.162 in.

(g) The capacitive reactance due to spacing factor is

$$X'_d = 0.06836 \log(D_m)$$

$$= 0.06836 \log 10(31.498)$$

$$= 0.102423 \ \text{M}\Omega \cdot \text{mi}$$

(h) The capacitive reactance per mile is

$$X_c = X'_a + X'_d$$

$$= 0.089894 + 0.102423$$

$$= 0.192317 \ \text{M}\Omega \cdot \text{mi}$$

(i) The total capacitive reactance of the line is

$$X_c = \frac{X'_a + X'_d}{\ell}$$

$$= \frac{0.089894 + 0.102423}{100 \ \text{mi}}$$

$$= \frac{0.192317 \ \text{M}\Omega \cdot \text{mi}}{100 \ \text{mi}}$$

$$= 0.00192317 \ \text{M}\Omega$$

(j) The total line impedance is

$$\sum Z_L = (R_a + jX_L)\ell$$

$$= (0.1185 + j0.8116 \ \Omega/\text{mi})\,100 \ \text{mi}$$

$$= 11.85 + j81.16$$

$$\cong 82\angle 81.7° \ \Omega$$

4.11 EQUIVALENT CIRCUITS FOR TRANSMISSION LINES

An OH line or a cable can be represented as a distributed constant circuit, as shown in Figure 4.15. The resistance, inductance, capacitance, and leakage conductance of a distributed constant circuit are distributed uniformly along the line length. In the figure, L represents the inductance of a line conductor to neutral per-unit length, r represents the ac resistance of a line conductor per-unit length, C is the capacitance of a line conductor to neutral per-unit length, and G is the leakage conductance per-unit length.

4.12 SHORT TRANSMISSION LINES (UP TO 50 mi, OR 80 km)

The modeling of a short transmission line is the most simplistic one. Its shunt capacitance is so small that it can be omitted entirely with little loss of accuracy. (Its shunt admittance is neglected since the current is the same throughout the line.) Thus, its capacitance and leakage resistance to the earth are usually neglected, as shown in Figure 4.16. Therefore, the transmission line can be treated as a simple, lumped, and constant impedance, that is,

$$\mathbf{Z} = R + jX_L$$
$$= zl$$
$$= rl + jxl \ \Omega \tag{4.160}$$

where
  $\mathbf{Z}$ is the total series impedance per phase in ohms
  z is the series impedance of one conductor in ohms per-unit length
  X_L is the total inductive reactance of one conductor in ohms
  x is the inductive reactance of one conductor in ohms per-unit length
  l is the length of line

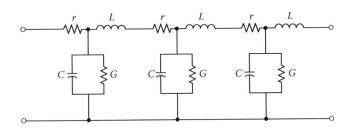

FIGURE 4.15 Distributed constant equivalent circuit of line.

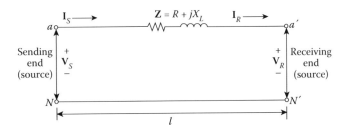

FIGURE 4.16 Equivalent circuit of short transmission line.

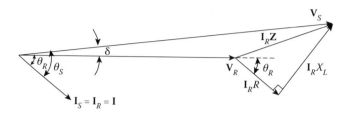

FIGURE 4.17   Phasor diagram of short transmission line to inductive load.

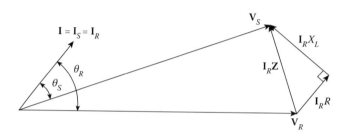

FIGURE 4.18   Phasor diagram of short transmission line connected to capacitive load.

The current entering the line at the sending end of the line is equal to the current leaving at the receiving end. Figures 4.17 and 4.18 show vector (or phasor) diagrams for a short transmission line connected to an inductive load and a capacitive load, respectively. It can be observed from the figures that

$$\mathbf{V}_S = \mathbf{V}_R + \mathbf{I}_R\mathbf{Z} \tag{4.161}$$

$$\mathbf{I}_S = \mathbf{I}_R = \mathbf{I} \tag{4.162}$$

$$\mathbf{V}_R = \mathbf{V}_S - \mathbf{I}_R\mathbf{Z} \tag{4.163}$$

where
    $\mathbf{V}_S$ is the sending-end phase (line-to-neutral) voltage
    $\mathbf{V}_R$ is the receiving-end phase (line-to-neutral) voltage
    $\mathbf{I}_S$ is the sending-end phase current
    $\mathbf{I}_R$ is the receiving-end phase current
    $\mathbf{Z}$ is the total series impedance per phase

Therefore, using $\mathbf{V}_R$ as the reference, Equation 4.161 can be written as

$$\mathbf{V}_S = \mathbf{V}_R + \left(I_R\cos\theta_R \pm jI_R\sin\theta_R\right)\left(R+jX\right) \tag{4.164}$$

where the plus or minus sign is determined by θ_R, the PF angle of the receiving end or load. If the PF is lagging, the minus sign is employed. On the other hand, if it is leading, the plus sign is used.

However, if Equation 4.163 is used, it is convenient to use $\mathbf{V}_S$ as the reference. Therefore,

$$\mathbf{V}_R = \mathbf{V}_S - \left(I_S\cos\theta_S \pm jI_S\sin\theta_S\right)\left(R+jX\right) \tag{4.165}$$

where θ_S is the sending-end PF angle that determines, as before, whether the plus or minus sign will be used. Also, from Figure 4.17, using $\mathbf{V}_R$ as the reference vector,

$$V_S = \left[\left(V_R + IR\cos\theta_R + IX\sin\theta_R \right)^2 + \left(IX\cos\theta_R \pm IR\sin\theta_R \right)^2 \right]^{1/2} \qquad (4.166)$$

and load angle

$$\delta = \theta_S - \theta_R \qquad (4.167)$$

or

$$\delta = \arctan\left(\frac{IX\cos\theta_R \pm IR\sin\theta_R}{V_R + IR\cos\theta_R + IX\sin\theta_R} \right) \qquad (4.168)$$

The generalized constants, or ABCD parameters, can be determined by inspection of Figure 4.16. Since

$$\begin{bmatrix} \mathbf{V}_S \\ \mathbf{I}_S \end{bmatrix} = \begin{bmatrix} \mathbf{A} & \mathbf{B} \\ \mathbf{C} & \mathbf{D} \end{bmatrix} \begin{bmatrix} \mathbf{V}_R \\ \mathbf{I}_R \end{bmatrix} \qquad (4.169)$$

and $\mathbf{AD} - \mathbf{BC} = 1$, where

$$\mathbf{A} = 1, \ \mathbf{B} = \mathbf{Z}, \ \mathbf{C} = 0, \ \mathbf{D} = 1 \qquad (4.170)$$

then

$$\begin{bmatrix} \mathbf{V}_S \\ \mathbf{I}_S \end{bmatrix} = \begin{bmatrix} 1 & \mathbf{Z} \\ 0 & 1 \end{bmatrix} \begin{bmatrix} \mathbf{V}_R \\ \mathbf{I}_R \end{bmatrix} \qquad (4.171)$$

and

$$\begin{bmatrix} \mathbf{V}_R \\ \mathbf{I}_R \end{bmatrix} = \begin{bmatrix} 1 & \mathbf{Z} \\ 0 & 1 \end{bmatrix}^{-1} \begin{bmatrix} \mathbf{V}_S \\ \mathbf{I}_S \end{bmatrix} = \begin{bmatrix} 1 & -\mathbf{Z} \\ 0 & 1 \end{bmatrix} \begin{bmatrix} \mathbf{V}_S \\ \mathbf{I}_S \end{bmatrix}$$

The transmission efficiency of the short line can be expressed as

$$\eta = \frac{\text{Output}}{\text{Input}}$$

$$= \frac{\sqrt{3}V_R I\cos\theta_R}{\sqrt{3}V_S I\cos\theta_S}$$

$$= \frac{V_R\cos\theta_R}{V_S\cos\theta_S} \qquad (4.172)$$

Equation 4.172 is applicable whether the line is single phase.

The transmission efficiency can also be expressed as

$$\eta = \frac{\text{Output}}{\text{Output} + \text{losses}}$$

For a single-phase line,

$$\eta = \frac{V_R I \cos\theta_R}{V_R I \cos\theta_R + 2I^2 R} \tag{4.173}$$

For a three-phase line,

$$\eta = \frac{\sqrt{3}V_R I \cos\theta_R}{\sqrt{3}V_R I \cos\theta_R + 3I^2 R} \tag{4.174}$$

4.12.1 STEADY-STATE POWER LIMIT

Assume that the impedance of a short transmission line is given as $Z = Z\angle\theta$. Therefore, the real power delivered, at a steady state, to the receiving end of the transmission line can be expressed as

$$P_R = \frac{V_S \times V_R}{Z}\cos(\theta - \delta) - \frac{V_R^2}{Z}\cos\theta \tag{4.175}$$

and similarly, the reactive power delivered can be expressed as

$$Q_R = \frac{V_S \times V_R}{Z}\sin(\theta - \delta) - \frac{V_R^2}{Z}\sin\theta \tag{4.176}$$

If V_S and V_R are the line-to-neutral voltages, Equations 4.175 and 4.176 give P_R and Q_R values per phase. Also, if the obtained P_R and Q_R values are multiplied by 3 or the line-to-line values of V_S and V_R are used, the equations give the three-phase real and reactive power delivered to a balanced load at the receiving end of the line.

If, in Equation 4.175, all variables are kept constant with the exception of δ, so that the real power delivered, P_R, is a function of δ only, P_R is maximum when $\delta = \theta$, and the maximum powers* obtainable at the receiving end for a given regulation can be expressed as

$$P_{R,\max} = \frac{V_R^2}{Z^2}\left(\frac{V_S}{V_R}Z - R\right) \tag{4.177}$$

where V_S and V_R are the phase (line-to-neutral) voltages whether the system is single phase or three phase.

The equation can also be expressed as

$$P_{R,\max} = \frac{V_S \times V_R}{Z} - \frac{V_R^2 \times \cos\theta}{Z} \tag{4.178}$$

---

* Also called the *steady-state power limit*.

If $V_S = V_R$,

$$P_{R,\max} = \frac{V_R^2}{Z}\left(1 - \cos\theta\right) \tag{4.179}$$

or

$$P_{R,\max} = \left(\frac{V_R}{Z}\right)^2 \left(Z - R\right) \tag{4.180}$$

and similarly, the corresponding reactive power delivered to the load is given by

$$Q_{R,\max} = -\frac{V_R^2}{Z}\sin\theta \tag{4.181}$$

As can be observed, both Equations 4.180 and 4.181 are independent of V_S voltage. The negative sign in Equation 4.181 points out that the load is a sink of *leading vars*,* that is, going to the load or a source of *lagging vars* (i.e., *from the load to the supply*). The total three-phase power transmitted on the three-phase line is three times the power calculated by using the aforementioned equations. If the voltages are given in volts, the power is expressed in watts or vars. Otherwise, if they are given in kilovolts, the power is expressed in megawatts or megavars.

In a similar manner, the real and reactive powers for the sending end of a transmission line can be expressed as

$$P_S = \frac{V_S^2}{Z}\cos\theta - \frac{V_S \times V_R}{Z}\cos\left(\theta + \delta\right) \tag{4.182}$$

and

$$Q_S = \frac{V_S^2}{Z}\sin\theta - \frac{V_S \times V_R}{Z}\sin\left(\theta + \delta\right) \tag{4.183}$$

If, in Equation 4.182, as before, all variables are kept constant with the exception of δ, so that the real power at the sending end, P_S, is a function of δ only, P_S is a maximum when

$$\theta + \delta = 180°$$

Therefore, the maximum power at the sending end, the maximum input power, can be expressed as

$$P_{S,\max} = \frac{V_S^2}{Z}\cos\theta + \frac{V_S \times V_R}{Z} \tag{4.184}$$

or

$$P_{S,\max} = \frac{V_S^2 \times R}{Z^2} + \frac{V_S \times V_R}{Z} \tag{4.185}$$

---

* For many decades, the electrical utility industry has declined to recognize two different kinds of reactive power, *leading* and *lagging vars*. Only *magnetizing vars* are recognized, printed on varmeter scale plates, bought, and sold. Therefore, in the following sections, the leading or lagging vars will be referred to as magnetizing vars.

However, if $V_S = V_R$,

$$P_{S,\text{max}} = \left(\frac{V_S}{Z}\right)^2 (Z + R) \tag{4.186}$$

and similarly, the corresponding reactive power at the sending end, the maximum input vars, is given by

$$Q_S = \frac{V_S^2}{Z} \sin\theta \tag{4.187}$$

As can be observed, both Equations 4.186 and 4.187 are independent of V_R voltage, and Equation 4.187 has a positive sign this time.

4.12.2 Percent Voltage Regulation

The voltage regulation of the line is defined by the rise in voltage when full load is removed, that is,

$$\text{Percentage of voltage regulation} = \frac{|\mathbf{V}_S| - |\mathbf{V}_R|}{|\mathbf{V}_R|} \times 100 \tag{4.188}$$

or

$$\text{Percentage of voltage regulation} = \frac{|\mathbf{V}_{R,\text{NL}}| - |\mathbf{V}_{R,\text{FL}}|}{|\mathbf{V}_{R,\text{FL}}|} \times 100 \tag{4.189}$$

where
$|\mathbf{V}_S|$ is the magnitude of the sending-end phase (line-to-neutral) voltage at no load
$|\mathbf{V}_R|$ is the magnitude of the receiving-end phase (line-to-neutral) voltage at full load
$|\mathbf{V}_{R,\text{NL}}|$ is the magnitude of the receiving-end voltage at no load
$|\mathbf{V}_{R,\text{FL}}|$ is the magnitude of the receiving-end voltage at full load with constant $|\mathbf{V}_S|$

Therefore, if the load is connected at the receiving end of the line,

$$|\mathbf{V}_S| = |\mathbf{V}_{R,\text{NL}}|$$

and

$$|\mathbf{V}_R| = |\mathbf{V}_{R,\text{FL}}|$$

An approximate expression for percentage of voltage regulation is

$$\text{Percentage of voltage regulation} \cong I_R \times \frac{(R\cos\Phi_R \pm X\sin\Phi_R)}{V_R} \times 100 \tag{4.190}$$

Example 4.8

A three-phase, 60 Hz OH short transmission line has a line-to-line voltage of 23 kV at the receiving end, a total impedance of $2.48 + j6.57$ Ω/phase, and a load of 9 MW with a receiving-end lagging PF of 0.85.

    (a) Calculate the line-to-neutral and line-to-line voltages at the sending end.
    (b) Calculate the load angle.

Solution

Method I. Using complex algebra

    (a) The line-to-neutral reference voltage is

$$\mathbf{V}_{R(L\text{-}N)} = \frac{\mathbf{V}_{R(L\text{-}L)}}{\sqrt{3}}$$

$$= \frac{23 \times 10^3 \angle 0°}{\sqrt{3}} = 13{,}294.8 \angle 0° \text{ V}$$

The line current is

$$\mathbf{I} = \frac{9 \times 10^6}{\sqrt{3} \times 23 \times 10^3 \times 0.85} \times (0.85 - j0.527)$$

$$= 266.1(0.85 - j0.527)$$

$$= 226.19 - j140.24 \text{ A}$$

Therefore,

$$\mathbf{IZ} = (226.19 - j140.24)(2.48 + j6.57)$$

$$= (266.1 \angle -31.8°)(7.02 \angle 69.32°)$$

$$= 1868.95 \angle 37.52° \text{ V}$$

Thus, the line-to-neutral voltage at the sending end is

$$\mathbf{V}_{S(L\text{-}N)} = \mathbf{V}_{R(L\text{-}N)} + \mathbf{IZ}$$

$$= 14{,}820 \angle 4.4° \text{ V}$$

The line-to-line voltage at the sending end is

$$\mathbf{V}_{S(L\text{-}L)} = \sqrt{3}\mathbf{V}_{S(L\text{-}N)}$$

$$= 25{,}640 \angle 4.4° + 30° = 25{,}640 \angle 34.4° \text{ V}$$

    (b) The load angle is 4.4°.

Method II. Using the current as the reference phasor

    (a)

$$V_R \cos\theta_R + IR = 13{,}294.8 \times 0.85 + 266.1 \times 2.48 = 11{,}960 \text{ V}$$

$$V_R \sin\theta_R + IX = 13{,}294.8 \times 0.527 + 266.1 \times 6.57 = 8{,}754 \text{ V}$$

Then

$$V_{S(L-N)} = \left(11{,}960.5^2 + 8754.66^2\right)^{1/2} = 14{,}820 \ \text{V/phase}$$

$$V_{S(L-L)} = 25{,}640 \ \text{V}$$

(b)

$$\theta_S = \theta_R + \delta = \tan^{-1}\left(\frac{8{,}754}{11{,}960}\right) = 36.2°$$

$$\delta = \theta_S - \theta_R = 36.2 - 31.8 = 4.4°$$

Method III. Using the receiving-end voltage as the reference phasor

(a)

$$V_{S(L-N)} = \left[\left(V_R + IR\cos\theta_R + IX\sin\theta_R\right)^2 + \left(IX\cos\theta_R - IR\sin\theta_R\right)^2\right]^{1/2}$$

$$IR\cos\theta_R = 266.1 \times 2.48 \times 0.85 = 560.9$$

$$IR\sin\theta_R = 266.1 \times 2.48 \times 0.527 = 347.8$$

$$IX\cos\theta_R = 266.1 \times 6.57 \times 0.85 = 1486$$

$$IX\sin\theta_R = 266.1 \times 6.57 \times 0.527 = 921$$

Therefore,

$$V_{S(L-N)} = \left[\left(13{,}294.8 + 560.9 + 921.0\right)^2 + \left(1{,}486 - 347.8\right)^2\right]^{1/2}$$

$$= \left[14{,}776.7^2 + 1{,}138.2^2\right]^{1/2}$$

$$= 14{,}820 \ \text{V}$$

$$V_{S(L-L)} = \sqrt{3}V_{S(L-N)} = 25{,}640 \ \text{V}$$

(b)

$$\delta = \tan^{-1}\left(\frac{1{,}138.2}{14{,}776.7}\right) = 4.4°$$

Method IV. Using power relationships

Power loss in the line is

$$P_{loss} = 3I^2R$$

$$= 3 \times 266.1^2 \times 2.48 \times 10^{-6} = 0.527 \text{ MW}$$

Total input power to the line is

$$P_T = P + P_{loss}$$

$$= 9 + 0.527 = 9.527 \text{ MW}$$

Var loss in the line is

$$Q_{loss} = 3I^2X$$

$$= 3 \times 266.1^2 \times 6.57 \times 10^{-6} = 1.396 \text{ Mvar lagging}$$

Total megavar input to the line is

$$Q_T = \frac{P \sin\theta_R}{\cos\theta_R} + Q_{loss}$$

$$= \frac{9 \times 0.527}{0.85} + 1.396 = 6.976 \text{ Mvar lagging}$$

Total megavolt-ampere input to the line is

$$S_T = \left(P_T^2 + Q_T^2\right)^{1/2}$$

$$= \left(9.527^2 + 6.976^2\right)^{1/2} = 11.81 \text{ MVA}$$

(a)

$$V_{S(L-L)} = \frac{S_T}{\sqrt{3}I}$$

$$= \frac{11.81 \times 10^6}{\sqrt{3} \times 266.1} = 25,640 \text{ V}$$

$$V_{S(L-N)} = \frac{V_{S(L-L)}}{\sqrt{3}} = 14,820 \text{ V}$$

(b)

$$\cos\theta_S = \frac{P_T}{S_T} = \frac{9,527}{11.81} = 0.807 \text{ lagging}$$

Therefore,

$$\theta_S = 36.2°$$

$$\delta = 36.2° - 31.8° = 4.4°$$

Method V. Treating the three-phase line as a single-phase line and having V_S and V_R represent line-to-line voltages, not line-to-neutral voltages

    (a) Power delivered is 4.5 MW

$$I_{line} = \frac{4.5 \times 10^6}{23 \times 103 \times 0.85} = 230.18 \ A$$

$$R_{loop} = 2 \times 2.48 = 4.96 \ \Omega$$

$$X_{loop} = 2 \times 6.57 = 13.14 \ \Omega$$

$$V_R \cos\theta_R = 23 \times 10^3 \times 0.85 = 19{,}550 \ V$$

$$V_R \sin\theta_R = 23 \times 103 \times 0.527 = 12{,}121 \ V$$

$$IR = 230.18 \times 4.96 = 1141.7 \ V$$

$$IX = 230.18 \times 13.14 = 3024.6 \ V$$

Therefore,

$$
\begin{aligned}
V_{S(L-L)} &= \left[\left(V_R \cos\theta_R + IR \right)^2 + \left(V_R \sin\theta_R + IX \right)^2 \right]^{1/2} \\
&= \left[\left(19{,}550 + 1{,}141.7 \right)^2 + \left(12{,}121 + 3{,}024.6 \right)^2 \right]^{1/2} \\
&= \left[20{,}691.7^2 + 15{,}145.6^2 \right]^{1/2} \\
&= 25{,}640 \ V
\end{aligned}
$$

Thus,

$$V_{S(L-N)} = \frac{V_{S(L-L)}}{\sqrt{3}} = 14{,}820 \ V$$

    (b)

$$\theta_s = \tan^{-1} \frac{15{,}145.6}{20{,}691.7} = 36.20°$$

and

$$\delta = 36.2° - 31.8° = 4.4°$$

Example 4.9

Calculate percentage of voltage regulation for the values given in Example 4.8:

    (a) Using Equation 4.188
    (b) Using Equation 4.190

Solution

(a) Using Equation 4.188,

$$\text{Percentage of voltage regulation} = \frac{|\mathbf{V}_S| - |\mathbf{V}_R|}{|\mathbf{V}_R|} \times 100$$

$$= \frac{14{,}820 - 13{,}294.8}{13{,}294.8} \times 100$$

$$= 11.5$$

(b) Using Equation 4.190,

$$\text{Percentage of voltage regulation} \cong I_R \times \frac{(R\cos\theta_R \pm X\sin\theta_R)}{V_R} \times 100$$

$$= 266.1 \times \frac{2.48 \times 0.85 + 6.57 \times 0.527}{13{,}294.8} \times 100$$

$$= 1.2$$

4.12.3 REPRESENTATION OF MUTUAL IMPEDANCE OF SHORT LINES

Figure 4.19a shows a circuit of two lines, x and y, that have self-impedances of $\mathbf{Z}_{xx}$ and $\mathbf{Z}_{yy}$ and mutual impedance of $\mathbf{Z}_{zy}$. Its equivalent circuit is shown in Figure 4.19b. Sometimes, it may be required to preserve the electrical identity of the two lines, as shown in Figure 4.20. The mutual impedance $\mathbf{Z}_{xy}$ can be in either line and transferred to the other by means of a transformer that has a 1:1 turns ratio. This technique is also applicable for three-phase lines.

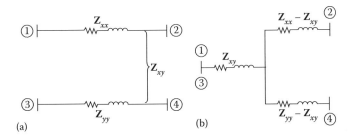

FIGURE 4.19 Representation of mutual impedance: (a) between two circuits and (b) its equivalent circuit.

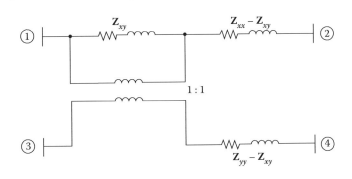

FIGURE 4.20 Representation of mutual impedance between two circuits by means of 1:1 transformer.

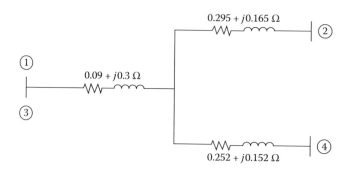

FIGURE 4.21   Resultant equivalent circuit.

Example 4.10

Assume that the mutual impedance between two parallel feeders is $0.09 + j0.3$ Ω/mi per phase. The self-impedances of the feeders are $0.604\angle50.4°$ and $0.567\angle52.9°$ Ω/mi per phase, respectively. Represent the mutual impedance between the feeders as shown in Figure 4.19b.

Solution

$$\mathbf{Z}_{xy} = 0.09 + j0.3 \ \Omega$$

$$\mathbf{Z}_{xx} = 0.604\angle50.4° = 0.385 + j0.465 \ \Omega$$

$$\mathbf{Z}_{yy} = 0.567\angle52.9° = 0.342 + j0.452 \ \Omega$$

Therefore,

$$\mathbf{Z}_{xx} - \mathbf{Z}_{xy} = 0.295 + j0.165 \ \Omega$$

$$\mathbf{Z}_{yy} - \mathbf{Z}_{xy} = 0.252 + j0.152 \ \Omega$$

Hence, the resulting equivalent circuit is shown in Figure 4.21.

4.13   MEDIUM-LENGTH TRANSMISSION LINES (UP TO 150 mi, OR 240 km)

As the line length and voltage increase, the use of the formulas developed for the short transmission lines gives inaccurate results. Thus, *the effect of the current leaking through the capacitance must be taken into account for a better approximation.* Thus, the shunt admittance is *lumped* at a few points along the line and represented by forming either a *T* or a *π* network, as shown in Figures 4.22 and 4.23.

In the figures,

$$\mathbf{Z} = \mathbf{z}l$$

For the *T* circuit shown in Figure 4.7,

$$\mathbf{V}_S = \mathbf{I}_S \times \frac{1}{2}\mathbf{Z} + \mathbf{I}_R \times \frac{1}{2}\mathbf{Z} + \mathbf{V}_R$$

$$= \left[\mathbf{I}_R + \left(\mathbf{V}_R + \mathbf{I}_R \times \frac{1}{2}\mathbf{Z}\right)\mathbf{Y}\right]\frac{1}{2}\mathbf{Z} + \mathbf{V}_R + \mathbf{I}_R\frac{1}{2}\mathbf{Z}$$

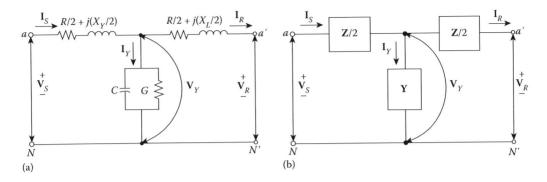

FIGURE 4.22   Nominal-*T* circuit: (a) actual circuit and (b) its equivalent lumped circuit.

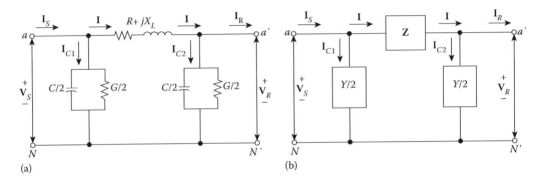

FIGURE 4.23   Nominal-*π* circuit: (a) actual circuit and (b) its equivalent lumped circuit.

or

$$\mathbf{V}_S = \underbrace{\left(1 + \frac{1}{2}\mathbf{Z}\mathbf{Y}\right)}_{A}\mathbf{V}_R + \underbrace{\left(\mathbf{Z} + \frac{1}{4}\mathbf{Y}\mathbf{Z}^2\right)}_{B}\mathbf{I}_R \tag{4.191}$$

and

$$\mathbf{I}_S = \mathbf{I}_R + \left(\mathbf{V}_R + \mathbf{I}_R \times \frac{1}{2}\mathbf{Z}\right)\mathbf{Y}$$

or

$$\mathbf{I}_S = \underbrace{\mathbf{Y}}_{C} \times \mathbf{V}_R + \underbrace{\left(1 + \frac{1}{2}\mathbf{Z}\mathbf{Y}\right)}_{D}\mathbf{I}_R \tag{4.192}$$

Alternatively, neglecting conductance so that

$$\mathbf{I}_C = \mathbf{I}_Y$$

and

$$\mathbf{V}_C = \mathbf{V}_Y$$

yields

$$\mathbf{I}_C = \mathbf{V}_C \times \mathbf{Y}$$

$$\mathbf{V}_C = \mathbf{V}_R + \mathbf{I}_R \times \frac{1}{2}\mathbf{Z}$$

Hence,

$$\mathbf{V}_S = \mathbf{V}_C + \mathbf{I}_S \times \frac{1}{2}\mathbf{Z}$$

$$= \mathbf{V}_R + \mathbf{I}_R \times \frac{1}{2}\mathbf{Z} + \left[\mathbf{V}_R\mathbf{Y} + \mathbf{I}_R\left(1 + \frac{1}{2}\mathbf{YZ}\right)\right]\left(\frac{1}{2}\mathbf{Z}\right)$$

or

$$\mathbf{V}_S = \underbrace{\left(1 + \frac{1}{2}\mathbf{YZ}\right)}_{A}\mathbf{V}_R + \underbrace{\left(\mathbf{Z} + \frac{1}{4}\mathbf{YZ}^2\right)}_{B}\mathbf{I}_R \qquad (4.193)$$

Also,

$$\mathbf{I}_S = \mathbf{I}_R + \mathbf{I}_C$$

$$= \mathbf{I}_R + \mathbf{V}_C \times \mathbf{Y}$$

$$= \mathbf{I}_R + \left(\mathbf{V}_R + \mathbf{I}_R \times \frac{1}{2}\mathbf{Z}\right)\mathbf{Y}$$

Again,

$$\mathbf{I}_S = \underbrace{\mathbf{Y}}_{C} \times \mathbf{V}_R + \underbrace{\left(1 + \frac{1}{2}\mathbf{YZ}\right)}_{D}\mathbf{I}_R \qquad (4.194)$$

Since

$$A = 1 + \frac{1}{2}\mathbf{YZ} \qquad (4.195)$$

$$B = \mathbf{Z} + \frac{1}{4}\mathbf{YZ}^2 \qquad (4.196)$$

$$C = \mathbf{Y} \qquad (4.197)$$

$$D = 1 + \frac{1}{2}\mathbf{YZ} \qquad (4.198)$$

for a nominal-*T* circuit, the *general circuit parameter matrix*, or *transfer matrix*, becomes

$$
\begin{bmatrix} \mathbf{A} & \mathbf{B} \\ \mathbf{C} & \mathbf{D} \end{bmatrix} = \begin{bmatrix} 1 + \dfrac{1}{2}\mathbf{YZ} & \mathbf{Z} + \dfrac{1}{4}\mathbf{YZ}^2 \\ \mathbf{Y} & 1 + \dfrac{1}{2}\mathbf{YZ} \end{bmatrix}
$$

Therefore,

$$
\begin{bmatrix} \mathbf{V}_S \\ \mathbf{I}_S \end{bmatrix} = \begin{bmatrix} 1 + \dfrac{1}{2}\mathbf{YZ} & \mathbf{Z} + \dfrac{1}{4}\mathbf{YZ}^2 \\ \mathbf{Y} & 1 + \dfrac{1}{2}\mathbf{YZ} \end{bmatrix} \begin{bmatrix} \mathbf{V}_R \\ \mathbf{I}_R \end{bmatrix}
\tag{4.199}
$$

and

$$
\begin{bmatrix} \mathbf{V}_R \\ \mathbf{I}_R \end{bmatrix} = \begin{bmatrix} 1 + \dfrac{1}{2}\mathbf{YZ} & \mathbf{Z} + \dfrac{1}{4}\mathbf{YZ}^2 \\ \mathbf{Y} & 1 + \dfrac{1}{2}\mathbf{YZ} \end{bmatrix}^{-1} \begin{bmatrix} \mathbf{V}_S \\ \mathbf{I}_S \end{bmatrix}
\tag{4.200}
$$

For the π circuit shown in Figure 4.23,

$$
\mathbf{V}_S = \left(\mathbf{V}_R \times \frac{1}{2}\mathbf{Y} + \mathbf{I}_R \right)\mathbf{Z} + \mathbf{V}_R
$$

or

$$
\mathbf{V}_S = \underbrace{\left(1 + \frac{1}{2}\mathbf{YZ} \right)}_{\mathbf{A}}\mathbf{V}_R + \underbrace{\mathbf{Z}}_{\mathbf{B}} \times \mathbf{I}_R
\tag{4.201}
$$

and

$$
\mathbf{I}_S = \frac{1}{2}\mathbf{Y} \times \mathbf{V}_S + \frac{1}{2}\mathbf{Y} \times \mathbf{V}_R + \mathbf{I}_R
\tag{4.202}
$$

By substituting Equation 4.199 into Equation 4.200,

$$
\mathbf{I}_S = \left[\left(1 + \frac{1}{2}\mathbf{YZ} \right)\mathbf{V}_R + \mathbf{ZI}_R \right]\frac{1}{2}\mathbf{Y} + \frac{1}{2}\mathbf{Y} \times \mathbf{V}_R + \mathbf{I}_R
$$

or

$$\mathbf{I}_S = \underbrace{\left(\mathbf{Y} + \frac{1}{4}\mathbf{Y}^2\mathbf{Z}\right)}_{C}\mathbf{V}_R + \underbrace{\left(1 + \frac{1}{2}\mathbf{YZ}\right)}_{D}\mathbf{I}_R \tag{4.203}$$

Alternatively, *neglecting conductance*,

$$\mathbf{I} = \mathbf{I}_{C2} + \mathbf{I}_R$$

where

$$\mathbf{I}_{C2} = \frac{1}{2}\mathbf{Y} \times \mathbf{V}_R$$

yields

$$\mathbf{I} = \frac{1}{2}\mathbf{Y} \times \mathbf{V}_R + \mathbf{I}_R \tag{4.204}$$

Also,

$$\mathbf{V}_S = \mathbf{V}_R + \mathbf{IZ} \tag{4.205}$$

By substituting Equation 4.204 into Equation 4.205,

$$\mathbf{V}_S = \mathbf{V}_R + \left(\frac{1}{2}\mathbf{Y} \times \mathbf{V}_R + \mathbf{I}_R\right)\mathbf{Z}$$

or

$$\mathbf{V}_S = \underbrace{\left(1 + \frac{1}{2}\mathbf{YZ}\right)}_{A}\mathbf{V}_R + \underbrace{\mathbf{Z}}_{B} \times \mathbf{I}_R \tag{4.206}$$

and

$$\mathbf{I}_{C1} = \frac{1}{2}\mathbf{Y} \times \mathbf{V}_S \tag{4.207}$$

By substituting Equation 4.206 into Equation 4.207,

$$\mathbf{I}_{C1} = \frac{1}{2}\mathbf{Y} \times \left(1 + \frac{1}{2}\mathbf{YZ}\right)\mathbf{V}_R + \frac{1}{2}\mathbf{Y} \times \mathbf{ZI}_R \tag{4.208}$$

and since

$$\mathbf{I}_S = \mathbf{I} + \mathbf{I}_{C1} \tag{4.209}$$

by substituting Equation 4.208 into Equation 4.209,

$$\mathbf{I}_S = \frac{1}{2}\mathbf{YV}_R + \mathbf{I}_R + \frac{1}{2}\mathbf{Y}\left(1 + \frac{1}{2}\mathbf{YZ}\right)\mathbf{V}_R + \frac{1}{2}\mathbf{YZI}_R$$

or

$$\mathbf{I}_S = \underbrace{\left(\mathbf{Y} + \frac{1}{4}\mathbf{Y}^2\mathbf{Z}\right)}_{\mathbf{C}}\mathbf{V}_R + \underbrace{\left(1 + \frac{1}{2}\mathbf{YZ}\right)}_{\mathbf{D}}\mathbf{I}_R \tag{4.210}$$

Since

$$\mathbf{A} = 1 + \frac{1}{2}\mathbf{YZ} \tag{4.211}$$

$$\mathbf{B} = \mathbf{Z} \tag{4.212}$$

$$\mathbf{C} = \mathbf{Y} + \frac{1}{4}\mathbf{Y}^2\mathbf{Z} \tag{4.213}$$

$$\mathbf{D} = 1 + \frac{1}{2}\mathbf{YZ} \tag{4.214}$$

for a nominal-π circuit, the general circuit parameter matrix becomes

$$\begin{bmatrix} \mathbf{A} & \mathbf{B} \\ \mathbf{C} & \mathbf{D} \end{bmatrix} = \begin{bmatrix} 1 + \frac{1}{2}\mathbf{YZ} & \mathbf{Z} \\ \mathbf{Y} + \frac{1}{4}\mathbf{Y}^2\mathbf{Z} & 1 + \frac{1}{2}\mathbf{YZ} \end{bmatrix} \tag{4.215}$$

Therefore,

$$\begin{bmatrix} \mathbf{V}_S \\ \mathbf{I}_S \end{bmatrix} = \begin{bmatrix} 1 + \frac{1}{2}\mathbf{YZ} & \mathbf{Z} \\ \mathbf{Y} + \frac{1}{4}\mathbf{Y}^2\mathbf{Z} & 1 + \frac{1}{2}\mathbf{YZ} \end{bmatrix} \begin{bmatrix} \mathbf{V}_R \\ \mathbf{I}_R \end{bmatrix} \tag{4.216}$$

and

$$\begin{bmatrix} \mathbf{V}_R \\ \mathbf{I}_R \end{bmatrix} = \begin{bmatrix} 1 + \frac{1}{2}\mathbf{YZ} & \mathbf{Z} \\ \mathbf{Y} + \frac{1}{4}\mathbf{Y}^2\mathbf{Z} & 1 + \frac{1}{2}\mathbf{YZ} \end{bmatrix}^{-1} \begin{bmatrix} \mathbf{V}_S \\ \mathbf{I}_S \end{bmatrix} \tag{4.217}$$

As can be proved easily by using a delta–wye transformation, *the nominal-T and nominal-π circuits are not equivalent to each other.* This result is to be expected since two different approximations are made to the actual circuit, neither of which is absolutely correct. More accurate results can be obtained by splitting the line into several segments, each given by its nominal-*T* or nominal-*π* circuits and cascading the resulting segments.

Here, the power loss in the line is given as

$$P_{\text{loss}} = I^2 R \tag{4.218}$$

which varies approximately as the square of the through-line current. The reactive powers absorbed and supplied by the line are given as

$$Q_L = Q_{\text{absorbed}} = I^2 X_L \tag{4.219}$$

and

$$Q_C = Q_{\text{supplied}} = V^2 b \tag{4.220}$$

respectively. The Q_L varies approximately as the square of the through-line current, whereas the Q_C varies approximately as the square of the mean line voltage. The result is that increasing transmission voltages decrease the reactive power absorbed by the line for heavy loads and increase the reactive power supplied by the line for light loads.

The percentage of voltage regulation for the medium-length transmission lines is given by Stevenson [3] as

$$\text{Percentage of voltage regulation} = \frac{\dfrac{\left|\mathbf{V}_S\right|}{\left|\mathbf{A}\right|} - \left|\mathbf{V}_{R,\text{FL}}\right|}{\left|\mathbf{V}_{R,\text{FL}}\right|} \times 100 \tag{4.221}$$

where
$\left|\mathbf{V}_S\right|$ is the magnitude of sending-end phase (line-to-neutral) voltage
$\left|\mathbf{V}_{R,\text{FL}}\right|$ is the magnitude of receiving-end phase (line-to-neutral) voltage at full load with constant $\left|\mathbf{V}_S\right|$
$\left|\mathbf{A}\right|$ is the magnitude of line constant *A*

Example 4.11

A three-phase 138 kV transmission line is connected to a 49 MW load at a 0.85 lagging PF. The line constants of the 52 mi long line are $\mathbf{Z} = 95\angle 78°$ Ω and $\mathbf{Y} = 0.001\angle 90°$ S. Using *nominal-T circuit representation*, calculate the following:

  (a) The **A**, **B**, **C**, and **D** constants of the line
  (b) Sending-end voltage
  (c) Sending-end current
  (d) Sending-end PF
  (e) Efficiency of transmission

Solution

$$V_{R(L-N)} = \frac{138 \text{ kV}}{\sqrt{3}} = 79{,}768.8 \text{ V}$$

Using the receiving-end voltage as the reference,

$$\mathbf{V}_{R(L-N)} = 79{,}768.8\angle 0° \text{ V}$$

The receiving-end current is

$$I_R = \frac{49 \times 10^6}{\sqrt{3} \times 138 \times 10^3 \times 0.85} = 241.17 \text{ A} \quad \text{or} \quad 241.17\angle -31.80° \text{ A}$$

(a) The **A**, **B**, **C**, and **D** constants for the nominal-T circuit representation are

$$\mathbf{A} = 1 + \frac{1}{2}\mathbf{YZ}$$

$$= 1 + \frac{1}{2}(0.001\angle 90°)(95\angle 78°)$$

$$= 0.9535 + j0.0099$$

$$= 0.9536\angle 0.6°$$

$$\mathbf{B} = Z + \frac{1}{4}\mathbf{YZ}^2$$

$$= 95\angle 78° + \frac{1}{4}(0.001\angle 90°)(95\angle 78°)^2$$

$$= 18.83 + j90.86$$

$$= 92.79\angle 78.3° \ \Omega$$

$$\mathbf{C} = Y = 0.001\angle 90° \ S$$

$$\mathbf{D} = 1 + \frac{1}{2}\mathbf{YZ} = \mathbf{A}$$

$$= 0.9536\angle 0.6°$$

(b)

$$\begin{bmatrix} \mathbf{V}_{S(L-N)} \\ \mathbf{I}_S \end{bmatrix} = \begin{bmatrix} 0.9536\angle 0.6° & 92.79\angle 78.3° \\ 0.001\angle 90° & 0.9536\angle 0.6° \end{bmatrix} \begin{bmatrix} 79{,}768.8\angle 0° \\ 241.46\angle -31.8° \end{bmatrix}$$

The sending-end voltage is

$$\mathbf{V}_{S(L-N)} = 0.9536\angle 0.6° \times 79{,}768.8\angle 0° + 92.79\angle 78.3° \times 241.46\angle -31.8°$$

$$= 91{,}486 + j17{,}048.6 = 93{,}060.9\angle 10.4° \text{ V}$$

or

$$\mathbf{V}_{S(L-L)} = 160{,}995.4\angle 40.4° \text{ V}$$

(c) The sending-end current is

$$\mathbf{I}_S = 0.001\angle 90° \times 79,768.8\angle 0° + 0.9536\angle 0.6° \times 241.46\angle -31.8°$$

$$= 196.95 - j39.5 = 200.88\angle -11.3° \text{ A}$$

(d) The sending-end PF is

$$\theta_s = 10.4° + 11.3° = 21.7°$$

$$\cos\Phi_s = 0.929$$

(e) The efficiency of transmission is

$$\eta = \frac{\text{Output}}{\text{Input}}$$

$$= \frac{\sqrt{3}V_R I_R \cos\Phi_R}{\sqrt{3}V_S I_S \cos\Phi_S} \times 100$$

$$= \frac{138 \times 10^3 \times 241.46 \times 0.85}{160,995.4 \times 200.88 \times 0.929} \times 100$$

$$= 94.27\%$$

Example 4.12

Repeat Example 4.11 using nominal-π circuit representation.

Solution

(a) The **A**, **B**, **C**, and **D** constants for the nominal-π circuit representation are

$$\mathbf{A} = 1 + \frac{1}{2}\mathbf{YZ}$$

$$= 0.9536\angle 0.6°$$

$$\mathbf{B} = Z = 95\angle 78° \text{ } \Omega$$

$$\mathbf{C} = \mathbf{Y} + \frac{1}{4}\mathbf{Y}^2\mathbf{Z}$$

$$= 0.001\angle 90° + \frac{1}{4}(0.001\angle 90°)^2(95\angle 78°)$$

$$= -4.9379 \times 10^{-6} + j102.375 \times 10^{-5} = 0.001\angle 90.3° \text{ S}$$

$$\mathbf{D} = 1 + \frac{1}{2}\mathbf{YZ} = \mathbf{A}$$

$$= 0.9536\angle 0.6°$$

(b)

$$\begin{bmatrix} \mathbf{V}_{S(L-N)} \\ \mathbf{I}_S \end{bmatrix} = \begin{bmatrix} 0.9536\angle 0.6° & 95\angle 78° \\ 0.001\angle 90.3° & 0.9536\angle 0.6° \end{bmatrix} \begin{bmatrix} 79,768.8\angle 0° \\ 241.46\angle -31.8° \end{bmatrix}$$

Therefore,

$$\mathbf{V}_{S(L-N)} = 0.9536\angle 0.6° \times 79{,}768.8\angle 0° + 95\angle 78° \times 241.46\angle -31.8°$$

$$= 91{,}940.2 + j17{,}352.8 = 93{,}563.5\angle 10.7° \text{ V}$$

or

$$\mathbf{V}_{S(L-L)} = 161{,}864.9\angle 40.7° \text{ V}$$

(c) The sending-end current is

$$\mathbf{I}_S = 0.001\angle 90.3° \times 79{,}768.8\angle 0° + 0.9536\angle 0.6° \times 241.46\angle -31.8°$$

$$= 196.53 - j139.51 = 200.46\angle -11.37° \text{ A}$$

(d) The sending-end PF is

$$\theta_S = 10.7° + 11.37° = 22.07°$$

and

$$\cos\theta_S = 0.927$$

(e) The efficiency of transmission is

$$\eta = \frac{\text{Output}}{\text{Input}}$$

$$= \frac{\sqrt{3}V_R I_R \cos\theta_R}{\sqrt{3}V_S I_S \cos\theta_S} \times 100$$

$$= \frac{138 \times 10^3 \times 241.46 \times 0.85}{161{,}864.9 \times 200.46 \times 0.927} \times 100$$

$$= 94.16\%$$

The discrepancy between these results and the results of Example 4.11 is due to the fact *that the nominal-T and nominal-π circuits of a medium-length line are not equivalent to each other.* In fact, neither the nominal-T nor the nominal-π equivalent circuit exactly represents the actual line due to the fact that the *line is not uniformly distributed.* However, it is possible to find the equivalent circuit of a long transmission line and to represent the line accurately.

4.14 LONG TRANSMISSION LINES (ABOVE 150 mi, OR 240 km)

A more accurate analysis of the transmission lines requires that the parameters of the lines are not lumped, as before, but are distributed uniformly throughout the length of the line.

Figure 4.24 shows a uniform long line with an incremental section dx at a distance x from the receiving end, its series impedance is $\mathbf{z}dx$, and its shunt admittance is $\mathbf{y}dx$, where $\mathbf{z}$ and $\mathbf{y}$ are the impedance and admittance per-unit length, respectively.

The voltage drop in the section is

$$d\mathbf{V}_x = \left(\mathbf{V}_x + d\mathbf{V}_x\right) - \mathbf{V}_x = d\mathbf{V}_x$$

$$= \left(\mathbf{I}_x + d\mathbf{I}_x\right)\mathbf{z}\ dx$$

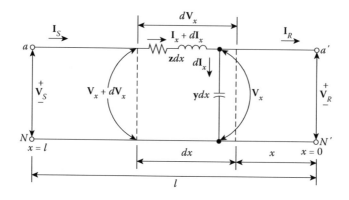

FIGURE 4.24   One phase and neutral connection of three-phase transmission line.

or

$$dV_x \cong I_x z \ dx \tag{4.222}$$

Similarly, the incremental charging current is

$$dI_x = V_x y \ dx \tag{4.223}$$

Therefore,

$$\frac{dV_x}{dx} = zI_x \tag{4.224}$$

and

$$\frac{dI_x}{dx} = yV_x \tag{4.225}$$

Differentiating Equations 4.224 and 4.225 with respect to x,

$$\frac{d^2V_x}{dx^2} = z\frac{dI_x}{dx} \tag{4.226}$$

and

$$\frac{d^2I_x}{dx^2} = y\frac{dV_x}{dx} \tag{4.227}$$

Substituting the values of dI_x/dx and dV_x/dx from Equations 4.222 and 4.226 in Equations 4.224 and 4.227, respectively,

$$\frac{d^2V_x}{dx^2} = yzV_x \tag{4.228}$$

and

$$\frac{d^2\mathbf{I}_x}{dx^2} = \mathbf{yzI}_x \tag{4.229}$$

At $x = 0$, $\mathbf{V}_x = \mathbf{V}_R$ and $\mathbf{I}_x = \mathbf{I}_R$. Therefore, the solution of the ordinary second-order differential Equations 4.228 and 4.229 gives

$$\mathbf{V}_{(x)} = \underbrace{\left(\cosh\sqrt{\mathbf{yz}}\,x\right)}_{A}\mathbf{V}_R + \underbrace{\left(\sqrt{\frac{\mathbf{z}}{\mathbf{y}}}\sinh\sqrt{\mathbf{yz}}\,x\right)}_{B}\mathbf{I}_R \tag{4.230}$$

Similarly,

$$\mathbf{I}_{(x)} = \underbrace{\left(\sqrt{\frac{\mathbf{y}}{\mathbf{z}}}\sinh\sqrt{\mathbf{yz}}\,x\right)}_{C}\mathbf{V}_R + \underbrace{\left(\cosh\sqrt{\mathbf{yz}}\,x\right)}_{D}\mathbf{I}_R \tag{4.231}$$

Equations 4.230 and 4.231 can be rewritten as

$$\mathbf{V}_{(x)} = \left(\cosh\gamma x\right)\mathbf{V}_R + \left(\mathbf{Z}_c\sinh\gamma x\right)\mathbf{I}_R \tag{4.232}$$

and

$$\mathbf{I}_{(x)} = \left(\mathbf{Y}_c\sinh\gamma x\right)\mathbf{V}_R + \left(\cosh\gamma x\right)\mathbf{I}_R \tag{4.233}$$

where
   γ is the propagation constant per-unit length, $= \sqrt{\mathbf{yz}}$
   $\mathbf{Z}_c$ is the characteristic (or surge or natural) impedance of line per-unit length, $= \sqrt{\mathbf{z}/\mathbf{y}}$
   $\mathbf{Y}_c$ is the characteristic (or surge or natural) admittance of line per-unit length, $= \sqrt{\mathbf{y}/\mathbf{z}}$

Further,

$$\gamma = \alpha + j\beta \tag{4.234}$$

where
   α is the attenuation constant (measuring decrement in voltage and current per-unit length in direction of travel) in nepers per-unit length
   β is the phase (or phase change) constant in radians per-unit length (i.e., change in phase angle between two voltages, or currents, at two points one per-unit length apart on infinite line)

When $x = l$, Equations 4.229 and 4.230 become

$$\mathbf{V}_S = \left(\cosh\gamma l\right)\mathbf{V}_R + \left(\mathbf{Z}_c\sinh\gamma l\right)\mathbf{I}_R \tag{4.235}$$

and

$$\mathbf{I}_S = \left(\mathbf{Y}_c\sinh\gamma l\right)\mathbf{V}_R + \left(\cosh\gamma l\right)\mathbf{I}_R \tag{4.236}$$

Equations 4.235 and 4.236 can be written in matrix form as

$$\begin{bmatrix} \mathbf{V}_S \\ \mathbf{I}_S \end{bmatrix} = \begin{bmatrix} \cosh \gamma l & \mathbf{Z}_c \sinh \gamma l \\ \mathbf{Y}_c \sinh \gamma l & \cosh \gamma l \end{bmatrix} \begin{bmatrix} \mathbf{V}_R \\ \mathbf{I}_R \end{bmatrix} \tag{4.237}$$

and

$$\begin{bmatrix} \mathbf{V}_R \\ \mathbf{I}_R \end{bmatrix} = \begin{bmatrix} \cosh \gamma l & \mathbf{Z}_c \sinh \gamma l \\ \mathbf{Y}_c \sinh \gamma l & \cosh \gamma l \end{bmatrix}^{-1} \begin{bmatrix} \mathbf{V}_S \\ \mathbf{I}_S \end{bmatrix} \tag{4.238}$$

or

$$\begin{bmatrix} \mathbf{V}_R \\ \mathbf{I}_R \end{bmatrix} = \begin{bmatrix} \cosh \gamma l & -\mathbf{Z}_c \sinh \gamma l \\ -\mathbf{Y}_c \sinh \gamma l & \cosh \gamma l \end{bmatrix} \begin{bmatrix} \mathbf{V}_S \\ \mathbf{I}_S \end{bmatrix} \tag{4.239}$$

Therefore,

$$\mathbf{V}_R = \left(\cosh \gamma l \right) \mathbf{V}_S - \left(\mathbf{Z}_c \sinh \gamma l \right) \mathbf{I}_S \tag{4.240}$$

and

$$\mathbf{I}_R = -\left(\mathbf{Y}_c \sinh \gamma l \right) \mathbf{V}_S + \left(\cosh \gamma l \right) \mathbf{I}_S \tag{4.241}$$

In terms of **ABCD** constants,

$$\begin{bmatrix} \mathbf{V}_S \\ \mathbf{I}_S \end{bmatrix} = \begin{bmatrix} \mathbf{A} & \mathbf{B} \\ \mathbf{C} & \mathbf{D} \end{bmatrix} \begin{bmatrix} \mathbf{V}_R \\ \mathbf{I}_R \end{bmatrix} = \begin{bmatrix} \mathbf{A} & \mathbf{B} \\ \mathbf{C} & \mathbf{A} \end{bmatrix} \begin{bmatrix} \mathbf{V}_R \\ \mathbf{I}_R \end{bmatrix} \tag{4.242}$$

and

$$\begin{bmatrix} \mathbf{V}_R \\ \mathbf{I}_R \end{bmatrix} = \begin{bmatrix} \mathbf{A} & -\mathbf{B} \\ -\mathbf{C} & \mathbf{D} \end{bmatrix} \begin{bmatrix} \mathbf{V}_S \\ \mathbf{I}_S \end{bmatrix} = \begin{bmatrix} \mathbf{A} & -\mathbf{B} \\ -\mathbf{C} & \mathbf{A} \end{bmatrix} \begin{bmatrix} \mathbf{V}_S \\ \mathbf{I}_S \end{bmatrix} \tag{4.243}$$

where

$$\mathbf{A} = \cosh \gamma l = \cosh \sqrt{\mathbf{YZ}} = \cosh \theta \tag{4.244}$$

$$\mathbf{B} = \mathbf{Z}_c \sinh \gamma l = \sqrt{\mathbf{Z/Y}} \, \sinh \sqrt{\mathbf{YZ}} = \mathbf{Z}_c \sinh \theta \tag{4.245}$$

$$\mathbf{C} = \mathbf{Y}_c \sinh \gamma l = \sqrt{\mathbf{Y/Z}} \, \sinh \sqrt{\mathbf{YZ}} = \mathbf{Y}_c \sinh \theta \tag{4.246}$$

$$\mathbf{D} = \mathbf{A} = \cosh \gamma l = \cosh \sqrt{\mathbf{YZ}} = \cosh \theta \tag{4.247}$$

$$\theta = \sqrt{\mathbf{YZ}} \qquad (4.248)$$

$$\sinh \gamma l = \frac{1}{2}\left(e^{\gamma l} - e^{-\gamma l}\right) \qquad (4.249)$$

$$\cosh \gamma l = \frac{1}{2}\left(e^{\gamma l} + e^{-\gamma l}\right) \qquad (4.250)$$

Also,

$$\sinh(\alpha + j\beta) = \frac{e^{\alpha}e^{j\beta} - e^{-\alpha}e^{-j\beta}}{2} = \frac{1}{2}\left[e^{\alpha}\angle\beta - e^{-\alpha}\angle - \beta\right]$$

and

$$\cosh(\alpha + j\beta) = \frac{e^{\alpha}e^{j\beta} + e^{-\alpha}e^{-j\beta}}{2} = \frac{1}{2}\left[e^{\alpha}\angle\beta + e^{-\alpha}\angle - \beta\right]$$

Note that β in these equations is the radian, and the radian is the unit found for β by computing the quadrature component of γ. Since 2π radians = 360°, one radian is 57.3°. Thus, the β is converted into degrees by multiplying its quantity by 57.3°. For a line length of l,

$$\sinh(\alpha l + j\beta l) = \frac{e^{\alpha l}e^{j\beta l} - e^{-\alpha l}e^{-j\beta l}}{2} = \frac{1}{2}\left[e^{\alpha l}\angle\beta l - e^{-\alpha l}\angle - \beta l\right]$$

and

$$\cosh(\alpha l + j\beta l) = \frac{e^{\alpha l}e^{j\beta l} + e^{-\alpha l}e^{-j\beta l}}{2} = \frac{1}{2}\left[e^{\alpha l}\angle\beta l + e^{-\alpha l}\angle - \beta l\right]$$

Equations 4.235 through 4.248 can be used if tables of complex hyperbolic functions or pocket calculators with complex hyperbolic functions are available.

Alternatively, the following expansions can be used:

$$\sinh \gamma l = \sinh(\alpha l + j\beta l) = \sinh \alpha l \cos \beta l + j\cosh \alpha l \sin \beta l \qquad (4.251)$$

$$\cosh \gamma l = \cosh(\alpha l + j\beta l) = \cosh \alpha l \cos \beta l + j\sinh \alpha l \sin \beta l \qquad (4.252)$$

The correct mathematical unit for βl is the radian, and the radian is the unit found for βl by computing the quadrature component of γl.

Furthermore, substituting for γl and $\mathbf{Z}_c$ in terms of $\mathbf{Y}$ and $\mathbf{Z}$, that is, the total line shunt admittance per phase and the total line series impedance per phase, in Equation 4.242 gives

$$\mathbf{V}_S = \left(\cosh \sqrt{\mathbf{YZ}}\right)\mathbf{V}_R + \left(\sqrt{\frac{\mathbf{Z}}{\mathbf{Y}}} \sinh \sqrt{\mathbf{YZ}}\right)\mathbf{I}_R \qquad (4.253)$$

and

$$\mathbf{I}_S = \left(\sqrt{\frac{\mathbf{Y}}{\mathbf{Z}}} \sinh \sqrt{\mathbf{YZ}} \right) \mathbf{V}_R + \left(\cosh \sqrt{\mathbf{YZ}} \right) \mathbf{I}_R \tag{4.254}$$

or, alternatively,

$$\mathbf{V}_S = \left(\cosh \sqrt{\mathbf{YZ}} \right) \mathbf{V}_R + \left(\frac{\sinh \sqrt{\mathbf{YZ}}}{\sqrt{\mathbf{YZ}}} \right) \mathbf{ZI}_R \tag{4.255}$$

and

$$\mathbf{I}_S = \left(\frac{\sinh \sqrt{\mathbf{YZ}}}{\sqrt{\mathbf{YZ}}} \right) \mathbf{YV}_R + \left(\cosh \sqrt{\mathbf{YZ}} \right) \mathbf{I}_R \tag{4.256}$$

The factors in parentheses in Equations 4.253 through 4.256 can readily be found by using Woodruff's charts, which are not included here but can be found in L. F. Woodruff, *Electric Power Transmission* (Wiley, New York, 1952).

The **ABCD** parameters in terms of infinite series can be expressed as

$$\mathbf{A} = 1 + \frac{\mathbf{YZ}}{2} + \frac{\mathbf{Y}^2\mathbf{Z}^2}{24} + \frac{\mathbf{Y}^3\mathbf{Z}^3}{720} + \frac{\mathbf{Y}^4\mathbf{Z}^4}{40,320} + \cdots \tag{4.257}$$

$$\mathbf{B} = \mathbf{Z} \left(1 + \frac{\mathbf{YZ}}{6} + \frac{\mathbf{Y}^2\mathbf{Z}^2}{120} + \frac{\mathbf{Y}^3\mathbf{Z}^3}{5,040} + \frac{\mathbf{Y}^4\mathbf{Z}^4}{362,880} + \cdots \right) \tag{4.258}$$

$$\mathbf{C} = \mathbf{Y} \left(1 + \frac{\mathbf{YZ}}{6} + \frac{\mathbf{Y}^2\mathbf{Z}^2}{120} + \frac{\mathbf{Y}^3\mathbf{Z}^3}{5,040} + \frac{\mathbf{Y}^4\mathbf{Z}^4}{362,880} + \cdots \right) \tag{4.259}$$

where
   $\mathbf{Z}$ = total line series impedance per phase
   $= \mathbf{z}l$
   $= (r + jx_L)l \ \Omega$
   $\mathbf{Y}$ = total line shunt admittance per phase
   $= \mathbf{y}l$
   $= (g + jb)l \ \mathrm{S}$

In practice, usually not more than three terms are necessary in Equations 4.257 through 4.259. Weedy [7] suggests the following approximate values for the **ABCD** constants if the OH transmission line is less than 500 km in length:

$$\mathbf{A} = 1 + \frac{1}{2}\mathbf{YZ} \tag{4.260}$$

$$B = Z\left(1 + \frac{1}{6}YZ\right) \tag{4.261}$$

$$C = Y\left(1 + \frac{1}{6}YZ\right) \tag{4.262}$$

However, the error involved may be too large to be ignored for certain applications.

The percentage of voltage regulation for the long-length transmission lines is given by Stevenson [3] as

$$\text{Percentage of voltage regulation} = \frac{\dfrac{|\mathbf{V}_S|}{|\mathbf{A}|} - |\mathbf{V}_{R,FL}|}{|\mathbf{V}_{R,FL}|} \times 100 \tag{4.263}$$

where
$|\mathbf{V}_S|$ is the magnitude of sending-end phase (line-to-neutral) voltage
$|\mathbf{V}_{R,FL}|$ is the magnitude of receiving-end phase (line-to-neutral) voltage at full load with constant $|\mathbf{V}_S|$
$|\mathbf{A}|$ is the magnitude of line constant A

Example 4.13

A single-circuit, 60 Hz, three-phase transmission line is 150 mi long. The line is connected to a load of 50 MVA at a lagging PF of 0.85 at 138 kV. The line constants are given as $R = 0.1858$ Ω/mi, $L = 2.60$ mH/mi, and $C = 0.012$ μF/mi. Calculate the following:

(a) **A, B, C,** and **D** constants of line
(b) Sending-end voltage
(c) Sending-end current
(d) Sending-end PF
(e) Sending-end power
(f) Power loss in line
(g) Transmission-line efficiency
(h) Percentage of voltage regulation
(i) Sending-end charging current at no load
(j) Value of receiving-end voltage rise at no load if sending-end voltage is held constant

Solution

$$\mathbf{z} = 0.1858 + j2\pi \times 60 \times 2.6 \times 10^{-3}$$

$$= 0.1858 + j0.9802$$

$$= 0.9977 \angle 79.27° \ \Omega/\text{mi}$$

$$\mathbf{y} = j2\pi \times 60 \times 0.012 \times 10^{-6}$$

$$= 4.5239 \times 10^{-6} \angle 90° \ \text{S/mi}$$

Thus, for the total line length,

$$\mathbf{Z} = \mathbf{z} \times \ell = \left(0.9977\angle 79.27° \ \Omega\right) \times 150 \ \text{mi}$$

$$= 149.655\angle 79.27° \ \Omega$$

and

$$\mathbf{Y} = \mathbf{y} \times \ell = \left(4.5239 \times 10^{-6}\angle 90° \ \text{S}\right) \times 150 \ \text{mi}$$

$$= 678.585\angle 90° \ \text{S}$$

The propagation constant of the line is

$$\gamma = \sqrt{\mathbf{yz}}$$

$$= \left[\left(4.5239 \times 10^{-6}\angle 90°\right)\left(0.9977\angle 79.27°\right)\right]^{1/2}$$

$$= \left[4.5135 \times 10^{-6}\right]^{1/2} \angle \left(\frac{90° + 79.27°}{2}\right) = 0.002144\angle 84.63°$$

$$= 0.0002007 + j0.0021346$$

Thus,

$$\gamma l = \alpha l + j\beta l$$

$$= (0.0002007 + j0.0021346)150$$

$$\cong 0.0301 + j0.3202$$

The characteristic impedance of the line is

$$\mathbf{Z}_C = \sqrt{\frac{\mathbf{z}}{\mathbf{y}}} = \left(\frac{0.9977\angle 79.27°}{4.5239 \times 10^{-6}\angle 90°}\right)^{1/2}$$

$$= \left(\frac{0.9977 \times 10^{6}}{4.5239}\right)^{1/2} \angle \left(\frac{79.27° - 90°}{2}\right) = 469.62\angle -5.37° \ \Omega$$

The receiving-end line-to-neutral voltage is

$$\mathbf{V}_{R(L-N)} = \frac{138 \ \text{kV}}{\sqrt{3}} = 79{,}674.34 \ \text{V}$$

Using the receiving-end voltage as the reference,

$$\mathbf{V}_{R(L-N)} = 79{,}674.34\angle 0° \ \text{V}$$

The receiving-end current is

$$\mathbf{I}_R = \frac{50 \times 10^{6}}{\sqrt{3} \times 138 \times 10^{3}} = 209.18 \ \text{A} \quad \text{or} \quad 209.18\angle -31.8° \ \text{A}$$

(a) The **A**, **B**, **C**, and **D** constants of the line

$$\mathbf{A} = \cosh \gamma l$$

$$= \cosh(\alpha + j\beta)l$$

$$= \frac{e^{\alpha l}e^{j\beta l} + e^{-\alpha l}e^{-j\beta l}}{2}$$

$$= \frac{e^{\alpha l}\angle \beta l + e^{-\alpha l}\angle -\beta l}{2}$$

Therefore,

$$\mathbf{A} = \frac{e^{0.0301}e^{j0.3202} + e^{-0.0301}e^{-j0.3202}}{2}$$

$$= \frac{e^{0.0301}\angle 18.35° + e^{-0.0301}\angle -18.35°}{2}$$

$$= \frac{1.0306\angle 18.35° + 0.9703\angle -18.35°}{2}$$

$$= 0.9496 + j0.0095 = 0.9497\angle 0.57°$$

Note that $e^{j0.3202}$ needs to be converted to degrees. Since 2π radians = 360°, one radian is 57.3°. Hence,

$$(0.3202 \text{ rad})(57.3°/\text{rad}) = 18.35°$$

and

$$\mathbf{B} = \mathbf{Z}_C \sinh \gamma l = \mathbf{Z}_C \sinh(\alpha + j\beta)l$$

$$= \mathbf{Z}_C \left[\frac{e^{\alpha l}e^{j\beta l} - e^{-\alpha l}e^{-j\beta l}}{2} \right]$$

$$= \mathbf{Z}_C \left[\frac{e^{\alpha l}\angle \beta l - e^{-\alpha l}\angle -\beta l}{2} \right]$$

$$= (469.62\angle -5.37°) \left[\frac{e^{0.0301}e^{j0.3202} - e^{-0.0301}e^{-j0.3202}}{2} \right]$$

$$= 469.62\angle -5.37° \left[\frac{1.0306\angle 18.35° - 0.9703\angle -18.35°}{2} \right]$$

$$= 469.62\angle -5.37° \left(\frac{0.0572 + j0.63}{2} \right)$$

$$= 469.62\angle -5.37° \left(\frac{0.6326\angle 84.81°}{2} \right)$$

$$= 469.62\angle -5.37° (0.3163\angle 84.81°)$$

$$= 148.54\angle 79.44° \ \Omega$$

and

$$\mathbf{C} = \mathbf{Y}_C \sinh \gamma l = \frac{1}{\mathbf{Z}_C} \sinh \gamma l$$

$$= \frac{1}{469.62\angle -5.37°} \times \left(\frac{0.6326\angle 84.81°}{2} \right)$$

$$= 0.00067\angle 90.18° \text{ S}$$

and

$$\mathbf{D} = \mathbf{A} = \cos \gamma l = 0.9497\angle 0.57°$$

(b)

$$\begin{bmatrix} \mathbf{V}_{S(L\text{-}N)} \\ I_S \end{bmatrix} = \begin{bmatrix} \mathbf{A} & \mathbf{B} \\ \mathbf{C} & \mathbf{D} \end{bmatrix} \begin{bmatrix} \mathbf{V}_{R(L\text{-}N)} \\ I_R \end{bmatrix}$$

$$= \begin{bmatrix} 0.9497\angle 0.57° & 148.54\angle 79.44° \\ 0.00067\angle 90.18° & 0.9497\angle 0.57° \end{bmatrix} \begin{bmatrix} 79,674.34\angle 0° \\ 209.18\angle -31.8° \end{bmatrix}$$

Thus, the sending-end voltage is

$$\mathbf{V}_{S(L\text{-}N)} = (0.9497\angle 0.57°)(79.674.34\angle 0°) + (148.54\angle 79.44°)(209.18\angle -31.8°)$$

$$= 99,470.05\angle 13.79° \text{ V}$$

and

$$\mathbf{V}_{S(L\text{-}L)} = \sqrt{3}\mathbf{V}_{S(L\text{-}N)}$$

$$= 172,287.18\angle 13.79° + 30° = 172,287.18\angle 43.79° \text{ V}$$

Note that an additional 30° is added to the angle since a line-to-line voltage is 30° ahead of its line-to-neutral voltage.

(c) The sending-end current is

$$\mathbf{I}_S = (0.00067\angle 90.18°)(79,674.34\angle 0°) + (0.9497\angle 0.57°)(209.18\angle -31.8°)$$

$$= 176.8084\angle -16.3° \text{ A}$$

(d) The sending-end PF is

$$\theta_S = 13.79° + 16.3° = 30.09°$$

$$\cos \theta_S = 0.8653$$

(e) The sending-end power is

$$P_S = \sqrt{3}V_{S(L\text{-}L)}I_S \cos \theta_S$$

$$= \sqrt{3} \times 172,287.18 \times 176.8084 \times 0.8653 \cong 45,654.46 \text{ kW}$$

(f) The receiving-end power is

$$P_R = \sqrt{3}V_{R(L-L)}I_R \cos\theta_R$$

$$= \sqrt{3} \times 138 \times 10^3 \times 209.18 \times 0.85 = 42,499 \text{ kW}$$

Therefore, the power loss in the line is

$$P_L = P_S - P_R = 3155.46 \text{ kW}$$

(g) The transmission-line efficiency is

$$\eta = \frac{P_R}{P_S} \times 100 = \frac{42,499}{45,654.46} \times 100 = 93.1\%$$

(h) The percentage of voltage regulation is

$$\text{Percentage of voltage regulation} = \frac{\dfrac{99,470.04}{0.9496} - 79,674.34}{79,674.34} \times 100$$

$$= \frac{104,738.4 - 79,674.34}{79,674.34} \times 100 = 31\%$$

(i) The sending-end charging current at no load is

$$I_C = \frac{1}{2}YV_{S(L-N)} = \frac{1}{2}\left(678.585 \times 10^{-6}\right)(99,470.05) = 33.75 \text{ A}$$

where

$$Y = y \times l = \left(4.5239 \times 10^{-6} \text{ S/mi}\right)(150 \text{ mi}) = 678.585 \times 10^{-6} \text{ S}$$

(j) The receiving-end voltage rise at no load is

$$\mathbf{V}_{R(L-N)} = \mathbf{V}_{S(L-N)} - I_C\mathbf{Z}$$

$$= 99,470.05\angle13.79° - (33.75\angle103.79°)(149.66\angle79.27°)$$

$$= 99,470.05\angle13.79° - 5,051.03\angle183.06°$$

$$= 99,470.05\angle13.79° + 5,051.03\angle183.06° - 180°$$

$$= 99,470.05\angle13.79° + 5,051.03\angle3.06°$$

$$= 104,436.74\angle13.27° \text{ V}$$

Therefore, the line-to-line voltage at the receiving end is

$$\mathbf{V}_{R(L-L)} = \sqrt{3}\mathbf{V}_{R(L-N)} = 180,889.74\angle13.27° + 30°$$

$$= 180,889.74\angle43.27° \text{ V}$$

Note that in a well-designed transmission line, the voltage regulation and the line efficiency should be not greater than about 5%.

4.14.1 Equivalent Circuit of Long Transmission Line

Using the values of the **ABCD** parameters obtained for a transmission line, it is possible to develop an exact π or an exact T, as shown in Figure 4.25.

For the equivalent-π circuit,

$$\mathbf{Z}_\pi = \mathbf{B} = \mathbf{Z}_C \sinh\theta \tag{4.264}$$

$$= \mathbf{Z}_C \sinh\gamma l \tag{4.265}$$

$$= \mathbf{Z}\left(\frac{\sinh\sqrt{\mathbf{YZ}}}{\sqrt{\mathbf{YZ}}}\right) \tag{4.266}$$

and

$$\frac{\mathbf{Y}_\pi}{2} = \frac{\mathbf{A}-1}{\mathbf{B}} = \frac{\cosh\theta-1}{\mathbf{Z}_C\sinh\theta} \tag{4.267}$$

or

$$\mathbf{Y}_\pi = \frac{2\tanh\left(\dfrac{\gamma l}{2}\right)}{\mathbf{Z}_C} \tag{4.268}$$

or

$$\frac{\mathbf{Y}_\pi}{2} = \frac{\mathbf{Y}}{2}\frac{2\tanh\left(\dfrac{\sqrt{\mathbf{YZ}}}{2}\right)}{\dfrac{\sqrt{\mathbf{YZ}}}{2}} \tag{4.269}$$

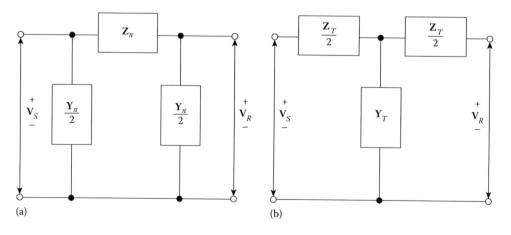

FIGURE 4.25 Equivalent-π and equivalent-T circuits for a long transmission line: (a) equivalent-π circuit and (b) equivalent-T circuit.

For the equivalent-T circuit,

$$\frac{\mathbf{Z}_T}{2} = \frac{\mathbf{A}-1}{\mathbf{C}} = \frac{\cosh\theta-1}{\mathbf{Y}_C \sinh\theta} \tag{4.270}$$

or

$$\mathbf{Z}_T = 2\mathbf{Z}_C \tanh\frac{\gamma l}{2} \tag{4.271}$$

or

$$\frac{\mathbf{Z}_T}{2} = \frac{\mathbf{Z}}{2}\left(\frac{\tanh\dfrac{\sqrt{\mathbf{YZ}}}{2}}{\dfrac{\sqrt{\mathbf{YZ}}}{2}}\right) \tag{4.272}$$

and

$$\mathbf{Y}_T = \mathbf{C} = \mathbf{Y}_C \sinh\theta \tag{4.273}$$

or

$$\mathbf{Y}_T = \frac{\sinh\gamma l}{\mathbf{Z}_C} \tag{4.274}$$

or

$$\mathbf{Y}_T = \mathbf{Y}\frac{\sinh\sqrt{\mathbf{YZ}}}{\sqrt{\mathbf{YZ}}} \tag{4.275}$$

Example 4.14

Find the equivalent-π and the equivalent-T circuits for the line described in Example 4.13 and compare them with the nominal-π and the nominal-T circuits.

Solution

Figures 4.26 and 4.27 show the equivalent-π and the nominal-π circuits, respectively. *For the equivalent-π circuit,*

$$\mathbf{Z}_\pi = \mathbf{B} = 148.54\angle 79.44°\ \Omega$$

$$\frac{\mathbf{Y}_\pi}{2} = \frac{\mathbf{A}-1}{\mathbf{B}} = \frac{0.9497\angle 0.57°-1}{148.54\angle 79.44°} = 0.000345\angle 89.89°\ \mathrm{S}$$

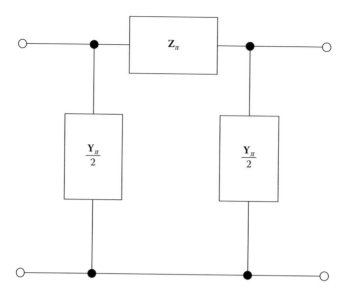

FIGURE 4.26 Equivalent-π circuit.

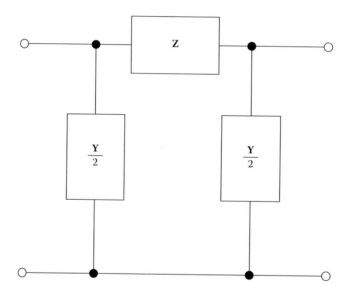

FIGURE 4.27 Nominal-π circuit.

For the nominal-π circuit,

$$Z = 150 \times 0.9977\angle79.27° = 149.655\angle79.27° \ \Omega$$

$$\frac{Y}{2} = \frac{150\left(4.5239\times10^{-6}\angle90°\right)}{2} = 0.000339\angle90° \ S$$

Figure 4.28a and b show the equivalent-T and nominal-T circuits, respectively. *For the equivalent-T circuit,*

$$\frac{Z_T}{2} = \frac{A-1}{C} = \frac{0.9497\angle0.57°-1}{0.00067\angle90.18°} = 76.57\angle79.15° \ \Omega$$

$$Y_T = C = 0.00067\angle90.18° \ S$$

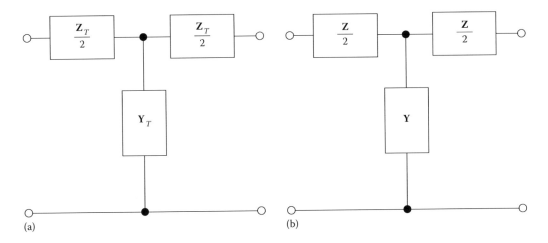

FIGURE 4.28   The T circuits: (a) equivalent *T* and (b) nominal *T*.

For the nominal-T circuit,

$$\frac{\mathbf{Z}}{2} = \frac{149.655\angle79.27°}{2} = 74.83\angle79.27° \ \Omega$$

$$\mathbf{Y} = 0.000678\angle90° \ \text{S}$$

As can be observed from the results, the difference between the values for the equivalent and nominal circuits is very small for a 150 mi long transmission line.

4.14.2   Incident and Reflected Voltages of Long Transmission Line

Previously, the propagation constant has been given as

$$\gamma = \alpha + j\beta \ \text{per-unit length} \tag{4.276}$$

and also

$$\cosh \gamma l = \frac{e^{\gamma l} + e^{-\gamma l}}{2} \tag{4.277}$$

$$\sinh \gamma l = \frac{e^{\gamma l} - e^{-\gamma l}}{2} \tag{4.278}$$

The sending-end voltage and current have been expressed as

$$\mathbf{V}_S = \left(\cosh \gamma l\right)\mathbf{V}_R + \left(\mathbf{Z}_C \sinh \gamma l\right)\mathbf{I}_R \tag{4.279}$$

and

$$\mathbf{I}_S = \left(\mathbf{Y}_C \sinh \gamma l\right)\mathbf{V}_R + \left(\cosh \gamma l\right)\mathbf{I}_R \tag{4.280}$$

By substituting Equations 4.276 through 4.278 in Equations 4.279 and 4.280,

$$\mathbf{V}_S = \frac{1}{2}\left(\mathbf{V}_R + \mathbf{I}_R\mathbf{Z}_C\right)e^{\alpha l}e^{j\beta l} + \frac{1}{2}\left(\mathbf{V}_R - \mathbf{I}_R\mathbf{Z}_C\right)e^{-\alpha l}e^{-j\beta l} \qquad (4.281)$$

and

$$\mathbf{I}_S = \frac{1}{2}\left(\mathbf{V}_R\mathbf{Y}_C + \mathbf{I}_R\right)e^{\alpha l}e^{j\beta l} - \frac{1}{2}\left(\mathbf{V}_R\mathbf{Y}_C - \mathbf{I}_R\right)e^{-\alpha l}e^{-j\beta l} \qquad (4.282)$$

In Equation 4.281, the first and the second terms are called the *incident voltage* and the *reflected voltage*, respectively. They act like *traveling waves* as a function of the line length *l*. The incident voltage increases in magnitude and phase as the *l* distance from the receiving end increases and decreases in magnitude and phase as the distance from the sending end toward the receiving end decreases, whereas the reflected voltage decreases in magnitude and phase as the *l* distance from the receiving end toward the sending end increases.

Therefore, for any given line length *l*, the voltage is the sum of the corresponding incident and reflected voltages. Here, the term $e^{\alpha l}$ changes as a function of *l*, whereas $e^{j\beta l}$ always has a magnitude of 1 and causes a phase shift of β radians per-unit length of line.

In Equation 4.281, when the two terms are 180° out of phase, a cancelation will occur. This happens when there is no load on the line, that is, when

$$\mathbf{I}_R = 0 \quad \text{and} \quad \alpha = 0$$

and when $\beta x = \pi/2$ radians, or one-quarter wavelengths.

The *wavelength A* is defined as the distance *l* along a line between two points to develop a phase shift of 2π radians, or 360°, for the incident and reflected waves. If β is the phase shift in radians per mile, the wavelength in miles is

$$\lambda = \frac{2\pi}{\beta} \qquad (4.283)$$

Since the propagation velocity is

$$v = \lambda f \quad \text{mi/s} \qquad (4.284)$$

and is approximately equal to the speed of light, that is, 186,000 mils, at a frequency of 60 Hz, the wavelength is

$$\lambda = \frac{186,000 \text{ mi/s}}{60 \text{ Hz}} = 3,100 \text{ mi}$$

whereas at a frequency of 50 Hz, the wavelength is approximately 6000 km. If a finite line is terminated by its characteristic impedance $\mathbf{Z}_C$, that impedance could be imagined replaced by an infinite line. In this case, there is no reflected wave of either voltage or current since

$$\mathbf{V}_R = \mathbf{I}_R\mathbf{Z}_C$$

in Equations 4.279 and 4.280, and the line is called an *infinite* (or *flat*) line.

Stevenson [3] gives the typical values of $\mathbf{Z}_C$ as 400 ft for a single-circuit line and 200 Ω for two circuits in parallel. The phase angle of $\mathbf{Z}_C$ is usually between 0 and −15° [3].

Example 4.15

Using the data given in Example 4.13, determine the following:

(a) Attenuation constant and phase change constant per mile of the line
(b) Wavelength and velocity of propagation
(c) Incident and reflected voltages at the receiving end of the line
(d) Line voltage at the receiving end of the line
(e) Incident and reflected voltages at the sending end of the line
(f) Line voltage at the sending end

Solution

(a) Since the propagation constant of the line is

$$\gamma = \sqrt{\mathbf{yz}} = 0.0002 + j0.0021$$

the attenuation constant is 0.0002 Np/mi, and the phase change constant is 0.0021 rad/mi.

(b) The wavelength of propagation is

$$\lambda = \frac{2\pi}{\beta} = \frac{2\pi}{0.0021} = 2{,}991.99 \ \text{mi}$$

and the velocity of propagation is

$$\upsilon = \lambda f = 2{,}991.99 \times 60 = 179{,}519.58 \ \text{mi/s}$$

(c) From Equation 4.281,

$$\mathbf{V}_S = \frac{1}{2}\left(\mathbf{V}_R + \mathbf{I}_R\mathbf{Z}_C\right)e^{\alpha l}e^{j\beta l} + \frac{1}{2}\left(\mathbf{V}_R - \mathbf{I}_R\mathbf{Z}_C\right)e^{-\alpha l}e^{-j\beta l}$$

Since, at the receiving end, $l = 0$,

$$\mathbf{V}_S = \frac{1}{2}\left(\mathbf{V}_R + \mathbf{I}_R\mathbf{Z}_C\right) + \frac{1}{2}\left(\mathbf{V}_R - \mathbf{I}_R\mathbf{Z}_C\right)$$

Therefore, the incident and reflected voltage at the receiving end are

$$\mathbf{V}_{R(\text{incident})} = \frac{1}{2}\left(\mathbf{V}_R + \mathbf{I}_R\mathbf{Z}_C\right)$$

$$= \frac{1}{2}\left[79{,}674.34\angle 0° + (209.18\angle -31.8°)(469.62\angle -5.37°)\right]$$

$$= 84{,}367.77\angle -20.59° \ \text{V}$$

and

$$\mathbf{V}_{R(\text{reflected})} = \frac{1}{2}\left(\mathbf{V}_R - \mathbf{I}_R\mathbf{Z}_C\right)$$

$$= \frac{1}{2}\left[79{,}674.34\angle 0° - (209.18\angle -31.8°)(469.62\angle -5.37°)\right]$$

$$= 29{,}684.15\angle 88.65° \ \text{V}$$

(d) The line-to-neutral voltage at the receiving end is

$$\mathbf{V}_{R(L-N)} = \mathbf{V}_{R(incident)} + \mathbf{V}_{R(reflected)} = 79,674\angle 0° \text{ V}$$

Therefore, the line voltage at the receiving end is

$$V_{R(L-L)} = \sqrt{3}V_{R(L-N)} = 138,000 \text{ V}$$

(e) At the sending end,

$$\mathbf{V}_{S(incident)} = \frac{1}{2}\left(\mathbf{V}_R + \mathbf{I}_R\mathbf{Z}_C\right)e^{\alpha l}e^{j\beta l}$$

$$= (84,367.77\angle -20.59°)e^{0.0301}\angle 18.35° = 86,946\angle -2.24° \text{ V}$$

and

$$\mathbf{V}_{S(reflected)} = \frac{1}{2}\left(\mathbf{V}_R - \mathbf{I}_R\mathbf{Z}_C\right)e^{-\alpha l}e^{-j\beta l}$$

$$= (29,684.15\angle 88.65°)e^{-0.0301}\angle -18.35° = 28,802.5\angle 70.3° \text{ V}$$

(f) The line-to-neutral voltage at the sending end is

$$\mathbf{V}_{S(L-N)} = \mathbf{V}_{S(incident)} + \mathbf{V}_{S(reflected)}$$

$$= 86,946\angle -2.24° + 28,802.5\angle 70.3° = 99,458.1\angle 13.8° \text{ V}$$

Therefore, the line voltage at the sending end is

$$V_{S(L-L)} = \sqrt{3}V_{S(L-N)} = 172,266.5 \text{ V}$$

4.14.3 Surge Impedance Loading of Transmission Line

In power systems, if the line *is lossless*,* the characteristic impedance Z_c of a line is sometimes called *surge impedance*. Therefore, for a loss-free line,

$$R = 0$$

and

$$\mathbf{Z}_L = jX_L$$

Thus,

$$Z_c = \sqrt{\frac{X_L}{Y_c}} \cong \sqrt{\frac{L}{C}} \ \Omega \tag{4.285}$$

---

* When dealing with high frequencies or with surges due to lightning, losses are often ignored [3].

and its series resistance and shunt conductance are zero. It is a function of the line inductance and capacitance as shown and is independent of the line length.

The SIL (or the *natural loading*) of a transmission line is defined as the power delivered by the line to a purely resistive load equal to its surge impedance. Therefore,

$$\text{SIL} = \frac{\left|kV_{R(\text{L-L})}\right|^2}{Z_c^*} \text{ MW} \tag{4.286}$$

or

$$\text{SIL} \cong \frac{\left|kV_{R(\text{L-L})}\right|^2}{\sqrt{\dfrac{L}{C}}} \text{ MW} \tag{4.287}$$

or

$$\text{SIL} = \sqrt{3}\left|\mathbf{V}_{R(\text{L-L})}\right|\left|\mathbf{I}_L\right| \text{ W} \tag{4.288}$$

where

$$\left|\mathbf{I}_L\right| = \frac{\left|\mathbf{V}_{R(\text{L-L})}\right|}{\sqrt{3} \times \sqrt{\dfrac{L}{C}}} \text{ A} \tag{4.289}$$

SIL is the surge impedance loading in megawatts or watts
$\left|kV_{R(\text{L-L})}\right|$ is the magnitude of line-to-line receiving-end voltage in kilovolts
$\left|\mathbf{V}_{R(\text{L-L})}\right|$ is the magnitude of line-to-line receiving-end voltage in volts
Z_c is the surge impedance in ohms $\cong \sqrt{L/C}$
$\mathbf{I}_L$ is the line current at SIL in amperes

In practice, the allowable loading of a transmission line may be given as a fraction of its SIL. Thus, SIL is used as a means of comparing the load-carrying capabilities of lines.

However, the SIL in itself is not a measure of the maximum power that can be delivered over a line. For the maximum delivered power, the line length, the impedance of sending- and receiving-end apparatus, and all of the other factors affecting stability must be considered.

Since the characteristic impedance of underground cables is very low, the SIL (or *natural load*) is far larger than the rated load of the cable. Therefore, *a given cable acts as a source of lagging vars.*

The best way of increasing the SIL of a line is to increase its voltage level, since, as it can be seen from Equation 4.284, the SIL increases with its square. However, increasing the voltage level is expensive. Therefore, instead, the surge impedance of the line is reduced. This can be accomplished by adding capacitors or induction coils. There are four possible ways of changing the line capacitance or inductance, as shown in Figures 4.29 and 4.30.

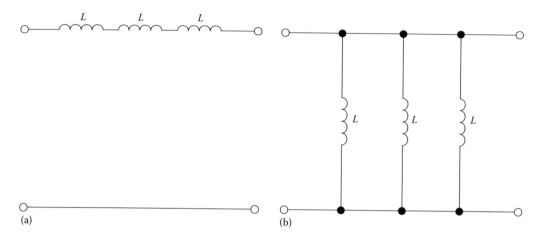

FIGURE 4.29 Transmission-line compensation by adding lump inductances in (a) series and (b) parallel (i.e., shunt).

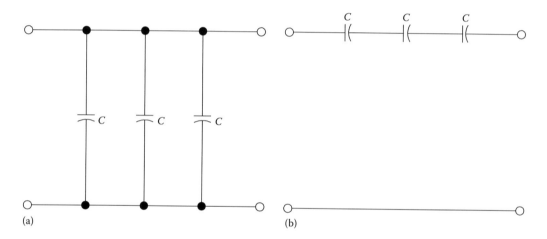

FIGURE 4.30 Transmission-line compensation by adding capacitances in (a) parallel (i.e., shunt) and (b) series.

For a lossless line, the characteristic impedance and the propagation constant can be expressed as

$$Z_c = \sqrt{\frac{L}{C}} \tag{4.290}$$

and

$$\gamma = \sqrt{LC} \tag{4.291}$$

Therefore, the addition of lumped inductances in series will increase the line inductance, and thus, the characteristic impedance and the propagation constant will be increased, which is not desirable.

The addition of lumped inductances in parallel will decrease the line capacitance. Therefore, the propagation constant will be decreased, but the characteristic impedance will be increased, which again is not desirable.

The addition of capacitances in parallel will increase the line capacitance. Hence, the characteristic impedance will be decreased, but the propagation constant will be increased, which affects negatively the system stability. However, for *the short lines, this method can be used effectively.*

Finally, the addition of capacitances in series will decrease the line inductance. Therefore, the characteristic impedance and the propagation constant will be reduced, which is desirable. Thus, *the SC compensation of transmission lines is used to improve stability limits and voltage regulation, to provide a desired load division, and to maximize the load-carrying capability of the system.* However, having the full line current going through the capacitors connected in series causes harmful overvoltages on the capacitors during short circuits. Therefore, they introduce special problems for line protective relaying.* Under fault conditions, they introduce an impedance discontinuity (negative inductance) and subharmonic currents, and when the capacitor protective gap operates, they impress high-frequency currents and voltages on the system. All of these factors result in incorrect operation of the conventional relaying schemes. The series capacitance compensation of distribution lines has been attempted from time to time for many years. However, it is not widely used.

Example 4.16

Determine the SIL of the transmission line given in Example 4.13.

Solution
The approximate value of the surge impedance of the line is

$$Z_c \cong \sqrt{\frac{L}{C}} = \left(\frac{2.6 \times 10^{-3}}{0.012 \times 10^{-6}}\right)^{1/2} = 465.5 \; \Omega$$

Therefore,

$$\text{SIL} \cong \frac{\left|kV_{R(L-L)}\right|^2}{\sqrt{\frac{L}{C}}} = \frac{\left|138\right|^2}{465.5} = 40.9 \; \text{MW}$$

which is an approximate value of the SIL of the line. The exact value of the SIL of the line can be determined as

$$\text{SIL} = \frac{\left|kV_{R(L-L)}\right|^2}{Z_c} = \frac{\left|138\right|^2}{465.5} = 40.9 \; \text{MW}$$

---

* The application of series compensation on the new EHV lines has occasionally caused a problem known as *subsynchronous resonance.* It can be briefly defined as an oscillation due to the interaction between an SC-compensated transmission system in electrical resonance and a turbine generator mechanical system in torsional mechanical resonance. As a result of the interaction, a negative resistance is introduced into the electric circuit by the turbine generator. If the effective resistance magnitude is sufficiently large to make the net resistance of the circuit negative, oscillations can increase until mechanical failures take place in terms of flexing or even breaking of the shaft. The event occurs when the electrical subsynchronous resonance frequency is equal or close to 60 Hz minus the frequency of one of the natural torsional modes of the turbine generator. The most well-known subsynchronous resonance problem took place at Mojave Generating Station [8–11].

4.15   GENERAL CIRCUIT CONSTANTS

Figure 4.31 shows a general two-port, four-terminal network consisting of passive impedances connected in some fashion. From the general network theory,

$$\mathbf{V}_S = \mathbf{A}\mathbf{V}_R + \mathbf{B}\mathbf{I}_R \tag{4.292}$$

and

$$\mathbf{I}_S = \mathbf{C}\mathbf{V}_R + \mathbf{D}\mathbf{I}_R \tag{4.293}$$

Also,

$$\mathbf{V}_R = \mathbf{D}\mathbf{V}_S - \mathbf{B}\mathbf{I}_S \tag{4.294}$$

and

$$\mathbf{I}_R = -\mathbf{C}\mathbf{V}_S + \mathbf{A}\mathbf{I}_S \tag{4.295}$$

It is always true that the determinant of Equations 4.290 and 4.291 or 4.292 and 4.293 is always unity, that is,

$$AD - BC = 1 \tag{4.296}$$

In these equations, **A**, **B**, **C**, and **D** are constants for a given network and are called general circuit constants. Their values depend on the parameters of the circuit concerned and the particular representation chosen. In general, they are complex numbers. For a network that has the symmetry of the uniform transmission line,

$$\mathbf{A} = \mathbf{D} \tag{4.297}$$

4.15.1   Determination of A, B, C, and D Constants

The **A**, **B**, **C**, and **D** constants can be calculated directly by network reduction. For example, when $\mathbf{I}_R = 0$, from Equation 4.132,

$$\mathbf{A} = \frac{\mathbf{V}_S}{\mathbf{V}_R} \tag{4.298}$$

and from Equation 4.291,

$$\mathbf{C} = \frac{\mathbf{I}_S}{\mathbf{V}_R} \tag{4.299}$$

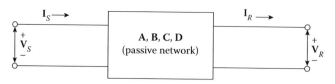

FIGURE 4.31   General two-port, four-terminal network.

Therefore, the **A** constant is the ratio of the sending- and receiving-end voltages, whereas the **C** constant is the ratio of sending-end current to receiving-end voltage when the receiving end is open-circuited. When $\mathbf{V}_R = 0$, from Equation 4.290,

$$\mathbf{B} = \frac{\mathbf{V}_S}{\mathbf{I}_R} \tag{4.300}$$

When $\mathbf{V}_R = 0$, from Equation 4.291,

$$\mathbf{D} = \frac{\mathbf{I}_S}{\mathbf{I}_R} \tag{4.301}$$

Therefore, the **B** constant is the ratio of the sending-end voltage to the receiving-end current when the receiving end is short-circuited, whereas the **D** constant is the ratio of the sending-end and receiving-end currents when the receiving end is short-circuited.

Alternatively, the **A**, **B**, **C**, and **D** generalized circuit constants can be calculated indirectly from a knowledge of the system impedance parameters as shown in the previous sections. Table 4.3 gives general circuit constants for different network types. Table 4.4 gives network conversion formulas to convert a given parameter set into another one.

As can be observed in Equations 4.132 and 4.133, the dimensions of the **A** and **D** constants are numeric. The dimension of the **B** constant is impedance in ohms, whereas the dimension of the **C** constant is admittance in Siemens.

4.15.2 A, B, C, and D Constants of Transformer

Figure 4.32 shows the equivalent circuit of a transformer *at no load*. Neglecting its series impedance,

$$\begin{bmatrix} \mathbf{V}_S \\ \mathbf{I}_S \end{bmatrix} = \begin{bmatrix} \mathbf{A} & \mathbf{B} \\ \mathbf{C} & \mathbf{D} \end{bmatrix} \begin{bmatrix} \mathbf{V}_R \\ \mathbf{I}_R \end{bmatrix} \tag{4.302}$$

where the transfer matrix is

$$\begin{bmatrix} \mathbf{A} & \mathbf{B} \\ \mathbf{C} & \mathbf{D} \end{bmatrix} = \begin{bmatrix} 1 & 0 \\ \mathbf{Y}_T & 1 \end{bmatrix} \tag{4.303}$$

since

$$\mathbf{V}_S = \mathbf{V}_R$$

and

$$\mathbf{I}_S = \mathbf{Y}_T \mathbf{V}_R + \mathbf{I}_R \tag{4.304}$$

and where $\mathbf{Y}_T$ is the magnetizing admittance of the transformer.

Figure 4.33 shows the equivalent circuit of a transformer *at full load* that has a transfer matrix of

$$\begin{bmatrix} \mathbf{A} & \mathbf{B} \\ \mathbf{C} & \mathbf{D} \end{bmatrix} = \begin{bmatrix} 1 + \dfrac{\mathbf{Z}_T \mathbf{Y}_T}{2} & \mathbf{Z}_T \left(1 + \dfrac{\mathbf{Z}_T \mathbf{Y}_T}{4} \right) \\ \mathbf{Y}_T & 1 + \dfrac{\mathbf{Z}_T \mathbf{Y}_T}{2} \end{bmatrix} \tag{4.305}$$

TABLE 4.3
General Circuit Contents for Different Network Types

Network Number	Type of Network	Equations for General Circuit Constants in Terms of Constants of Component Networks			
		$A =$	$B =$	$C =$	$D =$
1	Series impedance	1	Z	0	1
2	Shunt admittance	1	0	Y	1
3	Transformer	$1 + \dfrac{Z_T Y_T}{2}$	$Z_r\left(1 + \dfrac{Z_T Y_T}{4}\right)$	Y_T	$1 + \dfrac{Z_T Y_T}{2}$
4	Transmission line	$\cosh\sqrt{ZY} =$ $\left(1 + \dfrac{ZY}{2} + \dfrac{Z^2 Y^2}{24} + \cdots\right)$	$\sqrt{Z/Y}\,\sinh\sqrt{ZY} =$ $Z\left(1 + \dfrac{ZY}{6} + \dfrac{Z^2 Y^2}{120} + \cdots\right)$	$\sqrt{Y/Z}\,\sinh\sqrt{ZY} =$ $Y\left(1 + \dfrac{ZY}{6} + \dfrac{Z^2 Y^2}{120} + \cdots\right)$	Same as A
5	General network	A	B	C	D
6	General network and transformer impedance at receiving end	A_1	$B_1 + A_1 Z_{TR}$	C_1	$D_1 + C_1 Z_{TR}$
7	General network and transformer impedance at sending end	$A_1 + C_1 Z_{TS}$	$B_1 + D_1 Z_{TS}$	C_1	D_1

#	Network type	A	B	C	D
8	General network and transformer impedance at both ends—referred to HV	$A_1 + C_1 Z_{TS}$	$B_1 + A_1 Z_{TR} + D_1 Z_{TS} + C_1 Z_{TR} Z_{TS}$	C_1	$D_1 + C_1 Z_{TR}$
9	General network and transformer impedance at both ends—transformers having different ratios T_R and T_S—referred to LV	$\dfrac{T_R}{T_S}\left(A_1 + C_1 Z_{TS}\right)$	$\dfrac{1}{T_{RT} T_S}\left(B_1 + A_1 Z_{TR} + D_1 Z_{TS} + C_1 Z_{TR} Z_{TS}\right)$	$C_1 T_R T_S$	$\dfrac{T_S}{T_R}\left(D_1 + C_1 Z_{TR}\right)$
10	General network and shunt admittance at receiving end	$A_1 + B_1 Y_R$	B_1	$C_1 + D_1 Y_R$	D_1
11	General network and shunt admittance at sending end	A_1	B_1	$C_1 + A_1 Y_S$	$D_1 + B_1 Y_S$
12	General network and shunt admittance at both ends	$A_1 + B_1 Y_R$	B_1	$C_1 + A_1 Y_S + D_1 Y_R + B_1 Y_R Y_S$	$D_1 + B_1 Y_S$
13	Two general networks in series	$A_1 A_2 + C_1 B_2$	$B_1 A_2 + D_1 B_2$	$A_1 C_2 + C_1 D_2$	$B_1 C_2 + D_1 D_2$
14	Two general networks in series with intermediate impedance	$A_1 A_2 + C_1 B_2 + C_1 A_2 Z$	$B_1 A_2 + D_1 B_2 + D_1 A_2 Z$	$A_1 C_2 + C_1 D_2 + C_1 C_2 Z$	$B_1 C_2 + D_1 D_2 + B_1 D_2 Z$
15	Two general networks in series with intermediate shunt admittance	$A_1 A_2 + C_1 B_2 + A_1 B_2 Y$	$B_1 A_2 + D_1 B_2 + B_1 B_2 Y$	$A_1 C_2 + C_1 D_2 + A_1 D_2 Y$	$B_1 C_2 + D_1 D_2 + B_1 D_2 Z$

(continued)

TABLE 4.3 (continued)

General Circuit Contents for Different Network Types

Network Number	Type of Network	Equations for General Circuit Constants in Terms of Constants of Component Networks			
		$A =$	$B =$	$C =$	$D =$
16	Three general networks in series E_S $\boxed{A_3\ B_3\ C_3\ D_3}$ $\boxed{A_2\ B_2\ C_2\ D_2}$ $\boxed{A_1\ B_1\ C_1\ D_1}$ E_R	$A_3(A_1A_2 + C_1B_2) +$ $B_3(A_1C_2 + C_1D_2)$	$A_3(B_1A_2 + D_1B_2) +$ $B_3(B_1C_2 + D_1D_2)$	$C_3(A_1A_2 + C_1B_2) +$ $D_3(A_1C_2 + C_1D_2)$	$C_3(B_1A_2 + D_1B_2) +$ $D_3(B_1C_2 + D_1D_2)$
17	Two general networks in parallel E_S $\boxed{\begin{array}{l}A_1\ B_1\ C_1\ D_1\\ A_2\ B_2\ C_2\ D_2\end{array}}$ E_R	$\dfrac{A_1B_2 + B_1A_2}{B_1 + B_2}$	$\dfrac{B_1B_2}{B_1 + B_2}$	$C_1 + C_2 +$ $\dfrac{(A_1 - A_2) + (D_2 - D_1)}{B_1 + B_2}$	$\dfrac{B_1D_2 + D_1B_2}{B_1 + B_2}$

Source: Wagner, C.F. and Evans, R.D., *Symmetrical Components*, McGraw-Hill, New York, 1933. With permission.

Note: The exciting current of the receiving-end transformers should be added vectorially to the load current and the exciting current of the sending-end transformers should be added vectorially to the sending-end current.

General equations: $E_S = E_R A + I_R B$; $E_R = E_S D - I_S B$; $I_S = I_R D + E_R C$; $I_R = I_S A - E_S C$. As a check in the numerical calculation of the A, B, C, and D constants, note that to all cases, $AD - BC = 1$.

TABLE 4.4
Network Conversion Formulas

	To Convert from			Equivalent π	Equivalent T	To
	ABCD	**Admittance**	**Impedance**			
$A =$	*ABCD constants*	$\dfrac{Y_{11}}{Y_{12}}$	$-\dfrac{Z_{22}}{Z_{12}}$	$1 + ZY_R$	$1 + Z_S Y$	**ABCD**
$B =$	$E_2 = AE_1 + BI_1$ $I_2 = CE_1 + DI_1$	$\dfrac{1}{Y_{12}}$	$-\dfrac{Z_{11}Z_{22} - Z_{12}^2}{Z_{12}}$	Z	$Z_R + Z_S + YZ_R Z_S$	$P_1 + jQ_1 = \dfrac{\hat{A}}{\hat{B}}\bar{E}_1^2 - \dfrac{1}{\hat{B}}\hat{E}_1\hat{E}_2$
$C =$	$E_1 = DE_2 - BI_2$ $I_1 = CE_2 + AI_2$	$\dfrac{Y_{11}Y_{22} - Y_{12}^2}{Y_{12}}$	$-\dfrac{1}{Z_{12}}$	$Y_R + Y_S + ZY_RY_R$	Y	$P_2 + jQ_2 = \dfrac{\hat{D}}{\hat{B}}\bar{E}_2^2 - \dfrac{1}{\hat{B}}\hat{E}_1 E_2$
$D =$		$\dfrac{Y_{22}}{Y_{12}}$	$-\dfrac{Z_{11}}{Z_{12}}$	$1 + ZY_S$	$1 + Z_R Y$	
$Y_{11} =$	$\dfrac{A}{B}$	*Admittance constants*	$\dfrac{Z_{22}}{Z_{11}Z_{22} - Z_{12}^2}$	$Y_R + \dfrac{1}{Z}$	$\dfrac{1 + Z_S Y}{Z_R + Z_S + YZ_R Z_S}$	**Admittance**
$Y_{12} =$	$\dfrac{1}{B}$	$I_1 = Y_{11}E_1 - Y_{12}E_2$ $I_2 = Y_{22}E_2 - Y_{12}E_1$	$\dfrac{Z_{12}}{Z_{11}Z_{22} - Z_{12}^2}$	$\dfrac{1}{Z}$	$\dfrac{1}{Z_R + Z_S + YZ_R Z_S}$	$= \hat{Y}_{11}\bar{E}_1^2 - \hat{Y}_{12}\hat{E}_1\hat{E}_2$
$Y_{22} =$	$\dfrac{D}{B}$	$\dfrac{Y_{22}}{Y_{11}Y_{22} - Y_{12}^2}$	$\dfrac{Z_{11}}{Z_{11}Z_{22} - Z_{12}^2}$	$Y_S + \dfrac{1}{Z}$	$\dfrac{1 + YZ_R}{Z_R + Z_S + YZ_R Z_S}$	$= \hat{Y}_{22}\bar{E}_2^2 - \hat{Y}_{12}\hat{E}_1\hat{E}_2$
$Z_{11} =$	$\dfrac{D}{C}$	$\dfrac{Y_{22}}{Y_{11}Y_{22} - Y_{12}^2}$	*Impedance constants*	$\dfrac{1 + ZY_S}{Y_R + Y_S + ZY_R Y_S}$	$Z_R + \dfrac{1}{Y}$	**Impedance**
$Z_{12} =$	$\dfrac{1}{C}$	$-\dfrac{Y_{12}}{Y_{11}Y_{22} - Y_{12}^2}$		$\dfrac{1}{Y_R + Y_S + ZY_R Y_S}$	$-\dfrac{1}{Y}$	

(continued)

TABLE 4.4 (continued)
Network Conversion Formulas

	To Convert from					To
	ABCD	**Admittance**	**Impedance**	**Equivalent π**	**Equivalent T**	**Equivalent π**
$Z_{22}=$	$\dfrac{A}{C}$	$\dfrac{Y_{11}}{Y_{11}Y_{22}-Y_{12}^2}$	$E_1 = Z_{11}I_1 - Z_{12}I_2$ $E_2 = Z_{22}I_2 - Z_{12}I_1$	$\dfrac{1+ZY_R}{Y_R+Y_S+ZY_RY_S}$	$Z_S+\dfrac{1}{Y}$	$=Z_{11}I_1^2 - Z_{12}\hat{I}_1 I_2$ $=Z_{22}I_2^2 - Z_{12}I_1\hat{I}_2$
$Y_R=$	$\dfrac{A-1}{B}$	$Y_{11}-Y_{12}$	$\dfrac{Z_{22}+Z_{12}}{Z_{11}Z_{22}-Z_{12}^2}$	Equivalent π	$\dfrac{YZ_S}{Z_R+Z_S+YZ_RZ_S}$	
$Z=$	B	$\dfrac{1}{Y_{12}}$	$-\dfrac{Z_{11}Z_{22}-Z_{12}^2}{Z_{12}}$	[circuit diagram: Z series with Y_S, Y_R shunt]	$Z_R+Z_S+YZ_RZ_S$	
$Y_S=$	$\dfrac{D-1}{B}$	$Y_{22}-Y_{12}$	$\dfrac{Z_{11}+Z_{12}}{Z_{11}Z_{22}-Z_{12}^2}$		$\dfrac{YZ_R}{Z_R+Z_S+YZ_RZ_S}$	
$Z_R=$	$\dfrac{D-1}{C}$	$\dfrac{Y_{22}-Y_{12}}{Y_{11}Y_{22}-Y_{12}^2}$	$Z_{11}-Z_{12}$	$\dfrac{ZY_S}{Y_R+Y_S+ZY_RY_S}$	Equivalent T	**Equivalent T**
$Y=$	C	$\dfrac{Y_{11}Y_{22}-Y_{12}^2}{Y_{12}}$	$-\dfrac{1}{Z_{12}}$	$Y_R+Y_S+ZY_RY_S$	[circuit diagram: Z_S, Z_R series with Y shunt]	
$Z_S=$	$\dfrac{A-1}{C}$	$\dfrac{Y_{11}-Y_{12}}{Y_{11}Y_{22}-Y_{12}^2}$	$Z_{22}-Z_{12}$	$\dfrac{ZY_R}{Y_R+Y_S+ZY_RY_S}$		

Source: Wagner, C.F. and Evans, R.D., *Symmetrical Components*, McGraw-Hill, New York, 1933. With permission.

Note 1: P_1 and P_2 are positive in all cases for power flowing *into* the network from the point considered.

Note 2: P and Q of same sign indicate lagging PF; that is, $P + jQ = E\hat{I}$.

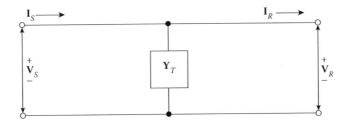

FIGURE 4.32 Transformer equivalent circuit *at no load.*

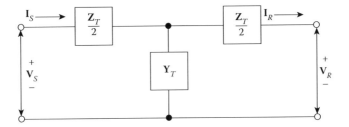

FIGURE 4.33 Transformer equivalent circuit *at full load.*

since

$$\mathbf{V}_S = \left(1 + \frac{\mathbf{Z}_T \mathbf{Y}_T}{2}\right)\mathbf{V}_R + \mathbf{Z}_T\left(1 + \frac{\mathbf{Z}_T \mathbf{Y}_T}{4}\right)\mathbf{I}_R \qquad (4.306)$$

and

$$\mathbf{I}_S = \left(\mathbf{Y}_T\right)\mathbf{V}_R + \left(1 + \frac{\mathbf{Z}_T \mathbf{Y}_T}{2}\right)\mathbf{I}_R \qquad (4.307)$$

where $\mathbf{Z}_T$ is the total equivalent series impedance of the transformer.

4.15.3 Asymmetrical π and T Networks

Figure 4.34 shows an asymmetrical π network that can be thought of as a series (or *cascade*, or *tandem*) connection of a shunt admittance, a series impedance, and a shunt admittance.

The equivalent transfer matrix can be found by multiplying together the transfer matrices of individual components. Thus,

$$\begin{bmatrix} \mathbf{A} & \mathbf{B} \\ \mathbf{C} & \mathbf{D} \end{bmatrix} = \begin{bmatrix} 1 & 0 \\ \mathbf{Y}_1 & 1 \end{bmatrix}\begin{bmatrix} 1 & \mathbf{Z} \\ 0 & 1 \end{bmatrix}\begin{bmatrix} 1 & 0 \\ \mathbf{Y}_2 & 1 \end{bmatrix}$$

$$= \begin{bmatrix} 1 + \mathbf{ZY}_2 & \mathbf{Z} \\ \mathbf{Y}_1 + \mathbf{Y}_2 + \mathbf{ZY}_1\mathbf{Y}_2 & 1 + \mathbf{ZY}_1 \end{bmatrix} \qquad (4.308)$$

When the π network is symmetrical,

$$\mathbf{Y}_1 = \mathbf{Y}_2 = \frac{\mathbf{Y}}{2}$$

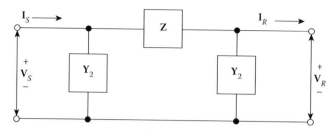

FIGURE 4.34 Asymmetrical-π network.

and the transfer matrix becomes

$$\begin{bmatrix} \mathbf{A} & \mathbf{B} \\ \mathbf{C} & \mathbf{D} \end{bmatrix} = \begin{bmatrix} 1 + \dfrac{\mathbf{ZY}}{2} & \mathbf{Z} \\ \mathbf{Y} + \dfrac{\mathbf{ZY}^2}{4} & 1 + \dfrac{\mathbf{ZY}}{2} \end{bmatrix} \tag{4.309}$$

which is the same as Equation 4.215 for a nominal-π circuit of a medium-length transmission line.

Figure 4.35 shows an asymmetrical T network that can be thought of as a cascade connection of a series impedance, a shunt admittance, and a series impedance.

Again, the equivalent transfer matrix can be found by multiplying together the transfer matrices of individual components. Thus,

$$\begin{bmatrix} \mathbf{A} & \mathbf{B} \\ \mathbf{C} & \mathbf{D} \end{bmatrix} = \begin{bmatrix} 1 & \mathbf{Z}_1 \\ 0 & 1 \end{bmatrix} \begin{bmatrix} 1 & 0 \\ \mathbf{Y} & 1 \end{bmatrix} \begin{bmatrix} 1 & \mathbf{Z}_2 \\ 0 & 1 \end{bmatrix}$$

$$= \begin{bmatrix} 1 + \mathbf{Z}_1\mathbf{Y} & \mathbf{Z}_1 + \mathbf{Z}_2 + \mathbf{Z}_1\mathbf{Z}_2\mathbf{Y} \\ \mathbf{Y} & 1 + \mathbf{Z}_2\mathbf{Y} \end{bmatrix} \tag{4.310}$$

When the T network is symmetrical,

$$\mathbf{Z}_1 = \mathbf{Z}_2 = \frac{\mathbf{Z}}{2}$$

and the transfer matrix becomes

$$\begin{bmatrix} \mathbf{A} & \mathbf{B} \\ \mathbf{C} & \mathbf{D} \end{bmatrix} = \begin{bmatrix} 1 + \dfrac{\mathbf{ZY}}{2} & \mathbf{Z} + \dfrac{\mathbf{Z}^2\mathbf{Y}}{4} \\ \mathbf{Y} & 1 + \dfrac{\mathbf{ZY}}{2} \end{bmatrix} \tag{4.311}$$

which is the same as the equation for a nominal-T circuit of a medium-length transmission line.

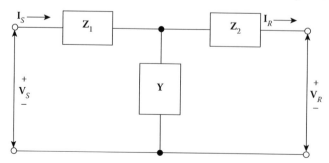

FIGURE 4.35 Asymmetrical T network.

4.15.4 NETWORKS CONNECTED IN SERIES

Two four-terminal transmission networks may be connected in series, as shown in Figure 4.36, to form a new four-terminal transmission network. For the first four-terminal network,

$$\begin{bmatrix} \mathbf{V}_S \\ \mathbf{I}_S \end{bmatrix} = \begin{bmatrix} \mathbf{A}_1 & \mathbf{B}_1 \\ \mathbf{C}_1 & \mathbf{D}_1 \end{bmatrix} \begin{bmatrix} \mathbf{V} \\ \mathbf{I} \end{bmatrix} \tag{4.312}$$

and for the second four-terminal network,

$$\begin{bmatrix} \mathbf{V} \\ \mathbf{I} \end{bmatrix} = \begin{bmatrix} \mathbf{A}_2 & \mathbf{B}_2 \\ \mathbf{C}_2 & \mathbf{D}_2 \end{bmatrix} \begin{bmatrix} \mathbf{V}_R \\ \mathbf{I}_R \end{bmatrix} \tag{4.313}$$

By substituting Equation 4.313 into Equation 4.312,

$$\begin{bmatrix} \mathbf{V}_S \\ \mathbf{I}_S \end{bmatrix} = \begin{bmatrix} \mathbf{A}_1 & \mathbf{B}_1 \\ \mathbf{C}_1 & \mathbf{D}_1 \end{bmatrix} \begin{bmatrix} \mathbf{A}_2 & \mathbf{B}_2 \\ \mathbf{C}_2 & \mathbf{D}_2 \end{bmatrix} \begin{bmatrix} \mathbf{V}_R \\ \mathbf{I}_R \end{bmatrix}$$

$$= \begin{bmatrix} \mathbf{A}_1\mathbf{A}_2 + \mathbf{B}_1\mathbf{C}_2 & \mathbf{A}_1\mathbf{B}_2 + \mathbf{B}_1\mathbf{D}_2 \\ \mathbf{C}_1\mathbf{A}_2 + \mathbf{D}_1\mathbf{C}_2 & \mathbf{C}_1\mathbf{B}_2 + \mathbf{D}_1\mathbf{D}_2 \end{bmatrix} \begin{bmatrix} \mathbf{V}_R \\ \mathbf{I}_R \end{bmatrix} \tag{4.314}$$

Therefore, the equivalent **A**, **B**, **C**, and **D** constants for two networks connected in series are

$$\mathbf{A}_{eq} = \mathbf{A}_1\mathbf{A}_2 + \mathbf{B}_1\mathbf{C}_2 \tag{4.315}$$

$$\mathbf{B}_{eq} = \mathbf{A}_1\mathbf{B}_2 + \mathbf{B}_1\mathbf{D}_2 \tag{4.316}$$

$$\mathbf{C}_{eq} = \mathbf{C}_3\mathbf{A}_2 + \mathbf{D}_1\mathbf{C}_2 \tag{4.317}$$

$$\mathbf{D}_{eq} = \mathbf{C}_1\mathbf{B}_2 + \mathbf{D}_1\mathbf{D}_2 \tag{4.318}$$

Example 4.17

Figure 4.37 shows two networks connected in cascade. Determine the equivalent **A**, **B**, **C**, and **D** constants.

Solution

For network 1,

$$\begin{bmatrix} \mathbf{A}_1 & \mathbf{B}_1 \\ \mathbf{C}_1 & \mathbf{D}_1 \end{bmatrix} = \begin{bmatrix} 1 & 10\angle 30° \\ 0 & 1 \end{bmatrix}$$

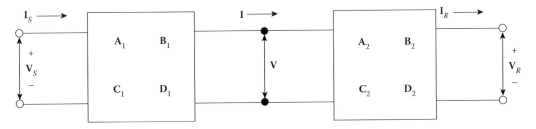

FIGURE 4.36 Transmission networks in series.

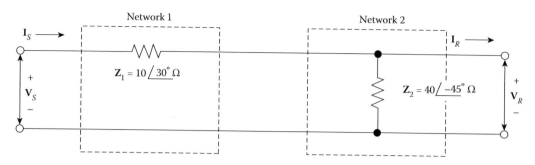

FIGURE 4.37 Network configurations for Example 4.17.

For network 2,

$$\mathbf{Y}_2 = \frac{1}{\mathbf{Z}_2} = \frac{1}{40\angle -45°} = 0.025\angle 45° \text{ S}$$

Then

$$\begin{bmatrix} \mathbf{A}_2 & \mathbf{B}_2 \\ \mathbf{C}_2 & \mathbf{D}_2 \end{bmatrix} = \begin{bmatrix} 1 & 0 \\ 0.025\angle 45° & 1 \end{bmatrix}$$

Therefore,

$$\begin{bmatrix} \mathbf{A}_{eq} & \mathbf{B}_{eq} \\ \mathbf{C}_{eq} & \mathbf{D}_{eq} \end{bmatrix} = \begin{bmatrix} 1 & 10\angle 30° \\ 0 & 1 \end{bmatrix} \begin{bmatrix} 1 & 0 \\ 0.025\angle 45° & 1 \end{bmatrix}$$

$$= \begin{bmatrix} 1.09\angle 12.8° & 10\angle 30° \\ 0.025\angle 45° & 1 \end{bmatrix}$$

4.15.5 NETWORKS CONNECTED IN PARALLEL

Two four-terminal transmission networks may be connected in parallel, as shown in Figure 4.38, to form a new four-terminal transmission network.

Since

$$\begin{aligned} \mathbf{V}_S &= \mathbf{V}_{S1} + \mathbf{V}_{S2} \\ \mathbf{V}_R &= \mathbf{V}_{R1} + \mathbf{V}_{R2} \end{aligned} \tag{4.319}$$

and

$$\begin{aligned} \mathbf{I}_S &= \mathbf{I}_{S1} + \mathbf{I}_{S2} \\ \mathbf{I}_R &= \mathbf{I}_{R1} + \mathbf{I}_{R2} \end{aligned} \tag{4.320}$$

for the equivalent four-terminal network,

$$\begin{bmatrix} \mathbf{V}_S \\ \mathbf{I}_S \end{bmatrix} = \begin{bmatrix} \dfrac{\mathbf{A}_1\mathbf{B}_2 + \mathbf{A}_2\mathbf{B}_1}{\mathbf{B}_1 + \mathbf{B}_2} & \dfrac{\mathbf{B}_1\mathbf{B}_2}{\mathbf{B}_1 + \mathbf{B}_2} \\ \mathbf{C}_2 + \mathbf{C}_2 + \dfrac{(\mathbf{A}_1 - \mathbf{A}_2)(\mathbf{D}_2 - \mathbf{D}_1)}{\mathbf{B}_1 + \mathbf{B}_2} & \dfrac{\mathbf{D}_1\mathbf{B}_2 + \mathbf{D}_2\mathbf{B}_1}{\mathbf{B}_1 + \mathbf{B}_2} \end{bmatrix} \begin{bmatrix} \mathbf{V}_R \\ \mathbf{I}_R \end{bmatrix} \tag{4.321}$$

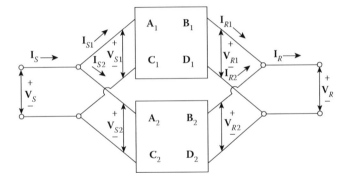

FIGURE 4.38   Transmission networks in parallel.

where the equivalent **A**, **B**, **C**, and **D** constants are

$$\mathbf{A}_{eq} = \frac{\mathbf{A}_1 \mathbf{B}_2 + \mathbf{A}_2 \mathbf{B}_1}{\mathbf{B}_1 + \mathbf{B}_2} \tag{4.322}$$

$$\mathbf{B}_{eq} = \frac{\mathbf{B}_1 \mathbf{B}_2}{\mathbf{B}_1 + \mathbf{B}_2} \tag{4.323}$$

$$\mathbf{C}_{eq} = \mathbf{C}_2 + \mathbf{C}_2 + \frac{(\mathbf{A}_1 - \mathbf{A}_2)(\mathbf{D}_2 - \mathbf{D}_1)}{\mathbf{B}_1 + \mathbf{B}_2} \tag{4.324}$$

$$\mathbf{D}_{eq} = \frac{\mathbf{D}_1 \mathbf{B}_2 + \mathbf{D}_2 \mathbf{B}_1}{\mathbf{B}_1 + \mathbf{B}_2} \tag{4.325}$$

Example 4.18

Assume that the two networks given in Example 4.17 are connected in parallel, as shown in Figure 4.39. Determine the equivalent **A**, **B**, **C**, and **D** constants.

Solution

Using the **A**, **B**, **C**, and **D** parameters found previously for networks 1 and 2, that is,

$$\begin{bmatrix} \mathbf{A}_1 & \mathbf{B}_1 \\ \mathbf{C}_1 & \mathbf{D}_1 \end{bmatrix} = \begin{bmatrix} 1 & 10\angle 30° \\ 0 & 1 \end{bmatrix}$$

and

$$\begin{bmatrix} \mathbf{A}_2 & \mathbf{B}_2 \\ \mathbf{C}_2 & \mathbf{D}_2 \end{bmatrix} = \begin{bmatrix} 1 & 0 \\ 0.025\angle 45° & 1 \end{bmatrix}$$

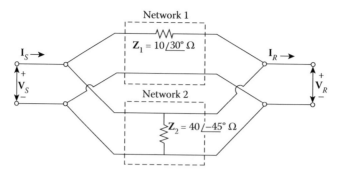

FIGURE 4.39   Transmission networks in parallel for Example 4.18.

the equivalent **A**, **B**, **C**, and **D** constants can be calculated as

$$\mathbf{A}_{eq} = \frac{\mathbf{A}_1\mathbf{B}_2 + \mathbf{A}_2\mathbf{B}_1}{\mathbf{B}_1 + \mathbf{B}_2}$$

$$= \frac{1\times 0 + 1\times 10\angle 30°}{10\angle 30° + 0} = 1$$

$$\mathbf{B}_{eq} = \frac{\mathbf{B}_1\mathbf{B}_2}{\mathbf{B}_1 + \mathbf{B}_2}$$

$$= \frac{1\times 0}{1 + 0} = 0$$

$$\mathbf{C}_{eq} = \mathbf{C}_2 + \mathbf{C}_2 + \frac{(\mathbf{A}_1 - \mathbf{A}_2)(\mathbf{D}_2 - \mathbf{D}_1)}{\mathbf{B}_1 + \mathbf{B}_2}$$

$$= 0 + 0.025\angle 45° + \frac{(1-1)(1-1)}{10\angle 30° - 0} = 0.025\angle 45°$$

$$\mathbf{D}_{eq} = \frac{\mathbf{D}_1\mathbf{B}_2 + \mathbf{D}_2\mathbf{B}_1}{\mathbf{B}_1 + \mathbf{B}_2}$$

$$= \frac{1\times 0 + 1\times 10\angle 30°}{10\angle 30° + 0} = 1$$

Therefore,

$$\begin{bmatrix} \mathbf{A}_{eq} & \mathbf{B}_{eq} \\ \mathbf{C}_{eq} & \mathbf{D}_{eq} \end{bmatrix} = \begin{bmatrix} 1 & 0 \\ 0.025\angle 45° & 1 \end{bmatrix}$$

4.15.6   Terminated Transmission Line

Figure 4.40 shows a four-terminal transmission network connected to (i.e., terminated by) a load $\mathbf{Z}_L$. For the given network,

$$\begin{bmatrix} \mathbf{V}_S \\ \mathbf{I}_S \end{bmatrix} = \begin{bmatrix} \mathbf{A} & \mathbf{B} \\ \mathbf{C} & \mathbf{D} \end{bmatrix} \begin{bmatrix} \mathbf{V}_R \\ \mathbf{I}_R \end{bmatrix} \tag{4.326}$$

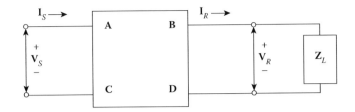

FIGURE 4.40 Terminated transmission line.

or

$$\mathbf{V}_S = \mathbf{A}\mathbf{V}_R + \mathbf{B}\mathbf{I}_R \qquad (4.327)$$

and

$$\mathbf{I}_S = \mathbf{C}\mathbf{V}_R + \mathbf{D}\mathbf{I}_R \qquad (4.328)$$

and also

$$\mathbf{V}_R = \mathbf{Z}_L\mathbf{I}_R \qquad (4.329)$$

Therefore, the input impedance is

$$\mathbf{Z}_{\text{in}} = \frac{\mathbf{V}_S}{\mathbf{I}_S}$$

$$= \frac{\mathbf{A}\mathbf{V}_R + \mathbf{B}\mathbf{I}_R}{\mathbf{C}\mathbf{V}_R + \mathbf{D}\mathbf{I}_R} \qquad (4.330)$$

or by substituting Equation 4.327 into Equation 4.328,

$$\mathbf{Z}_{\text{in}} = \frac{\mathbf{A}\mathbf{Z}_L + \mathbf{B}}{\mathbf{C}\mathbf{Z}_L + \mathbf{D}} \qquad (4.331)$$

Since for the symmetrical and long transmission line,

$$\mathbf{A} = \cosh\sqrt{\mathbf{YZ}} = \cosh\theta$$

$$\mathbf{B} = \sqrt{\frac{\mathbf{Z}}{\mathbf{Y}}}\,\sinh\sqrt{\mathbf{YZ}} = \mathbf{Z}_c\sinh\theta$$

$$\mathbf{C} = \sqrt{\frac{\mathbf{Y}}{\mathbf{Z}}}\,\sinh\sqrt{\mathbf{YZ}} = \mathbf{Y}_c\sinh\theta$$

$$\mathbf{D} = \mathbf{A} = \cosh\sqrt{\mathbf{YZ}} = \cosh\theta$$

The input impedance, from Equation 4.331, becomes

$$\mathbf{Z}_{in} = \frac{\mathbf{Z}_L \cosh\theta + \mathbf{Z}_c \sinh\theta}{\mathbf{Z}_L \mathbf{Y}_c \sinh\theta + \cosh\theta} \tag{4.332}$$

or

$$\mathbf{Z}_{in} = \frac{\mathbf{Z}_L \left[(\mathbf{Z}_c/\mathbf{Z}_L)\sinh\theta + \cosh\theta \right]}{(\mathbf{Z}_L/\mathbf{Z}_c)\sinh\theta + \cosh\theta} \tag{4.333}$$

If the load impedance is chosen to be equal to the characteristic impedance, that is,

$$\mathbf{Z}_L = \mathbf{Z}_c \tag{4.334}$$

the input impedance, from Equation 4.331, becomes

$$\mathbf{Z}_{in} = \mathbf{Z}_c \tag{4.335}$$

which is *independent* of θ and the line length. The value of the voltage is constant all along the line.

Example 4.19

Figure 4.41 shows a short transmission line that is terminated by a load of 200 kVA at a lagging PF of 0.866 at 2.4 kV. If the line impedance is $2.07 + j0.661\ \Omega$, calculate the following:

(a) Sending-end current
(b) Sending-end voltage
(c) Input impedance
(d) Real and reactive power loss in the line

Solution

(a) From Equation 4.326,

$$\begin{bmatrix} \mathbf{V}_S \\ \mathbf{I}_S \end{bmatrix} = \begin{bmatrix} \mathbf{A} & \mathbf{B} \\ \mathbf{C} & \mathbf{D} \end{bmatrix} \begin{bmatrix} \mathbf{V}_R \\ \mathbf{I}_R \end{bmatrix}$$

$$= \begin{bmatrix} 1 & \mathbf{Z} \\ 0 & 1 \end{bmatrix} \begin{bmatrix} \mathbf{V}_R \\ \mathbf{I}_R \end{bmatrix}$$

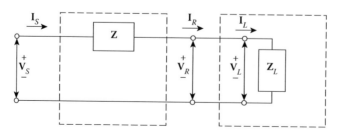

FIGURE 4.41   Transmission system for Example 4.19.

where

$$\mathbf{Z} = 2.07 + j0.661 = 2.173\angle 17.7° \ \Omega$$

$$\mathbf{I}_R = \mathbf{I}_S = \mathbf{I}_L$$

$$\mathbf{V}_R = \mathbf{Z}_L \mathbf{I}_R$$

Since

$$\mathbf{S}_R = 200\angle 30° = 173.2 + j100 \ \text{kVA}$$

and

$$\mathbf{V}_L = 2.4\angle 0° \ \text{kV}$$

then

$$\mathbf{I}_L^* = \frac{\mathbf{S}_R}{\mathbf{V}_L} = \frac{200\angle 30°}{2.4\angle 0°} = 83.33\angle 30° \ \text{A}$$

or

$$\mathbf{I}_L = 83.33\angle -30° \ \text{A}$$

Hence,

$$\mathbf{I}_S = \mathbf{I}_R = \mathbf{I}_L = 83.33\angle -30° \ \text{A}$$

(b)

$$\mathbf{Z}_L = \frac{\mathbf{V}_L}{\mathbf{I}_L} = \frac{2.4 \times 10^3 \angle 0°}{83.33\angle -30°} = 28.8\angle 30° \ \Omega$$

and

$$\mathbf{V}_R = \mathbf{Z}_L \mathbf{I}_R = 28.8\angle 30° \times 83.33\angle -30° = 2404\angle 0° \ \text{kV}$$

Thus,

$$\mathbf{V}_S = \mathbf{A}\mathbf{V}_R + \mathbf{B}\mathbf{I}_R$$
$$= 2400\angle 0° + 2.173\angle 17.7° \times 83.33\angle -30°$$
$$= 2576.9 - j38.58$$
$$= 2577.2\angle -0.9° \ \text{V}$$

(c) The input impedance is

$$\mathbf{Z}_{\text{in}} = \frac{\mathbf{V}_S}{\mathbf{I}_S} = \frac{\mathbf{A}\mathbf{V}_R + \mathbf{B}\mathbf{I}_R}{\mathbf{C}\mathbf{V}_R + \mathbf{D}\mathbf{I}_R}$$
$$= \frac{2577.2\angle -0.9°}{83.33\angle -30°} = 30.93\angle 29.1° \ \Omega$$

(d) The real and reactive power loss in the line is

$$\mathbf{S}_L = \mathbf{S}_S - \mathbf{S}_R$$

where

$$\mathbf{S}_S = \mathbf{V}_S \mathbf{I}_S^* = 2{,}577.2\angle -0.9° \times 83.33\angle 30° = 214{,}758\angle 29.1°\ \text{VA}$$

or

$$\mathbf{S}_S = \mathbf{I}_S \times \mathbf{Z}_{\text{in}} \times \mathbf{I}_S^* = 214{,}758\angle 29.1°\ \text{VA}$$

Thus,

$$\mathbf{S}_L = 214{,}758\angle 29.1° - 200{,}000\angle 30°$$

$$= 14{,}444.5 + j4{,}444.4\ \text{VA}$$

that is, the active power loss is 14,444.5 W, and the reactive power loss is 4,444.4 vars.

4.15.7 Power Relations Using A, B, C, and D Line Constants

For a given long transmission line, the complex power at the sending and receiving ends are

$$\mathbf{S}_S^* = P_S + jQ_S = \mathbf{V}_S \mathbf{I}_S^* \tag{4.336}$$

and

$$\mathbf{S}_R = P_R + jQ_R = \mathbf{V}_R \mathbf{I}_R^* \tag{4.337}$$

Also, the sending- and receiving-end voltages and currents can be expressed as

$$\mathbf{V}_S = \mathbf{A}\mathbf{V}_R + \mathbf{B}\mathbf{I}_R \tag{4.338}$$

$$\mathbf{I}_S = \mathbf{C}\mathbf{V}_R + \mathbf{D}\mathbf{I}_R \tag{4.339}$$

$$\mathbf{V}_R = \mathbf{A}\mathbf{V}_S - \mathbf{B}\mathbf{I}_S \tag{4.340}$$

$$\mathbf{I}_R = -\mathbf{C}\mathbf{V}_S + \mathbf{D}\mathbf{I}_S \tag{4.341}$$

where

$$\mathbf{A} = A\angle \alpha = \cosh\sqrt{\mathbf{YZ}} \tag{4.342}$$

$$\mathbf{B} = B\angle \beta = \sqrt{\frac{\mathbf{Z}}{\mathbf{Y}}}\sinh\sqrt{\mathbf{YZ}} \tag{4.343}$$

$$\mathbf{C} = C\angle\delta = \sqrt{\frac{\mathbf{Y}}{\mathbf{Z}}}\ \sinh\sqrt{\mathbf{YZ}} \qquad (4.344)$$

$$\mathbf{D} = \mathbf{A} = \cosh\sqrt{\mathbf{YZ}} \qquad (4.345)$$

$$\mathbf{V}_R = V_R\angle 0° \qquad (4.346)$$

$$\mathbf{V}_S = V_S\angle\delta \qquad (4.347)$$

From Equation 4.340,

$$\mathbf{I}_S = \frac{\mathbf{A}}{\mathbf{B}}\mathbf{V}_S - \frac{\mathbf{V}_R}{\mathbf{B}} \qquad (4.348)$$

or

$$\mathbf{I}_S = \frac{AV_S}{B}\angle\alpha + \delta - \beta - \frac{V_R\angle -\beta}{B} \qquad (4.349)$$

and

$$\mathbf{I}_S^* = \frac{AV_S}{B}\angle -\alpha - \delta + \beta - \frac{V_R\angle\beta}{B} \qquad (4.350)$$

and from Equation 4.338,

$$\mathbf{I}_R = \frac{\mathbf{V}_S}{\mathbf{B}} - \frac{\mathbf{A}}{\mathbf{B}}\mathbf{V}_R \qquad (4.351a)$$

or

$$\mathbf{I}_R = \frac{V_S}{B}\angle\delta - \beta - \frac{AV_R}{B}\angle\alpha - \beta \qquad (4.351b)$$

and

$$\mathbf{I}_R^* = \frac{V_S}{B}\angle -\delta + \beta - \frac{AV_R}{B}\angle -\alpha + \beta \qquad (4.352)$$

By substituting Equations 4.350a,b and 4.352 into Equations 4.334 and 4.335, respectively,

$$\mathbf{S}_S = P_S + jQ_S = \frac{AV_S^2}{B}\angle\beta - \alpha - \frac{V_S V_R}{B}\angle\beta + \delta \qquad (4.353)$$

and

$$\mathbf{S}_R = P_R + jQ_R = \frac{V_S V_R}{B} \angle \beta - \delta - \frac{A V_R^2}{B} \angle \beta - \alpha \qquad (4.354)$$

Therefore, the real and reactive powers at the sending end are

$$P_S = \frac{A V_S^2}{B} \cos(\beta - \alpha) - \frac{V_S V_R}{B} \cos(\beta + \delta) \qquad (4.355)$$

and

$$Q_S = \frac{A V_S^2}{B} \sin(\beta - \alpha) - \frac{V_S V_R}{B} \sin(\beta + \delta) \qquad (4.356)$$

and the real and reactive powers at the receiving end are

$$P_R = \frac{V_S V_R}{B} \cos(\beta - \delta) - \frac{A V_R^2}{B} \cos(\beta - \alpha) \qquad (4.357)$$

and

$$Q_R = \frac{V_S V_R}{B} \sin(\beta - \delta) - \frac{A V_R^2}{B} \sin(\beta - \alpha) \qquad (4.358)$$

For constant V_S and V_R, for a given line, the only variable in Equations 4.354 through 4.358 is δ, the power angle. Therefore, treating P_S as a function of δ only in Equation 4.351, P_S is maximum when $\beta + \delta = 180°$. Therefore, the maximum power at the sending end, the maximum input power, can be expressed as

$$P_{S,\max} = \frac{A V_S^2}{B} \cos(\beta - \alpha) + \frac{V_S V_R}{B} \qquad (4.359)$$

and similarly, the corresponding reactive power at the sending end, the maximum input vars, is

$$Q_{S,\max} = \frac{A V_S^2}{B} \sin(\beta - \alpha) \qquad (4.360)$$

On the other hand, P_R is maximum when $\delta = \beta$. Therefore, the maximum power obtainable (which is also called the *steady-state power limit*) at the receiving end can be expressed as

$$P_{R,\max} = \frac{V_S V_R}{B} - \frac{A V_R^2}{B} \cos(\beta - \alpha) \qquad (4.361)$$

and similarly, the corresponding reactive power delivered at the receiving end is

$$Q_{R,\max} = -\frac{A V_R^2}{B} \sin(\beta - \alpha) \qquad (4.362)$$

In these equations, V_S and V_R are the phase (line-to-neutral) voltages whether the system is single phase or three phase. Therefore, the total three-phase power transmitted on the three-phase line is three times the power calculated by using the aforementioned equations. If the voltages are given in volts, the power is expressed in watts or vars. Otherwise, if they are given in kilovolts, the power is expressed in megawatts or megavars.

For a given value of γ, the power loss P_L in a long transmission line can be calculated as the difference between the sending- and the receiving-end real powers,

$$P_L = P_S - P_R \tag{4.363}$$

and the lagging vars loss is

$$Q_L = Q_S - Q_R \tag{4.364}$$

Example 4.20

Figure 4.42 shows a three-phase, 345 kV ac transmission line with bundled conductors connecting two buses that are voltage regulated. Assume that SC and shunt-reactor compensation are to be considered. The bundled conductor line has two 795 kcmil ACSR conductors per phase. The subconductors are separated 18 in., and the phase spacing of the flat configuration is 24, 24, and 48 ft. The resistance inductive reactance and susceptance of the line are given as 0.059 Ω/mi per phase, 0.588 Ω/mi per phase, and 7.20×10^{-6} S phase to neutral per phase per mile, respectively. The total line length is 200 mi, and the line resistance may be neglected because simple calculations and approximate answers will suffice. First assume that there is no compensation in use; that is, both reactors are disconnected and the SC is bypassed. Determine the following:

(a) Total three-phase SIL of line in megavolt-amperes
(b) Maximum three-phase theoretical steady-state power flow limit in megawatts
(c) Total three-phase magnetizing var generation by line capacitance
(d) Open-circuit receiving-end voltage if line is open at the receiving end

Solution

(a) The surge impedance of the line is

$$Z_c = \left(x_L \times x_c \right)^{1/2} \tag{4.365}$$

where

$$x_c = \frac{1}{b_c} \ \Omega/\text{mi/phase} \tag{4.366}$$

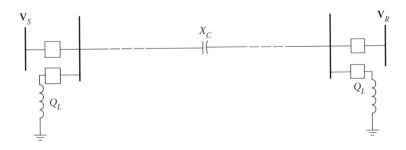

FIGURE 4.42 Figure for Example 4.20.

Thus,

$$Z_c = \left(\frac{x_L}{b_c}\right)^{1/2}$$

$$= \left(\frac{0.588}{7.20 \times 10^{-6}}\right)^{1/2} = 285.77 \ \Omega/\text{mi/phase} \tag{4.367}$$

Thus, the total three-phase SIL of the line is

$$\text{SIL} = \frac{\left|kV_{R(\text{L-L})}\right|^2}{Z_c}$$

$$= \frac{345^2}{285.77} = 416.5 \ \text{MVA/mi}$$

(b) Neglecting the line resistance,

$$P = P_S = P_R$$

or

$$P = \frac{V_S V_R}{X_L} \sin\delta \tag{4.368}$$

When $\delta = 90°$, the maximum three-phase theoretical steady-state power flow limit is

$$P_{\max} = \frac{V_S V_R}{X_L}$$

$$= \frac{(345 \ kV)2}{117.6} = 1012.1 \ \text{MW} \tag{4.369}$$

(c) Using a nominal-π circuit representation, the total three-phase magnetizing var generated by the line capacitance can be expressed as

$$Q_c = V_S^2 \frac{b_c l}{2} + V_R^2 \frac{b_c l}{2}$$

$$= V_S^2 \frac{B_c}{2} + V_R^2 \frac{B_c}{2}$$

$$= (345 \times 10^3)^2 \left(\frac{1}{2}(7.20 \times 10^{-6})200\right)$$

$$+ (345 \times 10^3)^2 \left(\frac{1}{2}(7.20 \times 10^{-6})200\right)$$

$$= 171.4 \ \text{Mvar} \tag{4.370}$$

(d) If the line is open at the receiving end, the open-circuit receiving-end voltage can be expressed as

$$\mathbf{V}_S = \mathbf{V}_{R(\text{oc})} \cosh\gamma l \tag{4.371}$$

or

$$\mathbf{V}_{R(oc)} = \frac{\mathbf{V}_S}{\cosh \gamma l} \qquad (4.372)$$

where

$$\gamma = j\omega\sqrt{LC}$$

$$= j\omega\left(\frac{x_L}{\omega}\frac{1}{\omega x_c}\right)^{1/2}$$

$$= j\left(\frac{x_L}{x_c}\right)^{1/2}$$

$$= j\left[(0.588)\left(7.20\times10^{-6}\right)\right]^{1/2} = 0.0021 \text{ rad/mi} \qquad (4.473)$$

and

$$\gamma l = j(0.0021)(200) = j0.4115 \text{ rad}$$

Thus,

$$\cosh \gamma l = \cosh(0 + j0.4115)$$

$$= \cosh(0)\cos(0.4115) + j\sinh(0)\sin(0.4115)$$

$$= 0.9164$$

and therefore,

$$V_{R(oc)} = \frac{345 \text{ kV}}{0.9165} = 376.43 \text{ kV}$$

Alternatively,

$$V_{R(oc)} = V_S \frac{X_c}{X_c + X_L}$$

$$= (345 \text{ kV})\left(\frac{-j1388.9}{-j1388.9 + j117.6}\right)$$

$$= 376.74 \text{ kV} \qquad (4.374)$$

Example 4.21

Use the data given in Example 4.20 and assume that the shunt compensation is now used. Assume also that the two shunt reactors are connected to absorb 60% of the total three-phase magnetizing var generation by line capacitance and that half of the total reactor capacity is placed at each end of the line. Determine the following:

(a) Total three-phase SIL of line in megavolt-amperes
(b) Maximum three-phase theoretical steady-state power flow limit in megawatts
(c) Three-phase megavolt-ampere rating of each shunt reactor
(d) Cost of each reactor at $10/kVA
(e) Open-circuit receiving-end voltage if line is open at receiving end

Solution

(a) SIL = 416.5, as before, in Example 4.20.

(b) P_{max} = 1012.1 MW, as before.

(c) The three-phase megavolt-ampere rating of each shunt reactor is

$$\frac{1}{2}Q_L = \frac{1}{2}0.60Q_c$$

$$= \frac{1}{2}0.60(171.4) = 51.42 \text{ MVA}$$

(d) The cost of each reactor at $10/kVA is

$$(51.42 \text{ MVA/reactor})(\$10/\text{kVA}) = \$514,200$$

(e) Since

$$\gamma l = j0.260 \text{ rad}$$

and

$$\cosh \gamma l = 0.9663$$

then

$$V_{R(oc)} = \frac{345 \text{ kV}}{0.9663} = 357.03 \text{ kV}$$

Alternatively,

$$V_{R(oc)} = V_S \frac{X_c}{X_c + X_L}$$

$$= (345 \text{ kV})\left(\frac{-j1,3472}{-j1,3472 + j117.6}\right)$$

$$= 357.1 \text{ kV}$$

Therefore, the inclusion of the shunt reactor causes the receiving-end open-circuit voltage to decrease.

4.16   BUNDLED CONDUCTORS

Bundled conductors are used at or above 345 kV. Instead of one large conductor per phase, two or more conductors of approximately the same total cross section are suspended from each insulator string. Therefore, by having two or more conductors per phase in close proximity compared with the spacing between phases, the voltage gradient at the conductor surface is significantly reduced. The bundles used at the EHV range usually have two, three, or four *subconductors*, as shown in Figure 4.43. The bundles used at the UHV range may also have 8, 12, and even 16 conductors.

Bundle conductors are also called *duplex*, *triplex*, and so on conductors, referring to the number of subconductors, and are sometimes referred to as grouped or multiple conductors. The advantages derived from the use of *bundled* conductors instead of single conductors per phase are (1) reduced line inductive reactance; (2) reduced voltage gradient; (3) increased corona critical voltage and, therefore, less corona power loss, AN, and RI; (4) more power may be carried per unit mass of

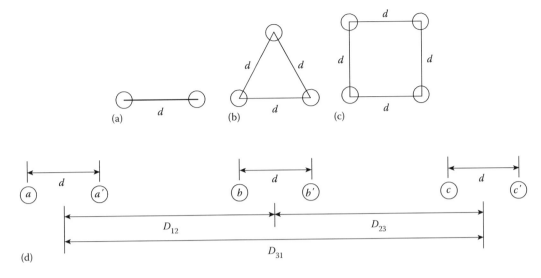

FIGURE 4.43 Bundle arrangements: (a) two-conductor bundle, (b) three-conductor bundle, (c) four-conductor bundle, and (d) cross section of bundled conductor three-phase line with horizontal tower configuration.

conductor; and (5) the amplitude and duration of high-frequency vibrations may be reduced. The disadvantages of bundled conductors include (1) increased wind and ice loading, (2) suspension is more complicated and duplex or quadruple insulator strings may be required, (3) the tendency to gallop is increased, (4) increased cost, (5) increased clearance requirements at structures, and (6) increased charging kilovolt-amperes.

If the subconductors of a bundle are transposed, the current will be divided exactly between the conductors of the bundle. The GMRs of bundled conductors made up of two, three, and four subconductors can be expressed, respectively, as

$$D_s^b = \left(D_s \times d\right)^{1/2} \tag{4.375}$$

$$D_s^b = \left(D_s \times d^2\right)^{1/3} \tag{4.376}$$

$$D_s^b = 1.09\left(D_s \times d_3\right)^{1/4} \tag{4.377}$$

where
  D_s^b is the GMR of bundled conductor
  D_s is the GMR of subconductors
  d is the distance between two subconductors

Therefore, the *average* inductance per phase is

$$L_a = 2 \times 10^{-7} \ln \frac{D_{eq}}{D_s^b} \text{ H/m} \tag{4.378}$$

and the inductive reactance is

$$X_L = 0.1213 \ln \frac{D_{eq}}{D_s^b} \text{ } \Omega/\text{mi} \tag{4.379}$$

where

$$D_{eq} \triangleq D_m = \left(D_{12} \times D_{23} \times D_{31} \right)^{1/3} \tag{4.380}$$

The modified GMRs (to be used in capacitance calculations) of bundled conductors made up of two, three, and four subconductors can be expressed, respectively, as

$$D_{sC}^b = \left(r \times d \right)^{1/2} \tag{4.381}$$

$$D_{sC}^b = \left(r \times d^2 \right)^{1/3} \tag{4.382}$$

$$D_{sC}^b = 1.09 \left(r \times d^3 \right)^{1/4} \tag{4.383}$$

where
D_{sC}^b is the modified GMR of bundled conductor
r is the outside radius of subconductors
d is the distance between two subconductors

Therefore, the line-to-neutral capacitance can be expressed as

$$C_N = \frac{2\pi \times 8.8538 \times 10^{-12}}{\ln \left(\dfrac{D_{eq}}{D_{sC}^b} \right)} \quad \text{F/m} \tag{4.384}$$

or

$$C_N = \frac{55.63 \times 10^{-12}}{\ln \left(\dfrac{D_{eq}}{D_{sC}^b} \right)} \quad \text{F/m} \tag{4.385}$$

For a two-conductor bundle, the maximum voltage gradient at the surface of a subconductor can be expressed as

$$E_0 = \frac{V_0 \left(1 + \dfrac{2r}{d} \right)}{2r \ln \left(\dfrac{D}{\sqrt{r \times d}} \right)} \tag{4.386}$$

Example 4.22

Consider the bundled-conductor three-phase 200 km line shown in Figure 4.43d. Assume that the power base is 100 MVA and the voltage base is 345 kV. The conductor used is 1113 kcmil ACSR, and the distance between two subconductors is 12 in. Assume that the distances D_{12}, D_{23}, and D_{31} are 26, 26, and 52 ft, respectively, and determine the following:

(a) Average inductance per phase in henries per meter
(b) Inductive reactance per phase in ohms per kilometer and ohms per mile

(c)   Series reactance of line in per units
(d)   Line-to-neutral capacitance of line in farads per meter
(e)   Capacitive reactance to neutral of line in ohm × kilometers ($\Omega \cdot$km) and ohmx per miles ($\Omega \cdot$mi)

Solution

(a)   From Table A.3, D_s is 0.0435 ft; therefore,

$$D_s^b = \left(D_s \times d\right)^{1/2}$$

$$= (0.0435 \times 0.3048 \times 12 \times 0.0254)^{1/2} = 0.0636 \text{ m}$$

$$D_{eq} = \left(D_{12} \times D_{23} \times D_{31}\right)^{1/3}$$

$$= \left(26 \times 26 \times 52 \times 0.3048^3\right)^{1/3} = 9.9846 \text{ m}$$

Thus, from Equation 4.478,

$$L_a = 2 \times 10^{-7} \ln \frac{D_{eq}}{D_s^b}$$

$$= 2 \times 10^{-7} \ln \left(\frac{9.9846}{0.0636}\right) = 1.0112 \text{ } \mu\text{H/m}$$

(b)

$$X_L = 2\pi f L_a$$

$$= 2\pi 60 \times 1.0112 \times 10^{-6} \times 10^3 = 0.3812 \text{ } \Omega\text{/km}$$

and

$$X_L = 0.3812 \times 1.609 = 0.6134 \text{ } \Omega\text{/mi}$$

(c)

$$Z_B = \frac{345^2}{100} = 1190.25 \text{ } \Omega$$

$$X_L = \frac{0.3812 \times 200}{1190.25} = 0.0641 \text{ pu}$$

(d)   From Table A.3, the outside diameter of the subconductor is 1.293 in.; therefore, its radius is

$$r = \frac{1.293 \times 0.3048}{2 \times 12} = 0.0164 \text{ m}$$

$$D_{sC}^b = (r \times d)^{1/2}$$

$$= (0.0164 \times 12 \times 0.0254)^{1/2} = 0.0707 \text{ m}$$

Thus, the line-to-neutral capacitance of the line is

$$C_N = \frac{55.63 \times 10^{-12}}{\ln\left(D_{eq}/D_{sC}^b\right)}$$

$$= \frac{55.63 \times 10^{-12}}{\ln(9.9846/0.0707)} = 11.238 \times 10^{-12} \ \text{F/m}$$

(c) The capacitive reactance to the neutral of the line is

$$X_c = \frac{1}{2\pi f C_N}$$

$$= \frac{10^{12} \times 10^{-3}}{2\pi 60 \times 11.238} = 0.236 \times 10^6 \ \Omega \cdot \text{km}$$

and

$$X_c = \frac{0.236 \times 10^6}{1.609} = 0.147 \times 10^6 \ \Omega \cdot \text{mi}$$

4.17 EFFECT OF GROUND ON CAPACITANCE OF THREE-PHASE LINES

Consider three-phase line conductors and their images below the surface of the ground, as shown in Figure 4.44. Assume that the line is transposed and that conductors a, b, and c have the charges q_a, q_b, and q_c, respectively, and their images have the charges $-q_a$, $-q_b$, and $-q_c$. The line-to-neutral capacitance can be expressed as [3]

$$C_N = \frac{2\pi \times 8.8538 \times 10^{-12}}{\ln\left(\dfrac{D_{eq}}{r}\right) - \ln\left(\dfrac{l_{12}l_{23}l_{31}}{h_{11}h_{22}h_{33}}\right)^{1/3}} \ \text{F/m} \qquad (4.387)$$

If the effect of the ground is not taken into account, the line-to-neutral capacitance is

$$C_N = \frac{2\pi \times 8.8538 \times 10^{-12}}{\ln\left(\dfrac{D_{eq}}{r}\right)} \ \text{F/m} \qquad (4.388)$$

As one can see, the effect of the ground increases the line capacitance. However, since the conductor heights are much larger than the distances between them, the effect of the ground is usually ignored for three-phase lines.

4.18 ENVIRONMENTAL EFFECTS OF OVERHEAD TRANSMISSION LINES

Recently, the importance of minimizing the environmental effects of OH transmission lines has increased substantially due to the increasing use of greater EHV and UHV levels. The magnitude and effect of RN, TVI, AN, electric field, and magnetic fields must not only be predicted and analyzed in the line design stage but also be measured directly. Measurements of corona-related phenomena must include radio and television station signal strengths and radio, television, and AN levels. To determine the effects of transmission line of these quantities, measurements should be

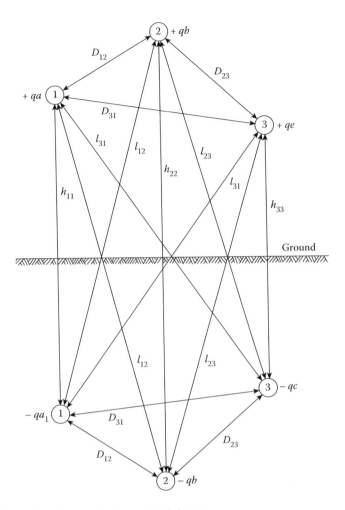

FIGURE 4.44 Three-phase line conductors and their images.

taken at three different times: (1) before construction of the line; (2) after construction, but before energization; and (3) after energization of the line. Noise measurements should be made at several locations along a transmission line. Also, at each location, measurements may be made at several points that might be of particular interest. Such points may include the point of maximum noise, the edge of the ROW, and the point 50 ft from the outermost conductor.

OH transmission lines and stations also produce EMFs, which have to be taken into account in the design process. The study of field effects (e.g., induced voltages and currents in conducting bodies) is becoming especially crucial as the operating voltage levels of transmission lines have been increasing due to the economics and operational benefits involved. Today, for example, such study at UHV level involves the following:

1. Calculation and measurement techniques for EMFs
2. Calculation and measurement of induced currents and voltages on objects of various shapes for all line voltages and design configurations
3. Calculation and measurement of currents and voltages induced in people as a result of various induction mechanisms
4. Investigation of sensitivity of people to various field effects
5. Study of conditions resulting in fuel ignition, corona from grounded objects, and other possible field effects [14]

Measurements of the transmission-line electric field must be made laterally at midspan and must extend at least to the edges of the ROW to determine the profile of the field. Further, related electric field effects such as currents and voltages induced in vehicles and fences should also be considered. Magnetic field effects are of much less concern than electric field effects for EHV and UHV transmission due to the fact that magnetic field levels for normal values of load current are low. The quantity and character of currents induced in the human body by magnetic effects have considerably less impact than those arising from electric induction. For example, the induced current densities in the human body are less than one-tenth those caused by electric field induction. Furthermore, most environmental measurements are highly affected by prevailing weather conditions and transmission-line geometry. The weather conditions include temperature, humidity, barometric pressure, precipitation levels, and wind velocity.

4.19 ADDITIONAL SOLVED NUMERICAL EXAMPLES FOR THE TRANSMISSION-LINE CALCULATIONS

Example 1 (for Short Line)

A 60 Hz, 30 MVA, 230 kV, 45 mi long, three-phase transmission line has 874.5 kcmil 54/3-strand ACSR conductors and is operating at 50°C. The conductors are spaced horizontally with $D_{ab} = 20$ ft, $D_{bc} = 20$ ft, and $D_{bc} = 40$ ft. Determine the following:

(a) Inductive reactance in ohms per mile
(b) Capacitive reactance in ohms per mile
(c) Total line resistance in ohms
(d) Total impedance of the line in ohms
(e) Total capacitive reactance of the line in ohms
(f) Receiving-end current
(g) Sending-end current
(h) The line voltage drop
(i) The line-to-neutral sending-end voltage
(j) The line-to-line sending-end voltage
(k) The efficiency of the line
(l) The total power loss of the line
(m) The voltage regulation

Solution

Since the line length is 45 mi, the short-line model will be used in the calculations. From Table A.3, it can be found that

$$D_s = 0.0386 \text{ ft}, \quad r = 0.1228 \ \Omega/\text{mi},$$

$$x_a = 0.395 \ \Omega/\text{mi}, \quad x_a' = 0.0903 \ \Omega/\text{mi}$$

Thus, the equivalent spacing factor is

$$D_{eq} = (20 \text{ ft} \times 20 \text{ ft} \times 40 \text{ ft})^{1/3} = 25.198 \text{ ft}$$

(a) The inductive reactance of the line, in ohms per mile, can be determined, after linear interpolation of the spacing factor as

$$X_d = 0.311 + \left(\frac{25.19 - 25.1}{25.2 - 25.1}\right)(0.3916 - 0.3911)$$

$$= 0.39155$$

$$\cong 0.3916 \ \Omega/\text{mi}.$$

Thus,

$$x_L = x_a + x_d$$

$$= 0.395 + 0.3916$$

$$= 0.7866 \ \Omega/\text{mi}$$

(b) The capacitive reactance of the line, in ohms per mile, is

$$x_c = x_a' + x_d'$$

$$= 0.0903 + 0.957$$

$$= 0.186 \ \text{M}\Omega \cdot \text{mi}$$

(c) The total line resistance of the line, in ohms, is

$$R = r \times l$$

$$= (0.1228 \ \Omega/\text{mi})(45 \ \text{mi})$$

$$= 5.526 \ \Omega$$

(d) The total impedance of the line, in ohms, is

$$\mathbf{Z} = R + j(X_L \times l)$$

$$= 5.526 + j(35.397 \ \Omega/\text{mi})(45 \ \text{mi})$$

$$= 5.526 + j35.397$$

$$\cong 35.826 \angle 81.13° \ \Omega$$

(e) The total capacitive reactance of the line, in ohms, is

$$X_c = \frac{x_c}{l}$$

$$= \frac{0.186 \ \text{M}\Omega \times \text{mi}}{45 \ \text{mi}}$$

$$= 0.00413 \ \text{M}\Omega$$

$$= 4.13 \ \text{k}\Omega$$

(f) The receiving-end current is

$$I_R = \frac{S_{3\phi}}{\sqrt{3}V_{R(\text{L-L})}}$$

$$= \frac{30 \ \text{MVA}}{\sqrt{3}(230 \ \text{kV})}$$

$$= 75.31 \ \text{A}$$

where

$$\mathbf{V}_{R(\text{L-N})} = \frac{\mathbf{V}_{R(\text{L-L})}}{\sqrt{3}} = \frac{230 \ \text{kV}}{\sqrt{3}} = 132.79 \ \text{kV}$$

$$\mathbf{I}_R = I \angle \cos^{-1}(0.95) = 75.31 \angle -18.195° \ \text{A}$$

(g) The sending-end current is

Since the line is a short line, $I_S = I_R = 75.31\angle -18.195°$ A

(h) The line voltage drop is

$$VD = I_R \times Z$$

$$= (75.31\angle -18.195° \ A)(35.826\angle 81.13° \ \Omega)$$

$$= 2.698\angle 62.9° \ kV$$

(i) The line-to-neutral sending-end voltage is

$$V_{S(L-N)} = V_R + VD = 134.04\angle 1.03° \ kV$$

(j) Since the line-to-line sending-end voltage is 30° ahead of line-to-neutral voltage and also $\sqrt{3}$ times greater than the line-to-neutral voltage,

$$V_{S(L-L)} = \sqrt{3}V_{S(L-N)}$$

$$= \sqrt{3}V_{S(L-N)}\angle \theta + 30°$$

$$= 134.04\angle 1.03 + 30°$$

$$= 232.164\angle 31.03° \ kV$$

(k) The efficiency of the line is

$$\%\mu = \frac{\text{Output}}{\text{Input}} \times 100$$

$$= \frac{\sqrt{3}V_R I \cos\theta_R}{\sqrt{3}V_S I \cos\theta_S} \times 100$$

$$= \frac{132.79 \times \cos(18.195°)}{134.04 \times \cos(18.195 + 1.03°)} \times 100$$

$$= 99.67\%$$

(l) The total power loss of the line is
(m)

$$\sum P_{\text{loss}(3\phi)} = 3I^2 R$$

$$= 3(75.31)^2 (5.526)$$

$$= 94.015 \ kW$$

or

$$\sum P_{\text{loss}(1\phi)} = I^2 R \quad \text{per phase}$$

$$= (75.31)^2 (5.526)$$

$$= \frac{94.015 \ kW}{3}$$

$$= 31.338 \ kW$$

(n) The voltage regulation is

$$\%VReg = \frac{232.164 - 230}{230} \times 100$$

$$= 0.907$$

Example 2 (for Medium-Length Line)

A three-phase, 60 Hz, 30 MVA, 230 kV, 55 mi long transmission line has 874.5 kcmil 54/3-strand ACSR conductors and is operating at 50°C. The conductors are spaced horizontally with $D_{ab} = 20$ ft, $D_{bc} = 20$ ft, and $D_{bc} = 40$ ft. Determine the following:

(a) Inductive reactance in ohms per mile
(b) Capacitive reactance in ohms per mile
(c) Total line resistance in ohms
(d) Total impedance of the line in ohms
(e) Total capacitive reactance of the line in ohms
(f) Receiving-end current
(g) Sending-end current
(h) The line voltage drop
(i) The line-to-neutral sending-end voltage
(j) The line-to-line sending-end voltage
(k) The efficiency of the line
(l) The total power loss of the line
(m) The voltage regulation

Solution

The line length is 55 mi. Since it is greater than 50 mi, the medium-line model will be used in the calculations. From Table A.3, it can be found that

$$D_s = 0.0386 \text{ ft}, \quad r = 0.1228 \ \Omega/\text{mi},$$

$$x_a = 0.395 \ \Omega/\text{mi}, \quad x_a' = 0.0903 \ M\Omega \cdot \text{mi}, \quad x_d' = 0.0957 \ M\Omega \cdot \text{mi}$$

Thus, the equivalent spacing factor is

$$D_{eq} = (20 \text{ ft} \times 20 \text{ ft} \times 40 \text{ ft})^{1/3} = 25.198 \text{ ft}$$

(a) The inductive reactance of the line, in ohms per mile, can be determined, after linear interpolation of the spacing factor as

$$X_d = 0.311 + \left(\frac{25.19 - 25.1}{25.2 - 25.1}\right)(0.3916 - 0.3911)$$

$$= 0.39155$$

$$\cong 0.3916 \ \Omega/\text{mi}.$$

Thus,

$$x_L = x_a + x_d$$

$$= 0.395 + 0.3916$$

$$= 0.7866 \ \Omega/\text{mi}$$

(b) The capacitive reactance of the line, in ohms per mile, is

$$x_c = x_a' + x_d'$$

$$= 0.0903 + 0.957$$

$$= 0.186 \ \text{M}\Omega \cdot \text{mi}$$

(c) The total line resistance of the line, in ohms, is

$$R = r \times l$$

$$= (0.1228 \ \Omega/\text{mi})(55 \ \text{mi})$$

$$= 6.754 \ \Omega$$

(d) The total impedance of the line, in ohms, is

$$\mathbf{Z} = R + j(X_L \times l)$$

$$= 6.754 + j(0.7866 \ \Omega/\text{mi})(55 \ \text{mi})$$

$$= 6.754 + j43.263$$

$$\cong 43.787 \angle 81.13° \ \Omega$$

(e) The total capacitive reactance of the line, in ohms, is

$$X_c = \frac{x_c}{l}$$

$$= \frac{0.186 \ \text{M}\Omega \cdot \text{mi}}{55 \ \text{mi}}$$

$$= 3.3818 \ \text{k}\Omega$$

(f) The receiving-end current is

$$\mathbf{I}_R = \frac{S_{3\phi}}{\sqrt{3}V_{R(L-L)}}$$

$$= \frac{30 \ \text{MVA}}{\sqrt{3}(230 \ \text{kV})} \angle - \cos PF$$

$$= \frac{30 \times 10^6 \ \text{VA}}{\sqrt{3}(230 \times 10^3 \ \text{V})} \angle - \cos(0.95)$$

$$= 75.31 \angle -18.195° \ \text{A}$$

or

$$\mathbf{I}_R = I_R \angle \cos^{-1}(0.95)$$

$$= 75.31 \angle -18.195° \ \text{A}$$

(g) For the sending-end current, first find the transmission-line parameters:

$$\mathbf{Y} = \frac{1}{-jX_c}$$

$$= \frac{1}{3.3818 \ \text{k}\Omega}$$

$$= j295.699 \times 10^{-6}$$

$$= 295.699 \times 10^{-6} \angle 90° \ \Omega$$

Therefore, the transmission-line parameters are

$$\mathbf{A} = 1 + \frac{\mathbf{YZ}}{2}$$

$$= 1 + \frac{\left(299.699 \times 10^{-6} \angle 90°\right)\left(43.787 \angle 81.13\right)}{2}$$

$$= 0.9936 \angle 0.05758°$$

$$\mathbf{B} = \mathbf{Z}$$

$$= 43.787 \angle 81.13° \ \Omega$$

$$\mathbf{C} = \mathbf{Y} + \frac{\mathbf{Y}^2 \mathbf{Z}}{4}$$

$$= j295.699 \times 10^{-6} + \frac{\left(295.699 \times 10^{-6} \angle 90°\right)^2 \left(43.787 \angle 81.13°\right)}{4}$$

$$= 294.753 \times 10^{-6} \angle 90.0287°$$

$$\mathbf{D} = \mathbf{A}$$

$$= 0.9936 \angle 0.05758°$$

Hence, the sending-end voltage and current can be found from

$$\begin{bmatrix} \mathbf{V}_S \\ \mathbf{I}_S \end{bmatrix} = \begin{bmatrix} \mathbf{A} & \mathbf{B} \\ \mathbf{C} & \mathbf{D} \end{bmatrix} \begin{bmatrix} \mathbf{V}_R \\ \mathbf{I}_R \end{bmatrix}$$

$$= \begin{bmatrix} 0.9936 \angle 0.05758° & 43.787 \angle 81.13° \\ 294.753 \times 10-6 \angle 90.0287° & 0.9936 \angle -0.5758° \end{bmatrix} \begin{bmatrix} 132.79 \angle 0° \ \text{kV} \\ 75.31 \angle -18.195° \end{bmatrix}$$

$$= \begin{bmatrix} 133.477 \times 103 \angle 1.317° \\ 72.833 \angle 12.568° \end{bmatrix}$$

Thus, the sending-end current is

$$\mathbf{I}_S = 72.833 \angle 12.568° \ \text{A}$$

(h) The line voltage drop is

$$\text{VD} = \mathbf{I} \times \mathbf{Z}$$

$$= \left(\frac{Y}{2} \times \mathbf{V}_R \right) \mathbf{Z}$$

$$= \left[\left(\frac{295.699 \times 10^{-6} \angle 90°}{2} \right) \left(132.79 \angle 0° \ \text{kV}\right) \right] \left(35.826 \angle 81.13° \ \Omega\right)$$

$$= \left[\left(147.8495 \times 10^{-6} \angle 90°\right)\left(132.79 \angle 0\right) \right] \left(35.826 \angle 81.13° \ \Omega\right)$$

$$= \left[19{,}632.93511 \times 10^{-6} \angle 90° \right] \left(35.826 \angle 81.13° \ \Omega\right)$$

$$= 0.7033695331 \ \text{kV}$$

$$\cong 703.37 \ \text{V}$$

(i) The line-to-neutral sending-end voltage is

$$\mathbf{V}_{S(L-N)} = 133.477\angle1.317° \text{ kV}$$

(j) The line-to-line sending-end voltage is 30° ahead of line-to-neutral voltage and also $\sqrt{3}$ times greater than the line-to-neutral voltage. Therefore,

$$\mathbf{V}_{S(L-L)} = \sqrt{3}\mathbf{V}_{S(L-N)}$$

$$= \sqrt{3}\mathbf{V}_{S(L-N)}\angle\theta + 30°$$

$$= \sqrt{3}(134.477\angle1.317° + 30°)$$

$$\cong 232.164\angle31.32° \text{ kV}$$

(k) The efficiency of the line is

$$\eta_{line} = \frac{\sqrt{3}V_R I \cos\theta_R}{\sqrt{3}V_S I \cos\theta_S} \times 100$$

$$= \frac{132.79 \times \cos(18.195°)}{134.477 \times \cos(11.257°)} \times 100$$

$$\cong 99.67\%$$

(l) The total power loss of the line is

$$P_{loss(3\phi)} = P_S - P_R$$

$$= \sqrt{3}V_{S(L-L)}I_S \cos\theta_S - \sqrt{3}V_{S(L-L)}I_S \cos\theta_S$$

$$= (28.604 - 28.5) \text{ MW}$$

$$= 104 \text{ kW}$$

(m) The voltage regulation is

$$\%\text{VReg} = \frac{\left|\dfrac{V_S}{A}\right| - |V_R|}{|V_R|} \times 100$$

$$= \frac{\dfrac{133.477}{0.9936} - 132.79}{132.79} \times 100 = 1.164$$

Example 3 (for Long Line)

A three-phase, 60 Hz, 30 MVA, 230 kV, 155 mi long transmission line has 874.5 kcmil 54/3-strand ACSR conductors and is operating at 50°C. The conductors are spaced horizontally with $D_{ab} = 20$ ft, $D_{bc} = 20$ ft, and $D_{bc} = 40$ ft. Determine the following:

(a) Inductive reactance in ohms per mile
(b) Capacitive reactance in ohms per mile

(c) Total line resistance in ohms
(d) Total impedance of the line in ohms
(e) Total capacitive reactance of the line in ohms
(f) Receiving-end current
(g) Sending-end current
(h) The line-to-neutral sending-end voltage
(i) The line-to-line sending-end voltage
(j) The efficiency of the line
(k) The total power loss of the line
(l) The voltage regulation

Solution

The line length is 155 mi. Since it is greater than 150 mi, the long-line model will be used in the calculations. From Table A.3, it can be found that

$$D_s = 0.0386 \text{ ft}, \quad r = 0.1228 \ \Omega/\text{mi},$$

$$x_a = 0.395 \ \Omega/\text{mi}, \quad x_a' = 0.0903 \ M\Omega \cdot \text{mi}, \quad x_d' = 0.0957 \ M\Omega \cdot \text{mi}$$

Thus, the equivalent spacing factor is

$$D_{eq} = (20 \text{ ft} \times 20 \text{ ft} \times 40 \text{ ft})^{1/3} = 25.198 \text{ ft}$$

(a) The inductive reactance of the line, in ohms per mile, can be determined, after linear interpolation of the spacing factor as

$$X_d = 0.311 + \left(\frac{25.19 - 25.1}{25.2 - 25.1}\right)(0.3916 - 0.3911)$$

$$= 0.39155$$

$$\cong 0.3916 \ \Omega/\text{mi}.$$

Thus,

$$x_L = x_a + x_d$$

$$= 0.395 + 0.3916$$

$$= 0.7866 \ \Omega/\text{mi}$$

(b) The capacitive reactance of the line, in ohms per mile, is

$$x_c = x_a' + x_d'$$

$$= 0.0903 + 0.957$$

$$= 0.186 \ M\Omega \cdot \text{mi}$$

(c) The total line resistance of the line, in ohms, is

$$R = r \times l$$

$$= (0.1228 \ \Omega/\text{mi})(155 \text{ mi})$$

$$= 19.034 \ \Omega$$

(d) The total impedance of the line, in ohms, is

$$\mathbf{Z} = R + j(X_L \times l)$$

$$= 19.034 + j(0.7866 \ \Omega/\text{mi})(155 \ \text{mi})$$

$$= 19.034 + j121.923$$

$$\cong 123.398\angle 81.13° \ \Omega$$

(e) The total capacitive reactance of the line, in ohms, is

$$X_c = \frac{x_c}{l}$$

$$= \frac{0.186 \ \text{M}\Omega \cdot \text{mi}}{155 \ \text{mi}}$$

$$= 1.2 \ \text{k}\Omega$$

(f) The receiving-end current is

$$\mathbf{I}_R = \frac{S_{3\phi}}{\sqrt{3}V_{R(\text{L-L})}}$$

$$= \frac{30 \ \text{MVA}}{\sqrt{3}(230 \ \text{kV})} \angle - \cos PF$$

$$= \frac{30 \times 10^6 \ \text{VA}}{\sqrt{3}(230 \times 10^3 \ \text{V})} \angle - \cos(0.95)$$

$$= 75.31\angle -18.195° \ \text{A}$$

or

$$\mathbf{I}_R = I_R \angle \cos^{-1}(0.95)$$

$$= 75.31\angle -18.195° \ \text{A}$$

(g) For the sending-end current, first find the transmission-line parameters:

$$\mathbf{Y} = \frac{1}{-jX_c}$$

$$= j\frac{1}{1.2 \ \text{k}\Omega}$$

$$= j0.00083$$

$$= 0.00083\angle 90° \ \text{S}$$

Therefore, the transmission-line parameters are

$$\mathbf{A} = \cosh\sqrt{\mathbf{YZ}}$$

$$= 0.9496 + j0.007797$$

$$\mathbf{B} = \sqrt{\frac{\mathbf{Z}}{\mathbf{Y}}} \sinh\sqrt{\mathbf{YZ}}$$

$$= 18.394 + j119.918$$

$$C = \sqrt{\frac{Y}{Z}} \sinh \sqrt{YZ}$$

$$= -2.1807 \times 10^{-6} + j0.81929 \times 10^{-3}$$

$$D = A$$

$$= 0.9496 + j0.007797$$

Hence, the sending-end voltage and current can be found from

$$\begin{bmatrix} V_S \\ I_S \end{bmatrix} = \begin{bmatrix} A & B \\ B & D \end{bmatrix} \begin{bmatrix} V_R \\ I_R \end{bmatrix}$$

$$= \begin{bmatrix} 0.9936\angle 0.05758° & 43.787\angle 81.13° \\ 294.753 \times 10^{-6}\angle 90.0287° & 0.9936\angle -0.5758° \end{bmatrix} \begin{bmatrix} 132.79\angle 0° \text{ kV} \\ 75.31\angle -18.195° \end{bmatrix}$$

$$= \begin{bmatrix} 130.559 \times 10^3 \angle 4.033° \\ 110.336\angle 52.063° \end{bmatrix}$$

Thus, the sending-end current is

$$I_S = 110.336\angle 52.063° \text{ A}$$

(h) The line-to-neutral sending-end voltage is

$$V_{S(L-N)} = 133.477\angle 1.317° \text{ kV}$$

(i) The line-to-line sending-end voltage is 30° ahead of line-to-neutral voltage and also $\sqrt{3}$ times greater than the line-to-neutral voltage. Therefore,

$$V_{S(L-L)} = \sqrt{3} V_{S(L-N)}$$

$$= \sqrt{3} V_{S(L-N)} \angle \theta + 30°$$

$$= \sqrt{3}(130.559\angle 4.0.33° + 30°)$$

$$\cong 226.136\angle 34.033° \text{ kV}$$

(j) The efficiency of the line is

$$\eta_{\text{line}} = \frac{\text{Output}}{\text{Input}} \times 100$$

$$= \frac{\sqrt{3} V_R I \cos\theta_R}{\sqrt{3} V_S I \cos\theta_S} \times 100$$

$$= \frac{28.5 \text{ MW}}{28.899 \text{ MW}}$$

$$\cong 98.62\%$$

(k) The total power loss of the line is

$$P_{\text{loss}(3\phi)} = P_S - P_R$$

$$= \sqrt{3}V_{S(L\text{-}L)}I_S\cos\theta_S - \sqrt{3}V_{S(L\text{-}L)}I_S\cos\theta_S$$

$$= (28.899 - 28.5)\ \text{MW}$$

$$\cong 399\ \text{kW}$$

(l) The voltage regulation is

$$\%\text{VReg} = \frac{\left|\dfrac{V_S}{A}\right| - |V_R|}{|V_R|} \times 100$$

$$= \frac{\dfrac{226.136}{0.9496} - 230}{230} \times 100$$

$$\cong 3.54\%$$

Note that this example is not realistic in the sense that the designated power is too small for such a long-line transmission line. Also, the distances between conductors are too small. The only reason for such exercises is to provide at least some comparison among the results of the different transmission-line lengths; however, they are too approximate and too simplistic.

PROBLEMS

4.1 Assume that the impedance of a line connecting buses 1 and 2 is $50\angle90°\ \Omega$ and that the bus voltages are $7560\angle10°$ and $7200\angle0°$ V per phase, respectively. Determine the following:
  (a) Real power per phase that is being transmitted from bus 1 to bus 2
  (b) Reactive power per phase that is being transmitted from bus 1 to bus 2
  (c) Complex power per phase that is being transmitted
4.2 Solve Problem 4.1 assuming that the line impedance is $50\angle26°\ \Omega$/phase.
4.3 Verify the following equations:
  (a) $V_{\text{pu}(L\text{-}N)} = V_{\text{pu}(L\text{-}L)}$
  (b) $\text{VA}_{\text{pu}(1\phi)} = \text{VA}_{\text{pu}(3\phi)}$
  (c) $Z_{\text{pu}(Y)} = Z_{\text{pu}(\Delta)}$
4.4 Verify the following equations:
  (a) Equation 4.24 for single-phase system
  (b) Equation 4.80 for three-phase system
4.5 Show that $Z_{B(\Delta)} = 3Z_{B(Y)}$.
4.6 Consider two three-phase transmission lines with different voltage levels that are located side by side in a close proximity. Assume that the bases of VA_B, $V_{B(1)}$, and $I_{B(1)}$ and the bases of VA_B, $V_{B(2)}$, and $I_{B(2)}$ are designated for the first and second lines, respectively. If the mutual reactance between the lines is $X_m\ \Omega$, show that this mutual reactance in per unit can be expressed as

$$X_{\text{pu}(m)} = \left(\text{physical } X_m\right)\frac{\text{MVA}_B}{\left[kV_{B(1)}kV_{B(2)}\right]}$$

4.7 Consider Example 4.3 and assume that the transformer is connected in delta–wye. Use a 25 MVA base and determine the following:

(a) New line-to-line voltage of the LV side

(b) New LV-side base impedance

(c) Turns ratio of windings

(d) Transformer reactance referred to the LV side in ohms

(e) Transformer reactance referred to the LV side in per units

4.8 Verify the following equations:

(a) Equation 4.92

(b) Equation 4.93

(c) Equation 4.94

(d) Equation 4.96

4.9 Verify the following equations:

(a) Equation 4.100

(b) Equation 4.102

4.10 Consider the one-line diagram given in Figure P4.10. Assume that the three-phase transformer T_1 has the nameplate ratings of 15,000 kVA, 7.97/13.8Y – 69Δ kV with leakage impedance of $0.01 + j0.08$ pu based on its ratings and that the three-phase transformer T_2 has the nameplate ratings of 1500 kVA, 7.97Δ kV – 277/480Y V with leakage impedance of $0.01 + j0.05$ pu based on its ratings. Assume that the three-phase generator G_1 is rated 10/12.5 MW/MVA, 7.97/13.8Y kV with an impedance of $0 + j1.10$ pu based on its ratings and that the three-phase generator G_2 is rated 4/5 MW/MVA, 7.62/13.2Y kV with an impedance of $0 + j0.90$ pu based on its ratings. Transmission line TL_{23} has a length of 50 mi and is composed of 4/0 ACSR conductors with an equivalent spacing (D_m) of 8 ft and has an impedance of $0.445 + j0.976$ Ω/mi. Its shunt susceptance is given as 5.78 μS/mi. The line connects buses 2 and 3. Bus 3 is assumed to be an infinite bus, that is, the magnitude of its voltage remains constant at a given value, and its phase position is unchanged regardless of the power and PF demands that may be put on it. Furthermore, it is assumed to have a constant frequency equal to the nominal frequency of the system studied. Transmission line TL_{14} connects buses 1 and 4. It has a line length of 2 mi and an impedance of $0.80 + j0.80$ Ω/mi.

Because of the line length, its shunt susceptance is assumed to be negligible. The load that is connected to bus 1 has a current magnitude $|\mathbf{I}_1|$ of 523 A and a lagging PF of 0.707. The load that is connected to bus 5 is given as $8000 + j6000$ kVA. Use the arbitrarily selected 5000 kVA as the three-phase kilovolt-ampere base and 39.84/69.00 kV as the line-to-neutral and line-to-line voltage base and determine the following:

(a) Complete Table P4.10 for the indicated values. Note the I_L means line current and I_ϕ means phase currents in delta-connected apparatus.

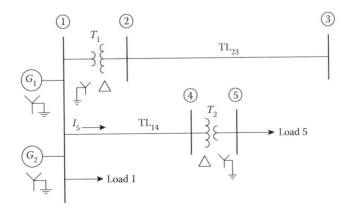

FIGURE P4.10 One-line diagram for Problem 4.10.

TABLE P4.10

Table for Problem 4.10

Quantity	Nominally 69 kV Circuits	Nominally 13 kV Circuits	Nominally 480 V Circuits
$kVA_B(3\phi)$	5000 kVA	5000 kVA	5000 kVA
$kV_{B(L-L)}$	69 kV		
$kV_{B(L-N)}$	39.84 kV		
$I_{B(L)}$			
IB(ϕ)			
Z_B			
Y_B			

(b) Draw a single-line positive-sequence network of this simple power system. Use the nominal-π circuit to represent the 69 kV line. Show the values of all impedances and susceptances in per units on the chosen bases. Show all loads in per unit $P + jQ$.

4.11 Assume that a 500 + j200 kVA load is connected to a load bus that has a voltage of 1.0∠0° pu. If the power base is 1000 kVA, determine the per-unit R and X of the load:
(a) When load is represented by parallel connection
(b) When load is represented by series connection

4.12 Assume that a three-phase transmission line is constructed of 700 kcmil, 37-strand copper conductors and the line length is 100 mi. The conductors are spaced horizontally with D_{ab} = 10 Ω, D_{bc} = 8 Ω, and D_{ca} = 18 Ω. Use 60 Hz and 25°C and determine the following line constants from tables in terms of
(a) Inductive reactance in ohms per mile
(b) Capacitive reactance in ohms per mile
(c) Total line resistance in ohms
(d) Total inductive reactance in ohms
(e) Total capacitive reactance in ohms

4.13 Redraw the phasor diagram shown in Figure 4.17 by using **I** as the reference vector and derive formulas to calculate the following:
(a) Sending-end phase voltage, V_S
(b) Sending-end PF angle, ϕ_S

4.14 A three-phase, 60 Hz, 15 mi long transmission line provides 10 MW at a PF of 0.9 lagging at a line-to-line voltage of 34.5 kV. The line conductors are made of 26-strand 300 kcmil ACSR conductors that operate at 25°C and are equilaterally spaced 3 ft apart. Calculate the following:
(a) Source voltage
(b) Sending-end PF
(c) Transmission efficiency
(d) Regulation of line

4.15 Repeat Problem 4.14 assuming the receiving-end PF of 0.8 lagging.

4.16 Repeat Problem 4.15 assuming the receiving-end PF of 0.8 leading.

4.17 A single-phase load is supplied by a $\left(34.5/\sqrt{3}\right)$ kV feeder whose impedance is 95 + j340 Ω and a $\left(34.5/\sqrt{3}\right)$/2.4 kV transformer whose equivalent impedance is 0.24 + j0.99 Ω referred to its LV side. The load is 200 kW at a leading PF of 0.85 and 2.25 kV. Calculate the following:
(a) Calculate the sending-end voltage of feeder.
(b) Calculate the primary-terminal voltage of transformer.
(c) Calculate the real and reactive power input at the sending end of feeder.

4.18 A short three-phase line has the series reactance of 15 Ω per phase. Neglect its series resistance. The load at the receiving end of the transmission line is 15 MW per phase and 12 Mvar lagging per phase. Assume that the receiving-end voltage is given as $115 + j0$ kV per phase and calculate:

(a) Sending-end voltage

(b) Sending-end current

4.19 A short 40 mi long three-phase transmission line has a series line impedance of $0.6 + j0.95$ Ω/mi per phase. The receiving-end line-to-line voltage is 69 kV. It has a full-load receiving-end current of $300\angle{-30°}$ A. Calculate the following:

(a) Calculate the percentage of voltage regulation.

(b) Calculate the **ABCD** constants of the line.

(c) Draw the phasor diagram of $\mathbf{V_S}$, $\mathbf{V_R}$, and $\mathbf{I}$.

4.20 Repeat Problem 4.19 assuming the receiving-end current of $300\angle{-45°}$ A.

4.21 A three-phase, 60 Hz, 12 MW load at a lagging PF of 0.85 is supplied by a three-phase, 138 kV transmission line of 40 mi. Each line conductor has a resistance of 41 Ω/mi and an inductance of 14 mH/mi. Calculate:

(a) Sending-end line-to-line voltage

(b) Loss of power in transmission line

(c) Amount of reduction in line power loss if load-PF were improved to unity

4.22 A three-phase, 60 Hz transmission line has sending-end voltage of 39 kV and receiving-end voltage of 34.5 kV. If the line impedance per phase is $18 + j57$ Ω, compute the maximum power receivable at the receiving end of the line.

4.23 A three-phase, 60 Hz, 45 mi long short line provides 20 MVA at a lagging PF of 0.85 at a line-to-line voltage of 161 kV. The line conductors are made of 19-strand 4/0 copper conductors that operate at 50°C. The conductors are equilaterally spaced with 4 ft spacing between them:

(a) Determine the percentage of voltage regulation of the line.

(b) Determine the sending-end PF.

(c) Determine the transmission-line efficiency if the line is single phase, assuming the use of the same conductors.

(d) Repeat Part (c) if the line is three phase.

4.24 A three-phase, 60 Hz, 15 MW load at a lagging PF of 0.9 is supplied by two parallel connected transmission lines. The sending-end voltage is 71 kV, and the receiving-end voltage on a full load is 69 kV. Assume that the total transmission-line efficiency is 98%. If the line length is 10 mi and the impedance of one of the lines is $0.7 + j1.2$ Ω/mi, compute the total impedance per phase of the second line.

4.25 Verify that $(\cosh \gamma l - 1)/\sinh \gamma l = \tanh(1/2) \gamma l$.

4.26 Derive Equations 4.198 and 4.199 from Equations 4.196 and 4.201.

4.27 Find the general circuit parameters for the network shown in Figure P4.27.

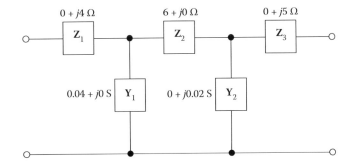

FIGURE P4.27 Network for Problem 4.27.

4.28 Find a T equivalent of the circuit shown in Figure P4.27.

4.29 Assume that the line is a 200 mi long transmission line and repeat Example 4.11.

4.30 Assume that the line is a 200 mi long transmission line and repeat Example 4.12.

4.31 Assume that the line is a short transmission line and repeat Example 4.11.

4.32 Assume that the line is a short transmission line and repeat Example 4.12.

4.33 Assume that the line in Example 4.13 is 75 mi long and the load is 100 MVA and repeat the example.

4.34 Develop the equivalent transfer matrix for the network shown in Figure P4.34 matrix manipulation.

4.35 Develop the equivalent transfer matrix for the network shown in Figure P4.35 matrix manipulation.

4.36 Verify Equations 4.282 through 4.285 without using matrix methods.

4.37 Verify Equations 4.289 through 4.292 without using matrix methods.

4.38 Assume that the line given in Example 4.11 is a 200 mi long transmission line. Use the other data given in Example 4.4 accordingly and repeat Example 4.15.

4.39 Use the data from Problem 4.38 and repeat Example 4.16.

4.40 Assume that the shunt compensation of Example 4.21 is to be retained and now 60% series compensation is to be used, that is, X_c is equal to 60% of the total series inductive reactance per phase of the transmission line. Determine the following:

    (a) Total three-phase SIL of line in megavolt-amperes

    (b) Maximum three-phase theoretical steady-state power flow limit in megawatts

4.41 Assume that the line given in Problem 4.40 is designed to carry a contingency peak load of 2 × SIL and that each phase of the SC bank is to be of series and parallel groups of two-bushing, 12 kV, 150 kvar shunt PF correction capacitors:

    (a) Specify the necessary series-parallel arrangements of capacitors for each phase.

    (b) Such capacitors may cost about $1.50/kvar. Estimate the cost of the capacitors in the entire three-phase SC bank. (Take note that the structure and the switching and protective equipment associated with the capacitor bank will add a great deal more cost.)

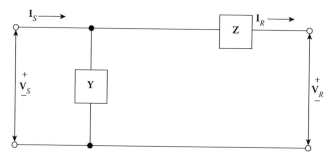

FIGURE P4.34   Network for Problem 4.34.

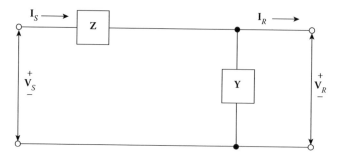

FIGURE P4.35   Network for Problem 4.35.

4.42 Use Table 5.7 for a 345 kV, pipe-type, three-phase, 1000 kcmil cable. Assume that the percent PF cable is 0.5 and maximum electric stress is 300 V/mil and that

$$\mathbf{V}_s = \frac{345{,}000}{\sqrt{3}} \angle 0° \text{ V}$$

Calculate the following:
(a) Susceptance b of cable
(b) Critical length of cable and compare with the value given in Table 5.7

4.43 Consider the cable given in Problem 4.42 and use Table 5.7 for the relevant data; determine the value of

$$\mathbf{I}_{l0} = \frac{\mathbf{V}_S}{\mathbf{Z}_c} \tanh \gamma l_0$$

accurately and compare it with the given value of cable ampacity in Table 5.7. (*Hint*: Use the exponential form of the tanh γl_0 function.)

4.44 Consider Equation 4.175 and verify that the maximum power obtainable (i.e., the steady-state power limit) at the receiving end can be expressed as

$$P_{R,\max} = \frac{|\mathbf{V}_S||\mathbf{V}_R|}{|X|} \sin \gamma$$

4.45 Repeat Problem 4.18 assuming that the given power is the sending-end power instead of the receiving-end power.

4.46 Assume that a three-phase transmission line is constructed of 700 kcmil, 37-strand copper conductors and the line length is 100 mi. The conductors are spaced horizontally with $D_{ab} = 10 \ \Omega$, $D_{bc} = 8 \ \Omega$, and $D_{ca} = 18 \ \Omega$. Use 60 Hz and 25°C and determine the following line constants from tables in terms of the following:
(a) Inductive reactance in ohms per mile
(b) Capacitive reactance in ohms per mile
(c) Total line resistance in ohms
(d) Total inductive reactance in ohms
(e) Total capacitive reactance in ohms

4.47 A 60 Hz, single-circuit, three-phase transmission line is 150 mi long. The line is connected to a load of 50 MVA at a logging PF of 0.85 at 138 kV. The line impedance and admittance are $\mathbf{z} = 0.7688 \angle 77.4° \ \Omega/\text{mi}$ and $\mathbf{y} = 4.5239 \times 10^{-6} \angle 90° \ \text{S/mi}$, respectively. Determine the following:
(a) Propagation constant of the line
(b) Attenuation constant and phase change constant, per mile, of the line
(c) Characteristic impedance of the line
(d) SIL of the line
(e) Receiving-end current
(f) Incident voltage at the sending end
(g) Reflected voltage at the sending end

4.48 Consider a three-phase transmission and assume that the following values are given:

$$\mathbf{V}_{R(L-N)} = 79{,}674.34 \angle 0° \text{ V}$$

$$\mathbf{I}_R = 209.18 \angle -31.8° \text{ A}$$

$$\mathbf{Z}_c = 469.62 \angle 5.37° \text{ } \Omega$$

$$\gamma l = 0.0301 + j0.3202$$

Determine the following:
(a) Incident and reflected voltages at the receiving end of the line.
(b) Incident and reflected voltages at the sending end of the line.
(c) Line voltage at the sending end of the line.

4.49 Repeat Example 4.18 assuming that the conductor used is 1431 kcmil ACSR and that the distance between two subconductors is 18 in. Also assume that the distances D_{72}, D_{23}, and D_{31} are 25, 25, and 50 ft, respectively.

REFERENCES

1. Elgerd, O. I. *Electric Energy Systems Theory: An Introduction*, McGraw-Hill, New York, 1971.
2. Neuenswander, J. R. *Modern Power Systems*, International Textbook Company, Scranton, PA, 1971.
3. Stevenson, W. D., Jr. *Elements of Power System Analysis*, 3rd edn., McGraw-Hill, New York, 1975.
4. Anderson, P. M. *Analysis of Faulted Power Systems*, Iowa State University Press, Ames, IA, 1973.
5. Fink, D. G. and Beaty, H. W. *Standard Handbook for Electrical Engineers*, 11th edn., McGraw-Hill, New York, 1978.
6. Wagner, C. F. and Evans, R. D. *Symmetrical Components*, McGraw-Hill, New York, 1933.
7. Weedy, B. M. *Electric Power Systems*, 2nd edn., Wiley, New York, 1972.
8. Concordia, C. and Rusteback, E. Self-excited oscillations in a transmission system using series capacitors, *IEEE Trans. Power Appar. Syst.* PAS-89(7), 1970, 1504–1512.
9. Elliott, L. C., Kilgore, L. A., and Taylor, E. R. The prediction and control of self-excited oscillations due to series capacitors in power systems, *IEEE Trans. Power Appar. Syst.* PAS-90(3), 1971, 1305–1311.
10. Farmer, R. G. et al. Solutions to the problems of subsynchronous resonance in power systems with series capacitors, *Proc. Am. Power Conf.* 35, 1973, 1120–1128.
11. Bowler, C. E. J., Concordia, C., and Tice, J. B. Subsynchronous torques on generating units feeding series-capacitor compensated lines, *Proc. Am. Power Conf.* 35, 1973, 1129–1136.
12. Schifreen, C. S. and Marble, W. C. Changing current limitations in operation of high-voltage cable lines, *Trans. Am. Inst. Electr. Eng.* 26, 1956, 803–817.
13. Wiseman, R. T. Discussions to charging current limitations in operation of high-voltage cable lines, *Trans. Am. Inst. Electr. Eng.* 26, 1956, 803–817.
14. Electric Power Research Institute. *Transmission Line Reference Book: 345 kV and Above*, EPRI, Palo Alto, CA, 1979.

GENERAL REFERENCES

Bowman, W. I. and McNamee, J. M. Development of equivalent Pi and T matrix circuits for long untransposed transmission lines, *IEEE Trans. Power Appar. Syst.* PAS-83, 1964, 625–632.
Clarke, E. *Circuit Analysis of A-C Power Systems*, vol. 1, General Electric Company, Schenectady, NY, 1950.
Cox, K. J. and Clark, E. Performance charts for three-phase transmission circuits under balance operations, *Trans. Am. Inst. Electr. Eng.* 76, 1957, 809–816.
Electric Power Research Institute. *Transmission Line Reference Book: 115–138 kV Compact Line Design*, EPRI, Palo Alto, CA, 1978.
Gönen, T. *Electric Power Distribution System Engineering*, McGraw-Hill, New York, 1986.
Gönen, T., Nowikowski, J., and Brooks, C. L. Electrostatic unbalances of transmission lines with "N" overhead ground wires—Part I, *Proceedings of Modeling and Simulation Conference*, Pittsburgh, PA, April 24–25, 1986, vol. 17 (Pt. 2), pp. 459–464.
Gönen, T., Nowikowski, J., and Brooks, C. L. Electrostatic unbalances of transmission lines with "N" overhead ground wires—Part II, *Proceedings of Modeling and Simulation Conference*, Pittsburgh, PA, April 24–25, 1986, vol. 17 (Pt. 2), pp. 465–470.

Gönen, T., Yousif, S., and Leng, X. Fuzzy logic evaluation of new generation impact on existing transmission system, *Proceedings of IEEE Budapest Tech'99 Conference*, Budapest, Hungary, August 29–September 2, 1999.

Gross, C. A. *Power System Analysis*, Wiley, New York, 1979.

Institute of Electrical and Electronics Engineers. Graphic symbols for electrical and electronics diagrams, IEEE Stand. 315-1971 for American National Standards Institute (ANSI) Y32.2-1971, IEEE, New York, 1971.

Kennelly, A. E. *The Application of Hyperbolic Functions to Electrical Engineering Problems*, 3rd edn., McGraw-Hill, New York, 1925.

Skilling, H. H. *Electrical Engineering Circuits*, 2nd edn., Wiley, New York. 1966.

Travis, I. Per unit quantities, *Trans. Am. Inst. Electr. Eng.* 56, 1937, 340–349.

Woodruf, L. F. *Electrical Power Transmission*, Wiley, New York, 1952.

Zaborsky, J. and Rittenhouse, J. W. *Electric Power Transmission*, Rensselaer Bookstore, Troy, NY, 1969.

5 Underground Power Transmission and Gas-Insulated Transmission Lines

A person is never happy except at the price of some ignorance.

Anatole France

5.1 INTRODUCTION

In the United States, a large percentage of transmission systems was installed during World War II between the mid-1950s and the mid-1970s, with limited construction in the past few decades. The equipment installed in the postwar period is now between 30 and 50 years old and is at the end of its expected life. For example, 70% of transmission lines and power transformers in this country are 25 years old or even older. Similarly, 60% of HV circuit breakers are 30 years old or older.

Even at a local level, transmission benefits are in danger. For the past 20 years, the growth of electricity demand has far exceeded the growth of transmission capacity. With limited new transmission capacity available, the loading of existing transmission lines has dramatically increased.

At the present time, the electric power industry is finally starting to invest more money on new transmission lines. This upgrading is usually accomplished by increasing the voltage levels, or by adding more wires, in terms of bundled conductors, to increase the current ratings. It is important that the new transmission construction be planned well, so that the existing electric power grid can be systematically transformed into a modern and adequate system rather than becoming a patchwork of incremental and isolated decisions and uncoordinated subsystems.

Today, 10 major metropolitan areas in the United States create almost 25% of the total electricity demand of the country. Because demand will continue to grow and become in remote sites, it becomes increasingly difficult to run OH power transmission lines through urban or heavily populated suburban areas. These considerations, in addition to the delay and cost complications associated with acquiring right-of-way, emphasize the need for advanced high-capacity underground power transmission systems.

This underground power transmission solution has the advantages of possible usage of existing rights-of-way of present OH transmission lines and decrease in waiting times for getting the necessary permissions. It goes without saying that the cost of building underground lines is much greater than building OH transmission lines.

Today, there are four main technical methods for underground transmission, namely, (1) using solidly insulated underground cables, (2) using gas-insulated lines (GILs), (3) using superconductive cables, and (4) using cryogenic cables.

The solidly insulated cables are used for underground power transmission since the very beginning of the installation of the transmission network. They are mostly used in cities or other applications where OH lines cannot be used. The use of solidly insulated cables is limited in length as well as in current rating, even though these values have been increased recently. The solidly insulated underground cables and their usage are further discussed extensively starting from the next section in this chapter.

The GILs are used for more than 30 years worldwide. They have been used in many projects providing a very high-power transmission capability similar to the OH lines and are practically not limited in length. For further discussions of the GIL, see Section 5.12.

The *superconductive cable* applications are still in their preliminary stages. The use of superconductive cable has been implemented so far only to a relatively few projects in the United States.

However, short experimental *superconducting lines* have been constructed and operated. It remains to be economical to be implemented. However, superconducting alternators have been built and operated. It is known that alternators with superconducting fields can be made 40% smaller in size, 1% more efficient, and up to 30% less expensive than typical alternators. The superconducting rotor is the reason for the low cost, size, and the greater efficiency. It is interesting to note that the magnetic field from the superconducting rotor windings is so strong that no magnetic core is required, even though a magnetic shield is needed to help contain the coolant and hold ac electricity and magnetic fields, from the stator, from reaching the rotor. Today, several superconducting alternators that are in the range of 20–50 MVA are in operation in the United States and abroad. However, larger superconducting alternators have been economically found to be less attractive.

It is important to note that *a cryogenic cable is not superconducting*. The conductor of such cable possesses a higher electrical conductivity at very low temperature than at ambient temperature. Because of this fact, a cryogenic conductor has a lower resistive loss. For example, at the temperature of liquid nitrogen, the conductivity of aluminum and copper improves by a factor of 10. However, it is usually aluminum that is used in such cables due to its low cost.

The technical feasibility of resistive cryogenic cable systems is large based on insulation performance under HV conditions at low temperature. Based on operational, technical, and economical reasons, the cable that is usually selected is liquid nitrogen–cooled flexible cable.

A cryogenic cable has a hollow former supporting a helically wound, stranded, transposed conductor made of aluminum. The conductor is taped with suitable electrical insulation impregnated with liquid nitrogen. An evacuated thermal insulation that is put on the cryogenic pipe reduces heat leak from the environment. Its refrigeration is facilitated by using a system of turbomachinery and neon as the cooling fluid. The ratio of refrigerator input power to refrigeration increases as the cryogenic refrigeration temperature decreases. Today, it is feasible to have an electrical insulation system for a cryogenic cable that is operating at a typical EHV voltage. For example, recent research results indicate successful performance in a liquid nitrogen environment at voltages up to the equivalent of 150% of a 500 kV system having a measured dielectric cable loss that is 300 times less than a typical EHV oil-filled underground cable.

5.2 UNDERGROUND CABLES

Underground cables may have one or more conductors within a protective sheath. The protective sheath is an impervious covering over insulation, and it usually is lead. The conductors are separated from each other and from the sheath by insulating materials. The insulation materials used are (1) rubber and rubberlike compounds, (2) varnished cambric, and (3) oil-impregnated paper.

Rubber is used in cables rated 600 V–35 kV, whereas polyethylene (PE), propylene (PP), and polyvinyl chloride (PVC) are used in cables rated 600 V–138 kV. The high-moisture resistance of rubber makes it ideal for submarine cables. Varnished cambric is used in cables rated 600 V–28 kV. Oil-impregnated paper is used in solid-type cables up to 69 kV and in pressurized cables up to 345 kV. In the solid-type cables, the pressure within the oil-impregnated cable is not raised above atmospheric pressure. In the pressurized cables, the pressure is kept above atmospheric pressure either by gas in gas pressure cables or by oil in oil-filled cables. Impregnated paper is used for higher voltages because of its low dielectric losses and lower cost. Cables used for 59 kV and below are either (1) low pressure, not over 15 psi, or (2) medium pressure, not over 45 psi. High-pressure cables, up to 200 psi, installed pipes are not economical for voltages of 69 kV and below.

Voids or cavities can appear as the result of faulty product or during the operation of the cable under varying load. Bending the cable in handling and on installation, and also the different thermal expansion coefficients of the insulating paper, the impregnating material and the lead sheath result in voids in the insulation of cable not under pressure. The presence of higher electrical field strength ionization that appears in the voids in the dielectric leads to destruction of the insulation. The presence of ionization can be detected by means of the power factor change as a test voltage is applied. The formation of voids is avoided in the case of the oil-filled cable. With the gas-filled cable, the pressure in the insulation is increased to such a value that existing voids or cavities are ionization free. Ionization increases with temperature and decreases with increasing pressure.

The conductors used in underground cables can be copper or aluminum. Aluminum dictates larger conductor sizes to carry the same current as copper. The need for mechanical flexibility requires stranded conductors to be used. The equivalent aluminum cable is lighter in weight and larger in diameter in comparison to copper cable. Stranded conductors can be in various configurations, for example, concentric, compressed, compact, and rope.

Cables are classified in numerous ways. For example, they can be classified as (1) underground, (2) submarine, and (3) aerial, depending on location. They can be classified according to the type of insulation, such as (1) rubber and rubberlike compounds, (2) varnished cambric, and (3) oil-impregnated paper. They can be classified as single conductor, two conductor (duplex), three conductor, etc., depending on the number of conductors in a given cable. Also, they can be classified as shielded (as in the Hochstadter or type H cable) or nonshielded (belted), depending on the presence or absence of metallic shields over the insulation. Shielded cables can be solid, oil filled, or gas filled. Further, they can be classified by their protective finish such as (1) metallic (e.g., a steel sheath) or (2) nonmetallic (e.g., plastic).

Insulation shields help to (1) confine the electric field within the cable; (2) protect cable better from induced potentials; (3) limit electromagnetic or electrostatic interference; (4) equalize voltage stress within the insulation, minimizing surface discharges; and (5) reduce shock hazard (when properly grounded) [1].

In general, shielding should be considered for nonmetallic covered cables operating at a circuit voltage over 2 kV and where any of the following conditions exist [2]:

1. Transition from conducting to nonconducting conduit
2. Transition from moist to dry earth
3. In dry soil, such as in the desert
4. In damp conduits
5. Connections to aerial lines
6. Where conducting pulling compounds are used
7. Where surface of cable collects conducting materials, such as soot, salt, cement deposits
8. Where electrostatic discharges are of low enough intensity not to damage cable but are sufficient in magnitude to interface with radio or television reception

In general, cables are pulled into underground ducts. However, if they have to be buried directly in the ground, the lead sheath (i.e., the covering over insulation) has to be protected mechanically by armor. The armor is to be made of two tapes overlapping each other or heavy steel wires.

Where heavy loads are to be handled, the usage of single-conductor cables is advantageous since they can be made in conductor sizes up to 3.5 kcmil or larger. They are also used where phase isolation is required or where balanced single-phase transformer loads are supplied. They are often used to terminate three-conductor cables in single-conductor potheads, such as at pole risers, to provide training in small manholes. They can be supplied triplexed or wound three in parallel on a reel, permitting installation of three-conductor cables in a single duct. Figure 5.1 shows a single-conductor, paper-insulated power cable.

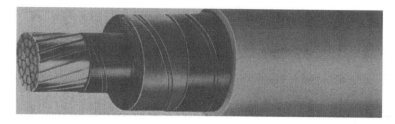

FIGURE 5.1   Single-conductor, paper-insulated power cable. (Courtesy of Okonite Company, Ramsey, NJ.)

The belted cable construction is generally used for three-phase low-voltage operation, up to 5 kV, or with the addition of conductor and belt shielding, in the 10–15 kV voltage range. It receives its name from the fact that a portion of the total insulation is applied over partially insulated conductors in the form of an insulating belt, which provides a smooth *cushion* for the lead sheath.

Even though this design is generally more economical than the shielded (or type H) construction, the electrical field produced by three-phase ac voltage is asymmetrical, and the fillers are also under electric stress. These disadvantages restrict the usage of this cable to voltages below 15 kV. Figure 5.2 shows a three-conductor, belted, compact sector, paper-insulated cable. They can have concentric round, compact round, or compact sector conductors.

The three-conductor shielded, or type H, construction with compact sector conductors is the design most commonly and universally used for three-phase applications at the 5–46 kV voltage range. Three-conductor cables in sizes up to 1 kcmil are standard, but for larger sizes, if overall size and weights are important factors, single-conductor cables should be preferred.

It confines the electric stress to the primary insulation, which causes the voltage rating (radial stress) to be increased and the dielectric losses to be reduced. The shielded paper–oil dielectric has the greatest economy for power cables at HVs where reliability and performance are of prime importance. Figure 5.3 shows a three-conductor, shielded (type H) compact sector, paper-insulated cable.

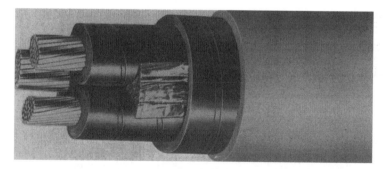

FIGURE 5.2   Three-conductor, belted compact sector, paper-insulated cable. (Courtesy of Okonite Company, Ramsey, NJ.)

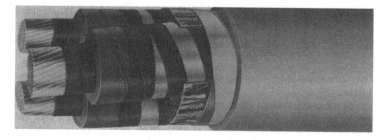

FIGURE 5.3   Three-conductor shielded (type H), compact sector, paper-insulated cable. (Courtesy of Okonite Company, Ramsey, NJ.)

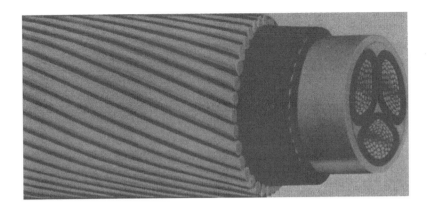

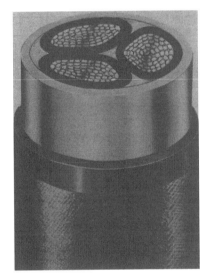
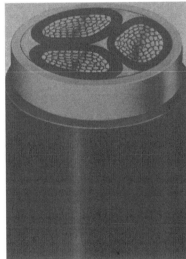

FIGURE 5.4 Various protective outer coverings for solid-type insulated cables. (Courtesy of Okonite Company, Ramsey, NJ.)

Figure 5.4 presents various protective outer coverings for solid-type cables, depending on installation requirements. Figure 5.5 shows the recommended voltage ranges for various types of paper-insulated power cables.

Most cable insulations are susceptible to deterioration by moisture to varying degrees. Paper and oil, which have had all the moisture completely extracted in the manufacture of a paper cable, will reabsorb moisture when exposed to the atmosphere, and prolonged exposure will degrade the exceptionally high electrical quantities. Because of this, it is mandatory in all paper cable splices and terminations to reduce exposure or the insulation to moisture and to construct and seal the accessories to ensure the complete exclusion of moisture for long and satisfactory service life.

Therefore, it is important that all cable ends are tested for moisture before splicing or potheading. The most reliable procedure is to remove rings of insulating paper from the section cut for the connector at the sheath, at the midpoint, and nearest the conductor and immerse the tape *loops* in clean oil or flushing compound heated to 280°F–300°F. If any traces of moisture are present, minute bubbles will exclude from the tape and form *froth* in the oil.

The shields and metallic sheaths of power cables must be grounded for safety and reliable operation. Without such grounding, shields would operate at a potential considerably above the ground potential. Therefore, they would be hazardous to touch and would incur rapid degradation of the

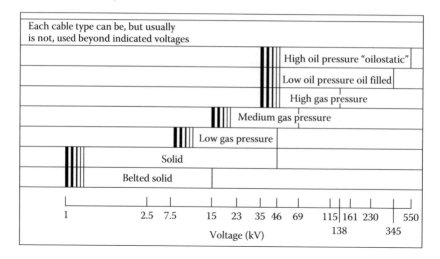

FIGURE 5.5 Recommended voltage ranges for various paper-insulated cables. (Courtesy of Okonite Company, Ramsey, NJ.)

jacket or other material that is between shield and ground. The grounding conductor and its attachment to the shield or metallic sheath, normally at a termination or splice, need to have an ampacity no lower than that of the shield. In the case of a lead sheath, the ampacity must be large enough to carry the available fault current and duration without overheating. Usually, the cable shield lengths are grounded at both ends such that the fault current would divide and flow to both ends, reducing the duty on the shield and therefore the chance of damage.

The capacitive charging current of the cable insulation, which is on the order of 1 mA/ft of conductor length, normally flows, at power frequency, between the conductor and the earth electrode of the cable, normally the shield. The shield, or metallic sheath, provides the fault return path in the event of insulation failure, permitting rapid operation of the protection devices [1].

5.3 UNDERGROUND CABLE INSTALLATION TECHNIQUES

There are a number of ways to install the underground cables such as the following:

1. Direct burial in the soil, as shown in Figure 5.6. The cable is laid in a trench that is usually dug by machine.
2. In ducts or pipes with concrete sheath, as shown in Figure 5.7. For secondary network systems, duct lines may have 6–12 ducts.
3. Wherever possible, in tunnels built for other purposes, for example, sewer lines, water mains, gas pipes, and duct lines for telephone and telegraph cables.

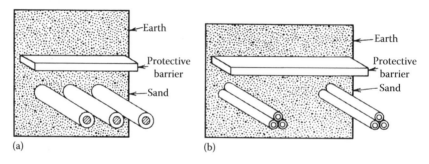

FIGURE 5.6 Direct burial (a) for single-conductor cables and (b) for triplexed cables.

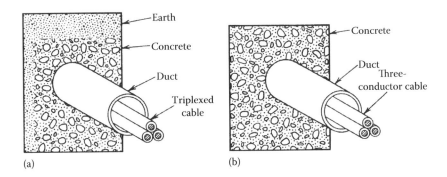

FIGURE 5.7 Burial in underground cuts (or duct bank) (a) for three single-conductor or triplexed cables and (b) for three-conductor cable.

In general, manholes are built at every junction point and corner. The spacing of manholes is affected by the types of circuits installed, allowable cable-pulling tensions, and utility company's standards and practice. Manholes give easily accessible and protected space in which cables and associated apparatus can be operated properly. For example, they should provide enough space for required switching equipment, transformers, and splices and terminations. Figure 5.8 shows a straight-type manhole. Figure 5.9 shows a typical street cable manhole, which is usually used to route cables at street intersections or other locations where cable terminations are required.

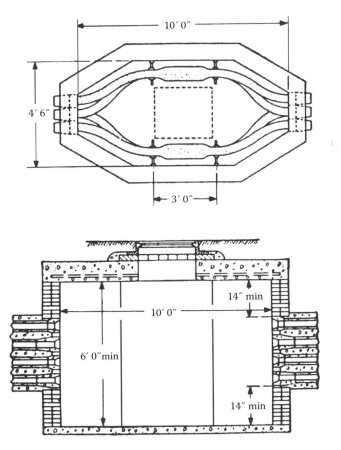

FIGURE 5.8 Straight-type manhole]. (From Fink, D.G. and Beaty, H.W., *Standard Handbook for Electrical Engineers*, 11th edn., McGraw-Hill, New York, 1978.)

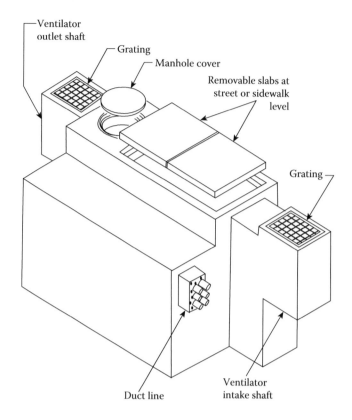

FIGURE 5.9   Street cable manhole. (From Skrotzki, B.G.A., ed., *Electric Transmission and Distribution*, McGraw-Hill, New York, 1954.)

5.4 ELECTRICAL CHARACTERISTICS OF INSULATED CABLES

5.4.1 Electric Stress in Single-Conductor Cable

Figure 5.10 shows a cross section of a single-conductor cable. Assume that the length of the cable is 1 m. Let the charge on the conductor surface be q coulomb per meter of length. Assume that the cable has a perfectly homogeneous dielectric and perfect symmetry between conductor and insulation. Therefore, according to Coulomb's law, the electric flux density at a radius of x is

$$D = \frac{q}{2\pi x} \text{ C/m}^2 \tag{5.1}$$

where

   D is the electric flux density at radius x in Coulombs per square meter
   q is the charge on conductor surface in Coulombs per square meter
   x is the distance from center of conductor in meters, where $r < x < R$

Since the absolute permittivity of the insulation is

$$\varepsilon = \frac{D}{E} \tag{5.2}$$

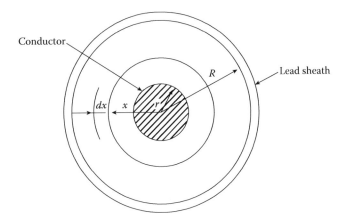

FIGURE 5.10 Cross section of single-conductor cable.

the electric field or potential gradient or electric stress or so-called dielectric stress E at radius x is

$$E = \frac{q}{2\pi\varepsilon x} \text{ V/m} \tag{5.3}$$

If the potential gradient at radius x is dV/dx, the potential difference V between conductor and lead sheath is

$$V = \int_r^R E \times dx \tag{5.4}$$

or

$$V = \int_r^R \frac{q}{2\pi\varepsilon x} \times dx \tag{5.5}$$

or

$$V = \frac{q}{2\pi\varepsilon} \times \ln\frac{R}{r} \text{ V} \tag{5.6}$$

From Equation 5.3,

$$\frac{q}{2\pi\varepsilon} = E \times x \tag{5.7}$$

Substituting it into Equation 5.6,

$$V = E \times x \times \ln\frac{R}{r} \text{ V} \tag{5.8}$$

Therefore,

$$E = \frac{V}{x \times \ln(R/r)} \ \text{V/m} \tag{5.9}$$

where
  E is the electric stress of cable in volts per meter
  V is the potential difference between conductor and lead sheath in volts
  x is the distance from center of conductor in meters
  R is the outside radius of insulation or inside radius of lead sheath in meters
  r is the radius of conductor in meters

Dielectric strength is the maximum voltage that a dielectric can stand in a uniform field before it breaks down. It represents the permissible voltage gradient through the dielectric. Average stress is the amount of voltage across the insulation material divided by the thickness of the insulation.

Maximum stress in a cable usually occurs at the surface of the conductor, while the minimum stress occurs at the outer surface of the insulation. Average stress is the amount of voltage across the insulation material divided by the thickness of the insulation. Therefore, the maximum electric stress in the cable shown in Figure 5.10 occurs at $x = r$; thus,

$$E_{\text{max}} = \frac{V}{r \times \ln(R/r)} \ \text{V/m} \tag{5.10}$$

and the minimum electric stress occurs at $x = R$; hence,

$$E_{\text{min}} = \frac{V}{R \times \ln(R/r)} \ \text{V/m} \tag{5.11}$$

Thus, for a given V and R, there is one particular radius that gives the minimum stress at the conductor surface. In order to get the smallest value of E_{max}, let

$$\frac{dE_{\text{max}}}{dr} = 0 \tag{5.12}$$

from which

$$\ln \frac{R}{r} = 1 \tag{5.13}$$

or

$$\frac{R}{r} = e \tag{5.14}$$

Thus,

$$R = 2.718r \tag{5.15}$$

and the insulation thickness is

$$R - r = 1.718r \tag{5.16}$$

and the actual stress at the conductor stress is

$$E_{max} = \frac{V}{r} \tag{5.17}$$

where r is the optimum conductor radius that satisfies Equation 5.15.

Example 5.1

A single-conductor belted cable of 5 km long has a conductor diameter of 2 cm and an inside diameter of lead sheath of 5 cm. The cable is used at 24.9 kV line-to-neutral voltage and 60 Hz frequency. Calculate the following:

(a) Maximum and minimum values of electric stress
(b) Optimum value of conductor radius that results in smallest (minimum) value of maximum stress

Solution

(a) From Equation 5.10,

$$E_{max} = \frac{V}{r \times \ln(R/r)} = \frac{24.9}{1 \times \ln 2.5} = 27.17 \text{ kV/cm}$$

and from Equation 5.11,

$$E_{min} = \frac{V}{r \times \ln(R/r)} = \frac{24.9}{2.5 \times \ln 2.5} = 10.87 \text{ kV/cm}$$

(b) From Equation 5.15, the optimum conductor radius is

$$r = \frac{R}{2.718} = \frac{2.5}{2.718} = 0.92 \text{ cm}$$

Therefore, the minimum value of the maximum stress is

$$E_{max} = \frac{24.9}{0.92 \ln(2.5/0.92)} = 27.07 \text{ kV/cm}$$

Example 5.2

Assume that a single-conductor belted cable has a conductor diameter of 2 cm and has insulation of two layers of different materials each 2 cm thick, as shown in Figure 5.11. The dielectric constants for the inner and the outer layers are 4 and 3, respectively. If the potential difference between the conductor and the outer lead sheath is 19.94 kV, calculate the potential gradient at the surface of the conductor.

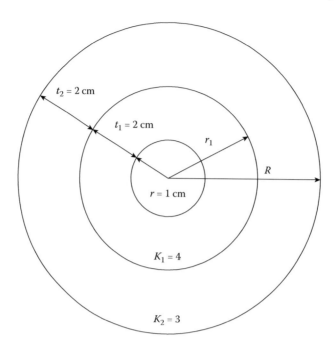

FIGURE 5.11   For Example 5.2.

Solution

$$R = 1 \text{ cm}$$

$$r_1 = r + t_1 = 3 \text{ cm}$$

$$R = r_1 + r_2 = 5 \text{ cm}$$

Since

$$E_1 = \frac{2q}{r \times K_1} \quad \text{and} \quad E_2 = \frac{2q}{r_1 \times K_2}$$

their division gives

$$\frac{E_1}{E_2} = \frac{r_1 \times t_2}{r \times t_1}$$

$$= \frac{3 \times 3}{1 \times 4} = 2.25$$

In addition,

$$E_1 = \frac{V_1}{r \times \ln(r_1/r)}$$

$$= \frac{V_1}{1 \times \ln(3/1)}$$

and

$$E_2 = \frac{V_2}{r_1 \times \ln(R/r_1)}$$

$$= \frac{19.94 - V_1}{3 \times \ln(5/3)}$$

or

$$\frac{E_1}{E_2} = \frac{V_1}{1 \times \ln(3/1)} \times \frac{3 \times \ln(5/3)}{19.94 - V_1}$$

or

$$\frac{E_1}{E_2} = \frac{1.532 V_1}{21.906 - 1.099 V_1}$$

but it was found previously that

$$\frac{E_1}{E_2} = 2.25$$

Therefore,

$$\frac{1.532 V_1}{21.906 - 1.099 V_1} = 2.25$$

from which

$$V_1 = 12.308 \text{ kV}$$

Hence,

$$E_1 = \frac{V_1}{1 \times \ln 3}$$

$$= \frac{12.308}{1 \ln 3}$$

$$= 11.20 \text{ kV/cm}$$

5.4.2 Capacitance of Single-Conductor Cable

Assume that the potential difference is V between the conductor and the lead sheath of the single-conductor cable shown in Figure 5.10. Let the charges on the conductor and sheath be $+q$ and $-q$ C/m of length. From Equation 5.6,

$$V = \frac{q}{2\pi\varepsilon} \times \ln\frac{R}{r} \text{ V} \tag{5.6}$$

where
  V is the potential difference between conductor and lead sheath in volts
  ε is the absolute permittivity of insulation
  R is the outside radius of insulation in meters
  r is the radius of conductor in meters

Therefore, the capacitance between conductor and sheath is

$$C = \frac{q}{V} \tag{5.18}$$

or

$$C = \frac{2\pi\varepsilon}{\ln(R/r)} \text{ F/m} \tag{5.19}$$

Since

$$\varepsilon = \varepsilon_0 \times K \tag{5.20}$$

thus,

$$C = \frac{2\pi\varepsilon_0 \times K}{\ln(R/r)} \text{ F/m} \tag{5.21}$$

where

$$\varepsilon_0 = \frac{1}{36\pi \times 10^9} \text{ F/m for air} \tag{5.22}$$

or

$$\varepsilon_0 = 8.85 \times 10^{-12} \text{ F/m} \tag{5.23}$$

and

$$K = \text{dielectric constant of cable insulation*}$$

Substituting Equation 5.22 into Equation 5.21,

$$C = \frac{10^{-9} K}{18 \ \ln(R/r)} \text{ F/m} \tag{5.24}$$

or

$$C = \frac{K}{18 \ \ln(R/r)} \ \mu\text{F/m} \tag{5.25}$$

or

$$C = \frac{0.0345 K}{\ln(R/r)} \ \mu\text{F/m} \tag{5.26}$$

or

$$C = \frac{0.0065 K}{10^6 \ \ln(R/r)} \text{ F/1000 ft} \tag{5.27}$$

---

* Note that there has been a shift in notation and K stands for dielectric constant.

or

$$C = \frac{0.0241K}{\log_{10}(R/r)} \ \mu\text{F/km} \tag{5.28}$$

or

$$C = \frac{0.0388K}{\log_{10}(R/r)} \ \mu\text{F/mi} \tag{5.29}$$

or

$$C = \frac{0.0073K}{10^6 \times \log_{10}(R/r)} \ \mu\text{F/1000 ft} \tag{5.30}$$

5.4.3 Dielectric Constant of Cable Insulation

The dielectric constant of any material is defined as the ratio of the capacitance of a condenser with the material as a dielectric to the capacitance of a similar condenser with air as the dielectric. It is also called the *relative permittivity* or *specific inductive capacity*. It is usually denoted by K. (It is also represented by ε_r or SIC.) Table 5.1 gives the typical values of the dielectric constants for various dielectric materials.

Using the symbol K, for example, in Equation 5.30, the formula for calculating the capacitance of a shielded or concentric neutral single-conductor cable becomes

$$C = \frac{0.0073K}{10^6 \log_{10}(D/d)} \ \text{F/1000 ft} \tag{5.31}$$

where
    C is the capacitance in farads per 1000 ft
    K is the dielectric constant of cable insulation
    D is the diameter over insulation in unit length
    d is the diameter over conductor shield in unit length

TABLE 5.1
Typical Values of Various Dielectric Materials

Dielectric Material	K
Air	1
Impregnated paper	3.3
PVC	3.5–8.0
Ethylene PP insulation	2.8–3.5
PE insulation	2.3
Cross-linked PE	2.3–6.0

5.4.4 Charging Current

By definition of susceptance,

$$b = \omega C \text{ S} \qquad (5.32)$$

or

$$b = 2\pi f C \text{ S} \qquad (5.33)$$

Then the admittance $\mathbf{Y}$ corresponding to C is

$$\mathbf{Y} = jb$$

or

$$\mathbf{Y} = j2\pi f C \text{ S} \qquad (5.34)$$

Therefore, the charging current is

$$\mathbf{I}_c = \mathbf{Y}\mathbf{V}_{\text{(L-N)}} \qquad (5.35)$$

or, ignoring j,

$$\mathbf{I}_c = 2\pi f C V_{\text{(L-N)}} \qquad (5.36)$$

For example, substituting Equation 5.31 into Equation 5.36, the charging current of a single-conductor cable is found as

$$I_c = \frac{2\pi f \times 0.0073 \times K \times V_{\text{(L-N)}}}{10^6 \times \log_{10}(D/d)} \qquad (5.37)$$

or

$$I_c = \frac{0.0459 \times f \times K \times V_{\text{(L-N)}}}{10^3 \times \log_{10}(D/d)} \text{ A/1000 ft} \qquad (5.38)$$

where
    f is the frequency in hertz
    D is the diameter over insulation in unit length
    d is the diameter over conductor shield in unit length
    K is the dielectric constant of cable insulation
    V is the line-to-neutral voltage in kilovolts

At 60 Hz frequency,

$$I_c = \frac{2.752 \times K \times V_{\text{(L-N)}}}{10^3 \times \log_{10}(D/d)} \text{ A/1000 ft} \qquad (5.39)$$

The charging current and the capacitance are relatively greater for insulated cables than in OH circuits because of closer spacing and the higher dielectric constant of the insulation of the cable. In general, the charging current is negligible for OH circuits at distribution voltages, contrary to HV transmission circuits.

5.4.5 DETERMINATION OF INSULATION RESISTANCE OF SINGLE-CONDUCTOR CABLE

Assume that the cable shown in Figure 5.12 has a length of 1 m. Then the incremental insulation resistance of the cylindrical element in the radial direction is

$$\Delta R_i = \frac{\rho}{2\pi \times x \times l} \times dx \tag{5.40}$$

Therefore, the total insulation resistance between the conductor and the lead sheath is

$$R_i = \int_r^R \frac{\rho}{2\pi \times l} \times \frac{dx}{x}$$

or

$$R_i = \frac{\rho}{2\pi \times l} \times \ln\left(\frac{R}{r}\right) \tag{5.41}$$

where
  R_i is the total insulation resistance in ohms
  ρ is the insulation (dielectric) resistivity in ohm meters
  l is the total length of cable in meters
  R is the outside radius of insulation or inside radius of lead sheath in meters
  r is the radius of conductor in meters

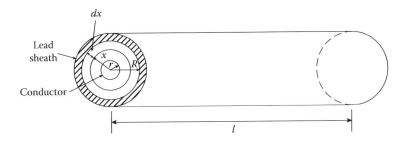

FIGURE 5.12 Cross section of single-conductor cable.

TABLE 5.2

Typical Values of r_{si}

Insulation Material	r_{si} (MΩ/1,000 ft)
Synthetic rubber	2,000
Ethylene PP insulation	20,000
PE	50,000
PVC	2,000
Cross-linked PE	20,000

A more practical version of Equation 5.41 is given by the Okonite Company* as

$$R_i = r_{si} \times \log_{10}\left(\frac{D}{d}\right) \text{ MΩ/1000 ft} \tag{5.42}$$

where

R_i is the total insulation resistance in megohms per 1000 ft for particular cable construction
r_{si} is the specific insulation resistance in megohms per 1000 ft at 60°F
D is the inside diameter of sheath
d is the outside diameter of conductor

Table 5.2 gives typical r_{si} values of various insulation materials. Equation 5.19 indicates that the insulation resistance is inversely proportional to the length of the insulated cable. An increase in insulation thickness increases the disruptive critical voltage of the insulation but does not give a proportional decrease in voltage gradient at the conductor surface. Therefore, it does not permit a proportional increase in voltage rating.

Example 5.3

A 250 kcmil, single-conductor, synthetic rubber, belted cable has a conductor diameter of 0.575 in. and an inside diameter of sheath of 1.235 in. The cable has a length of 6000 ft and is going to be used at 60 Hz and 115 kV. Calculate the following:

(a) Total insulation resistance in megohms at 60°F
(b) Power loss due to leakage current flowing through insulation resistance

Solution

(a) By using Equation 5.42,

$$R_i = r_{si} \times \log_{10}\left(\frac{D}{d}\right)$$

From Table 5.2, specific insulation resistance r_{si} is 2000 MΩ/1000 ft. Therefore, the total insulation resistance is

$$R_i = 6 \times 2000 \, \log\left(\frac{1.235}{0.575}\right)$$

$$= 3.984 \text{ MΩ}$$

---

* Engineering data for copper and aluminum conductor electrical cables, by the Okonite Company, Ramsey, NJ. Bulletin EHB-78. Used with permission.

(b) The power loss due to leakage current is

$$\frac{V^2}{R_i} = \frac{115,000^2}{3984 \times 10^6}$$

$$= 3.3195 \text{ W}$$

5.4.6 CAPACITANCE OF THREE-CONDUCTOR BELTED CABLE

As shown in Figure 5.13, two insulation thicknesses are to be considered in belted cables: (1) the conductor insulation of thickness T and (2) the belt insulation of thickness t. The belt insulation is required because with line voltage $\mathbf{V}_L$ between conductors, the conductor insulation is only adequate for $\mathbf{V}_L/2$ voltage, whereas the voltage between each conductor and ground (or earth) is $\mathbf{V}_L/\sqrt{3}$.

In the three-conductor belted cable, there are capacitances of C_c between conductors and capacitances of C_s between each conductor and the sheath, as shown in Figure 5.14. The arrangement of the capacitors, representing these capacitances per-unit length, is equivalent to a delta system connected in parallel with a wye system, as shown in Figure 5.15. Further, the delta system, representing the capacitances C_c, can be represented by an equivalent wye system of capacitance C_1, as shown in Figure 5.16. In the delta system, the capacitance between, say, conductors 1 and 2 is

$$C_c + \frac{C_c}{2} = \frac{3C_c}{2} \tag{5.43}$$

In the wye system, it is

$$\frac{C_1}{2} \tag{5.44}$$

Since the delta and wye systems are equivalent, the capacitance between the conductors must be the same:

$$\frac{3C_c}{2} = \frac{C_1}{2} \tag{5.45}$$

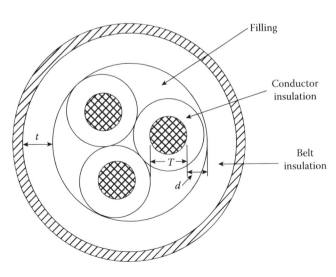

FIGURE 5.13 Three-conductor belted cable cross section.

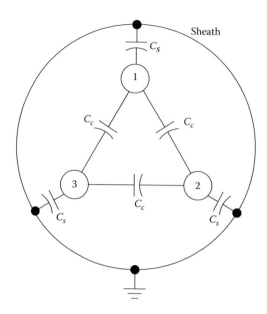

FIGURE 5.14   Effective capacitances.

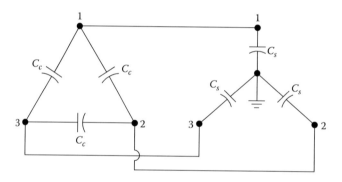

FIGURE 5.15   Equivalent circuit.

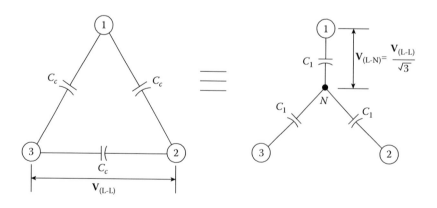

FIGURE 5.16   Equivalent delta and wye systems.

or

$$C_1 = 3C_c \qquad (5.46)$$

Alternatively, let the voltage across capacitor C_c in the delta system be $\mathbf{V}_{(L-L)}$, the line-to-line voltage. Therefore, the phase current through the capacitor is equal to $\omega C_c \mathbf{V}_{(L-L)}$, and the line current is

$$\mathbf{I}_L = 3\omega C_c \mathbf{V}_{(L-L)} \qquad (5.47)$$

On the other hand, in the equivalent wye systems, the line-to-neutral voltage is

$$\mathbf{V}_{(L-N)} = \frac{\mathbf{V}_{(L-L)}}{\sqrt{3}} \qquad (5.48)$$

and the phase current and the line current are the same. Therefore,

$$\mathbf{I}_L = \omega C_1 \times \frac{\mathbf{V}_{(L-L)}}{\sqrt{3}} \qquad (5.49)$$

Thus, for equivalent delta and wye systems, by equating Equations 5.47 and 5.49,

$$3\omega C_c \mathbf{V}_{(L-L)} = \omega C_1 \times \frac{\mathbf{V}_{(L-L)}}{3}$$

or

$$C_1 = 3C_c \qquad (5.50)$$

which is as same as Equation 5.46. Therefore, the delta system is converted to the wye system, as shown in Figure 5.16. All C_s capacitors are in wye connection with respect to the sheath, and all C_1 capacitors are in wye connection and in parallel with the first wye system of capacitors. The effective capacitance of each conductor to the grounded neutral is therefore

$$C_N = C_s + 3C_c \qquad (5.51)$$

The value of C_N can be calculated with usually acceptable accuracy by using the formula

$$C_N = \frac{0.048K}{\log_{10}\left\{1 + \left[\dfrac{T+t}{d}\right]\left[3.84 - \dfrac{1.7t}{T} + \dfrac{0.52t^2}{T^2}\right]\right\}} \; \mu\text{F/mi} \qquad (5.52)$$

where
  K is the dielectric constant of insulation
  T is the thickness of conductor insulation
  t is the thickness of belt insulation
  d is the diameter of conductor

In general, however, since the conductors are not surrounded by isotropic homogeneous insulation of one known permittivity, the C_c and C_s are not easily calculated and are generally obtained by measurements. The tests are performed at the working voltage, frequency, and temperature.
In determining the capacitances of this type of cable, the *common tests* are the following:

1. Measure the capacitance C_a between two conductors by means of a Schering bridge connecting the third conductor to the sheath to eliminate one of the C_s's, as shown in Figures 5.17 and 5.18. Therefore,

$$C_a = C_c + \frac{C_c + C_s}{2}$$ (5.53)

or

$$C_a = \frac{C_s + 3C_c}{2}$$ (5.54)

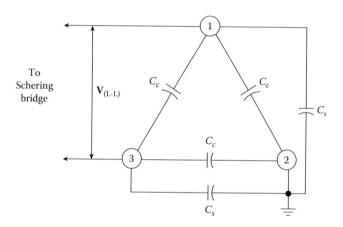

FIGURE 5.17 Measuring the capacitance C_a.

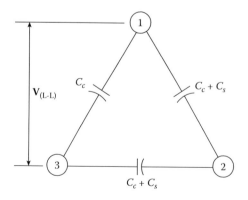

FIGURE 5.18 Measuring the capacitance C_a.

Substituting Equation 5.51 into Equation 5.54,

$$C_a = \frac{C_N}{2} \tag{5.55}$$

or

$$C_N = 2C_a \tag{5.56}$$

2. Measure the capacitance C_b between the sheath and all three conductors joined together to eliminate (or to short out) all three C_s's and to parallel all three C_s's, as shown in Figure 5.19. Therefore,

$$C_b = 3C_s \tag{5.57}$$

or

$$C_s = \frac{C_b}{3} \tag{5.58}$$

3. Connect two conductors to the sheath, as shown in Figure 5.20. Measure the capacitance C_d between the remaining single conductor and the two other conductors and the sheath. Therefore,

$$C_d = C_s + 2C_c \tag{5.59}$$

or

$$2C_c = C_d - C_s \tag{5.60}$$

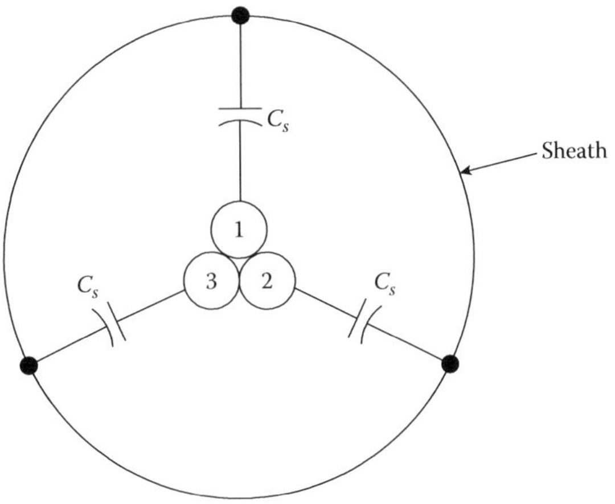

FIGURE 5.19 Measuring the capacitance C_b.

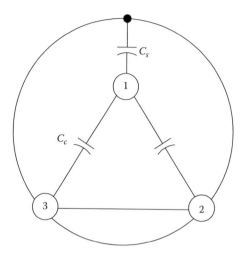

FIGURE 5.20   Connecting two conductors to the sheath.

Substituting Equation 5.58 into Equation 5.60,

$$C_c = \frac{C_d - \dfrac{C_b}{3}}{2} \tag{5.61}$$

Substituting this equation and Equation 5.58 into Equation 5.51, the effective capacitance to neutral is

$$C_N = \frac{9C_d - C_b}{6} \tag{5.62}$$

Example 5.4

A three-conductor three-phase cable has 2 mi of length and is being used at 34.5 kV, three phase, and 60 Hz. The capacitance between a pair of conductors on a single phase is measured to be 2 μF/mi. Calculate the charging current of the cable.

Solution

The capacitance between two conductors is given as

$$C_a = 2 \ \mu\text{F/mi}$$

or for total cable length,

$$C_a = (2 \ \mu\text{F/mi}) \times (2 \ \text{mi}) = 4 \ \mu\text{F}$$

The capacitance of each conductor to neutral can be found by using Equation 4.56,

$$C_N = 2C_a$$

$$= 8 \ \mu F$$

Therefore, the charging current is

$$I_c = \omega \times C_N \times V_{(L\text{-}N)}$$

$$= 27\pi \times 60 \times 8 \times 10^{-6} \times 19{,}942$$

$$= 60.14 \ A$$

Example 5.5

A three-conductor belted cable 4 mi long is used as a three-phase underground feeder and connected to a 13.8 kV, 60 Hz substation bus. The load, at the receiving end, draws 30 A at 0.85 lagging power factor. The capacitance between any two conductors is measured to be 0.45 μF/mi. Ignoring the power loss due to leakage current and also the line voltage drop, calculate the following:

(a) Charging current of feeder
(b) Sending-end current
(c) Sending-end power factor

Solution

The current phasor diagram is shown in Figure 5.21.

(a) The capacitance between two conductors is given as

$$C_a = 0.45 \ \mu F/mi$$

or for total feeder length,

$$C_a = 0.45 \ \mu F/mi \times 4 \ mi = 1.80 \ \mu F$$

The capacitance of each conductor to neutral can be found by using Equation 4.56,

$$C_N = 2C_a$$

$$3.6 \ \mu F$$

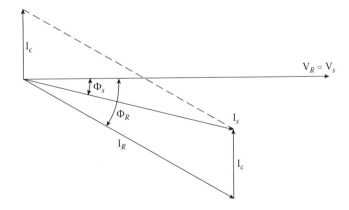

FIGURE 5.21 Current phasor diagram for Example 5.5.

Thus, the charging current is

$$I_c = \omega \times C_N \times V_{(L\text{-}N)}$$

$$= 2\pi \times 60 \times 3.6 \times 10^{-6} \times 13{,}800 \times \frac{1}{\sqrt{3}}$$

$$= 10.83 \text{ A}$$

or, in complex form,

$$\mathbf{I}_c = +j10.83 \text{ A}$$

(b) The receiving-end current is

$$\mathbf{I}_r = 30(\cos\phi_r - j\sin\phi_r)$$

$$= 30(0.85 - j0.5268)$$

$$= 25.5 - j15.803 \text{ A}$$

Therefore, the sending-end current is

$$\mathbf{I}_s = \mathbf{I}_r + \mathbf{I}_c$$

$$= 25.5 - j15.803 + j10.83$$

$$= 25.5 - j4.973$$

$$= 25.98 \angle -11.04° \text{ A}$$

(c) Hence, the sending-end power factor is

$$\cos\phi_s = \cos 11.04 = 0.98$$

and it is a lagging power factor.

5.4.7 CABLE DIMENSIONS

Overall diameter of a cable may be found from the following equations. They apply to conductors of circular cross section.

For a single-conductor cable,

$$D = d + 2T + 2S \tag{5.63}$$

For a two-conductor cable,

$$D = 2(d + 2T + t + S) \tag{5.64}$$

For a three-conductor cable,

$$D = 2.155(d + 2T) + 2(t + S) \tag{5.65}$$

For a four-conductor cable,

$$D = 2.414(d + 2T) + 2(t + S) \tag{5.66}$$

For a sector-type three-conductor cable,

$$D_{3s} = D - 0.35d \tag{5.67}$$

where
D is the overall diameter of cable with circular cross-sectional conductors
D_{3s} is the overall diameter of cable with sector-type three conductors
d is the diameter of conductor
S is the metal sheath thickness of cable
t is the belt insulation thickness of cable
T is the thickness of conductor insulation in inches

5.4.8 GEOMETRIC FACTORS

The geometric factor is defined as the relation in space between the cylinders formed by sheath internal surface and conductor external surface in a single-conductor belted cable. For a three-conductor belted cable, this relation (i.e., *geometric factor*) is sector shaped and by relative thicknesses of conductor insulation T and belt insulation t. For a single-conductor cable, the geometric factor G is given by

$$G = 2.303 \; \log_{10} \frac{D}{d} \tag{5.68}$$

where
D is the inside diameter of sheath
d is the outside diameter of conductor

Table 5.3 presents geometric factors for single-conductor and three-conductor belted cables. In this table, G indicates the geometric factor for a single-conductor cable, G_0 indicates the zero-sequence geometric factor, and G_1 indicates the positive-sequence geometric factor for three-conductor belted cables. Also, Figures 5.22 and 5.23 give geometric factors for single-conductor and three-conductor belted cables. In Figure 5.24, G_0 indicates the zero-sequence geometric factor, and G_1 indicates the positive-sequence geometric factor. In Table 5.3 and Figures 5.22 and 5.23,

T is the thickness of conductor insulation in inches
t is the thickness of belt insulation in inches
d is the outside diameter of conductor in inches

For single-conductor cables,

$$t = 0$$

Thus,

$$\frac{T+t}{d} = \frac{T}{d} \tag{5.69}$$

which is used to find the value of geometric factor G for a single-conductor cable.

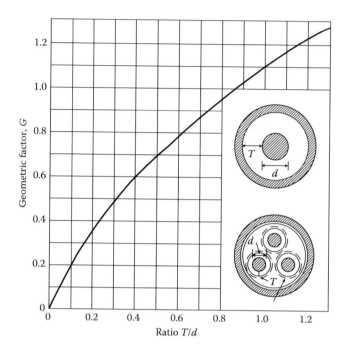

FIGURE 5.22 Geometric factor for single-conductor cables or three-conductor shielded cables having round conductors. (From Westinghouse Electric Corporation, *Electrical Transmission and Distribution Reference Book*, WEC, East Pittsburgh, PA, 1964.)

The geometric factor can be useful to calculate various cable characteristics such as capacitance, charging current, dielectric loss, leakage current, and heat transfer. For example, the general capacitance equation is given as [1]

$$C = \frac{0.0169 \times n \times K}{G} \ \mu F/1000 \ \text{ft} \tag{5.70}$$

where
  K is the dielectric constant of insulation
  n is the number of conductors
  G is the geometric factor

Also, the charging current of a three-conductor three-phase cable is given as [5]

$$I_c = \frac{3 \times 0.106 \times f \times K \times \mathbf{V}_{(L\text{-}N)}}{1000 \times G_1} \ A/1000 \ \text{ft} \tag{5.71}$$

where
  f is the frequency in hertz
  K is the dielectric constant of insulation
  $\mathbf{V}_{(L\text{-}N)}$ is the line-to-neutral voltage in kilovolts
  G_1 is the geometric factor for three-conductor cable from Table 5.3

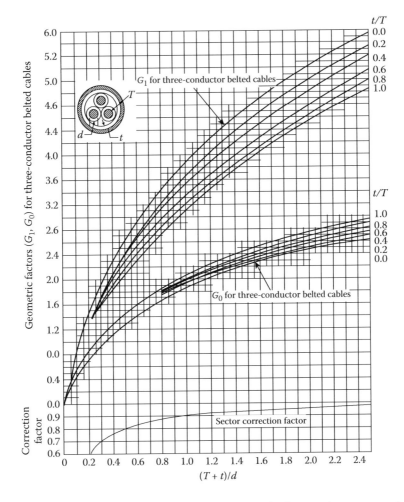

FIGURE 5.23   Geometric factor for three-conductor belted cables having round or sector conductors.

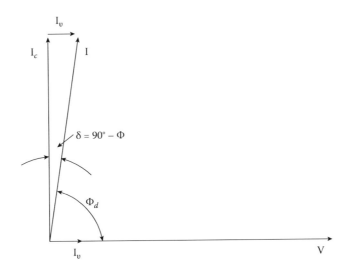

FIGURE 5.24   Phasor diagram for cable dielectric.

TABLE 5.3

Geometric Factors of Cables

Ratio $T + \dfrac{t}{d}$	Single Conductor, G	Sector Factor	Three-Conductor Cables					
			G_0 at Ratio t/T			G_1 at Ratio t/T		
			0	0.5	1.0	0	0.5	1.0
0.2	0.34		0.85	0.85	0.85	1.2	1.28	1.4
0.3	0.47	0.690	1.07	1.075	1.03	1.5	1.65	1.85
0.4	0.59	0.770	1.24	1.27	1.29	1.85	2.00	2.25
0.5	0.69	0.815	1.39	1.43	1.46	2.10	2.30	2.60
0.6	0.79	0.845	1.51	1.57	1.61	2.32	2.55	2.95
0.7	0.88	0.865	1.62	1.69	1.74	2.35	2.80	3.20
0.8	0.96	0.880	1.72	1.80	1.86	2.75	3.05	3.45
0.9	1.03	0.895	1.80	1.89	1.97	2.96	3.25	3.70
1.0	1.10	0.905	1.88	1.98	2.07	3.13	3.44	3.87
1.1	1.16	0.915	1.95	2.06	2.15	3.30	3.60	4.03
1.2	1.22	0.921	2.02	2.13	2.23	3.45	3.80	4.25
1.3	1.28	0.928	2.08	2.19	2.29	3.60	3.95	4.40
1.4	1.33	0.935	2.14	2.26	2.36	3.75	4.10	4.60
1.5	1.39	0.938	2.20	2.32	2.43	3.90	4.25	4.75
1.6	1.44	0.941	2.26	2.38	2.49	4.05	4.40	4.90
1.7	1.48	0.944	2.30	2.43	2.55	4.17	4.52	5.05
1.8	1.52	0.946	2.35	2.49	2.61	4.29	4.65	5.17
1.9	1.57	0.949	2.40	2.54	2.67	4.40	4.76	5.30
2.0	1.61	0.952	2.45	2.59	2.72	4.53	4.88	5.42

Example 5.6

A 60 Hz, 138 kV, three-conductor, paper-insulated, belted cable is going to be installed at 138 kV and used as a three-phase underground feeder. The cable has three 250 kcmil sector-type conductors each with 11/64 in. of conductor insulation and 5/64 in. of belt insulation. Calculate the following:

(a) Geometric factor of cable using Table 5.3
(b) Charging current in amperes per 1000 ft

Solution

(a) $T = 0.172$ in., $t = 0.078$, $d = 0.575$, $t/T = 0.454$:

$$\frac{t}{T} = 0.454$$

and

$$\frac{T+t}{d} = \frac{0.172+0.078}{0.575} = 0.435$$

From Table 5.3, by interpolation,

$$G_1 = 2.09$$

Since the cable has sector-type conductors, to find the real geometric factor G_1', G_1 has to be multiplied by the sector factor obtained for $(T + t)/d = 0.435$ from Table 5.3, by interpolation,

$$G_1' = G_1 \times (\text{sector factor})$$
$$= 2.09 \times 0.7858$$
$$= 1.642$$

(b)

$$V_{(L\text{-}N)} = \frac{V_{(L\text{-}L)}}{\sqrt{3}}$$
$$= \frac{138 \text{ kV}}{\sqrt{3}} = 79.6743 \text{ kV}$$

For impregnated paper cable, K is 3.3. Therefore, using Equation 5.71, the charging current is

$$I_c = \frac{3 \times 0.106 \times f \times K \times \mathbf{V}_{(L\text{-}N)}}{1000 \times G_1}$$
$$= \frac{3 \times 0.106 \times 60 \times 3.3 \times 79.6743}{1000 \times 1.642}$$
$$= 3.055 \text{ A}/1000 \text{ ft}$$

5.4.9 Dielectric Power Factor and Dielectric Loss

When a voltage is applied across a perfect dielectric, there is no dielectric loss because of the existence of an induced capacitance current I_c located 90° ahead of the voltage V. However, in practice, since a perfect dielectric cannot be achieved, there is a small current component I_V that is in phase with voltage V. Therefore, the summation of these two current vectors gives the current vector $\mathbf{I}$ that leads the voltage V by less than 90°, as shown in Figure 5.24. The cosine of the angle Φ_d is the power factor of the dielectric, which provides a useful measure of the quality of the cable dielectric. The power factor of a dielectric is

$$\cos \Phi_d = \frac{\text{losses in dielectric (W)}}{\text{apparent power (VA)}} \tag{5.72}$$

The power factor of an impregnated paper dielectric is very small, approximately 0.003. The *dielectric power factor* should not be confused with the regular (supply) power factor. The dielectric power factor represents loss, and therefore, an attempt to reduce it should be made. Conversely, an attempt should be made to increase the supply power factor toward unity. Since for a good dielectric insulation, Φ_d is close to 90°, δ is sometimes called the *dielectric loss angle*. Therefore, δ is, in radians,

$$\delta \approx \tan \delta = \sin \delta = \cos \Phi_d \tag{5.73}$$

since $\delta = 90° - \Phi_d$ and $\delta < 0.5°$ for most cables.

Here, $\cos \Phi_d$ should be held very small under all operating conditions. If it is large, the power loss is large, and the insulation temperature T rises considerably. The rise in temperature causes a rise in power loss in the dielectric, which again results in additional temperature rise. If the cable is to operate under conditions where $\partial(\cos \Phi_d)/\partial T$ is significantly large, the temperature continues to increase until the insulation of the cable is damaged.

When an ac $V_{(L\text{-}N)}$ voltage is applied across the effective cable capacitance C, the power loss in the dielectric, P_{dl}, is

$$P_{dl} = \omega \times C \times V_{(L\text{-}N)}^2 \times \cos \Phi_d \tag{5.74}$$

This is larger than the dielectric power loss if the applied voltage is dc. The increase in the power loss is due to dielectric hysteresis, and it usually is much greater than leakage loss. The dielectric hysteresis loss cannot be measured separately. The total dielectric loss, consisting of dielectric hysteresis loss and the power loss due to leakage current flowing through the insulation resistance, can be measured by means of the Schering bridge. These losses depend on voltage, frequency, and the state of the cable dielectric. Therefore, the test has to be made at rated voltage and frequency for a given cable.

For a balanced three-phase circuit, the dielectric loss at rated voltage and temperature is

$$P_{dl} = \omega \times C \times V_{(L\text{-}N)}^2 \times \cos\Phi_d \text{ W}/1000 \text{ ft} \tag{5.75}$$

where

P_{dl} is the cable dielectric loss in watts per 1000 ft
$\omega = 2\pi f$
C is the positive-sequence capacitance to neutral in farads per 1000 ft
$V_{(L\text{-}N)}$ is the line-to-neutral voltage in kilovolts
$\cos\Phi_d$ is the power factor of dielectric (insulation) at given temperature

Example 5.7

A single-conductor belted cable has a conductor diameter of 0.814 in., inside diameter of sheath of 2.442 in., and a length of 3.5 mi. The cable is to be operated at 60 Hz and 7.2 kV. The dielectric constant is 3.5, the power factor of the dielectric on open circuit at a rated frequency and temperature is 0.03, and the dielectric resistivity of the insulation is 1.3×10^7 MΩ-cm. Calculate the following:

(a) Maximum electric stress occurring in cable dielectric
(b) Capacitance of cable
(c) Charging current of cable
(d) Insulation resistance
(e) Power loss due to leakage current flowing through insulation resistance
(f) Total dielectric loss
(g) Dielectric hysteresis loss

Solution

(a) By using Equation 5.10,

$$E_{max} = \frac{V}{r \times \ln(R/r)}$$

$$= \frac{7.2}{0.407 \times 2.54 \ln 3}$$

$$= 6.34 \text{ kV/cm}$$

(b) From Equation 5.29,

$$C = \frac{0.0388K}{\log_{10}\left(\dfrac{R}{r}\right)}$$

$$= \frac{0.0388 \times 3.5}{\log_{10} 3}$$

$$= 0.2846 \text{ µF/mi}$$

or the capacitance of the cable is

$$0.2846 \text{ µF/mi} \times 3.5 \text{ mi} = 0.9961 \text{ µF}$$

(c) By using Equation 5.36,

$$I_c = 2\pi \times f \times C \times V_{(L\text{-}N)}$$

$$= \frac{2\pi \times 60 \times 0.9961 \times 7.2}{10^3}$$

$$= 2.704 \text{ A}$$

(d) From Equation 5.41,

$$R_i = \frac{\rho}{2\pi \times l} \times \ln\left(\frac{R}{r}\right)$$

$$= \frac{1.3 \times 107}{2\pi \times 3.5 \times 5280 \times 12 \times 2.54} \times \ln 3$$

$$= 4 \text{ M}\Omega$$

(e) The power loss due to leakage current flowing through the insulation is

$$P_{lc} = \frac{V^2}{R_i} = \frac{7200^2}{4 \times 10^6} = 12.85 \text{ W}$$

(f) The total dielectric loss is

$$P_{dl} = V_{(L\text{-}N)} I \cos \Phi_d$$

or

$$P_{dl} = V_{(L\text{-}N)} I \sin \delta$$

or

$$P_{dl} = \omega \times C \times V_{(L\text{-}N)}^2 \times \sin \delta$$

or

$$P_{dl} = \omega \times C \times V_{(L\text{-}N)}^2 \times \delta$$

$$= 2\pi \times 60 \times 0.9961 \times 7200^2 \times 0.03$$

$$= 584.01 \text{ W}$$

(g) The dielectric hysteresis loss is

$$P_{dh} = P_{dl} - P_{lc}$$

$$= 584.01 - 12.85$$

$$= 571.16 \text{ W}$$

5.4.10 Effective Conductor Resistance

The factors that determine effective ac resistance R_{eff} of each conductor of a cable are dc resistance, skin effect, proximity effect, sheath losses, and armor losses if there is any armor. Therefore, the effective resistance R_{eff} in ac resistance can be given as

$$R_{\text{eff}} = \left(\lambda_1 + \lambda_2 + \lambda_3 + \lambda_4 \right) R_{dc} \qquad (5.76)$$

where
R_{dc} is the dc resistance of conductor
λ_1 is the constant (or resistance increment) due to skin effect
λ_2 is the constant (or resistance increment) due to proximity effect
λ_3 is the constant (or resistance increment) due to sheath losses
λ_4 is the constant (or resistance increment) due to armor losses

For example, λ_3 constant can be calculated as follows; since

$$\text{Sheath loss} = \lambda_3 \times (\text{conductor loss})$$

$$\lambda_3 = \frac{\text{Sheath loss}}{\text{Conductor loss}}$$

Similarly, since

$$\text{Armor loss} = \lambda_4 \times (\text{conductor loss})$$

then

$$\lambda_4 = \frac{\text{Armor loss}}{\text{Conductor loss}}$$

5.4.11 DC Resistance

The dc resistance R_{dc} of a conductor is

$$R_{\text{dc}} = \frac{\rho l}{A}$$

where
ρ is the resistivity of conductor
l is the conductor length
A is the cross-sectional area

The units used must be of a consistent set. In practice, several different sets of units are used in the calculation of resistance. For example, in the SI units, l is in meters, A is in square meters, and ρ is in ohms per meter. Whereas in power systems in the United States, ρ is in ohm-circular mils per foot (Ω-cmil/ft), or ohms per circular mil-foot, l is usually in feet, and A is in circular mils (cmil). Resistivity ρ is 10.66 Ω-cmil/ft, or 1.77×10^{-8} Ω-m, at 20°C for hard-drawn copper and 10.37 Ωcmil/ft at 20°C for standard annealed copper. For hard-drawn aluminum at 20°C, ρ is 17.00 Ω-cmil/ft or 2.83×10^{-8} Ω-m. The dc resistance of a conductor in terms of temperature is given by

$$\frac{R_2}{R_1} = \frac{T_0 + t_2}{T_0 + t_1}$$

where
    R_1 is the conductor resistance at temperature t_1
    R_2 is the conductor resistance at temperature t_2
    t_1, t_2 is the conductor temperatures in degrees Celsius
    T_0 = constant varying with conductor material
        = 234.5 for annealed copper
        = 241 for hard-drawn copper
        = 228 for hard-drawn aluminum

The *maximum allowable conductor temperatures* are given by the Insulated Power Cable Engineers Association (IPCEA) for PE and cross-linked PE-insulated cables as follows:

Under normal operation
    PE-insulated cables: 75°C
    Cross-linked PE-insulated cables: 90°C

Under emergency operation
    PE-insulated cables: 90°C
    Cross-linked PE-insulated cables: 130°C

The maximum conductor temperatures for impregnated paper-insulated cables are given in Table 5.4.

5.4.12 Skin Effect

For dc currents, a uniform current distribution is assumed throughout the cross section of a conductor. This is not true for ac. As the frequency of ac current increases, the nonuniformity of current becomes greater. The current tends to flow more densely near the outer surface of the conductor than near the center. The phenomenon responsible for this nonuniform distribution is called *skin effect*.

Skin effect is present because the magnetic flux linkages of current near the center of the conductor are relatively greater than the linkages of current flowing near the surface of the conductor. Since the inductance of any element is proportional to the flux linkages per ampere, the inner areas of the conductor offer greater reactance to current flow. Therefore, the current follows the outer paths of lower reactance, which in turn reduces the effective path area and increases the effective resistance of the cable.

Skin effect is a function of conductor size, frequency, and the relative resistance of the conductor material. It increases as the conductor size and the frequency increase. It decreases as the material's relative resistance decreases. For example, for the same size conductors, the skin effect is larger for copper than for aluminum.

The effective resistance of a conductor is a function of power loss and the current in the conductor. Thus,

$$R_{\text{eff}} = \frac{P_{\text{loss in conductor}}}{|I|^2}$$

where
    P_{loss} is the power loss in conductor in watts
    I is the current in conductor in amperes

TABLE 5.4

Maximum Conductor Temperatures for Impregnated Paper-Insulated Cable

Rated Voltage (kV)	Conductor Temperature (°C)		
	Normal Operation	Emergency Operation	
Solid-type multiple conductor belted			
1	85	105	
2–9	80	100	
10–15	75	95	
Solid-type multiple conductor shielded and single conductor			
1–9	85	105	
10–17	80	100	
18–29	75	95	
30–39	70	90	
40–49	65	85	
50–59	60	75	
60–69	55	70	
Low-pressure gas filled			
8–17	80	100	
18–29	75	95	
30–39	70	90	
40–46	65	85	
Low-pressure oil filled and high-pressure pipe type			
		100 h	300 h
15–17	85	105	100
18–39	80	100	95
40–162	75	95	90
163–230	70	90	85

Sources: Fink, D.G. and Beaty, H.W., *Standard Handbook for Electrical Engineers*, 11th edn., McGraw-Hill, New York, 1978.; Insulated Power Cable Engineers Association, *Current Carrying Capacity of Impregnated Paper, Rubber, and Varnished Cambric Insulated Cables*, 1st edn., Publ. no. P-29-226. IPCEA, New York, 1965.

Skin effect increases this effective resistance. Also, it can decrease reactance as internal flux linkages decrease. Stranding the conductor considerably reduces the skin effect. In an underground cable, the central conductor strands are sometimes omitted since they carry small current. For example, some large cables are sometimes built over a central core of nonconducting material.

5.4.13 PROXIMITY EFFECT

The proximity effect is quite similar in nature to the skin effect. An increase in resistance is present due to nonuniformity in current density over the conductor section caused by the magnetic flux linkages of current in the other conductors. The result, as in the case of skin effect, is a crowding of the current in both conductors toward the portions of the cross sections that are immediately adjacent to each other. It can cause a significant change in the effective ac resistance of multiconductor cables or cables located in the same duct.

TABLE 5.5

DC Resistance and Correction Factors for AC Resistance

Conductor Size (AWG or kcmil)	DC Resistance, Ω/1000 ft at 25°C[a]		AC Resistance Multiplier			
			Single-Conductor Cables[b]		Multiconductor Cables[c]	
	Copper	Aluminum	Copper	Aluminum	Copper	Aluminum
8	0.6532	1.071	1.000	1.000	1.00	1.00
6	0.4110	0.6741	1.000	1.000	1.00	1.00
4	0.2584	0.4239	1.000	1.000	1.00	1.00
2	0.1626	0.2666	1.000	1.000	1.01	1.00
1	0.1289	0.2114	1.000	1.000	1.01	1.00
10	0.1022	0.1676	1.000	1.000	1.02	1.00
20	0.08105	0.1329	1.000	1.001	1.03	1.00
30	0.06429	0.1054	1.000	1.001	1.04	1.01
40	0.05098	0.08361	1.000	1.001	1.05	1.01
250	0.04315	0.07077	1.005	1.002	1.06	1.02
300	0.03595	0.05897	1.006	1.003	1.07	1.02
350	0.03082	0.05055	1.009	1.004	1.08	1.03
500	0.02157	0.03538	1.018	1.007	1.13	1.06
750	0.01438	0.02359	1.039	1.015	1.21	1.12
1000	0.01079	0.01796	1.067	1.026	1.30	1.19
1500	0.00719	0.01179	1.142	1.058	1.53	1.36
2000	0.00539	0.00885	1.233	1.100	1.82	1.56

Source: Adapted from Fink, D.G. and Beaty, H.W., *Standard Handbook for Electrical Engineers*, 11th edn., McGraw-Hill, New York, 1978. With permission.

[a] To correct to other temperatures, use the following:

For copper: $R_T = R_{25} \times (234.5 + T)/259.5$

For aluminum: $R_T = R_{25} \times (228 + T)/253$

where R_T is the new resistance at temperature T and R_{25} is the tabulated resistance.

[b] Includes only skin effect (use for cables in separate ducts).

[c] Includes skin effect and proximity effect (use for triplex, multiconductor, or cables in the same duct).

This phenomenon is called *proximity effect*. It is greater for a given size conductor in single-conductor cables than in three-conductor belted cables. Table 5.5 gives the dc resistance and skin effect and proximity effect multipliers for copper and aluminum conductors at 25°C. Additional tables of electrical characteristics are supplied by the manufacturers for their cables.

Example 5.8

A single-conductor, paper-insulated, belted cable will be used as an underground feeder of 3 mi. The cable has a 2000 MCM (2000 kcmil) copper conductor:

(a) Calculate the total dc resistance of the conductor at 25°C.
(b) Using Table 5.5, determine the effective resistance and the skin effect on the effective resistance in percent if the conductor is used at 60 Hz ac.
(c) Calculate the percentage of reduction in cable ampacity in part (b).

Solution

(a) From Table 5.5, the dc resistance of the cable is

$$R_{dc} = 0.00539 \ \Omega/1000 \ \text{ft}$$

or the total dc resistance is

$$R_{dc} = 0.00539 \times 5280 \times 3 = 0.0854 \ \Omega$$

(b) From Table 5.5, the skin effect coefficient is 1.233; therefore, the effective resistance at 60 Hz is

$$R_{eff} = (\text{skin effect coefficient}) \times R_{dc}$$

$$= (1.233) \times 0.0854$$

$$= 0.1053 \ \Omega$$

or it is 23.3% greater than for dc.

(c) The reduct ion in the cable ampacity is also 23.3%.

5.5 SHEATH CURRENTS IN CABLES

The flow of ac current in the conductors of single-conductor cables induces ac voltages in the cable sheaths. When the cable sheaths are bonded together at their ends, the voltages induced give rise to sheath (*eddy*) currents, and therefore, additional I^2R losses occur in the sheath. These losses are taken into account by increasing the resistance of the relevant conductor. For a single-conductor cable with bonded sheaths operating in three phase and arranged in equilateral triangular formation, the increase in conductor resistance is

$$\Delta r = r_s \times \frac{X_m^2}{r_s^2 + X_m^2} \tag{5.77}$$

where
  X_m is the mutual reactance between conductors and sheath per phase in ohms per mile
  r_s is the sheath resistance per phase in ohms per mile

The mutual reactance between conductors and sheath can be calculated from

$$X_m = 0.2794 \left(\frac{f}{60} \right) \log_{10} \left(\frac{2S}{r_0 + r_i} \right) \tag{5.78}$$

and the sheath resistance of a metal sheath cable can be determined from

$$r_s = \frac{0.2}{\left(r_0 + r_i \right)\left(r_0 - r_i \right)} \tag{5.79}$$

where
  f is the frequency in hertz
  S is the spacing between conductor centers in inches
  r_0 is the outer radius of metal sheath in inches
  r_i is the inner radius of metal sheath in inches

In Equation 5.78,

$$\text{GMR} = D_s = \frac{r_0 + r_i}{2} \tag{5.80}$$

and

$$\text{GMD} = D_m = S$$

Therefore, for other conductor arrangements, that is, other than equilateral triangular formation,

$$X_m = 0.2794 \left(\frac{f}{60} \right) \log_{10} \left(\frac{D_m}{D_s} \right) \ \Omega/\text{mi/phase} \tag{5.81}$$

and if the frequency used is 60 Hz,

$$X_m = 0.2794 \times \log_{10} \left(\frac{D_m}{D_s} \right) \tag{5.82}$$

or

$$X_m = 0.1213 \times \ln \left(\frac{D_m}{D_s} \right) \tag{5.83}$$

Hence, in single-conductor cables, the total resistance to positive- or negative-sequence current flow, including the effect of sheath current, is

$$r_a = r_c + \frac{r_s X_m^2}{r_s^2 + X_m^2} \ \Omega/\text{mi/phase} \tag{5.84}$$

where
r_a is the total positive- or negative-sequence resistance, including sheath current effects
r_c is the ac resistance of conductor, including skin effect

The sheath loss due to sheath currents is

$$P_s = I^2 \Delta r \tag{5.85}$$

or

$$P_s = I^2 \left(\frac{r_s X_m^2}{r_s^2 + X_m^2} \right) \tag{5.86}$$

or

$$P_s = r_s \left(\frac{I^2 X_m^2}{r_s^2 + X_m^2} \right) \ \text{W/mi/phase} \tag{5.87}$$

where
r_s is the sheath resistance per phase in ohms per mile
I is the current in one conductor in amperes
X_m is the mutual reactance between conductors and sheath per phase in ohms per mile

For a *three-conductor cable* with *round conductors*, the increase in conductor resistance due to sheath currents is

$$\Delta r = 0.04416 \left(\frac{S^2}{r_s \left(r_o + r_i\right)^2} \right) \ \Omega/\text{mi/phase} \tag{5.88}$$

where

$$S = \frac{d + 2T}{\sqrt{3}} \tag{5.89}$$

and

r_s is the sheath resistance, from Equation 5.79
r_o is the outer radius of lead sheath in inches
r_i is the inner radius of lead sheath in inches
S is the distance between conductor center and sheath center for three-conductor cable made of round conductors
d is the conductor diameter in inches
T is the conductor insulation thickness in inches

For *sector-shaped conductors*, use Equations 5.88 and 5.82 but conductor diameter is

$d = 82\%-86\%$ of diameter of round conductor having same cross-sectional area

Sheaths of single-conductor cables may be operated short-circuited or open-circuited. If the sheaths are short-circuited, they are usually bonded and grounded at every manhole. This decreases the sheath voltages to zero but allows the flow of sheath currents. There are various techniques of operating with the sheaths open-circuited:

1. When a ground wire is used, one terminal of each sheath section is bound to the ground wire. The other terminal is left open so that no current can flow in the sheath.
2. With cross bonding, at each section, connections are made between the sheaths of cables *a*, *b*, and *c*, as shown in Figure 5.25, so that only the sheaths are transposed electrically. The sheaths are bonded together and grounded at the end of each complete transposition. Thus, the sum of sheath voltages induced by the positive-sequence currents becomes zero.
3. With impedance bonding, impedances are added in each cable sheath to limit sheath currents to predetermined values without eliminating any sequence currents.
4. With bonding transformers [5].

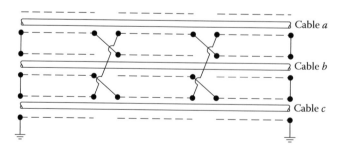

FIGURE 5.25   Cross bonding of single-conductor cables.

Example 5.9

Assume that three 35 kV, 350 kcmil, single-conductor belted cables are located in touching equilateral formation with respect to each other and the sheaths are bounded to ground at several points. The cables are operated at 34.5 kV and 60 Hz. The cable has a conductor diameter of 0.681 in., insulation thickness of 345 cmil, metal sheath thickness of 105 cmil, and a length of 10 mi. Conductor ac resistance is 0.190 Ω/mi per phase at 50°C. Calculate the following:

(a) Mutual reactance between conductors and sheath
(b) Sheath resistance of cable
(c) Increase in conductor resistance due to sheath currents
(d) Total resistance of conductor including sheath loss
(e) Ratio of sheath loss to conductor loss
(f) Total sheath losses of feeder in watts if current in conductor is 400 A

Solution

(a) By using Equation 5.78,

$$X_m = 0.2794\left(\frac{f}{60}\right)\log_{10}\left(\frac{2S}{r_0 + r_i}\right) \ \Omega/\text{mi/phase}$$

where

$$r_i = \frac{0.681}{2} + 0.345 = 0.686 \ \text{in.}$$

$$r_0 = r_i + 0.105 = 0.791 \ \text{in.}$$

$$S = 1.582 \ \text{in.}$$

Therefore,

$$X_m = 0.2794\log_{10}\left(\frac{2 \times 1.582}{0.791 + 0.686}\right)$$

$$= 0.09244 \ \Omega/\text{mi}$$

or

$$X_m = 0.9244 \ \Omega/\text{phase}$$

(b) By using Equation 5.79,

$$r_s = \frac{0.2}{\left(r_0 + r_i\right)\left(r_0 - r_i\right)}$$

$$= \frac{0.2}{(0.791 + 0.686)(0.791 - 0.686)}$$

$$= 1.2896 \ \Omega/\text{mi}$$

or

$$r_s = 12.896 \ \Omega/\text{phase}$$

(c) Using Equation 5.77,

$$\Delta r = r_s \times \frac{X_m^2}{r_s^2 + X_m^2}$$

$$= 1.2896 \times \frac{0.09244^2}{1.2896^2 + 0.09244^2}$$

$$= 0.00659 \ \Omega/\text{mi}$$

or

$$\Delta r = 0.0659 \ \Omega/\text{phase}$$

(d) Using Equation 5.84,

$$r_a = r_c + \frac{r_s X_m^2}{r_s^2 + X_m^2}$$

$$= 0.190 + 0.00659$$

$$= 0.19659 \ \Omega/\text{mi}$$

or

$$r_a = 1.9659 \ \Omega/\text{phase}$$

(e)

$$\frac{\text{Sheath loss}}{\text{Conductor loss}} = \frac{I^2 r_s X_m^2}{r_s^2 + X_m^2} \times \frac{1}{I^2 r_c}$$

$$= \frac{0.00659}{0.190}$$

$$= 0.0347$$

That is,

$$\text{Sheath loss} = 3.47\% \times \text{conductor } I^2 R \text{ loss}$$

(f) Using Equation 5.87,

$$P_s = r_s \left(\frac{I^2 X_m^2}{r_s^2 + X_m^2} \right) \text{W/mi}$$

or, for three-phase loss,

$$P_s = 3I^2 \left(\frac{r_s X_m^2}{r_s^2 + X_m^2} \right)$$

$$= 3 \times 400^2 \times 0.00659$$

$$= 3163.2 \ \text{W/mi}$$

or, for total feeder length,

$$P_s = 31,632 \ \text{W/mi}$$

5.6 POSITIVE- AND NEGATIVE-SEQUENCE REACTANCES

5.6.1 SINGLE-CONDUCTOR CABLES

The positive- and negative-sequence reactances for single-conductor cables when sheath currents are present can be determined as

$$X_1 = X_2 = 0.1213\left(\frac{f}{60}\right) \times \ln\left(\frac{D_m}{D_s}\right) - \frac{X_m^3}{X_m^2 + r_s^2} \quad \Omega/\text{mi} \tag{5.90}$$

or

$$X_1 = X_2 = 0.2794\left(\frac{f}{60}\right) \times \log_{10}\left(\frac{D_m}{D_s}\right) - \frac{X_m^3}{X_m^2 + r_s^2} \quad \Omega/\text{mi} \tag{5.91}$$

or

$$X_1 = X_2 = 0.2794\left(\frac{f}{60}\right) \times \log_{10}\left(\frac{D_m}{0.7788r}\right) - \frac{X_m^3}{X_m^2 + r_s^2} \quad \Omega/\text{mi} \tag{5.92}$$

where r is the outside of the radius of the conductors. For cables, it is convenient to express D_m, D_s, and r in inches. In Equation 5.91,

X_1 is the positive-sequence reactance per phase in ohms per mile
X_2 is the negative-sequence reactance per phase in ohms per mile
f is the frequency in hertz
D_m is the GMD among conductors
D_s is the GMR, or self-GMD, of one conductor
X_m is the mutual reactance between conductors and sheath per phase in ohms per mile
r_s is the sheath resistance per phase in ohms per mile

Equation 5.91 can be also expressed as

$$X_1 = X_2 = X_a + X_d - \frac{X_m^3}{X_m^2 + r_s^2} \quad \Omega/\text{mi} \tag{5.93}$$

where

$$X_a = 0.2794\left(\frac{f}{60}\right) \times \log_{10}\left(\frac{12}{D_s}\right) \tag{5.94}$$

and

$$X_d = 0.2794\left(\frac{f}{60}\right) \times \log_{10}\left(\frac{D_m}{12}\right) \tag{5.95}$$

Here, X_a and X_d are called *conductor component of reactance* and *separation component of reactance*, respectively. If the frequency is 60 Hz, Equations 5.94 and 5.95 may be written as

$$X_a = 0.2794 \times \log_{10}\left(\frac{12}{D_s}\right) \ \Omega/\text{mi} \tag{5.96}$$

or

$$X_a = 0.1213 \times \ln\left(\frac{12}{D_s}\right) \ \Omega/\text{mi} \tag{5.97}$$

and

$$X_d = 0.2794 \times \log_{10}\left(\frac{D_m}{12}\right) \ \Omega/\text{mi} \tag{5.98}$$

or

$$X_d = 0.1213 \times \ln\left(\frac{D_m}{12}\right) \ \Omega/\text{mi} \tag{5.99}$$

In Equation 5.93, the last term symbolizes the correction for the existence of sheath currents. The negative sign is there because the current in the sheath is in a direction opposite to that in the conductor, therefore inclining to restrict the flux to the region between the conductor and the sheath. The last term is taken from Equation 5.77, with X_m substituted for r_s, and is derived by considering the current in the sheath and the component of voltage it induces in the conductor in quadrature to the conductor current.

5.6.2 THREE-CONDUCTOR CABLES

The positive- and negative-sequence reactances for three-conductor cables can be determined as

$$X_1 = X_2 = 0.2794\left(\frac{f}{60}\right) \times \log_{10}\left(\frac{D_m}{D_s}\right) \ \Omega/\text{mi} \tag{5.100}$$

or

$$X_1 = X_2 = X_a + X_d \tag{5.101}$$

where D_m is the GMD among the three conductors. If the frequency is 60 Hz, X_a and X_d can be calculated from Equations 5.96 or 5.97 and 5.98 or 5.99, respectively. Equations 5.100 and 5.101 can be used for both shielded and nonshielded cables because of negligible sheet current effects.

5.7 ZERO-SEQUENCE RESISTANCE AND REACTANCE

The return of the zero-sequence currents flowing along the phase conductors of a three-phase cable is in either the ground, or the sheaths, or the parallel combination of both ground and sheaths.

5.7.1 THREE-CONDUCTOR CABLES

Figure 5.26 shows an actual circuit of a single-circuit three-conductor cable with solidly bonded and grounded sheath. It can be observed that

$$\left(\mathbf{I}_{a0} + \mathbf{I}_{b0} + \mathbf{I}_{c0}\right) + \left(\mathbf{I}_{0(s)} + \mathbf{I}_{0(g)}\right) = 0 \tag{5.102}$$

Figure 5.27 shows the equivalent circuit of this actual circuit in which $\mathbf{Z}_c$ represents the impedance of a composite conductor consisting of three single conductors. The zero-sequence current $\mathbf{I}_{0(a)}$ in the composite conductor can be expressed as [7]

$$\mathbf{I}_{0(a)} = 3\mathbf{I}_{a0} \tag{5.103}$$

First, assume that there is no return (zero-sequence) current flowing in the sheath, and therefore, it is totally in the ground. Hence, the zero-sequence impedance of the composite conductor can be written as

$$\mathbf{Z}_{0(a)} = (r_a + r_e) + j0.36396\left(\frac{f}{60}\right) \times \ln\left(\frac{D_e}{D_{aa}}\right) \quad \Omega/\text{mi/phase} \tag{5.104}$$

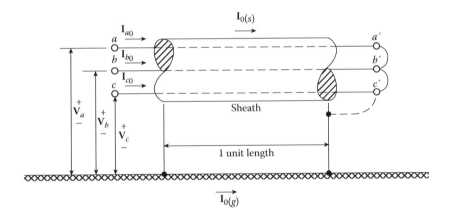

FIGURE 5.26 Actual circuit of three-conductor lead-sheathed cable.

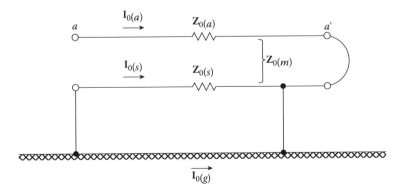

FIGURE 5.27 Equivalent circuit of three-conductor cable.

or

$$\mathbf{Z}_{0(a)} = (r_a + r_e) + j0.8382\left(\frac{f}{60}\right) \times \log_{10}\left(\frac{D_e}{D_{aa}}\right) \ \Omega/\text{mi/phase} \tag{5.105}$$

since the GMR, or the self-GMD, of this composite conductor is

$$D_{aa} = D_s^{1/3} \times D_{eq}^{2/3} \tag{5.106}$$

and since for three-conductor cables made of round conductors,

$$D_{eq} = D_m = d + 2T \tag{5.107}$$

where
 d is the conductor diameter in inches
 T is the conductor insulation thickness in inches

Equations 5.104 and 5.105 for 60 Hz frequency can be expressed as

$$\mathbf{Z}_{0(a)} = (r_a + r_e) + j0.36396 \ \ln\frac{D_e}{D_s^{1/3} \times D_{eq}^{2/3}} \ \Omega/\text{mi/phase} \tag{5.108}$$

and

$$\mathbf{Z}_{0(a)} = (r_a + r_e) + j0.8382\left(\frac{f}{60}\right) \ \ln\frac{D_e}{D_s^{1/3} \times D_{eq}^{2/3}} \ \Omega/\text{mi/phase} \tag{5.109}$$

Equations 5.108 and 5.109 are sometimes written as

$$\mathbf{Z}_{0(a)} = (r_a + r_e) + j0.1213 \ \ln\frac{D_e^3}{D_s \times D_{eq}^2} \ \Omega/\text{mi/phase} \tag{5.110}$$

and

$$\mathbf{Z}_{0(a)} = (r_a + r_e) + j0.2794\left(\frac{f}{60}\right)\log_{10}\frac{D_e^3}{D_s \times D_{eq}^2} \ \Omega/\text{mi/phase} \tag{5.111}$$

or

$$\mathbf{Z}_{0(a)} = (r_a + r_e) + j(X_a + X_e - 2X_d) \ \Omega/\text{mi/phase} \tag{5.112}$$

where

$$X_a = 0.1213 \ \ln\left(\frac{12}{D_s}\right) \ \Omega/\text{mi} \tag{5.113}$$

$$X_e = 3 \times 0.1213 \ \ln\left(\frac{D_e}{12}\right) \ \Omega/\text{mi} \tag{5.114}$$

$$X_d = 0.1213 \ \ln\left(\frac{D_{eq}}{12}\right) \ \Omega/\text{mi} \tag{5.115}$$

where
r_a is the ac resistance of one conductor in ohms per mile
r_e is the ac resistance of earth return
$\quad = 0.00476 \times f \ \Omega/\text{mi}$
D_e is the equivalent depth of earth return path
$\quad = 25920\sqrt{\rho/f} \ \text{in.}$
D_{eq} is the equivalent, or geometric, mean distance among conductor centers in inches
D_s is the GMR, or self-GMD, of one conductor in inches
X_a is the reactance of individual phase conductor at 12 in. spacing in ohms per mile

Second, consider only ground return path and sheath return path but not the composite conductor. Hence, the *zero-sequence impedance of the sheath* to zero-sequence currents is

$$\mathbf{Z}_{0(s)} = \left(3r_s + r_e\right) + j0.36396 \times \left(\frac{f}{60}\right) \times \ln\left(\frac{2D_e}{r_0 + r_i}\right) \ \Omega/\text{mi/phase} \tag{5.116}$$

or

$$\mathbf{Z}_{0(s)} = \left(3r_s + r_e\right) + j0.8382 \times \left(\frac{f}{60}\right) \times \log_{10}\left(\frac{2D_e}{r_0 + r_i}\right) \ \Omega/\text{mi/phase} \tag{5.117}$$

or, *at* 60 Hz *frequency,*

$$\mathbf{Z}_{0(s)} = \left(3r_s + r_e\right) + j0.36396 \times \ln\left(\frac{2D_e}{r_0 + r_i}\right) \ \Omega/\text{mi/phase} \tag{5.118}$$

or

$$\mathbf{Z}_{0(s)} = \left(3r_s + r_e\right) + j0.8382 \times \log_{10}\left(\frac{2D_e}{r_0 + r_i}\right) \ \Omega/\text{mi/phase} \tag{5.119}$$

or

$$\mathbf{Z}_{0(s)} = \left(3r_s + r_e\right) + j(3X_s + X_e + X_e) \ \Omega/\text{mi/phase} \tag{5.120}$$

where

$$r_s = \frac{0.2}{\left(r_o + r_i\right)\left(r_o - r_i\right)} \ \text{for lead sheaths, } \Omega/\text{mi} \tag{5.121}$$

$$X_s = 0.1213 \ \ln\left(\frac{24}{r_o + r_i}\right) \ \Omega/\text{mi} \tag{5.122}$$

$$X_e = 3 \times 0.1213 \ \ln\left(\frac{D_e}{12}\right) \ \Omega/\text{mi} \tag{5.123}$$

where
  r_s is the sheath resistance of metal sheath cable in ohms per mile
  r_e is the ac resistance of earth return in ohms per mile
  r_0 is the outer radius of metal sheath in inches
  r_i is the inner radius of metal sheath in inches
  X_s is the reactance of metal sheath in ohms per mile

The *zero-sequence mutual impedance between the composite conductor and sheath* can be expressed as

$$\mathbf{Z}_{0(m)} = r_e + j0.36396 \times \left(\frac{f}{60}\right) \times \ln\left(\frac{2D_e}{r_0 + r_i}\right) \ \Omega/\text{mi/phase} \tag{5.124}$$

or

$$\mathbf{Z}_{0(m)} = r_e + j0.8382 \times \left(\frac{f}{60}\right) \times \log_{10}\left(\frac{2D_e}{r_0 + r_i}\right) \ \Omega/\text{mi/phase} \tag{5.125}$$

or, at 60 Hz frequency,

$$\mathbf{Z}_{0(m)} = r_e + j0.36396 \times \ln\left(\frac{2D_e}{r_0 + r_i}\right) \ \Omega/\text{mi/phase} \tag{5.126}$$

or

$$\mathbf{Z}_{0(m)} = r_e + j0.8382 \times \log_{10}\left(\frac{2D_e}{r_0 + r_i}\right) \ \Omega/\text{mi/phase} \tag{5.127}$$

or

$$\mathbf{Z}_{0(m)} = r_e + j(3X_s + X_e) \tag{5.128}$$

The equivalent circuit shown in Figure 5.27 can be modified as shown in Figure 5.28. *Total zero-sequence impedance* can be calculated for three different cases as follows:

1. *When both ground and sheath return paths are present,*

$$\mathbf{Z}_{00} = \mathbf{Z}_0 = \left(\mathbf{Z}_{0(a)} - \mathbf{Z}_{0(m)}\right) + \frac{\left(\mathbf{Z}_{0(s)} - \mathbf{Z}_{0(m)}\right)\mathbf{Z}_{0(m)}}{\mathbf{Z}_{0(s)}} \tag{5.129}$$

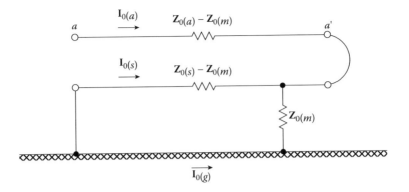

FIGURE 5.28   Modified equivalent circuit.

or

$$\mathbf{Z}_{00} = \mathbf{Z}_{0(a)} + \frac{\mathbf{Z}_{0(m)}^2}{\mathbf{Z}_{0(s)}} \ \Omega/\text{mi/phase} \tag{5.130}$$

or

$$\mathbf{Z}_{00} = \left[(r_a + r_e) + j(X_a + X_e - 2X_d) \right]$$
$$- \frac{[r_e + j(3X_s + X_e)]^2}{\left[(3r_s + r_e) + j(3X_s + X_e) \right]} \tag{5.131}$$

2. *When there is only sheath return path,*

$$\mathbf{Z}_{00} = \left(\mathbf{Z}_{0(a)} - \mathbf{Z}_{0(m)} \right) + \left(\mathbf{Z}_{0(s)} - \mathbf{Z}_{0(m)} \right) \ \Omega/\text{mi/phase} \tag{5.132}$$

or

$$\mathbf{Z}_{00} = \mathbf{Z}_{0(a)} + \mathbf{Z}_{0(s)} - 2\mathbf{Z}_{0(m)} \ \Omega/\text{mi/phase} \tag{5.133}$$

or

$$\mathbf{Z}_{00} = [(r_a + r_e) + j(X_a + X_e - 2X_d)] + [(3r_s + r_e) + j(3X_s + X_e)]$$
$$- 2[r_e + j(3X_s + X_e)] \tag{5.134}$$

or

$$\mathbf{Z}_{00} = (r_a + 3r_s) + j(X_a - 2X_d - 3X_s) \ \Omega/\text{mi/phase} \tag{5.135}$$

3. *When there is only ground return path (e.g., nonsheathed cables),*

$$\mathbf{Z}_{00} = \left(\mathbf{Z}_{0(a)} - \mathbf{Z}_{0(m)} \right) + \mathbf{Z}_{0(m)} \ \Omega/\text{mi/phase} \tag{5.136}$$

TABLE 5.6

D_e, r_e, and X_e for Various Earth Resistivities at 60 Hz

Earth Resistivity (Ω-m)	Equivalent Depth of Earth Return, D_e		Equivalent Earth Resistance, r_e (Ω/m)	Equivalent Earth Reactance, X_e (Ω/m)
	in.	ft		
1	3.36×10^3	280	0.286	2.05
5	7.44×10^3	620	0.286	2.34
10	1.06×10^4	880	0.286	2.47
50	2.40×10^4	2,000	0.286	2.76
100	3.36×10^4	2,800	0.286	2.89
500	7.44×10^4	6,200	0.286	3.18
1,000	1.06×10^5	8,800	0.286	3.31
5,000	2.40×10^5	20,000	0.286	3.60
10,000	3.36×10^5	28,000	0.286	3.73

Source: Westinghouse Electric Corporation, *Electrical Transmission and Distribution Reference Book*, WEC, East Pittsburgh, PA, 1964.

or

$$\mathbf{Z}_{00} = \mathbf{Z}_{0(a)} \ \Omega/\text{mi/phase} \tag{5.137}$$

$$\mathbf{Z}_{00} = (r_a + r_e) + j(X_a + X_e - 2X_d) \ \Omega/\text{mi/phase} \tag{5.138}$$

In the case of shielded cables, the zero-sequence impedance can be computed as if the shielding tapes were not present, with very small error. In general, calculating only the zero-sequence impedance for all return current in the sheath and none in the ground is sufficient. Table 5.6 offers the values of D_e, r_e, and X_e for various earth resistivities.

5.7.2 Single-Conductor Cables

The actual circuit of three single-conductor cables with solidly bonded and grounded sheath in a perfectly transposed three-phase circuit is shown in Figure 5.29. It can be observed from the figure that

$$\left(\mathbf{I}_{a0} + \mathbf{I}_{b0} + \mathbf{I}_{c0}\right) + \left(3\mathbf{I}_{0(s)} + \mathbf{I}_{0(g)}\right) = 0 \tag{5.139}$$

In general, the equivalent circuits shown in Figures 5.27 and 5.28 are still applicable. The *zero-sequence impedance of the composite conductor* at 60 Hz frequency can be expressed as before:

$$\mathbf{Z}_{0(a)} = \left(r_a + r_e\right) + j0.36396 \ \ln \frac{D_e}{D_s^{1/3} \times D_{\text{eq}}^{2/3}} \ \Omega/\text{mi/phase} \tag{5.140}$$

or

$$\mathbf{Z}_{0(a)} = \left(r_a + r_e\right) + j0.8382 \ \log_{10} \frac{D_e}{D_s^{1/3} \times D_{\text{eq}}^{2/3}} \ \Omega/\text{mi/phase} \tag{5.141}$$

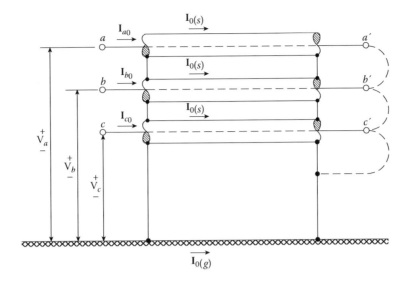

FIGURE 5.29   Actual circuit of three single-conductor lead-sheathed cables.

$$\mathbf{Z}_{0(a)} = (r_a + r_e) + j(X_a + X_e - 2X_d) \tag{5.142}$$

where

$$D_{eq} = (D_{ab} \times D_{bc} \times D_{ca})^{1/3} = D_m \text{ in.}$$

$$= \text{GMD among conductor centers}$$

The *zero-sequence impedance of the sheath* to zero-sequence currents is

$$\mathbf{Z}_{0(s)} = (r_s + r_e) + j0.36396 \ \ln \frac{D_e}{D_{s(3s)}} \tag{5.143}$$

or

$$\mathbf{Z}_{0(s)} = (r_s + r_e) + j0.8382 \ \log_{10} \frac{D_e}{D_{s(3s)}} \tag{5.144}$$

or

$$\mathbf{Z}_{0(s)} = (r_s + r_e) + j(X_s + X_e - 2X_d) \tag{5.145}$$

where

$$D_{s(3s)} = \left(D_m^2 \times \frac{r_o + r_i}{2} \right)^{1/3} \text{ in.}$$

$$= \text{GMR, or self-GMD, of conducting path composed of three sheaths in parallel} \tag{5.146}$$

The *zero-sequence mutual impedance between conductors and the sheaths* can be expressed as

$$\mathbf{Z}_{0(m)} = r_e + j0.36396 \ln \frac{D_e}{D_{m(3c-3s)}} \tag{5.147}$$

or

$$\mathbf{Z}_{0(m)} = r_e + j0.8382 \ \log_{10} \frac{D_e}{D_{m(3c-3s)}} \tag{5.148}$$

or

$$\mathbf{Z}_{0(m)} = r_e + j(X_e + X_s - 2X_d) \tag{5.149}$$

where

$$D_{m(3c-3s)} = \left(D_m^6 \times \left(\frac{r_o + r_i}{2} \right)^3 \right)^{1/9} \text{ in.} \tag{5.150}$$

or

$$D_{m(3c-3s)} = \left(D_m^2 \times \frac{r_o + r_i}{2} \right)^{1/3} \text{ in.}$$

$$= \text{GMD of all distances between conductors and sheaths} \tag{5.151}$$

Total zero-sequence impedance can be calculated, from Figure 5.29, for three different cases:

1. *When both ground and sheath return paths are present,*

$$\mathbf{Z}_{00} = \mathbf{Z}_{0(a)} + \frac{\mathbf{Z}_{0(m)}^2}{\mathbf{Z}_{0(s)}} \ \Omega/\text{mi/phase} \tag{5.152}$$

or

$$\mathbf{Z}_{00} = \left[(r_a + r_e) + j\left(X_a + X_e - 2X_d \right) \right] - \frac{[r_e + j(X_e + X_s) - 2X_d]^2}{\left[(r_s + r_e) + j(X_e + X_s - 2X_d) \right]} \tag{5.153}$$

2. *When there is only a sheath return path,*

$$\mathbf{Z}_{00} = \mathbf{Z}_{0(a)} - \mathbf{Z}_{0(s)} + 2\mathbf{Z}_{0(m)} \ \Omega/\text{mi/phase} \tag{5.154}$$

or

$$\mathbf{Z}_{00} = [(r_a + r_e) + j(X_e + X_s - 2X_d)] + [(r_s + r_e) + j(X_s + X_e - 2X_d)]$$
$$- 2[r_e + j(X_e + X_s - 2X_d)] \tag{5.155}$$

or

$$\mathbf{Z}_{00} = (r_a + r_s) + j(X_a - X_s) \tag{5.156}$$

or

$$\mathbf{Z}_{00} = (r_a + r_s) + j0.36396 \ \ln \frac{D_{s(3s)}}{D_s^{1/3} \times D_{eq}^{2/3}} \tag{5.157}$$

or

$$\mathbf{Z}_{00} = (r_a + r_s) + j0.8382 \ \log_{10} \frac{D_{s(3s)}}{D_s^{1/3} \times D_{eq}^{2/3}} \tag{5.158}$$

3. *When there is only a ground return path,*

$$\mathbf{Z}_{00} = (\mathbf{Z}_{0(a)} - \mathbf{Z}_{0(m)}) + \mathbf{Z}_{0(m)} \tag{5.159}$$

or

$$\mathbf{Z}_{00} = \mathbf{Z}_{0(a)}$$

or

$$\mathbf{Z}_{00} = (r_a + r_e) + j(X_a + X_e - 2X_d) \tag{5.160}$$

Example 5.10

A three-phase, 60 Hz, 23 kV cable of three 250 kcmil, concentric strand, paper-insulated single-conductor cables with solidly bonded and grounded metal sheath connected between a sending bus and receiving bus, as shown in Figures 5.29 and 5.30. The conductor diameter is 0.575 in., insulation thickness is 245 mils, and metal sheath thickness is 95 mils. The conductor resistance is 0.263 Ω/mi per phase and the earth resistivity is 100 Ω-rn. The GMR of one conductor is 0.221 in. Sheath resistance is 1.72 Ω/mi. Calculate the total zero-sequence impedance:

(a) When both ground and return paths are present
(b) When there is only sheath return path
(c) When there is only ground return path

Solution

$$T = \text{insulation thickness } 245 \text{ mils}$$

$$= \frac{245 \text{ mils}}{1000} = 0.245 \text{ in.}$$

$$\text{Lead sheath thicknes} = \frac{95 \text{ mils}}{1000} = 0.095 \text{ in.}$$

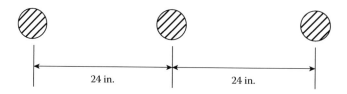

FIGURE 5.30   For Example 5.10.

Therefore,

$$r_i = \frac{\text{Conductor diameter}}{2} + \text{Insulation thickness}$$

$$= \frac{0.575}{2} + 0.245 = 0.5325 \text{ in.}$$

and

$$r_0 = r_i + \text{lead sheath thickness}$$

$$= 0.5325 + 0.095 = 0.6275 \text{ in.}$$

By using Equation 5.140,

$$\mathbf{Z}_{0(a)} = (r_a + r_e) + j0.36396 \ln \frac{D_e}{D_s^{1/3} \times D_{eq}^{2/3}} \ \Omega/\text{mi/phase}$$

where
  $r_a = 0.263 \ \Omega/\text{mi}$
  $r_e = 0.00476 f = 0.2856 \ \Omega/\text{mi}$

$$D_e = 25{,}920 \sqrt{\frac{\rho}{60}} = 33{,}462.6 \text{ in.}$$

  $D_s = 0.221$ in.

$$D_{eq} = D_m = (D_{ab} \times D_{bc} \times D_{ca})^{1/3} = 30.24 \text{ in.}$$

Therefore,

$$\mathbf{Z}_{0(a)} = (0.263 + 0.2856) + j0.36396 \ln \left(\frac{33{,}462.6}{\sqrt{0.221 \times 30.24}} \right)$$

$$= 0.5486 + j3.1478 = 3.1952 \angle 80.1° \ \Omega/\text{mi}$$

By using Equation 5.143,

$$\mathbf{Z}_{0(s)} = (r_s + r_e) + j0.36396 \ln \frac{D_e}{D_{s(3s)}}$$

where
  $r_s = 1.72 \ \Omega/\text{mi}$
  $r_e = 0.2856 \ \Omega/\text{mi}$
  $D_e = 33{,}462.6$ in.

$$D_{s(3s)} = \left(D_{eq}^2 \times \frac{r_0 + r_i}{2} \right)^{1/3}$$

$$= \left(30.242 \times \frac{0.5325 + 0.6275}{2} \right)^{1/3} = 8.09 \text{ in.}$$

Therefore,

$$\mathbf{Z}_{0(s)} = (1.72 + 0.2856) + j0.36396 \ln \left(\frac{33,462.6}{8.09} \right)$$

$$= 2.006 + j3.03 = 3.634 \angle 56.5° \ \Omega/\text{mi}$$

By using Equation 5.147,

$$\mathbf{Z}_{0(m)} = r_e + j0.36396 \ln \frac{D_e}{D_{m(3c-3s)}}$$

where

$$D_{m(3c-3s)} = D_{s(3s)} = 8.09 \text{ in.}$$

Hence,

$$\mathbf{Z}_{0(m)} = 0.2856 + j0.36396 \ln \left(\frac{33,462.6}{8.09} \right)$$

$$= 0.2856 + j3.03 = 3.04 \angle 84.6° \ \Omega/\text{mi}$$

Therefore, the *total zero-sequence impedances* are as follows:

(a) *When both ground and return paths are present,*

$$\mathbf{Z}_{00} = \mathbf{Z}_{0(a)} + \frac{\mathbf{Z}_{0(m)}^2}{\mathbf{Z}_{0(s)}}$$

$$= 0.5486 + j3.1478 - \frac{(3.04 \angle 84.6°)^2}{3.634 \angle 56.5°}$$

$$= 1.534 + j0.796 = 1.728 \angle 27.4° \ \Omega/\text{mi}$$

(b) *When there is only sheath return path,*

$$\mathbf{Z}_0 = \mathbf{Z}_{0(a)} + \mathbf{Z}_{0(s)} - 2\mathbf{Z}_{0(m)})$$

$$= (0.5486 + 2.006 - 2 \times 0.2856) + j(3.1478 + 3.03 - 2 \times 3.03)$$

$$= 1.983 + j0.117 = 1.987 \angle 3.4° \ \Omega/\text{mi}$$

(c) *When there is only ground return path,*

$$\mathbf{Z}_0 = \mathbf{Z}_{0(a)}$$

$$= 0.5486 + j3.1478 = 3.1952 \angle 80.1° \ \Omega/\text{mi}$$

5.8 SHUNT CAPACITIVE REACTANCE

Tables A.12 through A.19 give shunt capacitive reactances directly in ohms mile. Also, the following formulas give the shunt capacitance, shunt capacitive reactance, and charging current [2]:

1. *For single-conductor and three-conductor shielded cables,*

$$C_0 = C_1 = C_2 = \frac{0.0892K}{G} \ \mu\text{F/mi/phase} \tag{5.161}$$

$$X_0 = X_1 = X_2 = \frac{1.79G}{f \times K} \ \text{M}\Omega/\text{mi/phase} \tag{5.162}$$

$$I_0 = I_1 = I_2 = \frac{0.323 \times f \times K \times V_{(L-N)}}{1000 \times G} \ \text{A/mi/phase} \tag{5.163}$$

2. *For three-conductor belted cables with no conductor shielding,*

$$C_0 = \frac{0.0892K}{G_0} \ \mu\text{F/mi/phase} \tag{5.164}$$

$$C_1 = C_2 = \frac{0.267K}{G_1} \ \mu\text{F/mi/phase} \tag{5.165}$$

$$X_0 = \frac{1.79G_0}{G_1} \ \text{M}\Omega/\text{mi/phase} \tag{5.166}$$

$$X_1 = X_2 = \frac{0.597 \times G_1}{f \times K} \ \text{M}\Omega/\text{mi/phase} \tag{5.167}$$

$$I_0 = \frac{0.323 \times f \times K \times V_{(L-N)}}{1000 \times G_0} \ \text{A/mi/phase} \tag{5.168}$$

$$I_1 = I_2 = \frac{0.97 \times f \times K \times V_{(L-N)}}{1000 \times G_1} \ \text{A/mi/phase} \tag{5.169}$$

where
  C_0 is the zero-sequence capacitance in microfarads per mile per phase
  C_1 is the positive-sequence capacitance in microfarads per mile per phase
  C_2 is the negative-sequence capacitance in microfarads per mile
  K is the dielectric constant of insulation, from Table 5.1
  G is the geometric factor, from Figure 5.23
  G_1 is the geometric factor, from Figure 5.24
  f is the frequency in hertz
  $V_{(L-N)}$ is the line-to-neutral voltage in kilovolts

Here,

$$X = \frac{X, \ \Omega/\text{phase/mi}}{l, \ \text{mi}} \ \Omega/\text{phase} \tag{5.170}$$

Example 5.11

A 60 Hz, 15 kV, three-conductor, paper-insulated, shielded cable will be used at 13.8 kV as a three-phase underground feeder of 10 mi. The cable has three 350 kcmil compact sector-type conductors with a diameter of 0.539 in. and a dielectric constant of 3.7. The insulation thickness is 175 mils. Calculate the following:

(a) Shunt capacitance for zero, positive, and negative sequences
(b) Shunt capacitive reactance for zero, positive, and negative sequences
(c) Charging current for zero, positive, and negative sequences

Solution

$$T = \text{Insulation thickness}$$

$$= \frac{175\,\text{mils}}{1000} = 0.175\,\text{in.}$$

where
d = conductor diameter = 0.539 in.
$D = d + 2T = 0.539 + 2 \times 0.175 = 0.889$ in.
G = geometric factor from Figure 5.23
   = 0.5

or, by using Equation 5.68,

$$G = 2.303 \log_{10} \frac{D}{d}$$

$$= 2.303 \log_{10} \frac{0.889}{0.539} = 0.5005$$

Since the conductors are compact sector type, from Table 5.3, for

$$\frac{T + t}{d} = 0.3247$$

the sector factor is found to be 0.710.

(a) By using Equation 5.161,

$$C_0 = C_1 = C_2 = \frac{0.0892K}{G} \; \mu\text{F/mi/phase}$$

$$= \frac{0.0892 \times 3.7}{0.5005 \times 0.710} = 0.93 \; \mu\text{F/mi/phase}$$

(b) By using Equation 5.162,

$$X_0 = X_1 = X_2 = \frac{1.79G}{f \times K} \; \text{M}\Omega/\text{mi/phase}$$

$$= \frac{1.79 \times 0.5005 \times 0.710}{60 \times 3.7}$$

$$= 2.86 \; \text{k}\Omega/\text{mi/phase}$$

(c) By using Equation 5.163,

$$I_0 = I_1 = I_2 = \frac{0.323 \times f \times K \times V_{(L-N)}}{1000 \times G} \text{ A/mi/phase}$$

$$= \frac{0.323 \times 60 \times 3.7 \times (13.8/\sqrt{3})}{1000 \times 0.5005 \times 0.710}$$

$$= 1.609 \text{ A/mi/phase}$$

5.9 CURRENT-CARRYING CAPACITY OF CABLES

Tables A.12 through A.19 give current-carrying capacities of paper-insulated cables. The earth temperature is assumed to be uniform and at 20°C. In general, the calculation of ampacities of cables is very complex due to the characteristics of the thermal circuit, skin and proximity effects, and the nature of the insulation.

5.10 CALCULATION OF IMPEDANCES OF CABLES IN PARALLEL

5.10.1 SINGLE-CONDUCTOR CABLES

Figure 5.31 shows a three-phase circuit consisting of three single-conductor cables with concentric neutrals. Therefore, there are six circuits, each with ground return, three for the phase conductors and three for the concentric neutrals. Here x, y, and z indicate the concentric neutrals, and a, b, and c indicate the phases.

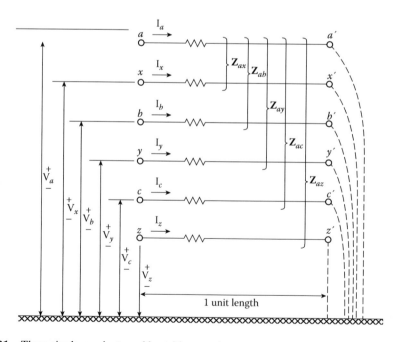

FIGURE 5.31   Three single-conductor cables with ground return.

Hence, the voltage drop equations in the direction of current flow can be written as

$$
\begin{bmatrix} \mathbf{V}_a \\ \mathbf{V}_b \\ \mathbf{V}_c \\ \mathbf{V}_x \\ \mathbf{V}_y \\ \mathbf{V}_z \end{bmatrix} = \begin{bmatrix} \mathbf{V}_{aa'} \\ \mathbf{V}_{bb'} \\ \mathbf{V}_{cc'} \\ \mathbf{V}_{xx'} \\ \mathbf{V}_{yy'} \\ \mathbf{V}_{zz'} \end{bmatrix} = \begin{bmatrix} \mathbf{V}_a - \mathbf{V}_{a'} \\ \mathbf{V}_b - \mathbf{V}_{b'} \\ \mathbf{V}_c - \mathbf{V}_{c'} \\ \mathbf{V}_x - \mathbf{V}_{x'} \\ \mathbf{V}_y - \mathbf{V}_{y'} \\ \mathbf{V}_z - \mathbf{V}_{z'} \end{bmatrix} = \begin{bmatrix} \mathbf{Z}_{aa} & \mathbf{Z}_{ab} & \mathbf{Z}_{ac} & \mathbf{Z}_{ax} & \mathbf{Z}_{ay} & \mathbf{Z}_{az} \\ \mathbf{Z}_{ba} & \mathbf{Z}_{bb} & \mathbf{Z}_{bc} & \mathbf{Z}_{bx} & \mathbf{Z}_{by} & \mathbf{Z}_{bz} \\ \mathbf{Z}_{ca} & \mathbf{Z}_{cb} & \mathbf{Z}_{cc} & \mathbf{Z}_{cx} & \mathbf{Z}_{cy} & \mathbf{Z}_{cz} \\ \mathbf{Z}_{xa} & \mathbf{Z}_{xb} & \mathbf{Z}_{xc} & \mathbf{Z}_{xx} & \mathbf{Z}_{xy} & \mathbf{Z}_{xz} \\ \mathbf{Z}_{ya} & \mathbf{Z}_{yb} & \mathbf{Z}_{yc} & \mathbf{Z}_{yx} & \mathbf{Z}_{yy} & \mathbf{Z}_{yz} \\ \mathbf{Z}_{za} & \mathbf{Z}_{zb} & \mathbf{Z}_{zc} & \mathbf{Z}_{zx} & \mathbf{Z}_{zy} & \mathbf{Z}_{zz} \end{bmatrix} \begin{bmatrix} \mathbf{I}_a \\ \mathbf{I}_b \\ \mathbf{I}_c \\ \mathbf{I}_x \\ \mathbf{I}_y \\ \mathbf{I}_z \end{bmatrix}
\tag{5.171}
$$

By taking advantage of symmetry, the voltage matrix equation (5.171) can be written in partitioned form as

$$
\begin{bmatrix} \mathbf{V}_{abc} \\ \hline \mathbf{V}_{xyz} \end{bmatrix} = \begin{bmatrix} \mathbf{Z}_S & \mathbf{Z}_M \\ \hline \mathbf{Z}_M^t & \mathbf{Z}_N \end{bmatrix} \begin{bmatrix} \mathbf{I}_{abc} \\ \mathbf{I}_{xyz} \end{bmatrix}
\tag{5.172}
$$

where

$$
\mathbf{Z}_s = \begin{bmatrix} \mathbf{Z}_{aa} & \mathbf{Z}_{ab} & \mathbf{Z}_{ac} \\ \mathbf{Z}_{ba} & \mathbf{Z}_{bb} & \mathbf{Z}_{bc} \\ \mathbf{Z}_{ca} & \mathbf{Z}_{cb} & \mathbf{Z}_{cc} \end{bmatrix}
\tag{5.173}
$$

$$
\mathbf{Z}_N = \begin{bmatrix} \mathbf{Z}_{xx} & \mathbf{Z}_{xy} & \mathbf{Z}_{xz} \\ \mathbf{Z}_{yx} & \mathbf{Z}_{yy} & \mathbf{Z}_{yz} \\ \mathbf{Z}_{zx} & \mathbf{Z}_{zy} & \mathbf{Z}_{zz} \end{bmatrix}
\tag{5.174}
$$

$$
\mathbf{Z}_M = \begin{bmatrix} \mathbf{Z}_{ax} & \mathbf{Z}_{ay} & \mathbf{Z}_{az} \\ \mathbf{Z}_{bx} & \mathbf{Z}_{by} & \mathbf{Z}_{bz} \\ \mathbf{Z}_{cx} & \mathbf{Z}_{cy} & \mathbf{Z}_{cz} \end{bmatrix}
\tag{5.175}
$$

and

$$
\mathbf{Z}_M^t = \begin{bmatrix} \mathbf{Z}_{xa} & \mathbf{Z}_{xb} & \mathbf{Z}_{xc} \\ \mathbf{Z}_{ya} & \mathbf{Z}_{yb} & \mathbf{Z}_{yc} \\ \mathbf{Z}_{za} & \mathbf{Z}_{zb} & \mathbf{Z}_{zc} \end{bmatrix}
\tag{5.176}
$$

Since the $[\mathbf{V}_{xyz}]$ submatrix for the voltage drops in the neutral conductors to ground will be a zero matrix due to having all its terms zero, Equation 5.172 can be rewritten as

$$
\begin{bmatrix} \mathbf{V}_{abc} \\ \hline 0 \end{bmatrix} = \begin{bmatrix} \mathbf{Z}_S & \mathbf{Z}_M \\ \hline \mathbf{Z}_M^t & \mathbf{Z}_N \end{bmatrix} \begin{bmatrix} \mathbf{I}_{abc} \\ \mathbf{I}_{xyz} \end{bmatrix}
\tag{5.177}
$$

By Kron reduction,

$$\left[\mathbf{V}_{abc}\right] = \left[\mathbf{Z}_{new}\right]\left[\mathbf{I}_{abc}\right] \tag{5.178}$$

where

$$\left[\mathbf{Z}_{new}\right] = \left[\mathbf{Z}_S\right] - \left[\mathbf{Z}_M\right]\left[\mathbf{Z}_N\right]^{-1}\left[\mathbf{Z}_M^t\right] \tag{5.179}$$

Once the impedance matrix for the three-phase cable configuration is known, the sequence impedances can be computed by similarity transformation as

$$\left[\mathbf{Z}_{012}\right] = \left[\mathbf{A}\right]^{-1}\left[\mathbf{Z}_{new}\right]\left[\mathbf{A}\right] \tag{5.180}$$

where

$$\left[\mathbf{A}\right]^{-1} = \frac{1}{3}\begin{bmatrix} 1 & 1 & 1 \\ 1 & a & a^2 \\ 1 & a^2 & a \end{bmatrix} \tag{5.181}$$

and

$$\left[\mathbf{A}\right] = \begin{bmatrix} 1 & 1 & 1 \\ 1 & a^2 & a \\ 1 & a & a^2 \end{bmatrix} \tag{5.182}$$

and

$$\left[\mathbf{Z}_{012}\right] = \begin{bmatrix} \mathbf{Z}_{00} & \mathbf{Z}_{01} & \mathbf{Z}_{02} \\ \mathbf{Z}_{10} & \mathbf{Z}_{11} & \mathbf{Z}_{12} \\ \mathbf{Z}_{20} & \mathbf{Z}_{21} & \mathbf{Z}_{22} \end{bmatrix} \tag{5.183}$$

where the diagonal elements ($\mathbf{Z}_{00}$, $\mathbf{Z}_{11}$, and $\mathbf{Z}_{22}$) are self-impedances, or simply the sequence impedances, and the off-diagonal elements ($\mathbf{Z}_{01}$, $\mathbf{Z}_{02}$, or $\mathbf{Z}_{12}$) are mutual impedances. For completely symmetrical or transposed circuits, the mutual terms are all zero.

Thus, the sequence voltage drops can be computed from

$$[\mathbf{V}_{012}] = [\mathbf{Z}_{012}][\mathbf{I}_{012}] \tag{5.184}$$

or

$$\begin{bmatrix} \mathbf{V}_{0(a)} \\ \mathbf{V}_{1(a)} \\ \mathbf{V}_{2(a)} \end{bmatrix} = \begin{bmatrix} \mathbf{Z}_{00} & \mathbf{Z}_{01} & \mathbf{Z}_{02} \\ \mathbf{Z}_{10} & \mathbf{Z}_{11} & \mathbf{Z}_{12} \\ \mathbf{Z}_{20} & \mathbf{Z}_{21} & \mathbf{Z}_{22} \end{bmatrix}\begin{bmatrix} \mathbf{I}_{0(a)} \\ \mathbf{I}_{1(a)} \\ \mathbf{I}_{2(a)} \end{bmatrix} \tag{5.185}$$

where

$$\left[\mathbf{V}_{012}\right] = \left[\mathbf{A}\right]^{-1}\left[\mathbf{V}_{abc}\right] \tag{5.186}$$

or

$$\begin{bmatrix} \mathbf{V}_{0(a)} \\ \mathbf{V}_{1(a)} \\ \mathbf{V}_{2(a)} \end{bmatrix} = \frac{1}{3} \begin{bmatrix} 1 & 1 & 1 \\ 1 & a & a^2 \\ 1 & a^2 & a \end{bmatrix} \begin{bmatrix} \mathbf{V}_a \\ \mathbf{V}_b \\ \mathbf{V}_c \end{bmatrix} \tag{5.187}$$

and

$$[\mathbf{I}_{012}] = [\mathbf{A}]^{-1} [\mathbf{I}_{abc}] \tag{5.188}$$

or

$$\begin{bmatrix} \mathbf{I}_{0(a)} \\ \mathbf{I}_{1(a)} \\ \mathbf{I}_{2(a)} \end{bmatrix} = \frac{1}{3} \begin{bmatrix} 1 & 1 & 1 \\ 1 & a & a^2 \\ 1 & a^2 & a \end{bmatrix} \begin{bmatrix} \mathbf{I}_a \\ \mathbf{I}_b \\ \mathbf{I}_c \end{bmatrix} \tag{5.189}$$

However, when the three conductors involved are identical and the circuit is completely symmetrical or transposed so that the mutual impedances between phases are identical, that is,

$$\mathbf{Z}_{ab} = \mathbf{Z}_{bc} = \mathbf{Z}_{ca}$$

the expressions to calculate the sequence impedances directly are

$$\mathbf{Z}_{00} = \mathbf{Z}_{aa} + 2\mathbf{Z}_{ab} - \frac{\left(\mathbf{Z}_{ax} + 2\mathbf{Z}_{ab}\right)^2}{\mathbf{Z}_{xx} + 2\mathbf{Z}_{ab}} \tag{5.190}$$

and

$$\mathbf{Z}_{11} = \mathbf{Z}_{22} = \mathbf{Z}_{aa} - \mathbf{Z}_{ab} - \frac{\left(\mathbf{Z}_{ax} - \mathbf{Z}_{ab}\right)^2}{\mathbf{Z}_{xx} - \mathbf{Z}_{ab}} \tag{5.191}$$

in which case Equation 5.183 becomes

$$[\mathbf{Z}_{012}] = \begin{bmatrix} \mathbf{Z}_{00} & 0 & 0 \\ 0 & \mathbf{Z}_{11} & 0 \\ 0 & 0 & \mathbf{Z}_{22} \end{bmatrix} \tag{5.192}$$

In case of distribution cables, Equations 5.190 and 5.191 are also valid for the asymmetrical case if the average value $\mathbf{Z}_{ab}$ in the equations is set equal to

$$\mathbf{Z}_{ab(\text{avg})} = \mathbf{Z} = \frac{1}{3}(\mathbf{Z}_{ab} + \mathbf{Z}_{bc} + \mathbf{Z}_{ca}) \tag{5.193}$$

When the concentric neutral conductors are not present or open-circuited, the neutral currents are zero:

$$[\mathbf{I}_{xyz}] = [0]$$

Therefore, the sequence impedance can be calculated from

$$\mathbf{Z}_{00} = \mathbf{Z}_{aa} + 2\mathbf{Z}_{ab} \tag{5.194}$$

$$\mathbf{Z}_{11} = \mathbf{Z}_{22} = \mathbf{Z}_{aa} - \mathbf{Z}_{ab} \tag{5.195}$$

When the neutral conductors are connected together but not grounded, if the circuit is completely symmetrical or transposed, the positive- and negative-sequence impedances are not affected due to lack of ground return current. However, in the case of zero sequence, due to symmetry,

$$\mathbf{I}_{0(x)} = \mathbf{I}_{0(y)} = \mathbf{I}_{0(z)} = -\mathbf{I}_{0(a)} = -\mathbf{I}_{0(b)}$$

$$= -\mathbf{I}_{0(c)} = -1 \tag{5.196}$$

Thus, in Equation 5.7, the matrix $[\mathbf{V}_{xyz}]$ is not a null matrix, that is,

$$[\mathbf{V}_{xyz}] \neq [0]$$

Hence,

$$\mathbf{Z}_{00} = \mathbf{Z}_{aa} + \mathbf{Z}_{xx} - 2\mathbf{Z}_{ax} \tag{5.197}$$

which is the same as the impedance of a single conductor with its own neutral. If the conductor arrangement is not a symmetrical one, the usage of Equation 5.197 to calculate zero-sequence impedance would still be valid.

5.10.2 BUNDLED SINGLE-CONDUCTOR CABLES

At times, it might be necessary to use two three-phase cable circuits to connect a sending bus to a receiving one, as shown in Figure 5.32. Each phase has two paralleled and unsheathed (or with open-circuited sheaths) single conductors. There is no ground return current. Therefore, before *bundling*, that is, connecting two conductors per phase, the voltage drop equations can be expressed as

$$
\begin{bmatrix} \mathbf{V}_a \\ \mathbf{V}_b \\ \mathbf{V}_c \\ \mathbf{V}_x \\ \mathbf{V}_y \\ \mathbf{V}_z \end{bmatrix} = \begin{bmatrix} \mathbf{Z}_{aa} & \mathbf{Z}_{ab} & \mathbf{Z}_{ac} & \mathbf{Z}_{ax} & \mathbf{Z}_{ay} & \mathbf{Z}_{az} \\ \mathbf{Z}_{ba} & \mathbf{Z}_{bb} & \mathbf{Z}_{bc} & \mathbf{Z}_{bx} & \mathbf{Z}_{by} & \mathbf{Z}_{bz} \\ \mathbf{Z}_{ca} & \mathbf{Z}_{cb} & \mathbf{Z}_{cc} & \mathbf{Z}_{cx} & \mathbf{Z}_{cy} & \mathbf{Z}_{cz} \\ \mathbf{Z}_{xa} & \mathbf{Z}_{xb} & \mathbf{Z}_{xc} & \mathbf{Z}_{xx} & \mathbf{Z}_{xy} & \mathbf{Z}_{xz} \\ \mathbf{Z}_{ya} & \mathbf{Z}_{yb} & \mathbf{Z}_{yc} & \mathbf{Z}_{yx} & \mathbf{Z}_{yy} & \mathbf{Z}_{yz} \\ \mathbf{Z}_{za} & \mathbf{Z}_{zb} & \mathbf{Z}_{zc} & \mathbf{Z}_{zx} & \mathbf{Z}_{zy} & \mathbf{Z}_{zz} \end{bmatrix} \begin{bmatrix} \mathbf{I}_a \\ \mathbf{I}_b \\ \mathbf{I}_c \\ \mathbf{I}_x \\ \mathbf{I}_y \\ \mathbf{I}_z \end{bmatrix} \quad \text{V/unit/length} \tag{5.198}
$$

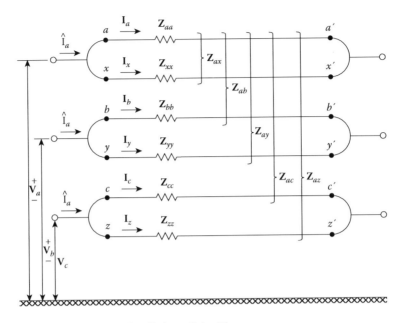

FIGURE 5.32 Equivalent circuit for bundled parallel cables.

The assumption of not having ground return current simplifies the calculation of the self-impedance and mutual impedance elements of the impedance matrix.

Self-impedances:

$$Z_{aa} = l(r_a + jX_a) \ \Omega \tag{5.199}$$

where

$$X_a = j0.1213 \ \ln \frac{12}{D_s} \ \Omega/\text{mi} \tag{5.200}$$

where
   r_a is the ac resistance of conductor a in ohms per mile
   X_a is the reactance of individual phase conductor at 12 in. spacing in ohms per mile
   D_s is the GMR or self-GMD of conductor a in inches

Based on the respective conductor characteristics, the self-impedances for conductors b, c, r, x, y, and z can be computed in a similar manner.

Mutual impedances:

$$\mathbf{Z}_{ab} = l\left(0.1213 \ \ln \frac{12}{D_{eq}} \right)$$

$$= jl \times X_d \ \Omega/\text{mi} \tag{5.201}$$

where D_{eq} is the equivalent, or geometric, mean distance among conductor centers in inches; based on the D_{eq}, other mutual impedances can be calculated similarly.

After bundling, the constraining equations can be written as

$$\mathbf{V}_x - \mathbf{V}_a = 0$$
$$\mathbf{V}_y - \mathbf{V}_b = 0 \qquad\qquad (5.202)$$
$$\mathbf{V}_x - \mathbf{V}_a = 0$$

and it is also possible to define

$$\hat{\mathbf{I}}_a = \mathbf{I}_a + \mathbf{I}_x$$
$$\hat{\mathbf{I}}_b = \mathbf{I}_b + \mathbf{I}_y \qquad\qquad (5.203)$$
$$\hat{\mathbf{I}}_c = \mathbf{I}_c + \mathbf{I}_z$$

By taking advantage of symmetry, the voltage matrix equation (5.198) can be expressed in partitioned form as

$$\left[\begin{array}{c} \mathbf{V}_{abc} \\ \hline \mathbf{V}_{xyz} \end{array} \right] = \left[\begin{array}{c|c} \mathbf{Z}_S & \mathbf{Z}_M \\ \hline \mathbf{Z}_M^t & \mathbf{Z}_N \end{array} \right] \left[\begin{array}{c} \mathbf{I}_{abc} \\ \hline \mathbf{I}_{xyz} \end{array} \right] \qquad (5.204)$$

If the bundled cabled did not consist of two identical cables, the two $[\mathbf{Z}_s]$ matrices would be different. When the $\mathbf{V}_x$, $\mathbf{V}_y$, and $\mathbf{V}_z$ equations in (5.25) are replaced by a new equation calculated from equation set (5.202) and the $\mathbf{I}_{abc}$ submatrix is replaced by $\hat{\mathbf{I}}_{abc}$,

$$\left[\begin{array}{c} \mathbf{V}_a \\ \mathbf{V}_b \\ \mathbf{V}_c \\ \hline \hat{0} \\ \hat{0} \\ \hat{0} \end{array} \right] = \left[\begin{array}{ccc|ccc} \mathbf{Z}_{aa} & \mathbf{Z}_{ab} & \mathbf{Z}_{ac} & \mathbf{Z}_{ax} - \mathbf{Z}_{aa} & \mathbf{Z}_{ay} - \mathbf{Z}_{ab} & \mathbf{Z}_{ax} - \mathbf{Z}_{ac} \\ \mathbf{Z}_{ba} & \mathbf{Z}_{bb} & \mathbf{Z}_{bc} & \mathbf{Z}_{bx} - \mathbf{Z}_{ba} & \mathbf{Z}_{by} - \mathbf{Z}_{bb} & \mathbf{Z}_{bz} - \mathbf{Z}_{bc} \\ \mathbf{Z}_{ca} & \mathbf{Z}_{cb} & \mathbf{Z}_{cc} & \mathbf{Z}_{cx} - \mathbf{Z}_{ca} & \mathbf{Z}_{cy} - \mathbf{Z}_{cb} & \mathbf{Z}_{cz} - \mathbf{Z}_{cc} \\ \hline \mathbf{Z}_{xa} - \mathbf{Z}_{aa} & \mathbf{Z}_{xb} - \mathbf{Z}_{ab} & \mathbf{Z}_{xc} - \mathbf{Z}_{ac} & \hat{\mathbf{Z}}_{xx} & \hat{\mathbf{Z}}_{xy} & \hat{\mathbf{Z}}_{xz} \\ \mathbf{Z}_{ya} - \mathbf{Z}_{ba} & \mathbf{Z}_{yb} - \mathbf{Z}_{bb} & \mathbf{Z}_{yc} - \mathbf{Z}_{bc} & \hat{\mathbf{Z}}_{yx} & \hat{\mathbf{Z}}_{yy} & \hat{\mathbf{Z}}_{yz} \\ \mathbf{Z}_{za} - \mathbf{Z}_{ca} & \mathbf{Z}_{zb} - \mathbf{Z}_{cb} & \mathbf{Z}_{zc} - \mathbf{Z}_{cc} & \hat{\mathbf{Z}}_{zx} & \hat{\mathbf{Z}}_{zy} & \hat{\mathbf{Z}}_{zz} \end{array} \right] \left[\begin{array}{c} \mathbf{I}_a + \mathbf{I}_x \\ \mathbf{I}_b + \mathbf{I}_y \\ \mathbf{I}_c + \mathbf{I}_z \\ \hline \hat{\mathbf{I}}_x \\ \hat{\mathbf{I}}_y \\ \hat{\mathbf{I}}_z \end{array} \right]$$

$$(5.205)$$

where all elements in the lower right position can be computed from

$$\hat{\mathbf{Z}}_{pq} = \mathbf{Z}_{pq} - \mathbf{Z}_{iq} - \mathbf{Z}_{pk} + \mathbf{Z}_{ik} \qquad\qquad (5.206)$$

where $i, k = a, b, c$, and $p, q = x, y, z$ or, in matrix notation,

$$\left[\begin{array}{c} \mathbf{V}_{abc} \\ \hline 0 \end{array} \right] = \left[\begin{array}{c|c} \mathbf{Z}_s & \mathbf{Z}_m - \mathbf{Z}_s \\ \hline \mathbf{Z}_m^t - \mathbf{Z}_s & \mathbf{Z}_k \end{array} \right] \left[\begin{array}{c} \hat{\mathbf{I}}_{abc} \\ \hline \mathbf{I}_{xyz} \end{array} \right] \qquad (5.207)$$

where

$$[\mathbf{Z}_k] = [\mathbf{Z}_s] - [\mathbf{Z}_m] - \{[\mathbf{Z}_m]^t - [\mathbf{Z}_s]\} \qquad\qquad (5.208)$$

By Kron reduction,

$$[\mathbf{V}_{abc}] = [\mathbf{Z}_{new}][\mathbf{I}_{abc}]$$

where

$$[\mathbf{Z}_{new}] = [\mathbf{Z}_s] - \{[\mathbf{Z}_m] - [\mathbf{Z}_s]\}[\mathbf{Z}_k]^{-1}\{[\mathbf{Z}_m]^t - [\mathbf{Z}_s]\} \qquad (5.209)$$

Therefore, the sequence impedances and sequence voltage drops can be computed from

$$\left[\mathbf{Z}_{012}\right] = \left[\mathbf{A}\right]^{-1}\left[\mathbf{Z}_{new}\right]\left[\mathbf{A}\right] \qquad (5.210)$$

and

$$[\mathbf{V}_{012}] = [\mathbf{Z}_{012}][\mathbf{I}_{012}] \qquad (5.211)$$

respectively.

Example 5.12

A three-phase, 60 Hz bundled cable circuit is connected between a sending bus and a receiving bus using six single-conductor unsheathed cables as shown in Figures 5.32 and 5.33. Each phase has two paralleled single conductors. There is no ground return current. The cable circuit operates at 35 kV and 60 Hz. All of the single-conductor cables are of 350 kcmil copper, concentric strand, paper insulated, 10 mi long, and spaced 18 in. apart from each other, as shown in Figure 5.33. Assume that the conductor resistance is 0.19 Ω/mi and the GMR of one conductor is 0.262 in. and calculate the following:

(a) Phase impedance matrix $[\mathbf{Z}_{abc}]$
(b) Sequence impedance matrix $[\mathbf{Z}_{012}]$

Solution

(a)

$$\mathbf{Z}_{aa} = \mathbf{Z}_{bb} = \mathbf{Z}_{cc} = \cdots \mathbf{Z}_{zz} = l \times (r_a + jX_a)$$

where

$r_a = 0.19\ \Omega/\text{mi}$

$X_a = j0.1213\ \ln\dfrac{12}{D_s}$

$\qquad = j0.1213\ \ln\dfrac{12}{D_s} = 0.464\ \Omega/\text{mi}$

Hence,

$$\mathbf{Z}_{aa} = \mathbf{Z}_{bb} = \mathbf{Z}_{zz} = 10(0.19 + j0.464)$$
$$= 1.9 + j4.64\ \Omega$$

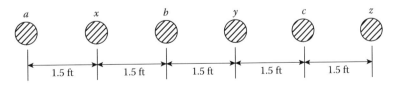

FIGURE 5.33 For Example 5.12.

$$Z_{ab} = Z_{bc} = Z_{xy} = Z_{yz} = -l\left(j0.1213 \ln\frac{12}{D_{eq}}\right)$$

$$= -10\left(j0.1213 \ln\frac{12}{54}\right)$$

$$= -j1.3326 \ \Omega$$

$$Z_{bz} = Z_{ay} = Z_{cx} = Z_{yz} = -10\left(j0.1213 \ln\frac{12}{54}\right)$$

$$= -j1.8214 \ \Omega$$

$$Z_{ac} = -10\left(j0.1213 \ln\frac{12}{72}\right)$$

$$= -j2.1734 \ \Omega$$

$$Z_{ax} = Z_{bx} = Z_{by} = Z_{cy} = Z_{cz} = -10\left(j0.1213 \ln\frac{12}{18}\right)$$

$$= -j0.4918 \ \Omega$$

$$Z_{az} = -10\left(j0.1213 \ln\frac{12}{90}\right)$$

$$= -j2.4441 \ \Omega$$

Therefore,

$$\left[\mathbf{Z}_{abcxyz}\right] = \begin{bmatrix} 1.9 + j4.64 & -j1.3326 & -j2.1734 & -j0.4918 & -j1.8244 & -j2.4441 \\ -j1.3326 & 1.9 + 14.64 & -j1.3326 & -j0.4918 & -j0.4918 & -j1.8244 \\ -j2.1734 & -j1.3326 & 1.9 + j4.64 & -j1.8244 & -j0.4918 & -j0.4918 \\ -j0.4918 & -j0.4918 & -j1.8244 & 1.9 + j4.64 & -j1.3326 & -j2.1734 \\ -j1.8244 & -j0.4918 & -j0.4918 & -j1.3326 & 1.9 + j4.64 & -j1.3326 \\ -j2.4441 & -j1.8244 & -j0.4918 & -j2.1734 & -j1.3326 & 1.9 + j4.64 \end{bmatrix}$$

By Kron reduction,

$$[\mathbf{Z}_{new}] = [\mathbf{Z}_s] - \{[\mathbf{Z}_m] - [\mathbf{Z}_s]\}[\mathbf{Z}_k]^{-1}\{[\mathbf{Z}_m]^t - [\mathbf{Z}_s]\}$$

or

$$\left[\mathbf{Z}_{abc}\right] = \begin{bmatrix} 4.521 + j2.497 & 1.594 - j2.604 & 1.495 - j3.090 \\ 1.594 - j2.604 & 2.897 + j3.802 & 0.930 - j1.929 \\ 1.495 - j3.090 & 0.930 - j1.929 & 2.897 + j3.802 \end{bmatrix}$$

(b) By doing the similarity transformation,

$$[\mathbf{Z}_{012}] = [\mathbf{A}]^{-1}[\mathbf{Z}_{abc}][\mathbf{A}] \ \Omega$$

or

$$\left[\mathbf{Z}_{012}\right] = \begin{bmatrix} 6.118 - j1.716 & 0.887 - j0.770 & 0.606 - j0.713 \\ 0.606 - j0.713 & 2.099 + j5.908 & -0.149 + j0.235 \\ 0.887 - j0.770 & 0.412 + j0.121 & 2.099 + j5.908 \end{bmatrix}$$

5.11 EHV UNDERGROUND CABLE TRANSMISSION

As discussed in the previous sections, the inductive reactance of an OH HVAC line is much greater than its capacitive reactance, whereas the capacitive reactance of an underground HVAC cable is much greater than its inductive reactance due to the fact that the three-phase conductors are located very close to each other in the same cable. The approximate values of the resultant vars (reactive power) that can be generated by ac cables operating at the phase-to-phase voltages of 132, 220, and 400 kV are 2,000, 5,000, and 15,000 kVA/mi, respectively. This var generation, due to the capacitive charging currents, sets a practical limit to the possible noninterrupted length of an underground ac cable.

This situation can be compensated for by installing appropriate inductive shunt reactors along the line. This *critical length* of the cable can be defined as the length of cable line that has a three-phase charging reactive power equal in magnitude to the thermal rating of the cable line. For example, the typical critical lengths of ac cables operating at the phase-to-phase voltages of 132, 200, and 400 kV can be given approximately as 40, 25, and 15 mi, respectively.

The study done by Schifreen and Marble [9] illustrated the limitations in the operation of HVAC cable lines due to the charging current. For example, Figure 5.34 shows that the magnitude of the maximum permissible power output decreases as a result of an increase in cable length. Figure 5.35 shows that increasing lengths of cable line can transmit full-rated current (1.0 pu) only if the load

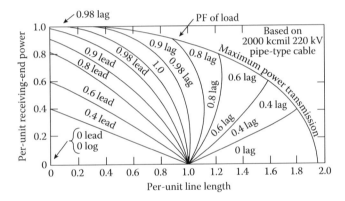

FIGURE 5.34 Power transmission limits of HVAC cable lines. Curved lines: sending-end current equal to rated or base current of cable. Horizontal lines: receiving-end current equal to rated or base current of cable. (From Schifreen, C.S. and Marble, W.C., Changing current limitations in operation of high-voltage cable lines, *Trans. Am. Inst. Electr. Eng.*, 26, 803–817, 1956. Used with permission. Copyright 1956 IEEE.)

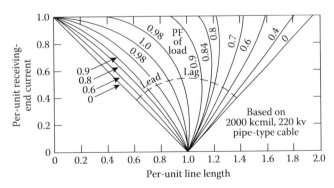

FIGURE 5.35 Receiving-end current limits of HVAC cable lines. Curved lines: sending-end current equal to rated or base current of cable. (From Schifreen, C.S. and Marble, W.C., Changing current limitations in operation of high-voltage cable lines, *Trans. Am. Inst. Electr. Eng.*, 26, 803–817, 1956. Used with permission. Copyright 1956 IEEE.)

TABLE 5.7
Characteristics of 345 kV Pipe-Type Cable

Characteristics	Maximum Electric Stress (300 V/mil) — Power Factor (%)				Maximum Electric Stress (350 V/mil) — Power Factor (%)			
Conductor size, thousand (cmils)	1000	1250	1500	2000	1000	1230	1300	2000
Insulation thickness, mils	1250	1173	1110	1035	980	915	885	835
E_R kV, 200 kV								
I_T A (0.3)	383 / 653	638 / 721	680 / 780	730 / 860	576 / 637	623 / 724	636 / 776	688 / 847
Rated three-phase MVA (0.3)	350 / 390	381 / 431	406 / 466	436 / 516	344 / 393	372 / 432	392 / 463	413 / 508
Z Ω/mi	0.403 ∠78.0	0.381 ∠78.8	0.363 ∠80.0	0.338 ∠80.0	0.377 ∠77.2	0.355 ∠78.5	0.367 ∠79.4	0.319 ∠80.0
Y S (mi ×10^{-4})	1.08 ∠89.7	1.20 ∠89.7	1.32 ∠89.7	1.53 ∠89.7	1.26 ∠89.7	1.41 ∠89.7	1.54 ∠89.7	1.78 ∠89.7
A numeric/mi ×10^{-8}	6.6 ∠83.9	6.8 ∠84.3	6.9 ∠84.9	7.19 ∠84.8	6.9 ∠83.5	7.1 ∠84.1	7.5 ∠84.6	7.54 ∠84.8
Z_0 Ω	61.2 ∠5.9	56.4 ∠5.5	52.5 ∠4.9	67.1 ∠6.9	54.7 ∠6.3	50.1 ∠3.6	48.9 ∠3.2	42.3 ∠4.9
0 A/mi	21.6	24.1	26.5	30.5	25.1	28.1	30.8	3.37
3Φ charging kVA/mi	12,900	14,400	13,800	18,300	15,000	16,800	18,000	21,300
S_4 (mi) (0.5 / 0.3)	27.1 / 30.3	26.5 / 30.0	25.7 / 29.3	24.0 / 28.2	22.9 / 26.2	22.2 / 25.7	21.3 / 25.2	19.4 / 23.9
Nominal pipe size (in)								
10^8/in earth resistivity (thermal ohm cm)	80	80	80	80	80	80	80	80
Conductor temperature (°C)	70	70	70	70	70	70	70	70
3Φ dielectric loss (W/ft) (0.5 / 0.3)	12.2 / 7.3	13.7 / 81	14.9 / 9.0	17.3 / 10.3	14.2 / 8.5	15.8 / 9.5	17.3 / 10.4	20.1 / 12.0
3Φ total loss (w/ft) (0.5 / 0.3)	29.0 / 28.3	30.8 / 29.9	32.2 / 31.8	34.3 / 33.8	30.5 / 29.7	32.1 / 31.5	33.5 / 33.0	35.2 / 34.8
Ratio watts dielectric loss Φ totla loss (0.5 / 0.3)	42.0 / 38.8	44.5 / 36.9	46.0 / 35.3	50.5 / 30.5	46.3 / 35.0	49.3 / 33.1	52.6 / 31.7	37.0 / 34.5

Source: Wiseman, R.T., Discussions to charging current limitations in operation of high-voltage cable lines, *Trans. Am. Inst. Electr. Eng.*, 26, 803–817, 1956. Used with permission. Copyright (1956) IEEE.

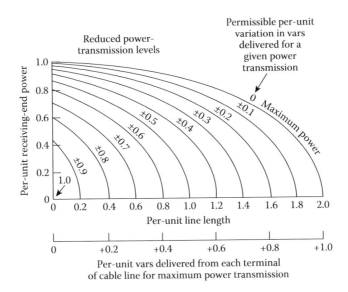

FIGURE 5.36   Permissible variations in per-unit vars delivered to electric system at each terminal of ac cable line for given power transmission. (From Schifreen, C.S. and Marble, W.C., Changing current limitations in operation of high-voltage cable lines, *Trans. Am. Inst. Electr. Eng.*, 26, 803–817, 1956. Used with permission. Copyright 1956 IEEE.)

power factor is decreased to resolve lagging values. Note that the critical length is used as the base length in the figures. Table 5.7 [10] gives characteristics of a 345 kV pipe-type cable. Figure 5.36 shows the permissible variation in per-unit vars delivered to the electric system at each terminal of cable line for a given power transmission.

Example 5.13

Consider an HV open-circuit three-phase insulated power cable of length l shown in Figure 5.37. Assume that a fixed sending-end voltage is to be supplied; the receiving-end voltage floats, and it is an overvoltage. Furthermore, assume that at some critical length ($l = l_0$), the sending-end current $\mathbf{I}_S$ is equal to the ampacity of the cable circuit, $\mathbf{I}_{l0}$. Therefore, if the cable length is l_0, no load, whatever of 1.0 or leading power factor, can be supplied without overloading the sending end of the cable. Use the general long-transmission-line equations, which are valid for steady-state sinusoidal operation, and verify that the approximate critical length can be expressed as

$$l_0 \cong \frac{I_{l0}}{V_s b}$$

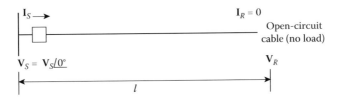

FIGURE 5.37   For Example 5.13.

Solution

The long-transmission-line equations can be expressed as

$$\mathbf{V}_S = \mathbf{V}_R \cosh \gamma l + \mathbf{I}_R \mathbf{Z}_C \sinh \gamma l \tag{5.212}$$

and

$$\mathbf{I}_S = \mathbf{I}_R \cosh \gamma l + \mathbf{V}_R \mathbf{Y}_C \sinh \gamma l \tag{5.213}$$

Since at critical length, $l = l_0$ and

$$\mathbf{I}_R = 0 \quad \text{and} \quad \mathbf{I}_S = \mathbf{I}_{l0}$$

from Equation 5.379, the sending-end current can be expressed as

$$\mathbf{I}_{l0} = \mathbf{V}_R \mathbf{Y}_c \sinh \gamma l_0 \tag{5.214}$$

or

$$\mathbf{I}_{l0} = \mathbf{V}_R \mathbf{Y}_c \left(\frac{e^{\gamma l_0} - e^{-\gamma l_0}}{2} \right) \tag{5.215}$$

$$\mathbf{I}_{l0} = \mathbf{V}_R \mathbf{Y}_c \left(\frac{\left[1 + \gamma l_0 + \left(\gamma l_0 \right)^2 / 2! + \cdots \right] - \left[1 - \gamma l_0 + \left(\gamma l_0 \right)^2 / 2! - \cdots \right]}{2} \right)$$

or

$$\mathbf{I}_{l0} = \mathbf{V}_R \mathbf{Y}_c \left(\gamma l_0 + \frac{\left(\gamma l_0 \right)^3}{3!} + \cdots \right) \tag{5.216}$$

Neglecting $(\gamma l_0)^3/3!$ and higher powers of γl_0,

$$\mathbf{I}_{l0} = \mathbf{V}_R \mathbf{Y}_c \gamma l_0 \tag{5.217}$$

Similarly, from Equation 5.378, the sending-end voltage for the critical length can be expressed as

$$\mathbf{V}_S = \mathbf{V}_R \cosh \gamma l_0 \tag{5.218}$$

or

$$\mathbf{V}_S = \mathbf{V}_R \left(\frac{e^{\gamma l_0} + e^{-\gamma l_0}}{2} \right) \tag{5.219}$$

or

$$\mathbf{V}_S = \mathbf{V}_R \left(\frac{\left[1 + \gamma l_0 + \left(\gamma l_0 \right)^2 / 2! + \cdots \right] + \left[1 - \gamma l_0 + \left(\gamma l_0 \right)^2 / 2! - \cdots \right]}{2} \right)$$

or

$$\mathbf{V}_S = \mathbf{V}_R \left(1 + \frac{\left(\gamma l_0 \right)^2}{2!} + \cdots \right) \tag{5.220}$$

Neglecting higher powers of γl_0,

$$\mathbf{V}_S \cong \mathbf{V}_R \left(1 + \frac{\left(\gamma l_0 \right)^2}{2!} \right) \tag{5.221}$$

Therefore,

$$\mathbf{V}_R = \frac{\mathbf{V}_S}{1 + \dfrac{\left(\gamma l_0 \right)^2}{2!} + \cdots} \tag{5.222}$$

Substituting Equation 5.222 into Equation 5.218,

$$\mathbf{I}_{l0} = \left(\frac{\mathbf{V}_S}{1 + \dfrac{\left(\gamma l_0 \right)^2}{2!} + \cdots} \right) \mathbf{Y}_c \gamma l_0 \tag{5.223}$$

or

$$\mathbf{I}_{l0} = \mathbf{V}_S \mathbf{Y}_c \gamma l_0 \left(1 + \frac{\left(\gamma l_0 \right)^2}{2!} \right)^{-1}$$

$$= \mathbf{V}_S \mathbf{Y}_c \gamma l_0 \left(1 - \frac{\left(\gamma l_0 \right)^2}{2!} + \cdots \right) \tag{5.224}$$

or

$$\mathbf{I}_{l0} = \mathbf{V}_S \mathbf{Y}_c \gamma l_0 - \frac{\mathbf{V}_S \mathbf{Y}_c \left(\gamma l_0 \right)^3}{2!} \tag{5.225}$$

Neglecting the second term,

$$\mathbf{I}_{l0} \cong \mathbf{V}_S \mathbf{Y}_c \gamma l_0 \tag{5.226}$$

Therefore, the critical length can be expressed as

$$l_0 \cong \frac{\mathbf{I}_{I0}}{\mathbf{V}_S\mathbf{Y}_c\gamma} \tag{5.227}$$

where

$$\mathbf{Y}_c = \sqrt{\frac{\mathbf{y}}{\mathbf{z}}}$$

$$\gamma = \sqrt{\mathbf{z} \times \mathbf{y}}$$

Thus,

$$\mathbf{y} = \mathbf{Y}_c\gamma \tag{5.228}$$

or

$$\mathbf{y} = g + jb \tag{5.229}$$

Therefore, the critical length can be expressed as

$$l_0 \cong \frac{\mathbf{I}_{I0}}{\mathbf{V}_S \times \mathbf{y}} \tag{5.230}$$

or

$$l_0 \cong \frac{\mathbf{I}_{I0}}{\mathbf{V}_S \times g + jb} \tag{5.231}$$

Since, for cables, $g \ll b$,

$$\mathbf{y} \cong b \angle 90°$$

and assuming

$$\mathbf{I}_{I0} \cong I_{I0} \angle 90°$$

from Equation 5.231, the critical length can be expressed as

$$l_0 \cong \frac{\mathbf{I}_{I0}}{\mathbf{V}_S \times b} \tag{5.232}$$

Example 5.14

Figure 5.38a shows an open-circuit HV-insulated ac underground cable circuit. The critical length of uncompensated cable is l_0 to for which $\mathbf{I}_S = \mathbf{I}_0$ is equal to cable ampacity rating. Note that $Q_0 = 3V_S I_0$, where the sending-end voltage $\mathbf{V}_S$ is regulated and the receiving-end voltage $\mathbf{V}_R$ floats. Here, the $|\mathbf{V}_R|$ differs little from $|\mathbf{V}_S|$ because of the low series inductive reactance of cables. Based on the given information, investigate the performances with $\mathbf{I}_R = 0$ (i.e., *zero load*):

(a) Assume that one shunt inductive reactor sized to absorb Q_0 magnetizing vars is to be purchased and installed as shown in Figure 5.38b. Locate the reactor by specifying l_1 and l_2 in terms of l_0. Place arrowheads on the four short lines, indicated by a solid line, to show the directions of magnetizing var flows. Also show on each line the amounts of var flow, expressed in terms of Q_0.
(b) Assume that one reactor size $2Q_0$ can be afforded and repeat part (a) on a new diagram.
(c) Assume that two shunt reactors, each of size $2Q_0$, are to be installed, as shown in Figure 5.38c, hoping, as usual, to extend the feasible length of cable. Repeat part (a).

Solution

The answers for parts (a), (b), and (c) are given in Figure 5.39a, b, and c, respectively.

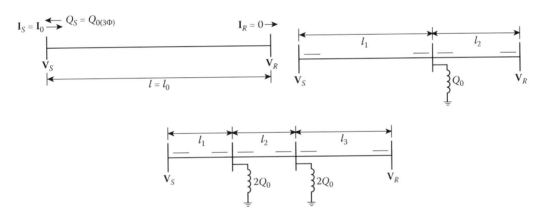

FIGURE 5.38   Insulated HV underground cable circuit for Example 5.14.

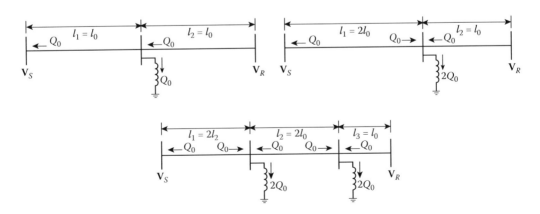

FIGURE 5.39   Solution for Example 5.14.

5.12   GAS-INSULATED TRANSMISSION LINES

The gas-insulated transmission lines (GILs) are a system for transmitting electric power at bulk power ratings over long distances. Its first application has taken place in 1974 to connect the electric generator of a hydro pump storage plant in Germany. For that application of the GIL, a tunnel was built in the mountain for a 420 kV OH line. To this day, a total of more than 100 km of GILs have been built worldwide at HV levels ranging from 135 to 550 kV. The GILs have also been built at power plants having adverse environmental conditions. Thus, in situations where OH lines are not feasible, the GIL may be an acceptable alternative since it provides a solution for a line without reducing transmission capacity under any kinds of climate conditions. This is due to the fact that GIL transmission system is independent of environmental conditions since it is completely sealed inside a metallic enclosure.

Applications of GIL include connecting HV transformers with HV switchgear within power plants, connecting HV transformers inside the cavern power plants to OH lines on the outside, connecting gas-insulated switchgear (GIS) with OH lines, and serving as a bus duct within GIS.

At the beginning, GIL system was only used in special applications due to its high cost. Today, the second-generation GIL system is used for high-power transmission over long distances due to substantial reduction in its cost. This is accomplished not only by its much lower cost but also by the use of N_2–SF_6 gas mixture for electrical insulation. The advantages of GIL system include low losses, low magnetic field emissions, greater reliability with high transmission capacity, no negative impacts on the environment or the landscape, and underground laying with a transmission capacity that is equal to an OH transmission line.

Example 5.15

Consider transmitting 2100 MVA electric power across 50 km by using an OH transmission line versus by using a GIL. The resulting power losses at peak load are 820 and 254 kW/km for the OH transmission and the GILs, respectively. Assume that the annual load factor and the annual power loss factor are the same and are equal to 0.7 for both alternatives. Also assume that the cost of electric energy is $0.10 per kWh. Determine the following:

(a) The power loss of the OH line at peak load.
(b) The power loss of the GIL.
(c) The total annual energy loss of the OH transmission line at peak load.
(d) The total annual energy loss of the GIL at peak load.
(e) The average energy loss of the OH transmission line.
(f) The average energy loss of the GIL at peak load.
(g) The average annual cost of losses of the OH transmission line.
(h) The average annual cost of losses of the GIL.
(i) The annual resultant savings in losses using the GIL.
(j) Find the break-even (or payback) period when the GIL alternative is selected, if the investment cost of the GIL is $200,000,000.

Solution

(a) The power loss of the OH transmission line at peak load is

$$\left(\text{Power loss}\right)_{\text{OH line}} = \left(829 \text{ kW/km}\right)50 \text{ km} = 41,000 \text{ kW}$$

(b) The power loss of the GIL transmission line at peak load is

$$\left(\text{Power loss}\right)_{\text{GIL line}} = \left(254 \text{ kW/km}\right)50 \text{ km} = 12,700 \text{ kW}$$

(c) The total annual energy loss of the OH transmission line at peak load is

$$(\text{Total annual energy loss})_{\text{at peak}} = (41{,}000 \text{ kW})(8760 \text{ h/year})$$
$$= 35{,}916 \times 10^4 \text{ kWh/year}$$

(d) The total annual energy loss of the GIL at peak load is

$$(\text{Total annual energy loss})_{\text{at peak}} = (12{,}700 \text{ kW})(8760 \text{ h/year})$$
$$= 11{,}125.2 \times 10^4 \text{ kWh/year}$$

(e) The total annual energy loss of the OH transmission line at peak load is

$$(\text{Average annual energy loss})_{\text{OH line}} = 0.7(35{,}916 \times 10^4 \text{ kWh/year})$$
$$= 25{,}141.2 \times 10^4 \text{ kWh/year}$$

(f) The average energy loss of the GIL at peak load is

$$(\text{Average annual energy loss})_{\text{GIL line}} = 0.7(11{,}125.2 \text{ kWh/year})$$
$$= 7{,}787.64 \times 10^4 \text{ kWh/year}$$

(g) The average annual cost of losses of the OH transmission line is

$$(\text{Average annual cost of losses})_{\text{OH line}} = (\$0.10/\text{kWh})(25{,}141.2 \times 10^4 \text{ kWh/year})$$
$$= \$25{,}141.2 \times 10^3/\text{year}$$

(h) The average annual cost of losses of the GIL is

$$(\text{Average annual cost of losses})_{\text{GIL line}} = (\$0.10/\text{kWh})(7{,}787.64 \times 10^4 \text{ kWh/year})$$
$$= \$7{,}787.64 \times 10^3/\text{year}$$

(i) The annual resultant savings in power losses using the GIL is

$$\text{Annual savings in losses} = (\text{Annual cost of losses})_{\text{OH line}} - (\text{Annual cost of losses})_{\text{GIL line}}$$
$$= \$25{,}141.2 \times 10^3 - \$7{,}781.64 \times 10^3$$
$$= \$17{,}353.56 \times 10^3/\text{year}$$

(j) If the GIL alternative is selected,

$$\text{Breakeven period} = \frac{\text{Total investment cost}}{\text{Savings per year}}$$
$$= \frac{\$200{,}000{,}000}{\$17{,}353.56 \times 10^3} \cong 11.5 \text{ years}$$

Example 5.16

The NP&NL power utility company is required to build a 500 kV line to serve a nearby town. There are two possible routes for the construction of the necessary power line. Route A is 50 mile long and goes around a lake. It has been estimated that the required OH transmission line will cost $1 million per mile to build and $500 per mile per year to maintain. Its salvage value will be $2000 per mile at the end of 40 years.

On the other hand, route B is 30 mile long and is an underwater (submarine) line that goes across the lake. It has been estimated that the required underwater line using submarine power cables will cost $4 million to build per mile and $1500 per mile per year to maintain. Its salvage value will be $6,000 per mile at the end of 40 years.

It is also possible to use GIL in the route C that goes across the lake. The route C is 20 mile in length. It has been estimated that the required GIL transmission will cost $7.6 million per mile to build and $200 per mile to maintain. Its salvage value will be $1000 per mile at the end of 40 years. It has also been estimated that if the GIL alternative is elected, the relative savings in power losses will be $17.5 ×10^6 per year in comparison to the other two alternatives.

Assume that the fixed charge rate is 10% and that the annual ad valorem (property) taxes are 3% of the first costs of each alternative. The cost of energy is $0.10 per kWh. Use any engineering economy interest tables* and determine the economically preferable alternative.

Solution

OH transmission

The first cost of the 500 kV OH transmission line is

$$P = (\$1,000,000/\text{mile})(50 \text{ miles}) = \$50,000,000$$

and its estimated salvage value is

$$F = (\$2,000/\text{mile})(50 \text{ miles}) = \$100,000$$

The annual equivalent cost of capital invested in the line is

$$A_1 = \$50,000,000(A/P)_{40}^{10\%} - \$100,000(A/F)_{40}^{10\%}$$

$$= \$50,000,000(0.10226) - \$100,000(0.00226)$$

$$= \$5,113,000 - \$266 = \$5,112,774$$

The annual equivalent cost of the tax and maintenance is

$$A_2 = (\$50,000,000)(0.03) + (\$500/\text{mile})(50 \text{ miles}) = \$1,525,000$$

The total annual equivalent cost of the OH transmission line is

$$A = A_1 + A_2 = \$5,112,774 + \$1,525,000$$

$$= \$6,637,774$$

Submarine transmission

The first cost of the 500 kV submarine power transmission line is

$$P = (\$4,000,000/\text{mile})(30 \text{ miles}) = \$120,000,000$$

and its estimated salvage value is

$$F = (\$6,000/\text{mile})(30 \ \text{miles}) = \$180,000$$

The annual equivalent cost of capital invested in the line is

$$A_1 = \$120,000,000(A/P)_{40}^{10\%} - \$180,000(A/F)_{40}^{10\%}$$

$$= \$120,000,000(0.10296) - \$180,000(0.00296)$$

$$= \$12,270,667$$

The annual equivalent cost of the tax and maintenance is

$$A_2 = (\$120,000,000)(0.03) + (\$1,500/\text{mile})(30 \ \text{miles}) = \$3,645,000$$

The total annual equivalent cost of the OH transmission line is

$$A = A_1 + A_2 = \$12,270,667.20 + \$3,645,000$$

$$= \$15,915,667$$

GIL transmission
The first cost of the 500 kV GIL transmission line is

$$P = (\$7,600,000/\text{mile})(20 \ \text{miles}) = \$152,000,000$$

and its estimated salvage value is

$$F = (\$1,000/\text{mile})(20 \ \text{miles}) = \$20,000$$

The annual equivalent cost of capital invested in the GIL line is

$$A_1 = \$152,000,000(A/P)_{40}^{10\%} - \$20,000(A/F)_{40}^{10\%}$$

$$= \$152,000,000(0.10226) - \$20,000(0.00226)$$

$$= \$15,543,520 - \$45 = \$15,543,475$$

The annual equivalent cost of the tax and maintenance is

$$A_2 = (\$152,000,000)(0.03) + (\$200/\text{mile})(20 \ \text{miles}) = \$4,564,000$$

The total annual equivalent cost of the GIL transmission line is

$$A = A_1 + A_2 = \$15,543,475 + \$4,564,000$$

$$= \$20,107,475$$

Since the relative savings in power losses is $17,500,000, the total net annual equivalent cost of the GIL transmission is

$$A_{net} = \$20,107,475 - \$17,500,000$$

$$= \$2,607,475$$

The results show that the use of GIL transmission for this application is the best choice. The next best alternative is the OH transmission. However, this example is only a rough and very simplistic estimate. In real applications, there are many other cost factors that need to be included in such comparisons.

5.13 LOCATION OF FAULTS IN UNDERGROUND CABLES

There are various methods for locating faults in underground cables. The method used for locating any particular fault depends on the nature of the fault and the extent of the experience of the testing engineer. Cable faults can be categorized as (1) conductor failures or (2) insulation failures.

In general, conductor failures are located by comparing the capacity of the insulated conductors. On the other hand, insulation failures are located by fault tests that compare the resistance of the conductors. In short cables, the fault is usually located by inspection, that is, looking for smoking manholes or listening for cracking sound when the *kenetront** is applied to the faulty cable. The location of ground faults on cables of known length can be determined by means of the balanced-bridge principle.

5.13.1 FAULT LOCATION BY USING MURRAY LOOP TEST

It is the simplest of the bridge methods for locating cable failures between conductors and ground in any cable where there is a second conductor of the same size as the one with the fault. It is one of the best methods of locating high-resistance faults in low-conductor-resistance circuits. Figure 5.40 shows a Murray loop.

The faulty conductor is looped to an unfaulted conductor of the same cross-sectional area, and a slide-wire resistance box with two sets of coils is connected across the open ends of the loop. Obviously, the Murray loop cannot be established if the faulty conductor is broken at any point.

Therefore, the continuity of the loop should be tested before applying the bridge principle. In order to avoid the effects of earth currents, the galvanometer is connected as shown in the figure. A battery energizes the bridge between the sliding contact or resistance box center and the point at which the faulty line is grounded. Balance is obtained by adjustment of the sliding contact

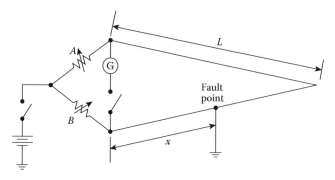

FIGURE 5.40 Murray loop.

---

* It is a two-electrode high-vacuum tube. They are used as power rectifiers for applications requiring low currents at high dc voltages, such as for electronic dust precipitation and high-voltage test equipment.

or resistance. If the nongrounded (unfaulted) line and the grounded (faulted) line have the same resistance per-unit length and if the slide wire is of uniform cross-sectional area,

$$\frac{A}{B} = \frac{2L - X}{X}$$

or

$$X = \frac{2L}{1 + \dfrac{A}{B}} \text{ units of length} \tag{5.233}$$

or

$$X = \frac{2LB}{A + B} \text{ units of length} \tag{5.234}$$

where
  X is the distance from measuring end to fault point
  L is the length of each looped conductor
  A is the resistance of top left-hand side bridge arm in balance
  B is the resistance of bottom left-hand side bridge arm in balance

Therefore, the distance X from the measuring end to the fault can be found directly in terms of the units used to measure the distance L.

5.13.2 FAULT LOCATION BY USING VARLEY LOOP TEST

It can be used for faults to ground where there is a second conductor of the same size as the one with the fault. It is particularly applicable in locating faults in relatively high-resistance circuits. Figure 5.41 shows a Varley loop.

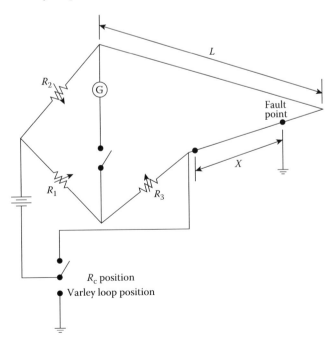

FIGURE 5.41 Varley loop.

The resistance per-unit length of the unfaulted conductor and the faulted conductor must be known. Therefore, if the conductors have equal resistances per-unit length (e.g., r_c Ω), the resistance $(2L - X)r_c$ constitutes one arm of the bridge and the resistance

$$\frac{R_1}{R_2} = \frac{R_3 + X \times r_c}{(2L - X)r_c}$$

or

$$X = \frac{2L\left(\dfrac{R_1}{R_2}\right) - \dfrac{R_3}{r_c}}{1 + \dfrac{R_1}{R_2}} \text{ units of length} \tag{5.235}$$

or

$$X = \frac{R_2}{R_1 + R_2}\left(2L\frac{R_1}{R_2} - \frac{R_3}{r_c}\right) \text{ units of length} \tag{5.236}$$

where
  X is the distance from measuring end to fault point
  L is the length of each looped conductor
  R_1 is the resistance of bottom left-hand side bridge arm in balance
  R_2 is the resistance of top left-hand bridge arm in balance
  R_3 is the adjustable resistance of known magnitude
  r_c is the conductor resistance in ohms per-unit length

If the conductor resistance is not known, it can easily be found by changing the switch to the r_c position and measuring the resistance of the conductor $2L$ by using the Wheatstone bridge method.

5.13.3 Distribution Cable Checks

Newly installed cables should be subjected to a nondestructive test at higher than normal use values. Megger testing is a common practice. The word *Megger* is the trade name of a line of ohmmeters manufactured by the James G. Biddle Company. Certain important information regarding the quality and condition of insulation can be determined from regular Megger readings that is a form of preventive maintenance.

For example, Figure 5.42 shows a portable high-resistance bridge for cable fault–locating work. Faults can be between two conductors or between a conductor and its conducting sheath, concentric neutral, or ground. Figure 5.43 shows a heavy-duty cable test and fault-locating system, which can be used for either grounded or ungrounded neutral 15 kV cables. The full 100 mA output current allows rapid reduction of high-resistance faults on cables rated 35 kV ac or higher to the level of 25 kV or lower for fault-locating purposes. Figure 5.44 shows a lightweight battery-operated cable route trace that can be used to locate, trace, and measure the depth of buried energized power cables. Figure 5.45 shows an automatic digital radar cable test set that requires no distance calculations, insulation calibrations, or zero pulse alignments.

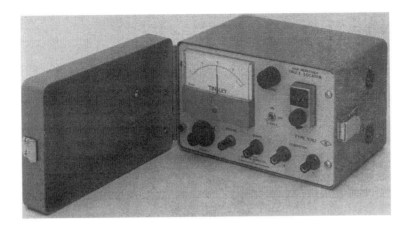

FIGURE 5.42 Portable Murray loop resistance bridge for cable fault–locating work. (Courtesy of James G. Biddle Company, Philadelphia, PA.)

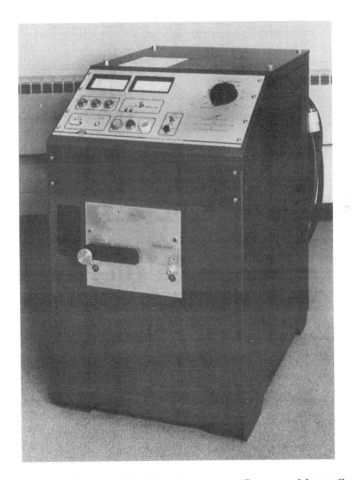

FIGURE 5.43 Heavy-duty cable test and fault-locating system. (Courtesy of James G. Biddle Company, Philadelphia, PA.)

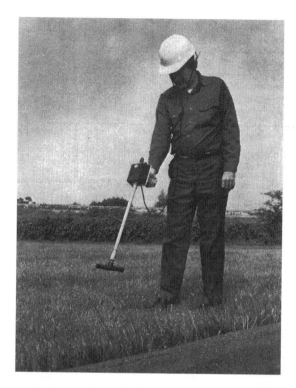

FIGURE 5.44　Lightweight battery-operated cable route tracer. (Courtesy of James G. Biddle Company, Philadelphia, PA.)

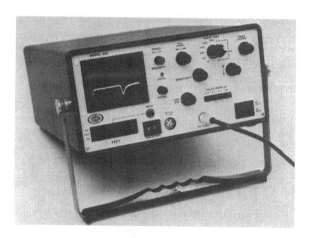

FIGURE 5.45　Automatic digital radar cable test set. (Courtesy of James G. Biddle Company, Philadelphia, PA.)

PROBLEMS

5.1　Assume that a 7.2 kV, 60 Hz, single-conductor, belted cable has a conductor diameter of 2 cm and a lead sheath with inside diameter of 4 cm. The resistivity of the insulation is 1.2×10^8 MΩ-cm, and the length of the cable is 3.5 mi. Calculate the following:

(a)　Total insulation resistance in megohms

(b)　Power loss due to leakage current flowing through insulation resistance

5.2　Assume that a 2 mi long, three-conductor, belted cable is connected to a 24.9 kV, three-phase, 60 Hz bus. A test result shows that the capacitance between bunch conductors and sheath is

0.8 µF/mi, and the capacitance between two conductors bunched together with the sheath and third conductor is 0.60 µF/mi. Find the charging current per conductor.

5.3   Assume that a single-conductor belted cable has a conductor diameter of 0.681 in., inside diameter of sheath of 1.7025 in., and a length of 8000 ft. The cable is to be operated at 12.47 kV. The dielectric constant is 4.5, and the power factor of the dielectric at a rated frequency and temperature is 0.05. Calculate the following:
   (a) Capacitance of cable
   (b) Charging current
   (c) Dielectric loss of cable
   (d) Equivalent resistance of insulation

5.4   Assume that a single-conductor belted cable has a conductor diameter of 2 cm and an inside diameter of sheath of 5 cm. Its insulation resistance is given as 275 MΩ/mi. Find the dielectric resistivity of the insulation.

5.5   Assume that a test has been conducted by means of a Schering bridge on a three-conductor belted cable at a rated voltage and frequency of 12.47 kV and 60 Hz, respectively. The capacitance between the two conductors when the third one is connected to the lead sheath was found to be 1.2 µF. Also, the capacitance between the three conductors connected together and the lead sheath was measured as 1.4 µF. Calculate the following:
   (a) Effective capacitance to neutral
   (b) Charging current per conductor
   (c) Total charging current of cable
   (d) Capacitance between each conductor and sheath
   (e) Capacitance between each pair of conductors

5.6   Assume that a single-phase concentric cable is 3 mi long and is connected to 60 Hz, 7.2 kV bus bars. The conductor diameter is 0.630 in., and the radial thickness of uniform insulation is 0.425 in. The relative permittivity of the dielectric is 4. Find the charging kilovolt-amperes.

5.7   Assume that a single-phase voltage of 7.97 kV at 60 Hz frequency is applied between two of the conductors of a three-phase belted cable. The capacitances between conductors and between a conductor and a sheath are measured as 0.30 and 0.2 µF, respectively. Calculate the following:
   (a) Potential difference between third conductor and sheath
   (b) Total charging current of cable

5.8   Assume that a three-conductor, paper-insulted, belted cable is used as a three-phase underground feeder of 18 mi. It is operated at 60 Hz and 33 kV. The cable has three 350 kcmil sector-type conductors each with $\dfrac{10}{32}$ in. of conductor insulation and $\dfrac{5}{32}$ in. of belt insulation. Calculate the following:
   (a) Geometric factor of cable using Table 5.3
   (b) Total charging current of line
   (c) Total charging kilovolt-ampere of line

5.9   Assume that a three-conductor, paper-insulted, belted cable is used as a three-phase underground feeder of 5000 ft. The cable is operated at 15 kV, 60 Hz, and 75°C. The cable has a 350 kcmil copper conductor. Calculate the effective resistance of the cable.

5.10 Repeat Problem 5.9 assuming the conductor is aluminum.

5.11 Repeat Problem 5.9 assuming three single-conductor cables are located in the separate ducts.

5.12 Repeat Example 5.9 assuming the spacing between conductor centers is 4.125 in. and the cables are located in the same horizontal plane.

5.13 Consider Example 5.12 and assume that the phase voltages are balanced and have a magnitude of 34.5 kV. Calculate the sequence voltage drop matrix $[\mathbf{V}_{012}]$.

5.14 A 60 Hz, 15 kV three-conductor, paper-insulated cable is used at 13.8 kV as a three-phase underground feeder of 10 mi. The cable has three 350 kcmil compact sector-type conductors with a diameter of 0.539 in. and a dielectric constant of 3.78. Calculate, for the zero, positive, and negative sequences, the shunt capacitance, shunt capacitive reactance, and charging current by using the formulas given in Section 5.9:

(a) For three-conductor shielded cables (insulation thickness 175 mils)
(b) For three-conductor belted cables with no conductor shielding (conductor insulation thickness 155 mils, belt insulation thickness 75 mils)

REFERENCES

1. IEEE Industrial Applications Society. *IEEE Recommended Practice for Electrical Power Distribution for Industrial Plants* (Red Book), IEEE Stand. 141-1976, IEEE, New York.
2. Westinghouse Electric Corporation. *Electrical Transmission and Distribution Reference Book*, WEC, East Pittsburgh, PA, 1964.
3. Special report. Underground cable systems, *Electr. World* 89, 1976, 44–58.
4. Fink, D. G. and Beaty, H. W. *Standard Handbook for Electrical Engineers*, 11th edn., McGraw-Hill, New York, 1978.
5. Clark, E. *Circuit Analysis of A-C Power Systems*, vol. 2, General Electric Company, Schenectady, NY, 1960.
6. Insulated Power Cable Engineers Association. *Current Carrying Capacity of Impregnated Paper, Rubber, and Varnished Cambric Insulated Cables*, 1st edn., Publ. no. P-29-226, IPCEA, New York, 1965.
7. Carson, J. R. Ground return impedance: Underground wire with earth return, *Bell Syst. Tech. J.* 8, 1929, 94.
8. Skrotzki, B. G. A., ed. *Electric Transmission and Distribution*, McGraw-Hill, New York, 1954.
9. Schifreen, C. S. and Marble, W. C. Changing current limitations in operation of high-voltage cable lines, *Trans. Am. Inst. Electr. Eng.* 26, 1956, 803–817.
10. Wiseman, R. T. Discussions to charging current limitations in operation of high-voltage cable lines, *Trans. Am. Inst. Electr. Eng.* 26, 1956, 803–817.

GENERAL REFERENCES

Anderson, P. M. *Analysis of Faulted Power Systems*, Iowa State University Press, Ames, IA, 1973.
Edison Electric Institute. *Underground Systems Reference Book*, 2nd edn., EEI, New York, 1957.
Gönen, T. *Engineering Economy for Engineering Managers*, Wiley, New York, 1990.
Gönen, T. High-temperature superconductors, a technical article in *McGraw-Hill Encyclopedia of Science & Technology*, 7th edn., vol. 7, 1992, pp. 127–129.
Gönen, T. *Electric Power Distribution System Engineering*, CRC Press, Boca Raton, FL, 2008.
Gooding, H. T. Cable-fault location on power systems, *Proc. Inst. Electr. Eng.* 113(1),1966, 111–119.
Shackleton, H. Underground cable fault location, *Electr. Rev.* (*London*) 28, 1955, 057–1061.
Stanforth, B. L. Locating faults in underground cables, *Electr. Times* 143(16), 1963, 581.

6 Direct-Current Power Transmission

By all means marry. If you get a good wife, you'll be happy.
If you get a bad one, you'll become a philosopher.

Socrates

6.1 BASIC DEFINITIONS

Converter. A machine, device, or system for changing ac power to dc power or vice versa.

Rectifier. A converter for changing ac to dc.

Inverter. A converter for changing dc to ac.

Arc-back. A malfunctioning phenomenon in which a valve conducts in the reverse direction.

Pulse number (*p*). The number of pulsations (i.e., *cycles of ripple*) of the direct voltage per cycle of alternating voltage (e.g., pulse numbers for three-phase one-way and three-phase two-way rectifier bridges are 3 and 6, respectively).

Ripple. The ac component from dc power supply arising from sources within the power supply. It is expressed in peak, peak-to-peak, rms volts, or percent rms. Since HVDC converters have large dc smoothing reactors, approximately 1 H, the resultant dc is constant (i.e., free from ripple). However, the direct voltage on the valve side of the smoothing reactor has ripple.

Ripple amplitude. The maximum value of the instantaneous difference between the average and instantaneous value of a pulsating unidirectional wave.

Reactor. An inductive reactor between the dc output of the converter and the load. It is used to smooth the ripple in the dc adequately, to reduce harmonic voltages and currents in the dc line, and to limit the magnitude of fault current. It is also called a *smoothing reactor*.

Commutation. The transfer of current from one valve to another in the same row.

Delay angle (α). The time, expressed in electrical degrees, by which the starting point of commutation is delayed. It cannot exceed 180°. It is also called *ignition angle* or *firing angle*.

Overlap angle (*u*). The time, expressed in degrees, during which the current is commutated between two rectifying elements. It is also called *commutation time*. In normal operation, it is less than 60° and is usually somewhere between 20° and 25° at full load.

Extinction angle (δ). The sum of the delay angle a and the overlap angle *u* of a rectifier and is expressed in degrees.

Ignition angle (β). The delay angle of an inverter and is equal to $\pi - \alpha$ electrical degrees.

Extinction (advance) angle (γ). The extinction angle of an inverter and is equal to $\pi - \gamma$ electrical degrees. It is defined as the time angle between the end of conduction and the reversal of the sign of the sinusoidal commutation voltage of the source.

Commutation margin angle (ζ). The time angle between the end of conduction and the reversal of the sign of the nonsinusoidal voltage across the outgoing valve of an inverter. Under normal operating conditions, the commutation margin angle is equal to the extinction advance angle.

Equivalent commutating resistance (R_c). The ratio of drop of direct voltage to dc. However, it does not consume any power.

Thyristor (*SCR*). A thyristor (silicon-controlled rectifier) is a semiconductor device with an anode, a cathode terminal, and a gate for the control of the firing.

6.2 INTRODUCTION

For the most part, electric power is transmitted worldwide by means of ac. However, there are certain applications where dc transmission offers distinct economic and/or performance advantages. These applications include long-distance overhead transmission, underwater or underground transmission, and asynchronous ties between power systems. The first practical application of dc transmission was in Sweden in 1954. But the wider applications of HVDC started after 1960.

Today, HVDC lines are used all over the world to transmit increasingly large amounts of energy over long distances. In the United States, one of the best-known HVDC transmission line is the Pacific HVDC Intertie, which interconnects California with Oregon. Additionally, there is the ±400 kV Coal Creek–Dicken lines as a good example for HVDC system. In Canada, Vancouver Island is supplied through an HVDC cable. Another famous HVDC system is the interconnection between England and France, which uses underwater cables.

Typically, in an HVDC system, the ac voltage is rectified and a dc transmission line transmits the energy. An inverter that is located at the end of the dc transmission line converts the dc voltage to ac, for example, the Pacific HVDC Intertie that operates with ±500 kV voltage and interconnects Southern California with the hydro station in Oregon. The bundled conductors are also used in HVDC transmission lines.

6.3 OVERHEAD HVDC TRANSMISSION

Figure 6.1 shows some of the typical circuit arrangements (*links*) for HVDC transmissions. In the monopolar arrangement, shown in Figure 6.1a, there is only one insulated transmission conductor (*pole*) installed and ground return is used. It is the least expensive arrangement but has certain disadvantages. For example, it causes the corrosion of buried pipes, cable sheaths, ground electrodes, etc., due to the electrolysis phenomenon caused by the ground return current. It is used in dc systems that have low power ratings, primarily with cable transmission. In order to eliminate the aforementioned electrolysis phenomenon, a metallic return (*conductor*) can be used, as shown in Figure 6.1b.

The bipolar circuit arrangement has two insulated conductors used as plus and minus poles. The two poles can be used independently if both neutrals are grounded. *Under normal operation*, the currents flowing in each pole are equal, and therefore, there is no ground current.

Under emergency operation, the ground return can be used to provide for increased transmission capacity. For example, if one of the two poles is out of order, the other conductor with ground return can carry up to the total power of the link. In that case, the transmission line losses are doubled. As shown in Figure 6.1c, the rated voltage of a bipolar arrangement is given as $\pm V_d$ (e.g., ±500 kV, which is read as *plus and minus* 500 kV). Figure 6.2 shows a dc transmission system operating in the bipolar mode.

It is possible to have two or more poles all having the same polarity and always having a ground return. This arrangement is known as the *homopolar arrangement* and is used to transmit power in dc systems that have very large ratings. The dc tower normally carries only two insulated conductors, and the ground return can be used as the additional conductor.

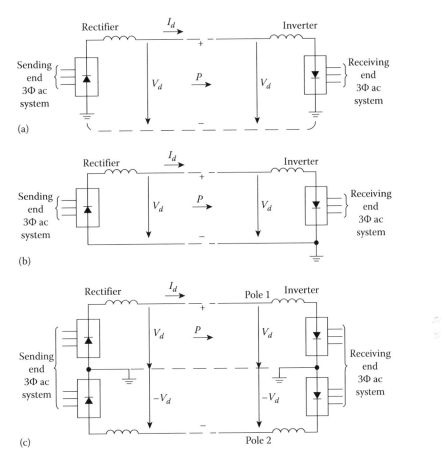

FIGURE 6.1 Typical circuit arrangements for HVDC transmissions: (a) monopolar arrangement with ground return, (b) monopolar arrangement with metallic return grounded at one end, and (c) bipolar arrangement.

6.4 COMPARISON OF POWER TRANSMISSION CAPACITY OF HVDC AND HVAC

Assume that there are two comparable transmission lines: one is the ac and the other the dc line. Assume that both lines have the same length and are made of the same conductor sizes and that the loading of both lines is thermally limited so that current I_d equals the rms ac I_L. Also assume that the ac line has three phase and three wires and has a power factor of 0.945 and the dc line is a bipolar circuit arrangement with two conductors. Furthermore, assume that the ac and dc insulators withstand the same crest voltage to ground so that the voltage V_d is equal to $\sqrt{2}$ times the rms ac voltage. Therefore, it can be shown that the dc power per conductor is

$$P_{(dc)} = V_d I_d \qquad (6.1)$$

and the ac power per conductor is

$$P_{(ac)} = V_{(L\text{-}N)} I_L \cos\theta \text{ W/conductor} \qquad (6.2)$$

where
V_d is the line-to-ground dc voltage in volts
$V_{(L\text{-}N)}$ is the line-to-neutral ac voltage in volts
I_d is the dc line current in amperes
I_L is the ac line current in amperes

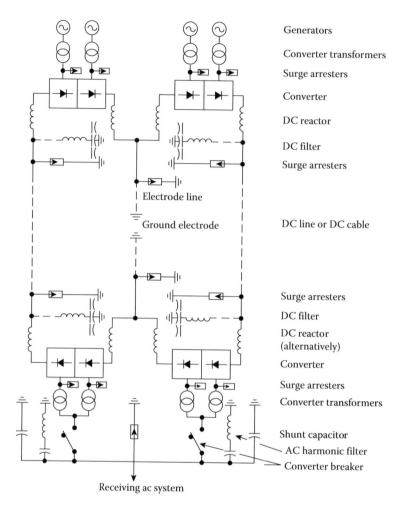

Generators

Converter transformers

Surge arresters

Converter

DC reactor

DC filter

Surge arresters

Electrode line

Ground electrode

DC line or DC cable

Surge arresters

DC filter

DC reactor
(alternatively)

Converter

Surge arresters

Converter transformers

Shunt capacitor

AC harmonic filter

Converter breaker

Receiving ac system

FIGURE 6.2 A dc transmission system operating in bipolar mode. (From Fink, D.G. and Beaty, H.W., *Standard Handbook for Electrical Engineers*, 11th edn., McGraw-Hill, New York, 1978.)

Therefore, the ratio of the dc power per conductor to the ac power per conductor (phase) can be expressed as

$$\frac{P_{(dc)}}{P_{(ac)}} = \frac{V_d I_d}{V_{(L-N)} I_L \cos\theta} \tag{6.3}$$

or

$$\frac{P_{(dc)}}{P_{(ac)}} = \frac{\sqrt{2}}{\cos\theta} \tag{6.4}$$

but since

$$\cos\theta = 0.945$$

then

$$\frac{P_{(dc)}}{P_{(ac)}} = 1.5 \tag{6.5}$$

or

$$P_{(dc)} = 1.5 \, P_{(ac)} \text{ W/conductor} \tag{6.6}$$

Furthermore, the total power transmission capabilities for the dc and ac lines can be expressed as

$$P_{(dc)} = 2p_{(dc)} \text{ W} \tag{6.7}$$

and

$$P_{(ac)} = 3p_{(ac)} \text{ W} \tag{6.8}$$

Therefore, their ratio can be expressed as

$$\frac{P_{(dc)}}{P_{(ac)}} = \frac{2}{3} \times \frac{p_{(dc)}}{p_{(ac)}} \tag{6.9}$$

Substituting Equation 6.5 into Equation 6.9,

$$\frac{P_{(dc)}}{P_{(ac)}} = \frac{2}{3} \times \frac{3}{2} = 1$$

or

$$P_{(dc)} = P_{(ac)} \text{ W} \tag{6.10}$$

Thus, both lines have the same transmission capability and can transmit the same amount of power. However, the dc line has two conductors rather than three and thus requires only two-thirds as many insulators. Therefore, the required towers and rights of way are narrower in the dc line than the ac line. Even though the power loss per conductor is the same for both lines, the total power loss of the dc line is only two-thirds that of the ac line.

Thus, studies indicate that a dc line generally costs about 33% less than an ac line of the same capacity. Furthermore, if a two-pole (homopolar) dc line is compared with a double-circuit three-phase ac line, the dc line costs would be about 45% less than the ac line. In general, the cost advantage of the dc line increases at higher voltages. The power losses due to the corona phenomena are smaller for dc than for ac lines.

The reactive powers generated and absorbed by an HVAC transmission line can be expressed as

$$Q_c = X_c V^2 \text{ vars/unit length} \tag{6.11}$$

or

$$Q_c = \omega C V^2 \text{ vars/unit length} \tag{6.12}$$

and

$$Q_L = X_L I^2 \text{ vars/unit length} \tag{6.13}$$

or

$$Q_L = \omega L I^2 \text{ vars/unit length} \tag{6.14}$$

where
X_c is the capacitive reactance of line in ohms per-unit length
X_L is the inductive reactance of line in ohms per-unit length
C is the shunt capacitance of line in farads per-unit length
L is the series inductance of line in farads per-unit length
V is the line-to-line operating voltage in volts
I is the line current in amperes

If the reactive powers generated and absorbed by the line are equal to each other,

$$Q_c = Q_L$$

or

$$\omega_c V^2 = \omega L I^2$$

from which the surge impedance of the line can be found as

$$Z_c = \frac{V}{I}$$

$$= \sqrt{\frac{L}{C}} \ \Omega \tag{6.15}$$

Therefore, the power transmitted by the line at the surge impedance can be expressed as

$$\text{SIL} = \frac{V_{L\text{-}L}^2}{Z_c} \text{ W} \tag{6.16}$$

Note that this surge impedance loading (or *natural load*) is a function of the voltage and line inductance and capacitance. However, it is not a function of the line length. In general, the economical load of a given overhead transmission line is larger than its SIL. In which case, the net reactive power absorbed by the line must be provided from one or both ends of the line and from intermediate series capacitors.

Hence, the costs of necessary series capacitor and shunt reactor compensation should be taken into account in the comparison of ac versus dc lines. The dc line itself does not require any reactive power. However, the converters at both ends of the line require reactive power from the ac systems.

Underground cables used for ac transmission can also be used for dc, and they can normally carry more dc power than ac due to the absence of capacitive charging current and better utilization of insulation and less dielectric wear. However, an HVDC transmission cable is designed somewhat differently than that of an ac transmission cable. Since a power cable employed for dc power transmission does not have capacitive leakage currents, the power transmission is restricted by the I^2R losses only.

Furthermore, submarine or underground ac cables are always operated at a load that is far less than the surge impedance load in order to prevent overheating. As a result of this practice, the reactive power generated by charging the shunt capacitance is greater than that absorbed by the series inductance. Thus, compensating shunt reactors are to be provided at regular intervals (approximately 20 mi). Contrarily, dc cables do not have such restrictions. Thus, the power transmission using dc cable is much cheaper than ac cable.

The major advantages of the dc transmission can be summarized as follows:

1. If the high cost of converter stations is excluded, the dc overhead lines and cables are less expensive than ac overhead lines and cables. The break-even distance is about 500 mi for the overhead lines, somewhere between 15 and 30 mi for submarine cables and 30 and 60 mi for underground cables. Therefore, in the event that the transmission distance is less than the break-even distance, the ac transmission is less expensive than dc; otherwise, the dc transmission is less expensive. The exact break-even distance depends on local conditions, line performance requirements, and connecting ac system characteristics.
2. A dc link is asynchronous; that is, it has no stability problem in itself. Therefore, the two ac systems connected at each end of the dc link do not have to be operating in synchronism with respect to each other or even necessarily at the same frequency.
3. The corona loss and RI conditions are better in the dc than the ac lines.
4. The power factor of the dc line is always unity, and therefore, no reactive compensation is needed.
5. Since the synchronous operation is not demanded, the line length is not restricted by stability.
6. The interconnection of two separate ac systems via a dc link does not increase the short-circuit capacity, and thus the circuit breaker ratings, of either system.
7. The le line loss is smaller than for the comparable ac line.

The major disadvantages of the dc transmission can be summarized as follows:

1. The converters generate harmonic voltages and currents on both ac and dc sides, and therefore, filters are required.
2. The converters consume reactive power.
3. The dc converter stations are expensive.
4. The dc circuit breakers have disadvantages with respect to the ac circuit breakers because the dc does not decrease to zero twice a cycle, contrary to the ac.

According to Hingorani and Ellert [2], the potential applications for HVDC transmission in the United States are as follows:

1. Long-distance overhead transmission
2. Power in-fed into urban areas by overhead transmission lines or underground cables
3. Asynchronous ties
4. Underground cable connections
5. East–west and north–south interconnecting overlays
6. DC networks with tapped lies
7. Stabilization of ac systems
8. Reduction of shorter-circuit currents in receiving ac systems

In the future, the application of HVDC transmission in the United States will increase due to the following two basic reasons:

1. The availability and ever-increasing prices of important oil imports are making coal and hydro more attractive. However, most of such coal and hydro power plants are located remotely from load centers. Their utilizations are often to be facilitated by the use of long-distance transmission lines.
2. The ever-increasing pressures by the environmental concerns to locate new power plants remotely from densely populated urban areas. Hence, obtaining sites for new power plants are becoming extremely difficult. Because of this difficulty, utility companies will be forced to locate them several hundred miles away from their load centers. Thus, the need for economical long-distance transmission of large blocks of electric energy will increasingly dictate the use of HVDC transmission lines.

6.5 HVDC TRANSMISSION LINE INSULATION

The factors that affect the insulation of the HVDC overhead transmission lines are (1) steady-state operating voltages, (2) switching surge overvoltages, and (3) lightning overvoltages. The factors must be restricted to values that cannot cause puncture or flashover of the insulation. The steady-state operating voltage affects the selection of leakage distance, particularly when there is considerable pollution in the environment. The switching surge and lightning overvoltages influence the required insulator chain length and strike distance [6].

Consider the transmission line conductor configurations shown in Figure 6.3 for the comparable ac and dc systems. For the steady-state operating voltages, it can be shown that the factor K given by the following equation relates the dc and ac voltages to ground that may be applied to a given insulation:

$$K = \frac{V_d/2}{E_p} \tag{6.17}$$

or

$$\frac{1}{2}V_d = KE_p \tag{6.18}$$

where

V_d is the line-to-line dc voltage in volts
$\frac{1}{2}V_d$ is the line-to-ground dc voltage in volts
E_p is the line-to-neutral ac voltage in volts

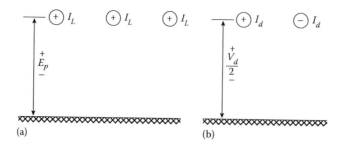

FIGURE 6.3 Transmission line conductor configuration for high voltage: (a) ac system and (b) dc system.

Typical values of factor K are as follows:

$K = \sqrt{2}$ for indoor porcelain
$K = 1$ for outdoor porcelain
$2 \leq K \leq 6$ for insulated power cables

The given data for factor K imply that conventional insulators have inferior wet flashover performance when used in the high-voltage service. Therefore, the HVDC lines require special insulators.

Typically, the following approximate insulation levels are required to withstand switching surges on overhead lines:

For HVAC lines,

$$\text{ac insulation level} = K_1 E_p$$
$$\cong 2.5 E_p \tag{6.19}$$

and for HVDC lines,

$$\text{dc insulation level} = K_2 \left(\frac{1}{2} V_d \right)$$
$$\cong 1.7 \left(\frac{1}{2} V_d \right) \tag{6.20}$$

Therefore, for a fixed value of insulation level, the following operating voltages can be used from the standpoint of switching surge performance:

$$K_1 E_p = K_2 \left(\frac{1}{2} V_d \right) \tag{6.21}$$

If $K_1 = 2.5$ and $K_2 = 1.7$,

$$2.5 E_p = 1.7 \left(\frac{1}{2} V_d \right)$$

or

$$\left(\frac{1}{2} V_d \right) = 1.47 E_p \tag{6.22}$$

On overhead lines, the maximum steady-state operating voltage or the minimum conductor size is also restricted by the power losses and RI due to corona. But in cables, the restricting factor is usually the normal steady-state operating voltage.

Example 6.1

Assume that the overhead ac and dc lines shown in Figure 6.3 have the same line length and are made of the same size conductors that transmit the same amount of power and have the same total I^2R losses. Assume that the ac line is three phase, has three wires, and has a unity power factor and that the dc line has two wires plus ground return. Furthermore, assume that the factors K_1 and K_2 are 2.5 and 1.7, respectively, and determine the following:

    (a) Line-to-line dc voltage of V_d in terms of line-to-neutral voltage E_p
    (b) The dc line current I_d in terms of ac line current I_L
    (c) Ratio of dc insulation level to ac insulation level

Solution

(a) Since the power losses are the same in either system,

$$P_{\text{loss(dc)}} = P_{\text{loss(ac)}}$$

or

$$2I_d^2 R_{\text{(dc)}} = 3I_L^2 R_{\text{(ac)}} \tag{6.23}$$

where, ignoring the skin effects,

$$R_{\text{(dc)}} = R_{\text{(ac)}}$$

so that

$$I_d = \sqrt{\frac{3}{2}} I_L$$

or

$$I_d = 1.225 I_L \tag{6.24}$$

(b) Since

$$P_{\text{(dc)}} = P_{\text{(ac)}}$$

or

$$V_d I_d = 3E_p I_L \tag{6.25}$$

$$V_d = 2.45 E_p \tag{6.26}$$

(c) The ratio is

$$\frac{\text{dc insulation level}}{\text{ac insulation level}} = \frac{K_2(V_d/2)}{K_1 E_p} \tag{6.27}$$

where

$$K_1 = 2.5 \quad K_2 = 1.7$$

Therefore, substituting Equation 6.26 into Equation 6.27,

$$\frac{\text{dc insulation level}}{\text{ac insulation level}} = 8.8328 \tag{6.28}$$

or

$$\text{dc insulation level} = 0.8328 \text{ (ac insulation level)} \tag{6.29}$$

Example 6.2

Consider an existing three-phase high-voltage cable circuit made of three single-conductor insulated power cables. The loading of the circuit is thermally limited at the cable rms ampacity current I_L. Assume that the normal ac operating voltage is E_p. Investigate the merits of converting the cable circuit to HVDC operation wherein one of the three existing cables is used either as a spare or as the grounded neutral conductor. Assume that factor K is 3 and determine the following:

(a) Maximum operating V_d in terms of voltage E_p
(b) Maximum power transmission capability ratio, that is, ratio of $P_{\text{(dc)}}$ to $P_{\text{(ac)}}$
(c) Ratio of total I^2R losses, that is, ratio of $P_{\text{loss(dc)}}$ to $P_{\text{loss(ac)}}$, that accompany maximum power flow. (Assume that the power factor for the ac operation is unity and that the skin effect is negligible.)

Solution

(a) From Equation 6.18,

$$\frac{1}{2}V_d = KE_p$$

$$= 3E_p$$

Therefore,

$$V_d = 6E_p \tag{6.30}$$

(b) The maximum power transmission capability ratio is

$$\frac{P_{(dc)}}{P_{(ac)}} = \frac{V_d I_d}{3E_p I_L} \tag{6.31}$$

Since the circuit is thermally limited,

$$I_d = I_L \tag{6.32}$$

Therefore, substituting Equations 6.30 and 6.32 into Equation 6.31,

$$\frac{P_{(dc)}}{P_{(ac)}} = 2 \tag{6.33}$$

or

$$P_{(dc)} = 2P_{(ac)} \tag{6.34}$$

(c) The ratio of total I^2R losses is

$$\frac{P_{loss(dc)}}{P_{loss(ac)}} = \frac{2I_d^2 R}{3I_L^2 R} \tag{6.35}$$

Since

$$R_{(dc)} = R_{(ac)} \tag{6.36}$$

Substituting Equations 6.32 and 6.36 into Equation 6.35 yields

$$\frac{P_{loss(dc)}}{P_{loss(ac)}} = \frac{2}{3} \tag{6.37}$$

or

$$P_{loss(dc)} = \frac{2}{3} P_{loss(ac)} \tag{6.38}$$

6.6 THREE-PHASE BRIDGE CONVERTER

The energy conversion from ac to dc is called *rectification* and the conversion from dc to ac is called *inversion*. A converter can operate as a rectifier or as an inverter provided that it has grid control. A valve, whether it is a mercury arc valve or a solid-state (*thyristor*) valve, can conduct in only one direction (*the forward direction*), from anode to cathode. The resultant arc voltage drop is less than 50 V. The valve can endure a considerably high voltage in the negative (*inverse*) direction without conducting. Any arc-back in mercury arc rectifiers can be stopped by grid control and by a bypass valve.

Presently, the thyristors have converter current ratings up to 2000 A. Their typical voltage rating is 3000 V. A solid-state valve has a large number of thyristors connected in series to provide proper voltage division among the thyristors. The thyristors are also connected in parallel, depending on the valve current rating. The thyristors are grouped in modules, each having 2–10 thyristors with all auxiliary circuits. Some of the advantages of thyristors are as follows:

1. There is no possibility of arc-back.
2. They have lower maintenance requirements.
3. They have less space requirements.
4. They have shorter deionization time.
5. There is no need for degassing facilities.
6. There is no need for bypass valves.

In this chapter, the term *valve* includes the solid-state devices as well as the mercury arc valves.

6.7 RECTIFICATION

In a given bridge rectifier, the transfer of current from one valve to another in the same row is called *commutation*. The time during which the current is commutated between two rectifying elements is known as the *overlap angle* or *commutation time*. Therefore, if two valves conduct simultaneously, there is no overlap, that is, *commutation delay*. The time during which the starting point of commutation is delayed is called the *delay angle*. The delay angle is governed by the grid control setting.

Neglecting overlap angle, the average direct voltage for a given delay angle a can be expressed as

$$V_d = \frac{3\sqrt{3}}{\pi} E_m \cos\alpha \tag{6.39}$$

or

$$V_d = V_{d0} \cos\alpha \tag{6.40}$$

since

$$V_{d0} = \frac{3\sqrt{3}}{\pi} E_m \tag{6.41}$$

where
V_{d0} is the ideal no-load direct voltage
E_m is the maximum value of phase-neutral alternating voltage
α is the delay angle

However, if there is no delay, that is, $\alpha = 0$, the average direct voltage can be expressed as

$$V_{d0} = \frac{3\sqrt{3}}{\pi} E_m \tag{6.42}$$

or

$$V_{d0} = \frac{3\sqrt{6}}{\pi} E_{(L\text{-}N)}$$
$$= 2.34 E_{(L\text{-}N)} \tag{6.43}$$

or

$$V_{d0} = \frac{3\sqrt{2}}{\pi} E_{(L\text{-}L)}$$
$$= 1.35 E_{(L\text{-}L)} \tag{6.44}$$

where
  $E_{(L\text{-}N)}$ is the rms line-to-neutral alternating voltage
  $E_{(L\text{-}L)}$ is the rms line-to-line alternating voltage

From Equation 6.40, one can observe that the delay angle α can change the average direct voltage by the factor $\cos \alpha$. Since α can take values from 0 to almost 180°, the average direct voltage can take values from positive V_{d0} to negative V_{d0}. However, the negative direct voltage V_d with positive current I_d causes the power to flow in the opposite direction. Hence, the converter operates as an inverter rather than as a rectifier. Note that since the current can only flow from anode to cathode, the direction of current I_d remains the same.

It can be shown that the rms value of the fundamental-frequency component of ac is

$$I_{L1} = \frac{\sqrt{6}}{\pi} I_d \tag{6.45}$$

or

$$I_{L1} = 0.780 I_d \tag{6.46}$$

When losses are disregarded, the active ac power can be set equal to the dc power, that is,

$$P_{(ac)} = P_{(dc)} \tag{6.47}$$

where

$$P_{(ac)} = 3 E_{(L\text{-}N)} I_{L1} \cos \theta \tag{6.48}$$

$$P_{(dc)} = V_d I_d \tag{6.49}$$

Substituting Equation 6.45 into Equation 6.48,

$$P_{(ac)} = \frac{3\sqrt{6}}{\pi} E_{(L\text{-}N)} I_d \cos \theta \tag{6.50}$$

Also substituting Equations 6.40 and 6.43 simultaneously into Equation 6.49,

$$P_{(dc)} = \frac{3\sqrt{6}}{\pi} E_{(L\text{-}N)} I_d \cos \alpha \tag{6.51}$$

Thus, by substituting Equations 6.50 and 6.51 into Equation 6.47, it can be shown that

$$\cos \theta = \cos \alpha \tag{6.52}$$

where
  $\cos \theta$ is the displacement factor (or vector power factor)
  θ is the angle by which fundamental-frequency component of alternating line current lags line-to-neutral source voltage
  α is the delay angle

Thus, the delay angle α displaces the fundamental component of the current by an angle θ. Therefore, the converter draws reactive power from the ac system: "The rectifier is said to take lagging current from the ac system, and the inverter is said either to take lagging current or to deliver leading current to the ac system" [3].

When there is an overlap angle (u), it causes the ac in each phase to lag behind its voltage. Therefore, the corresponding decrease in direct voltage due to the commutation delay can be expressed as

$$\Delta V_d = \frac{V_{d0}}{2}[\cos\alpha - \cos(\alpha + u)] \tag{6.53}$$

Thus, the associated average direct voltage can be expressed as

$$V_d = V_{d0}\cos\alpha - \Delta V_d \tag{6.54}$$

or

$$V_d = \frac{1}{2}V_{d0}[\cos\alpha + \cos(\alpha + u)] \tag{6.55}$$

Note that the extinction angle δ is

$$\delta \triangleq \alpha + u \tag{6.56}$$

Thus, substituting Equation 6.56 into Equations 6.53 and 6.55,

$$\Delta V_d = \frac{1}{2}V_{d0}(\cos\alpha - \cos\delta) \tag{6.57}$$

and

$$V_d = \frac{1}{2}V_{d0}(\cos\alpha + \cos\delta) \tag{6.58}$$

The overlap angle u is due to the fact that the ac supply source has inductance. Thus, the currents in it cannot change instantaneously. Therefore, the current transfer from one phase to another takes a certain time, which is known as the commutation time or overlap time (u/ω). In normal operation, the overlap angle is $0° < u < 60°$. Whereas in the abnormal operation mode, it is $60° < u < 120°$. The commutation delay takes place when two phases of the supplying ac source are short-circuited. Therefore, it can be shown that at the end of the commutation,

$$I_d = I_{s2}[\cos\alpha - \cos(\alpha + u)] \tag{6.59}$$

but

$$I_{s2} = \frac{\sqrt{3}E_m}{2\omega L_c} \tag{6.60}$$

Substituting Equation 6.60 into Equation 6.59,

$$I_d = \frac{\sqrt{3}E_m}{2\omega L_c}[\cos\alpha - \cos(\alpha + u)] \tag{6.61}$$

where
I_{s2} is the maximum value of current in line-to-line short circuit on ac source
L_c is the series inductance per phase of ac source

By dividing Equations 6.53 and 6.59 side by side,

$$\frac{\Delta V_d}{I_d} = \frac{V_{d0}[\cos\alpha - \cos(\alpha + u)]}{2I_{s2}[\cos\alpha - \cos(\alpha + u)]}$$

or

$$\frac{\Delta V_d}{I_d} = \frac{V_{d0}}{2I_{s2}} \tag{6.62}$$

so that

$$\Delta V_d = \frac{I_d}{2I_{s2}}V_{d0} \tag{6.63}$$

substituting Equation 6.63 into Equation 6.54,

$$V_d = V_{d0}\left(\cos\alpha - \frac{I_d}{2I_{s2}}\right) \tag{6.64}$$

or

$$V_d = V_{d0}\cos\alpha - R_c I_d \tag{6.65}$$

where R_c is the equivalent commutation resistance per phase (it does not consume any power and represents voltage drop due to commutation)

$$R_c = \frac{3}{\pi}X_c \tag{6.66}$$

or

$$R_c = \frac{3}{\pi}\omega L_c \tag{6.67}$$

or

$$R_c = 6fL_c \tag{6.68}$$

Figure 6.4 shows two different representations of the equivalent circuit of a bridge rectifier based on Equation 6.65. The direct voltage V_d can be controlled by changing the delay angle α or by varying the no-load direct voltage using a transformer tap changer.

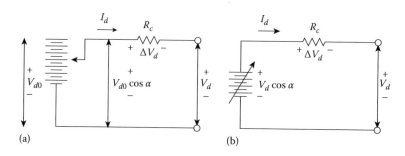

FIGURE 6.4 Equivalent circuit representations of bridge rectifier where the direct voltage V_d can be controlled: (a) by changing the delay angle or (b) by varying the no-load direct voltage using a transformer tap changer.

Example 6.3

Figure 6.5 shows that a rectifier transformer with a tap changer underload is connected to a large ac network. Assume that the Thévenin equivalent voltage of the ac network is given as 92.95/161Y kV and that the impedance of the rectifier transformer is 0.10 pu Ω based on transformer ratings. The subtransient Thévenin impedances of the ac system are to be computed from the three-phase short-circuit data given in the figure for the faults occurring at the bus.

Assume zero power factor faults in circuits of this size. The bridge rectifier ratings are given as 125 kV and 1600 A for the maximum continuous no-load direct voltage (i.e., V_{dr0}) and maximum continuous current (i.e., I_d), respectively. Use the given data and specify the rectifier transformer in terms of the following:

(a) Three-phase kilovolt-ampere rating
(b) Wye-side kilovolt rating

Solution

(a) The three-phase kilovolt-ampere rating of a rectifier transformer can be determined from

$$S_{(B)} = 1.047 V_{d0} I_d \qquad (6.69)$$

where

$$V_{d0} = V_{dr0} = 125 \text{ kV}$$

Therefore,

$$S_{(B)} = 1.047(125 \text{ kV}) (1600 \text{ A}) = 209,400 \text{ kVA}$$

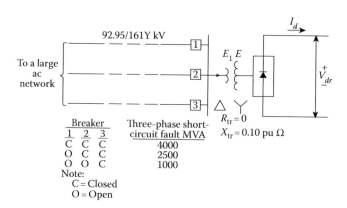

| Breaker | | | Three-phase short- |
1	2	3	circuit fault MVA
C	C	C	4000
O	C	C	2500
O	O	C	1000

Note:
  C = Closed
  O = Open

FIGURE 6.5 System for Example 6.3.

(b) Since

$$V_{d0} = 2.34E_{(L-N)}$$

then

$$E_{(L-N)} = \frac{V_{d0}}{2.34}$$

$$= \frac{125 \text{ kV}}{2.34} = 53.4188 \text{ kV}$$

Example 6.4

Use the results of Example 6.3 and determine the commutating reactance X_c, in ohms, referred to the wye side for all three possible values of ac system reactance.

Solution

(a) *When all three breakers are closed*
The system reactance can be calculated from

$$X_{sys} = \frac{\left[\text{Nominal kV}_{(L-L)}\right]^2}{\text{Short-circuit MVA}}$$

$$= \frac{\left[\sqrt{3}E_{(L-N)}\right]^2}{4000 \text{ MVA}}$$

$$= \frac{\left[\sqrt{3} \times 53.4188 \text{ kV}\right]^2}{4000 \text{ MVA}} = 2.14 \ \Omega \tag{6.70}$$

The rms value of the wye-side phase current is

$$I_{(1\phi)} \cong \sqrt{\frac{2}{3}} I_d$$

$$= 0.816 \times (1600 \text{ A}) = 1305.6 \text{ A} \tag{6.71}$$

Also, the associated reactance base is

$$X_{(B)} = \frac{E_{(L-N)}}{I_{(3\phi)}} \tag{6.72}$$

or

$$X_{(B)} = \frac{E_{(L-N)}}{\sqrt{\frac{2}{3}} I_d}$$

$$= \frac{53,418.8 \text{ V}}{1,305.6 \text{ A}} = 40.915 \ \Omega \tag{6.73}$$

Therefore, the reactance of the rectifier transformer is

$$X_{tr} = X_{tr} \times X_{(B)} = (0.10 \text{ pu } \Omega)(40.915 \ \Omega) = 4.0915 \ \Omega$$

Thus, the commutating reactance is

$$X_c = X_{sys} + X_{tr} = 2.14 + 4.0915 = 6.2315 \ \Omega \tag{6.74}$$

(b) *When breaker 1 is open*
     The system reactance is

$$X_{sys} = \frac{\left[\sqrt{3}E_{(L-N)}\right]^2}{2500 \text{ MVA}}$$

$$= \frac{[\sqrt{3} \times 53.4188 \text{ kV}]^2}{2500 \text{ MVA}} = 3.4243 \ \Omega$$

Thus, the commutating reactance is

$$X_c = X_{sys} + X_{tr} = 3.4243 + 4.0915 = 7.5158 \ \Omega$$

(c) *When breakers 1 and 2 are open*
     The system reactance is

$$X_{sys} = \frac{\left[\sqrt{3}E_{(L-N)}\right]^2}{1000 \text{ MVA}}$$

$$= 8.5607 \ \Omega$$

Therefore, the commutating reactance is

$$X_c = X_{sys} + X_{tr} = 8.5607 + 4.0915 = 12.6522 \ \Omega$$

Example 6.5

Use the results of Example 6.4 and assume that all three breakers are closed, the load tap changer (LTC) is on neutral, the delay angle *a* is zero, and the maximum continuous current I_d is 1600 A. Determine the following:

(a) Overlap angle *u* of rectifier
(b) The dc voltage V_{dr} of rectifier
(c) Displacement (i.e., power) factor of rectifier
(d) Magnetizing var input to rectifier

Solution

(a) Since the delay angle is zero, the overlap angle u can be expressed as

$$u = \delta$$

$$= \cos^{-1}\left(1 - \frac{2X_c I_d}{\sqrt{3}E_m}\right) \tag{6.75}$$

where

$$E_m = \sqrt{2}E_{(L-N)}$$

Therefore,

$$u = \cos^{-1}\left(1 - \frac{2X_c I_d}{\sqrt{6}E_{(L-N)}}\right)$$

$$= \cos^{-1}\left(1 - \frac{2(6.2315 \ \Omega)(1,600 \text{ A})}{\sqrt{6}(53,418.8 \text{ V})}\right) = 32.1° \tag{6.76}$$

(b) The dc voltage of the rectifier can be expressed as

$$V_d = V_{dr}$$

$$= V_{s0} \cos\alpha - R_c I_d$$

where

$$R_c = \frac{3}{\pi} X_c$$

Thus,

$$V_d = V_{d0} \cos\alpha - \frac{3}{\pi} X_c I_d$$

$$= (125,000 \text{ V})(1.0) - \frac{3}{\pi}(6.2315 \text{ }\Omega)(1,600 \text{ A})$$

$$= 115,479 \text{ V}$$

(c) The displacement or power factor of the rectifier can be expressed as

$$\cos\theta \cong \frac{V_d}{V_{d0}}$$

$$= \frac{115,479 \text{ V}}{125,000 \text{ V}} = 0.924 \qquad (6.77)$$

and

$$\theta = 22.5°$$

(d) The magnetizing var input can be expressed as

$$Q_r = P_{r(dc)}\tan\theta \qquad (6.78)$$

or

$$Q_r = V_d I_d \tan\theta$$

$$= (115,479 \text{ V})(1,600 \text{ A})(0.414)$$

$$\cong 76.532 \text{ Mvar} \qquad (6.79)$$

Example 6.6

Assume that all three breakers given in Example 6.3 are closed, the LTC is on neutral, the dc voltage of the rectifier is 100 kV, and the maximum continuous dc of the rectifier is 1600 A. Determine the following:

(a) Firing angle α
(b) Overlap angle u
(c) Power factor
(d) Magnetizing var input

Solution

(a) The firing angle α can be determined from

$$V_d = V_{d0}\cos\alpha - R_c I_d$$

or

$$\cos\alpha = \frac{V_d + R_c I_d}{V_{d0}} \tag{6.80}$$

where

$$R_c = \frac{3}{\pi}X_c$$

Therefore,

$$\cos\alpha = \frac{V_d + R_c I_d}{V_{d0}}$$

$$= \frac{100,000 + \dfrac{3}{\pi}(6.2315)(1,600)}{125,000}$$

$$= 0.876 \tag{6.81}$$

and

$$\alpha = 28.817°$$

(b) The overlap angle u can be determined from

$$V_d = \frac{1}{2}V_{d0}(\cos\alpha + \cos\delta)$$

or

$$\cos\delta = \frac{2V_d}{V_{d0}} - \cos\alpha$$

$$= \frac{2\times100,000}{125,000} - 0.876 = 0.724 \tag{6.82}$$

and

$$\delta = 43.627°$$

Since

$$\delta = \alpha + u$$

the overlap angle u is

$$u = \delta - \alpha = 43.627° - 28.817° = 14.81°$$

(c) The associated power factor is

$$\cos\theta \cong \frac{V_d}{V_{d0}}$$

$$= \frac{125\,kV}{100\,kV} = 0.8$$

and

$$\theta = 36.87°$$

(d) The magnetizing var input is

$$Q_r = V_d I_d \tan\theta$$

$$= 100,000 \times 1,600 \times 0.75 = 120\,Mvar$$

Example 6.7

Use the setup and data of Example 6.3 and assume that the worst possible second-contingency outage in the ac system has occurred, that is, two of the ac breakers are open.

  (a) Determine whether or not a dc of 1600 A causes the rectifier to operate at the second mode.
  (b) If so, at what I_d does the first-mode operation cease? If not, what is

$$V_{dr} \text{ when the dc is 1600 A?}$$

Solution

  (a) From Example 6.4, when two breakers are open, the commutating reactance is

$$X_c = 12.6522$$

and

$$\alpha = 0$$

so that

$$u = \delta$$

$$= \cos^{-1}\left(1 - \frac{2X_c I_d}{\sqrt{6}E_{(L\text{-}N)}}\right)$$

$$= \cos^{-1}\left(1 - \frac{2(12.6522)(1,600)}{\sqrt{6}(53,440)}\right) = 46.3°$$

Since

$$u < 60°$$

the rectifier operates at the first mode, the normal operating mode.

(b) Since the rectifier does not operate at the second mode,

$$V_{dr} = V_{d0} \cos\alpha - \frac{3}{\pi} X_c I_d$$

$$= (125,000)(1.0) - \frac{3}{\pi}(12.6522)(1,600)$$

$$= 105,668.9 \text{ V}$$

Note that the commutating reactance causes a dc voltage drop.

6.8 PER-UNIT SYSTEMS AND NORMALIZING

The per-unit value of any quantity is its ratio to the chosen base quantity of the same dimensions. Therefore, a per-unit quantity is a *normalized* quantity with respect to a selected base value. Figure 6.6 shows a one-line diagram of a single-bridge converter system connected to a transformer with a tap changer underload. The figure also shows the fundamental ac and dc system quantities. The base quantities are indicated by the subscript B.

All ac voltages indicated in Figure 6.6 are line-to-neutral voltages. Therefore,

$$E = E_{(L\text{-}N)}$$

$$= \frac{E_m}{\sqrt{2}} \tag{6.83}$$

The ratio of base ac voltages is a fixed value and is defined as

$$a \triangleq \frac{E_{1(B)}}{E_{(B)}} = \frac{I_{(B)}}{I_{(B)}} \tag{6.84}$$

On the other hand, the turns ratio in use is a variable that is changeable by the LTC position and is defined as

$$n \triangleq \frac{n_1}{n_2} = \frac{E_1}{E} = \frac{I}{I_1} \tag{6.85}$$

Therefore, the per-unit voltage on the ac side of the converter transformer is

$$E_{1(\text{pu})} = \frac{E_1}{E_{1(B)}} \text{ pu V} \tag{6.86}$$

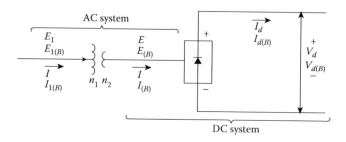

FIGURE 6.6 One-line diagram of a single-bridge converter system.

and the per-unit voltage on the dc side of the converter transformer is

$$E_{(pu)} = \frac{E}{E_{(B)}} \text{ pu V} \tag{6.87}$$

where

$$E = \frac{E_1}{n} \text{ V} \tag{6.88}$$

$$E_{(B)} = \frac{E_{1(B)}}{a} \text{ V} \tag{6.89}$$

thus, Equation 6.87 can be expressed as

$$E_{(pu)} = \left(\frac{a}{n}\right) E_1 \text{ pu V} \tag{6.90}$$

Note that when the LTC is on neutral,

$$n = a$$

and

$$E_{pu} < E_{1(pu)} \quad n > a$$

Thus, when the voltage on the dc side of the converter transformer is lowered with respect to the voltage on the ac side of the converter transformer by using the LTC of the transformer, the dc voltage V_d decreases.

6.8.1 AC System Per-Unit Bases

The per-unit bases for the quantities that are located on the ac side of the converter transformer are as follows:

$E_{1(B)}$ is the arbitrarily chosen voltage value
$S_{1(B)}$ is the arbitrarily chosen volt-ampere value

$$I_{1(B)} = \frac{S_{(B)}}{E_{1(B)}} \text{ A} \tag{6.91}$$

$$Z_{1(B)} = \frac{E_{1(B)}}{I_{1(B)}} \text{ } \Omega \tag{6.92}$$

$$L_{1(B)} = \frac{Z_{1(B)}}{\omega_{(B)}} \text{ H} \tag{6.93}$$

where

$$\omega_{(B)} = \omega = 377 \quad \text{if } f = 60 \text{ Hz}$$

On the other hand, the per-unit bases for the quantities that are located on the dc side of the converter transformer are

$$E_{(B)} = \frac{E_{1(B)}}{a} \text{ V} \tag{6.94}$$

$S(B)$ = arbitrarily chosen volt-ampere value (same as before)
  = $S_{1(B)}$

$$I_{(B)} = aI_{1(B)} \text{ A} \tag{6.95}$$

$$Z_{(B)} = \frac{Z_{1(B)}}{a^2} \text{ } \Omega \tag{6.96}$$

$$L_{(B)} = \frac{L_{1(B)}}{a^2} \text{ H} \tag{6.97}$$

6.8.2 DC System Per-Unit Bases

The dc system per-unit bases are constrained by the bridge circuit steady-state equations to be related to the chosen ac system per-unit bases. Note the analogy to the selection of ac bases on the two sides of a transformer, wherein such bases must be related by the transformer turns ratio.

When the firing angle α, overlap angle u, and dc I_d are zero, the dc voltage base is

$$V_{d(B)} \triangleq V_{d0}$$

or

$$V_{d(B)} = \frac{3\sqrt{6}}{\pi} E_{(B)} \tag{6.98}$$

or substituting Equation 6.94 into Equation 6.98, the dc voltage base can be expressed as

$$V_{d(B)} = \frac{3\sqrt{6}}{\pi} \times \frac{E_{1(B)}}{a} \tag{6.99}$$

The dc base can be expressed as

$$I_{d(B)} = \sqrt{\frac{3}{2}} I_{(B)} \tag{6.100}$$

or substituting Equation 6.95 into Equation 6.100,

$$I_{d(B)} = \sqrt{\frac{3}{2}} \left(aI_{1(B)} \right) \tag{6.101}$$

which is exact only if $u = 0$. However, it is an approximate relation with a maximum error of 4.3% at $u = 60°$ and only 1.1% at $u \leq 30°$ (i.e., the *normal operating range*).

The dc resistance base in the dc system can be expressed as

$$R_{d(B)} = \frac{V_{d(B)}}{I_{d(B)}}$$ (6.102)

or substituting Equations 6.99 and 6.101 into Equation 6.102,

$$R_{d(B)} = \frac{6}{\pi} \times \frac{Z_{1(B)}}{a^2}$$ (6.103)

or

$$R_{d(B)} = \frac{6}{\pi} \times Z_{(B)}$$ (6.104)

Similarly, the dc inductance base in the dc system can be expressed as

$$L_{d(B)} = \frac{6}{\pi} \times L_{(B)} \text{ H}$$ (6.105)

or

$$L_{d(B)} = \frac{6}{\pi} \times \frac{L_{1(B)}}{a^2} \text{ H}$$ (6.106)

Example 6.8

Normalize the steady-state rectifier equation of

$$V_d = V_{d0} \cos \alpha - \frac{3}{\pi} \omega L_c I_d$$ (6.107)

Solution
Since

$$V_{d0} = \frac{3\sqrt{6}}{\pi} \times E_{(L\text{-}N)}$$

the steady-state rectifier equation can be expressed as

$$V_d = \frac{3\sqrt{6}}{\pi} E_{(L\text{-}N)} \cos \alpha - \frac{3}{\pi} \omega L_c I_d$$ (6.108)

Dividing both sides of the equation by $V_{d(B)}$,

$$\frac{V_d}{V_{d(B)}} = \frac{3\sqrt{6}}{\pi} \times \frac{E}{V_{d(B)}} \cos \alpha - \frac{3}{\pi} \frac{\omega L_c I_d}{V_{d(B)}}$$ (6.109)

Substituting Equation 6.98 into Equation 6.108 and simplifying the resultant,

$$V_{d(pu)} = \frac{a}{n} E_{1(pu)} \cos \alpha - \frac{1}{2} L_{c(pu)} I_{d(pu)} \text{ pu V}$$ (6.110)

Example 6.9

Assume that the steady-state rectifier equation given in Example 6.8 can be modified by the substitution of

$$R_c = \frac{3}{\pi} \omega L_c$$

(a) Determine the normalized form of the modified steady-state rectifier equation.
(b) Find cos a from the normalized equation derived in part (a).

Solution

(a) From Equation 6.107,

$$V_d = V_{d0} \cos \alpha - \frac{3}{\pi} \omega L_c I_d$$

or

$$V_d = V_{d0} \cos \alpha - R_c I_d \ \text{V} \tag{6.65}$$

Since, in per units,

$$R_{c(pu)} = \frac{R_c}{R_{d(B)}} \ \text{pu} \tag{6.111}$$

or

$$R_c = R_{c(pu)} R_{d(B)} \ \Omega \tag{6.112}$$

and

$$I_{d(pu)} = \frac{I_d}{I_{d(B)}} \ \text{A} \tag{6.113}$$

or

$$I_d = I_{d(pu)} I_{d(B)} \ \text{A} \tag{6.114}$$

substituting Equations 6.112 and 6.114 into Equation 6.65 and dividing both sides of the resultant equation by $V_{d(B)}$ yields

$$V_{d(pu)} = E_{(pu)} \cos \alpha - R_{c(pu)} I_{d(pu)} \ \text{pu V} \tag{6.115}$$

or, alternatively,

$$V_{d(pu)} = \frac{a}{n} E_{1(pu)} \cos \alpha - R_{c(pu)} I_{d(pu)} \ \text{pu V} \tag{6.116}$$

(b) From Equation 6.116,

$$\cos \alpha = \frac{V_{d(pu)} + R_{c(pu)} I_{d(pu)}}{\dfrac{a}{n} \times E_{1(pu)}} \tag{6.117}$$

Example 6.10

Assume that all three breakers given in Example 6.3 are closed, the dc voltage of the rectifier is 100 kV, the maximum continuous dc of the rectifier is 1600 A, and the firing angle is zero. Assume that the LTC of the rectifier transformer is used to reduce the dc voltage to 100 kV. Use the per-unit quantities and relations and determine the following:

(a) Open-circuit dc voltage
(b) Open-circuit ac voltage on wye side of transformer
(c) Overlap angle u
(d) Power factor of rectifier
(e) Magnetizing var input to rectifier
(f) Number of 0.625% steps of buck required on LTC of transformer

Solution

(a) Since, in per units,

$$V_{d(pu)} = E_{(pu)} \cos \alpha - R_{c(pu)} I_{d(pu)} \text{ pu V}$$

from which

$$E_{(pu)} = \frac{V_{d(pu)} + R_{c(pu)} I_{d(pu)}}{\cos \alpha}$$

where

$$R_c = \frac{3}{n} X_c = \frac{3}{n}(6.2315) = 5.95 \ \Omega$$

the dc and voltage bases are

$$I_{d(B)} = 1600 \text{ A}$$

and

$$V_{d(B)} = 125{,}000 \text{ V}$$

The resistance base can be determined as

$$R_{d(B)} = \frac{V_{d(B)}}{I_{d(B)}} = \frac{125{,}000 \text{ V}}{1{,}600 \text{ A}} = 78.125 \ \Omega$$

Therefore,

$$V_{d(pu)} = \frac{V_d}{V_{d(B)}} = \frac{100{,}000 \text{ V}}{125{,}000 \text{ V}} = 0.8 \text{ pu V}$$

$$I_{d(pu)} = \frac{I_d}{I_{d(B)}} = \frac{1600 \text{ A}}{1600 \text{ A}} = 1.0 \text{ pu A}$$

$$R_{c(pu)} = \frac{R_c}{R_{c(B)}} = \frac{5.95 \ \Omega}{78.125 \ \Omega} = 0.0762 \text{ pu } \Omega$$

Thus,

$$E_{(pu)} = \frac{0.8 + (0.0762)(1.0)}{1.0} = 0.8762 \text{ pu V}$$

However,

$$E_{(pu)} = \frac{V_{d0}}{V_{d(B)}}$$

from which

$$V_{d0} = E_{(pu)}V_{d(B)} = (0.8762)\ (125,000) = 109,520 \text{ V}$$

(b) The open-circuit ac voltage on the wye side can be found from

$$V_{d0} = 2.34E$$

or

$$E = \frac{V_{d0}}{2.34} = \frac{109,520 \text{ V}}{2.34} = 46,803 \text{ V}$$

(c) Since

$$\cos\delta = \cos\alpha - \frac{X_{c(pu)} \times I_{d(pu)}}{\dfrac{a}{n} \times E_{1(pu)}}$$

where

$$a = n = \frac{E_{I(L-N)}}{E_{(L-N)}} = \frac{92.95 \text{ kV}}{53.44 \text{ kV}} = 1.74$$

$$X_{c(pu)} = 2R_{c(pu)} = 2(0.0762) = 0.1524 \text{ pu}$$

$$E_{1(pu)} = \frac{E_1}{E_{1(B)}} = \frac{92.95 \text{ kV}}{92.95 \text{ kV}} = 1.0$$

then

$$\cos\delta = 1.0 - \frac{(0.1524)(1.0)}{(1.74/1.74)(1.0)} = 0.8476$$

and

$$\delta = 32.04°$$

where

$$\delta = u + \alpha \quad \alpha = 0$$

so that the overlap angle is

$$u = \delta = 32.04°$$

(d) The power factor of the rectifier is

$$\cos\theta \cong \frac{V_d}{V_{d0}} = \frac{100,000 \text{ V}}{109,520 \text{ V}} = 0.913$$

and

$$\theta = 24.07°$$

(e) The magnetizing var input to the rectifier is

$$Q_r = V_d I_d \tan\theta$$

$$= (100,000 \text{ V}) (1600 \text{ A}) (0.4466)$$

$$= 71.458 \text{ Mvar}$$

(f) Since the necessary change in voltage is

$$\Delta V = 53,440 - 46,803 = 6,637 \text{ V}$$

and one buck step can change

$$(5/8\%)E_{(L\text{-}N)} = 0.00625(53,440 \text{ V})$$

$$= 334 \text{ V/step}$$

the number of 0.625% steps of buck required is

$$\text{Number of bucks} = \frac{6637 \text{ V}}{334 \text{ V/step}} = 20 \text{ steps}$$

6.9   INVERSION

In a given converter, the current flow is always from anode to cathode, that is, the unidirectional inside a rectifying valve or thyristor, so that the cathode remains the positive terminal. Therefore, the current direction in the converter cannot be reversed. When it is required to operate the converter as an inverter in order to reverse the direction of power flow, the direction of the average direct voltage must be reversed. This can be obtained by using the grid control to change the delay angle α until the average direct voltage V_d becomes negative. If there is no overlap, the voltage V_d decreases as the delay angle α is advanced, and it becomes zero when α is 90°. With further increase in the delay angle α, the average direct voltage becomes negative.

Therefore, it can be said that the rectification and inversion processes occur when $0° < \alpha < 90°$ and $90° < \alpha < 180°$, respectively. If there is an overlap, the inversion process may start at a value of the delay angle that is less than 90°. Therefore,

$$\alpha = \pi - \delta \tag{6.118}$$

or

$$\alpha = \frac{1}{2}(\pi - u) \tag{6.119}$$

where
   α is the delay angle in electrical degrees
   δ is the extinction angle in electrical degrees
   u is the overlap angle in electrical degrees

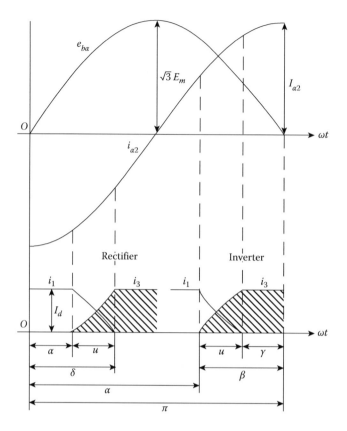

FIGURE 6.7 Relations among angles used in converter theory. (From Kimbark, E.W., *Direct Current Transmission*, vol. 1, Wiley, New York, 1971.)

Figure 6.7 shows relations among angles used in converter theory and the reason the curvature of the front of a current pulse of an inverter differs from that of a rectifier. Kimbark [3] gives the relations among the various inverter angles as

$$\beta = \pi - \alpha \tag{6.120}$$

$$\gamma = \pi - \delta \tag{6.121}$$

$$u = \delta - \alpha \tag{6.122}$$

$$u = \beta - \gamma \tag{6.123}$$

where
   β is the inverter ignition angle in electrical degrees
   γ is the inverter extinction angle in electrical degrees

In order to provide adequate time for the deionization of the arc for the appropriate valve, the minimum value of the inverter extinction angle γ_0 must be in the range of 1°–8°. If the value of γ_0 is not adequate, the valve starts to conduct again. This is called *commutation failure*.

The rectifier equations can be used to describe the inverter operation by substituting α and δ by $\pi - \beta$ and $\beta - \gamma$, respectively. In order to differentiate the inverter equations from the rectifier equations, it is customary to use the subscripts i and r to signify the inverter and rectifier operations, respectively. Therefore, it can be expressed that

$$I_{di} = I_{s2} (\cos \gamma - \cos \beta) \tag{6.124}$$

or substituting Equation 6.60 into Equation 6.124,

$$I_{di} = \frac{\sqrt{3}E_m}{2\omega L_c} I_{s2} (\cos \gamma - \cos \beta) \tag{6.125}$$

In general, it is customary to express the inverter voltage as negative when it is used in conjunction with a rectifier voltage in a given equation. Otherwise, when it is used alone, it is customary to express it as positive. Therefore, it can be expressed that

$$V_{di} = \frac{V_{d0i}}{2} V(\cos \gamma + \cos \beta) \tag{6.126}$$

Furthermore, for inverters with constant-ignition-angle (CIA) control,

$$V_{di} = V_{d0i} \cos \beta + R_c I_d \tag{6.127}$$

or

$$V_{di} = V_{d0i} \cos \beta + \frac{3}{\pi} X_c I_d \tag{6.128}$$

and for inverters with constant-extinction-angle (CEA) control,

$$V_{di} = V_{d0i} \cos \gamma - R_c I_d \tag{6.129}$$

or

$$V_{di} = V_{d0i} \cos \gamma - \frac{3}{\pi} X_c I_d \tag{6.130}$$

Note that it is preferable to operate inverters with CEA control rather than with CIA control. Figure 6.8 shows the corresponding equivalent inverter circuit representations.

It can be said that an inverter has a leading power factor, contrary to a rectifier, which has a lagging power factor. This is due to the fact that the lagging reactive power is provided to the inverter by the ac system into which the inverter is feeding active power. Therefore, this is equivalent to the inverter feeding current to the ac system at a leading power factor. The required additional reactive power by the inverter is provided by the synchronous capacitors or by static shunt capacitors.

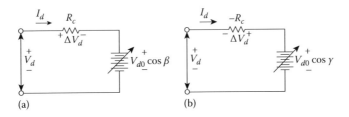

FIGURE 6.8 Equivalent circuits of inverter: (a) with constant β and (b) with constant γ.

Furthermore, harmonic filters are needed on both ac and dc sides of converters in order to prevent the harmonics generated by the rectifier and inverter from entering into the ac and dc systems. The order of harmonics in the direct voltage are expressed by

$$N = pq$$

and the order of harmonics in the ac are given by

$$N = pq \pm 1$$

where
    p is the pulse number
    q is the integer number

Example 6.11

Consider a single-bridge inverter and do the following:

(a) Verify that the power factor of the fundamental component of the inverter ac line current can be expressed as

$$\cos\theta_{1i} \cong \frac{1}{2}(\cos\beta + \cos\gamma)$$

(b) Explain the approximation involved in part (a).
(c) Explain the effect of increasing the ignition advance angle β on the power factor in part (a).
(d) Explain the effect of increasing the extinction angle γ on the power factor in part (a).
(e) Explain whether or not the power factor that can be found using the equation given in part (a) is greater or less than the power factor that would be measured in terms of the readings of the switchboard wattmeter, voltmeter, and ammeter.

Solution

(a) From Equation 6.126, inverter voltage can be expressed as

$$V_{di} = V_{d0i}\left[\frac{1}{2}(\cos\beta + \cos\gamma)\right]$$

where

$$V_{d0i} = \frac{3\sqrt{6}}{\pi} \times E_{(L\text{-}N)} \tag{6.43}$$

Therefore,

$$V_{di} = \frac{3\sqrt{6}}{\pi}\left[\frac{1}{2}(\cos\beta + \cos\gamma)\right]E_{(L\text{-}N)} \tag{6.131}$$

When losses are disregarded, the active ac power can be set equal to the dc power:

$$P_{(ac)} = P_{(dc)}$$

where

$$P_{(ac)} = 3E_{(L\text{-}N)}I_{L1}\cos\theta_{1i} \tag{6.132}$$

and

$$P_{(dc)} = V_{di}I_d$$

or

$$P_{(dc)} = \frac{3\sqrt{6}}{\pi}\left[\frac{1}{2}(\cos\beta + \cos\gamma)\right] E_{(L\text{-}N)} I_d \qquad (6.133)$$

Thus, from Equations 6.132 and 6.133,

$$3E_{(L\text{-}N)}I_{L1}\cos\Phi_{1i} = \frac{3\sqrt{6}}{\pi}\left[\frac{1}{2}(\cos\beta + \cos\gamma)\right] E_{(L\text{-}N)} I_d \qquad (6.134)$$

or

$$I_{L1}\cos\theta_{1i} = \frac{\sqrt{6}}{\pi}\left[\frac{1}{2}(\cos\beta + \cos\gamma)\right] I_d \qquad (6.135)$$

However,

$$I_{L1} \cong \frac{\sqrt{6}}{\pi} \times I_d \qquad (6.136)$$

which is an approximation. Therefore,

$$\cos\theta_{1i} \cong \frac{1}{2}(\cos\beta + \cos\gamma) \qquad (6.137)$$

which is also an approximation.

(b) Equations 6.136 and 6.137 would be exact only if $u = 0$. Otherwise, there will be some approximate values with a maximum error of 4.3% at $u = 60°$. At normal operating range (i.e., $u \leq 30°$), the error involved is less than 1.1%.
(c) An increase in the ignition advance angle β causes the power factor to decrease.
(d) An increase in the extinction angle γ causes the power factor to decrease.
(e) The power factor determined based on the readings can be expressed as

$$\cos\theta = \frac{W_{\text{reading}}}{\sqrt{3}\left(V_{(L\text{-}L)\text{reading}}\right)\left(I_{\text{reading}}\right)}$$

Therefore, the power factor calculated from Equation 6.137 is greater than the power factor determined from the readings because of the harmonics involved.

Example 6.12

Consider the single-bridge inverter in Example 6.11 and verify that the power factor of the fundamental component of the inverter ac line current can be expressed as

$$\cos\theta_{1i} \cong \frac{V_{di}}{V_{d0i}}$$

Solution

The inverter's direct voltage is

$$V_{di} = V_{d0i}\cos\beta - \Delta V_{di} \qquad (6.138)$$

where

$$\Delta V_{di} = \frac{1}{2}V_{d0i}(\cos\beta - \cos\gamma) \qquad (6.139)$$

Therefore,

$$V_{di} = V_{d0i}\cos\beta - \frac{1}{2}V_{d0i}(\cos\beta - \cos\gamma)$$

or

$$V_{di} = \frac{1}{2}V_{d0i}(\cos\beta + \cos\gamma) \tag{6.140}$$

Thus,

$$\frac{\cos\beta + \cos\gamma}{2} = \frac{V_{di}}{V_{d0i}} \tag{6.141}$$

$$\cos\theta_{1i} = \frac{\cos\beta + \cos\gamma}{2} \tag{6.142}$$

Therefore,

$$\cos\theta_{1i} = \frac{V_{di}}{V_{d0i}} \tag{6.143}$$

Alternatively, from Equation 6.126,

$$V_{di} = V_{d0i}\frac{\cos\beta + \cos\gamma}{2}$$

from which

$$\frac{\cos\beta + \cos\gamma}{2} = \frac{V_{di}}{V_{d0i}}$$

Therefore,

$$\cos\theta_{1i} \cong \frac{V_{di}}{V_{d0i}}$$

Example 6.13

Consider the single-bridge inverter in Example 6.11 and verify that the magnetizing var input to the inverter can be expressed as

$$Q_i \cong P_{(dc)}\left[\left(\frac{V_{d0i}}{V_{di}}\right)^2 - 1\right]^{1/2} \quad \text{var}$$

Solution

From Figure 6.9b,

$$Q_i \cong P_{(dc)}\tan\Phi_{1i} \tag{6.144}$$

From Figure 6.9a,

$$\tan\theta_{1i} = \frac{\left(V_{d0i}^2 - V_{di}^2\right)^{1/2}}{V_{di}} \tag{6.145}$$

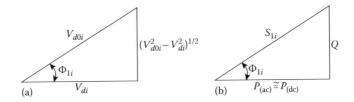

FIGURE 6.9 Voltage and power triangles: (a) voltage triangle and (b) power triangle.

or

$$\tan\Phi_{1i} = \left[\frac{V_{d0i}^2}{V_{di}^2} - 1\right]^{1/2} \tag{6.146}$$

Therefore,

$$Q_i = P_{(dc)}\left[\left(\frac{V_{d0i}}{V_{di}}\right)^2 - 1\right]^{1/2} \text{ var} \tag{6.147}$$

Example 6.14

Consider the single-bridge inverter of Example 6.13 and do the following:

(a) Verify that the volt-ampere load due to the fundamental component of inverter ac line current can be expressed as

$$S_{1i} \cong P_{(dc)}\frac{V_{di0}}{V_{di}} \text{ VA}$$

(b) Explain whether or not the total volt-ampere load is larger or smaller than the S_{1i} in part (a).

Solution

(a) From Figure 6.4b,

$$\cos\theta_{1i} \cong \frac{P_{(dc)}}{S_{1i}} \tag{6.148}$$

from which

$$S_{1i} \cong P_{(dc)}\left(\frac{1}{\cos\theta_{1i}}\right) \tag{6.149}$$

But from Example 6.12,

$$\cos\theta_{1i} \cong \frac{V_{di}}{V_{d0i}} \tag{6.143}$$

Therefore, substituting Equation 6.143 into Equation 6.149,

$$S_{1i} \cong P_{(dc)}\frac{V_{d0i}}{V_{di}} \text{ VA} \tag{6.150}$$

(b) The total volt-ampere load is larger than the one found in part (a) because in part (a), the effects of harmonics are ignored and only the fundamental component of the inverter ac line current is considered.

6.10 MULTIBRIDGE (*B*-BRIDGE) CONVERTER STATIONS

Figure 6.10 shows 800 kV dc terminals of a converter station. Figure 6.11 shows 800 kV disconnect switch on the ac side at the same converter station. Figure 6.12 shows 800 kV risers on the ac side at the same converter station.

Figure 6.13 shows a typical converter station layout. For such a station, the general arrangement of a converter station with 12-pulse converters is shown in Figure 6.14. Figure 6.15 shows a one-line diagram for a *B*-bridge converter (rectifier) station and the supplying ac network. The ac network system is represented by the Thévenin equivalent E_1 voltage and $X_{1(sys)}$ reactance. The E_1 voltage can be assumed to be sinusoidal due to the ac filter connected at the ac bus.

The converter bank is made of two or more three-phase bridges, and each bridge contains up to six mercury arc valves or thyristors. Note that there are *B*-bridges in the figure. The number of bridges required is dictated by the direct voltage level selected for economical transmission.

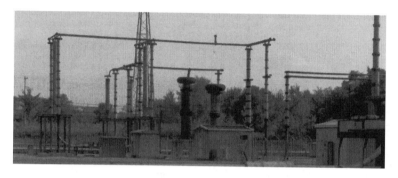

FIGURE 6.10   800 kV dc terminals of a converter station.

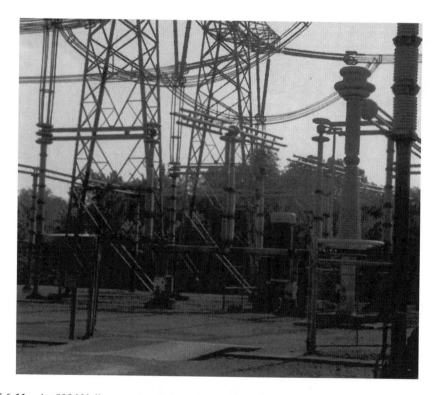

FIGURE 6.11   An 800 kV disconnect switch on the ac side at the same converter station.

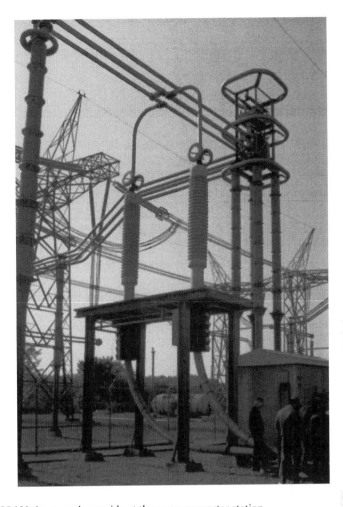

FIGURE 6.12   800 kV risers on the ac side at the same converter station.

In order to eliminate certain harmonics, the transformer connections are arranged in a certain way so that one-half of the bridge transformers has 0° phase shift and the other half has 30° phase shift. This arrangement gives 12-pulse operation. The two sets of transformer banks are connected either one set in wye–wye and the other set in wye–delta with 30° phase shift or one set in delta–delta with 0° phase shift and the other in wye–delta with 30° phase shift (or from one three-winding bank connected wye–wye–delta).

As a result of this arrangement, the two halves of the bridges do not commutate simultaneously. The current on the dc side of the converter is almost completely smoothed due to the dc reactors (L_d) connected. As can be seen from Figure 6.15, the B-bridges are connected in series on the dc side and in parallel on the ac side. Therefore, the direct voltage can be expressed as

$$V_d = \left(\frac{3\sqrt{6}}{\pi} \right) B \times n \times E_{(\text{L-N})} \cos \theta \tag{6.151}$$

or

$$V_d = 2.34 B \times n \times E_{(\text{L-N})} \cos \theta \tag{6.152}$$

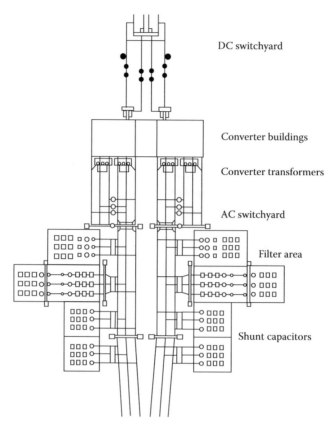

FIGURE 6.13 Typical converter station layout. (From Fink, D.G. and Beaty, H.W., *Standard Handbook for Electrical Engineers*, 11th edn., McGraw-Hill, New York, 1978.)

or

$$V_d = 1.35 B \times n \times E_{(\text{L-L})} \cos \theta \tag{6.153}$$

where
   B is the number of bridges
   n is the turns ratio in use
   $E_{(\text{L-N})}$ is the line-to-neutral voltage in volts
   $E_{(\text{L-L})}$ is the line-to-line voltage in volts
   $\cos \theta$ is the power factor of fundamental component of ac line current

The fundamental component of the ac line current can be expressed as

$$I_{1(a)} = \frac{\sqrt{6}}{\pi} B \times n \times I_d \tag{6.154}$$

or

$$I_{1(a)} = 0.78 B \times n \times I_d \tag{6.155}$$

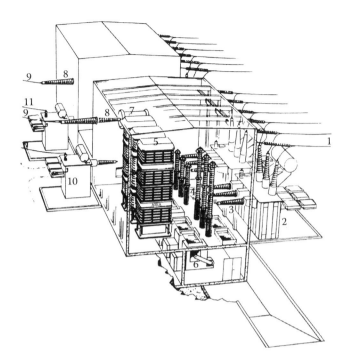

FIGURE 6.14 General arrangement of converter station with 12-pulse converters: (1) ac bus bar, (2) converter transformer, (3) valve-side bushing of converter transformer, (4) surge arresters, (5) quadruple valves, (6) valve-cooling fans, (7) air core reactor, (8) wall bushing, (9) outgoing dc bus work, (10) smoothing reactor, and (11) outgoing electrode line connection. (From Fink, D.G. and Beaty, H.W., *Standard Handbook for Electrical Engineers*, 11th edn., McGraw-Hill, New York, 1978.)

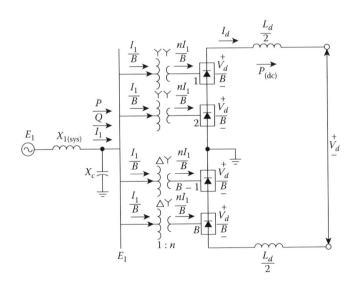

FIGURE 6.15 One-line diagram for *B*-bridge converter (rectifier) station.

The active ac power is equal to dc power, ignoring losses:

$$P_{(ac)} = P_{(dc)} \text{ W}$$

where

$$P_{(dc)} = V_d I_d \text{ W} \tag{6.156}$$

and

$$P_{(ac)} = 3E_{(L\text{-}N)}I_{1(a)}\cos \Phi \text{ W} \tag{6.157}$$

6.11 PER-UNIT REPRESENTATION OF *B*-BRIDGE CONVERTER STATIONS

Figure 6.16 shows a one-line diagram representation of two ac systems connected by a dc transmission link. The system has two *B*-bridge converter stations: the one on the left operates as a rectifier and the one on the right operates as an inverter. It is possible to reverse the direction of power flow by interchanging the functions of the converter stations.

In this section, only the first-mode operation is to be reviewed; that is, the overlap angle u is less than 30° so that the one-half of the bridges with 0° phase and the other half of the bridges with 30° phase shift do not commutate simultaneously.

The notation that will be used is largely defined in the illustration. As before, the subscript B designates the base value. An additional subscript in terms of r or i may be added to define the

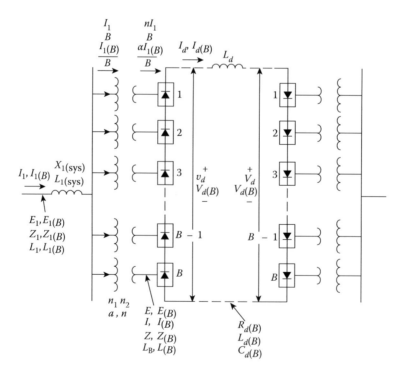

FIGURE 6.16 One-line diagram representation of two *B*-bridge converter stations connecting two ac systems over a dc transmission link.

rectifier or inverter operation involved, respectively. Assume that all ac voltages given are line-to-neutral voltages. The following notation is applicable for each transformer:

S_{tr} is the transformer nameplate rated in three-phase volt-amperes

a is the ratio of base ac voltages:

$$= \frac{E_{1(B)}}{E_{(B)}} = \frac{BI_{(B)}}{I_{1(B)}} \tag{6.158}$$

n is the turns ratio in use (variable changeable with LTC position):

$$= \frac{n_1}{n_2} = \frac{E_1}{E} = \frac{I}{I_1} \tag{6.159}$$

X_{tr} is the leakage reactance referred to the dc side in ohms:

$$= n^2 X_{tr} \tag{6.160}$$

$X_{1(tr)}$ is the leakage reactance referred to the ac side in ohms:

$$= n^2 X_{tr}$$

L_{tr} is the leakage inductance referred to the dc side in henries

$L_{1(tr)}$ is the inductance referred to the ac side in henries:

$$= n^2 L_{(tr)} \tag{6.161}$$

$X_{tr(pu)}$ is the per-unit leakage reactance (when LTC is on neutral):

$$= \frac{X_{(tr)}}{Z_{(B)}} = \frac{a^2 X_{tr}}{a^2 Z_{(B)}} = \frac{X_{1(tr)}}{Z_{1(B)}} \tag{6.162}$$

$L_{tr(pu)}$ is the per-unit leakage inductance:

$$= X_{tr(pu)}$$

If there is a significant amount of ac system impedance, the following notation is applicable:

$X_{1(sys)}$ is the ac system reactance referred to the ac side in ohms

X_{sys} is the ac system reactance referred to the dc side in ohms:

$$= \frac{X_{1(sys)}}{n^2} \tag{6.163}$$

$L_{1(sys)}$ is the ac system inductance referred to the ac side in henries

L_{sys} is the ac system inductance referred to the dc side in henries:

$$= \frac{L_{1(sys)}}{n^2} \tag{6.164}$$

6.11.1   AC System Per-Unit Bases

The per-unit bases for the quantities located on the ac side of the converter transformer are as follows:

$E_{1(B)}$ is the arbitrarily chosen voltage value

$S_{1(B)}$ is the arbitrarily chosen volt-ampere value

$$I_{1(B)} = \frac{S_{1(B)}}{3E_{1(B)}} \text{ A} \tag{6.165}$$

$$Z_{1(B)} = \frac{E_{1(B)}}{I_{1(B)}} \text{ } \Omega \tag{6.166}$$

$$L_{1(B)} = \frac{Z_{1(B)}}{\omega_{(B)}} \text{ H} \tag{6.167}$$

$$C_{1(B)} = \frac{1}{\omega_{(B)}Z_{1(B)}} \text{ F} \tag{6.168}$$

where

$$\omega_{(B)} = \omega = 377 \quad \text{if} \quad f = 60 \text{ Hz}$$

On the other hand, the per-unit bases for the quantities located on the dc side of the converter transformer are

$$E_{(B)} = \frac{E_{1(B)}}{a} \tag{6.169}$$

$$S_{(B)} = S_{1(B)} \tag{6.170}$$

$$I_{(B)} = aI_{1(B)} \tag{6.171}$$

$$Z_{(B)} = \frac{Z_{1(B)}}{a^2} \tag{6.172}$$

$$L_{(B)} = \frac{L_{1(B)}}{a^2} \tag{6.173}$$

$$C_{(B)} = a^2 C_{1(B)} \tag{6.174}$$

Note that the per-unit size of each transformer is

$$S_{\text{tr(pu)}} = \frac{1}{B} \text{ pu VA} \tag{6.175}$$

provided that

$$S_{(B)} = BS_{\text{tr}} \text{ VA} \tag{6.176}$$

is selected. For example, the per-unit size of each transformer of a four-bridge converter station is

$$
\begin{aligned}
S_{tr(pu)} &= \frac{S_{tr}}{S_{(B)}} \\
&= \frac{S_{tr}}{4S_{tr}} \\
&= 0.25 \ \text{pu VA}
\end{aligned}
$$

6.11.2   DC System Per-Unit Bases

The dc system per-unit bases for a B-bridge converter are selected somewhat differently than the previous bases used for a single-bridge converter in Section 6.7.

When the firing angle α, overlap angle u, and dc I_d are zero, the ratio of base ac voltages a and turns ratio in use n are equal, and

$$
E_{(pu)} = E_{1(pu)} = 1.0 \ \text{pu V}
$$

the dc voltage base is

$$
V_{d(B)} \triangleq V_{d0}
$$

or

$$
V_{d(B)} = \frac{3\sqrt{6}}{\pi} \times B \times E_{(B)} \tag{6.177}
$$

or

$$
V_{d(B)} = \frac{3\sqrt{6}}{\pi} \times \frac{B \times E_{1(B)}}{a} \tag{6.178}
$$

By forcing the ac and dc power bases to be exactly equal,

$$
3E_{(B)}I_{(B)} = V_{d(B)}I_{d(B)} \tag{6.179}
$$

so that

$$
I_{d(B)} = \frac{3E_{(B)}I_{(B)}}{V_{d(B)}} \tag{6.180}
$$

Substituting Equations 6.177 and 6.178 into Equation 6.180 separately,

$$
I_{d(B)} = \frac{\pi}{\sqrt{6}} \times \frac{I_{(B)}}{B} \tag{6.181}
$$

and

$$
I_{d(B)} = \frac{\pi}{\sqrt{6}} \times \frac{a \times I_{1(B)}}{B} \tag{6.182}
$$

The fundamental component of the ac per line to a bridge having no overlap is

$$I_{1(a)} = \frac{\sqrt{6}}{\pi} \times I_d \tag{6.183}$$

or

$$I_{1(a)} = 0.78 \times I_d \tag{6.184}$$

whereas the total rms ac is

$$I_{(a)} = \sqrt{\frac{2}{3}} \times I_d \tag{6.185}$$

or

$$I_{(a)} = 0.8165\, I_d \tag{6.186}$$

Note that, in the bases discussed in Section 6.7, the constant $\sqrt{3/2}$ was in the definition of $I_{d(B)}$ and that $P_{d(B)}$ was not exactly equal to the ac power base. However, in the present bases, the constant $\sqrt{6}/\pi$ is in the definition of $I_{d(B)}$, and ac and dc power bases are exactly equal.

The dc resistance base in the dc system can be expressed as

$$R_{d(B)} = \frac{V_{d(B)}}{I_{d(B)}} \tag{6.187}$$

or

$$R_{d(B)} = \frac{18B^2 \times Z_{(B)}}{\pi^2} \tag{6.188}$$

or

$$R_{d(B)} = \frac{18B^2 \times Z_{1(B)}}{\pi^2 \times a^2} \tag{6.189}$$

The dc inductance base in the dc system can be expressed as

$$L_{d(B)} = \frac{V_{d(B)} t_{(B)}}{I_{d(B)}} \tag{6.190}$$

or

$$L_{d(B)} = \frac{R_{d(B)}}{\omega_{(B)}} \tag{6.191}$$

where

$$t_{(B)} = \frac{1}{\omega_{(B)}} \tag{6.192}$$

Similarly, the dc capacitance base in the dc system can be expressed as

$$C_{d(B)} = \frac{1}{R_{d(B)}\omega_{(B)}} \text{ F} \tag{6.193}$$

6.12   OPERATION OF DC TRANSMISSION LINK

Figure 6.17 shows the equivalent circuit for a simple dc transmission link. Here, the dc link may be a transmission line, a cable, or a link with negligible length. The subscripts r and i signify rectifier and inverter, respectively.

The dc I_d that flows from the rectifier to the inverter can be expressed as

$$I_d = \frac{V_{dr} - V_{di}}{R_L} \tag{6.194}$$

and the sending-end power can be expressed as

$$P_{(dc)} = V_{dr}I_d \tag{6.195}$$

Since it is possible for a converter to become a rectifier or an inverter by grid control, the direction of the power flow can be reversible. This can be accomplished by reversing the direct voltage, as previously explained. Figure 6.18 illustrates this reversion in power flow direction. It can be shown, from Kirchhoff's voltage law, that

$$V_{ab} = I_dR_L + V_{cd} \tag{6.196}$$

Therefore, when the V_{ab} and V_{cd} voltages represent the average direct voltages of a rectifier and an inverter, respectively, Equation 6.196 can be expressed as

$$V_{dr} = I_dR_L - V_{di} \tag{6.197}$$

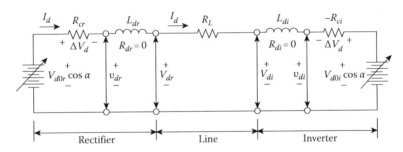

FIGURE 6.17   Equivalent circuit of dc link.

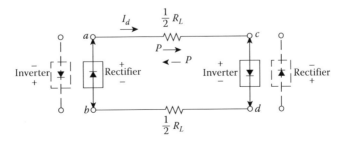

FIGURE 6.18   Illustration of reversion in power flow direction.

Similarly, when the V_{ab} and V_{cd} voltages represent the average direct voltages of an inverter and a rectifier, respectively, Equation 6.196 can be expressed as

$$V_{di} = I_d R_L - V_{dr} \tag{6.198}$$

Therefore, it can be shown in either case that

$$I_d R_L = V_{dr} + V_{di} \tag{6.199}$$

where

$$V_{dr} = V_{d0r} \cos\alpha - \frac{3}{\pi}\omega L_{cr} I_d \tag{6.200}$$

$$V_{di} = -V_{d0i} \cos\alpha + \frac{3}{\pi}\omega L_{ci} I_d \tag{6.201}$$

Thus,

$$I_d = \frac{V_{d0r}\cos\alpha - V_{d0i}\cos\gamma}{R_L + \dfrac{3}{\pi}\omega L_{cr} - \dfrac{3}{\pi}\omega L_{ci}} \tag{6.202}$$

or

$$I_d = \frac{V_{d0r}\cos\alpha - V_{d0i}\cos\gamma}{R_L + R_{cr} - R_{ci}} \tag{6.203}$$

where

$$R_{cr} = \frac{3}{\pi}\omega L_{cr} \tag{6.204}$$

$$R_{ci} = \frac{3}{\pi}\omega L_{ci} \tag{6.205}$$

The value of the dc I_d can be controlled by changing either V_{d0r} and V_{d0i} values or delay angle α or extinction angle γ. The values of V_{d0r} and V_{d0i} can be governed by using the LTCs of the supply transformers to change the ratio between the dc and ac voltages. Unfortunately, this method is very slow to be practical, whereas the delay angle α can be controlled very fast by using the grid control system. However, this method causes the converter to consume an excessively large amount of reactive power. Therefore, it is usual to operate the rectifier with minimum delay angle and the inverter with minimum extinction angle in order to achieve the control with minimum amount of reactive power consumption. Thus, it is a better practice to operate the rectifier with a constant-current (CC) characteristic and the inverter with a constant-voltage characteristic, as shown in Figure 6.19. As succinctly put by Kimbark [3], "the rectifier controls the direct current and the inverter controls the direct voltage." In practice, the values of the delay angle α and the extinction angle γ are usually selected in the ranges of 12°–18° and 15°–18°, respectively. Since a converter can be operating as a rectifier or inverter depending on the direction of power flow, it is necessary that each converter has dual-control systems, as shown in Figure 6.20.

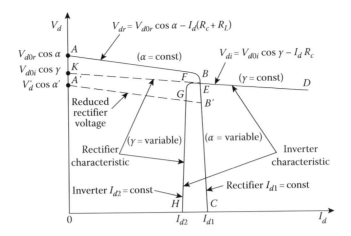

FIGURE 6.19   Inverter and rectifier operation characteristics with CC compounding.

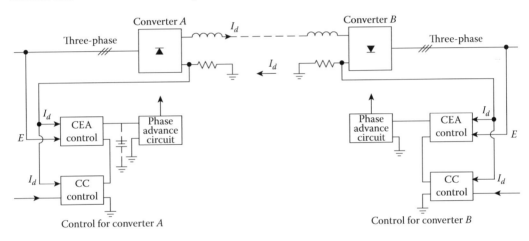

FIGURE 6.20   Schematic control diagram of HVDC system with CEA and CC controls. (From Weedy, B.M., *Electric Power Systems*, 3rd edn., Wiley, New York, 1979.)

Note that, in Figure 6.19, the normal operation point is E, where the characteristics of rectifier and inverter intersect. The rectifier characteristic has two line segments: the AB segment, at which the minimum delay angle α is constant, and the BC segment, at which the rectifier current I_{d1} is constant. Similarly, the inverter characteristic has two segments: the DF segment, at which the minimum extinction angle γ is constant, and the FH segment, at which the inverter current I_{d2} is constant. Normally, the current regulator of the inverter is set at a lower current value than the one of the rectifier. Hence, the difference in currents is

$$\Delta I_d = I_{d1} - I_{d2} \tag{6.206}$$

where
   ΔI_d is the current margin (usually 10%–15% of rated current)
   I_{d1} is the CC of rectifier
   I_{d2} is the CC of inverter

As aforementioned, under normal operating conditions, the operation point is E, at which the rectifier controls the dc and the inverter controls the direct voltage.

However, under emergency conditions, the operation point may change. For example, if the rectifier voltage characteristic is shifted down due to a large dip in rectifier voltage, it intersects the FH CC segment of the inverter characteristic at a new operation point G, where the inverter controls the dc and the rectifier controls the direct voltage.

Note that if the inverter were not equipped with the CC (*control*) regulator, it would have the characteristic DFK, as shown in Figure 6.19. Therefore, it can be seen that the shifted rectifier characteristic $A'B'$ would not have intersected the inverter characteristic. Consequently, the current and power would have decreased to zero.

Under normal operation, if the current is required to increase, the current setting is increased first at the rectifier and second at the inverter. On the other hand, if the current is required to decrease, the order of the operation is reversed; the current setting is decreased first at the inverter and second at the rectifier. This keeps the sign of the current margin the same and thus prevents any unexpected reversing in the direction of power flow.

Furthermore, the current margin between such points E and G shown in Figure 6.19 has to be adequate in order to prevent both inverter and rectifier current regulators operating at the same time. Note also that the voltage margin indicated by BE is due to a trade-off between minimum reactive compensations by holding the delay angle α as low as possible and preventing inverter control, which affects current.

6.13 STABILITY OF CONTROL

As aforementioned, the control system is made of CC control of the rectifier and CEA control of the inverter. An inappropriate control system can make oscillations by various disturbances, that is, converter faults and line-to-ground faults, and can cause *instability*. Kimbark [3] gives the following approximate method to study this phenomenon.

Figure 6.21 shows an equivalent circuit of a dc link for analysis of stability of control. Note that the rectifier on a CC control shows a large resistance $K + R_{c1}$ (where K is the gain of the CC regulator). But the inverter on a CEA control shows a low negative resistance, $-R_{c2}$.

Therefore, it can be written in the s domain that

$$E_{1(s)} = Z_{1(s)}I_{1(s)} - Z_{m(s)}I_{2(s)} \tag{6.207}$$

$$E_{2(s)} = Z_{m(s)}I_{1(s)} - Z_{2(s)}I_{2(s)} \tag{6.208}$$

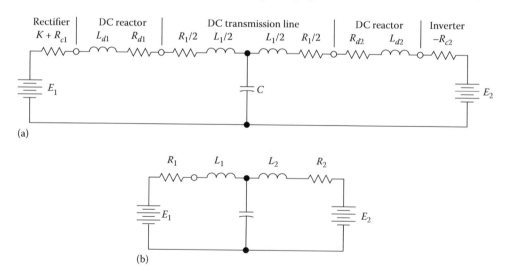

(a)

(b)

FIGURE 6.21 Equivalent circuit of dc link for analysis of stability of control: (a) before combination of line with terminal equipment and (b) after combination. (From Kimbark, E.W., *Direct Current Transmission*, vol. 1, Wiley, New York, 1971.)

or, in matrix notation,

$$\begin{bmatrix} Z_{1(s)} & -Z_{m(s)} \\ Z_{m(s)} & -Z_{2(s)} \end{bmatrix} \begin{bmatrix} I_{1(s)} \\ I_{2(s)} \end{bmatrix} = \begin{bmatrix} E_{1(s)} \\ E_{2(s)} \end{bmatrix} \tag{6.209}$$

Since the transient response is being studied,

$$\begin{bmatrix} Z_{1(s)} & -Z_{m(s)} \\ Z_{m(s)} & -Z_{2(s)} \end{bmatrix} \begin{bmatrix} I_{1(s)} \\ I_{2(s)} \end{bmatrix} = 0$$

But

$$\begin{bmatrix} I_{1(s)} \\ I_{2(s)} \end{bmatrix} \neq 0$$

Therefore,

$$\begin{bmatrix} Z_{1(s)} & -Z_{m(s)} \\ Z_{m(s)} & -Z_{2(s)} \end{bmatrix} = 0$$

Thus, the characteristic equation of the circuit can be expressed as

$$-Z_1(s)Z_2(s) + Z_m^2(s) = 0 \tag{6.210}$$

where

$$Z_1(s) = R_1 + L_1 s + \frac{1}{Cs} \tag{6.211}$$

$$Z_2(s) = R_2 + L_2 s + \frac{1}{Cs} \tag{6.212}$$

$$Z_m(s) = \frac{1}{Cs} \tag{6.213}$$

where
s = complex frequency
$= \sigma + j\omega$

Substituting Equations 6.211 through 6.213 into Equation 6.210,

$$-\left(R_1 + L_1 s + \frac{1}{Cs} \right)\left(R_2 + L_2 s + \frac{1}{Cs} \right) + \left(\frac{1}{Cs} \right)^2 = 0 \tag{6.214}$$

or

$$CL_1 L_2 s^3 + C(R_1 L_2 + R_2 L_1)s^2 + (L_1 + L_2 + R_1 D_2 C)s + (R_1 + R_2) = 0 \tag{6.215}$$

Assume that $R_1 \gg L_1 s$ and that $L_1 = 0$. Thus, Equation 6.125 becomes

$$CR_1 L_2 s^2 + (L_2 + R_1 R_2 C)s + (R_1 + R_2) = 0 \tag{6.216}$$

or

$$s^2 + \left(\frac{1}{R_1 C} + \frac{R_2}{L_2}\right)s + \frac{R_1 + R_2}{C R_1 L_2} = 0 \tag{6.217}$$

However, since $R_1 \gg R_2$,

$$R_1 + R_2 \cong R_1 \tag{6.218}$$

substituting Equation 6.218 into Equation 6.217,

$$s^2 + \left(\frac{1}{R_1 C} + \frac{R_2}{L_2}\right)s + \frac{1}{C L_2} = 0 \tag{6.219}$$

Comparing Equation 6.219 with the standard equation of

$$s^2 + 2\zeta\omega_n s + \omega_n^2 = 0 \tag{6.220}$$

the undamped natural frequency can be expressed as

$$\omega_n \cong \frac{1}{\sqrt{C L_2}} \tag{6.221}$$

Since

$$2\zeta\omega_n = \frac{1}{R_1 C} + \frac{R_2}{L_2} \tag{6.222}$$

the damping coefficient can be expressed as

$$\sigma = \zeta\omega_n$$
$$= \frac{1}{2}\left(\frac{1}{R_1 C} + \frac{R_2}{L_2}\right) \tag{6.223}$$

from which the damping ratio can be found as

$$\zeta = \frac{1}{2R_1}\sqrt{\frac{L_2}{C}} + \frac{R_2}{2}\sqrt{\frac{C}{L_2}} \tag{6.224}$$

From Equation 6.224,

$$R_1 \cong \frac{L_2}{2\zeta\sqrt{L_2 C} - R_2 C} \tag{6.225}$$

In general, a positive, but less than critical, damping (i.e., $\zeta = 1$) is required. For example, when $\zeta = 0.7$,

$$R_1 \cong \frac{L_2}{14\sqrt{L_2 C} - R_2 C}$$

Note that at critical damping,

$$R_1 \cong \frac{L_2}{2\sqrt{L_2 C} - R_2 C} \tag{6.226}$$

Applying Routh's criterion to the characteristic equation of the HVDC link given by Equation 6.215 and assuming equal dc smoothing reactors (i.e., $L_{d1} = L_{d2} = L_d$), it can be found that

$$R_1 = -\frac{L_d}{R_2 C} \tag{6.227}$$

or

$$R_1 = -\frac{L_d}{\left(-R_2\right)C} \tag{6.228}$$

or since

$$L_2 \cong L_d$$

then

$$R_1 = -\frac{L_2}{\left(-R_2\right)C} \tag{6.229}$$

Therefore, in order to have a stable system or oscillations to be damped, the maximum value of R_1 must be

$$R_{1(max)} < \frac{L_2}{\left|R_2\right|C} \tag{6.230}$$

But

$$R_{1(max)} = K_{(max)} + R_{c1} + R_{d1} + \frac{1}{2}R_1 \tag{6.231}$$

Therefore, there is a maximum value of K for which the system is stable. However, note that if $R_2 < 0$,

$$R_{1(max)} > \frac{L_1}{L_2}\left|R_2\right| \tag{6.232}$$

6.14　USE OF FACTS AND HVDC TO SOLVE BOTTLENECK PROBLEMS IN THE TRANSMISSION NETWORKS

The control of power flows and the bottleneck problems of power flows can be solved by the use of electronic equipment in the ac transmission network by using FACTS and HVDC equipment. Here, FACTS stands for *flexible ac transmission system*, which is able to control via electronic valves (thyristors) the power flows in a transmission line. Similarly, HVDC stands for *high-voltage dc*. It also uses electronic valves for power flow control with a dc transmission line between the two HVDC converter stations at its ends. This electronic control can prevent outages in cases when the power flow can be rerouted without creating new overload sections and bottleneck problems.

6.15　HIGH-VOLTAGE POWER ELECTRONIC SUBSTATIONS

According to Juette and Mukherjee [5], the extensive developments in power electronics in the past decades caused significant progress in electric power transmission technology. As a result, there are special transmission systems that require the use of special kinds of substations. Among them are the converter stations for HVDC transmission systems and converter stations for the FACTS.

FACTS are the applications of power electronics for control of ac system to improve the power flow, operation, and control of the ac system. The use of FACTS allows parallel circuits in a network to be loaded up to their full thermal capacity and/or enforce a pattern of power flows that are required for economic operation. Due to their fast speed of operation, FACTS devices can also be used to control system dynamics and especially for transient stability problems.

In some sense, the high-voltage power electronic substations are basically made of the main power electronic equipment, that is, converter valves and FACTS controllers with their dedicated cooling systems, in addition to the conventional substation equipment [5].

They also have converter transformers and reactive power compensation equipment in addition to harmonic filters, buildings, and auxiliaries. Most of high-voltage power electronic substations are air insulated, even though some of them have some combinations of air and gas insulation. All the requirements and concerns for the traditional power substations also apply for these substations, including substation grounding, lightning protection, seismic protection, and general fire protection requirements.

Also, these substations may emit electric and acoustic noise, which require special shielding. Furthermore, these substations dictate to have extra fire protection due to the high power density in the electronic circuits [5].

6.16　ADDITIONAL COMMENDS ON HVDC CONVERTER STATIONS

The exchange of power between systems that have different constants or variable frequencies is possible by using power converters. The most common type of converter stations are ac–dc converters, which are used for HVDC transmission. The two types of HVDC converter stations used are the *back-to-back ac–dc–ac converter stations* and the terminal stations for the long-distance dc transmission lines.

In general, the *back-to-back converters* are used to transmit power between nonsynchronous ac systems, for example, the converter stations that are used between the western and eastern grids of North America or the ones used between the 50 and 60 Hz power grids in South America, as well as in Quebec or Japan.

Figure 6.22 shows the schematic diagram of an HVDC back-to-back converter station with a dc smoothing reactor and reactance power compensation, including ac harmonic filters, on both ac buses. Note that here the term *back-to-back* describes the fact that both the *rectifier* (*ac to dc*) and *inverter* (*dc to ac*) are located in the same station [5].

Typically, long-distance HVDC overhead transmission lines or cables are terminated at the HVDC converter stations and are linked to ac buses or systems. The voltages of the converters are determined by transmission efficiency of the lines. These voltages often can be one million volt

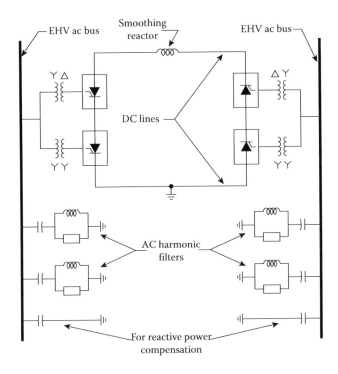

FIGURE 6.22 A schematic diagram of an HVDC back-to-back converter station.

(i.e., ±500 kV) or greater. The power that is involved may be greater than several thousands of megawatts. Also, the two poles of a bipolar system can be operated independently. In the event of a fault on one of the poles, the remaining pole can carry the total power as before. Figure 6.23 shows the schematic diagram of such an operation.

Today, most HVDC converters are line-commutated 12-pulse converters. Figure 6.24 illustrates a typical 12-pulse bridge circuit that employs delta- and wye-connected transformers. These

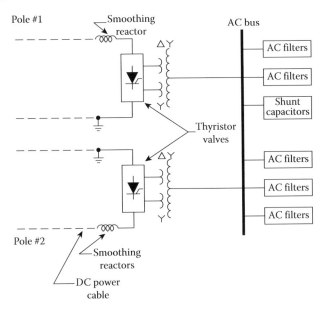

FIGURE 6.23 A schematic diagram of the Auchencrosh terminal station of the Scotland–Ireland HVDC cable.

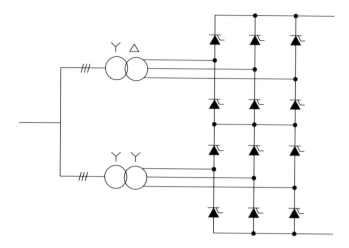

FIGURE 6.24   A typical 12-pulse converter bridge using delta and wye transformer windings.

transformers eliminate some of the harmonics that are typical for a 6-pulse Graetz bridge converter. The remaining harmonics are absorbed by the ac harmonic passive filters. These filters are made of capacitors, reactors, and resistors.

PROBLEMS

6.1   Assume that the following data are given for the overhead ac line discussed in Example 6.1:
    Steady-state operating voltage = 200/346 kV
    Line current = 1000 A
    Power = 600 MVA
    Insulation level = 500 kV
Use the assumptions and results given in the example, and determine the following for the comparable dc line:
    (a) Line-to-line dc voltage in kilovolts
    (b) Line-to-ground dc voltage in kilovolts
    (c) The dc line current in amperes
    (d) Associated dc power in megavolt-amperes
    (e) The dc line power loss in kilowatts
    (f) The dc insulation level
6.2   Assume that factor K is 4 and repeat Example 6.2.
6.3   Assume that factor K is 5 and repeat Example 6.2.
6.4   A three-conductor dc overhead line with equal conductor sizes is considered to be employed to transmit three-phase, three-conductor ac energy at a 0.92 power factor (see Figure P6.4). If maximum voltages to ground line and transmission efficiencies are the same for both dc and ac and the load is balanced, determine the change in the power transmitted in percent.
6.5   Derive Equation 6.110 from Equation 6.109.

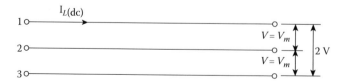

FIGURE P6.4   For Problem 6.4.

6.6   Derive Equations 6.188 and 6.189.

6.7   Derive Equation 6.193.

6.8   Verify the following equations:

(a) $L_{d(B)} = \dfrac{18B^2 Z_{(B)}}{\pi^2 \omega_{(B)}}$ H

(b) $L_{d(B)} = \dfrac{18B^2 Z_{1(B)}}{\pi^2 a^2 \omega_{(B)}}$ H

6.9   Verify the following equations:

(a) $C_{d(B)} = \dfrac{\pi^2}{18B^2 Z_{(B)} \omega_{(B)}}$ F

(b) $C_{d(B)} = \dfrac{\pi^2 a^2}{18B^2 Z_{1(B)} \omega_{(B)}}$ F

6.10 Derive the equation

$$V_{d(pu)} = \frac{a}{n} E_{1(pu)} \cos\alpha - R_{c(pu)} I_{d(pu)}$$

from Equation 6.65

6.11 Verify Equation 6.65.

6.12 Consider a B-bridge converter station and use the angles α and δ, which imply rectifier action. Consider only the first-mode operation, ($u \le 30°$). Apply the following equation:

$$I_d = \frac{\sqrt{3} E_m}{2\omega L_c} (\cos\alpha - \cos\delta)$$

which gives the average dc in any one bridge if E_m is properly interpreted. Also apply the following equation:

$$V_d = V_{d0} \cos\alpha - \Delta V_d$$

which gives the average dc terminal voltage of one bridge if $B = 1$ bridge is being analyzed.

(a) Redefine V_d, V_{d0}, and ΔV_{d0} to designate total voltages for B-bridges in series on the dc sides and show that

$$V_d = V_{d0} \cos a - \frac{3}{\pi} \omega B L_c I_d$$

is valid for the pole-to-pole voltage of the B-bridge station.

(b) Define V_d, in part (a), in terms of B, E, and E_1.

6.13 Review Problem 6.12 carefully to ensure that the definition and meaning of L_c are clearly in mind. Remember further that only first-mode operation is being studied. For the treatment of the LTC transformers, consider the following information that is taken from General Electric Company's Bulletin GET-1285: "In an actual transformer, tests will show that changing the taps on a specific winding will not materially affect the per unit short-circuit impedance of the transformer, based on the new voltage base, as determined by the tap position."

(a) Determine the L_c inductance of the rectifier referred to the dc side in henries.

(b) Determine the L_{c1} inductance of the rectifier referred to the ac side in henries.

(c) Repeat part (a) in per units.

(d) Repeat part (b) in per units.

6.14 Explain two different circumstances under which L_{s1} (i.e., the system common to all bridges) may be negligibly small.

6.15 Normalize the dc average terminal voltage equation for a B-bridge converter station using the per-unit system bases given in Section 6.11. This time, formalize the treatment of radian frequency with

$$\omega = \omega_{(pu)}\omega_{(B)}$$

where, ordinarily, $\omega_{(pu)} = 1.00$ and $\omega_{(B)} = 377$ rad/s. Show that the result is

$$V_{d(pu)} = \frac{a}{n}E_{1(pu)}\cos\alpha - \frac{\pi\omega_{(pu)}}{6B}\left(L_{(tr)pu} + \frac{B}{2}L_{(sys)pu}\right)\left(\frac{a}{n}\right)^2 I_{d(pu)}$$

6.16 An HVDC transmission link consists of two four-bridge converter stations operating as a rectifier and an inverter, similar to the setup given in Figure 6.13. The maximum continuous V_{d0r} and V_{d0i} voltages are 125 kV and that the maximum continuous dc I_d is 1200 A for all eight bridges involved. Each converter transformer has a continuous rating $S_{(tr)}$ of 157.05 MVA and a LTC range of $\pm 20\%$ in 32 steps of 1.25%. The rated transformer voltages for the rectifier station have been given as 199.2/345 kV for the ac side and 53.44/92.56 kV for the dc side.

Similarly, the rated transformer voltages for the inverter station have been given as 288.67/500 kV for the ac side and 53.44/92.56 kV for the dc side. The leakage reactances have been given as 0.14 pu for the 345 kV transformers and 0.16 pu for the 500 kV transformers.

The voltage ratings and the reactances given are correct when the LTC is in the neutral position. The arbitrary ac system bases are 500 MVA for three-phase volt-ampere and 199.2 and 288.67 kV for the $E_{1(B)r}$ and $E_{1(B)i}$ line-to-neutral rectifier and inverter voltages, respectively. Determine the following:
(a) Base voltage ratios of a_r for a_i for rectifier and inverter, respectively
(b) The ac side rectifier per-unit system bases of $I_{1(B)r}$, $I_{(B)r}$, $Z_{1(B)r}$, $Z_{(B)r}$, $L_{1(B)r}$, and $L_{(B)r}$
(c) The ac side inverter per-unit system bases of $I_{1(B)i}$, $I_{(B)i}$, $Z_{1(B)i}$, $Z_{(B)i}$, $L_{1(B)i}$, and $L_{(B)i}$
(d) The dc side per-unit system bases of $V_{d(B)}$, $I_{d(B)}$, $R_{d(B)}$, $L_{d(B)}$, and $C_{d(B)}$

6.17 In Problem 6.16, the three-phase short-circuit fault duties are given as 20,000 MVA on the 500 kV inverter bus and 10,000 MVA on the 345 kV rectifier bus. Determine the following:
(a) Commutating inductances of rectifier and inverter in per units
(b) Commutating inductances of rectifier and inverter referred to the dc sides in henries
(c) Commutating inductances of rectifier and inverter referred to the ac sides in per units

6.18 In Problem 6.17, the dc transmission line has three-conductor bundles of 1590 kcmil ACSR conductor, with 18 in. equilateral triangular configuration of bundles and 32 in. pole-to-pole spacing. Use 50° resistances for the 400 mi transmission line. The HVDC link is being operated at reduced capacity so that the current I_d is 1000 A and the inverter station power P_{di} is 400 MW and the voltages $E_{1(pu)r}$ and $E_{1(pu)i}$ are 1 pu. The minimum extinction angle of the inverter γ_{min} is desired as 10° in the interest of minimum var consumption by the inverter station. Use normalized equations and per-unit variables.
(a) Determine if the CEA control and γ_{min} will prevail during this reduced-load operation. If so, find the corresponding value of a_i/n_i. How many steps of LTC buck or boost is this? If γ_{min} cannot be used, find the best value of γ and the corresponding a_i/n_i and LTC position.
(b) Find the rectifier station terminal voltage $V_{d(pu)r}$.

6.19 In Problem 6.18, assume the CIA operation of the rectifier station with 1000 A as the set value of the CC I_d and 15° as the set value of the ignition angle. For this particular problem, assume the rectifier CC characteristic is vertical. The rectifier station LTCs are so positioned that terminal voltage $V_{d(r)}$ is 450 kV when CIA control changes to the CC control. Assume that the rectifier LTCs retain the position described.

(a) Find a_r/n_r for the rectifier.
(b) Find the rectifier LTC positions and specify them in terms of the number of steps of buck or boost.
(c) Find the ignition angle a that prevails during the reduced-load operation being studied.
(d) Find $V_{dr0}\cos \alpha_{set}$ and V_{d0r} in kilovolts.

6.20 The curves shown in Figure P6.20 are for a simple single-bridge rectifier–inverter link. Assume that the rectifier and inverter stations have identical apparatus and parameters and that the steady-state operating point at the rectifier terminal voltage $V_{d(r)}$ is 100 kV. The dc line has a total loop resistance of 5.00 Ω, a pole-to-pole capacitance of 0.010 μF/m, and a loop inductance of 3.20 mH/mi. Use dimensional one-bridge equations.

(a) Determine the rectifier commutating resistance R_c.
(b) Determine the inverter dc average terminal voltage $V_{d(i)}$.
(c) Determine the rectifier firing angle α at the operating point E.
(d) The line length is 50 mi, and the current margin ΔI_d is 200 A. Find the necessary inverter station dc smoothing inductance L_{d2} if the damping ratio is desired to be 0.70. Use the necessary simplifying assumptions.

6.21 Consider the rectifier CC control and inverter CEA control. Use the steps and notation of Figure 6.18, but simplify by setting the dc smoothing reactor resistances to zero, that is, $R_{d1} = R_{d2} = 0$. When the dc transmission line is relatively long but $\frac{1}{2}R_L + R_{c2} < 0$, it appears that there may be some difficulty in achieving both a desirably large damping ratio and a desirably small value of ΔI_d. Show how this problem can arise by approximating R_1

$$R_1 \cong \frac{1}{2\zeta}\sqrt{\frac{L_2}{C}}\ \Omega$$

and then modifying the approximate R_1 equation to contain system parameters and line length X explicitly. Show the nature of the possible problem described and discuss the possible remedies.

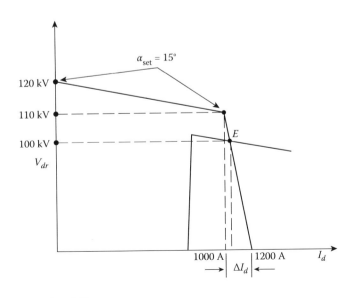

FIGURE P6.20 For Problem 6.20.

REFERENCES

1. Fink, D. G. and Beaty, H. W. *Standard Handbook for Electrical Engineers*, 11th edn., McGraw-Hill, New York, 1978.
2. Hingorani, N. G. and Ellert, F. H. General trends in the development of ± 400-kV to ± 1200-kV HVDC systems and areas of applications, *Proc. Am. Power Conf.* 36, 1976, 82–91.
3. Kimbark, E. W. *Direct Current Transmission*, vol. 1, Wiley, New York, 1971.
4. Weedy, B. M. *Electric Power Systems*, 3rd edn., Wiley, New York, 1979.
5. Juette, G. and Mukherjee, A. High-voltage power electronic substations, chapter 5 in *Electric Power Substations Engineering*, 2nd edn., J. D. MacDonald, ed., CRC Press, Boca Raton, FL, 2007.
6. Electric Power Research Institute. *Transmission Line Reference Book: HVDC to ± 600 kV*, EPRI, Palo Alto, CA, 1978.

GENERAL REFERENCES

Bergstrom, L. Simulator study of multiterminal HVDC system performance, *IEEE Trans. Power Appar. Syst.* PAS-97 (6), 1978, 2057–2066.

Bowles, J. P. Multiterminal HVDC transmission systems incorporating diode rectifier stations, *IEEE Trans. Power Appar. Syst.* PAS-100 (4), 1981, 1674–1678.

Braunagel, D. A. et al. Inclusion of DC converter and transmission equations directly in a Newton power flow, *IEEE Trans. Power Appar. Syst.* PAS-95 (1), 1976, 76–88.

Carrol, D. P. and Krause, P. C. Stability analysis of a DC power system, *IEEE Trans. Power Appar. Syst.* PAS-51 (6), 1970, 1112–1119.

D'Amore, M. New similarity laws for corona loss prediction on HVDC transmission lines, *IEEE Trans. Power Appar. Syst.* PAS-95 (2), 1976, 550–559.

Dougherty, J. J. Application range and economy of DC transmission systems, *Proc. Underground Trans. Conf.* 1972, 173–180.

Ekstrom, A. and Danfors, P. Future HVDC converter station design based on experience with the World's first thyristor installation, *Proc. Am. Power Conf.* 35, 1973, 1153–1159.

Ellert, F. J. and Hingorani, N. G. HVDC for the long run, *IEEE Spectrum.* 13(8), 1976, 36.

El-Serafi, A. M. and Shehata, S. A. Digital simulation of an AC/DC system in direct-phase quantities, *IEEE Trans. Power Appar. Syst.* PAS-95(2), 1976, 731–742.

Fink, J. L. and Wilson, D. D. Economic and technical progress in HVDC, *IEEE Power Eng. Soc. Summer Meet.*, 1974, paper no. C74 460-2.

Gönen, T. *Electric Power Distribution System Engineering*, McGraw-Hill, New York, 1986.

Harrison, R. E. et al. A proposed test specification for HVDC thyristor valves, *IEEE Trans. Power Appar. Syst.* PAS-97 (6), 1978, 2207–2218.

Hill, H. L. *Transmission Line Reference Book HVDC To ± 600 kV*, Electric Power Research Institute, Palo Alto, CA, 1976.

Hingorani, N. G. and Burbery, M. F. Simulation of AC system impedance in HVDC system studies, *IEEE Trans. Power Appar. Syst.* PAS-89(5/6), 1970, 451–460.

Hwang, H. H., Imai, R. M., and Simmons, T. C. Bibliography on high voltage direct current transmission 1969–1976: Part A, *IEEE Power Eng. Soc. Summer Meet.*, 1977, paper no. A 77 541-6.

Hwang, H. H., Imai, R. M., and Simmons, T. C. Bibliography on high voltage direct current transmission 1969–1976: Part B, *IEEE Power Eng. Soc. Summer Meet.*, 1977, paper no. 77 542-4.

Kaiser, F. D. Solid-state HVDC, *IEEE Spectrum.* 3, 1966, 25–31.

Knudsen, N. Contribution to the electrical design of EHVDC overhead lines, *IEEE Trans. Power Appar. Syst.* PAS-93(1), 1974, 233–239.

Lasseter, R. H. et al. Transient overvoltages on the neutral bus of HVDC transmission systems, *Power Eng. Soc. Summer Meet.*, 1978, paper no. A 78 607-4.

Lips, H. P. Aspects of multiple infeed of HVDC inverter stations into a common AC system, *IEEE Trans. Power Appar. Syst.* PAS-92, 1973, 775–779.

Lips, H. P. Compact HVDC converter station design considerations, *IEEE Trans. Power Appar. Syst.* PAS-95(3), 1976, 894–902.

Lips, H. P. and Ring, H. The performance of AC systems with predominant power supply by HVDC inverters, *IEEE Trans. Power Appar. Syst.* PAS-94 (2), 1975, 408–415.

Morgan, M. The DC breaker key to HVDC expansion, *Electr. Light Power* 53, 1975, 43–45.

Nakata, R. et al. An underground high voltage direct current transmission line, *Proc. Underground Transmission Distrib. Conf.*, 1974, 111–120.

Pelly, B. R. *Thyristor Phase-Controlled Converters and Cycloconverters*, Wiley (Interscience), New York, 1971.

Prabhakara, F. S. and Shah, K. R. A simplified method of calculation of telephone interference from HVDC lines, *IEEE Power Eng. Soc. Winter Meet.*, 1976, paper no. A76 198-2.

Uhlmann, E. *Power Transmission by DC*, Springer-Verlag, Berlin, Germany, 1975.

7 Transient Overvoltages and Insulation Coordination

An education isn't how much you have committed to memory, or even how much you know. It's being able to differentiate between what you do know and what you don't.

Anatole France

7.1 INTRODUCTION

By definition, a transient phenomenon is an aperiodic function of time and has a short duration. Examples for such transient* phenomena are voltage or current surges. A voltage surge is introduced by a sudden change in voltage at a point in a power system. Its velocity depends on the medium in which the surge is traveling. Such voltage surge always has an associated current surge with which it travels. The current surges are made up of charging or discharging capacitive currents that are introduced by the change in voltages across the shunt capacitances of the transmission system. The surge voltages can be caused by lightning, switching, faults, etc. HV surges on power systems can be very destructive to system equipment, and thus, they must be limited to safe levels.

When lightning strikes a phase conductor or shield wire (OHGW), the current of the lightning stroke tends to divide, half going in each direction. If the OHGW is struck at the tower, current will also flow in the tower, including its footings and counterpoise. The current of the lightning stroke will see the surge impedance of the conductor or conductors so that a voltage will be built up. As stated earlier, both the voltage and the current will move along the conductor as traveling waves.

Studies of transient disturbances on a transmission system have shown that lightning strokes and switching operations are followed by a traveling wave of a steep wave front. When a voltage wave of this type reaches a power transformer, for example, it causes an unequal stress distribution along its windings and may lead to breakdown of the insulation system.

Therefore, it is required that the insulation behavior be studied under such impulse voltages. An impulse voltage is a unidirectional voltage that rises quickly to a maximum value and then decays slowly to zero. The wave shape is referred to as $T_1 \times T_2$, where both values are given in microseconds. For example, for the international standard[†] wave shape (which is also the new US standard waveform), the $T_1 \times T_2$ is 1.2×50, as shown in Figure 7.1. Note that the crest (peak) value of the voltage is reached in 1.2 µs and the 50% point on the tail of the wave is reached in 50 µs. Not all of the voltage waves caused by lightning can conform to this specification.

7.2 TRAVELING WAVES

To study transient problems on a transmission line in terms of traveling waves, the line can be represented as incremental sections, as shown in Figure 7.2a. The two-wire line is shown with one phase and neutral return. The parameters L and C are inductance and capacitance of the line (OH or cable) per-cable length, respectively. To simplify the analysis, the line is assumed to be lossless, that is, its resistance R and conductance G are zero.

---

* It is often that the words *transients* and *surges* are used interchangeably to describe the same phenomenon.
† It is a standard set by the International Electrotechnical Commission (IEC).

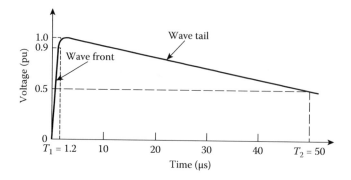

FIGURE 7.1 Standard impulse voltage waveform.

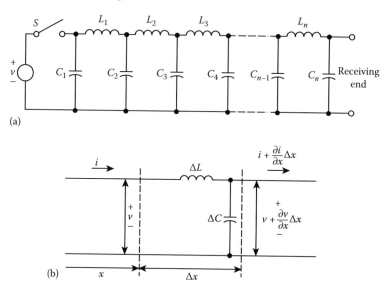

FIGURE 7.2 Representation of two-wire transmission line for application of traveling waves: (a) lumpy representation and (b) elemental section of line.

Any disturbance on the line can be represented by the closing or opening of the switch S, as shown in Figure 7.2a. For example, when the line is suddenly connected to a voltage source, the whole of the line is not energized instantaneously. In other words, if the voltage v is applied to the sending end of the line by closing switch S, the voltage does not appear instantaneously at the receiving end. When switch S is closed, the first capacitor becomes charged immediately to the instantaneous applied voltage. However, because of the first series inductor (since it acts as an open circuit), the second capacitor does not respond immediately but is delayed. Similarly, the third capacitor is delayed still more by the existence of the second inductor. Therefore, the farther away from the sending end of the line, the greater is the delay. This gradual buildup of voltage over the transmission-line conductors can be regarded as though a voltage wave is traveling from one end to the other end, and the gradual charging of the capacitances is due to the associated current wave.

If the applied voltage is in the form of a surge, starting from zero and returning again to zero, it can be seen that the voltages on the intermediate capacitors rise to some maximum value and return again to zero. The disturbance of the applied surge is therefore propagated along the line in the form of a wave. Thus, such a propagation of the sending-end voltage and current conditions along the line is called *traveling waves*. Therefore, the voltage and current are functions of both x and t:

$$v = v(x,t) \quad \text{and} \quad i = i_j(x,t)$$

Thus, the series voltage drop along the elemented length of line can be expressed as

$$\Delta v(\Delta x,t) = v_j(x,t) - v_j(x+\Delta x,t)$$
$$= \int_x^{x+\Delta x} L \frac{\partial i}{\partial t} dt \tag{7.1}$$

or in the limit as Δx approaches to zero,

$$\frac{\partial v_j(x,t)}{\partial x} = -L \frac{\partial i_j(x,t)}{\partial t} \tag{7.2}$$

or

$$\frac{\partial v}{\partial x} = -L \frac{\partial v}{\partial t} \tag{7.3}$$

Similarly, the current to charge the infinitesimal capacitance can be expressed as

$$\frac{\partial i_j(x,t)}{\partial x} = -C \frac{\partial i_j(x,t)}{\partial t} \tag{7.4}$$

or

$$\frac{\partial i}{\partial x} = -C \frac{\partial v}{\partial t} \tag{7.5}$$

Note that the negative signs in Equations 7.2 through 7.5 are due to the direction of progress, at distance x, along the line. Figure 7.2 shows that x is increasing to the right. Therefore, based on the given current direction, both voltage v and current i will decrease with increasing x.

The i can be eliminated from Equations 7.3 and 7.5 by taking the partial derivative of Equation 7.3 with respect to x and Equation 7.5 with respect to t so that

$$\frac{\partial^2 v}{\partial x^2} = -L \frac{\partial^2 i}{\partial x \partial t} \tag{7.6}$$

and

$$\frac{\partial^2 i}{\partial x \partial t} = -C \frac{\partial^2 v}{\partial t^2} \tag{7.7}$$

Substituting Equation 7.7 into Equation 7.6,

$$\frac{\partial^2 v}{\partial x^2} = LC \frac{\partial^2 v}{\partial t^2} \tag{7.8}$$

Similarly, it can be shown that

$$\frac{\partial^2 i}{\partial x^2} = LC \frac{\partial^2 i}{\partial t^2} \tag{7.9}$$

Equations 7.8 and 7.9 are known as *transmission-line wave equations*. They can be expressed as

$$\frac{\partial^2 v}{\partial x^2} = \frac{1}{v^2}\frac{\partial^2 v}{\partial t^2} \tag{7.10}$$

and

$$\frac{\partial^2 i}{\partial x^2} = \frac{1}{v^2}\frac{\partial^2 i}{\partial t^2} \tag{7.11}$$

where

$$v \triangleq \frac{1}{\sqrt{LC}} \ \text{m/s} \tag{7.12}$$

Here, v represents the velocity of the voltage and current (wave) propagation along the line in the positive direction. The dimensions of L and C are in henries per meter and farads per meter.

It can be shown that Equation 7.8 can be satisfied by

$$v_f = v_1(x - vt) \tag{7.13}$$

and

$$v_b = v_2(x + vt) \tag{7.14}$$

where
v_f denotes a forward-traveling wave (i.e., *incident wave*)
v_b denotes a backward-traveling wave (i.e., *reflected wave*)

Therefore, the general solution of Equation 7.8 can be expressed as

$$v(x,t) = v_f + v_b \tag{7.15}$$

or

$$v(x,t) = v_1(x - vt) + v_2(x + vt) \tag{7.16}$$

that is, the value of a voltage wave, at a given time t and location x along the line, is the sum of forward- and backward-traveling waves. The actual shape of each component is defined by the initial and boundary (*terminal*) conditions of a given problem.

The relationships between the traveling voltage and current waves can be expressed as

$$v_f = Z_c i_f \tag{7.17}$$

and

$$v_b = -Z_c i_b \tag{7.18}$$

where Z_c is the surge (or *characteristic*) impedance of the line. Since

$$Z_c = \left(\frac{L}{C}\right)^{1/2} \tag{7.19}$$

Therefore,

$$i_f = \frac{v_f}{Z_c} \qquad (7.20)$$

and

$$i_b = -\frac{v_b}{Z_c} \qquad (7.21)$$

Hence, the general solution of Equation 7.9 can be expressed as

$$i(x,t) = i_f + i_b \qquad (7.22)$$

or

$$i(x,t) = Z_c(v_f - v_b)$$

$$= \frac{1}{Z_c}[v_1(x - vt) - v_2(x + vt)] \qquad (7.23)$$

or

$$i(x,t) = \left(\frac{C}{L}\right)^{1/2}\left[v_1\left(t - vx\right) - v_2\left(t + vx\right)\right] \qquad (7.24)$$

7.2.1 Velocity of Surge Propagation

The velocity of propagation of any electromagnetic disturbance in air is equal to the speed of light, that is, about 300,000 km/s.* As stated earlier, the velocity of surge propagation along the line can be expressed as

$$v \triangleq \frac{1}{\sqrt{LC}} \text{ m/s} \qquad (7.25)$$

Since inductance of a single-phase OH line conductor, assuming zero ground resistivity, is

$$L = 2 \times 10^{-7} \ln\left(\frac{2h}{r}\right) \text{ H/m} \qquad (7.26)$$

its capacitance is

$$C = \frac{1}{18 \times 10^9 \ln\left(2h/r\right)} \text{ F/m} \qquad (7.27)$$

where
  h is the height of conductor above ground in meters
  r is the radius of conductor in meters

---

* To travel a distance of 2500 km, an electric wave requires 1/120 s, which is equal to a half-period of the 60 Hz ac frequency.

Thus, the surge velocity in a single-phase OH line can be found as

$$v = \frac{1}{\sqrt{LC}}$$

$$= \left[\left(\frac{2 \times 10^{-7} \ln\left(2h/r\right)}{18 \times 10^9 \ln\left(2h/r\right)} \right)^{1/2} \right]^{-1}$$

$$= 3 \times 10^8 \text{ m/s}$$

Hence, its surge velocity is the same as that of light. If the surge velocity in a three-phase OH line is calculated, it can be seen that it is the same as for the single-phase OH line. Furthermore, the surge velocity is independent of the conductor size and spacing between the conductors.

Similarly, the surge velocity in cables can be expressed as

$$v = \frac{1}{\sqrt{LC}}$$

$$= 3 \times 10^8 \sqrt{K} \text{ m/s}$$

where K is the dielectric constant of the cable insulation, and let's say its value varies from 2.5 to 4.0. Thus, taking it as 4.0, the surge velocity in a cable can be found as 1.5×10^8 m/s. In other words, the surge velocity in a cable is half the one in an OH line conductor.*

7.2.2 Surge Power Input and Energy Storage

Consider the two-wire transmission line shown in Figure 7.2. When switch S is closed, a surge voltage and surge current wave of magnitudes v and i, respectively, travel toward the open end of the line at a velocity of v (m/s). Therefore, the surge power input to the line can be expressed as

$$P = vi \text{ W} \tag{7.28}$$

Since the receiving end of the line is open-circuited and the line is assumed to be lossless, energy input per second is equal to energy stored per second. The energy stored is, in turn, equal to the sum of the electrostatic and electromagnetic energies stored. The electrostatic component is determined by the voltage and capacitance per-unit length as

$$W_s = \frac{1}{2} C v^2 \tag{7.29}$$

Similarly, the electromagnetic component is determined by the current and inductance per-unit length as

$$W_m = \frac{1}{2} L i^2 \tag{7.30}$$

---

* Note that in 1/120 s, the surge travels 1250 km in a cable contrary to 2500 km that it can travel in an overhead line.

Since the two components of energy storage are equal, the total energy content stored per-unit length is

$$W = W_s + W_m \tag{7.31}$$

or

$$W = 2W_s = 2W_m \tag{7.32}$$

that is,

$$W = Cv^2 = Li^2 \tag{7.33}$$

Therefore, the surge power can be expressed in terms of energy content and surge velocity as

$$P = Wv \tag{7.34}$$

or

$$P = \frac{Li^2}{\sqrt{LC}} = i^2 Z_c \tag{7.35}$$

or

$$P = \frac{v^2}{Z_c} \tag{7.36}$$

It is interesting to note that for a given voltage level, the surge power is greater in cables than in OH line conductors due to the smaller surge impedance of the cables.

Example 7.1

Assume that a surge voltage of 1000 kV is applied to an OH line with its receiving end open. If the surge impedance of the line is 500 Ω, determine the following:

(a) Total surge power in-line
(b) Surge current in-line

Solution

(a) The total surge power is

$$P = \frac{v^2}{Z_c}$$

$$= \frac{1 \times 10^6}{500} = 2000 \text{ MW} \tag{7.37}$$

(b) Therefore, the surge current is

$$i = \frac{v}{Z_c}$$

$$= \frac{1 \times 10^6}{500} = 2000 \text{ A}$$

Example 7.2

Repeat Example 7.1 assuming a cable with surge impedance of 50 Ω.

Solution

(a) The total surge power is

$$P = \frac{v^2}{Z_c}$$

$$= \frac{1 \times 10^{12}}{50} = 20,000 \text{ MW}$$

(b) Thus, the surge current is

$$i = \frac{v}{Z_c}$$

$$= \frac{1 \times 10^6}{50} = 20,000 \text{ A}$$

7.2.3 Superposition of Forward- and Backward-Traveling Waves

Figure 7.3a shows forward-traveling voltage and current waves. Note that x is increasing to the right in the positive direction, as before, according to the sign convention. Figure 7.3b shows backward-traveling voltage and current waves. Figure 7.3c shows the superposition of forward and backward

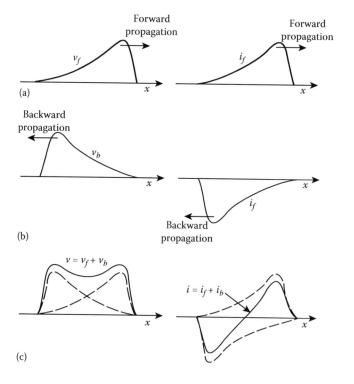

FIGURE 7.3 Representation of voltage and current waves: (a) in forward direction, (b) in backward direction, and (c) in superposition of waves.

waves of voltage and current, respectively. It can be shown that on loss-free transmission lines, the voltage and current waves have the same shape, being related to each other by the characteristic impedance of the line, and travel is undistorted. Furthermore, when two waves meet, they do not affect each other but appear to pass through each other without any distortion.

7.3 EFFECTS OF LINE TERMINATIONS

Assume that v_f and i_f and v_b and i_b are the instantaneous voltage and current of the forward and backward waves, respectively, at the point of discontinuity (i.e., at the end of the line). Hence, the instantaneous voltage and current at the point of discontinuity can be expressed as

$$v = v_f + v_b \tag{7.38}$$

$$i = i_f + i_b \tag{7.39}$$

Substituting Equations 7.20 and 7.21 into Equation 7.39,

$$i = \frac{v_f}{Z_c} - \frac{v_b}{Z_c} \tag{7.40}$$

or

$$iZ_c = v_f - v_b \tag{7.41}$$

Adding Equations 7.38 and 7.41,

$$v + iZ_c = 2v_f \tag{7.42}$$

or

$$v_f = \frac{1}{2}\left(v + iZ_c\right) \tag{7.43}$$

Similarly, subtracting Equation 7.41 from Equation 7.38,

$$v_b = \frac{1}{2}\left(v - iZ_c\right) \tag{7.44}$$

Alternatively, from Equation 7.42,

$$v = 2v_f - iZ_c \tag{7.45}$$

Substituting Equation 7.45 into Equation 7.44,

$$v_b = v_f - iZ_c \tag{7.46}$$

7.3.1 LINE TERMINATION IN RESISTANCE

Assume that the receiving end of the line is terminated in a pure resistance so that

$$v = iR \tag{7.47}$$

Substituting this equation into Equation 7.42,

$$i = \left(\frac{2}{R + Z_c}\right) v_f \tag{7.48}$$

and from Equation 7.47,

$$v = \left(\frac{2R}{R + Z_c}\right) v_f \tag{7.49}$$

or

$$v_f = \frac{R + Z_c}{2R} \tag{7.50}$$

Similarly, substituting Equations 7.48 and 7.49 into Equation 7.44,

$$v_b = \left(\frac{R - Z_c}{R + Z_c}\right) v_f \tag{7.51}$$

The power transmitted to the termination point by the forward wave is

$$P_f = \frac{v_f^2}{Z_c} \tag{7.52}$$

On the other hand, the power transmitted from the termination point by the backward wave is

$$P_b = \frac{v_b^2}{Z_c} \tag{7.53}$$

Hence, the power absorbed by the resistor R is

$$P_R = \frac{v^2}{R} \tag{7.54}$$

or

$$P_R = \frac{(v_f + v_b)^2}{R} \tag{7.55}$$

so that

$$P_f = P_b + P_R \tag{7.56}$$

7.3.2 Line Termination in Impedance

In the general case of a line of characteristic impedance Z_c terminated in an impedance Z,

$$i = \left(\frac{2}{Z + Z_c}\right) v_f \tag{7.57}$$

$$v = \left(\frac{2Z}{Z + Z_c}\right) v_f \tag{7.58}$$

or

$$v = \tau \times v_f \tag{7.59}$$

where τ is the *refraction coefficient* or *transmission factor* or simply *coefficient τ*. Thus, for voltage waves,

$$\tau \triangleq \frac{2Z}{Z + Z_c} \tag{7.60}$$

The value of τ varies between zero and two depending on the relative values of Z and Z_c. Alternatively,

$$v_f = \left(\frac{Z + Z_c}{2Z}\right) v \tag{7.61}$$

Similarly,

$$v_b = \left(\frac{Z - Z_c}{Z + Z_c}\right) v_f \tag{7.62}$$

or

$$v_b = \rho \times v_f \tag{7.63}$$

where ρ is the *reflection coefficient*. Therefore, for voltage waves,

$$\rho \triangleq \frac{Z - Z_c}{Z + Z_c} \tag{7.64}$$

The ρ can be positive or negative depending on the relative values of Z and Z_c. For example, when the line is terminated with its characteristic impedance (i.e., $Z = Z_c$), then $\rho = 0$, that is, no reflection. Thus, $v_b = 0$ and $i_b = 0$. In other words, the line acts as if it is infinitely long. When the line is terminated in an impedance that is larger than its characteristic impedance (i.e., $Z > Z_c$), then v_b is positive and i_b is negative. Therefore, the reflected surges consist of increased voltage and reduced current, as shown in Figure 7.4. On the other hand, when the line is terminated in an impedance that is smaller than its characteristic impedance (i.e., $Z < Z_c$), then v_b is negative and i_b is positive. Thus, the reflected surges consist of reduced voltage and increased current, as shown in Figure 7.5.

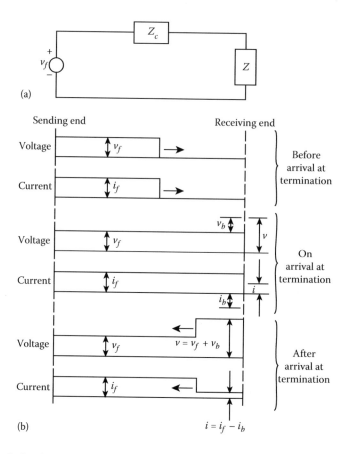

FIGURE 7.4 Analysis of traveling waves when $Z > Z_c$: (a) circuit diagram and (b) voltage and current distributions.

If Z_s and Z_r are defined as the sending-end and receiving-end Thévenin equivalent impedances, respectively, the sending-end reflection coefficient is

$$\rho_s = \frac{Z_s - Z_c}{Z_s + Z_c} \qquad (7.65)$$

and the receiving-end reflection coefficient is

$$\rho_s = \frac{Z_s - Z_c}{Z_s + Z_c} \qquad (7.66)$$

Note that waves traveling back toward the sending end will result in new reflections as determined by the reflection coefficient at the sending end ρ_s. Furthermore, note that the reflection coefficient for current is always the negative of the reflection coefficient for voltage.

Example 7.3

Consider Equations 7.60 and 7.62 and verify that

(a) $i_b = \rho \times i_f$

(b) $\tau = \rho + 1$

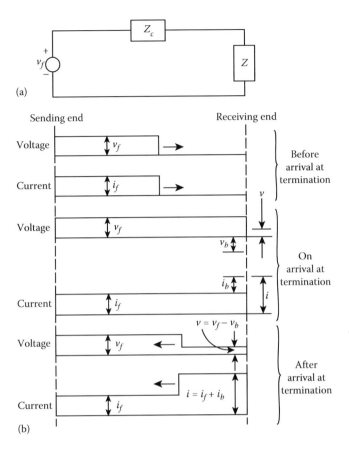

FIGURE 7.5 Analysis of traveling waves when $Z < Z_c$: (a) circuit diagram and (b) voltage and current distributions.

Solution

(a) Since

$$i_f = \frac{v_f}{Z_c} \quad \text{and} \quad i_b = -\frac{v_b}{Z_c}$$

then

$$v_f = Z_c \times i_f \quad \text{and} \quad v_b = -Z_c \times i_b$$

Substituting them into Equation 7.62,

$$-Z_c i_b = \rho Z_c i_f$$

Therefore,

$$i_b = -\rho i_f \tag{7.67}$$

(b) Since

$$\rho_s = \frac{Z_s - Z_c}{Z_s + Z_c}$$

then

$$\rho + 1 = \frac{Z - Z_0}{Z + Z_0} + 1$$

$$= \frac{2Z}{Z + Z_0}$$

Therefore,

$$\tau = \rho + 1 \qquad\qquad\qquad\qquad (7.68)$$

Example 7.4

A line has a characteristic impedance of 400 Ω and a resistance of 500 Ω. Assume that the magnitudes of forward-traveling voltage and current waves are 5000 V and 12.5 A, respectively. Determine the following:

(a) Reflection coefficient of voltage wave
(b) Reflection coefficient of current wave
(c) Backward-traveling voltage wave
(d) Voltage at the end of the line
(e) Refraction coefficient of voltage wave
(f) Backward-traveling current wave
(g) Current flowing through the resistor
(h) Refraction coefficient of current wave

Solution

(a)

$$\rho = \frac{R - Z_c}{R + Z_c} = \frac{500 - 400}{500 + 400} = 0.1111$$

(b)

$$\rho = -\frac{R - Z_c}{R + Z_c} = -\frac{500 - 400}{500 + 400} = -0.1111$$

(c)

$$v_b = \rho \times v_f = 0.1111 \times 5000 = 555.555 \text{ V}$$

(d)

$$v = v_f + v_b = 5000 + 555.555 = 5555.555 \text{ V}$$

or

$$v = \left(\frac{2R}{R + Z_c}\right) v_f = \left(\frac{2 \times 500}{500 + 400}\right) \times 5000 = 5555.555 \text{ V}$$

(e)

$$\tau = \frac{2R}{R + Z_c} = \frac{2 \times 500}{500 + 400} = 1.1111$$

(f)

$$i_b = -\frac{v_b}{Z_c} = -\frac{555.555}{400} = -1.3889\,\text{A}$$

or

$$i_b = -\rho i_f = -0.1111 \times 12.5 \cong -1.3889\,\text{A}$$

(g)

$$i = \frac{v}{R} = \frac{5555.555}{500} = 11.1111\,\text{A}$$

(h)

$$\tau = \frac{2Z_c}{R + Z_c} = \frac{2 \times 400}{500 + 400} = 0.8889$$

7.3.3 Open-Circuit Line Termination

The boundary condition for current is

$$i = 0 \tag{7.69}$$

Hence,

$$i_f = -i_b \tag{7.70}$$

Substituting this in Equations 7.17 and 7.18,

$$v_b = Z_c \times i_b = Z \times i_f = v_f \tag{7.71}$$

Thus, the total voltage at the receiving end is

$$v = v_f + v_b = 2v_f \tag{7.72}$$

Therefore, the voltage at the open end of the line is twice the forward voltage wave, as shown in Figure 7.6a.

7.3.4 Short-Circuit Line Termination

The boundary condition for voltage at the short-circuited receiving end is

$$v = 0 \tag{7.73}$$

Hence,

$$v_f = -v_b \tag{7.74}$$

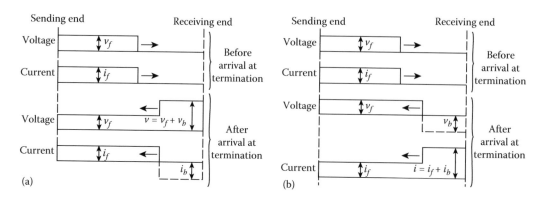

FIGURE 7.6 Analysis of traveling waves for (a) open-circuit line termination and (b) short-circuit line termination.

Substituting this in Equations 7.20 and 7.21,

$$i_f = \frac{v_f}{Z_c} = -\frac{v_b}{Z_c} = i_b \tag{7.75}$$

Thus, the total current at the receiving end is

$$i = i_f + i_b = 2i_f \tag{7.76}$$

Therefore, the current at the short-circuited end of the line is twice the forward current wave, as shown in Figure 7.6b.

7.3.5 OVERHEAD LINE TERMINATION BY TRANSFORMER

It is a well-known fact that at high frequencies, the voltage distribution across each winding is modified due to the capacitive currents between the transformer windings, between the turns of each winding, and between each winding and the grounded iron core. The impact of high velocity of a surge on a transformer is similar. Therefore, the resulting capacitive voltage distribution can be represented in the same manner as the one for a string of suspension insulators. Thus, the maximum voltage gradient takes place at the winding turns nearest to the line conductor. Because of this, when wye-connected transformers are employed in grounded neutral systems, their winding insulations are graded by more heavily insulating the winding turns closer to the line. Furthermore, the magnitude of the voltage surge can be reduced before it arrives at the transformer by putting in a short cable between the OH line and the transformer. In addition to the reduction in the magnitude of the voltage wave, the steepness is also reduced due to the capacitance of the cable. Therefore, the voltage distribution along the windings of the apparatus is further reduced.

7.4 JUNCTION OF TWO LINES

Figure 7.7 shows a simple junction between two lines. Assume that $Z_{c1} > Z_{c2}$ where Z_{c1} and Z_{c2} are the characteristic impedances of the first and second lines, respectively. For example, Figure 7.7 might represent the junction between an OH line and an underground cable. If a voltage surge of step function form and amplitude v_f approaches the junction along the OH line, the current wave will have the same shape and an amplitude of

$$i_f = \frac{v_f}{Z_{c1}} \tag{7.77}$$

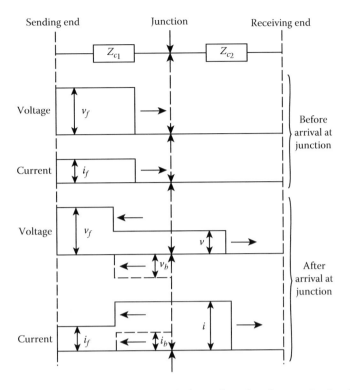

FIGURE 7.7 Traveling voltage and current waves being reflected and transmitted at junction between two lines.

Therefore, after the arrival at the junction,

$$i_b = \frac{v_b}{Z_{c1}} \tag{7.78}$$

$$i = \frac{v}{Z_{c2}} \tag{7.79}$$

Since

refracted or transmitted wave = forward wave + backward wave (7.80)

then

$$v_f + v_b = v \tag{7.81}$$

$$i_f + i_b = 1 \tag{7.82}$$

Substituting Equations 7.77 through 7.79 into Equation 7.82,

$$\frac{v_f}{Z_{c1}} - \frac{v_b}{Z_{c1}} = \frac{v}{Z_{c2}} \tag{7.83}$$

by multiplying Equation 7.83 by Z_{c1} and adding the resulting equation and Equation 7.82 side by side yields

$$2v_f = \left(1 + \frac{Z_{c1}}{Z_{c2}}\right)v \tag{7.84}$$

Thus, the transmitted (i.e., *refracted*) voltage and current waves can be expressed as

$$v = \left(\frac{2Z_{c2}}{Z_{c1} + Z_{c2}}\right)v_f \tag{7.85}$$

and

$$i = \left(\frac{2Z_{c1}}{Z_{c1} + Z_{c2}}\right)i_f \tag{7.86}$$

The reflected (i.e., *backward*) voltage and current waves can be expressed as

$$v_b = \left(\frac{Z_{c2} - Z_{c1}}{Z_{c1} + Z_{c2}}\right)v_f \tag{7.87}$$

and

$$i_b = \left(\frac{Z_{c1} - Z_{c2}}{Z_{c1} + Z_{c2}}\right)i_f \tag{7.88}$$

The sign change between Equations 7.87 and 7.82 is because of the negative sign in Equation 7.20. The power in the forward wave arriving at the junction is

$$P_f = \frac{v_f^2}{Z_{c1}} \tag{7.89}$$

and the transmitted wave power is

$$P = \frac{v^2}{Z_{c2}} \tag{7.90}$$

Similarly, the power in the backward wave is

$$P_b = \frac{v_b^2}{Z_{c1}} \tag{7.91}$$

Example 7.5

Assume that an OH line is connected in series with an underground cable. The surge (i.e., characteristic) impedances of the OH line and cable are 400 and 40 Ω, respectively. The forward-traveling surge voltage is 200 kV and is traveling toward the junction from the sending end of the OH line.

(a) Determine the magnitude of the forward current wave.
(b) Determine the reflection coefficient.
(c) Determine the refraction coefficient.
(d) Determine the surge voltage transmitted forward into the cable.
(e) Determine the surge current transmitted forward into the cable.
(f) Determine the surge voltage reflected back along the OH line.
(g) Determine the surge current reflected back along the OH line.
(h) Plot voltage and current surges showing them after arriving at the junction.

Solution

(a)

$$i_f = \frac{v_f}{Z_{c1}} = \frac{200,000}{400} = 500\,A$$

(b)

$$\rho = \frac{Z_{c2} - Z_{c1}}{Z_{c1} + Z_{c2}} = \frac{40 - 400}{400 + 40} = -0.8182$$

(c)

$$\tau = \frac{2Z_{c2}}{Z_{c1} + Z_{c2}} = \frac{2 \times 40}{400 + 40} = 0.1818$$

(d)

$$v = \tau \times v_f = 0.1818 \times 200 = 36.36\ kV$$

(e)

$$i = \frac{v}{Z_{c2}} = \frac{36,360}{40} = 909\,A$$

(f)

$$v_b = \rho v_f = -0.8182 \times 200 = -163.64\ kV$$

(g)

$$i_b = -\rho i_f = 0.8182 \times 500 = 409\ A$$

(h) Figure 7.8 shows the plot of the voltage and current surges after arriving at the junction.

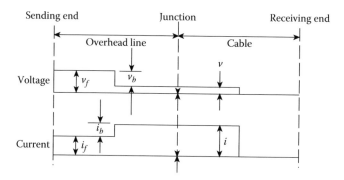

FIGURE 7.8   The plot for Example 7.5.

7.5   JUNCTION OF SEVERAL LINES

Figure 7.9a shows the analysis of a traveling voltage wave encountering a line bifurcation made of two lines having equal surge impedances Z_{c2}. Figure 7.9b shows the corresponding equivalent circuit. Figure 7.9c shows the traveling voltage wave being reflected and transmitted at the junction J. Note that at the junction, the impedance seen is that due to the two equal surge impedances Z_{c2} in parallel. Therefore, equations developed in the previous section are applicable as long as Z_{c2} is replaced by $(1/2)Z_{c2}$. For example, the transmitted (i.e., *refracted*) voltage and current can be expressed as

$$v = \left(\frac{2v_f}{Z_{c1} + \left(Z_{c2}/2 \right)} \right) \frac{Z_{c2}}{2} \tag{7.92}$$

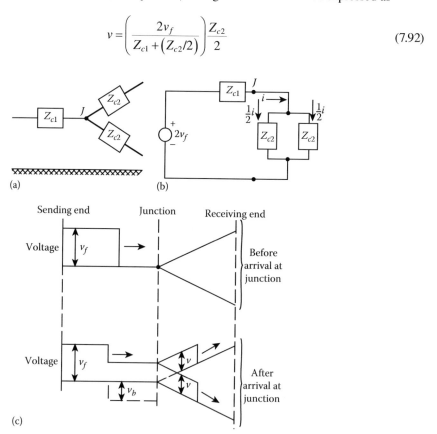

FIGURE 7.9   Traveling voltage wave encountering line bifurcation: (a) system, (b) equivalent circuit, and (c) traveling voltage wave reflected and transmitted at junction of three lines.

and

$$i = \left(\frac{2Z_{c1}}{Z_{c1} + \left(Z_{c2}/2 \right)} \right) i_f \tag{7.93}$$

where

$$i_f = \left(\frac{2v_f}{Z_{c1} + \left(Z_{c2}/2 \right)} \right) \tag{7.94}$$

7.6 TERMINATION IN CAPACITANCE AND INDUCTANCE

7.6.1 TERMINATION THROUGH CAPACITOR

Assume that a line is terminated in a capacitor, as shown in Figure 7.10a. Figure 7.10b shows its equivalent circuit. From Equation 7.60, the refraction coefficient can be expressed as

$$\tau = \frac{2Z}{Z + Z_c} \tag{7.95}$$

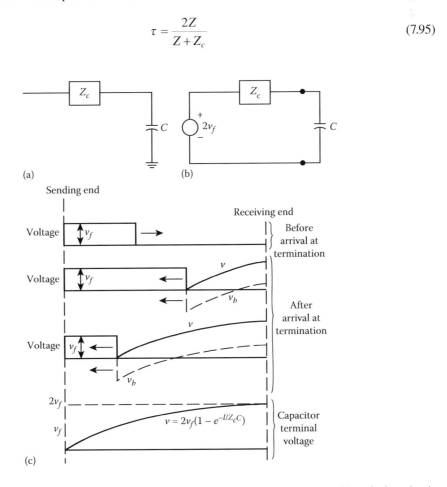

FIGURE 7.10 Traveling voltage wave on line with capacitive termination: (a) system, (b) equivalent circuit, and (c) disposition of wave at various instants.

or in a Laplace transform as

$$\tau = \frac{2(1/Cs)}{Z_c + (1/Cs)} \tag{7.96}$$

where s is the Laplace transform operator. Therefore, the refracted voltage can be found as

$$v = \tau \times v_f$$

or

$$v(s) = \left(\frac{2(1/Cs)}{Z_c + (1/Cs)} \right) \left(\frac{v_f}{s} \right)$$

$$= \left(\frac{2v_f}{s} \right) \left(\frac{1}{Z_c Cs + 1} \right)$$

$$= \left(\frac{2v_f}{s} \right) \left(\frac{1/Z_c}{s + (1/Z_c)} \right)$$

$$= 2v_f \left(\frac{1}{s} \right) - \frac{1}{s + (1/Z_c C)} \tag{7.97}$$

so that

$$v(t) = 2v_f \left(1 - e^{-t/Z_c C} \right) \tag{7.98}$$

where $v_f(t)$ is not a traveling wave but the voltage that will be impressed across the capacitor.
The current flowing through capacitor C is

$$i(t) = \frac{2v_f}{Z_c} e^{-t/Z_c C} \tag{7.99}$$

The reflected voltage wave can be expressed as

$$V_b(t) = v_f \left(1 - 2e^{-t/Z_c C} \right) \tag{7.100}$$

Figure 7.10c shows the disposition of the voltage wave at various instants. Succinctly put, the capacitor acts as a short circuit at the instant of arrival of the forward wave. At this moment, the reflected voltage wave is negative because the terminal voltage is momentarily zero, and the current of the forward wave is momentarily doubled. As the capacitor becomes fully charged, it behaves as an open circuit. Thus, its terminal current becomes zero and its voltage becomes equal to twice of the forward voltage wave.

7.6.2 Termination through Inductor

Assume that the capacitor C shown in Figure 7.10a and b has been replaced by an inductor L. The circuit behaves like an open-circuited line initially (since a current cannot flow through the inductor instantaneously) but finally acts like a short-circuited line. Therefore, the inductive termination is the dual of the capacitive termination. From the equivalent circuit, the voltage across the inductor is

$$v(t) = 2v_f 2e^{-(Z_c/L)t} \tag{7.101}$$

Its voltage starts at a value twice that of the forward wave and eventually becomes zero. At that time, the current flowing through the inductor is

$$i(t) = \frac{2v_f}{Z_c}\left(1 - e^{-(Z_c/L)t}\right) \tag{7.102}$$

The reflected voltage wave is

$$v_b(t) = v(t) - v_f(t) \tag{7.103}$$

or

$$v_b(t) = v_f\left(2e^{-(Z_c/L)t} - 1\right) \tag{7.104}$$

7.7 BEWLEY LATTICE DIAGRAM

The *bounce diagram*, developed by Bewley [1], determines the voltages at a given point and time in a transmission system. It is a useful visual aid to keep track of traveling voltage or current wave as it reflects back and forth from the ends of the line, as shown in Figure 7.11.

Figure 7.11a shows the circuit diagram where Z_s and Z_r represent internal source impedance and impedance connected at the end of the line, respectively. In the lattice diagram, the distance between the sending and receiving ends is represented by the horizontal line drawn to scale, and time is represented by the two vertical lines scaled in time. T is the time for a wave to travel the line length. The diagonal zigzag line represents the wave as it travels back and forth between the ends or discontinuities. The slopes of the zigzag lines give the times corresponding to the distances traveled.

The reflections are determined by multiplying the incident waves by the appropriate reflection coefficient. The voltage at a given point in time and distance is found by adding all terms that are directly above that point. For example, the voltage at $t = 5.5T$ and $x = (1/4)l$ is

$$v\left(\frac{1}{4}l, 5.5T\right) = v_f\left(1 + \rho_r + \rho_s\rho_r + \rho_s\rho_r^2 + \rho_s^2\rho_r^2\right)$$

whereas the voltage at $t = 6.5T$ and $x = (3/4)l$ is

$$v\left(\frac{3}{4}l, 6.5T\right) = v_f\left(1 + \rho_r + \rho_s\rho_r^2 + \rho_s^2\rho_r^2 + \rho_s^2\rho_r^3\right)$$

Lattice diagrams for current can also be drawn. However, the fact that the reflection coefficient for current is always the negative of the reflection coefficient for voltage should be taken into account.

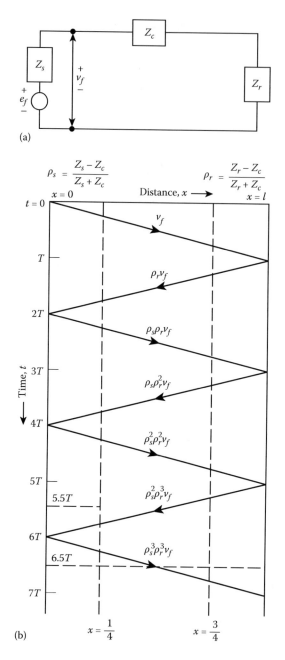

FIGURE 7.11 Bewley lattice diagram: (a) circuit diagram and (b) lattice diagram.

Example 7.6

Consider the circuit diagram shown in Figure 7.11a and assume that the dc source is a 1000 V ideal voltage source so that its internal impedance Z_s is zero and it is connected to the sending end of an underground cable with characteristic impedance of 40 Ω. The cable is terminated in a 60 Ω resistor.

(a) Determine the reflection coefficient at the sending end.
(b) Determine the reflection coefficient at the receiving end.
(c) Draw the associated lattice diagram showing the value of each reflected voltage.

(d) Determine the value of voltage at $t = 6.5T$ and $x = 0.25l$.
(e) Plot the receiving-end voltage versus time.

Solution

(a)

$$\rho_s = \frac{Z_s - Z_c}{Z_s + Z_c} = \frac{0 - 40}{0 + 40} = -1$$

(b)

$$\rho_r = \frac{Z_r - Z_c}{Z_r + Z_c} = \frac{60 - 40}{60 + 40} = 0.2$$

(c) The lattice diagram is shown in Figure 7.12a.
(d) From Figure 7.12a, the voltage value is 1008 V.
(e) The plot of the receiving-end voltage versus time is shown in Figure 7.12b.

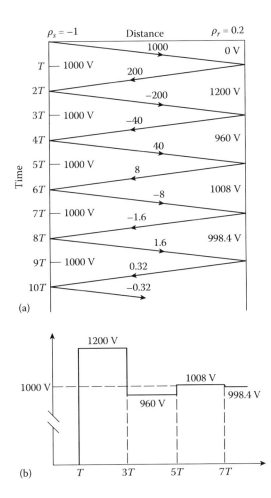

FIGURE 7.12 Lattice diagram for Example 7.6: (a) lattice diagram and (b) plot of the receiving and voltage versus time.

7.8 SURGE ATTENUATION AND DISTORTION

In general, in addition to the effects of reflections at transition points, traveling waves are also subject to both attenuation (*decrease in magnitude*) and distortion (*change in shape*) as they propagate along the line. They are caused by losses in the energy of the wave due to resistance, leakage, dielectric, and corona. Corona is the main cause of attenuation at HVs. It reduces the magnitude and the steepness of the wave fronts within a few miles to a safe voltage. If the attenuation cannot be neglected, then, in Figure 7.11, the amplitude of the wave after each reflection should be reduced by factor of e^{-al} due to the fact that the wave is attenuated by that amount of each transit.

The values of voltage and current waves can be found by taking the power and losses into account as they travel over a length dx of a line. The power loss in the differential element dx can be expressed as

$$dp = i^2 R dx + v^2 G dx \tag{7.105}$$

where R and G are the resistance and conductance of per-unit length of the line, respectively. Since

$$p = vi = i^2 Z_c$$

then the differential power is

$$dp = -2iZ_c di \tag{7.106}$$

The negative sign reflects the fact that the dp represents reduction in power. Thus, substituting Equation 7.106 into Equation 7.105,

$$-2iZ_c di = i^2 R dx + v^2 G dx$$

or

$$\frac{di}{i} = -\frac{R + GZ_c^2 dx}{2Z_c}$$

At $x = 0$, $i = i_f$, so that

$$i = i_f \exp\left(-\frac{R + GZ_c^2}{2Z_c}x\right) \tag{7.107}$$

Similarly,

$$v = v_f \exp\left(-\frac{R + GZ_c^2}{2Z_c}x\right) \tag{7.108}$$

7.9 TRAVELING WAVES ON THREE-PHASE LINES

Even though the basic traveling-wave equations remain unchanged when a three-phase system is considered, mutual coupling exists between the phases of the system and must be included in any calculation. In single-phase OH conductor applications, it can be seen that the presence of line losses attenuates and retards a traveling voltage wave along the line. In three-phase OH conductor applications, the situation is much more complex due to the fact that mutual coupling exists between the phases, which causes second-order changes of voltage on each phase to be functions of the voltages on the other conductors. The losses cannot be represented by simply attenuating and retarding the voltages in each phase. The solution to this problem can be found using an appropriate transformation matrix to diagonalize the matrix equations. Thus, the line can be represented by a number of modes of propagation so that the associated voltages travel uncoupled, that is, independently of each other. Hence, the losses can be introduced to each mode as it is done in the single-phase system.

For completely balanced lines, there are a number of simple transformation matrices that decouple the line equations. One such matrix for three-phase lines is the transformation matrix of the Clark components, that is, α, β, and 0 components. Since its elements are real, it is well suited for transient analyses. The phase voltages can be transformed into the modal domain using the modal transformation so that [2]

$$
\begin{bmatrix} \mathbf{v}_a \\ \mathbf{v}_b \\ \mathbf{v}_c \end{bmatrix} = \begin{bmatrix} \dfrac{1}{\sqrt{3}} & \dfrac{1}{\sqrt{6}} & \dfrac{1}{\sqrt{2}} \\ \dfrac{1}{\sqrt{3}} & \dfrac{-2}{\sqrt{6}} & 0 \\ \dfrac{1}{\sqrt{3}} & \dfrac{1}{\sqrt{6}} & \dfrac{-1}{\sqrt{2}} \end{bmatrix} \begin{bmatrix} \mathbf{v}_0 \\ \mathbf{v}_\alpha \\ \mathbf{v}_\beta \end{bmatrix}
\tag{7.109}
$$

or

$$
\begin{bmatrix} \mathbf{v}_{abc} \end{bmatrix} = \begin{bmatrix} T_c \end{bmatrix} \begin{bmatrix} \mathbf{v}_{0\alpha\beta} \end{bmatrix}
\tag{7.110}
$$

where the subscripts represent the modal quantities. Since the matrix $[T_c]$ is a unitary matrix, its inverse matrix can be found easily as

$$
\begin{bmatrix} T_c \end{bmatrix}^{-1} = \begin{bmatrix} T_c \end{bmatrix}^{t}
\tag{7.111}
$$

Similarly, it can be shown that

$$
\begin{bmatrix} \mathbf{i}_{abc} \end{bmatrix} = \begin{bmatrix} T_c \end{bmatrix} \begin{bmatrix} \mathbf{i}_{0\alpha\beta} \end{bmatrix}
\tag{7.112}
$$

Equation 7.109 can be expressed using the Laplace transforms as

$$
\begin{bmatrix} \mathbf{v}_a(s) \\ \mathbf{v}_b(s) \\ \mathbf{v}_c(s) \end{bmatrix} = \begin{bmatrix} \dfrac{1}{\sqrt{3}} & \dfrac{1}{\sqrt{6}} & \dfrac{1}{\sqrt{2}} \\ \dfrac{1}{\sqrt{3}} & \dfrac{-2}{\sqrt{6}} & 0 \\ \dfrac{1}{\sqrt{3}} & \dfrac{1}{\sqrt{6}} & \dfrac{-1}{\sqrt{2}} \end{bmatrix} \begin{bmatrix} \mathbf{v}_0(s) \\ \mathbf{v}_\alpha(s) \\ \mathbf{v}_\beta(s) \end{bmatrix}
\tag{7.113}
$$

or

$$
\begin{bmatrix} \mathbf{v}_{abc}(s) \end{bmatrix} = \begin{bmatrix} T_c \end{bmatrix} \begin{bmatrix} \mathbf{v}_{0\alpha\beta}(s) \end{bmatrix}
\tag{7.114}
$$

Similarly, Equation 7.112 can be expressed as

$$\begin{bmatrix} \mathbf{I}_a(s) \\ \mathbf{I}_b(s) \\ \mathbf{I}_c(s) \end{bmatrix} = \begin{bmatrix} \dfrac{1}{\sqrt{3}} & \dfrac{1}{\sqrt{6}} & \dfrac{1}{\sqrt{2}} \\ \dfrac{1}{\sqrt{3}} & \dfrac{-2}{\sqrt{6}} & 0 \\ \dfrac{1}{\sqrt{3}} & \dfrac{1}{\sqrt{6}} & \dfrac{-1}{\sqrt{2}} \end{bmatrix} \begin{bmatrix} \mathbf{I}_0(s) \\ \mathbf{I}_\alpha(s) \\ \mathbf{I}_\beta(s) \end{bmatrix} \tag{7.115}$$

or

$$\left[\mathbf{I}_{abc}(s) \right] = \left[T_c \right] \left[\mathbf{I}_{0\alpha\beta}(s) \right] \tag{7.116}$$

Hence,

$$\left[\mathbf{v}_{0\alpha\beta}(s) \right] = \left[\mathbf{Z}_{0\alpha\beta}(s) \right] \left[\mathbf{I}_{0\alpha\beta}(s) \right] \tag{7.117}$$

where the matrix $\left[\mathbf{Z}_{0\alpha\beta}(s) \right]$ is found using the similarity transformation.
Thus,

$$\left[\mathbf{Z}_{0\alpha\beta}(s) \right] = \left[T_c \right]^{-1} \left[\mathbf{Z}_{abc} \right] \left[T_c \right] \tag{7.118}$$

or

$$\left[\mathbf{Z}_{0\alpha\beta}(s) \right] = \left[T_c \right]^{t} \left[\mathbf{Z}_{abc} \right] \left[T_c \right] \tag{7.119}$$

If the line is completely balanced, the result of Equation 7.119 becomes

$$\begin{bmatrix} \mathbf{Z}_0(s) \\ \mathbf{Z}_\alpha(s) \\ \mathbf{Z}_\beta(s) \end{bmatrix} = \begin{bmatrix} \mathbf{Z}_0 & 0 & 0 \\ 0 & \mathbf{Z}_\alpha & 0 \\ 0 & 0 & \mathbf{Z}_\beta \end{bmatrix} \tag{7.120}$$

where

$$\mathbf{Z}_0 = \mathbf{Z}_s + 2\mathbf{Z}_m \tag{7.121}$$

$$\mathbf{Z}_\alpha = \mathbf{Z}_\beta = \mathbf{Z}_s - \mathbf{Z}_m \tag{7.122}$$

$$\mathbf{Z}_s = R_s + sL_s \tag{7.123}$$

$$\mathbf{Z}_m = R_m + sL_m \tag{7.124}$$

$$R_s = 2R \tag{7.125}$$

$$R_m = R \quad s = j\omega \tag{7.126}$$

Gross [2,3] shows that in the lossless case, the modal series impedances can be directly determined from sequence impedances as

$$\mathbf{Z}_0 = \frac{s}{j\omega} \mathbf{Z}_0 \qquad (7.127)$$

$$\mathbf{Z}_\alpha = \mathbf{Z}_\beta = \frac{s}{j\omega} \mathbf{Z}_1 \qquad (7.128)$$

After transforming terminal conditions into 0, α, β components, the 0, α, β decoupled line models can be developed, and therefore, the transient response of each mode can be determined separately from each other.

Hedman [4] shows that the multiphase reflection coefficient can be developed from a transmission line terminated in a resistive network. The equations that are applicable for a multiphase network are similar to those for the single-phase case, with the exception that each term is a matrix. Therefore,

$$[v] = [v_f] + [v_b] \qquad (7.129)$$

$$[i] = [i_f] + [i_b] \qquad (7.130)$$

$$[v_f] = [Z_l][i_f] \qquad (7.131)$$

$$[v_b] = -[Z_l][i_b] \qquad (7.132)$$

$$[v] = [Z][i] \qquad (7.133)$$

where the voltage and current matrices are column vectors and the impedance matrices are square matrices. Eliminating terms in Equations 7.129 through 7.133 and expressing the results in terms of $[v_f]$ and $[v_b]$ results in

$$[v_f] + [v_b] = [Z]\{[Z_1]^{-1}[v_f] - [Z_1]^{-1}[v_b]\} \qquad (7.134)$$

premultiplying by $[Z]^{-1}$ and getting coefficients for $[v_f]$ and $[v_b]$ results in

$$\{[Z_1]^{-1} - [Z]^{-1}[v_f] = [Z]^{-1} + [Z_1]^{-1}\}[v_b] \qquad (7.135)$$

The reflected voltage matrix in terms of forward voltages can be expressed as

$$[v_b] = \{[Z]^{-1} + [Z_1]^{-1}\}^{-1}([Z_1]^{-1} - [Z]^{-1})[v_f] \qquad (7.136)$$

Hence, the reflection coefficient for the multiphase case* can be determined from

$$[\rho] = \{[Z]^{-1} + [Z_1]^{-1}\}^{-1}\{[Z_1]^{-1} - [Z]^{-1}\} \qquad (7.137)$$

Today, there are various analog or digital computer techniques that have been developed to study the traveling-wave phenomenon on large systems. Existing digital computer programs are based

---

* Those who are interested in the application of matrix methods to the solution of traveling waves should also read Wedepohl [5], Uram et al. [6,7], Hedman [8,9], Virmani et al. [10], Dommel [11], and Dommel and Meyer [12].

on mathematical models using either differential equations or Fourier or Laplace transforms. It is interesting to note that the most rapid and least expensive computer solutions now known have been obtained with hybrid computers.

7.10 LIGHTNING AND LIGHTNING SURGES

7.10.1 LIGHTNING

By definition, lightning is an electrical discharge. It is the high-current discharge of an electrostatic electricity accumulation between cloud and earth or between clouds. The mechanism by which a cloud becomes electrically charged is not yet fully understood. However, it is known that the ice crystals in an active cloud are positively charged, while the water droplets usually carry negative charges. Therefore, a thundercloud has a positive center in its upper section and a negative charge center in its lower section. Electrically speaking, this constitutes a dipole. An interpretation of particle flow in relation to temperature and height is shown in Figure 7.13. Note that the charge separation is related to the supercooling, and occasionally even the freezing, of droplets. The disposition of charge concentrations is partially due to the vertical circulation in terms of updrafts and downdrafts.

As a negative charge builds up in the cloud base, a corresponding positive charge is induced on earth, as shown in Figure 7.14a. The voltage gradient in the air between charge centers in cloud (or clouds) or between cloud and earth is not uniform, but it is maximum where the charge concentration is greatest. When voltage gradients within the cloud build up to the order of 5–10 kV/cm, the air in the region breaks down and an ionized path called *leader* or *leader stroke* starts to form, moving from the cloud up to the earth, as shown in Figure 7.14b.

The tip of the leader has a speed between 10^5 and 2×10^5 m/s (i.e., less than one-thousandth of the speed of light of 3×10^8 m/s) and moves in jumps. If photographed by a camera, the lens of which

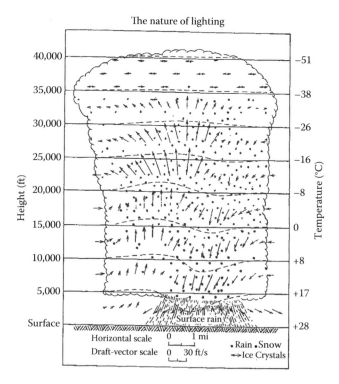

FIGURE 7.13 Idealized thunderstorm cloud cell in its mature state. (From Byers, H.R. and Braham, R.R., *The Thunderstorm*, U.S. Department of Commerce, Washington, DC, 1949.)

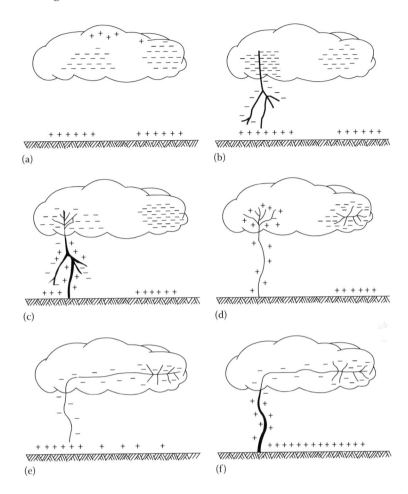

FIGURE 7.14 Charge distribution at various stages of lightning discharge: (a) charge centers in cloud and induced charge on ground, (b) leader stroke about to strike ground, (c) return stroke, (d) first charge center completely discharged, (e) dart leader, and (f) return stroke.

is moving from left to right, the leader stroke would appear as shown in Figure 7.15. Therefore, the formation of a lightning stroke is a progressive breakdown of the arc path instead of the complete and instantaneous breakdown of the air path from the cloud to the earth. As the leader strikes the earth, an extremely bright return streamer, called *return stroke*, propagates upward from the earth to the cloud following the same path, as shown in Figures 7.14c and 7.15.

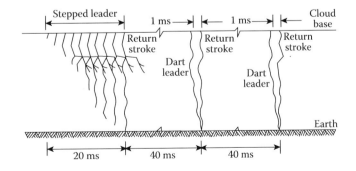

FIGURE 7.15 Mechanism of lightning flash.

In a sense, the return stroke establishes an electric short circuit between the negative charge disposited along the leader and the electrostatically induced positive charge in the ground. Therefore, the charge energy from the cloud is released into the ground, neutralizing the charge centers. The initial speed of the return stroke is 10^8 m/s. The current involved in the return stroke has a peak value from 1 to 200 kA, lasting about 100 μs. About 40 μs later, a second leader, called *dart leader*, may stroke usually following the same path taken by the first leader. The dart leader is much faster and has no branches and may be produced by discharge between two charge centers in the cloud, as shown in Figure 7.14e. Note the distribution of the negative charge along the stroke path. The process of dart leader and return stroke (Figure 7.14f) can be repeated several times. The complete process of successive strokes is called *lightning flash*. Therefore, a lightning flash may have a single stroke or a sequence of several discrete strokes (as many as 40) separated by about 40 ms, as shown in Figure 7.15.

7.10.2 Lightning Surges

The voltages produced on OH lines by lightning* may be due to indirect strokes or direct strokes. In the indirect stroke, induced charges can take place on the lines as a result of close by lightning strokes to ground. Even though the cloud and earth charges are neutralized through the established cloud-to-earth current path, a charge will be trapped on the line, as shown in Figure 7.16a. The magnitude of this trapped charge is a function of the initial cloud-to-earth voltage gradient and the closeness of the stroke to the line. Such voltage may also be induced as a result of lightning among clouds, as shown in Figure 7.16b. In any case, the voltage induced on the line propagates along the line as a traveling wave until it is dissipated by attenuation, leakage, insulation failure, or arrester operation.

In a direct stroke, the lightning current path is directly from the cloud to the line, causing the voltage to rise rapidly at the contact point. The contact point may be on the top of a tower, on the shield (OHGWs) wire, or on a line conductor. If lightning hits a tower top, some of the current may flow through the shield wires, and the remaining current flows through the tower to the earth. If the stroke is average in terms of both current magnitude and rate of rise, the current may flow into the ground without any harm provided that the tower and its footings have low resistance values. Otherwise, the lightning current will raise the tower to an HV above the ground, causing a flashover from the tower, over the line insulators, to one or more of the phase conductors.

On the other hand, when lightning strikes a line directly, the raised voltage, at the contact point, propagates in the form of a traveling wave in both directions and raises the potential of the line to

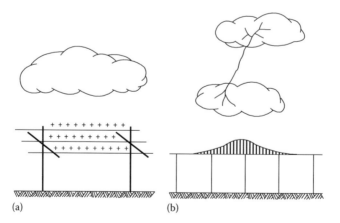

FIGURE 7.16 Induced line charges due to indirect lightning strokes: (a) trapped charge on the line and (b) voltage induced on the line due to a lighting among clouds.

---

* On EHV lines, lightning is the greatest single cause of outages.

the voltage of the downward leader. If the line is not properly protected against such overvoltage, such voltage may exceed the line-to-ground withstand voltage of line insulation and cause insulation failure. Therefore, such insulation failure, or preferably arrester operation, establishes a path from the line conductor to ground for the *lightning surge current.*

If the lightning strikes an OHGW somewhere between two adjacent towers, it causes traveling waves along the OHGW. The lightning current flows to the ground at the towers without causing any damage provided that the surge impedance of towers and the resistance tower footings are not too high.

Otherwise, the tower-top voltage is impressed across the line insulator strings and can cause a flashover, resulting in a *line outage.* It is possible that the arcing from the GW to the phase conductor may be sustained by the 60 Hz line voltage and can only be removed by deenergizing the line. This phenomenon is known as the *backflash.* It is most prevalent when footing resistances are high but can also occur on tall towers with low footing resistances.

7.10.3 USE OF OVERHEAD GROUND WIRES FOR LIGHTNING PROTECTION OF THE TRANSMISSION LINES

It is a well-known fact that a transmission line provides a protection shadow area on the earth beneath it so that any stroke normally hitting this area is drawn to the line instead.

The line itself is protected from direct stroke of lightning by one or two OHGWs.

The *OHGWs* are also called *shield wires* or *static wires.* These wires are conductors strung above the load-carrying conductors on transmission and distribution poles or towers to protect the load-carrying line conductors from lightning strikes. Since these shield wires are above the phase conductors, the lightning strokes hit them instead of the phase conductors below. Hence, the power-carrying line conductors are protected from the direct strokes of lightning by the shield wires. Almost all lines above 34.5 kV use shield wires.

These wires are directly connected to the tower, which means that they are electrically connected to the tower and are therefore at ground potential. Because of this, they are referred as the *OHGWs.* As a rule of thumb, the zone of protection is usually accepted to be about 30° on each side vertically beneath a GW. Hence, the transmission line must come within this 60° area.

In case of wood poles, they are grounded at every pole to provide a path for the lightning current. This lightning current is very high but lasts for only a few seconds. Because of this, the wires used for such shielding can be much smaller in diameter than phase conductors. The shield wires are made of either steel conductors, alumoweld strand conductors, or single-layer ACSR conductors.

Underground cables are, of course, immune to direct lightning strokes and can be protected against transients emanating on OH transmission lines.

In dc transmission lines, as in the case of ac OH transmission lines, an OHGW can be placed on top of the tower to protect against direct lightning strokes. However, the demand for GW in a dc line is usually for decreasing the resulting footing resistance per tower to ensure proper operation of the larger fault protection system. Hence, a larger protection angle is often accepted. Just like in ac applications that have less lightning exposures, the GWs can often be used close to the station.

7.10.4 LIGHTNING PERFORMANCE OF TRANSMISSION LINES

Figure 7.17 shows an isokeraunic map indicating the frequency of occurrence of thunderstorms throughout the United States. The contours represent the *isokeraunic* level, that is, the average number of thunderstorm days (i.e., days on which thunder could be heard) to be expected each year in different parts of the country.

However, the isokeraunic level can vary widely from year to year and does not differentiate between cloud-to-cloud lightning (which cause little harm) and cloud-to-earth lightning (which is very destructive). In a region of average storm intensity of 30 thunderstorm days per year, a 100 mi long transmission line will be struck on the average of 100 direct strokes per year.

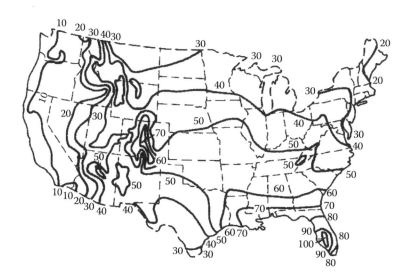

FIGURE 7.17 Isokeraunic map of the United States showing average number of thunderstorm days per year. (Courtesy of US Weather Bureau, College Park, MD.)

One of the most important parameters for the line design is the probability of the actual flashover rate exceeding some specified value in a given year. The probability of having exactly k no flashovers (*successes*) for n flashes to the line can be expressed, based on the binomial distribution, as

$$P_k = \frac{n!}{k!(n-k)!} p^k q^{n-k} \tag{7.138}$$

where

 p is the probability of having no flashover (*success*) for single flash
 q is the probability of having flashover (*failure*) for single flash, $= 1 - p$
 $n - k$ is the flashover rate

As stated earlier, n is the number of flashes to earth per square mile per year in the vicinity of the line. Anderson [16] gives the following equations to estimate the number of flashes to earth per square or per square miles per year, respectively, as

$$n = 0.12T \text{ flashes/km}^2\text{-year} \tag{7.139}$$

and

$$n = 0.31T \text{ flashes/mi}^2\text{-year} \tag{7.140}$$

where T is the keraunic level in thunderstorm days per year in the area.

It is a well-known fact that a transmission line provides a protective shadow area on the earth beneath it so that any stroke normally hitting this area is drawn to the line instead. The line itself is protected by the shield wires. The degree of protection afforded by shielding depends on the disposition of such OHGWs with respect to the phase conductors.

As said previously, the shield wires must have adequate clearance from the conductors, not only at the towers but throughout the span. Shield wires inevitably increase the number of strokes likely to terminate somewhere on the line, but this should not increase the number of outages.

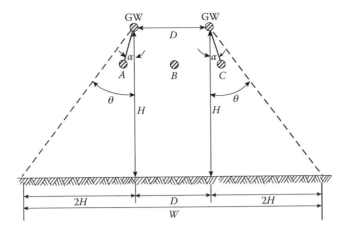

FIGURE 7.18 Width of ROW shielded from lightning strokes.

Figure 7.18 illustrates how such shadow can be determined for a single-circuit line with two GWs and horizontal configuration. The width of the shadow is

$$W = D + 4H \tag{7.141}$$

where
  D is the distance between the two GWs
  H is the *average* height of the GW

If there is only one GW, the distance D is zero. The average height H of the GW can be found from

$$H = H_t - \frac{2}{3}(H_t - H_{ms}) \tag{7.142}$$

where
  H_t is the height of the GWs at the tower
  H_{ms} is the height of the GWs at midspan with respect to ground

An improved version of Equation 7.141 is suggested by Whitehead [15] as

$$W = D + 4H^{1.09} \text{ m} \tag{7.143}$$

Therefore, the number of flashes to the line can be expressed as

$$n_{\text{line}} = 0.012T(D + 4H^{1.09}) \tag{7.144}$$

where
  n_{line} is the number of flashes to the line per 100 km per year
  T is the keraunic level in thunderstorm days per year

Note that, in Figure 7.18, θ is the *shadow angle* (usually assumed to be 63.5°), α is the *shield angle** between shield wire and phase conductor, W is the shadow width on the surface of the earth beneath the line, GW is the GW location, and A, B, and C are the phase conductors.

Besides receiving the shock of the direct strokes, the OHGW provides a certain amount of electrostatic screening as this reduces the voltage induced in the phase conductors by the discharge of a nearby cloud. For example, assume that E is the potential difference between the cloud and the

---

* Field experience indicates that a shield angle of 30° (from the vertical) reduces the direct stroke chance of a phase conductor by about a factor of 1000.

earth and that C_1 and C_2 are the capacitances of the cloud to line and the line to ground, respectively. Therefore, the induced voltage between the line to ground can be expressed as

$$v_{\text{L-G}} = E \times \frac{C_1}{C_1 + C_2} \qquad (7.145)$$

Thus, the presence of the GW above the line causes a considerable increase in C_2 and hence a reduction of the induced voltage of the line.

A properly located shield wire intercepts a great portion (probably above 95%) of the strokes that would otherwise hit a phase conductor. Shielding failure is defined as the situation when a stroke passes the shield wire and hits a phase conductor instead. Such shielding failures* might be due to the high wind accompanying the thunderstorm so that the phase conductor is blown out beyond the zone of protection of the shield wire.

An evaluation of tower clearances and conductor and OHGW configurations for an acceptable lightning protection design is based on theory and experience. The major factors affecting the lightning performance of a transmission line can be summarized as follows: (1) isokeraunic level, (2) magnitude and wave shape of the stroke current, (3) tower height, (4) resistance of tower and its footings, (5) number and location of OHGWs (shield angles to conductors), (6) span length, (7) midspan clearance between conductors and OHGWs, and (8) number of insulator units.

Since the basic inputs such as the lightning frequency, lightning current magnitude, wave front time, and incident rate are random variables, the prediction of lightning performance of a line is a probabilistic problem. Various probabilistic methods of computing the lightning flashover performance of lines have been developed.

Among the successful approaches is the Monte Carlo method used by Anderson [16]. In this method, deterministic relationships between surge voltage across the insulator string or air gap and variables such as lightning current magnitude, wave front time, stroke location, tower surge impedance, and footing resistance were determined by measurements in miniature physical models representing towers, ground, insulators, conductors, and the lightning path itself.

The results of these measurements with appropriate perturbations of the significant variables were then entered as input to a digital program together with statistical distributions of the input variables and estimates of the frequency of lightning strokes terminating on the transmission line. Flashover rates were then computed by Monte Carlo simulations.

Today, many digital computer programs exist to determine the response of the line to lightning strokes without requiring any miniature physical models. Based on such computer programs, generalized results in the form of design curves have been developed and published for specific tower types [17,18].

7.11 SHIELDING FAILURES OF TRANSMISSION LINES

Shielding failures take place when a flash misses the shield wires or tower and lands directly on the phase conductor of a given transmission line. When this happens overwhelmingly, HVs will rapidly developed at the contact point. These HVs will travel in both directions along the phase conductor until coming across one or more insulators and causing a flashover.

7.11.1 ELECTROGEOMETRIC THEORY

Young et al. [19] established the foundation of the electrogeometric (EGM) theory to analyze the frequency of the shielding failures on lines. This work was followed by Whitehead et al. [20,21],

---

* An excellent review of this topic is given by Anderson [14, p. 569].

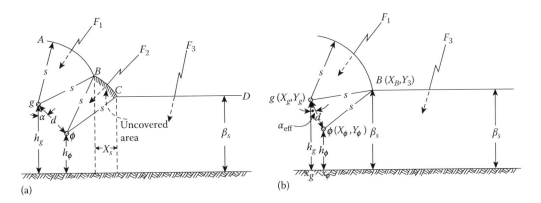

FIGURE 7.19 Electromagnetic model for shielding failures: (a) incomplete shielding and (b) effective shielding.

who have made important additional contributions to the theory in terms of both in fieldwork and in analytical evaluations.

Consider the shielding failure of one shield (i.e., OHGW) wire, g, and one phase conductor, ϕ, above a horizontal earth, as shown in Figure 7.19. Assume that there are three lightning flashes of equal current magnitude approaching the line, as shown in Figure 7.19a.

It is important to note that as a flash approaches within certain distance, s, of the earth and the line, it is influenced by what is below it and humps the distance s to make contact. This distance s is called the *strike distance* or *striking distance* and it is the fundamental concept in the EGM theory. Here, the strike distance is a function of the charge (and therefore the current) within the nearing flash. Return-stroke current (or simply stroke current), magnitude I, and strike distance s are interrelated. The following equations have been proposed for determining the stroke distance:

$$s = 9.4I^{2.3} \quad \text{Whitehead (1974)} \tag{7.146}$$

$$s = 2I + 30\left(1 - e^{-1/6.8}\right) \quad \text{Darveniza (1975)} \tag{7.147}$$

$$s = 3.3I^{0.78} \quad \text{Suzuki et al. (1981)} \tag{7.148}$$

$$s = 8I^{0.65} \quad \text{IEEE (1985)} \tag{7.149}$$

$$s = 10I^{0.65} \quad \text{Love (1987, 1993)} \tag{7.150}$$

where
  s is the strike distance in meters
  I is the return-stroke current in kiloamperes

It may be somewhat confusing to recognize that these equations vary by as much as a factor of 1–2. However, lightning experts now tend to be more favorable for the shorter strike distances that can be found by using Equation 7.149. These equations may also be expressed differently. For example, Equations 7.149 and 7.150 can, respectively, be expressed as

$$I = 0.041s^{1.54} \tag{7.151}$$

and

$$I = 0.029s^{1.54} \tag{7.152}$$

Complete shielding and effective shielding are illustrated in Figure 7.19a and b. For example, in Figure 7.19a, flash F_1 may make its final jump only to the shield wire because anywhere on the arc AB, the distance to the phase conductor ϕ exceeds s. Also, flash F_3 may jump only the distance βs to the earth because anywhere on the line CD, the distance to the phase conductor is too great.

Note that the coefficient permits for the strong likelihood that the final strike distance to the horizontal ground plane will be substantially different than the strike distance to a wire suspended above the grounds. Anderson [23] suggests 0.8 for EHV lines and 0.65 for UHV lines for the value of β.

On the other hand, flash F_2 as soon as it comes near the arc BC may jump only to the phase conductor ϕ. This is due to the fact that distances to the shield wire and earth will be greater than the strike distance. Therefore, for vertical flashes, the width x_s then provides the *uncovered area* of the earth in which flashes usually would reach the earth contact than the phase conductor instead. The width needs to be adjusted for the locations along the span due to sag, terrain, and nearby trees.

Anderson [23] suggests using only vertical flashes until further notice by the industry, average conductor height, that is, height at the tower minus two thirds of the sag. As illustrated in Figure 7.19b, in the event that the shield wire is moved more nearly over the phase conductor, the previously uncovered arc BC (and the unprotected width x_s) vanishes, and therefore, any incoming stroke cannot reach the phase conductor ϕ. As a result, there is an effective shielding angle α_{eff}. According to Anderson [23], in the event that the strike distance s is known and if $\beta s > y_\phi$, then the unshielded (to uncovered) width x_s can be expressed as

$$x_s = s\left[\cos\theta + \sin\left(\alpha_s - \omega\right)\right] \tag{7.153}$$

where

$$\theta = \sin^{-1}\left(\frac{\beta s - y_\phi}{s}\right) \tag{7.154}$$

$$\omega = \cos^{-1}\left(\frac{d}{2s}\right) \tag{7.155}$$

$$\alpha_s = \tan^{-1}\left(\frac{x_\phi - x_g}{y_g - y_\phi}\right) \tag{7.156}$$

In the event that $\beta s < y_\phi$, then $\cos\theta$ is set equal to unity and

$$x_s = s\left[1 + \sin\left(\alpha_s - \omega\right)\right] \tag{7.157}$$

7.11.2 Effective Shielding

In order to accomplished an effective shielding, as illustrated in Figure 7.19b, the phase conductor is usually kept fixed and the shield wire is moved horizontally until the unprotected width x_s disappears. For good shielding, setting $x_\phi = 0$, then the x_g coordinate of the shield wire becomes

$$x_g = \left[s^2 - \left(\beta s - y_\phi\right)^2\right]^{1/2} - \left[s^2 - \left(\beta s - y_g\right)^2\right]^{1/2} \tag{7.158}$$

and the effective shield angle becomes

$$\alpha_{\text{eff}} = \tan^{-1}\left(\frac{x_g}{y_\phi - y_g}\right) \tag{7.159}$$

Note that $x_g < 0$ for positive shield angles due to the fact that the shield wire is to the left of the phase conductor, as shown in Figure 7.19b [14].

7.11.3 Determination of Shielding Failure Rate

In the event that the line is not effectively shielded against lightning, shielding failures will take place. As said earlier, the uncovered width x_s can be found by using either Equation 7.153 or 7.157. In order to determine the shielding failure rate, one has to go through the following procedure:

1. Find out the magnitude of stroke current, $I_{\min}$, to the most exposed phase ϕ just adequate to flashover its insulator. This current can be found from

$$I_{\min} = \frac{2V_{\text{crit}}}{Z_c} \tag{7.160}$$

where
$I_{\min}$ is the minimum shielding failure stroke current in kiloamperes
V_{crit} is the insulator critical flashover (CFO) voltage in kilovolts
Z_c is the surge impedance of the phase conductor (including corona effects) in ohms

2. Substituting $I_{\min}$ found earlier into Equation 7.149, solve for the minimum strike distance $s_{\min}$ to that phase conductor.
3. After finding the minimum strike distance $s_{\min}$, determine the unshielded (or unprotected) width x_s from Equations 7.153 or 7.157.

Note that as the distance s in Figure 7.19a is increased, the arc that represents the unshielded (or unprotected) BC decreases. Also, if the distance s is adequately large, the arc BC becomes zero, and Figure 7.19a becomes equivalent to Figure 7.19b. For the maximum value of stroke current $I_{\max}$ that causes a shielding failure, the corresponding strike distance is $s_{\max}$.

According to the electromagnetic theory, only flashes that have stroke currents between $I_{\min}$ and $I_{\max}$ can cause a shielding failure. These currents have to terminate within the unprotected area. The value of $s_{\max}$ is determined from Equation 7.158.

However, according to Brown [24], the length OB, in Figure 7.20a, approaches $s_{\max}$ for most practical causes. If it is assumed that the line OB is approximately the same as $s_{\max}$, then the value of maximum strike distance can be found that

$$s_{\max} \cong y_0\left(\frac{B_s - \sqrt{B_s^2 + A_s C_s}}{A_s}\right) \tag{7.161}$$

or

$$s_{\max} \cong y_0 \times \bar{s} \tag{7.162}$$

where

$$y_0 = \frac{y_g + y_\phi}{2} \tag{7.163}$$

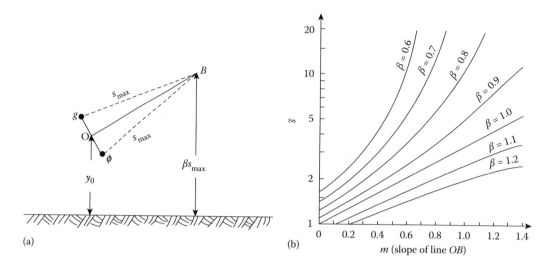

FIGURE 7.20   Determination of the maximum possible striking distance: (a) situational sketch and (b) the value of strike distance $\bar{s}$ by which y_0 must be multiplied to find s_{max}.

$$A_s = m^2 - m^2\beta^2 - \beta^2 \tag{7.164}$$

$$B_s = \beta\left(m^2 + 1\right) \tag{7.165}$$

$$C_s = \left(m^2 + 1\right) \tag{7.166}$$

where m is the slope of line OB from Figure 7.20a
or

$$m = \frac{X_\phi - X_g}{y_g - y_\phi} \tag{7.167}$$

where
   β is the coefficient
   y_0 is the height of midpoint of the distance between GW g and the phase conductor ϕ

The value of $\bar{s}$ is determined from Figure 7.20b based on the value of β and the slope of line OB. Anderson [16] suggests to use $\beta = 0.8$ for EHV lines and $\beta = 0.67$ for UHV lines. However, these values are not firmly established by industry. Note that the coefficient β permits for the strong probability that the final strike distance to the horizontal ground plane, with its attractive effects, will be significantly different from the strike distance to a conductor suspended above the ground plane.

Once the value of s_{max} is determined from Equation 7.161 or Equation 7.162, then one can use Equation 7.151 to determine the value of I_{max} as

$$I_{max} = 0.041 s_{max}^{1.54} \tag{7.168}$$

Note that for the maximum current I_{max}, the unshielded width x_s shrinks to zero. The average unshielded width is $x_s/2$ and this width, $\bar{x}_s$, is used for the shielding failure computation. According to Anderson [23], the number of flashes causing shielding failure is then found by calculating the most probable number of flashes per 100 per year falling between $\bar{x}_s$, determined by using Equation 7.139 and multiplying this number by the difference of the probabilities of the I_{min} and the I_{max} flashes occurring, or

$$n_{sf} = 0.012T\left(\frac{X_s}{2}\right)\left(P_{min} - P_{max}\right) \tag{7.169}$$

where
  n_{sf} is the number of shielding failures per 100 km per year
  T is the keraunic level (thunder-days)
  x_s is the unprotected width in meters
  P_{min} is the probability that a stroke will exceed I_{min}
  P_{max} is the probability that a stroke will exceed I_{max}

One has to recognize that Equation 7.169 is for one shield wire and one phase wire. If there are other phase wires that are also exposed, or if there is a phase wire that is exposed on both sides, then each such shielding failure rate is added separately to determine the total shielding failure rate. To find out the total number of strokes available to be used in back flashover computations, subtract the total shielding failure rate from the total number of strokes.

7.12 LIGHTNING PERFORMANCE OF UHV LINES

According to Anderson [16], UHV lines above 800 kV are practically lightning proof due to the large air gaps and insulator lengths, as long as proper shield angles are provided and footing resistances are maintained below 50 ohms. The determination of the value of β to use for proper shield angles is somewhat problematic. Anderson suggests to use $\beta = 0.64$ to be conservative.

7.13 STROKE CURRENT MAGNITUDE

As said in Section 7.11.1, the stroke current and striking distance are related. Thus, it may be of interest to know the distribution of stroke current magnitudes. According to Anderson [23], the median value of strokes to OHGW (*shields wire*), phase conductors, towers, other structures, and masts is about 31 kA. Hence, the probability that a certain peak current will be exceeded in any stroke can be expressed as

$$P\left(I\right) = \frac{1}{1 + \left(I/31\right)^{2.6}} \tag{7.170}$$

where
  $P(I)$ is the probability that the peak current in any stroke will exceed I
  I is the specified crest current of the stroke in kiloamperes

However, Mousa and Srivastava [25] have demonstrated that a median stroke current of 24 kA for strokes to flat ground results in the best correlation based on the field studies. Hence, based on

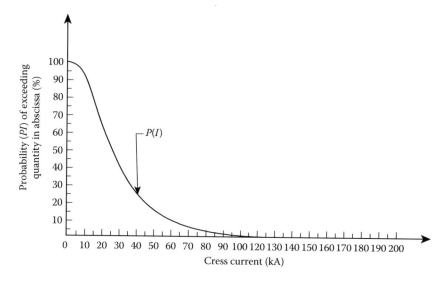

FIGURE 7.21   Probability of stroke current exceeding abscissa for strokes to flat ground.

this median value of stroke current, the probability that a certain peak current will be exceeded in any stroke can be expressed as

$$P(I) = \frac{1}{1 + (I/24)^{2.6}} \tag{7.171}$$

Figure 7.21 is a plot of Equation 7.171. It gives the probability of stroke current exceeding abscissa for strokes to flat ground.

7.14   SHIELDING DESIGN METHODS

There are two classic empirical design methods that have been used in the past to protect substations from direct lightning strokes: (1) fixed angles and (2) empirical curves [26].

7.14.1   FIXED-ANGLE METHOD

In the fixed-angle design method, vertical angles are used to determine the number, position, and height of shielding wires or masts. The method of fixed angle for shielding wires is illustrated in Figure 7.22. Similarly, the method fixed angles for shielding masts is illustrated in Figure 7.23. Note that the angles employed are determined by the degree of the importance of the substation, the physical terrain occupied by the substation, and the degree of lightning exposure. Also note that the value of the angle α that is usually used is 45°. The value of the angle β that is usually used is 30°or 45°.

7.14.2   EMPIRICAL METHOD (OR WAGNER METHOD)

The empirical curve method is also called the *Wagner method*. Wagner [27–29], based on field studies and laboratory model tests, determined empirical curves to determine the number, position, and height of shielding wires and masts. These curves were developed for shielding failure rates of 0.1%, 1.0%, 5%, 10%, and 15%. In general, a failure rate of 0.1% is used in designs.

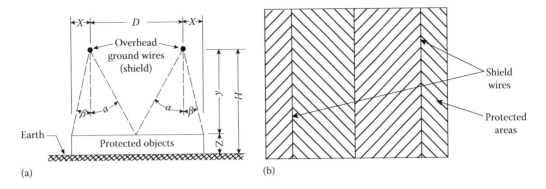

FIGURE 7.22   Fixed angles for shielding wires: (a) method and (b) protected areas.

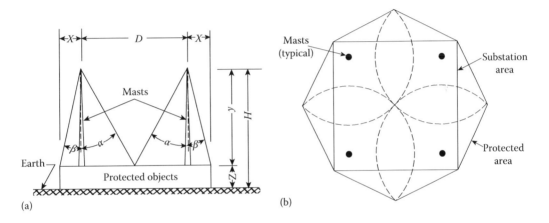

FIGURE 7.23   Fixed angles for shielding wires: (a) method and (b) protected areas.

7.14.3   ELECTROGEOMETRIC MODEL

In the past, shielding systems based on classical shielding methods to provide the necessary shielding for *direct stroke protection* of substations have been satisfactory. But the classical shielding methods have become less sufficient as structure and conductor heights have increased over the years as a result of increased voltage levels.

Anderson [16] developed a computer program for calculation of transmission-line lightning performance that uses the Monte Carlo method. This method showed good correlation with actual line performance. An earlier version of the EGM was developed in 1963 by Young et al. [19], but continuing research provided new models. For example, Whitehead [30] provided a theoretical model of a transmission system subject to direct strokes, development of analytical formulations of the line performance, and supporting field data that verified the theoretical model and analyses. The revised EGM was developed by Mousa and Srivastava [25], which differs from Whitehead's model in the following aspects:

1. The stroke is assumed to arrive in a vertical direction.
2. The differing strike distances to masts, wires, and the ground plane are taken into account.
3. A value of 24 kA is used as the median stroke current.
4. The model is not fixed to a specific form of the striking distance equation, given in Section 7.11.

In the revised EGM model, since the final striking distance is related to the magnitude of the stroke current, a coefficient k is introduced. This coefficient k provides for the different striking distances to a mast, a shield wire, and to the ground. Hence, the strike distance can be found from

$$s_m = 8\,kI^{0.65}$$

(7.172)

or

$$s_f = 26.25\,kI^{0.65}$$

(7.173)

where
s_m is the strike distance in meters
s_f is the strike distance in feets
I is the return-stroke current in kiloamperes
k is a coefficient to consider different striking distances to a mast, a shield wire, or the ground plane
k is 1, for strokes to wires or the ground plane
k is 1.2, for strokes to a lightning mast

Bus insulators are generally chosen to withstand a *basic lightning impulse level* (BIL). Insulators may also be selected based on other electrical characteristics, such as negative polarity *impulse* CFO voltage. Flashover takes place if the voltage developed by the lightning stroke current flowing through the surge impedance of the station bus exceeds the withstand value. The permissible stroke current is determined from

$$I_s = \text{BIL} \times \frac{1.1}{Z_s/2} = \text{BIL}\left(\frac{2.2}{Z_s}\right)$$

(7.174)

or

$$I_s = 0.94\left(\text{CFO}\right)\frac{1.1}{Z_s/2} = \frac{2.068\left(\text{CFO}\right)}{Z_s}$$

(7.175)

where
I_s is the permissible stroke current in kiloamperes
BIL is the basic lightning impulse level in kilovolts
CFO is the negative polarity CFO voltage through which the surge is passing in ohms
Z_s is the surge impedance of the conductor through which the surge is passing in ohms
1.1 is the factor to account for the reduction of stroke current terminating on a conductor as compared to zero-impedance earth

The withstand voltages in kV of insulator strings can be determined at 2 and 6 μs, respectively, as

$$V_2 = 0.94 \times 820w$$

(7.176)

and

$$V_6 = 0.94 \times 585 w \tag{7.177}$$

where
  w is the length of insulator string (or air gap) in meters
  0.94 is the ratio of withstand voltage to CFO voltage
  V_2 is the withstand voltage in kV at 2 μs
  V_6 is the withstand voltage in kV at 6 μs

The modified striking distance s can be found, if the permissible stroke current is determined from Equations 7.174 or 7.175 that are substituted in Equations 7.172 or 7.173 as

$$s_m = 8k \left[\frac{2.2(\text{BIL})}{Z_s} \right]^{0.65} \tag{7.178}$$

or

$$s_f = 26.25k \left[\frac{2.2(\text{BIL})}{Z_s} \right]^{0.65} \tag{7.179}$$

and

$$s_m = 8k \left[\frac{2.068(\text{CFO})}{Z_s} \right]^{0.65} \tag{7.180}$$

or

$$s_f = 26.25k \left[\frac{2.068(\text{CFO})}{Z_s} \right]^{0.65} \tag{7.181}$$

Note that BIL values of station post insulators can be from vendor catalogs.

Lee [31–33] developed a simplified technique for implementing the electromagnetic theory to the shielding of buildings and industrial plants. Orrell [34] extended the technique to include the protection of electrical substations.

The technique developed by Lee is known as the *rolling sphere method*. This method is based on the assumption that the striking distances to the ground, a mast, or a wire are the same. In the improved version of the rolling sphere method, an imaginary sphere of the radius s is rolled over the surface of substation. This sphere rolls up and over shield wires, substation fences, lightning masts, and other grounded metallic objects that can provide lightning shielding. Hence, any equipment that remains below the curved surface of the sphere is protected since the sphere is being elevated by shield wires or other devices.

As illustrated in Figure 7.24, any equipment that touches the sphere or penetrates its surface is not protected. *Increasing the shield mast height greater than strike distance s will provide additional protection in the case of lightning protection with a single mast.* However, *this is not necessarily true in the case of multiple masts and shield wires.* As the sphere is rolled around the mast, a 3D surface of protection is defined. This concept can be applied to multiple shielding masts, horizontal shield wires, or a combination of the two.

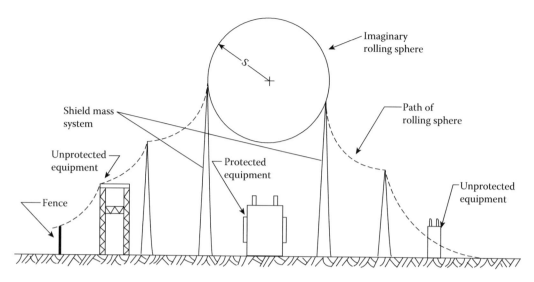

FIGURE 7.24   Principle of the rolling sphere.

7.15   SWITCHING AND SWITCHING SURGES

7.15.1   Switching

In an ac circuit, energy is continually exchanged cyclically between circuit inductances and capacitances. Depending on resistances present, losses will extract energy that will be supplied by various sources within the system. Each steady-state condition dictates its own unique set of energy storage and exchange rates in and among the various circuit elements. Therefore, redistribution of energy must take place among the various system elements to change from one steady-state condition to another. This change cannot take place instantaneously; a finite period of time, called *transient period*, prevails during which transient voltages and currents develop to enforce these changes.

Therefore, whenever a switch in an electric circuit is opened or closed, a switching transient may take place. This is true for transmission as well as distribution circuits. Table 7.1 presents various possible switching operations. Therefore, the interruption by a switching operation of a circuit having inductance and capacitance may result in transient oscillations that can cause overvoltages on the system.

Switching surges with high rates of voltage rise may produce repeated restriking of the arc between the opening contacts of a CB and thus impose such excessive duty on the CB as to result in its destruction. The interrupting ability of a CB depends on its capacity to increase the dielectric strength across its contacts at a more rapid rate than the rate at which the voltage is built up. Furthermore, switching surges may result in resonant oscillations in the windings of transformers or machines, and therefore, such windings may need to be protected using electrostatic shields.

As far as transmission-line insulation coordination is concerned, two particular types of switching operations are important: (1) energizing a line with no initial voltage and (2) high-speed reclosing following a line trip out. The main difference between these two switching operations is the fact that there may be energy trapped on the line from the previous opening. For example, the switching of a capacitance, such as disconnecting a line or a cable or a capacitor bank, may cause excessive overvoltages across the CB contacts, especially if restrikes occur in the switching device.

Restriking occurs if the recovery voltage across the CB builds up at a faster rate than the dielectric strength of the interrupting medium causing reestablishment of the arc across the interrupting contacts. Consider the circuit shown in Figure 7.25, where the current drawn by the capacitor leads the voltage by 90°. As the CB contacts separate from each other, an arc is established between the contacts, and current continues to flow. As the current goes through zero, the arc loses conductivity

TABLE 7.1
Various Possible Switching Operations

Switching Operation	System	Voltage across Contacts
1. Terminal short circuit		
2. Short line fault		
3. Two out-of-phase systems—voltage depends on grounding conditions in systems		
4. Small inductive currents, current chopped (unloaded transformer)	Transformer	
5. Interrupting capacitive currents—capacitor banks, lines, and cables on no load		
6. Evolving fault—e.g., flashover across transformer plus arc across contacts when interrupting transformer on no load	Transformer	
7. Switching—in unloaded EHV/UHV line (trapped charge)		

Source: Brown Boveri Review, December 1970. With permission.

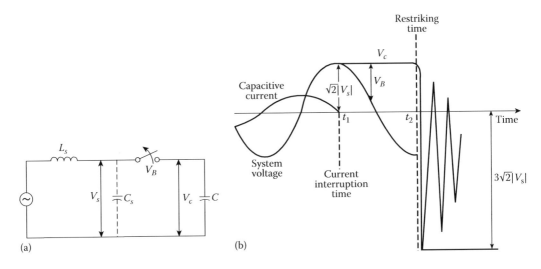

FIGURE 7.25   Restriking voltage transient caused by switch opening: (a) circuit and (b) restriking voltage transient.

and the current is interrupted. Note that C_s represents the stray capacitance. The arc cannot reignite due to the fact that the voltage across the contacts of the CB V_B (which is equal to $V_c - V_s$) is too small.

Therefore, the capacitor remains charged to a voltage equal to the peak value of the supply voltage, that is, -1.0 pu. In other words, the voltage *trapped* on the capacitor is 1.0 pu. As the supply voltage reverses, the recovery voltage V_s ($= V_c - V_s$) on the CB rises. Half a cycle later, when the source voltage V_s has changed to $+1.0$ pu, there will be a voltage of about 2.0 pu across the breaker. In the event that the breaker has regained enough dielectric strength to withstand this voltage, the switching operation will be successful.

Otherwise, there will be a *restrike*, which simply means that the insulation gap collapses and the breaker contacts are basically short-circuited. The restrike causes a fast oscillatory voltage in the *LC* circuit. Thus, the voltage overshoot on the capacitor will be as high as $+3.0$ pu $\left(\text{i.e., } 3\sqrt{2} \, |V_s| \right)$. When the voltage on the capacitor has reached its maximum, the transient discharge current will pass through zero, and arc may again extinguish, leaving the capacitor charged to $+3.0$ pu. Since the source voltage is V_s, the voltage across the breaker contacts after another half cycle will be -4.0 pu, which may cause another restrike, leaving the capacitor charged to -5.0 pu. This phenomenon may theoretically continue indefinitely, increasing the voltage by successive increments of 2.0 pu.

In practice, however, losses, stray capacitance, and possibly the resulting insulation failure will restrict the overvoltage. Voltages on the order of 2.5 times the V_s are more typical of field measurements. Switching overvoltages may rarely be determined by hand calculations, at least for realistic three-phase transmission-line circuits. Usually, they are determined by employing a transient network analyzer (TNA) or a digital computer program [11].

7.15.2 CAUSES OF SWITCHING SURGE OVERVOLTAGES

As mentioned in the previous section, the operation of CBs produces a transient overvoltage. However, the concept of switching should not be limited only to the intentional actions of opening and closing CBs and switches but may also include the arcing faults and even lightning.

The causes of switching surge overvoltages can be summarized as follows: (1) normal line energizing or deenergizing; (2) high-speed line reclosing; (3) switching cable circuits, capacitor banks, and shunt reactors; (4) load rejection; (5) out-of-phase switching, (6) reinsertion of SCs; (7) CB restriking; and (8) current chopping.

On the other hand, the 60 Hz voltages are caused by an abnormal condition that exists until change in the system alters or removes the condition. Examples of this condition are (1) voltages on the unfaulted phases during a phase-to-ground fault, (2) load rejection, (3) open end of a long energized line (Ferranti effect), and (4) ferroresonance.

7.15.3 CONTROL OF SWITCHING SURGES

IEEE Standard 399-1980 [35] recommends the following *philosophy of mitigation and control* of switching surges: (1) minimizing the number and severity of switching events, (2) restriction of the rate of exchange of energy that prevails among system elements during the transient periods, (3) extraction of energy, (4) provision of energy reservoirs to contain released or trapped energy within safe limits of current and voltage, (5) provision of preferred paths for elevated-frequency currents attending switching, and (6) shifting particularly offensive frequencies.

Furthermore, IEEE Standard 399-1980 [35] recommends the implementation of this control philosophy through the judicious use of the following means: (1) temporary insertion of resistance between circuit elements, for example, insertion resistors in CBs; (2) inrush control reactors; (3) damping resistors in filter circuits and surge-protective circuits; (4) tuning reactors; (5) surge capacitors; (6) filters; (7) surge arrestors; (8) necessary switching only, with properly maintained switching devices; and (9) proper switching sequences. Additional means of reducing switching overvoltages on EHV and UHF lines are given in Table 7.2.

TABLE 7.2

Means of Reducing Switching Overvoltages on EHV and UHV Lines

Means of Reducing Switching Overvoltages	Basic Diagram
1. HV shunt reactors connected to the line to reduce power-frequency overvoltage	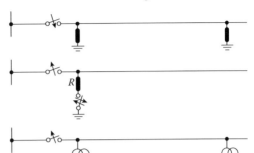
2. Eliminating or reducing trapped charge by 2.1 Line shunting after interruption	
2.2 Line discharge by magnetic potential transformers	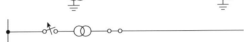
2.3 LV side disconnection of the line	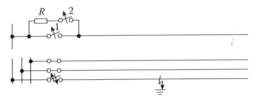
2.4 Opening, resistors	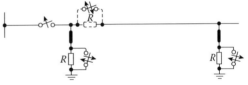
2.5 Single-phase reclosing	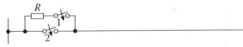
2.6 Damping of line voltage oscillation after disconnecting a line equipped with HV reactors	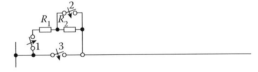
3. Damping the transient oscillation of the switching overvoltages 3.1 Single-stage closing resistor insertion	
3.2 Multistage closing resistor insertion	
3.3 Closing resistor in-line between CB and shunt reactor	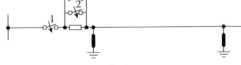
3.4 Closing resistor in-line on the line side of the shunt reactor	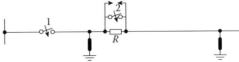
3.5 Resonance circuit (surge absorber) connected to the line	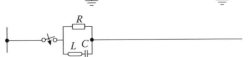

(continued)

TABLE 7.2 (continued)

Means of Reducing Switching Overvoltages on EHV and UHV Lines

Means of Reducing Switching Overvoltages	Basic Diagram

4. Switching at favorable switching moments
   4.1 Synchronized closing
   4.2 Reclosing at voltage minimum of a beat across the breaker
 	
 5. Simultaneous closing at both ends of the line
 	
 6. Limitation by surge arresters when (a) energizing line at no load, (b) disconnecting reactor-loaded transformers, and (c) disconnecting HV reactors
	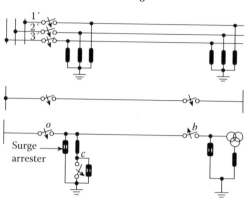

Source: *Brown Boveri Review*, December 1970. With permission.

Figure 7.26 shows a digital transient recorder that can be used for the continuous surveillance of a transmission network. The analysis is instantaneous through remote substation data acquisition units that transmit via telephone line or microwave link to the central station. The transient data are presented on a CRT screen. Waveform amplitude and timing information are derived automatically, without manual measurements and calculations.

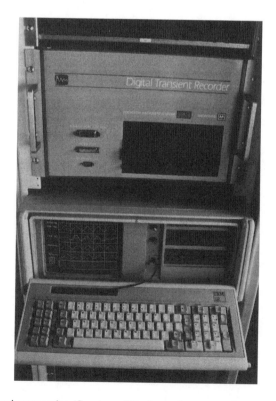

FIGURE 7.26   Digital transient recorder. (Courtesy of Rochester Instrument Systems Company, Rochester, N.Y.)

7.16   OVERVOLTAGE PROTECTION

In addition to the OHGWs or shield wires, air (rod and horn) gaps, surge diverters, and surge arresters are used to protect a power system against severe overvoltages. As stated earlier, the effectiveness of OHGWs for lightning protection depends on a low-impedance path to ground. Hence, all metal structures in transmission lines having OHGWs should be adequately grounded. If there are two OHGWs, they should be tied together at the top of each structure to reduce the impedance to ground. An array of GWs would be very effective but too expensive. Thus, the maximum number of GWs used is normally two, even on double-circuit lines.

The rod gap is the simplest form of a diverter. It has a preset air gap designed to flashover first if there is an excessive overvoltage. It is connected between a phase conductor and ground. Unfortunately, the rod gap cannot clear itself, and therefore, it will persist at the 60 Hz voltages. Also, its electrodes are damaged in the arcing process. Table 7.3 [36] gives flashover values of various air gaps. For a given air gap, the time for breakdown changes almost inversely with the applied voltage. However, the breakdown time for positive voltages are lower than those for negative.

In general, a *rod gap* is set to a breakdown voltage that is not less than 30% below the withstand voltage level of the protected power apparatus. Succinctly put, the surge diverters pass no current at the 60 Hz voltage, prevent the 60 Hz follow-on current after a flashover, and break down quickly after the arrival of the excessive overvoltage. The *surge diverter* derives its name from the fact that when an HV surge reaches its gap, sparkover takes place, and therefore, the surge energy is diverted to the earth.

Surge arresters are also called *lightning arresters*. They are applied on electric systems to protect equipment such as transformers, rotating machines, etc., against the effects of overvoltages resulting from lightning, switching surges, or other disturbances. Surge arresters are also connected in shunt with equipment to be protected. It has basically a nonlinear resistor so that its resistance decreases rapidly as the voltage across it rises.

After the surge ends and the voltage across the arrester returns to the normally 60 Hz line-to-neutral voltage level, the resistance becomes high enough to limit the arc current to a value that can be quenched by the series gap of the arrester. Therefore, the surge arrester provides both gap protection and nonlinear resistance. A disruptive discharge between the electrodes of a surge arrester is called *sparkover*. The highest value of applied voltage at which an arrester will not flash is the *withstand voltage*. Current that flows through an arrester, caused by the 60 Hz system voltage across it, during and after the flow of surge current is called *follow current*. Surge arresters, with their controlled breakdown characteristics, sparkover at voltages well below the withstand strength of system insulation.

7.17   INSULATION COORDINATION

7.17.1   BASIC DEFINITIONS

Basic impulse insulation level (BIL): Reference insulation levels expressed in impulse crest (peak) voltage with a standard wave not longer than a 1.2 × 50 μs wave. It is determined by tests made using impulses of a 1.2 × 50 μs wave shape. BIL is usually defined as a per unit of maximum value of the line-to-neutral voltage. For example, for 345 kV, it is

$$1\,\text{pu} = \sqrt{2}\left(\frac{345}{\sqrt{3}}\right) = 282\,\text{kV}$$

so that a BIL of 2.7 pu = 760 kV.

TABLE 7.3
Flashover Values of Air Gaps

Air Gap		Flashover		Air Gap		Flashover	
mm	in.	60 Hz Wet, kV	Positive Critical Impulse, kV	mm	in.	60 Hz Wet, kV	Positive Critical Impulse, kV
25	1		38	1295	51	438	814
51	2		60	1321	52	447	829
76	3		75	1346	53	455	843
102	4		91–95	1372	54	464	858
127	5		106–114	1397	55	472	872
152	6		128–141	1422	56	481	887
178	7		141–155	1448	57	489	901
203	8		159–166	1473	58	498	916
229	9		175–178	1499	59	506	930
254	10	80	190	1524	60	515	945
279	11	89	207	1549	61	523	960
305	12	98	224	1575	62	532	975
330	13	107	241	1600	63	540	990
356	14	116	258	1626	64	549	1005
381	15	125	275	1651	65	557	1020
406	16	134	290	1676	66	566	1035
432	17	143	305	1702	67	574	1050
457	18	152	320	1727	68	383	1065
483	19	161	335	1753	69	591	1080
508	20	170	350	1778	70	600	1095
533	21	178	365	1803	71	607	1109
559	22	187	381	1829	72	615	1124
584	23	195	396	1854	73	622	1138
610	24	204	412	1880	74	630	1153
635	25	212	427	1905	75	637	1167
660	26	221	443	1930	76	645	1182
686	27	229	458	1956	77	652	1196
711	28	238	474	1981	78	660	1211
737	29	246	489	2007	79	667	1225
762	30	255	505	2032	80	675	1240
787	31	264	519	2057	81	683	1254
813	32	273	534	2083	82	691	1269
838	33	282	548	2108	83	699	1283
864	34	291	563	2134	84	707	1298
889	35	300	577	2159	85	715	1312
914	36	309	592	2184	86	723	1327
940	37	318	606	2210	87	731	1341
965	38	327	621	2235	88	739	1356
991	39	336	635	2261	89	747	1370
1016	40	345	650	2286	90	755	1385
1041	41	353	665	2311	91	763	1399
1067	42	362	680	2337	92	771	1414
1092	43	370	695	2362	93	779	1428
1118	44	379	710	2388	94	787	1443
1143	45	387	725	2413	95	795	1457
1168	46	396	740	2438	96	803	1472

TABLE 7.3 (continued)
Flashover Values of Air Gaps

Air Gap		Flashover		Air Gap		Flashover	
mm	in.	60 Hz Wet, kV	Positive Critical Impulse, kV	mm	in.	60 Hz Wet, kV	Positive Critical Impulse, kV
1194	47	404	755	2464	97	811	1486
1219	48	413	770	2489	98	819	1501
1245	49	421	785	2515	99	827	1515
1270	50	430	800	2540	100	835	1530
2565	101	842	1544	3835	151	1176	2269
2591	102	848	1559	3861	152	1182	2284
2616	103	855	1573	3886	153	1188	2298
2642	104	862	1588	3912	154	1194	2313
2667	105	869	1602	3937	155	1200	2327
2692	106	875	1617	3962	156	1206	2342
2718	107	882	1631	3988	157	1212	2356
2743	108	889	1646	4013	158	1218	2371
2769	109	896	1660	4039	159	1224	2385
2794	110	902	1675	4064	160	1230	2400
2819	111	909	1689	4089	161	1236	2414
2845	112	916	1704	4115	162	1242	2429
2870	113	923	1718	4140	163	1248	2443
2896	114	929	1733	4166	164	1254	2458
2921	115	936	1747	4191	165	1260	2472
2946	116	943	1762	4216	166	1266	2487
2972	117	950	1776	4242	167	1272	2501
2997	118	956	1791	4267	168	1278	2516
3023	119	963	1805	4293	169	1284	2530
3048	120	970	1820	4318	170	1290	2545
3073	121	977	1834	4343	171	1296	2559
3099	122	984	1849	4369	172	1302	2574
3124	123	991	1863	4394	173	1308	2588
3150	124	998	1878	4420	174	1314	2603
3175	125	1005	1892	4445	175	1320	2617
3200	126	1012	1907	4470	176	1326	2632
3226	127	1019	1921	4496	177	1332	2646
3251	128	1026	1936	4521	178	1338	2661
3277	129	1033	1950	4547	179	1344	2675
3302	130	1040	1965	4572	180	1350	2690
3327	131	1047	1979	4597	181	1355	2704
3353	132	1054	1994	4623	182	1361	2719
3378	133	1061	2008	4648	183	1366	2733
3404	134	1068	2023	4674	184	1372	2748
3429	135	1075	2037	4699	185	1377	2762
3454	136	1082	2052	4724	186	1383	2777
3480	137	1089	2066	4750	187	1388	2191
3505	138	1096	2081	4775	188	1394	2806
3531	139	1103	2095	4801	189	1399	2820
3556	140	1110	2110	4826	190	1405	2835
3581	141	1116	2124	4851	191	1410	2849

(continued)

TABLE 7.3 (continued)
Flashover Values of Air Gaps

Air Gap		Flashover		Air Gap		Flashover	
mm	in.	60 Hz Wet, kV	Positive Critical Impulse, kV	mm	in.	60 Hz Wet, kV	Positive Critical Impulse, kV
3607	142	1122	2139	4877	192	1416	2864
3632	143	1128	2153	4902	193	1421	2878
3658	144	1134	2168	4928	194	1427	2893
3683	145	1140	2182	4953	195	1432	2907
3708	146	1146	2197	4978	196	1438	2922
3734	147	1152	2211	5004	197	1443	2936
3759	148	1158	2226	5029	198	1449	2951
3785	149	1164	2240	5055	199	1454	2965
3810	150	1170	2255	5090	200	1460	2980

Source: Farr, H.H., *Transmission Line Design Manual*, U.S. Department of the Interior, Water and Power Resources Service, Denver, CO, 1980.

Withstand voltage: The BIL that can be repeatedly applied to an equipment without any flashover, disruptive charge, puncture, or other electrical failure, under specified test conditions.

Chopped-wave insulation level: It is determined by tests using waves of the same shape to determine the BIL, with the exception that the wave is chopped after about 3 μs. If there is no information, the chopped-wave level is assumed to be 1.15 times the BIL for oil-filled equipment, for example, transformers. It is assumed to be equal to the BIL for dry-type insulation. The equipment manufacturer should be consulted for exact values.

CFO voltage: The peak voltage for a 50% probability of flashover or disruptive discharge.

Impulse ratio (for flashover or puncture of insulation): It is the ratio of impulse peak voltage to the peak value of the 60 Hz voltage to cause flashover or puncture. In other words, it is the ratio of breakdown voltage at surge frequency to breakdown voltage at normal system frequency.

7.17.2 Insulation Coordination

Insulation coordination is the process of determining the proper insulation levels of various components in a power system and their arrangement. In other words, it is the selection of an insulation structure that will withstand the voltage stresses to which the system or equipment will be subjected together with the proper surge arrester. This process is determined from the known characteristics of voltage surges and the characteristics of surge arresters.

There are three different voltage stresses to consider when determining *insulation and electrical clearance requirements* for the design of HV transmission lines:

1. The 60 Hz power voltage
2. Lightning surge voltage
3. Switching surge voltage

Thus, insulation for transmission systems must be chosen after a careful study of both the transient and power-frequency voltage stresses on each insulation element. In general, lightning impulse voltages have the highest values and the highest rates of voltage rise.

A *properly done insulation coordination* provides the following:

1. The assurance that the insulation provided will withstand all normal operating stresses and a majority of abnormal ones.
2. The efficient discharge of overvoltages due to the lightning and switching surges as well as other internal cause.
3. The breakdown will occur only due to the external flashover.
4. The positions at which breakdown takes place will be where breakdown may cause no or comparatively minor damage.

Thus, insulation coordination involves the following:

1. Determination of line insulation
2. Selection of the BIL and insulation levels of other apparatus
3. Selection of lightning arresters

For transmission lines up to 345 kV, the line insulation is determined by the lightning flashover rate. At 345 kV, the line insulation may be dictated by either switching surge considerations or by the lightning flashover rate. Above 345 kV, switching surges become the major factor in flashover considerations and will more likely control the insulation design.

The probability of flashover due to a switching surge is a function of the line insulation characteristics and the magnitude of the surges expected. The number of insulators used may be selected to keep the probability of flashover from switching surges very low.

Switching surge impulse insulation strength is based on tests that have been made on simulated towers. At EHV levels, an increase in insulation length does not provide a proportional increase in switching surge withstand strength. This is due to the electric field distortion caused by the proximity of the tower surfaces and is called the proximity effect. Since the proximity effect is not related to lightning impulses, switching surge considerations dictate the insulation values at the EHV levels.

The maximum switching surge level used in the design of a substation is either the maximum surge that can take place on the system or the protective level of the arrester, which is the maximum switching surge the arrester will allow into the station.

Hence, the *coordination of insulation in a substation* means the selection of the minimum arrester rating applicable to withstand the 60 Hz voltage and the choice of equipment having an insulation level that can be protected by the arrester. The results may be used to determine and coordinate proper impulse insulation and switching surge strength required in substation apparatus. The distance between the arrester location and the protected insulation affects the voltage imposed on insulation due to reflections.

The severity of the surge depends on how well the substation is shielded, the insulation level of the substation structure, and the incoming line insulation. For a traveling wave coming into a dead-end station, the discharge current in the arrester is determined by the maximum voltage that the line insulation can allow, by the surge impedance of the line, and by the voltage characteristic of the arrester. Hence, the discharge current of an arrester can be expressed as

$$I_{ar} = \frac{2V - V_{ar}}{Z_c} \tag{7.182}$$

where
  I_{ar} is arrester current
  V is magnitude of incoming surge voltage
  V_{ar} is arrester terminal voltage
  Z_c is surge impedance of line

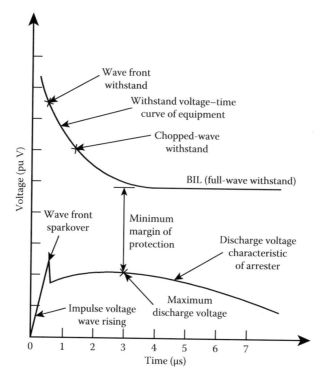

FIGURE 7.27 Illustration of insulation coordination between oil-filled equipment and surge arrester.

Figure 7.27 illustrates the insulation coordination between an oil-filled equipment (e.g., transformer) and a surge arrester. The arrester impulse sparkover voltage is compared to the chopped-wave test level of the transformer. A more meaningful comparison is to compare the arrester sparkover with the wave front test. The difference between arrester discharge characteristics and equipment withstand level, at any given instant of time, is called the *margin of protection* (MP) and is expressed as

$$MP = \frac{BIL_{equip} - V_{ar}}{BIL_{equip}} \tag{7.183}$$

where

BIL_{equip} is the BIL of the equipment
V_{ar} is the discharge of voltage of the arrester

The MP is a safety factor for the equipment protection and should not be less than 0.20. It also takes into account various possible errors and unknown factors. Figure 7.28 illustrates the insulation coordination in a 138 kV substation for 1.5 × 40 μs. The present US standard impulse wave is 1.2 × 50 μs.

7.17.3 INSULATION COORDINATION IN TRANSMISSION LINES

In transmission-line design, there are two basic insulations to be considered: the insulation string and air. Three types of voltage stresses need to be considered: (1) lightning impulse, (2) switching surges, and (3) power frequency. Switching surge performance is based on the probability of flashover following a CB operation. Lightning performance is measured by the number of trip outs per 161 km (i.e., 100 mi) of line per year. Power-frequency performance is measured in terms of the mean recurrence interval.

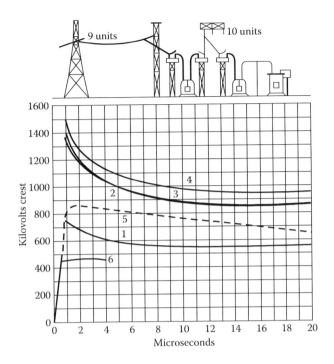

FIGURE 7.28 Insulation coordination in 138 kV substation for 1.5 × 40 μs wave: (1) transformer with 550 kV BIL, (2) line insulation of 9 suspension units, (3) disconnect switches on 4 apparatus insulators, (4) bus insulation of 10 suspension units, (5) maximum 1.5 × 40 μs wave permitted by line insulation, and (6) discharge of 121 kV arrester for maximum 1.2 × 40 μs full wave. (From Westinghouse Electric Corporation, *Electrical Transmission and Distribution Reference Book*, WEC, East Pittsburgh, PA, 1964.)

Insulation withstand has to be coordinated across the insulator string and the air gap. The following factors are included in an evaluation of the insulation withstand of an insulator string:

1. Maximum system operating voltage
2. Crest factor of the wave
3. Maximum switching surge overvoltage
4. Strength of air to switching surges in relation to the impulse strength of the insulators or the ratio of critical impulse to switching surge withstand
5. Percent allowance that is made between withstand voltage and CFO of air or ratio of withstand to CFO
6. Contaminated atmosphere (chemical, etc.)
7. Nonstandard air density (altitude)
8. Maximum fault voltage on unfaulted phases
9. Factor of safety

The maximum operating voltage can vary; however, a 5% overvoltage is generally accepted for this limit. The crest factor of the wave is $\sqrt{2}$. The maximum switching surge carries with breaker characteristics, line length, and the state of the system at the time of switching. The variation in the switching surges can be described by statistical distribution. These distributions will vary depending upon the proximity of grounded surfaces, humidity, and barometric pressure. It is suggested to use 2.8 as the switching surge value for a 115 kV line and 2.5 for 230 and 345 kV lines.

Usually, 1.175 is used as the ratio of the critical impulse strength for air to the switching surges. Also, 1.175 is used as the ratio of withstand to CFO voltage. A factor of 1.1 is used for contaminated atmosphere.

TABLE 7.4

Relative Air Density and Barometric Pressure

Elevation		Barometric Pressure		Relative Air Density	
m	ft	mm	in.	At 25°C	At 25°C
0	0	760	29.92	1.00	1.00
328.08	1,000	733	28.86	0.96	0.96
656.17	2,000	707	27.82	0.93	0.93
984.25	3,000	681	26.81	0.90	0.90
1312.34	4,000	656	25.84	0.86	0.86
1640.42	5,000	632	24.89	0.83	0.83
1968.50	6,000	609	23.98	0.80	0.80
2296.59	7,000	587	23.10	0.77	0.77
2652.76	8,000	564	22.22	0.74	0.74
2952.76	9,000	544	21.40	0.72	0.72
3280.84	10,000	523	20.58	0.69	0.69
3608.92	11,000	503	19.81	0.66	0.66
3937.01	12,000	484	19.05	0.64	0.64
4265.09	13,000	465	18.31	0.61	0.61
4593.18	14,000	447	17.58	0.59	0.59
4921.26	15,000	429	16.88	0.56	0.56
5249.34	16,000	412	16.21	0.54	0.54

Source: Farr, H.H., *Transmission Line Design Manual*, U.S. Department of the Interior, Water and Power Resources Service, Denver, CO, 1980.

An added altitude factor for nonstandard air is dependent upon the elevation of the given transmission line above the sea level. The relative air densities and barometric pressures at various elevations are given in Table 7.4.

Table 7.5 gives data for the barometric pressure versus elevation. A factor of 1.5 for contaminated atmosphere, 1.2 for the maximum fault voltage on unfaulted phases, and a safety factor of 1.25 are used when examining the insulation strength for power-frequency overvoltages.

Usually, for 115 kV wood-pole transmission-line construction, one extra insulator unit is added to allow for possible defective unit. However, for 115 kV steel structures, two extra units are added. For 230 kV steel construction, two extra units are added, one for a possible defective unit and one for hot-line maintenance. But for 345 kV steel construction, one extra unit is added as a combination of safety unit for defective unit and for hot-line maintenance safety.

The power insulation coordination is very important in transmission-line design. It prevents many unexplainable outages during the operation of the line. The insulation selection procedure for a 115 kV transmission line is given in Table 7.6. Similarly, the insulation selection procedures for 230 and 345 kV transmission lines are given in Tables 7.6 and 7.7, respectively.

7.18 GEOMAGNETIC DISTURBANCES AND THEIR EFFECTS ON POWER SYSTEM OPERATORS

It is well known that solar flares and other solar phenomena can cause transient fluctuations in the earth's magnetic field. When these fluctuations are severe, they are called *geomagnetic storms*. These storms can be seen visually as the *aurora borealis* in the northern and *aurora*

TABLE 7.5
Barometric Pressures versus Elevation

Nonstandard Air Factor	Barometric Pressure		Elevation		Nonstandard Air Factor	Barometric Pressure		Elevation	
	mm of Mercury	in. of Mercury[a]	m	ft		mm of Mercury	in. of Mercury[a]	m	ft
1.00	760	29.92	0	0	1.23	585	23.04	2154	7,068
1.01	752	29.62	85	280	1.24	578	22.74	2258	7,409
1.02	745	29.32	171	561	1.25	570	22.44	2362	7,750
1.03	737	29.02	256	841	1.26	562	22.14	2468	8,098
1.04	730	29.72	343	1126	1.27	555	21.84	2580	8,463
1.05	722	28.42	432	1417	1.28	547	21.54	2691	8,829
1.06	714	28.12	521	1709	1.29	540	21.24	2803	9,195
1.07	707	27.83	609	1999	1.30	532	20.94	2914	9,561
1.08	699	27.53	697	2287	1.31	524	20.64	2026	9,927
1.09	692	27.23	788	2584	1.32	517	20.35	4139	10,299
1.10	684	26.93	878	2881	1.33	509	20.05	4258	10,688
1.11	676	26.63	971	3186	1.34	502	19.75	4377	11,079
1.12	669	26.33	1065	3495	1.35	494	19.45	4497	11,474
1.13	661	29.03	1159	3804	1.36	486	19.15	4617	11,868
1.14	654	25.73	1253	4112	1.37	479	18.85	4740	12,270
1.15	646	25.43	1347	4418	1.38	471	18.55	4864	12,676
1.16	638	25.13	1440	4724	1.39	464	18.25	4987	13,082
1.17	631	24.83	1534	5034	1.40	456	17.74	4113	13,493
1.18	623	24.53	1638	5375	1.41	448	17.74	4238	13,904
1.19	616	24.24	1739	5705	1.42	441	17.74	4369	14,333
1.20	608	23.94	1843	6045	1.43	433	17.74	4501	14,768
1.21	600	23.64	1946	6386	1.44	426	16.74	4630	15,191
1.22	593	23.34	2050	6727	1.45	418	16.46	4765	15,632

[a] Barometric pressure = (29.92) (2 − nonstandard air factor).

australis in the southern hemisphere. These disturbances due to the effect of solar flares cause relatively rapid transient fluctuations in the earth's magnetic field, which is called *geomagnetic field*. The intensities of such geomagnetic storms are classified* from K-0 to K-9[+], according to the magnitude of the field fluctuations.

These geomagnetic field changes (i.e., the disturbances to the earth's magnetic field) induce an *earth surface potential* (ESP) that causes *geomagnetically induced current* (GIC) power systems. These GICs are near-dc currents, typically with a frequency that is less than 0.01 Hz. These GICs flow simultaneously through the power system, entering and exiting the many grounding points on the transmission network.

These grounding points are usually the grounded neutrals of wye-connected substation transformers that are located at opposite ends of long transmission lines. Since the earth is a spherical conductor in the large, the transient geomagnetic field variations produce an ESP that can be 3–6 V/km or even higher. The GICs have a fundamental period on the order of minutes.

---

* The classification is done by the Space Environment Services Center (SESC) in Boulder, Colorado. There are two indices that are commonly used to express levels of geomagnetic activity, namely, the K index and the A index. The index is a 3 h index of geomagnetic observations. The A index is a daily index obtained by averaging the eight 3 h K indices and assigning a numerical A-index number to the K number. An A < 50 is a *minor storm*, and an A > 50 is considered a *major storm* and is in the range that could produce noticeable power system effects. Geomagnetic field fluctuations are measured in units of nanoteslas (nT) or gammas (1 nT = 1 gamma = 10^{-9} T = 10^{-5} G.)

TABLE 7.6

Insulation Selection for a 115 kV Transmission Line

	Switching Surge Impulse, Positive Critical	Wet 60 Hz Flashover, kV
1. Overvoltage	1.05	1.05
2. Crest factor	1.414	
3. Switching surge[a]	2.8	
4. Ratio of critical impulse to switching surge	1.175	
5. Ratio of withstand to CFO voltage	1.175	1.175
6. Contaminated atmosphere	1.1	1.5
7. Factor of safety	1.2	1.25
8. Rise due to line faults		1.2
Total withstand multiplying factor (at sea level)[Product of (1) through (8)]	7.57	2.78
Normal line to neutral, $115/\sqrt{3} = 66.4$ kV		
Total withstand multiplying factor (at sea level) times		
Normal line-to-neutral voltage	503 kV	185 kV
Flashover of six insulator units, 146 by 254 mm (5 – 3/4 by 10 in.), from Table 2.4	610 kV	255 kV
Factor for nonstandard air density (altitude)	610/503 = 1.21	255/185 = 1.38
From Table 7.5, permissible elevation limit	1946 m (6386 ft)	3,864 m (12,676 ft)

Source: Farr, H.H., *Transmission Line Design Manual*, U.S. Department of the Interior, Water and Power Resources Service, Denver, CO, 1980.

[a] A switching surge value of 2.8 is more realistic value for 115 kV lines than the 2.5 value used for 230 and 345 kV lines.

Only a few amperes are necessary to disrupt transformer operation. However, over 300 A has been measured in the grounding connections of transformers in affected areas. These GICs, when they are present in transformers on the system, will produce half-cycle saturation on these transformers. And this is the root cause of all related problems in the electric power systems and will occur simultaneously throughout large portions of the interconnected network. This half-cycle saturation produces voltage regulation and harmonic distortion that affect each transformer in quantities that build cumulatively over the network.

The result can be enough to overwhelm the voltage regulation capability and the protection margins of equipment over large regions of the network. These widespread but correlated impacts can quickly lead to systemic failures of the network. The large continental grids, which have built due to reliability concerns, have become now in effect a large antenna to these storms.

When such geomagnetic storms taking place, they appear insignificant problem areas on ac lines, including increased inductive var requirements and also shifts in reactive power flow, system voltage fluctuations, generation of harmonics, protective relaying misoperations, and possible localized internal heating in transformers due to stray flux in the transformer from GIC-caused half-cycle saturation of the transformer magnetic core. Furthermore, reports of equipment damage have also included large electric generators and capacitor banks.

As mentioned in Section 1.11, power networks are operated using the *N – 1 operation criterion.* Accordingly, the system must always be operated to withstand the next substantial disturbance contingency without causing a cascading collapse of the system as a whole. This criterion is normally

TABLE 7.7
Insulation Selection for a 230 kV Transmission Line

	Switching Surge Impulse, Positive Critical	Wet 60 Hz Flashover, kV
1. Overvoltage	1.05	1.05
2. Crest factor	1.414	
3. Switching surge[a]	2.5	
4. Ratio of critical impulse to switching surge	1.175	
5. Ratio of withstand to CFO voltage	1.175	1.175
6. Contaminated atmosphere	1.1	1.5
7. Factor of safety	1.2	1.25
8. Rise due to line faults	1.2	
Total withstand multiplying factor (at sea level). [Product of (1) through (8)]	6.76	2.78
Normal line to neutral, $230/\sqrt{3} = 132.8\,\text{kV}$		
Total withstand multiplying factor (at sea level) times		
Normal line-to-neutral voltage	898 kV	369 kV
Flashover of 12 insulator units, 146 by 254 mm (5 – 3/4 by 10 in.), from Table 2.4	1105 kV	490 kV
Factor for nonstandard air density (altitude)	1105/898 = 1.23	490/369 = 1.32
From Table 7.5, permissible elevation limit	2154 m (7068 ft)	3,139 m (10,299 ft)

Source: Farr, H.H., *Transmission Line Design Manual*, U.S. Department of the Interior, Water and Power Resources Service, Denver, CO, 1980.

[a] A switching surge value of 2.8 is more realistic value for 115 kV lines than the 2.5 value used for 230 and 345 kV lines.

applicable for the well-known terrestrial environmental problems that usually spread out more slowly and are more geographically confined. They require a response time of 10–30 min, so that the system can be ready to survive the next possible contingency.

According to Kappenman [37], geomagnetic field disturbances during a severe geomagnetic storm can have a sudden onset and cover large geographic regions. They can therefore cause near-simultaneous, correlated, multipoint failures in power system infrastructures, allowing little or no time for meaningful human interventions that are intended within the framework of the $N - 1$ criterion, for example, in the collapse of the Hydro-Quebec power grid on March 13, 1989, when the system went from normal conditions to a situation where they sustained seen contingencies (i.e., $N - 7$) in an elapsed time of 92 s, from normal conditions to a complete collapse of the power grid, that black out the whole province. This was the result of a regional disturbance of 480 nT/min.

Kappenman [37] informs us that disturbance levels greater than 2000 nT/min have been observed even in contemporary storms on at least three occasions over the last 30 years in the North America that affected the power grid infrastructure. These levels of storms have also been observed in the similar world locations in August 1972, July 1982, and March 1989. He informs us that the past disturbances may have nearly reached the level of 5000 nT/min, which is ten times greater than the one that caused the Hydro-Quebec collapse. Figure 7.29 shows the comparison of GIC flows on the US transmission lines at various voltage levels. It is assumed that the field disturbance is uniform at 1.0 V/km and the grid resistance is average.

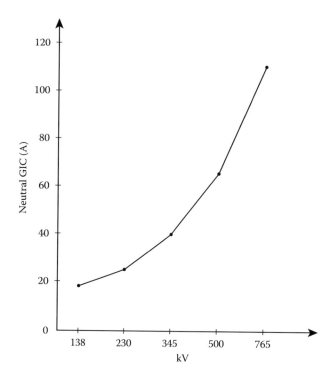

FIGURE 7.29 Average neutral GIC flows versus kilovolt ratings of 100 km long transmission lines.

PROBLEMS

7.1   Consider Figure 7.2 and derive Equation 7.5.
7.2   Consider Equations 7.2 and 7.16 and verify Equation 7.23 by using derivatives and integrals.
7.3   Consider Figure 7.2 and assume that switch S is closed and that the surge velocity is v. Verify that the electrostatic and electromagnetic energy storage (due to the surge phenomenon) are equal.
7.4   Repeat Example 7.1 assuming a surge impedance of 400 Ω.
7.5   Repeat Example 7.2 assuming a surge impedance of 40 Ω.
7.6   Repeat Example 7.2 assuming a surge voltage of 100 kV.
7.7   Consider an open-circuit line termination and verify the following:
   (a) $\tau = 2$ for voltage waves
   (b) $\tau = 0$ for current waves
   (c) $\rho = 1$ for voltage waves
   (d) $\rho = -1$ for current waves
7.8   Assume that a line is terminated in its characteristic impedance and verify the following:
   (a) $\tau = 1$ for voltage waves
   (b) $\tau = 1$ for current waves
   (c) $\rho = 0$ for voltage waves
   (d) $\rho = 0$ for current waves
7.9   Repeat Example 7.4 assuming that the line is terminated in a 200 Ω resistance and that the magnitudes for forward-traveling voltage and current waves are 2000 V and 5 A, respectively.

7.10 Repeat Example 7.4 assuming that the line is terminated in a 400 Ω resistance and that the magnitudes of forward-traveling voltage and current waves are 2000 V and 5 A, respectively.

7.11 A static charge on a line can be represented by the interaction of traveling waves, even though there are no transport phenomena involved. Assume that the line is open at both ends and charged to the voltage v. Determine the following:

(a) $i_b = -i_f$ for every point x along the line.

(b) $v_b = v_f = \frac{1}{2}v$ for every point x along the line.

(c) Plot the voltage and current distributions.

7.12 Assume that a dc source is supplying current to a resistance R over a transmission line having a characteristic impedance of Z_c and that the dc source voltage is v. Verify the following:

(a) $i_b = \dfrac{v}{R} - i_f$

(b) $v = 2Z_c i_f - \dfrac{Z_c}{R}v$

(c) $i_f = \left(1 + \dfrac{R}{Z_c}\right)\dfrac{i}{2}$

(d) $i_b = \left(1 - \dfrac{R}{Z_c}\right)\dfrac{i}{2}$

(e) $v_f = \left(1 + \dfrac{Z_c}{R}\right)\dfrac{v}{2}$

(f) $v_b = \left(1 - \dfrac{Z_c}{R}\right)\dfrac{v}{2}$

7.13 Consider Problem 7.11 and Figure 7.16a and assume that a static charge along a transmission line is built up below a cloud, which is suddenly released by a lightning discharge at time $t = 0$ into the cloud. The static charge existing in the line below the cloud at time $t = 0$ is essentially released by the lightning discharge and cannot remain static but must propagate along the line to permit transition to a new final steady-state solution. Use the results of Problem 7.11 and verify that

$$i_f = -i_b = \frac{v}{2Z_c}$$

7.14 Verify the following expressions:

(a) $\dfrac{P}{P_f} = \left(\dfrac{2}{\left(Z_{c1}/Z_{c2}\right)^{1/2} + \left(Z_{c2}/Z_{c1}\right)^{1/2}}\right)^2$

(b) $\dfrac{P_b}{P_f} = \left(\dfrac{Z_{c2} - Z_{c1}}{Z_{c1} + Z_{c2}}\right)^2$

7.15 Repeat Example 7.5 assuming that the 200 kV voltage surge is traveling toward the junction from the cable end.

7.16 Verify Equation 7.91 using Laplace transforms.

7.17 Use Laplace transforms and verify the following:

(a) Equation 7.101

(b) Equation 7.104

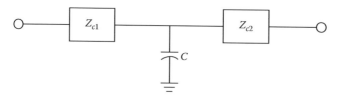

FIGURE P7.18   Figure for Problem 7.18.

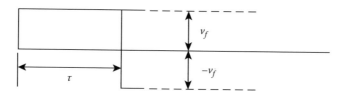

FIGURE P7.19   Figure for Problem 7.19.

7.18 Consider the junction between two lines with characteristic impedances of Z_{c1} and Z_{c2}, respectively. Assume that a shunt capacitor C is connected at the junction, as shown in Figure P7.18. Verify that the voltage across the capacitor is

$$v(t) = \frac{2v_f Z_{c2}}{Z_{c1} + Z_{c2}} \left[1 - \exp\left(-\frac{Z_{c1} + Z_{c2}}{Z_{c1} Z_{c2} C} \right) t \right]$$

7.19 Consider Problem 7.18 and assume that the traveling surge is of finite duration of τ, as shown in Figure P7.19, rather than of infinite length, and that its magnitude is v_f units. The wave can be decomposed into two waves as shown in the figure. Verify that the maximum voltage across the capacitor can be expressed as

$$v(t) = \frac{2v_f Z_{c2}}{Z_{c1} + Z_{c2}} \left[1 - \exp\left(-\frac{Z_{c1} + Z_{c2}}{Z_{c1} Z_{c2} C} \tau \right) \right]$$

7.20 Repeat Example 7.6 assuming that the cable is terminated in a 10 Ω resistor.

7.21 Assume that a new 100 mi long transmission line is built and that the line is designed to have a flashover rate of 1.0 per 100 mi per year. If the line is located in an area with a keraunic level such that 100 strokes (i.e., flashes) hit the line in an average year, determine the following:
(a) Probability of having zero flashover
(b) Probability of having one flashover
(c) Probability of having two flashovers
(d) Probability of having three flashovers
(e) Probability of having four flashovers

7.22 Assume that a 345 kV transmission is built in a location that has a keraunic level of 50 thunderstorm days per year. Each tower has two GWs separated from each other by 26 ft. The heights of the GWs at the tower and at the midspan are 57 and 48 ft, respectively. Determine the following:
(a) Average height of GW
(b) Width of protective shadow provided by line
(c) Number of flashes to line that can be expected per 100 km/year

7.23 Assume that a thyrite-type nonlinear lightning arrester has a characteristic of $RI^{0.72} = 57,000$. Determine the ratio of the voltages appearing at the end of a line having a surge impedance of 400 Ω due to a 400 kV surge when

(a) Line is open-circuited

(b) Line is terminated by arrester

REFERENCES

1. Bewley, L. V. *Traveling Waves on Transmission Systems*, Wiley, New York, 1951.
2. Gross, C. A. *Power System Analysis*, Wiley, New York, 1979.
3. Gross, C. A. Modal impedance of nontransposed power transmission lines, *Conf. Rec. Midwest Power Symp.* 1974.
4. Hedman, D. E. Attenuation of traveling waves on three-phase lines, *IEEE Trans. Power Appar. Syst.* PAS-90(3), 1971, 1312–1319.
5. Wedepohl, L. M. Application of matrix methods to the solution of traveling-wave phenomena in poly-phase systems, *Proc. Inst. Electr. Eng.* 110(12), 1963, 2200–2212.
6. Uram, R. and Miller, R. W. Mathematical analysis of transmission-line transients: I. Theory, *IEEE Trans. Power Appar. Syst.* PAS-83, 1964, 1116–1123.
7. Uram, R. and Feero, W. E. Mathematical analysis of transmission-line transients: II. Applications, *IEEE Trans. Power Appar. Syst.* PAS-83, 1964, 1123–1137.
8. Hedman, D. E. Propagation on overhead transmission lines: I. Theory of modal analysis, *IEEE Trans. Power Appar. Syst.* PAS-84, 1965, 200–205.
9. Hedman, D. E. Propagation on overhead transmission lines: II. Earth conduction effects and practical results, *IEEE Trans. Power Appar. Syst.* PAS-84, 1965, 205–211.
10. Virmani, S., Reitan, D. K., and Phadke, A. G. Computer analysis of switching transients on transmission lines-single line and lines on a common right-of-way, *IEEE Trans. Power Appar. Syst.* PAS-90(3), 1971, 1334–1346.
11. Dommel, H. W. Digital computer solution of electromagnetic transients in single- and multi-phase networks, *IEEE Trans. Power Appar. Syst.* PAS-88, 1969, 388–399.
12. Dommel, H. W. and Meyer, W. S. Computation of electromagnetic transients, *Proc. IEEE* 62(7), 1974, 983–993.
13. Byers, H. R. and Braham, R. R. *The Thunderstorm*, U.S. Department of Commerce, Washington, DC, 1949.
14. Electric Power Research Institute. *Transmission Line Reference Book- 345 kV and Above*, 2nd edn., EPRI, Palo Alto, CA, 1982.
15. Whitehead, E. R. Protection of transmission lines, in *Lightning*, R. H. Golde, ed., vol. 2, pp. 697–745, Academic Press, New York, 1977.
16. Anderson, J. G. Monte Carlo calculation of transmission line lightning performance, *Trans. Am. Inst. Electr. Eng.* part 3 vol., 1961, 414–420.
17. Westinghouse Electric Corporation. *Electrical Transmission and Distribution Reference Book*, WEC, East Pittsburgh, PA, 1964.
18. Edison Electric Institute. *EHV Transmission Line Reference Book*, EEI, New York, 1968.
19. Young, F. S., Clayton, J. M., and Hileman, A. R. Shielding of transmission lines, *AIEE Trans. PAS* Special Supplement, paper no. 63-640, 1963, 132–154.
20. Armstrong, H. P. and Whitehead, E. R. Field and analytical studies of transmission line shielding, *IEEE Trans. PAS* PAS-87, 1968, 270–281.
21. Brown, G. W. and Whitehead, E. R. Shielding of transmission lines, *IEEE Trans. PAS* PAS-88, 1969, 617–626.
22. Whitehead, E. R. CIGRÉ survey of the lightning performance of extra-high-voltage transmission lines, *Electra* 60, 1974, 69–89.
23. Anderson, J. G. Lightning performance of transmission lines, Chapter 12, in *Transmission Line Reference Book: 345 kV and Above*, 2nd edn., EPRI, Palo Alto, CA, 1987.
24. Brown, G. W. Lightning performance, II-updating backflash calculations, *IEEE Trans. PAS* PAS-97, 1978, 39–52.
25. Mousa, A. M. and Srivastava, K.D. The implications of the electromagnetic model regarding effect of height of structure on the median amplitude of collected lightning strokes, *IEEE Trans. Power Delivery* 4(2), 1989, 1450–1460.

26. IEEE Standard 998-1996, *Guide for Direct Lightning Strike Shielding of Substations*, 1996, IEEE, New York.
27. Wagner, C. F., McCann, G. D., and Beck, E. Field investigations of lightning, *AIEE Trans*. 60, 1941, 1222–1230.
28. Wagner, C. F., McCann, G. D., and Lear, C. M. Field investigations of lightning, *AIEE Trans*. 61, 1942, 96–100.
29. Wagner, C. F., McCann, G. D., and MacLane, G. L. Shielding transmission lines, *AIEE Trans*. 60, 1941, 313–328, 612–614.
30. Whitehead, E. R. *Mechanism of Lightning Flashover*, EEI Research Project, RP 50, Pub. 77-900, Illinois Institute of Technology, Chicago, IL, 1971.
31. Lee, R. H. Lightning protection of buildings, *IEEE Trans. Ind. Appl.* 15(3), 1979, 220–240.
32. Lee, R. H. Protection zone for buildings against lightning strokes using transmission line protection practice, *IEEE Trans. Ind. Appl.* 14(6), 1978, 465–470.
33. Lee, R. H. Protect your plant against lightning, *Instrum. Control Syst.* 55(2), 1982, 31–34.
34. Orrell, J. T. Direct stroke lightning protection, Paper presented at *EEI Electric System and Equipment Committee Meeting*, Washington, DC, 1988.
35. IEEE Std. 399-1980, *IEEE Recommended Practice for Power System Analysis*, IEEE, New York, 1980.
36. Farr, H. H. *Transmission Line Design Manual*, U.S. Department of the Interior, Water and Power Resources Service, Denver, CO, 1980.
37. Kappenman, J. G. Geomagnetic disturbances and impact upon power system operation, in *Electric Power Generation, Transmission, and Distribution*, L. L. Grigsby, ed., CRC Press, Boca Raton, FL, 2007.

GENERAL REFERENCES

Ametani, A. Modified traveling-wave techniques to solve electrical transients on lumped and distributed constant circuits, *Proc. Inst. Electr. Eng.* 120(4), 1973, 497–507.
Bickford, J. P. and Doepel, P. S. Calculation of switching transients with particular reference to line energization, *Proc. Inst. Electr. Eng.* 114(4), 1967, 465–474.
Brown, G. W. et al. Transmission line response to a surge with earth return, *IEEE Trans. Power Apparatus Syst.* PAS-90(3), 1971, 1112–1920.
Gönen, T. *Electric Power Distribution System Engineering*, 2nd edn., CRC Press, New York, 2008.
Greenwood, A. *Electrical Transients in Power Systems*, Wiley, New York, 1971.
Gridley, J. H. *Principles of Electrical Transmission Lines in Power and Communication*, Pergamon Press, New York, 1967.
Hylten-Cavallius, N. and Gjerlov, P. Distortion of traveling waves in high-voltage power lines, *ASEA Res.* 2, 1959, 147–180.
Lewis, W. W. *The Protection of Transmission System against Lightning*, Dover, New York, 1965.
Magnusson, P. C. *Transmission Lines and Wave Propagation*, 2nd edn., Allyn & Bacon, Boston, MA, 1970.
McElroy, A. J. and Smith, H. M. Propagation of switching-surge wavefronts, *Trans. Am. Inst. Electr. Eng.* 82, 1963, 983–998.
Metzger, G. and Vabre, J. E. *Transmission Lines with Pulse Excitation*, Academic Press, New York, 1969.
Moore, R. K. *Traveling-Wave Engineering*, McGraw-Hill, New York, 1960.
Peterson, H. A. *Transients in Power Systems*, Dover, New York, 1951.
Rüdenberg, R. *Transient Performance of Electric Power Systems-Phenomena in Lumped Networks*, McGraw-Hill, New York, 1950.
Rüdenberg, R. *Electrical Shock Waves in Power Systems*, Harvard University Press, Cambridge, MA, 1968.
Uman, M. A. *Lightning*, McGraw-Hill, New York, 1969.

8 Limiting Factors for Extrahigh- and Ultrahigh-Voltage Transmission
Corona, Radio Noise, and Audible Noise

To accomplish great things, we must not only act,
but also dream; not only plan, but also believe.

Anatole France

8.1 INTRODUCTION

A *corona* is a *partial discharge* and takes place at the surface of a transmission line conductor when the electrical stress, that is, the electric field intensity (or surface potential gradient), of a conductor exceeds the breakdown strength of the surrounding air. In such a nonuniform field, various visual manifestations of locally confined ionization and excitation processes can be viewed. These local breakdowns (i.e., corona or partial discharges) can be either of a transient (nonself-sustaining) or steady-state (self-sustaining) nature. These manifestations are called *coronas* due to the similarity between them and the glow or corona surrounding the sun (which can only be observed during a total eclipse of the sun). In nature, the corona phenomenon can also be observed between and within electrically charged clouds. According to a theory of cloud electrification, such a corona is not only the effect but also the cause of the appearance of charged clouds and thus of lightning and thunder storms.

A corona* on transmission lines causes power loss, RI and TVI, and AN (in terms of buzzing, hissing, or frying sounds) in the vicinity of the line. At extrahigh-voltage levels (i.e., at 345 kV and higher), the conductor itself is the major source of AN, RI, TVI, and corona loss. The AN is a relatively new environmental concern and is becoming more important with increasing voltage level.

For example, for transmission lines up to 800 kV, AN and electric field effects have become major design factors and have received considerable testing and study. It had been observed that the AN from the corona process mainly takes place in foul weather. In dry conditions, the conductors normally operate below the corona detection level, and therefore, very few corona sources exist. In wet conditions, however, water drops on the conductors cause a large number of corona discharges and a resulting burst of noise. At UHV levels (1000 kV and higher), such AN is the limiting environmental design factor.

---

* According to Nasser [1], "coronas have various industrial applications, such as in high-speed printout devices, in air purification devices by electronic precipitators, in dry-ore separation systems, as chemical catalysts, in radiation detectors and counters, and in discharging undesirable electric charges from airplanes and plastics. Coronas are used as efficient means of discharging other statically electrified surfaces of wool and paper in the manufacturing industry. They are also used successfully in the deemulsification of crude oil-brine mixtures."

8.2 CORONA

8.2.1 Nature of Corona

Succinctly put, a corona is a luminous partial discharge due to ionization of the air surrounding a conductor caused by electrical overstress. Many tests show that dry air at normal atmospheric pressure and temperature (25°C and 76 cm barometric pressure) breaks down at 29.8 kV/cm (maximum, or peak, value) or 21.1 kV/cm (rms, or effective, value). There are always a few free electrons in the air due to ultraviolet radiation from the sun, cosmic rays from outer space, radioactivity of the earth, etc.

As the conductor becomes energized on each half cycle of the ac voltage wave, the electrons in the air near its surface are accelerated toward the conductor on its positive half cycle and away from the conductor on its negative half cycle. The velocity attained by a free electron is dependent on the intensity of the electric field. If the intensity of the electric field exceeds a certain critical value, any free electron in this field will acquire a sufficient velocity and energy to knock one of the outer orbit electrons clear out of one of the two atoms of the air molecule. This process is called *ionization*, and the molecule with the missing electron is called a *positive ion*.

The initial electron, which lost most of its velocity in the collision, and the electron knocked out of the air molecule, which also has a low velocity, are both accelerated by the electric field, and therefore, each electron is capable of ionizing an air molecule at the next collision. After the second collision, there are now four electrons to repeat the process, and so on, the number of electrons doubling after each collision. All this time, the electrons are advancing toward the positive electrode, and after many collisions, their number has grown enormously. Thus, this process is called the *avalanche process*.* Note that each so-called electron avalanche is initiated by a single free electron that finds itself in an intense electrostatic field. Also note that the intensity of the electrostatic field around a conductor is nonuniform.

Hence, it has its maximum strength at the surface of the conductor, and its intensity diminishes inversely as the distance increases from the center of the conductor. Thus, as the voltage level in the conductor is increased, the critical field strength is approached, and the initial discharges take place only at or near the conductor surface.

For the positive half cycle, the electron avalanches move toward the conductor and continue to grow until they hit the surface. For the negative half cycle, the electron avalanches move away from the conductor surface toward a weaker field and cease to advance when the field becomes too weak to accelerate the electrons to ionizing velocity. Most of the early studies done by Trichel [3], Loeb [4–6], and others [7–9] have been on the negative nonuniform field corona processes. For example, Trichel [3,5] observed a type of negative corona from a point discontinuity. The corona consisted of a sequence of low-amplitude current pulses whose repetition rate depended on the sharpness of the point.

Figure 8.1 illustrates the fact that when the voltage across a point-to-plane gap is gradually increased, a current (in the order of 10^{-14} A) is measured. Here, there is no ionization that takes place, and this current is known as the *saturation current*. At a certain voltage, an abrupt current increase indicates the development of an ionization form that produces regular current pulses. These pulses were studied in great detail by Trichel in 1938 and are therefore called the *Trichel pulses*.

Figure 8.1 shows the onset voltage of different coronas plotted as a function of electrode separation *d* for a typical example of a cathode of 0.06. Early corona studies included the use of photographs of the coronas known as *Lichtenberg figures* [8,9]. The ac corona, viewed through a stroboscope, has the same appearance as the dc corona.

---

* It is also known as *Townsend's avalanche process*, after Townsend [2].

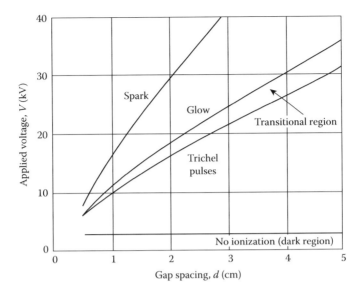

FIGURE 8.1 Basic negative corona modes and their regions in typical gap with cathode radius of 0.06 mm. (From Nasser, E., *Fundamentals of Gaseous Ionization and Plasma Electronics*, Wiley, New York, 1971.)

8.2.2 MANIFESTATIONS OF CORONA

Corona manifests itself by a *visual corona*, which appears as bluish (or violet-colored) tuffs and streamers and/or glows around the conductor, being more or less concentrated at irregularities on the conductor surface. This light is produced by the recombination of positive nitrogen ions with free electrons. This glow discharge is a very faint (or weak) light that appears to surround the conductor surface. It also may appear on critical regions of insulator surfaces during high-humidity conditions.

Figures 8.2 through 8.4 show various corona discharges at extrahigh-voltage levels. The streamer-type discharge is also known as the *brush discharge* and is projected radially from the conductor surfaces. The discharge resembling a plume is also known as the *plume discharge* and has a concentrated

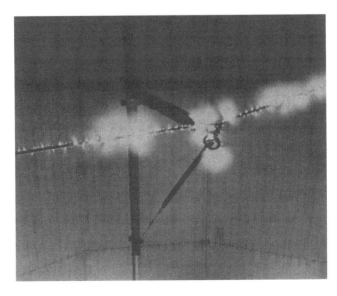

FIGURE 8.2 Corona testing of conductor in laboratory environment. (Courtesy of Ohio Brass Company, Wadsworth, OH.)

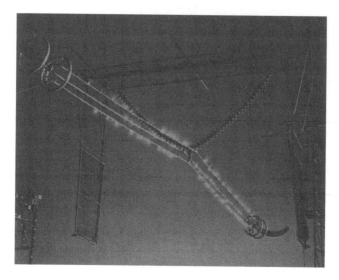

FIGURE 8.3 Corona testing on 500 kV triple-conductor support at elevated 60 Hz voltage for visual study of corona. (Courtesy of Ohio Brass Company, Wadsworth, OH.)

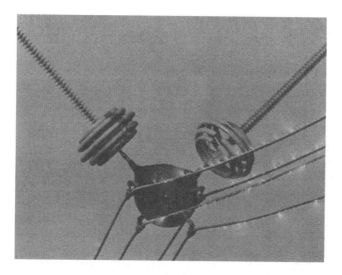

FIGURE 8.4 Corona testing of line with four bundled conductors. (Courtesy of Ohio Brass Company, Wadsworth, OH.)

stem that may be anywhere from a fraction of an inch long to several inches in length depending on the voltage level of the conductor. At its outer end, the stem branches many times and merges into a violet-colored treelike halo that has a length from a few inches at lower voltages to a foot or more at very high voltages.

The second manifestation of corona is known as the *audible corona*, which appears as a hissing or frying sound whenever the conductor is energized above its corona threshold voltage. The sound is produced by the disturbances set up in the air in the vicinity of the discharge, possibly by the movement of the positive ions as they are suddenly created in an intense electric field.

There is generally no sound associated with glow discharges. The corona phenomenon is also accompanied by the odor of ozone. In the presence of moisture, nitrous acid is produced, and if the corona is heavy enough, corrosion of the conductors will result. There is always a power loss associated with corona. Furthermore, the charging current under corona condition increases due to the fact that the corona introduces harmonic currents.

The last and perhaps most serious manifestation of the corona is the electrical effect that causes RI and/or TVI. The avalanches, being electrons in motion, actually constitute electric currents and therefore produce both magnetic and electrostatic fields in the vicinity. Since they are formed very suddenly and have short duration, these magnetic and electrostatic fields can induce high-frequency voltage pulses in nearby radio (or television) antennas and thus may cause RI (or TVI). These electrical disturbances are usually measured with a radiometer. It is interesting to note that corona will reduce the overvoltage on lung open-circuited lines due to lightning or switching surges.

8.2.3 FACTORS AFFECTING CORONA

As a rule of thumb, if the ratio of spacing between conductors to the radius is less than 15, flashover will take place between the conductors before corona phenomenon occurs. Since for overhead lines this ratio is much greater than 15, the flashover can be considered as impossible under normal circumstances. At a given voltage level, the factors affecting corona include line configuration, conductor type, condition of conductor surface, and weather.

In a horizontal configuration, the field near the middle conductor is larger than the field near the outer conductors. Therefore, the disruptive, critical voltage is lower for the middle conductor, causing larger corona loss than the ones for the two other conductors. If the conductors are not spaced equilaterally, the surface gradients of the conductors and therefore the corona losses are not equal.

Also, the conductor height affects the coronas loss, that is, the greater the height, the smaller the corona loss. The corona loss is proportional to the frequency of the voltage. Hence, the higher the frequency, the higher the corona losses. Thus, the corona loss at 60 Hz is greater than the one at 50 Hz. The corona loss at zero frequency, that is, dc, is far less than the one for ac.

The irregularity of the conductor surface in terms of scratches, raised strands, die burrs, die grease, and the particles of dust and dirt that clog the conductor can significantly increase the corona loss. The smoother the surface of a given cylindrical conductor, the higher the disruptive voltage.

For the same diameter, a stranded conductor is usually satisfactory for about 80%–85% of the voltage of a smooth conductor. As said before, the size of the conductors and their spacings also has considerable effect on corona loss. The larger the diameter, the less likelihood of corona. Thus, the use of conductors with large diameters or the use of hollow conductors or the use of bundled conductors increases the effective diameter by reducing the electric stress at the conductor surfaces.

The breakdown strength of air varies with atmospheric conditions. The breakdown strength of air is directly proportional to the density of the air. The air-density factor is defined as

$$\delta = \frac{3.9211 \times p}{273 + t} \tag{8.1}$$

where
  p is the barometric pressure in centimeters of mercury
  t is the ambient temperature in degrees Celsius

Table 8.1 gives barometric pressures as a function of altitude. Foul weather conditions (e.g., rain, snow, hoarfrost, sleet, and fog) all lower the critical voltage and increase the corona. Rain affects corona loss usually more than any other factor. For example, it may cause the corona loss to be produced on a conductor at voltages as low as 65% of the voltage at which the same loss takes place during fair weather.

Heavy winds have no effect on the disruptive critical voltage or on the loss, but presence of smoke lowers the critical voltage and increases the loss. Corona in fair weather may be negligible

TABLE 8.1
Standard Barometric Pressure as a Function of Altitude

Altitude (ft)	Pressure (cm Hg)	Altitude (ft)	Pressure (cm Hg)
−1000	78.79	5,000	63.22
−500	77.40	6,000	60.91
0	76.00	7,000	58.67
1000	73.30	8,000	56.44
2000	70.66	10,000	52.27
3000	68.10	15,000	42.88
4000	65.54	20,000	34.93

up to a voltage close to the disruptive critical voltage for a particular conductor. Above this voltage, the impacts of corona increase very quickly.

A transmission line should be designed to operate just below the disruptive critical voltage in fair weather so that corona only takes place during adverse atmospheric conditions. Thus, the calculated disruptive critical voltage is an indicator of corona performance of the line. However, a high value of the disruptive critical voltage is not the only criterion of satisfactory corona performance. The sensitivity of the conductor to foul weather should also be considered (e.g., corona increases more slowly on stranded conductors than on smooth conductors).

Due to the numerous factors involved, the precise calculation of the peak value of corona loss is extremely difficult, if not impossible. The minimum voltage at which the ionization occurs in fair weather is called the *disruptive critical voltage* and can be determined from

$$E_0 = \frac{V_0}{r \times \ln(D/r)} \tag{8.2}$$

as

$$V_0 = E_0 \times r \times \ln\frac{D}{r} \tag{8.3}$$

where
  E_0 is the value of electric stress (or *critical gradient*) at which disruption starts in kilovolts per centimeters
  V_0 is the disruptive critical voltage to neutral in kilovolts (rms)
  r is the radius of conductor in centimeters
  D is the spacing between two conductors in centimeters

Since, in fair weather, the E_0 of air is 21.1 kV/cm rms,

$$V_0 = 21.1 \times r \times \ln\frac{D}{r} \text{ kV} \tag{8.4}$$

which is correct for normal atmospheric pressure and temperature (76 cm Hg at 25°C). For other atmospheric pressures and temperatures,

$$V_0 = 21.1 \times \delta \times r \times \ln\frac{D}{t} \text{ kV} \tag{8.5}$$

where δ is the air-density factor given by Equation 8.1. Further, according to Peek [10], after making allowance for the surface condition of the conductor by using the irregularity factor, the disruptive critical voltage can be expressed as

$$V_0 = 21.1 \times \delta \times m_0 \times r \times \ln \frac{D}{r} \text{ kV} \tag{8.6}$$

where m is the irregularity factor ($0 < m_0 \le 1$): 1 for smooth, polished, solid, cylindrical conductors; 0.93–0.98 for weathered, solid, cylindrical conductors; 0.87–0.90 for weathered conductors with more than seven strands; and 0.80–0.87 for weathered conductors with up to seven strands.

Note that at the disruptive critical voltage V_0, there is no visible corona. In the event that the potential difference (or *critical gradient*) is further increased, a second point is reached at which a weak luminous glow of violet color can be seen to surround each conductor. The voltage value at this point is called the visual critical voltage and is given by Peek [10] as

$$V_v = 21.1 \times \delta \times m_v \times r \times \left(1 + \frac{0.3}{\sqrt{\delta \times r}}\right) \ln \frac{D}{r} \text{ kV} \tag{8.7}$$

where

V_v is the visual critical voltage in kilovolts (rms)

m_v is the irregularity factor for visible corona ($0 < m_v \le 1$): 1 for smooth, polished, solid, cylindrical conductors; 0.93–0.98 for local and general visual corona on weathered, solid, cylindrical conductors; 0.70–0.75 for local visual corona on weathered stranded conductors; and 0.80–0.85 for general visual corona on weathered, stranded conductors

Note that the voltage equations given in this section are for fair weather. For wet-weather voltage values, multiply the resulting fair-weather voltage values by 0.80. For a three-phase horizontal conductor configuration, the calculated disruptive critical voltage should be multiplied by 0.96 and 1.06 for the middle conductor and for the two outer conductors, respectively.

Example 8.1

A three-phase overhead transmission line is made up of three equilaterally spaced conductors, each with an overall diameter of 3 cm. The equilateral spacing between conductors is 5.5 m. The atmosphere pressure is 74 cm Hg and the temperature is 10°C. If the irregularity factor of the conductors is 0.90 in each case, determine the following:

(a) Disruptive critical rms line voltage
(b) Visual critical rms line voltage

Solution

(a) From Equation 8.1,

$$\delta = \frac{3.9211 \times p}{273 + t} = \frac{3.9211 \times 74}{273 + 10} = 1.0253$$

$$V_0 = 21.1 \times \delta \times m_0 \times r \times \ln \frac{D}{r}$$

$$= 21.1 \times 1.0253 \times 0.90 \times 1.5 \times \ln \frac{550}{1.5}$$

$$= 172.4 \text{ kV/phase}$$

Thus, the rms line voltage is

$$V_0 = \sqrt{3} \times 172.4 = 298.7 \text{ kV}$$

(b) The visual critical rms line voltage is

$$V_v = 21.1 \times \delta \times m_v \times r \times \left(1 + \frac{0.3}{\sqrt{\delta \times r}}\right) \ln \frac{D}{r}$$

$$= 21.1 \times 1.0253 \times 0.90 \times 1.5 \times \left(1 + \frac{0.3}{\sqrt{1.0253 \times 1.5}}\right) \ln \frac{550}{1.5}$$

$$= 214.2 \text{ kV/phase}$$

Therefore, the rms line voltage is

$$V_0 = \sqrt{3} \times 214.2 = 370.9 \text{ kV}$$

8.2.4 Corona Loss

According to Peek [10], the fair-weather corona loss per phase or conductor can be calculated from

$$P_c = \frac{241}{\delta}(f + 25)\left(\frac{r}{D}\right)^{1/2}(V - V_0)^2 \times 10^{-5} \text{ kW/km} \tag{8.8}$$

or

$$P_c = \frac{390}{\delta}(f + 25)\left(\frac{r}{D}\right)^{1/2}(V - V_0)^2 \times 10^{-5} \text{ kW/mi} \tag{8.9}$$

where
f is the frequency in hertz
V is the line-to-neutral operating voltage in kilovolts
V_0 is the disruptive critical voltage in kilovolts

The wet-weather corona can be calculated from these equations by multiplying V_0 by 0.80. Peek's equation gives a correct result if (1) the frequency is between 25 and 120 Hz, (2) the conductor radius is greater than 0.25 cm, and (3) the ratio of V to V_0 is greater than 1.8. From Equation 10.8 or 10.9, one can observe that the power loss due to the corona is

$$P_c \propto \left(\frac{r}{D}\right)^{1/2}$$

that is, the power loss is proportional to the square root of the size of the conductor. The larger the radius of the conductor, the larger the power loss. Also, the larger the spacing between conductors, the smaller the power loss. Similarly,

$$P_c \propto \left(V - V_0\right)^2$$

that is, for a given voltage level, the larger the conductor size, the larger the disruptive critical voltage and therefore the smaller the power loss.

According to Peterson [11], the fair-weather corona loss per phase or conductor* can be calculated from

$$P_c = \frac{1.11066 \times 10^{-4}}{\left[\ln\left(2D/d\right)\right]^2} \times f \times V^2 \times F \text{ kW/km} \tag{8.10}$$

---

* An additional and also popular method to calculate the fair-weather corona loss has been suggested by Carroll and Rockwell [12].

or

$$P_c = \frac{1.78738 \times 10^{-4}}{\left[\ln(2D/d)\right]^2} \times f \times V^2 \times F \ \text{kW/mi} \tag{8.11}$$

where

    d is the conductor diameter
    D is the spacing between conductors
    f is the frequency in hertz
    V is the line-to-neutral operating voltage in kilovolts
    F is the corona factor determined by test and is a function of ratio of V to V_0

Typically, for a fair-weather corona,*

$\frac{V}{V_0}$	0.6	0.8	1.0	1.2	1.4	1.6	1.8	2.0	2.2
F	0.012	0.018	0.05	0.08	0.3	1.0	3.5	6.0	8.0

In general, the corona losses due to fair weather conditions are not significantly large at extrahigh-voltage range. Therefore, their effects are not significant from technical and/or economic points of view. On the other hand, the corona losses due to foul weather conditions are very significant. For lines operating between 400 and 700 kV, the corona loss due to rainy weather is determined from the following expression [12–14]:

$$\text{TP}_{c,\text{RW}} = \text{TP}_{c,\text{FW}} + \left[\frac{V}{\sqrt{3}} \times j \times r^2 \times \ln(1+KR)\right] \sum_{i=1}^{n} E_i^m \tag{8.12}$$

where

    $\text{TP}_{c,\text{RW}}$ is the total three-phase corona losses due to rainy weather in kilowatts per kilometer
    $\text{TP}_{c,\text{FW}}$ is the total three-phase corona losses due to fair weather in kilowatts per kilometer
    V is the line-to-line operating voltage in kilovolts
    r is the conductor radius in centimeters
    n is the total number of conductors (number of conductors per bundle times 3)
    E_i is the voltage gradient on underside of conductor i in kilovolts (peak) per centimeter
    m is an exponent ($\cong 5$)
    j is the loss current constant ($\sim 4.37 \times 10^{-10}$ at 400 kV and 3.32×10^{-10} at 500 and 700 kV)[†]
    R is the rain rate in millimeters per hour or inches per hour
    K is the wetting coefficient (10 if R is in millimeter per hour or 254 if R is in inches per hour)

Note that the terms given in the square brackets are strictly due to the rain. The *EHV Transmission Line Reference Book* [13] gives a probabilistic method to determine the corona losses on the extrahigh voltage of various standard designs for different climatic regions of the United States.

    Figures 8.5 and 8.6 show corona loss curves for 69, 115, 161, and 230 kV lines designed for different elevations [15]. The curves are based on the Carroll–Rockwell method [12] and were developed

---

* The loss current constant j is approximately 7.04×10^{-10} at 400 kV and 5.35×10^{-10} at 500 and 700 kV if both the $\text{TP}_{c,\text{FW}}$ and $\text{TP}_{c,\text{RW}}$ are calculated in kilowatts per mile rather than in kilowatts per kilometer.
† For wet-weather corona, determine the factor F using $V/0.80V_0$.

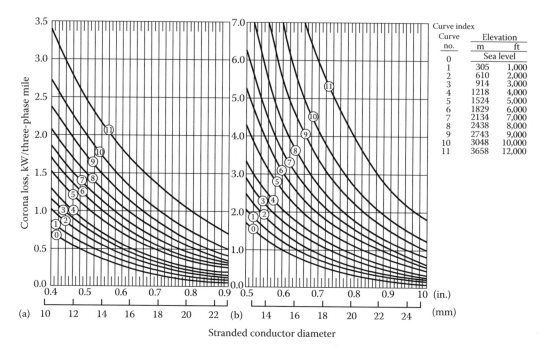

FIGURE 8.5 Corona loss curves for (a) 115 kV line with 12 ft horizontal spacing and (b) 161 kV line with 17 ft horizontal spacing. (From Farr, H.H., *Transmission Line Design Manual*, U.S. Department of the Interior, Water and Power Resources Service, Denver, CO, 1980.) All curves computed by the Carroll–Rockwell method for fair weather at 25°C (77°F).

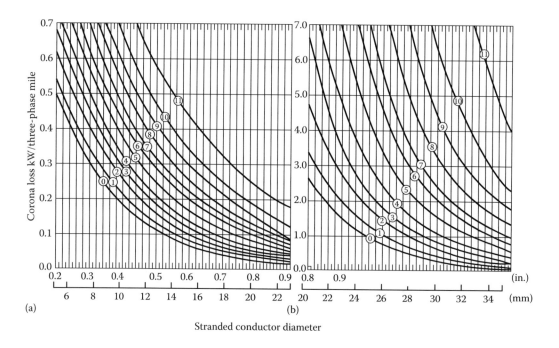

FIGURE 8.6 Corona loss curves for (a) 69 kV line with 10 ft horizontal spacing and (b) 230 kV line with 22 ft horizontal spacing. (From Farr, H.H., *Transmission Line Design Manual*, U.S. Department of the Interior, Water and Power Resources Service, Denver, CO, 1980.)

for fair-weather corona at 25°C (77°F) using ACSR conductors. Note that for a given conductor diameter, the curves give the fair-weather corona loss in kilowatts per three-phase mile.*

Example 8.2

Consider Example 8.1 and assume that the line operates at 345 kV at 60 Hz and the line length is 50 mi. Determine the total fair-weather corona loss for the line by using Peek's formula.

Solution

According to Peek, the fair-weather corona loss per phase is

$$P_c = \frac{390}{\delta}(f+25)\left(\frac{r}{D}\right)^{1/2}(V-V_0)^2 \times 10^{-5}$$

$$= \frac{390}{1.0253}(60+25)\left(\frac{1.5}{550}\right)^{1/2}(199.2-172.4)^2 \times 10^{-5}$$

$$= 12.1146 \text{ kW/mi/phase}$$

or, for the total line length,

$$P_c = 12.1146 \times 50 = 605.7 \text{ kW/phase}$$

Therefore, the total corona loss of the line is

$$P_c = 3 \times 605.7 = 1817.2 \text{ kW}$$

8.3 RADIO NOISE

RN (i.e., *electromagnetic interference*) from overhead power lines can occur due to partial electrical discharges (i.e., *corona*) or due to complete electrical discharges across small gaps (i.e., *gap discharges*, specifically *sparking*). The gap-type RN sources can take place in insulators, at tie wires between hardware parts, at small gaps between neutral or ground wires and hardware, in defective electrical apparatus, and on overhead power lines themselves. Typically, more than 90% of the consumer complaints are due to the gap-type RN.

Note the fact that RN is a general term that can be defined as "any unwanted disturbance within the radio frequency band, such as undesired electric waves in any transmission channel or device" [16]. The corona discharge process produces pulses of current and voltage on the line conductors. The frequency spectrum of such pulses is so large that it can include a significant portion of the RF band, which extends from 3 kHz to 30,000 MHz. Thus, the term *radio noise* is a general term that includes the terms *radio interference* and *television interference*. In the substations, continuously radiated RF noise and corona-induced AN can be controlled by using corona-free hardware and shielding for high-voltage conductors and equipment connections and by paying attention to conductor shapes to eliminate corners.

8.3.1 RADIO INTERFERENCE

The RI (also called the *radio influence*) is a noise type that occurs in the AM radio reception, including the standard broadcast band from 0.5 to 1.6 MHz. It does not take place in the FM band.

---

* For those readers interested in the design aspects of transmission lines, Farr [15] is highly recommended.

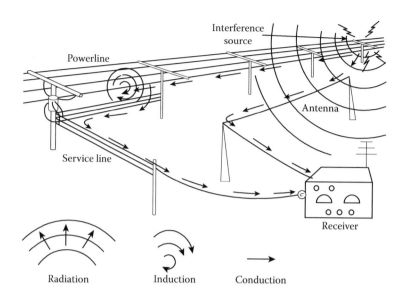

Radiation   Induction   Conduction

FIGURE 8.7   Paths by which interference energy travels from source to radio receiver. (From Chartier, V.L., Interference sources, complaint statistics, and limits, IEEE Tutorial Course: Location, Correction, and Prevention of RI and TVI Sources for Overhead Power Lines, IEEE Publ. No. 76 CH1163-5-PWR, IEEE, New York. Used with permission. © (1976) IEEE.)

Figure 8.7 illustrates the manner and paths by which such interference is transmitted to a radio receiver. As succinctly put by Chartier [17], "The *interference energy* can travel by one, or simultaneously, by two or three of the following means of transmission:

1. It travels *by conduction* via the transformer or by means of the neutral wire into the receiver power supply or wiring.
2. It travels *by induction* when the power line conductor or power supply lead carrying the interference energy is near enough to the antenna or some part of the receiver circuit to couple the interference energy into the receiver.
3. It travels *by radiation*, when the energy is launched into space by the overhead line or lines acting as a broadcasting antenna. In this instance, the energy can be reflected or reradiated from a nearby fence, power line, or metallic structure.

Transmission by the first two methods is most important at very low frequencies because conduction current decreases more slowly with distance along the line as the frequency is decreased. At higher frequencies, *radiation* becomes relatively more efficient and is more likely to be the cause of interference than the conduction currents or the induction fields.

In any case, however, power line interference tends to be roughly in inverse proportion to the frequency, that is, the higher the frequency, the lower the absolute interference level. Above a frequency of 100 MHz, conducted power line interference is very likely to have its source within a distance of 6–8 pole line spans of the receiver affected. However, in the case of *radiated* power line interference, there have been reports of objectionable interference originating from sources as far as 30 miles away."

According to a report published by the Iowa State University [17], 25% of all the cases of RI could be traced to household equipment, while 15% of the cases were in the receiver itself. The remaining cases are distributed as follows: 30%, industrial equipment; 17%, generation,

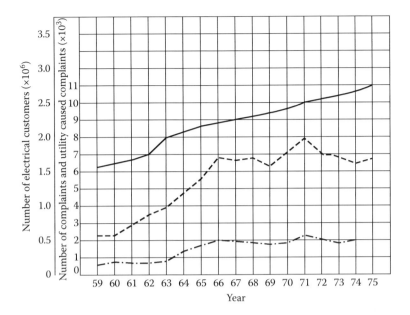

FIGURE 8.8 Radio and television interference complaints for 1959–1975 compared to the number of customers of Southern California Edison Company: ——, number of electrical customers; – – – –, total RI and TVI complaints; – · – · – utility-caused complaints. (From Nelson, W.R. and Schlinger, W.R., Construction practices for the elimination and mitigation of RI and TVI sources from overhead power lines, IEEE Tutorial Course: Location, Correction, and Prevention of RI and TVI Sources from Overhead Power Lines, IEEE Publ. No. 76 CH1163-5-PWR, IEEE, New York. Used with permission. © (1976) IEEE.)

transmission, and distribution equipment; and 13%, miscellaneous. Figure 8.8 shows the RI and TVI complaints for the years 1959–1975 compared to number of customers of Southern California Edison Company.

The RI properties of a transmission line conductor can be specified by *radio influence voltage* (RIV) generated on the conductor surface. This term refers to the magnitude of the line-to-ground voltage that exists on a device such as the power line or a station apparatus at any specified frequency below 30 MHz.

The threshold of RIV coincides with the appearance of visual corona. At the visual corona voltage, the RIV is negligibly small, but with the initial appearance of corona, RIV level increases quickly, reaching very high values for small increases above the visual corona voltages. The rate of increase in RI is affected by conductor surface and diameter, being higher for smooth conductors and large-diameter conductors. The corona and RI problems can be reduced or avoided by the correct choice of conductor size and the use of *conductor bundling*, often made necessary by other line design requirements.

Figure 8.9 shows typical values of conductor diameter that yield acceptable levels of electromagnetic interference. Precipitation increases RI, as does high humidity. Instrumentation to measure the electromagnetic interference field and to determine its frequency spectrum has been developed and standardized. The *quasi-peak* (*QP*) value of the electric field component obtained with a narrowband amplifier of standard gain is recognized as representing the disturbing effect of typical corona noise.

RN (RI or TVI) is usually expressed in millivolts per meter or in decibels above 1 μV/m. Figure 8.10 provides a comparison of measured fair-weather RN profile and computed heavy-rain RN profile for a 735 kV line. As conductors age, RN levels tend to decrease. Since corona is mainly a function of the potential gradients at the conductors and the RN is associated with the corona, the

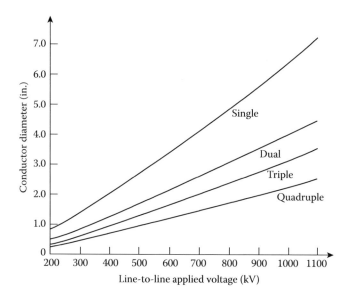

FIGURE 8.9 Typical values of conductor diameter that yield acceptable levels of interference.

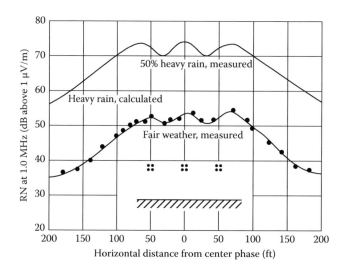

FIGURE 8.10 Comparison of measured fair-weather RN profile and computed heavy-rain RN profile for a 735 kV line. (From Anderson, J.C. et al., Ultra high voltage power transmission, *Proc. IEEE*, 59(11), 1548–1556. Used with permission. © (1971) IEEE.)

RN as well as corona will increase with higher voltage, other things being equal. The RN depends also on the layout of the line, including the number and location of the phase and ground conductors and the line length.

The RN is measured adjacent to a transmission line by an antenna equipped with an RN meter. The standard noise meter operates at 1 MHz (in the standard AM broadcast band) with a bandwidth of 5 kHz, using a QP detector having a charging time constant of 1 ms and a discharging time constant of 600 ms. For measurements in the RI range, a rod antenna is usually used for the determination of the electric field E, and a loop antenna is normally used for the determination of the magnetic field component H.

Succinctly put, RI generated by a corona streamer is caused by the movement of space charges in the electric field of the conductor. As explained before, these charges are due to the ionization of air in the immediate vicinity of the conductor. As a source of RI, the streamer is usually represented as a *current generator*. Therefore, the current injected from this generator into the conductor depends only on the characteristics of the streamer.

Adams [18–23] has done extensive research on the RI phenomenon and has demonstrated [18] that this representation was somewhat imperfect and that, in reality, the corona streamer induced currents in all conductors of a multiwire system and therefore not only in the conductor that produced it. These currents depend on the characteristics of the conductor under corona and the self-capacitance and mutual capacitance of the conductors. Thus, the RI currents in conductors of different lines are not necessarily equal from one line to the other, even if they are generated by identical corona streamers.

According to Adams [18], the term that expresses the characteristics of the corona streamer is *excitation function*. Later, to predict the RI associated with different line designs, measurements were taken in specially built *test cages* for various conductor bundles. From measurements of the RI produced within these short lengths of enclosed line, the effective noise current (i.e., the excitation function) being injected into each phase of the line was inferred.

Figure 8.11 shows this excitation function as a function of the maximum surface gradient for bundled conductors made up of conductors of the diameter shown. Therefore, the noise currents being injected into each phase of the line can be determined for the excitation function.* Once the excitation function of a conductor is known, the RI (or RN) of a line having the same conductor can be calculated.

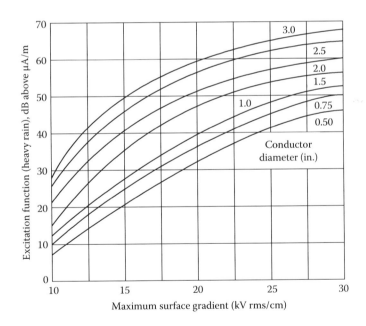

FIGURE 8.11 RI excitation function in heavy rain of different bundles as function of maximum surface gradient (add 7 dB for $n = 1$, 2 dB for $n = 2$, and 0 dB for $n = 3$, where n is number of subconductors). (From Anderson, J.C. et al., Ultra high voltage power transmission, *Proc. IEEE*, 59(11), 1548–1556. Used with permission. © (1971) IEEE.)

---

* For an excellent explanation of the physical meaning of the excitation function, see Gary [24].

The approximate value of the RI can be determined from the following empirical formula:

$$RI = 50 + K(E_m - 16.95) + 17.3686 \ln \frac{d}{3.93} + F_n + 13.8949 \ln \frac{20}{D} + F_{FW} \tag{8.13}$$

where

RI is the RN in decibels above 1 μV/m at 1 MHz

K is 3 for 750 kV class and 3.5 for others, gradient limits 15–19 kV/cm

E_m is the maximum electric field at conductor (gradient) in kilovolts per centimeter rms

d is the (sub)conductor diameter in centimeters

F_n is –4 dB for single conductor and $4.34221n$ $(n/4)$ for $n > 1$, n is the number of conductors in bundle

D is the radial distance from conductor to antenna in meters, $= (h^2 + R^2)^{1/2}$

h is the line height in meters

R is the lateral distance from antenna to nearest phase in meters

F_{FW} is 17 for foul weather and 0 for fair weather

Alternatively, the RI of a transmission line can also be determined from a method adopted by the BPA [25]. The method relates the RI of any given line to that of an RI (under the same meteorological conditions) for which the RI is known through measurement. Therefore, the RI of the given line can be determined from

$$RI = RI_0 + 120 \log_{10} \left(\frac{g}{g_0} \right) + 40 \log_{10} \left(\frac{d}{d_0} \right) + 20 \log_{10} \frac{hD_0^2}{h_0 D^2} \tag{8.14}$$

where

RI_0 is the RI of reference line

g is the average maximum (bundle) gradient in kilovolts per centimeter

d is the (sub) conductor in millimeters

h is the line height in meters

D is the direct (radial) distance from conductor to antenna in meters

8.3.2 Television Interference

In general, power line RN sources disturbing television reception are due to noncorona sources. Such power line interference in the VHF (30–300 MHz) and UHF (300–3000 MHz) bands is almost always caused by *sparking*. TVI can be categorized as fair-weather TVI and foul-weather TVI. Since the sparks are usually shorted out during rain, sparking is considered to be a fair-weather problem rather than a foul weather one.

The foul-weather TVI is basically from water droplet corona on the bottom side of the conductors, and therefore, it does not require *source locating*. If the RI of a transmission line is known, its foul-weather TVI can be determined from the following [14]:

$$TVI = RI - 20 \log_{10} \left[f \left(\frac{1 + (R/h)^2}{1 + (15/h)^2} \right) \right] + 3.2 \tag{8.15}$$

where

TVI is the television interference, in decibels (QP) above 1 μV/m at a frequency f in megahertz

RI is the radio interference in decibels (QP) above 1 μV/m at 1 MHz and at standard reference location of 15 m laterally from outermost phase

f is the frequency in megahertz

R is the lateral distance from antenna to nearest phase in meter

h is the height of closest phase in meters

Alternatively, the foul-weather TVI of a transmission line can also be determined from a method adopted by the BPA [25]. The method relates the TVI of any given line to that of a reference line (under the same meteorological conditions) for which the TVI is known through measurement. Therefore, the TVI of the given line can be determined from

$$\text{TVI} = \text{TVI}_0 + 120\log_{10}\left(\frac{g}{g_0}\right) + 40\log_{10}\left(\frac{d}{d_0}\right) + 20\log_{10}\left(\frac{D}{D_0}\right) \tag{8.16}$$

where

TVI_0 is the TVI of reference line

g is the average maximum (bundle) gradient in kilovolts per centimeter rms

d is the (sub)conductor diameter in millimeters

D is the direct (radial) distance from conductor to antenna in meters

8.4   AUDIBLE NOISE

With increasing transmission system voltages, AN produced by corona on the transmission line conductors has become a significant design factor. AN from transmission lines occurs primarily in foul weather. In fair weather, the conductors usually operate below the corona inception level, and very few corona sources exist. Therefore, the emission from well-designed UHV bundle conductor in fair weather is quite low.

In wet weather, however, water drops impinging or collecting on the conductors produce a large number of corona discharges, each of them creating a burst of noise. Therefore, the AN increases to such an extent that it represents one of the most serious limitations to the use of UHV.

It has been shown that the broadband component of random noise generated by corona may extend to frequencies well beyond the sonic range [26]. The noise manifests itself as a sizzle, crackle, or hiss. Additionally, corona creates low-frequency pure tones (hum), basically 120 and 240 Hz, which are caused by the movement of the space charge surrounding the conductor.

Figure 8.12 shows a typical random-noise portion of the AN frequency spectrum measured near a UHV test line having 4×2 in. conductors per phase. The plotted test results can be expressed by the following empirical equation [27]:

$$\text{AN} = k \times n \times d^{2.2} \times E^{3.6} \tag{8.17}$$

where

k is the coefficient of proportionality

n is the number of conductors

d is the diameter of conductors

E is the field strength at conductor surface (potential gradient)

It has been determined that the bundle diameter has relatively little effect on the noise produced. Figure 8.13 shows a direct comparison of noise predicted from cage tests and actual noise found during overhead line tests. Instrumentation and AN measurements have been described in the ANSI standards and procedures [26].

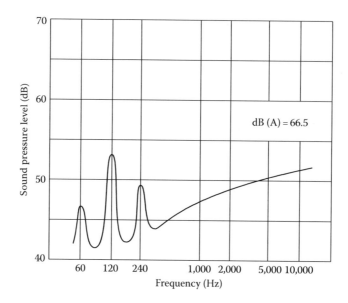

FIGURE 8.12 AN frequency spectrum during rain (1/10 octave bandwidth dB above 0.0002 μbar general radiometer) of a UHV line 4 × 2 in. bundle. (From Anderson, J.C. et al., Ultra high voltage power transmission, *Proc. IEEE*, 59(11), 1548–1556. Used with permission. © (1971) IEEE.)

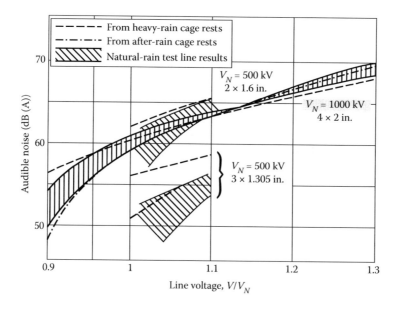

FIGURE 8.13 Comparison line between AN results with test lines under natural rain and computed values from cage tests with artificial rain. Line results are from two 500 kV lines of BPA (measuring point under outside phase) and from single-phase test line of Project UHV (measuring point at 100 ft from line). (From Anderson, J.C. et al., Ultra high voltage power transmission, *Proc. IEEE*, 59(11), 1548–1556. Used with permission. © (1971) IEEE.)

8.5 CONDUCTOR SIZE SELECTION

In the past, RI mitigation, rather than economic requirements, dictated the conductor size. This was due to the fact that (1) energy was inexpensive and (2) smaller conductor sizes would have facilitated an optimum balance between initial investment cost and operation cost. Today, due to increasing energy costs, the lower future energy and demand losses on a line more than offset the greater initial investment cost.

As conductor size increases, the investment cost increases, whereas the costs of energy and demand losses will decrease. Therefore, the total annual equivalent cost of a line with given conductor size for year n can be expressed as

$$\text{TAC}_n = \text{AIC}_n + \text{AEC}_n + \text{ADC}_n \ \text{\$/mi} \tag{8.18}$$

where
TAC_n is the total annual equivalent cost of line in dollars per mile
AIC_n is the annual equivalent investment cost of line in dollars per mile
AEC_n is the annual equivalent energy cost due to I^2R losses in line conductors in dollars per mile
ADC_n is the annual equivalent demand cost incurred to maintain adequate system capacity to supply I^2R losses in line conductors in dollars per mile

The annual equivalent investment of a given line for year n can be expressed as

$$\text{AIC}_n = \text{IC}_L \times \frac{i_L}{100} \ \text{\$/mi} \tag{8.19}$$

where
IC_L is the total investment cost of line in dollars per mile
i_L is the annual fixed charge rate applicable to line in percent

The annual equivalent energy cost due to I^2R losses in line conductors for year n can be expressed as

$$\text{AEC}_n = \frac{C_{\text{MWh}} \times \text{inf}_n}{10^6} \times I_L^2 \times \frac{R}{N_c} \times N_{ckt} \times N_p \times \frac{F_{\text{LS}}}{100} \times 8760 \ \text{\$/mi} \tag{8.20}$$

where
C_{MWh} is the cost of generating energy in dollars per megawatt
inf_n is the inflation cost factor for year n
I_L is the phase current in amperes per circuit
R is the single conductor resistance in ohms per mile
N_c is the number of conductors per phase
N_{ckt} is the number of circuits
N_p is the number of phases
F_{LS} is the loss factor in percent

The annual equivalent demand cost incurred to maintain adequate system capacity to supply the I^2R losses in the line conductors for year n can be expressed as

$$\text{ADC}_n = \frac{C_{\text{kW}} \times \inf_n}{1000} \left[1 + F_{\text{res}} \times I_L^2 \times \frac{R}{N_c} \times N_{ckt} \times N \right] \frac{i_G}{100} \; \text{\$/mi} \tag{8.21}$$

where
C_{kW} is the installed generation cost in dollars per kilowatts
F_{res} is the required generation reserve (factor) in percent
i_G is the generation fixed charge rate in percent

The *inflation cost factor* (also called *escalation cost factor*) for year n can be determined from

$$\inf_n = \left(1 + \frac{\inf}{100} \right)^{n-1} \tag{8.22}$$

where inf is inflation rate in percent. Therefore, the *present equivalent* (or *worth*) cost of the line can be expressed as

$$\text{PEC} = \sum_{i=1}^{N} \left(1 + \frac{i}{100} \right)^{-n} (\text{AIC}_n + \text{AEC}_n + \text{ADC}_n) \; \text{\$/mi} \tag{8.23}$$

where
PEC is the present equivalent cost of line in dollars per mile
N is the study period in years
i is the annual discount rate in percent

Thus, the present equivalent of revenue required is the sum of the present equivalent of levelized annual fixed charges on the total line capital investment plus annual expenses for line losses [28].

PROBLEMS

8.1 Repeat Example 8.2 using Peterson's formula.

8.2 Assume that a three-phase overhead transmission line is made up of three equilaterally spaced conductors each with an overall diameter of 2.5 cm. The equilateral spacing between conductors is 2.5 m. The 40-mi-long line is located at an altitude of 10,000 ft with an average air temperature of 20°C. If the irregularity factor of the conductors is 0.85 in each case, determine the following:
   (a) Disruptive critical rms line voltage
   (b) Visual critical rms line voltage

8.3 Consider the results of Problem 8.2 and assume that the line operates at 161 kV at 60 Hz. Determine the total fair-weather corona loss for the line using
   (a) Peek's formula
   (b) Peterson's formula

8.4 Solve Problem 8.2 assuming a conductor diameter of 1 cm.

8.5 Consider the results of Problem 8.4 and assume that the line operates at 69 kV at 60 Hz. Determine the total fair-weather corona loss for the line using Peek's formula.

8.6 Consider the results of Problem 8.4 and assume that the line operate at 69 kV at 60 Hz. Determine the total fair-weather corona loss for the line using Peterson's formula.

8.7 Determine the approximate greatest operating voltage that can be applied to a three-phase line having smooth, solid, and cylindrical conductors each 14 mm in diameter and spaced 3 m apart in equilateral configuration. Neglect conductor irregularity and assume that the electrical strength of air is 30 kV/cm.

8.8 Assume that a three-phase overhead transmission line has weathered solid cylindrical conductors of 14 mm in diameter and spaced 9 ft apart in an equilateral configuration. The regularity factor for the conductors is 0.95. Determine the maximum operating voltage at which the electrical stress at the surface of a conductor will not exceed the electrical strength of air at 30°C and 27 in. Hg.

8.9 Consider a three-phase 150 km long line with smooth and clean copper conductors having a diameter of 15 mm and spaced 4 m apart in equilateral configuration. The line-to-line operating voltage is 230 kV at 60 Hz. The barometric pressure is 73 cm Hg at –5°C. Use Peek's formula and determine the total corona losses of the line.

8.10 Consider a three-phase transmission line having stranded copper conductors 12 mm in diameter and spaced 4 m apart in equilateral configuration. The barometric pressure is 78 cm Hg at an air temperature of 29°C. Assume that the irregularity factors are 0.90, 0.72, and 0.82 for the disruptive critical voltage, local visual corona, and general visual corona, respectively. Determine the following:
(a) Disruptive critical rms line voltage
(b) The rms line voltage for local visual corona
(c) The rms line voltage for general visual corona

8.11 Solve Problem 8.9 assuming wet-weather corona.

8.12 Solve Problem 8.9 using Peterson's formula under the assumption of fair weather.

8.13 Solve Problem 8.9 using Peterson's formula under the assumption of wet weather.

8.14 Assume that a prediction of the foul-weather TVI is required for an antenna location 90 m from a three-phase 1100 kV transmission line and for a TV channel 6 signal (carrier frequency 83.25 MHz). The average foul-weather RI at the standard reference location of 15 m laterally from the outmost phase is 58 dB above 1 μV/m. If the height of the closest phase is 25 m, determine the foul-weather TVI of the line.

REFERENCES

1. Nasser, E. *Fundamentals of Gaseous Ionization and Plasma Electronics*, Wiley, New York, 1971.
2. Townsend, J. S. *Electricity in Gases*, Oxford University Press/Clarendon Press, London, U.K., 1915.
3. Trichel, G. W. The mechanism of the positive point-to-plane corona in air at atmospheric pressure, *Phys. Rev.* 55, 1939, 382.
4. Loeb, L. B. Recent developments in analysis of the mechanism of positive and negative coronas in air, *J. Appl. Phys.* 19, 1943, 882–897.
5. Loeb, L. B. *Electrical Coronas, Their Basic Physical Mechanisms*, University of California Press, Berkeley, CA, 1965.
6. Loeb, L. B. *Static Electrification*, Springer-Verlag, New York, 1958.
7. Ganger, B. *Der Elektrische Durchschlag von Gasen*, Springer-Verlag, Berlin, Germany, 1953.
8. Lichtenberg, G. C. *Novi Comment* 8, 1777, 168–169, Gottingen.
9. Nasser, E. and Loeb, L. B. Impulse streamer branching from Lichtenberg figure studies, *J. Appl. Phys.* 34, 1963, 3340.
10. Peek, F. W., Jr. *Dielectric Phenomena in High Voltage Engineering*, McGraw-Hill, New York, 1929.
11. Peterson, W. S. AIEE discussion, *Trans. Am. Inst. Electr. Eng.* (Part No. 3), 1933, 52, 62–65.
12. Carroll, J. S. and Rockwell, M. M. Empirical method of calculating corona loss from high-voltage transmission lines, *Am. Inst. Electr. Eng.* 56, 1937, 558–565.
13. Edison Electric Institute. *EHV Transmission Line Reference Book*, EEI, New York, 1968.
14. Electric Power Research Institute. *Transmission Line Reference Book: 345 kV and Above*, 2nd edn., EPRI, Palo Alto, CA, 1982.
15. Farr, H. H. *Transmission Line Design Manual*, U.S. Department of the Interior, Water and Power Resources Service, Denver, CO, 1980.

16. IEEE Standard Procedures for the Measurement of Radio Noise from Overhead Power Lines. IEEE Std. 430-1976, IEEE, New York, 1976.

17. Chartier, V. L. Interference sources, complaint statistics, and limits, IEEE Tutorial Course: Location, Correction, and Prevention of RI and TVI Sources for Overhead Power Lines, IEEE Publ. No. 76 CH1163-5-PWR, IEEE, New York, 1976.

18. Adams, G. E. The calculation of the radio interference level of high voltage transmission lines due to corona discharges, *Trans. Am. Inst. Electr. Eng.* 75 (Part No. 3), 1956, 411–419.

19. Adams, G. E. An analysis of the radio interference characteristics of bundled conductors, *Trans. Am. Inst. Electr. Eng.* 75 (Part No. 3), 1956, 1569–1583.

20. Adams, G. E. Recent radio interference investigations on high voltage transmission lines, *Proc. Power Conf.* 18, 1956, 432–448.

21. Adams, G. E. Radio interference from high voltage transmission lines as influenced by the line design, *Trans. Am. Inst. Electr. Eng.* 77 (Part No. 3), 1958, 54–63.

22. Adams, G. E. Radio interference and transmission line design, *Proc. CIGRE Conf.*, Paris, France, 1958, paper no. 305.

23. Adams, G. E. and Barthold, L. O. The calculation of attenuation constants for radio noise analysis of overhead lines, *Trans. Am. Inst. Electr. Eng.* 79 (Part No. 3), 1960, 975–981.

24. Gary, C. H. The theory of the excitation function: A demonstration of its physical meaning, *IEEE Trans. Power Apparatus Syst.* PAS-19 (1), 1972, 305–310.

25. Perry, D. E., Chartier, V. L., and Reiner, G. L. BPA 1100 kV transmission system development corona and electric field studies, *IEEE Trans. Power Appar. Syst.* PAS-98 (5), 1979, 1728–1738.

26. Juette, G. W. Evaluation of television interference from high voltage transmission lines, *IEEE Trans. Power Appar. Syst.* PAS-91 (3), 1972, 865–873.

27. Anderson, J. C. et al. Ultra high voltage power transmission, *Proc. IEEE* 59 (11), 1971, 1548–1556.

28. Electric Power Research Institute. *Transmission Line Reference Book: 115–138 kV Compact Line Design*, EPRI, Palo Alto, CA, 1978.

GENERAL REFERENCES

Bartenstein, R. and Rachel, E. A. *Die 400 kV Forschungsanlage Rheinau*, vol. 2, Koronamessung, Heidelberg, Germany, 1958.

Chartier, V. L., Taylor, E. R., and Rice, D. N. Audible noise and visual corona from EHV and EHV transmission lines and substation conductors laboratory tests, *IEEE Trans. Power Appar. Syst.* PAS-88(5), 1969, 666–679.

Coquard, A. and Gary, C. Audible noise produced by electrical power transmission lines at very high voltage, *Proc. CIGRE Conf.*, 1972, paper no. 36-03.

Grant, I. S. and Longo, V. J. Economic incentives for larger transmission conductors, *IEEE Trans. Power Appar. Syst.* PAS-100(9), 1981, 4291–4297.

IEEE Task Force Report. A guide for the measurement of audible noise from transmission lines, *IEEE Trans. Power Appar. Syst.* PAS-91(3), 1972, 853–865.

IEEE Working Group Report. CIGRE/IEEE survey on extra high voltage transmission line radio noise, *IEEE Trans. Power Appar. Syst.* PAS-92(3), 1973, 1019–1028.

Juette, G. W. and Zaffanella, L. E. Radio noise currents and audible noise on short sections of UHV bundle conductors, *IEEE Trans. Power Appar. Syst.* PAS-89, 1970, 902–908.

Juette, G. W. and Zaffanella, L. E. Radio noise, audible noise and corona loss of EHV and UHV transmission lines under rain: Predetermination based on cage tests, *IEEE Trans. Power Appar. Syst.* PAS-89, 1970, 1168–1178.

McNeely, J. K. *The Location and Elimination of Radio Interference*, vol. 30(7), Iowa State College of Agriculture and Mechanic Arts, Ames, IA, 1931.

Nelson, W. R. and Schlinger, W. R. Construction practices for the elimination and mitigation of RI and TVI sources from overhead power lines, IEEE Tutorial Course: Location, Correction, and Prevention of RI and TVI Sources from Overhead Power Lines, IEEE Publ. No. 76 CH1163-5-PWR, IEEE, New York, 1976.

Perry, D. E. An analysis of transmission line audible noise levels based upon field and three phase test line measurements, *IEEE Trans. Power Apparatus Syst.* PAS-91, 1972, 223–232.

9 Symmetrical Components and Fault Analysis

Some cause happiness wherever they go; others, whenever they go.

Oscar Wilde

9.1 INTRODUCTION

In general, it can be said that truly balanced three-phase systems exist only in theory. In reality, many systems are very nearly balanced and for practical purposes can be analyzed as if they were truly balanced systems. However, there are also emergency conditions (e.g., unsymmetrical faults, unbalanced loads, open conductors, or unsymmetrical conditions arising in rotating machines) where the degree of unbalance cannot be neglected. To protect the system against such contingencies, it is necessary to size protective devices, such as fuses and CBs, and set the protective relays. Therefore, to achieve this, currents and voltages in the system under such unbalanced operating conditions have to be known (and therefore calculated) in advance.

In 1918, Fortescue [1] proposed a method for resolving an unbalanced set of *n* related phasors into *n* sets of balanced phasors called the *symmetrical components* of the original unbalanced set. The phasors of each set are of equal magnitude and spaced 120° or 0° apart. The method is applicable to systems with any number of phases, but in this book, only three-phase systems will be discussed.

Today, the symmetrical component theory is widely used in studying unbalanced systems. Furthermore, many electrical devices have been developed and are operating based on the concept of symmetrical components. The examples include (1) the negative-sequence relay to detect system faults, (2) the positive-sequence filter to make generator voltage regulators respond to voltage changes in all three phases rather than in one phase alone, and (3) the Westinghouse-type HCB pilot wire relay using positive- and zero-sequence filters to detect faults.

9.2 SYMMETRICAL COMPONENTS

Any unbalanced three-phase system of phasors can be resolved into three balanced systems of phasors: (1) positive-sequence system, (2) negative-sequence system, and (3) zero-sequence system, as illustrated in Figure 9.1.

The *positive-sequence system* is represented by a balanced system of phasors having the same phase sequence (and therefore positive-phase rotation) as the original unbalanced system. The phasors of the positive-sequence system are equal in magnitude and displaced from each other by 120°, as shown in Figure 9.1b.

The *negative-sequence system* is represented by a balanced system of phasors having the opposite phase sequence (and therefore negative-phase rotation) to the original system. The phasors of the negative-sequence system are also equal in magnitude and displaced from each other by 120°, as shown in Figure 9.1c.

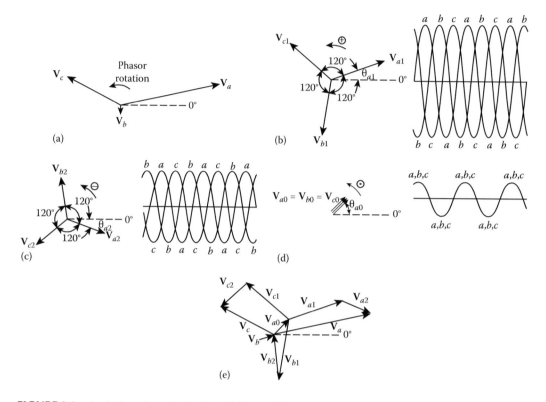

FIGURE 9.1   Analysis and synthesis of set of three unbalanced voltage phasors: (a) original system of unbalanced phasors, (b) positive-sequence components, (c) negative-sequence components, (d) zero-sequence components, (e) graphical addition of phasors to get original unbalanced phasors.

The zero-sequence system is represented by three single phasors that are equal in magnitude and angular displacements, as shown in Figure 9.1d. Note that, in the hook, the subscripts 0, 1, and 2 denote the zero sequence, positive sequence, and negative sequence, respectively. Therefore, three voltage phasors $\mathbf{V}_a$, $\mathbf{V}_b$, and $\mathbf{V}_c$ of an unbalanced set, as shown in Figure 9.1a, can be expressed in terms of their symmetrical components as the following:

$$\mathbf{V}_a = \mathbf{V}_{a1} + \mathbf{V}_{a2} + \mathbf{V}_{a0} \tag{9.1}$$

$$\mathbf{V}_b = \mathbf{V}_{b1} + \mathbf{V}_{b2} + \mathbf{V}_{b0} \tag{9.2}$$

$$\mathbf{V}_c = \mathbf{V}_{c1} + \mathbf{V}_{c2} + \mathbf{V}_{c0} \tag{9.3}$$

Figure 9.1e shows the graphical additions of the symmetrical components of Figure 9.1b through d to obtain the original three unbalanced phasors shown in Figure 9.1a.

9.3   OPERATOR a

Because of the application of the symmetrical components theory to three-phase systems, there is a need for a *unit phasor* (or *operator*) that will rotate another phasor by 120° in the counterclockwise direction (i.e., it will add 120° to the phase angle of the phasor) but leave its magnitude unchanged

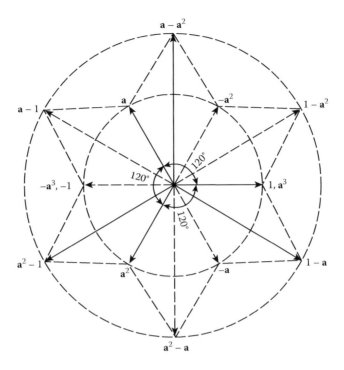

FIGURE 9.2 Phasor diagram of various powers and functions of operator **a**.

when it is multiplied by the phasor (see Figure 9.2). Such an operator is a complex number of unit magnitude with an angle of 120° and is defined by

$$\begin{aligned}
\mathbf{a} &= 1\angle 120° \\
&= 1e^{j(2\pi/3)} \\
&= 1(\cos\ 120° + j\sin\ 120°) \\
&= -0.5 + j0.866
\end{aligned}$$

where

$$j = \sqrt{-1}$$

It is clear that if operator **a** is designated as

$$\mathbf{a} = 1\angle 120°$$

then

$$\begin{aligned}
\mathbf{a}^2 &= \mathbf{a} \times \mathbf{a} \\
&= (1\angle 120°)(1\angle 120°) = 1\angle 240° = 1\angle -120°
\end{aligned}$$

$$\begin{aligned}
\mathbf{a}^3 &= \mathbf{a}^2 \times \mathbf{a} \\
&= (1\angle 240°)(1\angle 120°) = 1\angle 360° = 1\angle 0°
\end{aligned}$$

TABLE 9.1

Powers and Functions of Operator a

Power or Function	In Polar Form	In Rectangular Form
$\mathbf{a}$	$1\angle 120°$	$-0.5 + j0.866$
$\mathbf{a}^2$	$1\angle 240° = 1\angle -120°$	$-0.5 - j0.866$
$\mathbf{a}^3$	$1\angle 360° = 1\angle 0°$	$1.0 + j0.0$
$\mathbf{a}^4$	$1\angle 120°$	$-0.5 + j0.866$
$1 + \mathbf{a} = -\mathbf{a}^2$	$1\angle 60°$	$0.5 + j0.866$
$1 - \mathbf{a}$	$\sqrt{3}\angle -30°$	$1.5 - j0.866$
$1 + \mathbf{a}^2 = -\mathbf{a}$	$1\angle -60°$	$0.5 - j0.866$
$1 - \mathbf{a}^2$	$\sqrt{3}\angle 30°$	$1.5 + j0.866$
$\mathbf{a} - 1$	$\sqrt{3}\angle 150°$	$-1.5 + j0.866$
$\mathbf{a} + \mathbf{a}^2$	$1\angle 180°$	$-1.0 + j0.0$
$\mathbf{a} - \mathbf{a}^2$	$\sqrt{3}\angle 90°$	$0.0 + j1.732$
$\mathbf{a}^2 - \mathbf{a}$	$\sqrt{3}\angle -90°$	$0.0 - j1.732$
$\mathbf{a}^2 - 1$	$\sqrt{3}\angle -150°$	$-1.5 - j0.866$
$1 + \mathbf{a} + \mathbf{a}^2$	$0\angle 0°$	$0.0 + j0.0$

$$\mathbf{a}^4 = \mathbf{a}^3 \times \mathbf{a}$$
$$= (1\angle 0°)(1\angle 120°) = 1\angle 120° = \mathbf{a}$$

$$\mathbf{a}^5 = \mathbf{a}^3 \times \mathbf{a}^2$$
$$= (1\angle 0°)(1\angle 240°) = 1\angle 240° = \mathbf{a}^2$$

$$\mathbf{a}^6 = \mathbf{a}^3 \times \mathbf{a}^3$$
$$= (1\angle 0°)(1\angle 0°) = 1\angle 0° = \mathbf{a}^3$$

$$\vdots$$

$$\mathbf{a}^{n+3} = \mathbf{a}^n \times \mathbf{a}^3 = \mathbf{a}^n$$

Figure 9.2 shows a phasor diagram of the various powers and functions of the operator $\mathbf{a}$.

Various combinations of the operator $\mathbf{a}$ are given in Table 9.1. In manipulating quantities involving the operator $\mathbf{a}$, it is useful to remember that

$$1 + \mathbf{a} + \mathbf{a}^2 = 0 \tag{9.4}$$

9.4 RESOLUTION OF THREE-PHASE UNBALANCED SYSTEM OF PHASORS INTO ITS SYMMETRICAL COMPONENTS

In the application of the symmetrical component, it is customary to let the phase a be the reference phase. Therefore, using the operator $\mathbf{a}$, the symmetrical components of the positive-, negative-, and zero-sequence components can be expressed as

$$\mathbf{V}_{b1} = \mathbf{a}^2 \mathbf{V}_{a1} \tag{9.5}$$

$$\mathbf{V}_{c1} = \mathbf{a}\mathbf{V}_{a1} \tag{9.6}$$

$$\mathbf{V}_{b2} = \mathbf{a}\mathbf{V}_{a2} \tag{9.7}$$

$$\mathbf{V}_{c2} = \mathbf{a}^2\mathbf{V}_{a2} \tag{9.8}$$

$$\mathbf{V}_{b0} = \mathbf{V}_{c0} = \mathbf{V}_{a0} \tag{9.9}$$

Substituting the previous equations into Equations 9.2 and 9.3, as appropriate, the phase voltages can be expressed in terms of the sequence voltages as

$$\mathbf{V}_a = \mathbf{V}_{a1} + \mathbf{V}_{a2} + \mathbf{V}_{a0} \tag{9.10}$$

$$\mathbf{V}_b = \mathbf{a}^2\mathbf{V}_{a1} + \mathbf{a}\mathbf{V}_{a2} + \mathbf{V}_{a0} \tag{9.11}$$

$$\mathbf{V}_c = \mathbf{a}\mathbf{V}_{a1} + \mathbf{a}^2\mathbf{V}_{a2} + \mathbf{V}_{a0} \tag{9.12}$$

Equations 9.10 through 9.12 are known as the *synthesis equations*. Therefore, it can be shown that the sequence voltages can be expressed in terms of phase voltages as

$$\mathbf{V}_{a0} = \frac{1}{3}\left(\mathbf{V}_a + \mathbf{V}_b + \mathbf{V}_c\right) \tag{9.13}$$

$$\mathbf{V}_{a1} = \frac{1}{3}\left(\mathbf{V}_a + \mathbf{a}\mathbf{V}_b + \mathbf{a}^2\mathbf{V}_c\right) \tag{9.14}$$

$$\mathbf{V}_{a2} = \frac{1}{3}\left(\mathbf{V}_a + \mathbf{a}^2\mathbf{V}_b + \mathbf{a}\mathbf{V}_c\right) \tag{9.15}$$

which are known as the *analysis equations*. Alternatively, the synthesis and analysis equations can be written, respectively, in matrix form as

$$\begin{bmatrix} \mathbf{V}_a \\ \mathbf{V}_b \\ \mathbf{V}_c \end{bmatrix} = \begin{bmatrix} 1 & 1 & 1 \\ 1 & \mathbf{a}^2 & \mathbf{a} \\ 1 & \mathbf{a} & \mathbf{a}^2 \end{bmatrix} \begin{bmatrix} \mathbf{V}_{a0} \\ \mathbf{V}_{a1} \\ \mathbf{V}_{a2} \end{bmatrix} \tag{9.16}$$

and

$$\begin{bmatrix} \mathbf{V}_{a0} \\ \mathbf{V}_{a1} \\ \mathbf{V}_{a2} \end{bmatrix} = \frac{1}{3}\begin{bmatrix} 1 & 1 & 1 \\ 1 & \mathbf{a} & \mathbf{a}^2 \\ 1 & \mathbf{a}^2 & \mathbf{a} \end{bmatrix} \begin{bmatrix} \mathbf{V}_a \\ \mathbf{V}_b \\ \mathbf{V}_c \end{bmatrix} \tag{9.17}$$

or

$$[\mathbf{V}_{abc}] = [\mathbf{A}][\mathbf{V}_{012}] \tag{9.18}$$

and

$$[\mathbf{V}_{012}] = [\mathbf{A}]^{-1}[\mathbf{V}_{abc}] \tag{9.19}$$

where

$$[\mathbf{A}] = \begin{bmatrix} 1 & 1 & 1 \\ 1 & \mathbf{a}^2 & \mathbf{a} \\ 1 & \mathbf{a} & \mathbf{a}^2 \end{bmatrix} \tag{9.20}$$

$$[\mathbf{A}]^{-1} = \frac{1}{3} \begin{bmatrix} 1 & 1 & 1 \\ 1 & \mathbf{a} & \mathbf{a}^2 \\ 1 & \mathbf{a}^2 & \mathbf{a} \end{bmatrix} \tag{9.21}$$

$$[\mathbf{V}_{abc}] = \begin{bmatrix} \mathbf{V}_a \\ \mathbf{V}_b \\ \mathbf{V}_c \end{bmatrix} \tag{9.22}$$

$$[\mathbf{V}_{012}] = \begin{bmatrix} \mathbf{V}_{a0} \\ \mathbf{V}_{a1} \\ \mathbf{V}_{a2} \end{bmatrix} \tag{9.23}$$

The synthesis and analysis equations in terms of phase and sequence currents can be expressed as

$$\begin{bmatrix} \mathbf{I}_a \\ \mathbf{I}_b \\ \mathbf{I}_c \end{bmatrix} = \begin{bmatrix} 1 & 1 & 1 \\ 1 & \mathbf{a}^2 & \mathbf{a} \\ 1 & \mathbf{a} & \mathbf{a}^2 \end{bmatrix} \begin{bmatrix} \mathbf{I}_{a0} \\ \mathbf{I}_{a1} \\ \mathbf{I}_{a2} \end{bmatrix} \tag{9.24}$$

and

$$\begin{bmatrix} \mathbf{I}_{a0} \\ \mathbf{I}_{a1} \\ \mathbf{I}_{a2} \end{bmatrix} = \frac{1}{3} \begin{bmatrix} 1 & 1 & 1 \\ 1 & \mathbf{a} & \mathbf{a}^2 \\ 1 & \mathbf{a}^2 & \mathbf{a} \end{bmatrix} \begin{bmatrix} \mathbf{I}_a \\ \mathbf{I}_b \\ \mathbf{I}_c \end{bmatrix} \tag{9.25}$$

or

$$[\mathbf{I}_{abc}] = [\mathbf{A}][\mathbf{I}_{012}] \tag{9.26}$$

and

$$[\mathbf{I}_{012}] = [\mathbf{A}]^{-1}[\mathbf{I}_{abc}] \tag{9.27}$$

Example 9.1

Determine the symmetrical components for the phase voltages of $\mathbf{V}_a = 7.3\angle 12.5°$, $\mathbf{V}_b = 0.4\angle -100°$, and $\mathbf{V}_c = 4.4\angle 154° \ V$.

Solution

$$
\begin{aligned}
\mathbf{V}_{a0} &= \frac{1}{3}\left(\mathbf{V}_a + \mathbf{V}_b + \mathbf{V}_c\right) \\
&= \frac{1}{3}(7.3\angle 12.5° + 0.4\angle -100° + 4.4\angle 154°) \\
&= 1.47\angle 45.1° \ V
\end{aligned}
$$

$$
\begin{aligned}
\mathbf{V}_{a1} &= \frac{1}{3}\left(\mathbf{V}_a + \mathbf{a}\mathbf{V}_b + \mathbf{a}^2\mathbf{V}_c\right) \\
&= \frac{1}{3}\left[7.3\angle 12.5° + (1\angle 120°)(0.4\angle -100°) + (1\angle 240°)(4.4\angle 154°)\right] \\
&= 3.97\angle 20.5° \ V
\end{aligned}
$$

$$
\begin{aligned}
\mathbf{V}_{a2} &= \frac{1}{3}\left(\mathbf{V}_a + \mathbf{a}^2\mathbf{V}_b + \mathbf{a}\mathbf{V}_c\right) \\
&= \frac{1}{3}\left[7.3\angle 12.5° + (1\angle 240°)(0.4\angle -100°) + (1\angle 20°)(4.4\angle 154°)\right] \\
&= 2.52\angle -19.7° \ V
\end{aligned}
$$

$$
\mathbf{V}_{b0} = \mathbf{V}_{a0} = 1.47\angle 45.1° \ V
$$

$$
\mathbf{V}_{b1} = \mathbf{a}^2\mathbf{V}_{a1} = (1\angle 240°)(3.97\angle 20.5°) = 3.97\angle 260.5° \ V
$$

$$
\mathbf{V}_{b2} = \mathbf{a}\mathbf{V}_{a2} = (1\angle 120°)(2.52\angle -19.7°) = 2.52\angle 100.3° \ V
$$

$$
\mathbf{V}_{c0} = \mathbf{V}_{a0} = 1.47\angle 45.1° \ V
$$

$$
\mathbf{V}_{c1} = \mathbf{a}\mathbf{V}_{a1} = (1\angle 120°)(3.97\angle 20.5°) = 3.97\angle 140.5° \ V
$$

$$
\mathbf{V}_{c2} = \mathbf{a}^2\mathbf{V}_{a2} = (1\angle 240°)(2.52\angle -19.7°) = 2.52\angle 220.3° \ V
$$

Note that the resulting values for the symmetrical components can be checked numerically (e.g., using Equation 9.11) or graphically, as shown in Figure 9.1e.

9.5 POWER IN SYMMETRICAL COMPONENTS

The three-phase complex power at any point of a three-phase system can be expressed as the sum of the individual complex powers of each phase so that

$$
\begin{aligned}
\mathbf{S}_{3\phi} &= P_{3\phi} + jQ_{3\phi} \\
&= \mathbf{S}_a + \mathbf{S}_b + \mathbf{S}_c \\
&= \mathbf{V}_a\mathbf{I}_a^* + \mathbf{V}_b\mathbf{I}_b^* + \mathbf{V}_c\mathbf{I}_c^*
\end{aligned}
\tag{9.28}
$$

or, in matrix notation,

$$\mathbf{S}_{3\phi} = \begin{bmatrix} \mathbf{V}_a & \mathbf{V}_b & \mathbf{V}_c \end{bmatrix} \begin{bmatrix} \mathbf{I}_a \\ \mathbf{I}_b \\ \mathbf{I}_c \end{bmatrix}^* = \begin{bmatrix} \mathbf{V}_a \\ \mathbf{V}_b \\ \mathbf{V}_c \end{bmatrix}^t \begin{bmatrix} \mathbf{I}_a \\ \mathbf{I}_b \\ \mathbf{I}_c \end{bmatrix}^* \tag{9.29}$$

or

$$\mathbf{S}_{3\phi} = \begin{bmatrix} \mathbf{V}_{abc} \end{bmatrix}^t \begin{bmatrix} \mathbf{I}_{abc} \end{bmatrix}^* \tag{9.30}$$

where

$$\begin{bmatrix} \mathbf{V}_{abc} \end{bmatrix} = \begin{bmatrix} \mathbf{A} \end{bmatrix} \begin{bmatrix} \mathbf{V}_{012} \end{bmatrix}$$

$$\begin{bmatrix} \mathbf{I}_{abc} \end{bmatrix} = \begin{bmatrix} \mathbf{A} \end{bmatrix} \begin{bmatrix} \mathbf{I}_{012} \end{bmatrix}$$

and therefore,

$$\begin{bmatrix} \mathbf{V}_{abc} \end{bmatrix}^t = \begin{bmatrix} \mathbf{V}_{012} \end{bmatrix}^t \begin{bmatrix} \mathbf{A} \end{bmatrix}^t \tag{9.31}$$

$$\begin{bmatrix} \mathbf{I}_{abc} \end{bmatrix}^* = \begin{bmatrix} \mathbf{A} \end{bmatrix}^* \begin{bmatrix} \mathbf{I}_{012} \end{bmatrix}^* \tag{9.32}$$

Substituting Equations 9.31 and 9.32 into Equation 9.30,

$$\mathbf{S}_{3\phi} = \begin{bmatrix} \mathbf{V}_{012} \end{bmatrix}^t \begin{bmatrix} \mathbf{A} \end{bmatrix}^t \begin{bmatrix} \mathbf{A} \end{bmatrix}^* \begin{bmatrix} \mathbf{I}_{012} \end{bmatrix}^* \tag{9.33}$$

where

$$\begin{bmatrix} \mathbf{A} \end{bmatrix}^t \begin{bmatrix} \mathbf{A} \end{bmatrix}^* = \begin{bmatrix} 1 & 1 & 1 \\ 1 & \mathbf{a}^2 & \mathbf{a} \\ 1 & \mathbf{a} & \mathbf{a}^2 \end{bmatrix} \begin{bmatrix} 1 & 1 & 1 \\ 1 & \mathbf{a} & \mathbf{a}^2 \\ 1 & \mathbf{a}^2 & \mathbf{a} \end{bmatrix} = \begin{bmatrix} 3 & 0 & 0 \\ 0 & 3 & 0 \\ 0 & 0 & 3 \end{bmatrix} = 3 \begin{bmatrix} 1 & 0 & 0 \\ 0 & 1 & 0 \\ 0 & 0 & 1 \end{bmatrix}$$

Therefore,

$$\mathbf{S}_{3\phi} = 3 \begin{bmatrix} \mathbf{V}_{012} \end{bmatrix}^t \begin{bmatrix} \mathbf{I}_{012} \end{bmatrix}^* = 3 \begin{bmatrix} \mathbf{V}_{a0} & \mathbf{V}_{a1} & \mathbf{V}_{a2} \end{bmatrix} \begin{bmatrix} \mathbf{I}_{a0} \\ \mathbf{I}_{a1} \\ \mathbf{I}_{a2} \end{bmatrix}^* \tag{9.34a}$$

or

$$\mathbf{S}_{3\phi} = 3 \begin{bmatrix} \mathbf{V}_{a0}\mathbf{I}_{a0}^* + \mathbf{V}_{a1}\mathbf{I}_{a1}^* + \mathbf{V}_{a2}\mathbf{I}_{a2}^* \end{bmatrix} \tag{9.34b}$$

Note that there are no cross terms (e.g., $\mathbf{V}_{a0}\mathbf{I}_{a1}^*$ or $\mathbf{V}_{a1}\mathbf{I}_{a0}^*$) in this equation, which indicates that there is no coupling of power among the three sequences. Also note that the symmetrical components of voltage and current belong to the same phase.

Example 9.2

Assume that the phase voltages and currents of a three-phase system are given as

$$\left[\mathbf{V}_{abc}\right] = \begin{bmatrix} 0 \\ 50 \\ -50 \end{bmatrix} \quad \text{and} \quad \left[\mathbf{I}_{abc}\right] = \begin{bmatrix} -5 \\ j5 \\ -5 \end{bmatrix}$$

and determine the following:

(a) Three-phase complex power using Equation 9.30
(b) Sequence voltage and current matrices, that is, $[\mathbf{V}_{012}]$ and $[\mathbf{I}_{012}]$
(c) Three-phase complex power using Equation 9.34

Solution

(a)

$$\mathbf{S}_{3\phi} = \left[\mathbf{V}_{abc}\right]^t \left[\mathbf{I}_{abc}\right]^*$$

$$= \begin{bmatrix} 0 & 50 & -50 \end{bmatrix} \begin{bmatrix} -5 \\ -j5 \\ -5 \end{bmatrix} = 250 - j250 = 353.5534\angle -45°\ \text{VA}$$

(b)

$$\left[\mathbf{V}_{012}\right] = \left[\mathbf{A}\right]^{-1}\left[\mathbf{V}_{abc}\right]$$

$$= \frac{1}{3}\begin{bmatrix} 1 & 1 & 1 \\ 1 & \mathbf{a} & \mathbf{a}^2 \\ 1 & \mathbf{a}^2 & \mathbf{a} \end{bmatrix}\begin{bmatrix} 0 \\ 50 \\ -50 \end{bmatrix} = \begin{bmatrix} 0.0\angle 0° \\ 28.8675\angle 90° \\ 28.8675\angle -90° \end{bmatrix}\ \text{V}$$

$$\left[\mathbf{I}_{012}\right] = \left[\mathbf{A}\right]^{-1}\left[\mathbf{I}_{abc}\right]$$

$$= \frac{1}{3}\begin{bmatrix} 1 & 1 & 1 \\ 1 & \mathbf{a} & \mathbf{a}^2 \\ 1 & \mathbf{a}^2 & \mathbf{a} \end{bmatrix}\begin{bmatrix} -5 \\ j5 \\ -5 \end{bmatrix} = \begin{bmatrix} 3.7268\angle 153.4° \\ 2.3570\angle 165° \\ 2.3570\angle -75° \end{bmatrix}$$

(c)

$$\mathbf{S}_{3\phi} = 3\left[\mathbf{V}_{a0}\mathbf{I}_{a0}^* + \mathbf{V}_{a1}\mathbf{I}_{a1}^* + \mathbf{V}_{a2}\mathbf{I}_{a2}^*\right] = 353.5534\angle -45°\ \text{VA}$$

9.6 SEQUENCE IMPEDANCES OF TRANSMISSION LINES

9.6.1 Sequence Impedances of Untransposed Lines

Figure 9.3a shows a circuit representation of an untransposed transmission line with unequal self-impedances and unequal mutual impedances. Here,

$$[\mathbf{V}_{abc}] = [\mathbf{Z}_{abc}][\mathbf{I}_{abc}] \tag{9.35}$$

where

$$\left[\mathbf{Z}_{abc}\right] = \begin{bmatrix} \mathbf{Z}_{aa} & \mathbf{Z}_{ab} & \mathbf{Z}_{ac} \\ \mathbf{Z}_{ba} & \mathbf{Z}_{bb} & \mathbf{Z}_{bc} \\ \mathbf{Z}_{ca} & \mathbf{Z}_{cb} & \mathbf{Z}_{cc} \end{bmatrix} \tag{9.36}$$

in which the self- and mutual impedances in general are

$$\mathbf{Z}_{aa} \neq \mathbf{Z}_{bb} \neq \mathbf{Z}_{cc}$$

$$\mathbf{Z}_{ab} \neq \mathbf{Z}_{bc} \neq \mathbf{Z}_{ca}$$

Multiplying both sides of Equation 9.35 by $\left[\mathbf{A}\right]^{-1}$ and also substituting Equation 9.26 into Equation 9.35,

$$\left[\mathbf{A}\right]^{-1}\left[\mathbf{V}_{abc}\right] = \left[\mathbf{A}\right]^{-1}\left[\mathbf{Z}_{abc}\right]\left[\mathbf{A}\right]\left[\mathbf{I}_{012}\right] \tag{9.37}$$

where the similarity transformation is defined as

$$\left[\mathbf{Z}_{012}\right] \triangleq \left[\mathbf{A}\right]^{-1}\left[\mathbf{Z}_{abc}\right]\left[\mathbf{A}\right] \tag{9.38}$$

Therefore, the sequence impedance matrix of an untransposed transmission line can be calculated using Equation 9.38 and can be expressed as

$$\left[\mathbf{Z}_{012}\right] = \begin{bmatrix} \mathbf{Z}_{00} & \mathbf{Z}_{01} & \mathbf{Z}_{02} \\ \mathbf{Z}_{10} & \mathbf{Z}_{11} & \mathbf{Z}_{12} \\ \mathbf{Z}_{20} & \mathbf{Z}_{21} & \mathbf{Z}_{22} \end{bmatrix} \tag{9.39}$$

or

$$\left[\mathbf{Z}_{012}\right] = \begin{bmatrix} \left(\mathbf{Z}_{s0} + 2\mathbf{Z}_{m0}\right) & \left(\mathbf{Z}_{s2} - \mathbf{Z}_{m2}\right) & \left(\mathbf{Z}_{s1} - \mathbf{Z}_{m1}\right) \\ \left(\mathbf{Z}_{s1} - \mathbf{Z}_{m1}\right) & \left(\mathbf{Z}_{s0} - \mathbf{Z}_{m0}\right) & \left(\mathbf{Z}_{s2} + 2\mathbf{Z}_{m2}\right) \\ \left(\mathbf{Z}_{s2} - \mathbf{Z}_{m2}\right) & \left(\mathbf{Z}_{s1} + 2\mathbf{Z}_{m1}\right) & \left(\mathbf{Z}_{s0} - \mathbf{Z}_{m0}\right) \end{bmatrix} \tag{9.40}$$

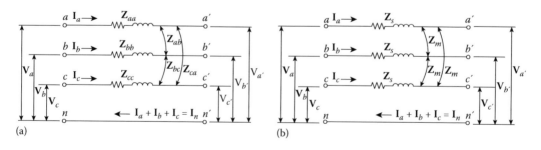

FIGURE 9.3 Transmission line circuit diagrams: (a) with unequal series and unequal impedances; (b) with equal series and equal mutual impedances.

where, by definition,

$$\mathbf{Z}_{s0} = \text{zero-sequence self-impedance}$$

$$\triangleq \frac{1}{3}\left(\mathbf{Z}_{aa} + \mathbf{Z}_{bb} + \mathbf{Z}_{cc}\right) \tag{9.41}$$

$$\mathbf{Z}_{s1} = \text{positive-sequence self-impedance}$$

$$\triangleq \frac{1}{3}\left(\mathbf{Z}_{aa} + \mathbf{a}\mathbf{Z}_{bb} + \mathbf{a}^2\mathbf{Z}_{cc}\right) \tag{9.42}$$

$$\mathbf{Z}_{s2} = \text{negative-sequence self-impedance}$$

$$\triangleq \frac{1}{3}\left(\mathbf{Z}_{aa} + \mathbf{a}^2\mathbf{Z}_{bb} + \mathbf{a}\mathbf{Z}_{cc}\right) \tag{9.43}$$

$$\mathbf{Z}_{m0} = \text{zero-sequence mutual impedance}$$

$$\triangleq \frac{1}{3}\left(\mathbf{Z}_{bc} + \mathbf{Z}_{ca} + \mathbf{Z}_{ab}\right) \tag{9.44}$$

$$\mathbf{Z}_{m1} = \text{positive-sequence mutual impedance}$$

$$\triangleq \frac{1}{3}\left(\mathbf{Z}_{bc} + \mathbf{a}\mathbf{Z}_{ca} + \mathbf{a}^2\mathbf{Z}_{ab}\right) \tag{9.45}$$

$$\mathbf{Z}_{m2} = \text{negative-sequence mutual impedance}$$

$$\triangleq \frac{1}{3}\left(\mathbf{Z}_{bc} + \mathbf{a}^2\mathbf{Z}_{ca} + \mathbf{a}\mathbf{Z}_{ab}\right) \tag{9.46}$$

Therefore,

$$\left[\mathbf{V}_{012}\right] = \left[\mathbf{Z}_{012}\right]\left[\mathbf{I}_{012}\right] \tag{9.47}$$

Note that the matrix in Equation 9.40 is not a symmetrical matrix, and therefore, the application of Equation 9.47 will show that there is a mutual coupling among the three sequences, which is not a desirable result.

9.6.2 SEQUENCE IMPEDANCES OF TRANSPOSED LINES

The remedy is either to completely transpose the line or to place the conductors with equilateral spacing among them so that the resulting mutual impedances* are equal to each other, that is, $\mathbf{Z}_{ab} = \mathbf{Z}_{bc} = \mathbf{Z}_{ca} = \mathbf{Z}_m$, as shown in Figure 9.3b. Furthermore, if the self-impedances of conductors are equal to each other, that is, $\mathbf{Z}_{aa} = \mathbf{Z}_{bb} = \mathbf{Z}_{cc} = \mathbf{Z}_s$, Equation 9.36 can be expressed as

$$\left[\mathbf{Z}_{abc}\right] = \begin{bmatrix} \mathbf{Z}_s & \mathbf{Z}_m & \mathbf{Z}_m \\ \mathbf{Z}_m & \mathbf{Z}_s & \mathbf{Z}_m \\ \mathbf{Z}_m & \mathbf{Z}_m & \mathbf{Z}_s \end{bmatrix} \tag{9.48}$$

---

* In passive networks $\mathbf{Z}_{ab} = \mathbf{Z}_{ba}$, $\mathbf{Z}_{bc} = \mathbf{Z}_{cb}$, etc.

where

$$\mathbf{Z}_s = \left[(r_a + r_e) + j0.1213 \ \ln\frac{D_e}{D_s} \right] l \quad \Omega \tag{9.49}$$

$$\mathbf{Z}_m = \left[r_e + j0.1213 \ \ln\frac{D_e}{D_{eq}} \right] l \quad \Omega \tag{9.50}$$

$$D_{eq} \triangleq D_m = \left(D_{ab} \times D_{bc} \times D_{ca} \right)^{1/3}$$

r_a is the resistance of a single conductor a per-unit length.

The r_e is the resistance of Carson's [2] equivalent (and fictitious) earth return conductor. It is a function of frequency and can be expressed as

$$r_e = 1.588 \times 10^{-3} f \quad \Omega/\text{mi} \tag{9.51}$$

or

$$r_e = 9.869 \times 10^{-4} f \quad \Omega/\text{km} \tag{9.52}$$

At 60 Hz, $r_e = 0.09528$ Ω/mi. The quantity D_e is a function of both the earth resistivity ρ and the frequency f and can be expressed as

$$D_e = 2160 \left(\frac{\rho}{f} \right)^{1/2} \text{ ft} \tag{9.53}$$

where ρ is the earth resistivity and is given in Table 9.2 for various earth types. If the actual earth resistivity is unknown, it is customary to use an average value of 100 Ω/m for ρ. Therefore, at 60 Hz, $D_e = 2788.55$ ft. The D_s is the GMR of the phase conductor as before. Therefore, by applying Equation 9.38,

$$\left[\mathbf{Z}_{012} \right] = \begin{bmatrix} (\mathbf{Z}_s + 2\mathbf{Z}_m) & 0 & 0 \\ 0 & (\mathbf{Z}_s - \mathbf{Z}_m) & 0 \\ 0 & 0 & (\mathbf{Z}_s - \mathbf{Z}_m) \end{bmatrix} \tag{9.54}$$

TABLE 9.2
Resistivity of Different Soils

Ground Type (Ω/m)	Resistivity, ρ
Seawater	0.01–1.0
Wet organic soil	10
Moist soil (average earth)	100
Dry soil	1000
Bedrock	10^4
Pure slate	10^7
Sandstone	10^9
Crushed rock	1.5×10^8

where, by definition,

$$\mathbf{Z}_0 = \text{zero-sequence impedance at 60 Hz}$$

$$\triangleq \mathbf{Z}_{00} = \mathbf{Z}_s + 2\mathbf{Z}_m \tag{9.55a}$$

$$= \left[\left(r_a + 3r_e\right) + j0.1213 \ \ln\frac{D_e^3}{D_s \times D_{eq}^2}\right] l \quad \Omega \tag{9.55b}$$

$$\mathbf{Z}_1 = \text{positive-sequence impedance at 60 Hz}$$

$$\triangleq \mathbf{Z}_{11} = \mathbf{Z}_s - \mathbf{Z}_m \tag{9.56a}$$

$$= \left[r_a + j0.1213 \ \ln\frac{D_{eq}}{D_s}\right] l \quad \Omega \tag{9.56b}$$

$$\mathbf{Z}_2 = \text{negative-sequence impedance at 60 Hz}$$

$$\triangleq \mathbf{Z}_{22} = \mathbf{Z}_s - \mathbf{Z}_m \tag{9.57a}$$

$$= \left[r_a + j0.1213 \ \ln\frac{D_{eq}}{D_s}\right] l \quad \Omega \tag{9.57b}$$

Thus, Equation 9.54 can be expressed* as

$$\left[\mathbf{Z}_{012}\right] = \begin{bmatrix} \mathbf{Z}_0 & 0 & 0 \\ 0 & \mathbf{Z}_1 & 0 \\ 0 & 0 & \mathbf{Z}_2 \end{bmatrix} \tag{9.58}$$

---

* Equations 9.55 and 9.57 can easily be modified so that they can give approximate sequence impedances at other frequencies. For example, their expressions at 50 Hz are given as

$$\mathbf{Z}_0 = \text{zero-sequence impedance at 50 Hz}$$

$$\triangleq \mathbf{Z}_{00} = \mathbf{Z}_s + 2\mathbf{Z}_m$$

$$= \left[\left(r_a + 3r_e\right) + j0.1213\left(\frac{50\ \text{Hz}}{60\ \text{Hz}}\right)\ln\frac{D_e^3}{D_s \times D_{eq}^2}\right] l\ \Omega$$

$$= \left[\left(r_a + 3r_e\right) + j0.10108 \ \ln\frac{D_e^3}{D_s \times D_{eq}^2}\right] l\ \Omega$$

$$\mathbf{Z}_1 = \text{positive-sequence impedance at 50 Hz}$$

$$\triangleq \mathbf{Z}_{11} = \mathbf{Z}_s - \mathbf{Z}_m$$

$$= \left[r_a + j0.10108 \ \ln\frac{D_{eq}}{D_s}\right] l\ \Omega$$

$$\mathbf{Z}_2 = \text{negative-sequence impedance at 50 Hz}$$

$$\triangleq \mathbf{Z}_{22} = \mathbf{Z}_s - \mathbf{Z}_m$$

$$= \left[r_a + j0.10108 \ \ln\frac{D_{eq}}{D_s}\right] l\ \Omega$$

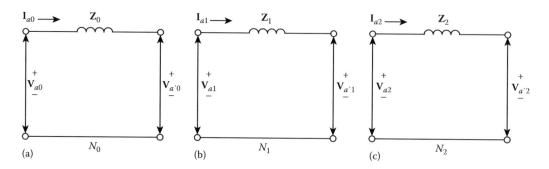

FIGURE 9.4 Sequence networks of a transmission line: (a) zero-sequence network, (b) positive-sequence network, (c) negative-sequence network.

Both Equations 9.54 and 9.58 indicate that there is no mutual coupling among the three sequences, which is the desirable result. Therefore, the zero-, positive-, and negative-sequence currents cause voltage drops only in the zero-, positive-, and negative-sequence networks, respectively, of the transmission line. Also note in Equation 9.54 that the positive- and negative-sequence impedances of the transmission line are equal to each other, but they are far less than the zero-sequence impedance of the line. Figure 9.4 shows the sequence networks of a transmission line.

9.6.3 ELECTROMAGNETIC UNBALANCES DUE TO UNTRANSPOSED LINES

If neither the line is transposed nor its conductors equilaterally spaced, Equation 9.48 cannot be used. Instead, use the following equation:

$$\left[\mathbf{Z}_{abc}\right] = \begin{bmatrix} \mathbf{Z}_{aa} & \mathbf{Z}_{ab} & \mathbf{Z}_{ac} \\ \mathbf{Z}_{ba} & \mathbf{Z}_{bb} & \mathbf{Z}_{bc} \\ \mathbf{Z}_{ca} & \mathbf{Z}_{cb} & \mathbf{Z}_{cc} \end{bmatrix} \tag{9.59}$$

where

$$\mathbf{Z}_{aa} = \mathbf{Z}_{bb} = \mathbf{Z}_{cc} = \left[\left(r_a + r_e\right) + j0.1213 \ \ln \frac{D_e}{D_s} \right] l \tag{9.60}$$

$$\mathbf{Z}_{ab} = \mathbf{Z}_{ba} = \left[r_e + j0.1213 \ \ln \frac{D_e}{D_{ab}} \right] l \tag{9.61}$$

$$\mathbf{Z}_{ac} = \mathbf{Z}_{ca} = \left[r_e + j0.1213 \ \ln \frac{D_e}{D_{ac}} \right] l \tag{9.62}$$

$$\mathbf{Z}_{bc} = \mathbf{Z}_{cb} = \left[r_e + j0.1213 \ \ln \frac{D_e}{D_{bc}} \right] l \tag{9.63}$$

The corresponding sequence impedance matrix can be found from Equation 9.38 as before. Therefore, the associated sequence admittance matrix can be found as

$$\left[\mathbf{Y}_{012}\right] = \left[\mathbf{Z}_{012}\right]^{-1} \tag{9.64a}$$

$$= \begin{bmatrix} \mathbf{Y}_{00} & \mathbf{Y}_{01} & \mathbf{Y}_{02} \\ \mathbf{Y}_{10} & \mathbf{Y}_{11} & \mathbf{Y}_{12} \\ \mathbf{Y}_{20} & \mathbf{Y}_{21} & \mathbf{Y}_{22} \end{bmatrix} \tag{9.64b}$$

Therefore,

$$\left[\mathbf{I}_{012}\right] = \left[\mathbf{Y}_{012}\right]\left[\mathbf{V}_{012}\right] \tag{9.65}$$

Since neither the line is transposed nor its conductors equilaterally spaced, there is an electromagnetic unbalance in the system. Such unbalance is determined from Equation 9.65 with only positive-sequence voltage applied. Therefore,

$$\begin{bmatrix} \mathbf{I}_{a0} \\ \mathbf{I}_{a1} \\ \mathbf{I}_{a2} \end{bmatrix} = \begin{bmatrix} \mathbf{Y}_{00} & \mathbf{Y}_{01} & \mathbf{Y}_{02} \\ \mathbf{Y}_{10} & \mathbf{Y}_{11} & \mathbf{Y}_{12} \\ \mathbf{Y}_{20} & \mathbf{Y}_{21} & \mathbf{Y}_{22} \end{bmatrix} \begin{bmatrix} 0 \\ \mathbf{V}_{a1} \\ 0 \end{bmatrix} \tag{9.66a}$$

$$= \begin{bmatrix} \mathbf{Y}_{01} \\ \mathbf{Y}_{11} \\ \mathbf{Y}_{21} \end{bmatrix} \mathbf{V}_{a1} \tag{9.66b}$$

According to Gross and Hesse [3], the per-unit unbalances for zero sequence and negative sequence can be expressed, respectively, as

$$\mathbf{m}_0 \triangleq \frac{\mathbf{I}_{a0}}{\mathbf{I}_{a1}} \, \text{pu} \tag{9.67a}$$

$$= \frac{\mathbf{Y}_{01}}{\mathbf{Y}_{11}} \, \text{pu} \tag{9.67b}$$

and

$$\mathbf{m}_2 \triangleq \frac{\mathbf{I}_{a2}}{\mathbf{I}_{a1}} \, \text{pu} \tag{9.68a}$$

$$= \frac{\mathbf{Y}_{21}}{\mathbf{Y}_{11}} \, \text{pu} \tag{9.68b}$$

Since, in physical systems [33],

$$\mathbf{Z}_{22} \gg \mathbf{Z}_{02} \quad \text{or} \quad \mathbf{Z}_{21}$$

and

$$\mathbf{Z}_{00} \gg \mathbf{Z}_{20} \quad \text{or} \quad \mathbf{Z}_{01}$$

the approximate values of the per-unit unbalances for zero and negative sequences can be expressed, respectively, as

$$\mathbf{m}_0 \cong -\frac{\mathbf{Z}_{01}}{\mathbf{Z}_{00}} \text{ pu} \tag{9.69a}$$

and

$$\mathbf{m}_2 \cong -\frac{\mathbf{Z}_{21}}{\mathbf{Z}_{22}} \text{ pu} \tag{9.69b}$$

Example 9.3

Consider the compact-line configuration shown in Figure 9.5. The phase conductors used are made up of 500 kcmil, 30/7 stand ACSR. The line length is 40 mi and the line is not transposed. Ignore the OH ground wire. If the earth has an average resistivity, determine the following:

(a) Line impedance matrix
(b) Sequence impedance matrix of line

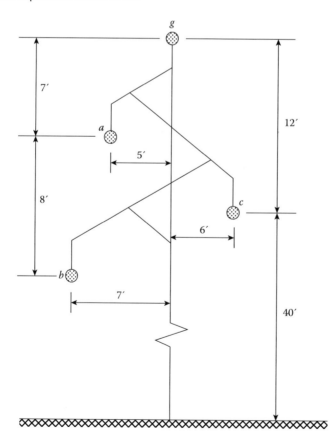

FIGURE 9.5 Compact-line configuration for Example 9.3.

Solution

(a) The conductor parameters can be found from Table A.3 as

$$r_a = r_b = r_c = 0.206 \ \Omega/\text{mi}$$

$$D_s = D_{sa} = D_{sb} = D_{sc} = 0.0311 \ \text{ft}$$

$$D_{ab} = (2^2 + 8^2)^{1/2} = 8.2462 \ \text{ft}$$

$$D_{bc} = (3^2 + 13^2)^{1/2} = 13.3417 \ \text{ft}$$

$$D_{ac} = (5^2 + 11^2)^{1/2} = 12.0830 \ \text{ft}$$

Since the earth has an average resistivity, $D_e = 2788.5$ ft. At 60 Hz, $r_e = 0.09528 \ \Omega/\text{mi}$. From Equation 9.60, the self-impedances of the line conductors are

$$\mathbf{Z}_{aa} = \mathbf{Z}_{bb} = \mathbf{Z}_{cc} = \left[(r_a + r_e) + j0.1213 \ \ln \frac{D_e}{D_s} \right] l$$

$$= \left[(0.206 + 0.09528) + j0.1213 \ \ln \frac{2788.5}{0.0311} \right] \times 40$$

$$= 12.0512 + j55.3495 \ \Omega$$

The mutual impedances calculated from Equations 9.61 through 9.63 are

$$\mathbf{Z}_{ab} = \mathbf{Z}_{ba} = \left[r_e + j0.1213 \ \ln \frac{D_e}{D_{ab}} \right] l$$

$$= \left[0.09528 + j0.1213 \ \ln \frac{2788.5}{8.2462} \right] \times 40$$

$$= 3.8112 + j28.2650 \ \Omega$$

$$\mathbf{Z}_{bc} = \mathbf{Z}_{cb} = \left[r_e + j0.1213 \ \ln \frac{D_e}{D_{bc}} \right] l$$

$$= \left[0.09528 + j0.1213 \ \ln \frac{2788.5}{13.3417} \right] \times 40$$

$$= 3.8112 + j25.9297 \ \Omega$$

$$\mathbf{Z}_{ac} = \mathbf{Z}_{ca} = \left[r_e + j0.1213 \ \ln \frac{D_e}{D_{ac}} \right] l$$

$$= \left[0.09528 + j0.1213 \ \ln \frac{2788.5}{12.0830} \right] \times 40$$

$$= 3.8112 + j26.4107 \ \Omega$$

Therefore,

$$[\mathbf{Z}_{abc}] = \begin{bmatrix} (12.0512 + j55.3495) & (3.8112 + j28.2650) & (3.8112 + j26.4107) \\ (3.8112 + j28.2650) & (12.0512 + j55.3495) & (3.8112 + j25.9297) \\ (3.8112 + j26.4107) & (3.8112 + j25.9297) & (12.0512 + j55.3495) \end{bmatrix}$$

(b) Thus, the sequence impedance matrix of the line can be found from Equation 9.38 as

$$[\mathbf{Z}_{012}] = [\mathbf{A}]^{-1}[\mathbf{Z}_{abc}][\mathbf{A}] = \begin{bmatrix} (19.67 + j109.09) & (0.54 + j0.47) & (-0.54 + j0.47) \\ (-0.54 + j0.47) & (8.24 + j28.48) & (-1.07 - j0.94) \\ (0.54 + j0.47) & (1.07 - j0.94) & (8.24 + j28.48) \end{bmatrix}$$

Example 9.4

Repeat Example 9.3 assuming that the line is completely transposed.

Solution

(a) From Equation 9.49,

$$\mathbf{Z}_s = \left[(r_a + r_e) + j0.1213 \ \ln\frac{D_e}{D_s} \right] l \ \Omega$$
$$= 12.0512 + j53.3495 \ \Omega \text{ as before}$$

From Equation 9.50,

$$\mathbf{Z}_m = \left[r_e + j0.1213 \ \ln\frac{D_e}{D_{eq}} \right] l \ \Omega$$

where

$$D_{eq} = (8.2462 \times 13.3417 \times 12.0830)^{1/3} = 11 \text{ ft}$$

Thus,

$$\mathbf{Z}_m = \left[0.09528 + j0.1213 \ \ln\frac{2788.5}{11} \right] \times 40$$
$$= 3.8112 + j26.8684 \ \Omega$$

Therefore,

$$[\mathbf{Z}_{abc}] = \begin{bmatrix} \mathbf{Z}_s & \mathbf{Z}_m & \mathbf{Z}_m \\ \mathbf{Z}_m & \mathbf{Z}_s & \mathbf{Z}_m \\ \mathbf{Z}_m & \mathbf{Z}_m & \mathbf{Z}_s \end{bmatrix}$$
$$= \begin{bmatrix} (12.0512 + j55.3495) & (3.8112 + j26.8684) & (3.8112 + j26.8684) \\ (3.8112 + j26.8684) & (12.0512 + j55.3495) & (3.8112 + j26.8684) \\ (3.8112 + j26.8684) & (3.8112 + j26.8684) & (12.0512 + j55.3495) \end{bmatrix}$$

(b) From Equation 9.54,

$$[\mathbf{Z}_{012}] = \begin{bmatrix} (\mathbf{Z}_s + 2\mathbf{Z}_m) & 0 & 0 \\ 0 & (\mathbf{Z}_s - \mathbf{Z}_m) & 0 \\ 0 & 0 & (\mathbf{Z}_s - \mathbf{Z}_m) \end{bmatrix}$$

$$= \begin{bmatrix} 19.6736 + j109.086 & 0 & 0 \\ 0 & 8.2400 + j28.4811 & 0 \\ 0 & 0 & 8.2400 + j28.4811 \end{bmatrix}$$

or by substituting Equations 9.55b and 9.56b into Equation 9.58,

$$[\mathbf{Z}_{012}] = \begin{bmatrix} 19.6736 + j109.086 & 0 & 0 \\ 0 & 8.2400 + j28.4811 & 0 \\ 0 & 0 & 8.2400 + j28.4811 \end{bmatrix}$$

Example 9.5

Consider the results of Example 9.3 and determine the following:

(a) Per-unit electromagnetic unbalance for zero sequence
(b) Approximate value of per-unit electromagnetic unbalance for zero sequence
(c) Per-unit electromagnetic unbalance for negative sequence
(d) Approximate value of per-unit electromagnetic unbalance for negative sequence

Solution

The sequence admittance of the line can be found as

$$[\mathbf{Y}_{012}] = [\mathbf{Z}_{012}]^{-1}$$

$$= \begin{bmatrix} (1.60\times10^{-3} - j8.88\times10^{-3}) & (7.57\times10^{-5} + j1.93\times10^{-4}) & (-2.01\times10^{-4} + j6.15\times10^{-5}) \\ (-2.01\times10^{-4} + j6.15\times10^{-5}) & (9.44\times10^{-3} - j3.25\times10^{-2}) & (-4.55\times10^{-4} - j1.55\times10^{-3}) \\ (7.57\times10^{-5} + j1.93\times10^{-4}) & (1.60\times10^{-3} - j2.54\times10^{-4}) & (9.44\times10^{-3} - j3.25\times10^{-2}) \end{bmatrix}$$

(a) From Equation 9.67b,

$$\mathbf{m}_0 = \frac{\mathbf{Y}_{01}}{\mathbf{Y}_{11}} = \frac{7.57\times10^{-5} + j1.93\times10^{-4}}{9.44\times10^{-3} - j3.25\times10^{-2}} = 0.61\angle142.4°$$

(b) From Equation 9.69a,

$$\mathbf{m}_0 \cong -\frac{\mathbf{Z}_{01}}{\mathbf{Z}_{11}} = -\frac{0.54 + j0.47}{19.67 + j109.09} = 0.64\angle141.3°$$

(c) From Equation 9.68b,

$$\mathbf{m}_2 = \frac{\mathbf{Y}_{21}}{\mathbf{Y}_{11}} = \frac{1.60 \times 10^{-3} - j2.54 \times 10^{-4}}{9.44 \times 10^{-3} - j3.25 \times 10^{-2}} = 4.79 \angle 64.8°$$

(d) From Equation 9.69b,

$$\mathbf{m}_2 \cong -\frac{\mathbf{Z}_{21}}{\mathbf{Z}22} = \frac{1.07 - j0.94}{8.24 + j28.48} = 4.8 \angle 64.8°$$

9.6.4 Sequence Impedances of Untransposed Line with Overhead Ground Wire

Assume that the untransposed line shown in Figure 9.5 is *shielded* against direct lightning strikes by the OH ground wire u (used instead of g).

Therefore,

$$\left[\mathbf{V}_{abcu} \right] = \left[\mathbf{Z}_{abcu} \right]\left[\mathbf{I}_{abcu} \right] \tag{9.70}$$

but since for the ground wire $\mathbf{V}_u = 0$,

$$\begin{bmatrix} \mathbf{V}_a \\ \mathbf{V}_b \\ \mathbf{V}_c \\ 0 \end{bmatrix} = \begin{bmatrix} \mathbf{Z}_{aa} & \mathbf{Z}_{ab} & \mathbf{Z}_{ac} & \mathbf{Z}_{au} \\ \mathbf{Z}_{ba} & \mathbf{Z}_{bb} & \mathbf{Z}_{bc} & \mathbf{Z}_{bu} \\ \mathbf{Z}_{ca} & \mathbf{Z}_{cb} & \mathbf{Z}_{cc} & \mathbf{Z}_{cu} \\ \mathbf{Z}_{ua} & \mathbf{Z}_{ub} & \mathbf{Z}_{uc} & \mathbf{Z}_{uu} \end{bmatrix} \begin{bmatrix} \mathbf{I}_a \\ \mathbf{I}_b \\ \mathbf{I}_c \\ \mathbf{I}_u \end{bmatrix} \tag{9.71}$$

The matrix $\left[\mathbf{Z}_{abcu} \right]$ can be determined using Equations 9.59 through 9.63, as before, and also using the following equations:

$$\mathbf{Z}_{au} = \mathbf{Z}_{ua} = \left[r_e + j0.1213 \; \ln \frac{D_e}{D_{au}} \right] l \tag{9.72}$$

$$\mathbf{Z}_{bu} = \mathbf{Z}_{ub} = \left[r_e + j0.1213 \; \ln \frac{D_e}{D_{bu}} \right] l \tag{9.73}$$

$$\mathbf{Z}_{cu} = \mathbf{Z}_{uc} = \left[r_e + j0.1213 \; \ln \frac{D_e}{D_{cu}} \right] l \tag{9.74}$$

$$\mathbf{Z}_{uu} = \mathbf{Z}_{uu} = \left[(r_e + r_u) + j0.1213 \; \ln \frac{D_e}{D_{uu}} \right] l \tag{9.75}$$

where r_u and D_{uu} are the resistance and GMR of the OH ground wire, respectively.

The matrix $\left[\mathbf{Z}_{abcu} \right]$ given in Equation 9.71 can be reduced to $\left[\mathbf{Z}_{abc} \right]$ by using *the Kron reduction technique*. Therefore, Equation 9.71 can be reexpressed as

$$\begin{bmatrix} \mathbf{V}_{abc} \\ \hline 0 \end{bmatrix} = \begin{bmatrix} \mathbf{Z}_1 & \mathbf{Z}_2 \\ \hline \mathbf{Z}_3 & \mathbf{Z}_4 \end{bmatrix} \begin{bmatrix} \mathbf{I}_{abc} \\ \mathbf{I}_u \end{bmatrix} \tag{9.76}$$

where the submatrices $[\mathbf{Z}_1]$, $[\mathbf{Z}_2]$, $[\mathbf{Z}_3]$, and $[\mathbf{Z}_4]$ are specified in the partitioned matrix $[\mathbf{Z}_{abcu}]$ in Equation 9.71. Therefore, after the reduction,

$$[\mathbf{V}_{abc}] = [\mathbf{Z}_{abc}][\mathbf{I}_{abc}] \tag{9.77}$$

where

$$\left[\mathbf{Z}_{abc}\right] \triangleq \left[\mathbf{Z}_1\right] - \left[\mathbf{Z}_2\right]\left[\mathbf{Z}_4\right]^{-1}\left[\mathbf{Z}_3\right] \tag{9.78}$$

Therefore, the sequence impedance matrix can be found from

$$\left[\mathbf{Z}_{012}\right] = \left[\mathbf{A}\right]^{-1}\left[\mathbf{Z}_{abc}\right]\left[\mathbf{A}\right] \tag{9.79}$$

Thus, the sequence admittance matrix becomes

$$\left[\mathbf{Y}_{012}\right] = \left[\mathbf{Z}_{012}\right]^{-1} \tag{9.80}$$

9.7 SEQUENCE CAPACITANCES OF TRANSMISSION LINE

9.7.1 THREE-PHASE TRANSMISSION LINE WITHOUT OVERHEAD GROUND WIRE

Consider Figure 4.29, showing the mirror reaction of the charged conductors, and assume that the three-phase conductors are charged. Therefore, for sinusoidal steady-state analysis, both voltage and charge density can be represented by phasors. Thus,

$$\left[\mathbf{V}_{abc}\right] = \left[P_{abc}\right]\left[Q_{abc}\right] \tag{9.81}$$

or

$$\begin{bmatrix} \mathbf{V}_a \\ \mathbf{V}_b \\ \mathbf{V}_c \end{bmatrix} = \begin{bmatrix} p_{aa} & p_{ab} & p_{ac} \\ p_{ba} & p_{bb} & p_{bc} \\ p_{ca} & p_{cb} & p_{cc} \end{bmatrix} \begin{bmatrix} q_a \\ q_b \\ q_c \end{bmatrix} \tag{9.82}$$

where $\left[P_{abc}\right]$ is the matrix of potential coefficients.
  Considering Figure 4.29,

$$p_{aa} = \frac{1}{2\pi\varepsilon} \ln \frac{h_{11}}{r_a} \ \mathrm{F^{-1}m} \tag{9.83}$$

$$p_{bb} = \frac{1}{2\pi\varepsilon} \ln \frac{h_{22}}{r_b} \ \mathrm{F^{-1}m} \tag{9.84}$$

$$p_{cc} = \frac{1}{2\pi\varepsilon} \ln \frac{h_{33}}{r_c} \ \mathrm{F^{-1}m} \tag{9.85}$$

$$p_{ab} = p_{ba} = \frac{1}{2\pi\varepsilon} \ln \frac{l_{12}}{D_{12}} \ \text{F}^{-1}\text{m} \tag{9.86}$$

$$p_{bc} = p_{cb} = \frac{1}{2\pi\varepsilon} \ln \frac{l_{23}}{D_{23}} \ \text{F}^{-1}\text{m} \tag{9.87}$$

$$p_{ac} = p_{ca} = \frac{1}{2\pi\varepsilon} \ln \frac{l_{31}}{D_{31}} \ \text{F}^{-1}\text{m} \tag{9.88}$$

Therefore, from Equation 9.81,

$$\left[Q_{abc}\right] = \left[P_{abc}\right]^{-1}\left[V_{abc}\right] \text{C/m} \tag{9.89a}$$

$$= \left[C_{abc}\right]\left[V_{abc}\right] \text{C/m} \tag{9.89b}$$

since

$$\left[C_{abc}\right] = \left[P_{abc}\right]^{-1} \text{F/m} \tag{9.90}$$

or

$$\left[C_{abc}\right] = \begin{bmatrix} C_{aa} & -C_{ab} & C_{ac} \\ -C_{ba} & C_{bb} & -C_{bc} \\ -C_{ca} & -C_{cb} & C_{cc} \end{bmatrix} \text{F/m} \tag{9.91}$$

where $[C_{abc}]$ is the *matrix of Maxwell's coefficients*, the diagonal terms are *Maxwell's* (or *capacitance*) *coefficients*, and the off-diagonal terms are *electrostatic induction coefficients*.

Therefore, the sequence capacitances can be found by using the similarity transformation as

$$\left[C_{012}\right] \triangleq \left[\mathbf{A}\right]^{-1}\left[C_{abc}\right]\left[\mathbf{A}\right] \text{F/m} \tag{9.92a}$$

$$= \begin{bmatrix} C_{00} & C_{01} & C_{02} \\ C_{10} & C_{11} & C_{12} \\ C_{20} & C_{21} & C_{22} \end{bmatrix} \text{F/m} \tag{9.92b}$$

Note that if the line is *transposed*, the matrix of potential coefficients can be expressed in terms of self-potential and mutual potential coefficients as

$$\left[P_{abc}\right] = \begin{bmatrix} p_s & p_m & p_m \\ p_m & p_s & p_m \\ p_m & p_m & p_s \end{bmatrix} \tag{9.93}$$

Therefore, using the similarity transformation,

$$\left[P_{012}\right] \triangleq \left[\mathbf{A}\right]^{-1}\left[P_{abc}\right]\left[\mathbf{A}\right] \tag{9.94a}$$

$$= \begin{bmatrix} p_0 & 0 & 0 \\ 0 & p_1 & 0 \\ 0 & 0 & p_2 \end{bmatrix} \tag{9.94b}$$

Thus,

$$\left[C_{012}\right] \triangleq \left[P_{012}\right]^{-1} \tag{9.95a}$$

$$= \begin{bmatrix} 1/p_0 & 0 & 0 \\ 0 & 1/p_1 & 0 \\ 0 & 0 & 1/p_2 \end{bmatrix} \tag{9.95b}$$

$$= \begin{bmatrix} C_0 & 0 & 0 \\ 0 & C_1 & 0 \\ 0 & 0 & C_2 \end{bmatrix} \tag{9.95c}$$

Alternatively, the sequence capacitances can approximately be calculated without using matrix algebra. For example, the zero-sequence capacitance can be calculated [4] from

$$C_0 = \frac{29.842}{\ln\left(\dfrac{H_{aa}}{D_{aa}}\right)} \text{ nF/mi} \tag{9.96}$$

where
H_{aa} = GMD between three conductors and their images

$$= \left[h_{11} \times h_{22} \times h_{33}\left(l_{12} \times l_{23} \times l_{31}\right)^2 \right]^{1/9} \tag{9.97}$$

D_{aa} is the self-GMD of OH conductors as composite group but with D_s of each conductor taken as its radius

$$D_{aa} = \left[r_a \times r_b \times r_c \left(D_{12} \times D_{23} \times D_{31}\right)^2 \right]^{1/9} \tag{9.98}$$

Note that D_s has been replaced by the conductor radius since all charge on a conductor resides on its surface. The positive- and negative-sequence capacitances of a line are the same owing to the fact that the physical parameters do not vary with a change in sequence of the applied voltage. Therefore, they are the same as the line-to-neutral capacitance C_n and can be calculated from

$$C_1 = C_2 = C_n = \frac{2\pi \times 8.8538 \times 10^{-12}}{\ln\left(\dfrac{D_{eq}}{r}\right) - \ln\left(\dfrac{l_{12} \times l_{23} \times l_{31}}{h_{11} \times h_{22} \times h_{33}}\right)^{1/3}} \text{ F/m}$$

But without taking the effects of the ground into account,

$$C_1 = C_2 = C_n = \frac{2\pi \times 8.8538 \times 10^{-12}}{\ln\left(\dfrac{D_{eq}}{r}\right)} \text{ F/m}$$

Hence, as a result, the positive- and negative-sequence capacitances are increased. But since in the line design, $l_{ij} \ll h_{ii}$, ignore the ground's effects.

Note that the mutual capacitances of the line can be found from Equation 9.91. The capacitances to ground can be expressed as

$$\begin{bmatrix} C_{ag} \\ C_{bg} \\ C_{cg} \end{bmatrix} = \begin{bmatrix} C_{aa} & C_{ab} & -C_{ac} \\ -C_{ab} & -C_{bb} & C_{bc} \\ -C_{ac} & C_{bc} & -C_{cc} \end{bmatrix} \begin{bmatrix} 1 \\ -1 \\ -1 \end{bmatrix} \tag{9.99}$$

If the line is transposed, the capacitance to ground is an average value that can be determined from

$$C_{g,avg} = \frac{1}{3}\left(C_{ag} + C_{bg} + C_{cg}\right) \tag{9.100}$$

Also note that the shunt admittance matrix of the line is

$$\begin{bmatrix} \mathbf{Y}_{abc} \end{bmatrix} = j\omega \begin{bmatrix} C_{abc} \end{bmatrix} \tag{9.101}$$

Therefore,

$$\begin{bmatrix} \mathbf{Y}_{012} \end{bmatrix} = \begin{bmatrix} \mathbf{A} \end{bmatrix}^{-1} \begin{bmatrix} \mathbf{Y}_{abc} \end{bmatrix} \begin{bmatrix} \mathbf{A} \end{bmatrix} \tag{9.102}$$

Thus,

$$\begin{bmatrix} C_{012} \end{bmatrix} = \frac{\begin{bmatrix} \mathbf{Y}_{012} \end{bmatrix}}{j\omega} \tag{9.103}$$

Hence,

$$\begin{bmatrix} \mathbf{I}_{012} \end{bmatrix} = j\omega \begin{bmatrix} C_{012} \end{bmatrix} \begin{bmatrix} \mathbf{V}_{012} \end{bmatrix} = j\begin{bmatrix} B_{012} \end{bmatrix} \begin{bmatrix} \mathbf{V}_{012} \end{bmatrix} \tag{9.104}$$

and

$$\begin{bmatrix} \mathbf{I}_{abc} \end{bmatrix} = \begin{bmatrix} \mathbf{A} \end{bmatrix} \begin{bmatrix} \mathbf{I}_{012} \end{bmatrix} \tag{9.105}$$

or

$$\begin{bmatrix} \mathbf{I}_{abc} \end{bmatrix} = j\omega \begin{bmatrix} C_{abc} \end{bmatrix} \begin{bmatrix} \mathbf{V}_{abc} \end{bmatrix} = j\begin{bmatrix} B_{abc} \end{bmatrix} \begin{bmatrix} \mathbf{V}_{abc} \end{bmatrix} \tag{9.106}$$

9.7.2 THREE-PHASE TRANSMISSION LINE WITH OVERHEAD GROUND WIRE

Consider Figure 9.6a and assume that the line is transposed and that the OH ground wire is denoted by u and that there are nine capacitances involved. The voltages and charge densities involved can be represented by phasors. Therefore,

$$\left[\mathbf{V}_{abcu} \right] = \left[P_{abcu} \right] \left[Q_{abcu} \right] \tag{9.107}$$

but since, for the ground wire, $\mathbf{V}_u = 0$,

$$
\begin{bmatrix} \mathbf{V}_a \\ \mathbf{V}_b \\ \mathbf{V}_c \\ 0 \end{bmatrix} =
\begin{bmatrix}
p_{aa} & p_{ab} & p_{ac} & p_{au} \\
p_{ba} & p_{bb} & p_{bc} & p_{bu} \\
p_{ca} & p_{cb} & p_{cc} & p_{cu} \\
p_{ua} & p_{ub} & p_{uc} & p_{uu}
\end{bmatrix}
\begin{bmatrix} q_a \\ q_b \\ q_c \\ q_u \end{bmatrix} \tag{9.108}
$$

The matrix $[P_{abcu}]$ can be calculated as before. The corresponding matrix of the Maxwell coefficients can be found as

$$\left[C_{abcu} \right] = \left[P_{abcu} \right]^{-1} \tag{9.109}$$

The corresponding equivalent circuit is shown in Figure 9.6a. Such equivalent circuit representation is convenient to study switching transients, traveling waves, overvoltages, etc.

The matrix $[P_{abcu}]$ given in Equation 9.108 can be reduced to $[P_{abc}]$ by using the Kron reduction technique. Therefore, Equation 9.97 can be reexpressed as

$$
\begin{bmatrix} \mathbf{V}_{abc} \\ \hline 0 \end{bmatrix} =
\begin{bmatrix} P_1 & P_2 \\ \hline P_3 & P_4 \end{bmatrix}
\begin{bmatrix} Q_{abc} \\ \hline Q_u \end{bmatrix} \tag{9.110}
$$

where the submatrices $[P_1]$, $[P_2]$, $[P_3]$, and $[P_4]$ are specified in the partitioned matrix $[P_{abcu}]$ in Equation 3.108. Thus, after the reduction,

$$\left[\mathbf{V}_{abc} \right] = \left[P_{abc} \right] \left[Q_{abc} \right] \tag{9.111}$$

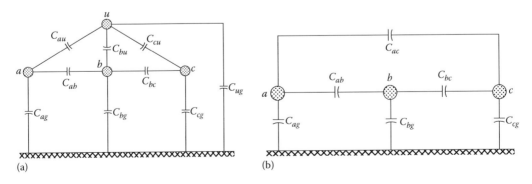

FIGURE 9.6 Three-phase line with one OH ground wire u: (a) equivalent circuit showing ground wire; (b) equivalent circuit without showing ground wire.

where

$$\left[P_{abc} \right] \triangleq \left[P_1 \right] - \left[P_2 \right] \left[P_4 \right]^{-1} \left[P_3 \right] \tag{9.112}$$

Thus, the corresponding matrix of the Maxwell coefficients can be found as

$$\left[C_{abc} \right] = \left[P_{abc} \right]^{-1} \tag{9.113}$$

as before. The corresponding equivalent circuit is shown in Figure 9.6b, and such representation is convenient to study a load-flow problem. Of course, the average capacitances to ground can be found as before.

Alternatively, the sequence capacitances can approximately be calculated without using the matrix algebra. For example, the zero-sequence capacitance can be calculated [4] from

$$C_0 = \frac{29.842 \ \ln\left(\dfrac{h_{gg}}{D_{gg}} \right)}{\ln\left(\dfrac{H_{aa}}{D_{aa}} \right) \times \ln\left(\dfrac{H_{gg}}{D_{gg}} \right) - \left[\ln\left(\dfrac{H_{ag}}{D_{ag}} \right) \right]^2} \quad \text{nF/mi} \tag{9.114}$$

where
  H_{aa} is given by Equation 9.97
  D_{aa} is given by Equation 9.98
  h_{gg} is the GMD between ground wires and their images
  D_{gg} is the self-GMD of ground wires with $D_s = r_g$
  H_{ag} is the GMD between phase conductors and images of ground wires
  D_{ag} is the GMD between phase conductors and ground wires

If the transmission line is untransposed, both electrostatic and electromagnetic unbalances exist in the system. If the system neutral is (solidly) grounded, in the event of an electrostatic unbalance, there will be a neutral residual current flow in the system due to the unbalance in the charging currents of the line. Such residual current flow is continuous and independent of the load. Since the neutral is grounded, $V_n = V_{a0} = 0$, and the *zero-sequence displacement* or *unbalance* is

$$\mathbf{d}_0 \triangleq \frac{\mathbf{C}_{01}}{\mathbf{C}_{11}} \tag{9.115}$$

and the *negative-sequence unbalance* is

$$\mathbf{d}_2 \triangleq -\frac{\mathbf{C}_{21}}{\mathbf{C}_{11}} \tag{9.116}$$

If the *system neutral is not grounded*, there will be the neutral voltage $V_n \neq 0$, and therefore, the neutral point will be shifted. Such *zero-sequence neutral displacement* or *unbalance* is defined as

$$\mathbf{d}_0 \triangleq -\frac{\mathbf{C}_{01}}{\mathbf{C}_{00}} \tag{9.117}$$

Example 9.6

Consider the line configuration shown in Figure 9.5. Assume that the 115 kV line is not transposed and its conductors are made up of 500 kcmil, 30/7-strand ACSR conductors. Ignore the OH ground wire and determine the following:

(a) Matrix of potential coefficients
(b) Matrix of Maxwell's coefficients
(c) Matrix of sequence capacitances
(d) Zero- and negative-sequence electrostatic unbalances, assuming that the system neutral is solidly grounded

Solution

(a) The corresponding potential coefficients are calculated using Equations 9.83 through 9.88. For example, let r_a to be the radius of the cable and then

$$p_{aa} = \frac{1}{2\pi\varepsilon} \ln\left(\frac{h_{11}}{r_a}\right)$$

$$= 11.185 \ \ln\left(\frac{90}{\dfrac{0.904}{2\times12}}\right) = 11.185 \ \ln\left(\frac{90}{0.037667}\right) = 87.0058 \ \text{F}^{-1}/\text{m}$$

$$p_{ab} = \frac{1}{2\pi\varepsilon} \ln\left(\frac{l_{12}}{D_{12}}\right) = 11.185 \ \ln\left(\frac{82.0244}{8.2462}\right) = 25.6949 \ \text{F}^{-1}/\text{m}$$

where

$$\varepsilon = \varepsilon_0 \times K = \frac{1}{36\pi\times10^9} = 8.85\times10^{-12}$$

$$K = 1, \ \text{for air}$$

$$l_{12} = \left[2^2 + (45+37)^2\right]^{1/2} = 82.0244 \ \text{ft}$$

$$D_{12} = \left(2^2 + 8^2\right)^{1/2} = 8.2462 \ \text{ft}$$

The others can also be found similarly. Therefore,

$$[P_{abc}] = \begin{bmatrix} 87.0058 & 25.6949 & 21.9132 \\ 25.6949 & 84.8164 & 19.7635 \\ 21.9132 & 19.7635 & 85.6884 \end{bmatrix}$$

(b)

$$[C_{abc}] = [P_{abc}]^{-1}$$

$$= \begin{bmatrix} 1.31\times10^{-2} & -3.38\times10^{-3} & -2.58\times10^{-3} \\ -3.38\times10^{-3} & 133\times10^{-2} & -2.21\times10^{-3} \\ -2.58\times10^{-3} & -2.21\times10^{-3} & 1.28\times10^{-2} \end{bmatrix}$$

(c)

$$[\mathbf{C}_{012}] = [\mathbf{A}]^{-1}[\mathbf{C}_{abc}][\mathbf{A}]$$

$$= \begin{bmatrix} 7.66 \times 10^{-3} + j0.0 & -2.38 \times 10^{-4} + j8.94 \times 10^{-5} & -2.38 \times 10^{-4} - j8.94 \times 10^{-5} \\ -2.38 \times 10^{-4} - j8.94 \times 10^{-5} & 1.58 \times 10^{-2} + j0.0 & 5.33 \times 10^{-4} - j6.02 \times 10^{-4} \\ -2.38 \times 10^{-4} + j8.94 \times 10^{-4} & 5.33 \times 10^{-4} + j6.02 \times 10^{-4} & 1.58 \times 10^{-2} + j.0.0 \end{bmatrix}$$

(d) From Equation 9.115,

$$\mathbf{d}_0 = \frac{\mathbf{C}_{01}}{\mathbf{C}_{11}} = \frac{-2.38 \times 10^{-4} + j8.94 \times 10^{-5}}{1.58 \times 10^{-2}} = 0.016 \angle 159.4° \text{ or } 1.6\%$$

and from Equation 9.116,

$$\mathbf{d}_2 = -\frac{\mathbf{C}_{21}}{\mathbf{C}_{11}} = -\frac{5.33 \times 10^{-4} + j6.02 \times 10^{-4}}{1.58 \times 10^{-2}} = 0.0508 \angle 311.5° \text{ or } 5.08\%$$

9.8 SEQUENCE IMPEDANCES OF SYNCHRONOUS MACHINES

In general, the impedances to positive-, negative-, and zero-sequence currents in synchronous machines (as well as other rotating machines) have different values. The positive-sequence impedance of the synchronous machine can be selected to be its *subtransient* (X_d''), *transient* (X_d'), or synchronous* (X_d) reactance depending on the time assumed to elapse from the instant of fault initiation to the instant at which values are desired (e.g., for relay response, breaker opening, or sustained fault conditions). Usually, however, in fault studies, the subtransient reactance is taken as the positive-sequence reactance of the synchronous machine.

The negative-sequence impedance of a synchronous machine is usually determined from

$$\mathbf{Z}_2 = jX_2 = j\left(\frac{X_d'' + X_q''}{2}\right) \tag{9.118}$$

In a cylindrical-rotor synchronous machine, the subtransient and negative-sequence reactances are the same, as shown in Table 9.3.

The zero-sequence impedance of a synchronous machine varies widely and depends on the pitch of the armature coils. It is much smaller than the corresponding positive- and negative-sequence reactances. It can be measured by connecting the three armature windings in series and applying a single-phase voltage. The ratio of the terminal voltage of one phase winding to the current is the zero-sequence reactance. It is approximately equal to the zero-sequence reactance. Table 9.3 [5] gives typical reactance values of three-phase synchronous machines. Note that in the previous discussion, the resistance values are ignored because they are much smaller than the corresponding reactance values.

Figure 9.7 shows the equivalent circuit of a cylindrical-rotor synchronous machine with constant field current. Since the coil groups of the three-phase stator armature windings are displaced from each other by 120 electrical degrees, balanced three-phase sinusoidal voltages are induced in the stator windings. Furthermore, the three self-impedances and mutual impedances are equal to each

---

* It is also called the *direct-axis synchronous reactance*. It is also denoted by X_s.

TABLE 9.3
Typical Reactances of Three-Phase Synchronous Machines

	Turbine Generators						Salient-Pole Generators						Synchronous Condensers					
	Two Pole			Four Pole			With Dampers			Without Dampers			Air Cooled			Hydrogen Cooled		
	Low	Avg.	High	Low	Avg.	High	Low	Avg.	High	Low	Avg.	High	Low	Avg.	High	Low	Avg.	High
X_d	0.95	1.2	1.45	1.00	1.2	1.45	0.6	1.25	1.5	0.6	1.25	1.5	1.25	1.85	2.2	1.5	2.2	2.65
X'_d	0.12	0.15	0.21	0.2	0.23	0.28	0.2	0.3	0.5	0.2	0.3	0.5	0.3	0.4	0.5	0.36	0.48	0.6
X''_d	0.07	0.09	0.14	0.12	0.14	0.17	0.13	0.2	0.32	0.2	0.3	0.5	0.19	0.27	0.3	0.23	0.32	0.36
X_q	0.92	1.16	1.42	0.92	1.16	1.42	0.4	0.7	0.8	0.4	0.7	0.8	0.95	1.15	1.3	1.1	1.35	1.55
X_2	0.07	0.09	0.14	0.12	0.14	0.17	0.13	0.2	0.32	0.35	0.48	0.65	0.18	0.26	0.4	0.22	0.31	0.48
X_0	0.01	0.03	0.08	0.015	0.08	0.14	0.03	0.18	0.23	0.03	0.19	0.24	0.025	0.12	0.15	0.03	0.14	0.18

Source: Westinghouse Electric Corporation, *Electrical Transmission and Distribution Reference Book*, WEC, East Pittsburgh, PA, 1964.

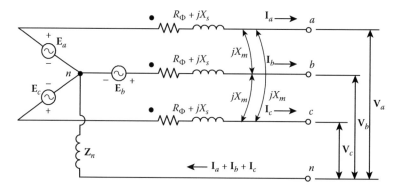

FIGURE 9.7 Equivalent circuit of cylindrical-rotor synchronous machine.

other, respectively, owing to the machine symmetry. Therefore, taking into account the neutral impedance $\mathbf{Z}_n$ and applying KVL, it can be shown that

$$\mathbf{E}_a = \left(R_\phi + jX_s + \mathbf{Z}_n \right)\mathbf{I}_a + \left(jX_m + \mathbf{Z}_n \right)\mathbf{I}_b + \left(jX_m + \mathbf{Z}_n \right)\mathbf{I}_c + \mathbf{V}_a \qquad (9.119)$$

$$\mathbf{E}_b = \left(jX_m + \mathbf{Z}_n \right)\mathbf{I}_a + \left(R_\phi + jX_s + \mathbf{Z}_n \right)\mathbf{I}_b + \left(jX_m + \mathbf{Z}_n \right)\mathbf{I}_c + \mathbf{V}_b \qquad (9.120)$$

$$\mathbf{E}_c = \left(jX_m + \mathbf{Z}_n \right)\mathbf{I}_a + \left(jX_m + \mathbf{Z}_n \right)\mathbf{I}_b + \left(R_\phi + jX_s + \mathbf{Z}_n \right)\mathbf{I}_c + \mathbf{V}_c \qquad (9.121)$$

or, in matrix form,

$$\begin{bmatrix} \mathbf{E}_a \\ \mathbf{E}_b \\ \mathbf{E}_c \end{bmatrix} = \begin{bmatrix} \mathbf{Z}_s & \mathbf{Z}_m & \mathbf{Z}_m \\ \mathbf{Z}_m & \mathbf{Z}_s & \mathbf{Z}_m \\ \mathbf{Z}_m & \mathbf{Z}_m & \mathbf{Z}_s \end{bmatrix} \begin{bmatrix} \mathbf{I}_a \\ \mathbf{I}_b \\ \mathbf{I}_c \end{bmatrix} + \begin{bmatrix} \mathbf{V}_a \\ \mathbf{V}_b \\ \mathbf{V}_c \end{bmatrix} \qquad (9.122)$$

where

$$\mathbf{Z}_s = R_\phi + jX_s + \mathbf{Z}_n \qquad (9.123)$$

$$\mathbf{Z}_m = jX_m + \mathbf{Z}_n \qquad (9.124)$$

$$\mathbf{E}_a = \mathbf{E}_a \qquad (9.125)$$

$$\mathbf{E}_b = \mathbf{a}^2\mathbf{E}_a \qquad (9.126)$$

$$\mathbf{E}_c = \mathbf{a}\mathbf{E}_a \qquad (9.127)$$

Alternatively, Equation 9.122 can be written in shorthand matrix notation as

$$\left[\mathbf{E}_{abc} \right] = \left[\mathbf{Z}_{abc} \right]\left[\mathbf{I}_{abc} \right] + \left[\mathbf{V}_{abc} \right] \qquad (9.128)$$

Multiplying both sides of this equation by $\left[\mathbf{A}\right]^{-1}$ and also substituting Equation 9.26 into it,

$$\left[\mathbf{A}\right]^{-1}\left[\mathbf{E}_{abc}\right]=\left[\mathbf{A}\right]^{-1}\left[\mathbf{Z}_{abc}\right]\left[\mathbf{A}\right]\left[\mathbf{I}_{012}\right]+\left[\mathbf{A}\right]^{-1}\left[\mathbf{V}_{abc}\right] \qquad (9.129)$$

where

$$\left[\mathbf{A}\right]^{-1}\left[\mathbf{E}_{abc}\right]=\frac{1}{3}\begin{bmatrix} 1 & 1 & 1 \\ 1 & a & a^2 \\ 1 & a^2 & a \end{bmatrix}\begin{bmatrix} \mathbf{E} \\ a^2\mathbf{E} \\ a\mathbf{E} \end{bmatrix}=\begin{bmatrix} 0 \\ \mathbf{E} \\ 0 \end{bmatrix} \qquad (9.130)$$

$$\left[\mathbf{Z}_{012}\right]\triangleq\left[\mathbf{A}\right]^{-1}\left[\mathbf{Z}_{abc}\right]\left[\mathbf{A}\right] \qquad (9.38)$$

$$\left[\mathbf{V}_{012}\right]=\left[\mathbf{A}\right]^{-1}\left[\mathbf{V}_{abc}\right] \qquad (9.19)$$

Also, due to the symmetry of the machine,

$$\left[\mathbf{Z}_{012}\right]=\begin{bmatrix} \mathbf{Z}_s+2\mathbf{Z}_m & 0 & 0 \\ 0 & \mathbf{Z}_s-\mathbf{Z}_m & 0 \\ 0 & 0 & \mathbf{Z}_s-\mathbf{Z}_m \end{bmatrix} \qquad (9.131)$$

or

$$\left[\mathbf{Z}_{012}\right]=\begin{bmatrix} \mathbf{Z}_{00} & 0 & 0 \\ 0 & \mathbf{Z}_{11} & 0 \\ 0 & 0 & \mathbf{Z}_{22} \end{bmatrix} \qquad (9.132)$$

where

$$\mathbf{Z}_{00}=\mathbf{Z}_s+2\mathbf{Z}_m=R_\phi+j\left(X_s+2X_m\right)+3\mathbf{Z}_n \qquad (9.133)$$

$$\mathbf{Z}_{11}=\mathbf{Z}_s-\mathbf{Z}_m=R_\phi+j\left(X_s-X_m\right) \qquad (9.134)$$

$$\mathbf{Z}_{22}=\mathbf{Z}_s-\mathbf{Z}_m=R_\phi+j\left(X_s-X_m\right) \qquad (9.135)$$

Therefore, Equation 9.128 in terms of the symmetrical components can be expressed as

$$\begin{bmatrix} 0 \\ \mathbf{E}_a \\ 0 \end{bmatrix}=\begin{bmatrix} \mathbf{Z}_{00} & 0 & 0 \\ 0 & \mathbf{Z}_{11} & 0 \\ 0 & 0 & \mathbf{Z}_{22} \end{bmatrix}\begin{bmatrix} \mathbf{I}_{a0} \\ \mathbf{I}_{a1} \\ \mathbf{I}_{a2} \end{bmatrix}+\begin{bmatrix} \mathbf{V}_{a0} \\ \mathbf{V}_{a1} \\ \mathbf{V}_{a2} \end{bmatrix} \qquad (9.136)$$

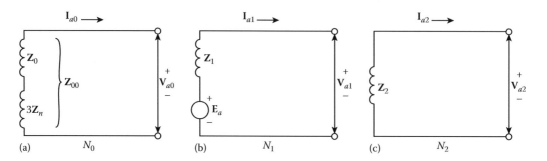

FIGURE 9.8 Sequence networks of synchronous machine: (a) zero-sequence network, (b) positive-sequence network, (c) negative-sequence network.

or, in shorthand matrix notation,

$$\left[\mathbf{E}\right]=\left[\mathbf{Z}_{012}\right]\left[\mathbf{I}_{012}\right]+\left[\mathbf{V}_{012}\right] \tag{9.137}$$

Similarly,

$$\begin{bmatrix}\mathbf{V}_{a0}\\\mathbf{V}_{a1}\\\mathbf{V}_{a2}\end{bmatrix}=\begin{bmatrix}0\\\mathbf{E}_a\\0\end{bmatrix}-\begin{bmatrix}\mathbf{Z}_{00}&0&0\\0&\mathbf{Z}_{11}&0\\0&0&\mathbf{Z}_{22}\end{bmatrix}\begin{bmatrix}\mathbf{I}_{a0}\\\mathbf{I}_{a1}\\\mathbf{I}_{a2}\end{bmatrix} \tag{9.138}$$

or

$$\left[\mathbf{V}_{012}\right]=\left[\mathbf{E}\right]-\left[\mathbf{Z}_{012}\right]\left[\mathbf{I}_{012}\right] \tag{9.139}$$

Note that the machine sequence impedances in these equations are

$$\mathbf{Z}_0\triangleq\mathbf{Z}_{00}-3\mathbf{Z}_n \tag{9.140}$$

$$\mathbf{Z}_1\triangleq\mathbf{Z}_{11} \tag{9.141}$$

$$\mathbf{Z}_2\triangleq\mathbf{Z}_{22} \tag{9.142}$$

The expression given in Equation 9.140 is due to the fact that the impedance $\mathbf{Z}_n$ is external to the machine. Figure 9.8 shows the sequence networks of a synchronous machine.

9.9 ZERO-SEQUENCE NETWORKS

It is important to note that the zero-sequence system, in a sense, is not a three-phase system but a single-phase system. This is because the zero-sequence currents and voltages are equal in magnitude and in phase at any point in all the phases of the system. However, the Lero-sequence currents can only exist in a circuit if there is a complete path for their flow. Therefore, if there is no complete path for zero-sequence currents in a circuit, the zero-sequence impedance is infinite. In a zero-sequence network drawing, this infinite impedance is indicated by an open circuit.

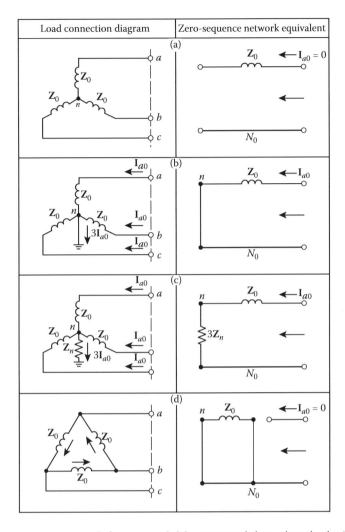

FIGURE 9.9 Zero-sequence network for wye- and delta-connected three-phase loads: (a) wye-connected load with undergrounded neutral, (b) wye-connected load with grounded neutral, (c) wye-connected load grounded through neutral impedance, (d) delta-connected load.

Figure 9.9 shows zero-sequence networks for wye- and delta-connected three-phase loads. Note that a wye-connected load with an ungrounded neutral has infinite impedance to zero-sequence currents since there is no return path through the ground or a neutral conductor, as shown in Figure 9.9a. On the other hand, a wye-connected load with solidly grounded neutral, as shown in Figure 9.9b, provides a return path for the zero-sequence currents flowing through the three phases and their sum, $3\mathbf{I}_{a0}$, flowing through the ground. If the neutral is grounded through some impedance $\mathbf{Z}_n$ as shown in Figure 9.9c, an impedance of $3\mathbf{Z}_n$ should be inserted between the neutral point n and the zero-potential bus N_0 in the zero-sequence network. The reason for this is that a current of $3\mathbf{I}_{a0}$ produces a zero-sequence voltage drop of $3\mathbf{I}_{a0}\mathbf{Z}_n$ between the neutral point n and the ground. Therefore, in order to reflect this voltage drop in the zero-sequence network where the zero-sequence current $3\mathbf{I}_{a0}$ flows, the neutral impedance should be $3\mathbf{Z}_n$. A delta-connected load, as shown in Figure 9.9d, provides no path for zero-sequence currents flowing in the line. Therefore, its zero-sequence impedance, as seen from its terminals, is infinite. Yet it is possible to have zero-sequence currents circulating within the delta circuit. However, they have to be produced in the delta by zero-sequence voltages or by induction from an outside source.

9.10 SEQUENCE IMPEDANCES OF TRANSFORMERS

A three-phase transformer may be made up of three identical single-phase transformers. If this is the case, it is called a three-phase *transformer bank*. Alternatively, it may be built as a three-phase transformer having a single common core (either with shell-type or core-type design) and a tank. For the sake of simplicity, here only the three-phase transformer banks will be reviewed. The impedance of a transformer to both positive- and negative-sequence currents is the same. Even though

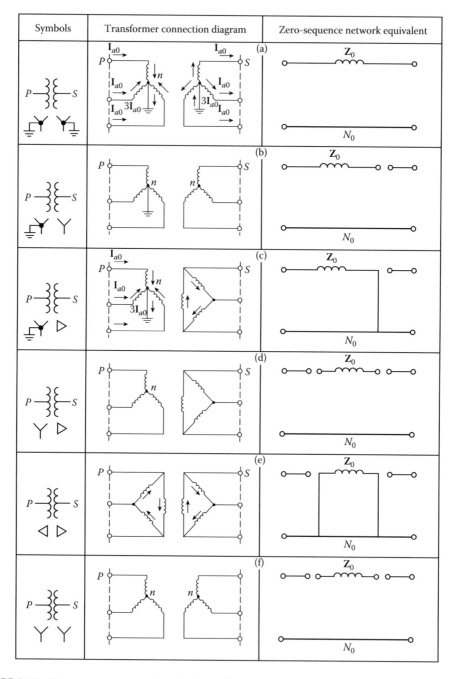

FIGURE 9.10 Zero-sequence network equivalents of three-phase transformer banks made of three identical single-phase transformers with two windings.

the zero-sequence series impedances of three-phase units are little different than the positive- and negative-sequence series impedances, it is often assumed in practice that series impedances of all sequences are the same without paying attention to the transformer type

$$\mathbf{Z}_0 = \mathbf{Z}_1 = \mathbf{Z}_2 = \mathbf{Z}_{\text{trf}} \qquad (9.143)$$

If the flow of zero-sequence current is prevented by the transformer connection, $\mathbf{Z}_0$ is infinite.

Figure 9.10 shows zero-sequence network equivalents of three-phase transformer banks made up of three identical single-phase transformers having two windings with excitation currents neglected. The possible paths for the flow of zero-sequence current are indicated on the connection diagrams, as shown in Figure 9.10a, c, and e. If there is no path shown on the connection diagram, this means that the transformer connection prevents the flow of the zero-sequence current by not providing path for it, as indicated in Figure 9.10b, d, and f.

Note that even though the delta–delta bank can have zero-sequence currents circulating within its delta windings, it also prevents the flow of the zero-sequence current outside the delta windings by not providing a return path for it, as shown in Figure 9.10e.

Also note that if the neutral point n of the wye winding (shown in Figure 9.10a or c) is grounded through $\mathbf{Z}_n$, the corresponding zero-sequence impedance $\mathbf{Z}_0$ should be replaced by $\mathbf{Z}_0 + 3\mathbf{Z}_n$.

If the wye winding is *solidly grounded*, the $\mathbf{Z}_n$ is zero, and therefore, $3\mathbf{Z}_n$ should be replaced by a short circuit. On the other hand, if the connection is *ungrounded*, the $\mathbf{Z}_n$ is infinite, and therefore, $3\mathbf{Z}_n$ should be replaced with an open circuit. It is interesting to observe that the type of grounding only affects the zero-sequence network, not the positive- and negative-sequence networks.

It is interesting to note that there is no path for the flow of zero-sequence current in a wye-grounded–wye-connected three-phase transformer bank, as shown in Figure 9.10b. This is because there is no zero-sequence current in any given winding on the wye side of the transformer bank since it has an ungrounded wye connection. Therefore, because of the lack of equal and opposite ampere turns in the wye side of the transformer bank, there cannot be any zero-sequence current in the corresponding winding on the wye-grounded side of the transformer, with the exception of a negligible small magnetizing current.

Figure 9.11 shows zero-sequence network equivalents of three-phase transformer banks made of three identical single-phase transformers with three windings. The impedances of the three-winding transformer between primary, secondary, and tertiary terminals, indicated by P, S, and T, respectively, taken two at a time with the other winding open, are $\mathbf{Z}_{PS}$, $\mathbf{Z}_{PT}$, and $\mathbf{Z}_{ST}$, the subscripts indicating the terminals between which the impedances are measured. Note that only the wye–wye connection with delta tertiary, shown in Figure 9.11a, permits zero-sequence current to flow in from either wye line (as long as the neutrals are grounded).

Example 9.7

Consider the power system shown in Figure 9.12 and the associated data given in Table 9.4. Assume that each three-phase transformer bank is made of three single-phase transformers. Do the following:

  (a) Draw the corresponding positive-sequence network.
  (b) Draw the corresponding negative-sequence network.
  (c) Draw the corresponding zero-sequence network.

Solution

  (a) The positive-sequence network is shown in Figure 9.13a.
  (b) The negative-sequence network is shown in Figure 9.13b.
  (c) The zero-sequence network is shown in Figure 9.13c.

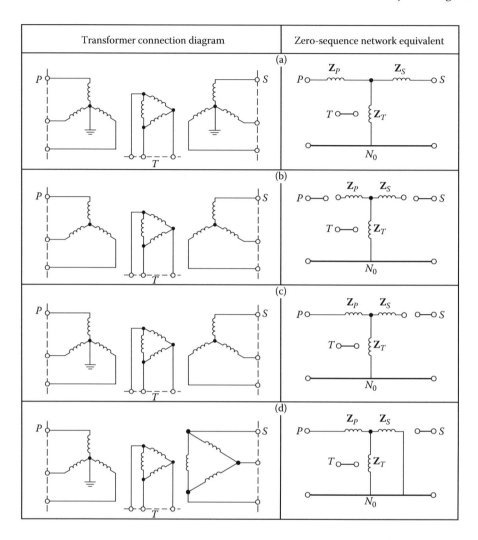

FIGURE 9.11 Zero-sequence network equivalents of three-phase transformer banks made of three identical single-phase transformers with three windings.

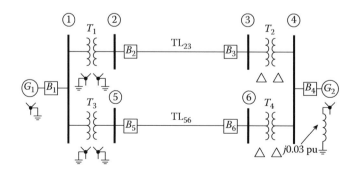

FIGURE 9.12 Power system for Example 9.7.

TABLE 9.4
System Data for Example 9.7

Network Component	MVA Rating	Voltage Rating (kV)	X_1 (pu)	X_2 (pu)	X_0 (pu)
G_1	200	20	0.2	0.14	0.06
G_2	200	13.2	0.2	0.14	0.06
T_1	200	20/230	0.2	0.2	0.2
T_2	200	13.2/230	0.3	0.3	0.3
T_3	200	20/230	0.25	0.25	0.25
T_4	200	13.2/230	0.35	0.35	0.35
TL_{23}	200	230	0.15	0.15	0.3
TL_{56}	200	230	0.22	0.22	0.5

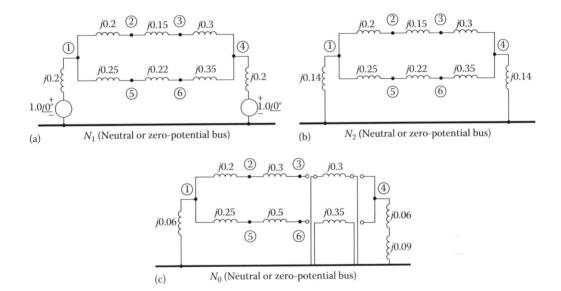

FIGURE 9.13 The sequence networks for Example 9.7.

Example 9.8

Consider the power system given in Example 9.7 and assume that there is a fault on bus 3. Reduce the sequence networks drawn in Example 9.7 to their Thévenin equivalents *looking in* at bus 3.

(a) Show the steps of the positive-sequence network reduction.
(b) Show the steps of the negative-sequence network reduction.
(c) Show the steps of the zero-sequence network reduction.

Solution

(a) Figure 9.14 shows the steps of the positive-sequence network reduction.
(b) Figure 9.15 shows the steps of the negative-sequence network reduction.
(c) Figure 9.16 shows the steps of the zero-sequence network reduction.

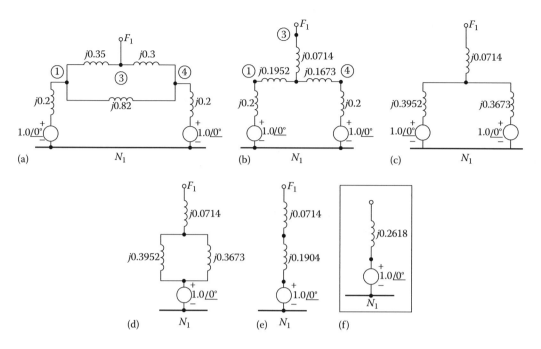

FIGURE 9.14 The reduction steps for positive-sequence network of Example 9.8.

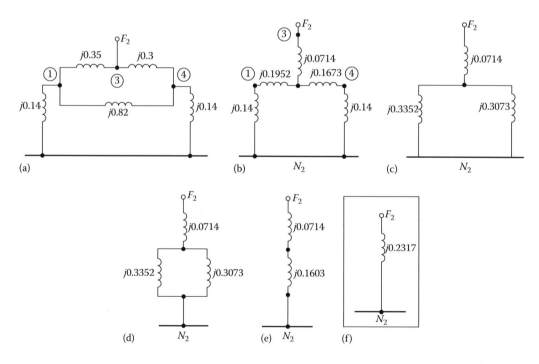

FIGURE 9.15 The reduction steps for negative-sequence network of Example 9.8.

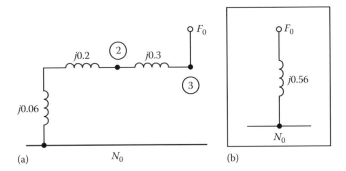

FIGURE 9.16 The reduction steps for zero-sequence network of Example 9.8.

9.11 ANALYSIS OF UNBALANCED FAULTS

Most of the faults that occur on power systems are not the balanced (i.e., *symmetrical*) three-phase faults but the unbalanced (i.e., *unsymmetrical*) faults, specifically the SLG faults. For example, Ref. [5] gives the typical frequency of occurrence for the three-phase, single line-to ground, line-to-line, and double line-to-ground (DLG) faults as 5%, 70%, 15%, and 10%, respectively.

In general, the three-phase fault is considered to be the most severe one. However, it is possible that the SLG fault may be more severe than the three-phase fault under two circumstances: (1) the generators involved in the fault have solidly grounded neutrals or low-impedance neutral impedances, and (2) it occurs on the wye-grounded side of delta–wye-grounded transformer banks. The line-to-line fault current is about 86.6% of the three-phase fault current.

The faults can be categorized as the shunt faults (*short circuits*), series faults (*open conductor*), and simultaneous faults (*having more than one fault occurring at the same time*). The unbalanced faults can be easily solved by using the symmetrical components of an unbalanced system of currents or voltages. Therefore, an unbalanced system can be converted to three fictitious networks: the positive-sequence (the only one that has a driving voltage), the negative-sequence, and the zero-sequence networks interconnected to each other in a particular fashion depending on the fault type involved. In this book, only shunt faults are reviewed.

9.12 SHUNT FAULTS

The voltage to ground of phase a at the fault point F before the fault occurred is V_F, and it is usually selected as $1.0 \angle 0°$ pu. However, it is possible to have a V_F value that is not $1.0 \angle 0°$ pu. If so, Table 9.5 [8] gives formulas to calculate the fault currents and voltages at the fault point F and their corresponding symmetrical components for various types of faults. Note that the positive-, negative-, and zero-sequence impedances are viewed from the fault point as Z_1, Z_2, and Z_0, respectively. In the table, Z_f is the fault impedance and Z_{eq} is the equivalent impedance to replace the fault in the positive-sequence network. Also, note that the value of the impedance Z_g is zero in Table 9.5.

9.12.1 SINGLE LINE-TO-GROUND FAULT

In general, the SLG fault on a transmission system occurs when one conductor falls to ground or contacts the neutral wire. Figure 9.17a shows the general representation of an SLG fault at a

TABLE 9.5

Fault Currents and Voltages at Fault Point F and Their Corresponding Symmetrical Components for Various Types of Faults

	Three-Phase Fault through Three-Phase Fault Impedance (Z_f)	Line-to-Line, Phases b and c Shorted through Fault Impedance (Z_f)	Line-to-Ground Fault, Phase a Grounded through Fault Impedance (Z_f)	DLG Fault, Phases b and c Shorted and Then Grounded through Fault Impedance (Z_f)
I_{a1}	$I_{a1} = \dfrac{V_f}{Z_1 + Z_f}$	$I_{a1} = -I_{a2}$ $= \dfrac{V_f}{Z_1 + Z_2 + Z_f}$	$I_{a1} = I_{a2} = I_{a0}$ $= \dfrac{V_f}{Z_0 + Z_1 + Z_2 + 3Z_f}$	$I_{a1} = -(I_{a2} + I_{a0}) = \dfrac{V_f}{Z_1 + \dfrac{Z_2(Z_0 + 3Z_f)}{Z_2 + Z_0 + 3Z_f}}$
I_{a2}	$I_{a2} = 0$	$I_{a2} = -I_{a1}$	$I_{a2} = I_{a1}$	$I_{a2} = -I_{a1}\dfrac{Z_0 + 3Z_f}{Z_2 + Z_0 + 3Z_f}$
I_{a0}	$I_{a0} = 0$	$I_{a0} = 0$	$I_{a0} = I_{a1}$	$I_{a0} = -I_{a1}\dfrac{Z_2}{Z_2 + Z_0 + 3Z_f}$
V_{a1}	$V_{a1} = I_{a1}Z_f$	$V_{a1} = V_{a2} + I_{a1}Z_f$ $= I_{a1}(Z_2 + Z_f)$	$V_{a1} = -(V_{a2} + V_{a2} + V_{a0}) + I_{a1}(3Z_f)$ $= I_{a1}(Z_0 + Z_2 + 3Z_f)$	$V_{a1} = V_{a2} = V_{a0} - 3I_{a0}Z_f$ $= I_{a1}\dfrac{Z_2(Z_0 + 3Z_f)}{Z_2 + Z_0 + 3Z_f}$
V_{a2}	$V_{a2} = 0$	$V_{a2} = -I_{a2}Z_2 = I_{a1}Z_2$	$V_{a2} = -I_{a2}Z_2 = -I_{a1}Z_2$	$V_{a2} = -I_{a2}Z_2 = I_{a1}\dfrac{Z_2(Z_0 + 3Z_f)}{Z_2 + Z_0 + 3Z_f}$
V_{a0}	$V_{a0} = 0$	$V_{a0} = 0$	$V_{a0} = -I_{a0}Z_0 = I_{a1}Z_0$	$V_{a0} = -I_{a0}Z_0 = I_{a1}\dfrac{Z_0 Z_2}{Z_2 + Z_0 + 3Z_f}$
Z_{eq}	$Z_{eq} = Z_f$	$Z_{eq} = Z_2 + Z_f$	$Z_{eq} = Z_0 + Z_2 + 3Z_f$	$Z_{eq} = \dfrac{Z_2(Z_0 + 3Z_f)}{Z_2 + Z_0 + 3Z_f}$
I_{af}	$\dfrac{V_f}{Z_1 + Z_f}$	0	$\dfrac{3V_f}{Z_0 + Z_1 + Z_2 + 3Z_f}$	0

I_{bf}	$\dfrac{a^2 V_f}{Z_1 + Z_f}$	$-j\sqrt{3}\,\dfrac{V_f}{Z_1 + Z_2 + Z_f}$	0	$-j\sqrt{3}V_f\,\dfrac{Z_0 + 3Z_f - aZ_2}{Z_1 Z_2 + (Z_1 + Z_2)(Z_0 + 3Z_f)}$
I_{cf}	$\dfrac{a V_f}{Z_1 + Z_f}$	$j\sqrt{3}\,\dfrac{V_f}{Z_1 + Z_2 + Z_f}$	0	$j\sqrt{3}V_f\,\dfrac{Z_0 + 3Z_f - a^2 Z_2}{Z_1 Z_2 + (Z_1 + Z_2)(Z_0 + 3Z_f)}$
V_{af}	$V_f\,\dfrac{Z_f}{Z_1 + Z_f}$	$V_f\,\dfrac{2Z_2 + Z_f}{Z_1 + Z_2 + Z_f}$	$V_f\,\dfrac{3Z_f}{Z_0 + Z_1 + Z_2 + 3Z_f}$	$V_f\,\dfrac{3Z_2\left(Z_0 + 2Z_f\right)}{Z_1 Z_2 + (Z_1 + Z_2)(Z_0 + 3Z_f)}$
V_{bf}	$V_f\,\dfrac{a^2 Z_f}{Z_1 + Z_f}$	$V_f\,\dfrac{a^2 Z_f - Z_2}{Z_1 + Z_2 + Z_f}$	$V_f\,\dfrac{3a^2 Z_f - j\sqrt{3}\left(Z_2 - aZ_0\right)}{Z_0 + Z_1 + Z_2 + 3Z_f}$	$V_f\,\dfrac{-3Z_f Z_2}{Z_1 Z_2 + (Z_1 + Z_2)(Z_0 + 3Z_f)}$
V_{cf}	$V_f\,\dfrac{a Z_f}{Z_1 + Z_f}$	$V_f\,\dfrac{a Z_f - Z_2}{Z_1 + Z_2 + Z_f}$	$V_f\,\dfrac{3a Z_f + j\sqrt{3}\left(Z_2 - a^2 Z_0\right)}{Z_0 + Z_1 + Z_2 + 3Z_f}$	$V_f\,\dfrac{-3Z_f Z_2}{Z_1 Z_2 + (Z_1 + Z_2)(Z_0 + 3Z_f)}$
V_{bc}	$j\sqrt{3}V_f\,\dfrac{Z_f}{Z_1 + Z_f}$	$j\sqrt{3}V_f\,\dfrac{Z_f}{Z_1 + Z_2 + Z_f}$	$j\sqrt{3}V_f\,\dfrac{3Z_f + Z_0 + 2Z_2}{Z_0 + Z_1 + Z_2 + 3Z_f}$	0
V_{ca}	$j\sqrt{3}V_f\,\dfrac{a^2 Z_f}{Z_1 + Z_f}$	$j\sqrt{3}V_f\,\dfrac{a^2 Z_f - j\sqrt{3}Z_2}{Z_1 + Z_2 + Z_f}$	$j\sqrt{3}V_f\,\dfrac{a^2\left(3Z_f + Z_0\right) - Z_2}{Z_0 + Z_1 + Z_2 + 3Z_f}$	$\sqrt{3}V_f\,\dfrac{\sqrt{3}Z_2\left(Z_0 + 3Z_f\right)}{Z_1 Z_2 + (Z_1 + Z_2)(Z_0 + 3Z_f)}$
V_{ab}	$j\sqrt{3}V_f = \dfrac{a^2 Z_f}{Z_1 + Z_f}$	$j\sqrt{3}V_f\,\dfrac{a Z_f + j\sqrt{3}Z_2}{Z_1 + Z_2 + Z_f}$	$j\sqrt{3}V_f\,\dfrac{a\left(3Z_f + Z_0\right) - Z_2}{Z_0 + Z_1 + Z_2 + 3Z_f}$	$-\sqrt{3}V_f\,\dfrac{\sqrt{3}Z_2\left(Z_0 + 3Z_f\right)}{Z_1 Z_2 + (Z_1 + Z_2)(Z_0 + 3Z_f)}$

Source: Clarke, E., *Circuit Analysis of A-C Power Systems*, vol. 2, General Electric Co., Schenectady, NY, 1960. Note that Clarke only considers Z_g and calls it Z_f. At the same time, the regular Z_f that is used in this book is totally ignored in her treatment of fault analysis. Also, Clarke treats DLG fault differently. She lets $Z_g = Z_f$. Her fault impedance Z_f for the variables in the last column.

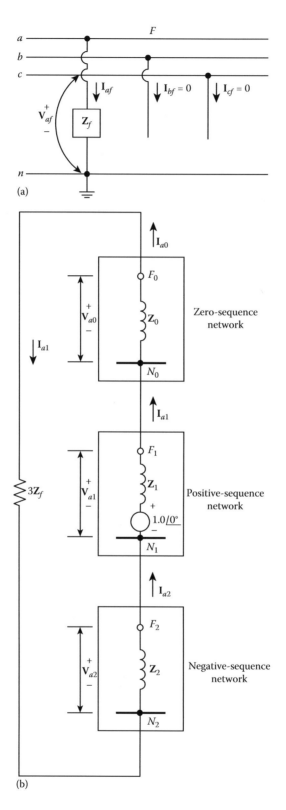

FIGURE 9.17   SLG fault: (a) general representation; (b) interconnection of sequence networks.

fault point F with a fault impedance $\mathbf{Z}_f$.* Usually, the fault impedance $\mathbf{Z}_f$ is ignored in fault studies. Figure 9.17b shows the interconnection of the resulting sequence networks. For the sake of simplicity in fault calculations, the faulted phase is usually assumed to be phase a, as shown in Figure 9.17b.

However, if the faulted phase in reality is other than phase a (e.g., phase b), the phases of the system can simply be relabeled (i.e., a, b, c becomes c, a, b) [4]. A second method involves the use of the *generalized fault diagram* of Atabekov [9] further developed by Anderson [4]. From Figure 9.17b, it can be observed that the zero-, positive-, and negative-sequence currents are equal to each other. Therefore,

$$\mathbf{I}_{a0} = \mathbf{I}_{a1} = \mathbf{I}_{a2} = \frac{1.0\angle 0^\circ}{\mathbf{Z}_0 + \mathbf{Z}_1 + \mathbf{Z}_2 + 3\mathbf{Z}_f} \tag{9.144}$$

Since

$$\begin{bmatrix} \mathbf{I}_{af} \\ \mathbf{I}_{bf} \\ \mathbf{I}_{cf} \end{bmatrix} = \begin{bmatrix} 1 & 1 & 1 \\ 1 & \mathbf{a}^2 & \mathbf{a} \\ 1 & \mathbf{a} & \mathbf{a}^2 \end{bmatrix} \begin{bmatrix} \mathbf{I}_{a0} \\ \mathbf{I}_{a1} \\ \mathbf{I}_{a2} \end{bmatrix} \tag{9.145}$$

the fault current for phase a can be found as

$$\mathbf{I}_{af} = \mathbf{I}_{a0} + \mathbf{I}_{a1} + \mathbf{I}_{a2}$$

or

$$\mathbf{I}_{af} = 3\mathbf{I}_{a0} = 3\mathbf{I}_{a1} = 3\mathbf{I}_{a2} \tag{9.146}$$

From Figure 9.17a,

$$\mathbf{V}_{af} = \mathbf{Z}_f \mathbf{I}_{af} \tag{9.147}$$

Substituting Equation 9.145 into Equation 9.147, the voltage at faulted phase a can be expressed as

$$\mathbf{V}_{af} = 3\mathbf{Z}_f \mathbf{I}_{a1} \tag{9.148}$$

But

$$\mathbf{V}_{af} = \mathbf{V}_{a0} + \mathbf{V}_{a1} + \mathbf{V}_{a2} \tag{9.149}$$

Therefore,

$$\mathbf{V}_{a0} + \mathbf{V}_{a1} + \mathbf{V}_{a2} = 3\mathbf{Z}_f \mathbf{I}_{a1} \tag{9.150}$$

which justifies the interconnection of sequence networks in series, as shown in Figure 9.17b.

---

* The fault impedance $\mathbf{Z}_f$ may be thought of as the impedances in the arc (in the event of having a flashover between the line and a tower), the tower, and the tower footing.

Once the sequence currents are found, the zero-, positive-, and negative-sequence voltages can be found from

$$
\begin{bmatrix} \mathbf{V}_{a0} \\ \mathbf{V}_{a1} \\ \mathbf{V}_{a2} \end{bmatrix} = \begin{bmatrix} 0 \\ 1.0\angle 0^\circ \\ 0 \end{bmatrix} - \begin{bmatrix} \mathbf{Z}_0 & 0 & 0 \\ 0 & \mathbf{Z}_1 & 0 \\ 0 & 0 & \mathbf{Z}_2 \end{bmatrix} \begin{bmatrix} \mathbf{I}_{a0} \\ \mathbf{I}_{a1} \\ \mathbf{I}_{a2} \end{bmatrix}
\tag{9.151}
$$

as

$$
\mathbf{V}_{a0} = -\mathbf{Z}_0 \mathbf{I}_{a0}
\tag{9.152}
$$

$$
\mathbf{V}_{a1} = 1.0 - \mathbf{Z}_1 \mathbf{I}_{a1}
\tag{9.153}
$$

$$
\mathbf{V}_{a2} = -\mathbf{Z}_2 \mathbf{I}_{a2}
\tag{9.154}
$$

In the event of having an SLG fault on phase b or c, the voltages related to the known phase a voltage components can be found from

$$
\begin{bmatrix} \mathbf{V}_{af} \\ \mathbf{V}_{bf} \\ \mathbf{V}_{cf} \end{bmatrix} = \begin{bmatrix} 1 & 1 & 1 \\ 1 & \mathbf{a}^2 & \mathbf{a} \\ 1 & \mathbf{a} & \mathbf{a}^2 \end{bmatrix} \begin{bmatrix} \mathbf{V}_{a0} \\ \mathbf{V}_{a1} \\ \mathbf{V}_{a2} \end{bmatrix}
\tag{9.155}
$$

as

$$
\mathbf{V}_{bf} = \mathbf{V}_{a0} + \mathbf{a}^2 \mathbf{V}_{a1} + \mathbf{a} \mathbf{V}_{a2}
\tag{9.156}
$$

and

$$
\mathbf{V}_{cf} = \mathbf{V}_{a0} + \mathbf{a} \mathbf{V}_{a1} + \mathbf{a}^2 \mathbf{V}_{a2}
\tag{9.157}
$$

Example 9.9

Consider the system described in Examples 9.7 and 9.8, and assume that there is an SLG fault, involving phase a, and that the fault impedance is $5 + j0\ \Omega$. Also assume that $\mathbf{Z}_0$, $\mathbf{Z}_1$, and $\mathbf{Z}_2$ are $j0.56$, $j0.2618$, and $j0.3619\ \Omega$, respectively.

(a) Show the interconnection of the corresponding equivalent sequence networks.
(b) Determine the sequence and phase currents.
(c) Determine the sequence and phase voltages.
(d) Determine the line-to-line voltages.

Solution

(a) Figure 9.18 shows the interconnection of the resulting equivalent sequence networks.
(b) The impedance base on the 230 kV line is

$$
\mathbf{Z}_B = \frac{230^2}{200} = 264.5\ \Omega
$$

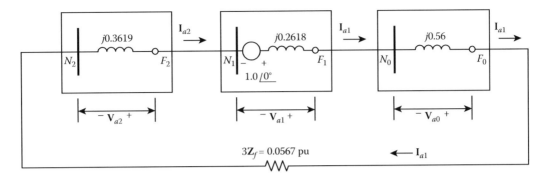

FIGURE 9.18 The interconnection of resultant equivalent sequence networks of Example 9.9.

Therefore,

$$\mathbf{Z}_f = \frac{5\ \Omega}{264.5\ \Omega} = 0.0189\ \text{pu}\ \Omega$$

Thus, the sequence currents and the phase currents are

$$\mathbf{I}_{a0} = \mathbf{I}_{a1} = \mathbf{I}_{a2} = \frac{1.0\angle 0°}{\mathbf{Z}_0 + \mathbf{Z}_1 + \mathbf{Z}_2 + 3\mathbf{Z}_f}$$

$$= \frac{1.0\angle 0°}{j0.56 + j0.2618 + j0.3619 + 0.0567}$$

$$= 0.8438\angle -87.2571°\ \text{pu A}$$

and

$$\begin{bmatrix} \mathbf{I}_{af} \\ \mathbf{I}_{bf} \\ \mathbf{I}_{cf} \end{bmatrix} = \begin{bmatrix} 1 & 1 & 1 \\ 1 & \mathbf{a}^2 & \mathbf{a} \\ 1 & \mathbf{a} & \mathbf{a}^2 \end{bmatrix} \begin{bmatrix} 0.8438\angle -87.3° \\ 0.8438\angle -87.3° \\ 0.8438\angle -87.3° \end{bmatrix} = \begin{bmatrix} 2.5315\angle -87.2571° \\ 0 \\ 0 \end{bmatrix} \text{pu A}$$

(c) The sequence and phase voltages are

$$\begin{bmatrix} \mathbf{V}_{a0} \\ \mathbf{V}_{a1} \\ \mathbf{V}_{a2} \end{bmatrix} = \begin{bmatrix} 0 \\ 1.0\angle 0° \\ 0 \end{bmatrix} - \begin{bmatrix} j0.56 & 0 & 0 \\ 0 & j0.2618 & 0 \\ 0 & 0 & j0.3619 \end{bmatrix} \begin{bmatrix} 0.8438\angle -87.3° \\ 0.8438\angle -87.3° \\ 0.8438\angle -87.3° \end{bmatrix}$$

$$= \begin{bmatrix} 0.4726\angle -177.7° \\ 0.7794\angle -0.8° \\ 0.3054\angle -177.7° \end{bmatrix} \text{pu V}$$

and

$$\begin{bmatrix} \mathbf{V}_{af} \\ \mathbf{V}_{bf} \\ \mathbf{V}_{cf} \end{bmatrix} = \begin{bmatrix} 1 & 1 & 1 \\ 1 & \mathbf{a}^2 & \mathbf{a} \\ 1 & \mathbf{a} & \mathbf{a}^2 \end{bmatrix} \begin{bmatrix} 0.4725\angle -177.7° \\ 0.7794\angle -0.8° \\ 0.3054\angle -177.7° \end{bmatrix} = \begin{bmatrix} 0.0479\angle -87.26° \\ 1.1827\angle -126.6° \\ 1.1709\angle 127.4919° \end{bmatrix} \text{pu V}$$

(d) The line-to-line voltages at the fault point are

$$\mathbf{V}_{abf} = \mathbf{V}_{af} - \mathbf{V}_{bf}$$
$$= 0.0479\angle - 87.2571° - 1.1827\angle - 126.6°$$
$$= 1.146\angle 51.85° \text{ pu V}$$

$$\mathbf{V}_{bcf} = \mathbf{V}_{bf} - \mathbf{V}_{cf}$$
$$= 1.1827\angle - 126.6° - 1.1709\angle 127.4919°$$
$$= 1.878\angle - 89.785° \text{ pu V}$$

$$\mathbf{V}_{caf} = \mathbf{V}_{cf} - \mathbf{V}_{af}$$
$$= 1.1709\angle 127.4919° - 0.0479\angle - 87.2571°$$
$$= 1.2107\angle 126.2° \text{ pu V}$$

Example 9.10

Consider the system given in Figure 9.19a and assume that the given impedance values are based on the same megavolt-ampere value. The two three-phase transformer banks are made of three single-phase transformers. Assume that there is an SLG fault, involving phase a, at the middle of the transmission line TL_{23}, as shown in the figure.

(a) Draw the corresponding positive-, negative-, and zero-sequence networks, without reducing them, and their corresponding interconnections.
(b) Determine the sequence currents at fault point F.
(c) Determine the sequence currents at the terminals of generator G_1.
(d) Determine the phase currents at the terminals of generator G_1.
(e) Determine the sequence voltages at the terminals of generator G_1.
(f) Determine the phase voltages at the terminals of generator G_1.
(g) Repeat parts (c) through (f) for generator G_2.

Solution

(a) Figure 9.19b shows the corresponding sequence networks.
(b) The sequence currents at fault point F are

$$\mathbf{I}_{a0} = \mathbf{I}_{a1} = \mathbf{I}_{a2} = \frac{1.0\angle 0°}{\mathbf{Z}_0 + \mathbf{Z}_1 + \mathbf{Z}_2}$$
$$= \frac{1.0\angle 0°}{j0.2619 + j0.25 + j0.25}$$
$$= -j1.3125 \text{ pu A}$$

(c) Therefore, the sequence current contributions of generator G_1 can be found by symmetry as

$$\mathbf{I}_{a1,G_1} = \frac{1}{2} \times \mathbf{I}_{a1} = -j0.6563 \text{ pu A}$$

and

$$\mathbf{I}_{a2,G_1} = \frac{1}{2} \times \mathbf{I}_{a2} = -j0.6563 \text{ pu A}$$

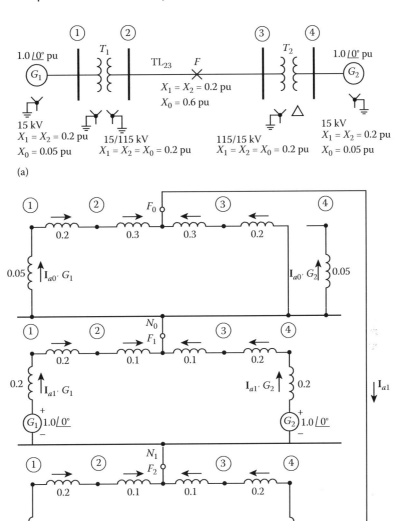

FIGURE 9.19   The system and the solution for Example 9.10.

and by current division

$$\mathbf{I}_{a0,G_1} = \frac{0.5}{0.55+0.5} \times \mathbf{I}_{a0} = -j0.6250 \text{ pu A}$$

(d) The phase currents at the terminals of generator G_1 are

$$\begin{bmatrix} \mathbf{I}_{af} \\ \mathbf{I}_{bf} \\ \mathbf{I}_{cf} \end{bmatrix} = \begin{bmatrix} 1 & 1 & 1 \\ 1 & \mathbf{a}^2 & \mathbf{a} \\ 1 & \mathbf{a} & \mathbf{a}^2 \end{bmatrix} \begin{bmatrix} 0.6250\angle -90° \\ 0.6563\angle -90° \\ 0.6563\angle -90° \end{bmatrix} = \begin{bmatrix} 1.9375\angle -90° \\ 0.0312\angle 90° \\ 0.0312\angle 90° \end{bmatrix} \text{ pu A}$$

(e)　The sequence voltages at the terminals of generator G_1 are

$$
\begin{bmatrix} \mathbf{V}_{a0} \\ \mathbf{V}_{a1} \\ \mathbf{V}_{a2} \end{bmatrix} = \begin{bmatrix} 0 \\ 1.0\angle 0° \\ 0 \end{bmatrix} - \begin{bmatrix} j0.2619 & 0 & 0 \\ 0 & j0.25 & 0 \\ 0 & 0 & j0.25 \end{bmatrix} \begin{bmatrix} 0.6250\angle -90° \\ 0.6563\angle -90° \\ 0.6563\angle -90° \end{bmatrix}
$$

$$
= \begin{bmatrix} 0.1637\angle 180° \\ 0.8359\angle 0° \\ 0.1641\angle 180° \end{bmatrix} \text{pu V}
$$

(f)　Therefore, the phase voltages are

$$
\begin{bmatrix} \mathbf{V}_{af} \\ \mathbf{V}_{bf} \\ \mathbf{V}_{cf} \end{bmatrix} = \begin{bmatrix} 1 & 1 & 1 \\ 1 & a^2 & a \\ 1 & a & a^2 \end{bmatrix} \begin{bmatrix} 0.1641\angle 180° \\ 0.8359\angle 0° \\ 0.1641\angle 180° \end{bmatrix} \cong \begin{bmatrix} 0.5082\angle 0° \\ 0.9998\angle -120° \\ 0.9998\angle 120° \end{bmatrix} \text{pu V}
$$

(g)　Similarly, for generator G_2, by symmetry,

$$
\mathbf{I}_{a1,G_2} = \frac{1}{2} \times \mathbf{I}_{a1} = -j0.6563 \text{ pu A}
$$

and

$$
\mathbf{I}_{a2,G_2} = \frac{1}{2} \times \mathbf{I}_{a2} = -j0.6563 \text{ pu A}
$$

and by inspection

$$
\mathbf{I}_{a0,G_2} = 0
$$

However, *since transformer T_2 has wye–delta connections and the US standard terminal markings provide that $\mathbf{V}_{a1(HV)}$ leads $\mathbf{V}_{a1(LV)}$ by 30° and $\mathbf{V}_{a2(HV)}$ lags $\mathbf{V}_{a2(LV)}$ by 30°, regardless of which side has the delta-connected windings,* taking into account the 30° phase shifts,

$$
\mathbf{I}_{a1,G_2} = 0.6563\angle -90° -30°
$$
$$
= 0.6563\angle -120° \text{ pu A}
$$

and

$$
\mathbf{I}_{a2,G_2} = 0.6563\angle -90° +30°
$$
$$
= 0.6563\angle -60° \text{ pu A}
$$

This is because generator G_2 is on the LV side of the transformer. Therefore,

$$
\begin{bmatrix} \mathbf{I}_{af} \\ \mathbf{I}_{bf} \\ \mathbf{I}_{cf} \end{bmatrix} = \begin{bmatrix} 1 & 1 & 1 \\ 1 & a^2 & a \\ 1 & a & a^2 \end{bmatrix} \begin{bmatrix} 0 \\ 0.6563\angle -120° \\ 0.6563\angle -60° \end{bmatrix} = \begin{bmatrix} 1.1367\angle -90° \\ 1.1366\angle 90° \\ 0 \end{bmatrix} \text{pu A}
$$

The positive- and negative-sequence voltages on the G_2 side are the same as on the G_1 side. Thus,

$$\mathbf{V}_{a1} = 0.8434\angle 0° \text{ pu V}$$

$$\mathbf{V}_{a2} = 0.1641\angle 180° \text{ pu V}$$

Again, taking into account the 30° phase shifts,

$$\mathbf{V}_{a1} = 0.8434\angle 0° - 30°$$
$$= 0.8434\angle - 30° \text{ pu V}$$

$$\mathbf{V}_{a2} = 0.1641\angle 180° + 30°$$
$$= 0.1641\angle 210° \text{ pu V}$$

Obviously,

$$\mathbf{V}_{a0} = 0$$

Therefore, the phase voltages at the terminals of generator G_2 are

$$\begin{bmatrix} \mathbf{V}_{af} \\ \mathbf{V}_{bf} \\ \mathbf{V}_{cf} \end{bmatrix} = \begin{bmatrix} 1 & 1 & 1 \\ 1 & \mathbf{a}^2 & \mathbf{a} \\ 1 & \mathbf{a} & \mathbf{a}^2 \end{bmatrix} \begin{bmatrix} 0 \\ 0.8434\angle - 30° \\ 0.1641\angle 210° \end{bmatrix} \cong \begin{bmatrix} 0.7672\angle - 40.673° \\ 0.7671\angle - 139.33° \\ 1.0000\angle 90° \end{bmatrix} \text{pu V}$$

9.12.2 LINE-TO-LINE FAULT

In general, a *line-to-line* (L-L) fault on a transmission system occurs when two conductors are short-circuited.* Figure 9.20a shows the general representation of a line-to-line fault at fault point F with a fault impedance $\mathbf{Z}_f$. Figure 9.20b shows the interconnection of resulting sequence networks. It is assumed, for the sake of symmetry, that the line-to-line fault is between phases b and c. It can be observed from Figure 9.20a that

$$\mathbf{I}_{af} = 0 \tag{9.158}$$

$$\mathbf{I}_{bf} = -\mathbf{I}_{cf} \tag{9.159}$$

$$\mathbf{V}_{bc} = \mathbf{V}_b - \mathbf{V}_c = \mathbf{Z}_f \mathbf{I}_{bf} \tag{9.160}$$

From Figure 9.20b, the sequence currents can be found as

$$\mathbf{I}_{a0} = 0 \tag{9.161}$$

$$\mathbf{I}_{a1} = -\mathbf{I}_{a2} = \frac{1.0\angle 0°}{\mathbf{Z}_1 + \mathbf{Z}_2 + \mathbf{Z}_f} \tag{9.162}$$

---

* Note that $\left|\mathbf{I}_{f,\text{L-L}}\right| = 0.866 \left|\mathbf{I}_{f,3\phi}\right|$. Therefore, if the magnitude of the three-phase fault current is known, the magnitude of the line-to-line fault current can readily be found.

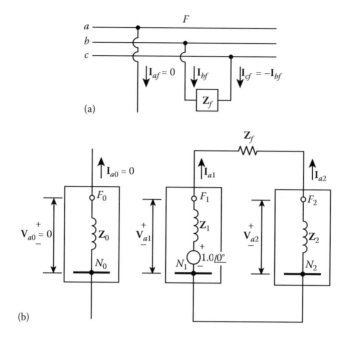

FIGURE 9.20   Line-to-line fault: (a) general representation; (b) interconnection of sequence networks.

If $\mathbf{Z}_f = 0$,

$$\mathbf{I}_{a1} = -\mathbf{I}_{a2} = \frac{1.0\angle 0°}{\mathbf{Z}_1 + \mathbf{Z}_2} \tag{9.163}$$

Substituting Equations 9.161 and 9.162 into Equation 9.145, the fault currents for phases a and b can be found as

$$\mathbf{I}_{bf} = -\mathbf{I}_{cf} = \sqrt{3}\mathbf{I}_{a1}\angle -90° \tag{9.164}$$

Similarly, substituting Equations 9.161 and 9.162 into Equation 9.151, the sequence voltages can be found as

$$\mathbf{V}_{a0} = 0 \tag{9.165}$$

$$\mathbf{V}_{a1} = 1.0 - \mathbf{Z}_1\mathbf{I}_{a1} \tag{9.166}$$

$$\mathbf{V}_{a2} = -\mathbf{Z}_2\mathbf{I}_{a2} = \mathbf{Z}_2\mathbf{I}_{a1} \tag{9.167}$$

Also, substituting Equations 9.165 through 9.167 into Equation 9.155,

$$\mathbf{V}_{af} = \mathbf{V}_{a1} + \mathbf{V}_{a2} \tag{9.168}$$

or

$$\mathbf{V}_{af} = 1.0 + \mathbf{I}_{a1}(\mathbf{Z}_2 - \mathbf{Z}_1) \tag{9.169}$$

and

$$\mathbf{V}_{bf} = \mathbf{a}^2\mathbf{V}_{a1} + \mathbf{a}\mathbf{V}_{a2} \tag{9.170}$$

or

$$\mathbf{V}_{bf} = \mathbf{a}^2 + \mathbf{I}_{a1}(\mathbf{a}\mathbf{Z}_2 - \mathbf{a}^2\mathbf{Z}_1) \tag{9.171}$$

and

$$\mathbf{V}_{cf} = \mathbf{a}\mathbf{V}_{a1} + \mathbf{a}^2\mathbf{V}_{a2} \tag{9.172}$$

or

$$\mathbf{V}_{cf} = \mathbf{a} + \mathbf{I}_{a1}(\mathbf{a}^2\mathbf{Z}_2 - \mathbf{a}\mathbf{Z}_1) \tag{9.173}$$

Thus, the line-to-line voltages can be expressed as

$$\mathbf{V}_{ab} = \mathbf{V}_{af} - \mathbf{V}_{bf} \tag{9.174}$$

or

$$\mathbf{V}_{ab} = \sqrt{3}\left(\mathbf{V}_{a1}\angle 30° + \mathbf{V}_{a2}\angle -30°\right) \tag{9.175}$$

and

$$\mathbf{V}_{bc} = \mathbf{V}_{bf} - \mathbf{V}_{cf} \tag{9.176}$$

or

$$\mathbf{V}_{bc} = \sqrt{3}\left(\mathbf{V}_{a1}\angle -90° + \mathbf{V}_{a2}\angle 90°\right) \tag{9.177}$$

and

$$\mathbf{V}_{ca} = \mathbf{V}_{cf} - \mathbf{V}_{af} \tag{9.178}$$

or

$$\mathbf{V}_{ca} = \sqrt{3}\left(\mathbf{V}_{a1}\angle 150° + \mathbf{V}_{a2}\angle -150°\right) \tag{9.179}$$

Example 9.11

Repeat Example 9.9 assuming that there is a line-to-line fault, involving phases b and c, at bus 3.

Solution

(a) Figure 9.21 shows the interconnection of the resulting equivalent sequence networks.
(b) The sequence and the phase currents are

$$\mathbf{I}_{a0} = 0$$

$$\mathbf{I}_{a1} = -\mathbf{I}_{a2} = \frac{1.0\angle 0°}{\mathbf{Z}_1 + \mathbf{Z}_2 + \mathbf{Z}_f}$$

$$= \frac{1.0\angle 0°}{j0.2618 + j0.3619 + 0.0189}$$

$$= 1.6026\angle -88.3° \text{ pu A}$$

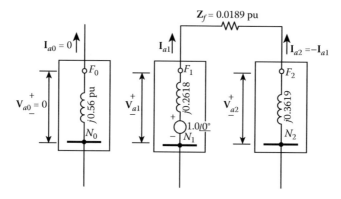

FIGURE 9.21   The interconnection of resultant equivalent sequence networks of Example 9.11.

and

$$
\begin{bmatrix} \mathbf{I}_{af} \\ \mathbf{I}_{bf} \\ \mathbf{I}_{cf} \end{bmatrix} = \begin{bmatrix} 1 & 1 & 1 \\ 1 & a^2 & a \\ 1 & a & a^2 \end{bmatrix} \begin{bmatrix} 0 \\ 1.6026\angle -88.3° \\ 1.6026\angle 91.7° \end{bmatrix} = \begin{bmatrix} 0 \\ 2.7757\angle -178.3° \\ 2.7757\angle 1.74° \end{bmatrix} \text{pu A}
$$

(c) The sequence and phase voltages are

$$
\begin{bmatrix} \mathbf{V}_{a0} \\ \mathbf{V}_{a1} \\ \mathbf{V}_{a2} \end{bmatrix} = \begin{bmatrix} 0 \\ 1.0\angle 0° \\ 0 \end{bmatrix} - \begin{bmatrix} j0.56 & 0 & 0 \\ 0 & j0.2618 & 0 \\ 0 & 0 & j0.3619 \end{bmatrix} \begin{bmatrix} 0 \\ 1.6026\angle -88.3° \\ 1.6026\angle 91.7° \end{bmatrix}
$$
$$
= \begin{bmatrix} 0 \\ 0.5808\angle -1.26° \\ 0.5800\angle 1.74° \end{bmatrix} \text{pu V}
$$

and

$$
\begin{bmatrix} \mathbf{V}_{af} \\ \mathbf{V}_{bf} \\ \mathbf{V}_{cf} \end{bmatrix} = \begin{bmatrix} 1 & 1 & 1 \\ 1 & a^2 & a \\ 1 & a & a^2 \end{bmatrix} \begin{bmatrix} 0 \\ 0.5808\angle -1.2° \\ 0.5800\angle 1.7° \end{bmatrix} = \begin{bmatrix} 1.1604\angle 0.24° \\ 0.6064\angle -179.3° \\ 0.5540\angle -179.83° \end{bmatrix} \text{pu V}
$$

(d) The line-to-line voltages at the fault point are

$$
\mathbf{V}_{abf} = \mathbf{V}_{af} - \mathbf{V}_{bf} = 0.5546 + j0.0073 \cong 1.7668\angle 0.26° \text{ pu V}
$$

$$
\mathbf{V}_{bcf} = \mathbf{V}_{bf} - \mathbf{V}_{cf} = 0.0509 - j0.0013 \cong 0.0525\angle -178.3° \text{ pu V}
$$

$$
\mathbf{V}_{caf} = \mathbf{V}_{cf} - \mathbf{V}_{af} = -0.6055 - j0.006 \cong 1.7143\angle -179.8° \text{ pu V}
$$

9.12.3 Double Line-to-Ground Fault

In general, the DLG fault on a transmission system occurs when two conductors fall and are connected through ground or when two conductors contact the neutral of a three-phase grounded system. Figure 9.22a shows the general representation of a DLG fault at a fault point F with a fault impedance $\mathbf{Z}_f$ and the impedance from line-to-ground $\mathbf{Z}_g$ (which can be equal to zero or infinity). Figure 9.22b shows the interconnection of resultant sequence networks. As before, it is assumed, for the sake of symmetry, that the DLG fault is between phases b and c. It can be observed from Figure 9.22a that

$$\mathbf{I}_{af} = 0 \tag{9.180}$$

$$\mathbf{V}_{bf} = (\mathbf{Z}_f + \mathbf{Z}_g)\mathbf{I}_{bf} + \mathbf{Z}_g\mathbf{I}_{cf} \tag{9.181}$$

$$\mathbf{V}_{cf} = (\mathbf{Z}_f + \mathbf{Z}_g)\mathbf{I}_{cf} + \mathbf{Z}_g\mathbf{I}_{bf} \tag{9.182}$$

From Figure 9.22b, the positive-sequence current can be found as

$$\mathbf{I}_{a1} = \frac{1.0\angle 0^\circ}{\left(\mathbf{Z}_1 + \mathbf{Z}_f\right) + \dfrac{\left(\mathbf{Z}_2 + \mathbf{Z}_f\right)\left(\mathbf{Z}_0 + \mathbf{Z}_f + 3\mathbf{Z}_g\right)}{\left(\mathbf{Z}_2 + \mathbf{Z}_f\right) + \left(\mathbf{Z}_0 + \mathbf{Z}_f + 3\mathbf{Z}_g\right)}} \tag{9.183a}$$

$$= \frac{1.0\angle 0^\circ}{\left(\mathbf{Z}_1 + \mathbf{Z}_f\right) + \dfrac{\left(\mathbf{Z}_2 + \mathbf{Z}_f\right)\left(\mathbf{Z}_0 + \mathbf{Z}_f + 3\mathbf{Z}_g\right)}{\mathbf{Z}_0 + \mathbf{Z}_2 + 2\mathbf{Z}_f + 3\mathbf{Z}_g}} \tag{9.183b}$$

The negative- and zero-sequence currents can be found, by using current division, as

$$\mathbf{I}_{a2} = -\left[\frac{\left(\mathbf{Z}_0 + \mathbf{Z}_f + 3\mathbf{Z}_g\right)}{\left(\mathbf{Z}_2 + \mathbf{Z}_f\right) + \left(\mathbf{Z}_0 + \mathbf{Z}_f + 3\mathbf{Z}_g\right)}\right]\mathbf{I}_{a1} \tag{9.184}$$

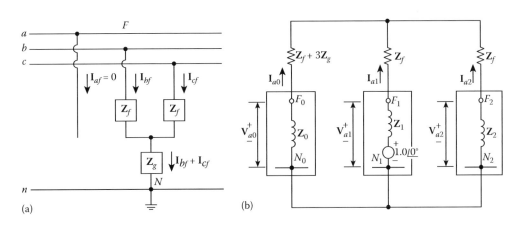

FIGURE 9.22 DLG fault: (a) general representation; (b) interconnection of sequence networks.

and

$$\mathbf{I}_{a0} = -\left[\frac{\left(\mathbf{Z}_2 + \mathbf{Z}_f\right)}{\left(\mathbf{Z}_2 + \mathbf{Z}_f\right) + \left(\mathbf{Z}_0 + \mathbf{Z}_f + 3\mathbf{Z}_g\right)}\right]\mathbf{I}_{a1} \tag{9.185}$$

or as an alternative method, since

$$\mathbf{I}_{af} = 0 = \mathbf{I}_{a0} + \mathbf{I}_{a1} + \mathbf{I}_{a2}$$

then if $\mathbf{I}_{a1}$ and $\mathbf{I}_{a2}$ are known,

$$\mathbf{I}_{a0} = -(\mathbf{I}_{a1} + \mathbf{I}_{a2}) \tag{9.186}$$

Note that in the event of having $\mathbf{Z}_f = 0$ and $\mathbf{Z}_g = 0$, the positive, negative, and zero sequences can be expressed as

$$\mathbf{I}_{a1} = \frac{1.0\angle 0^\circ}{\mathbf{Z}_1 + \dfrac{\mathbf{Z}_0 \times \mathbf{Z}_2}{\mathbf{Z}_0 + \mathbf{Z}_2}} \tag{9.187}$$

and

$$\mathbf{I}_{a2} = -\left[\frac{\mathbf{Z}_0}{\mathbf{Z}_0 + \mathbf{Z}_2}\right]\mathbf{I}_{a1} \tag{9.188}$$

$$\mathbf{I}_{a0} = -\left[\frac{\mathbf{Z}_2}{\mathbf{Z}_0 + \mathbf{Z}_2}\right]\mathbf{I}_{a1} \tag{9.189}$$

Note that the fault current for phase a is already known to be

$$\mathbf{I}_{af} = 0$$

the fault currents for phases a and b that can be found by substituting Equations 9.183 through 9.185 into Equation 9.145 so that

$$\mathbf{I}_{bf} = \mathbf{I}_{a0} + \mathbf{a}^2\mathbf{I}_{a1} + \mathbf{a}\mathbf{I}_{a2} \tag{9.190}$$

and

$$\mathbf{I}_{cf} = \mathbf{I}_{a0} + \mathbf{a}\mathbf{I}_{a1} + \mathbf{a}^2\mathbf{I}_{a2} \tag{9.191}$$

It can be shown that the total fault current flowing into the neutral is

$$\mathbf{I}_n = \mathbf{I}_{bf} + \mathbf{I}_{cf} = 3\mathbf{I}_{a0} \tag{9.192}$$

The sequence voltages can be found from Equation 9.151 as

$$\mathbf{V}_{a0} = -\mathbf{Z}_0 \mathbf{I}_{a0} \tag{9.193}$$

$$\mathbf{V}_{a1} = 1.0 - \mathbf{Z}_1 \mathbf{I}_{a1} \tag{9.194}$$

$$\mathbf{V}_{a2} = -\mathbf{Z}_2 \mathbf{I}_{a2} \tag{9.195}$$

Similarly, the phase voltages can be found from Equation 9.155 as

$$\mathbf{V}_{af} = \mathbf{V}_{a0} + \mathbf{V}_{a1} + \mathbf{V}_{a2} \tag{9.196}$$

$$\mathbf{V}_{bf} = \mathbf{V}_{a0} + \mathbf{a}^2 \mathbf{V}_{a1} + \mathbf{a} \mathbf{V}_{a2} \tag{9.197}$$

$$\mathbf{V}_{cf} = \mathbf{V}_{a0} + \mathbf{a} \mathbf{V}_{a1} + \mathbf{a}^2 \mathbf{V}_{a2} \tag{9.198}$$

or, alternatively, the phase voltages $\mathbf{V}_{bf}$ and $\mathbf{V}_{cf}$ can be determined from Equations 9.181 and 9.182, respectively. As before, the line-to-line voltages can be found from

$$\mathbf{V}_{ab} = \mathbf{V}_{af} - \mathbf{V}_{bf} \tag{9.199}$$

$$\mathbf{V}_{bc} = \mathbf{V}_{bf} - \mathbf{V}_{cf} \tag{9.200}$$

$$\mathbf{V}_{ca} = \mathbf{V}_{cf} - \mathbf{V}_{af} \tag{9.201}$$

Note that in the event of having $\mathbf{Z}_f = 0$ and $\mathbf{Z}_g = 0$, the sequence voltages become

$$\mathbf{V}_{a0} = \mathbf{V}_{a1} = \mathbf{V}_{a2} = 1.0 - \mathbf{Z}_1 \mathbf{I}_{a1} \tag{9.202}$$

where the positive-sequence current is found by using Equation 9.187. Once the sequence voltages are determined from Equation 9.202, the negative- and zero-sequence currents can be determined from

$$\mathbf{I}_{a2} = -\frac{\mathbf{V}_{a2}}{\mathbf{Z}_2} \tag{9.203}$$

and

$$\mathbf{I}_{a0} = -\frac{\mathbf{V}_{a0}}{\mathbf{Z}_0} \tag{9.204}$$

Using the relationship given in Equation 9.202, the resultant phase voltages can be expressed as

$$\mathbf{V}_{af} = \mathbf{V}_{a0} + \mathbf{V}_{a1} + \mathbf{V}_{a2} = 3\mathbf{V}_{a1} \tag{9.205}$$

$$\mathbf{V}_{bf} = \mathbf{V}_{cf} = 0 \tag{9.206}$$

Therefore, the line-to-line voltages become

$$\mathbf{V}_{abf} = \mathbf{V}_{af} - \mathbf{V}_{bf} = \mathbf{V}_{af} \tag{9.207}$$

$$\mathbf{V}_{bcf} = \mathbf{V}_{bf} - \mathbf{V}_{cf} = 0 \tag{9.208}$$

$$\mathbf{V}_{caf} = \mathbf{V}_{cf} - \mathbf{V}_{af} = -\mathbf{V}_{af} \tag{9.209}$$

Example 9.12

Repeat Example 9.9 assuming that there is a DLG fault with $\mathbf{Z}_f = 5\ \Omega$ and $\mathbf{Z}_g = 10\ \Omega$, involving phases b and c, at bus 3.

Solution

(a) Figure 9.23 shows the interconnection of the resulting equivalent sequence networks.
(b) Since

$$\mathbf{Z}_f + 3\mathbf{Z}_g = \frac{5+30}{264.5} = 0.1323\ \text{pu}\ \Omega$$

the sequence currents are

$$\mathbf{I}_{a1} = \frac{1.0\angle 0°}{\left(\mathbf{Z}_1 + \mathbf{Z}_f\right) + \dfrac{\left(\mathbf{Z}_2 + \mathbf{Z}_f\right)\left(\mathbf{Z}_0 + \mathbf{Z}_f + 3\mathbf{Z}_g\right)}{\left(\mathbf{Z}_2 + \mathbf{Z}_f\right) + \left(\mathbf{Z}_0 + \mathbf{Z}_f + 3\mathbf{Z}_g\right)}}$$

$$= \frac{1.0\angle 0°}{(j0.2618 + 0.0189) + \dfrac{(j0.3619 + 0.0189)(j0.56 + 0.1323)}{j0.3619 + 0.0189 + j0.56 + 0.1323}}$$

$$\cong 2.0595\angle -84.57°\ \text{pu}\ \Omega$$

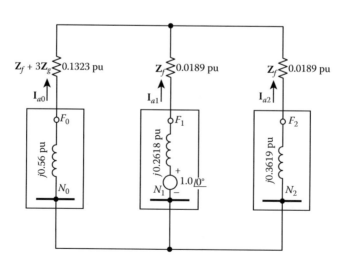

FIGURE 9.23   The interconnection of resultant equivalent sequence networks of Example 9.12.

$$\mathbf{I}_{a2} = -\left[\frac{\left(\mathbf{Z}_0 + \mathbf{Z}_f + 3\mathbf{Z}_g\right)}{\left(\mathbf{Z}_2 + \mathbf{Z}_f\right) + \left(\mathbf{Z}_0 + \mathbf{Z}_f + 3\mathbf{Z}_g\right)}\right]\mathbf{I}_{a1}$$

$$= -\left[\frac{0.5754\angle 76.7°}{0.9342\angle 80.7°}\right]\left(2.0597\angle -84.5°\right)$$

$$\cong -1.2685\angle 91.5° \text{ pu } \Omega$$

$$\mathbf{I}_{a0} = -\left[\frac{\left(\mathbf{Z}_2 + \mathbf{Z}_f\right)}{\left(\mathbf{Z}_2 + \mathbf{Z}_f\right) + \left(\mathbf{Z}_0 + \mathbf{Z}_f + 3\mathbf{Z}_g\right)}\right]\mathbf{I}_{a1}$$

$$= -\left[\frac{0.3624\angle 87°}{0.9342\angle 80.7°}\right]\left(2.0597\angle -84.5°\right)$$

$$\cong -0.7989\angle 101.76° \text{ pu } \Omega$$

and the phase currents are

$$\begin{bmatrix} \mathbf{I}_{af} \\ \mathbf{I}_{bf} \\ \mathbf{I}_{cf} \end{bmatrix} = \begin{bmatrix} 1 & 1 & 1 \\ 1 & a^2 & a \\ 1 & a & a^2 \end{bmatrix}\begin{bmatrix} -0.799\angle -78.2° \\ 2.0597\angle -84.5° \\ -1.2686\angle -88.5° \end{bmatrix} = \begin{bmatrix} 0 \\ 3.2673\angle 162.6° \\ 2.9650\angle 27.5° \end{bmatrix} \text{ pu A}$$

(c) The sequence and phase voltages are

$$\begin{bmatrix} \mathbf{V}_{a0} \\ \mathbf{V}_{a1} \\ \mathbf{V}_{a2} \end{bmatrix} = \begin{bmatrix} 0 \\ 1.0\angle 0° \\ 0 \end{bmatrix} - \begin{bmatrix} j0.56 & 0 & 0 \\ 0 & j0.2618 & 0 \\ 0 & 0 & j0.3619 \end{bmatrix}\begin{bmatrix} -0.799\angle -78.2° \\ 2.0597\angle -84.5° \\ -1.2686\angle -88.5° \end{bmatrix}$$

$$\cong \begin{bmatrix} 0.4474\angle 11.8° \\ 0.4660\angle -6.3° \\ 0.459\angle 1.5° \end{bmatrix} \text{ pu V}$$

and

$$\begin{bmatrix} \mathbf{V}_{af} \\ \mathbf{V}_{bf} \\ \mathbf{V}_{cf} \end{bmatrix} = \begin{bmatrix} 1 & 1 & 1 \\ 1 & a^2 & a \\ 1 & a & a^2 \end{bmatrix}\begin{bmatrix} 0.4474\angle 11.8° \\ 0.4662\angle -6.4° \\ 0.4591\angle 1.5° \end{bmatrix} \cong \begin{bmatrix} 1.3612\angle 2.2° \\ 0.1322\angle 126.1° \\ 0.1188\angle 74.8° \end{bmatrix} \text{ pu V}$$

(d) The line-to-line voltages at the fault point are

$$\mathbf{V}_{abf} = \mathbf{V}_{af} - \mathbf{V}_{bf} = 1.4386 - j0.0555 = 1.4386 \angle -2.2° \text{ pu } \Omega$$

$$\mathbf{V}_{bcf} = \mathbf{V}_{bf} - \mathbf{V}_{cf} = -0.1107 - j0.0077 = 0.111 \angle -176° \text{ pu } \Omega$$

$$\mathbf{V}_{caf} = \mathbf{V}_{cf} - \mathbf{V}_{af} = -1.3279 + j0.0632 = 1.3304 \angle 177.3° \text{ pu } \Omega$$

9.12.4 Three-Phase Fault

In general, the *three-phase* (3ϕ) fault is not an unbalanced (i.e., unsymmetrical) fault. Instead, the three-phase fault is a balanced (i.e., *symmetrical*) fault that could also be analyzed using symmetrical components. Figure 9.24a shows the general representation of a balanced three-phase fault at a fault point F with impedances $\mathbf{Z}_f$ and $\mathbf{Z}_g$. Figure 3.24b shows the lack of interconnection of resulting sequence networks. Instead, the sequence networks are short-circuited over their own fault impedances and are therefore isolated from each other. Since only the positive-sequence network is considered to have internal voltage source, the positive-, negative-, and zero-sequence currents can be expressed as

$$\mathbf{I}_{a1} = 0 \tag{9.210}$$

$$\mathbf{I}_{a2} = 0 \tag{9.211}$$

$$\mathbf{I}_{a1} = \frac{1.0\angle 0^\circ}{\mathbf{Z}_1 + \mathbf{Z}_f} \tag{9.212}$$

If the fault impedance $\mathbf{Z}_f$ is zero,

$$\mathbf{I}_{a1} = \frac{1.0\angle 0^\circ}{\mathbf{Z}_1} \tag{9.213}$$

Substituting Equations 9.210 through 9.212 into Equation 9.145,

$$\begin{bmatrix} \mathbf{I}_{af} \\ \mathbf{I}_{bf} \\ \mathbf{I}_{cf} \end{bmatrix} = \begin{bmatrix} 1 & 1 & 1 \\ 1 & \mathbf{a}^2 & \mathbf{a} \\ 1 & \mathbf{a} & \mathbf{a}^2 \end{bmatrix} \begin{bmatrix} 0 \\ \mathbf{I}_{a1} \\ 0 \end{bmatrix} \tag{9.214}$$

from which

$$\mathbf{I}_{af} = \mathbf{I}_{a1} = \frac{1.0\angle 0^\circ}{\mathbf{Z}_1 + \mathbf{Z}_f} \tag{9.215}$$

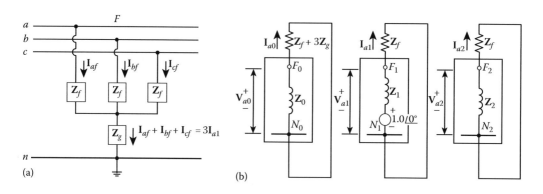

FIGURE 9.24   Three-phase fault: (a) general representation; (b) interconnection of sequence networks.

$$\mathbf{I}_{bf} = \mathbf{a}^2 \mathbf{I}_{a1} = \frac{1.0\angle 240°}{\mathbf{Z}_1 + \mathbf{Z}_f} \tag{9.216}$$

$$\mathbf{I}_{cf} = \mathbf{a}\mathbf{I}_{a1} = \frac{1.0\angle 120°}{\mathbf{Z}_1 + \mathbf{Z}_f} \tag{9.217}$$

Since the sequence networks are short-circuited over their own fault impedances,

$$\mathbf{V}_{a0} = 0 \tag{9.218}$$

$$\mathbf{V}_{a1} = \mathbf{Z}_f \mathbf{I}_{a1} \tag{9.219}$$

$$\mathbf{V}_{a2} = 0 \tag{9.220}$$

Therefore, substituting Equations 9.218 through 9.220 into Equation 9.155,

$$\begin{bmatrix} \mathbf{V}_{af} \\ \mathbf{V}_{bf} \\ \mathbf{V}_{cf} \end{bmatrix} = \begin{bmatrix} 1 & 1 & 1 \\ 1 & \mathbf{a}^2 & \mathbf{a} \\ 1 & \mathbf{a} & \mathbf{a}^2 \end{bmatrix} \begin{bmatrix} 0 \\ \mathbf{V}_{a1} \\ 0 \end{bmatrix} \tag{9.221}$$

Thus,

$$\mathbf{V}_{af} = \mathbf{V}_{a1} = \mathbf{Z}_f \mathbf{I}_{a1} \tag{9.222}$$

$$\mathbf{V}_{bf} = \mathbf{a}^2 \mathbf{V}_{a1} = \mathbf{Z}_f \mathbf{I}_{a1} \angle 240° \tag{9.223}$$

$$\mathbf{V}_{cf} = \mathbf{a}\mathbf{V}_{a1} = \mathbf{Z}_f \mathbf{I}_{a1} \angle 120° \tag{9.224}$$

Hence, the line-to-line voltages become

$$\mathbf{V}_{ab} = \mathbf{V}_{af} - \mathbf{V}_{bf} = \mathbf{V}_{a1}\left(1 - \mathbf{a}^2\right) = \sqrt{3}\mathbf{Z}_f \mathbf{I}_{a1} \angle 30° \tag{9.225}$$

$$\mathbf{V}_{bc} = \mathbf{V}_{bf} - \mathbf{V}_{cf} = \mathbf{V}_{a1}\left(\mathbf{a}^2 - \mathbf{a}\right) = \sqrt{3}\mathbf{Z}_f \mathbf{I}_{a1} \angle -90° \tag{9.226}$$

$$\mathbf{V}_{ca} = \mathbf{V}_{cf} - \mathbf{V}_{af} = \mathbf{V}_{a1}(\mathbf{a} - 1) = \sqrt{3}\mathbf{Z}_f \mathbf{I}_{a1} \angle 150° \tag{9.227}$$

Note that in the event of having $\mathbf{Z}_f = 0$,

$$\mathbf{I}_{af} = \frac{1.0\angle 0°}{\mathbf{Z}_1} \tag{9.228}$$

$$\mathbf{I}_{bf} = \frac{1.0\angle 240°}{\mathbf{Z}_1} \tag{9.229}$$

$$\mathbf{I}_{cf} = \frac{1.0\angle 120°}{\mathbf{Z}_1} \tag{9.230}$$

and

$$\mathbf{V}_{af} = 0 \tag{9.231}$$

$$\mathbf{V}_{bf} = 0 \tag{9.232}$$

$$\mathbf{V}_{cf} = 0 \tag{9.233}$$

and, of course,

$$\mathbf{V}_{a0} = 0 \tag{9.234}$$

$$\mathbf{V}_{a1} = 0 \tag{9.235}$$

$$\mathbf{V}_{a2} = 0 \tag{9.236}$$

Example 9.13

Repeat Example 9.9 assuming that there is a symmetrical three-phase fault with $\mathbf{Z}_f = 5\ \Omega$ and $\mathbf{Z}_g = 10\ \Omega$ at bus 3 where $\mathbf{Z}_B = 264.5\ \Omega$. Let $\mathbf{Z}_0 = j0.5$ pu Ω and $\mathbf{Z}_2 = j0.2317$ pu Ω.

Solution

(a) Figure 9.25 shows the interconnection of the resulting equivalent sequence networks.
(b) The sequence and phase currents are

$$\mathbf{I}_{a0} = \mathbf{I}_{a2} = 0$$

$$\mathbf{I}_{a1} = \frac{1.0\angle 0°}{\mathbf{Z}_1 + \mathbf{Z}_f} = \frac{1.0\angle 0°}{j0.2618 + 0.0189} = 3.8098\angle -85.9°\ \text{pu A}$$

and

$$\begin{bmatrix} \mathbf{I}_{af} \\ \mathbf{I}_{bf} \\ \mathbf{I}_{cf} \end{bmatrix} = \begin{bmatrix} 1 & 1 & 1 \\ 1 & a^2 & a \\ 1 & a & a^2 \end{bmatrix} \begin{bmatrix} 0 \\ 3.8098\angle -85.9° \\ 0 \end{bmatrix} \cong \begin{bmatrix} 3.8098\angle -85.87° \\ 3.8098\angle 154.13° \\ 3.8098\angle 34.13° \end{bmatrix} \text{pu A}$$

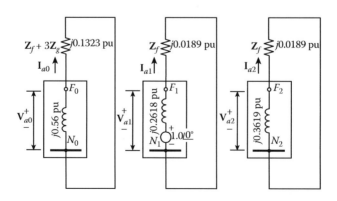

FIGURE 9.25   The interconnection of resultant equivalent sequence networks of Example 9.13.

(c) The sequence and phase voltages are

$$
\begin{bmatrix} \mathbf{V}_{a0} \\ \mathbf{V}_{a1} \\ \mathbf{V}_{a2} \end{bmatrix} = \begin{bmatrix} 0 \\ 1.0\angle 0° \\ 0 \end{bmatrix} - \begin{bmatrix} j0.5 & 0 & 0 \\ 0 & j0.2618 & 0 \\ 0 & 0 & j0.2317 \end{bmatrix} \begin{bmatrix} 0 \\ 3.8098\angle -85.9° \\ 0 \end{bmatrix}
$$

$$
= \begin{bmatrix} 0 \\ 0.072\angle -85.87° \\ 0 \end{bmatrix} \text{pu V}
$$

and

$$
\begin{bmatrix} \mathbf{V}_{af} \\ \mathbf{V}_{bf} \\ \mathbf{V}_{cf} \end{bmatrix} = \begin{bmatrix} 1 & 1 & 1 \\ 1 & \mathbf{a}^2 & \mathbf{a} \\ 1 & \mathbf{a} & \mathbf{a}^2 \end{bmatrix} \begin{bmatrix} 0 \\ 0.072\angle -85.9° \\ 0 \end{bmatrix} = \begin{bmatrix} 0.072\angle -85.87° \\ 0.072\angle 154.13° \\ 0.072\angle 34.13° \end{bmatrix} \text{pu V}
$$

(d) The line-to-line voltages at the fault point are

$$
\mathbf{V}_{abf} = \mathbf{V}_{af} - \mathbf{V}_{bf} = 0.0699 - j0.1033 = 0.1247\angle -55.87° \text{ pu V}
$$

$$
\mathbf{V}_{bcf} = \mathbf{V}_{bf} - \mathbf{V}_{cf} = -0.1244 - j0.0089 = 0.1247\angle -175.87° \text{ pu } \Omega
$$

$$
\mathbf{V}_{caf} = \mathbf{V}_{cf} - \mathbf{V}_{af} = 0.0545 + j0.1122 = 0.1247\angle 64.1° \text{ pu } V
$$

9.13   SERIES FAULTS

In general, the series (longitudinal) faults are due to an unbalanced series impedance condition of the lines. One or two broken lines, or an impedance inserted in one or two lines, may be considered as *series faults*. In practice, a series fault is encountered, for example, when line (or circuits) is controlled by CBs (or by fuses) or any device that does not open all three phases; one or two phases of the line (or the circuit) may be open, while the other phases or phase is closed.

Figure 9.26 shows a series fault due to one line (phase *a*) being open, which causes a series unbalance. In a series fault, contrary to a shunt fault, there are two fault points, *F* and *F'*, one on either side of the unbalance. The series line impedances **Z**'s can take any values between zero and infinity (in this case, obviously, the line impedance between points *F* and *F'* of phase *a* is infinity). The sequence networks include the symmetrical portions of the system, looking back to the left of *F* and to the right of *F'*. Since in series faults there is no connection between lines or between line(s) and neutral, only the sequence voltages of $\mathbf{V}_{aa'-0}$, $\mathbf{V}_{aa'-1}$, and $\mathbf{V}_{aa'-2}$ are of interest, not the sequence voltages of $\mathbf{V}_{a0}$, $\mathbf{V}_{a1}$, $\mathbf{V}_{a2}$, etc. (as it was the case with the shunt faults).

9.13.1   ONE LINE OPEN (OLO)

From Figure 9.26, it can be observed that the line impedance for the open-line conductor in phase *a* is infinity, whereas the line impedances for the other two phases have some finite values. Hence, the positive-, negative-, and zero-sequence currents can be expressed as

$$
\mathbf{I}_{a1} = \frac{\mathbf{V}_F}{\mathbf{Z} + \mathbf{Z}_1 + (\mathbf{Z} + \mathbf{Z}_0)(\mathbf{Z} + \mathbf{Z}_2)/(2\mathbf{Z} + \mathbf{Z}_0 + \mathbf{Z}_2)} \tag{9.237}
$$

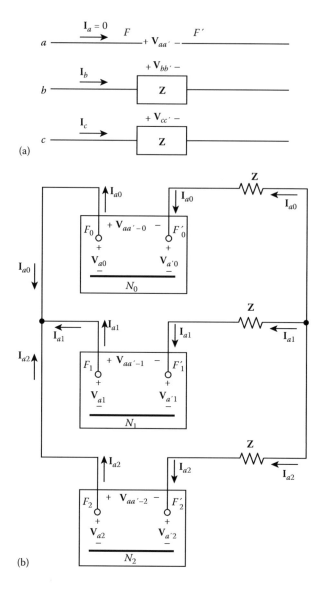

FIGURE 9.26 One line open: (a) general representation, (b) connection of sequence networks.

and by current division,

$$\mathbf{I}_{a2} = \left(-\frac{\mathbf{Z} + \mathbf{Z}_0}{2\mathbf{Z} + \mathbf{Z}_0 + \mathbf{Z}_2} \right) \mathbf{I}_{a1} \tag{9.238}$$

and

$$\mathbf{I}_{a0} = \left(-\frac{\mathbf{Z} + \mathbf{Z}_2}{2\mathbf{Z} + \mathbf{Z}_0 + \mathbf{Z}_2} \right) \mathbf{I}_{a1} \tag{9.239}$$

or simply

$$\mathbf{I}_{a0} = -\left(\mathbf{I}_{a1} + \mathbf{I}_{a2} \right) \tag{9.240}$$

9.13.2 Two Lines Open (TLO)

If two lines are open as shown in Figure 9.27, then the line impedances for OLO in phases b and c are infinity, whereas the line impedance of phase a has some finite value. Thus,

$$\mathbf{I}_b = \mathbf{I}_c = 0 \tag{9.241}$$

and

$$\mathbf{V}_{aa'} = \mathbf{ZI}_a \tag{9.242}$$

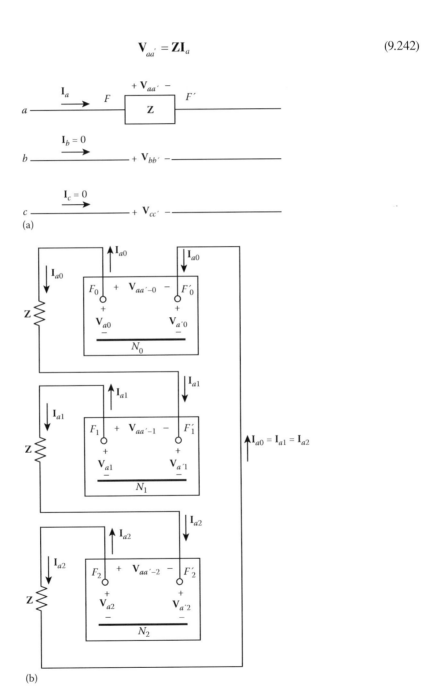

(a)

(b)

FIGURE 9.27 Two lines open: (a) general representation, (b) interconnection of sequence networks.

By inspection of Figure 9.27, the positive-, negative-, and zero-sequence currents can be expressed as

$$\mathbf{I}_{a1} = \mathbf{I}_{a2} = \mathbf{I}_{a0} = \frac{\mathbf{V}_F}{\mathbf{Z}_0 + \mathbf{Z}_1 + \mathbf{Z}_2 + 3\mathbf{Z}_f} \tag{9.243}$$

9.14 DETERMINATION OF SEQUENCE NETWORK EQUIVALENTS FOR SERIES FAULTS

Since the series faults have two fault pints (i.e., F and F'), contrary to the shunt faults having only one fault point, the direct application of the Thévenin theorem is not possible. Instead, what is needed is a two-port Thévenin equivalent of the sequence networks as suggested by Anderson [4].

9.14.1 BRIEF REVIEW OF TWO-PORT THEORY

Figure 9.28 shows a general two-port network for which it can be written that

$$\begin{bmatrix} \mathbf{V}_1 \\ \mathbf{V}_2 \end{bmatrix} = \begin{bmatrix} \mathbf{Z}_{11} & \mathbf{Z}_{12} \\ \mathbf{Z}_{21} & \mathbf{Z}_{22} \end{bmatrix} \begin{bmatrix} \mathbf{I}_1 \\ \mathbf{I}_2 \end{bmatrix} \tag{9.244}$$

where the *open-circuit impedance parameters* can be determined by leaving the ports open and expressed in terms of voltage and current as

$$\mathbf{Z}_{11} = \left. \frac{\mathbf{V}_1}{\mathbf{I}_1} \right|_{\mathbf{I}_2 = 0} \tag{9.245}$$

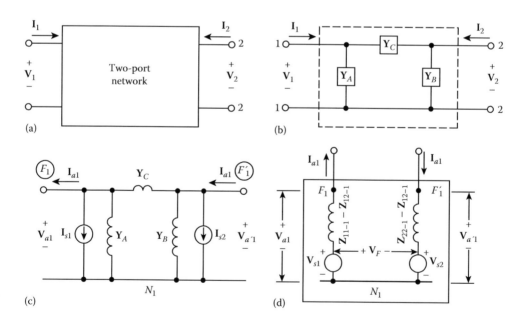

FIGURE 9.28 Application of two-port network theory for determining equivalent positive-sequence network for series faults: (a) general two-port network, (b) general π-equivalent positive-sequence network, (c) equivalent positive-sequence network, and (d) uncoupled positive-sequence network.

$$\mathbf{Z}_{12} = \left. \frac{\mathbf{V}_1}{\mathbf{I}_2} \right|_{\mathbf{I}_1 = 0} \tag{9.246}$$

$$\mathbf{Z}_{21} = \left. \frac{\mathbf{V}_2}{\mathbf{I}_1} \right|_{\mathbf{I}_2 = 0} \tag{9.247}$$

$$\mathbf{Z}_{22} = \left. \frac{\mathbf{V}_2}{\mathbf{I}_2} \right|_{\mathbf{I}_1 = 0} \tag{9.248}$$

Alternatively, it can be observed that

$$\begin{bmatrix} \mathbf{I}_1 \\ \mathbf{I}_2 \end{bmatrix} = \begin{bmatrix} \mathbf{Y}_{11} & \mathbf{Y}_{12} \\ \mathbf{Y}_{21} & \mathbf{Y}_{22} \end{bmatrix} \begin{bmatrix} \mathbf{V}_1 \\ \mathbf{V}_2 \end{bmatrix} \tag{9.249}$$

where the *short-circuit admittance parameters* can be determined (by short-circuiting the ports) from

$$\mathbf{Y}_{11} = \left. \frac{\mathbf{I}_1}{\mathbf{V}_1} \right|_{\mathbf{V}_2 = 0} \tag{9.250}$$

$$\mathbf{Y}_{21} = \left. \frac{\mathbf{I}_2}{\mathbf{V}_1} \right|_{\mathbf{V}_2 = 0} \tag{9.251}$$

$$\mathbf{Y}_{12} = \left. \frac{\mathbf{I}_1}{\mathbf{V}_2} \right|_{\mathbf{V}_1 = 0} \tag{9.252}$$

$$\mathbf{Y}_{22} = \left. \frac{\mathbf{I}_2}{\mathbf{V}_2} \right|_{\mathbf{V}_1 = 0} \tag{9.253}$$

Figure 9.28b shows a general π-equivalent of a two-port network in terms of admittances. The $\mathbf{Y}_A$, $\mathbf{Y}_B$, and $\mathbf{Y}_C$ admittances can be found from

$$\mathbf{Y}_A = \mathbf{Y}_{11} + \mathbf{Y}_{12} \tag{9.254}$$

$$\mathbf{Y}_B = \mathbf{Y}_{22} + \mathbf{Y}_{12} \tag{9.255}$$

$$\mathbf{Y}_C = -\mathbf{Y}_{12} \tag{9.256}$$

9.14.2 Equivalent Zero-Sequence Networks

By comparing the zero-sequence network shown in Figure 9.26 with the general two-port network shown in Figure 9.28a, it can be observed that

$$\mathbf{I}_1 = -\mathbf{I}_{a0} \tag{9.257}$$

$$\mathbf{I}_2 = \mathbf{I}_{a0} \tag{9.258}$$

$$\mathbf{V}_1 = \mathbf{V}_{a0} \tag{9.259}$$

$$\mathbf{V}_2 = \mathbf{V}_{a'0} \tag{9.260}$$

Hence, substituting Equations 9.257 through 9.260 into Equation 9.249, it can be expressed for the Thévenin equivalent of the zero-sequence network that

$$\mathbf{Y}_C = -\mathbf{Y}_{12-0} \tag{9.261a}$$

$$\begin{bmatrix} -\mathbf{I}_{a0} \\ \mathbf{I}_{a0} \end{bmatrix} = \begin{bmatrix} \mathbf{Y}_{11-0} & \mathbf{Y}_{12-0} \\ \mathbf{Y}_{21-0} & \mathbf{Y}_{22-0} \end{bmatrix} \begin{bmatrix} \mathbf{V}_{a0} \\ \mathbf{V}_{a'0} \end{bmatrix} \tag{9.261b}$$

9.14.3 EQUIVALENT POSITIVE- AND NEGATIVE-SEQUENCE NETWORKS

Figure 9.28c shows the equivalent positive-sequence network as an active two-port network with internal sources. Thus, it can be expressed for the two-port Thévenin equivalent of the positive-sequence network that

$$\begin{bmatrix} -\mathbf{I}_{a1} \\ \mathbf{I}_{a1} \end{bmatrix} = \begin{bmatrix} \mathbf{Y}_{11-1} & \mathbf{Y}_{12-1} \\ \mathbf{Y}_{21-1} & \mathbf{Y}_{22-1} \end{bmatrix} \begin{bmatrix} \mathbf{V}_{a1} \\ \mathbf{V}_{a'1} \end{bmatrix} + \begin{bmatrix} \mathbf{I}_{s1} \\ \mathbf{I}_{s2} \end{bmatrix} \tag{9.262}$$

or, alternatively,

$$\begin{bmatrix} \mathbf{V}_{a1} \\ \mathbf{V}_{a'1} \end{bmatrix} = \begin{bmatrix} \mathbf{Z}_{11-1} & \mathbf{Z}_{12-1} \\ \mathbf{Z}_{21-1} & \mathbf{Z}_{22-1} \end{bmatrix} \begin{bmatrix} -\mathbf{I}_{a1} \\ \mathbf{I}_{a1} \end{bmatrix} + \begin{bmatrix} \mathbf{V}_{s1} \\ \mathbf{V}_{s2} \end{bmatrix} \tag{9.263}$$

where $\mathbf{I}_{s1}$, $\mathbf{V}_{s1}$ and $\mathbf{I}_{s2}$, $\mathbf{V}_{s2}$ represent the internal sources 1 and 2, respectively. As before, the admittances $\mathbf{Y}_A$, $\mathbf{Y}_B$, and $\mathbf{Y}_C$ can be determined from

$$\mathbf{Y}_A = \mathbf{Y}_{11-1} + \mathbf{Y}_{12-1} \tag{9.264}$$

$$\mathbf{Y}_B = \mathbf{Y}_{22-1} + \mathbf{Y}_{12-1} \tag{9.265}$$

$$\mathbf{Y}_C = -\mathbf{Y}_{12-1} \tag{9.266}$$

The two-port Thévenin equivalent of the negative-sequence network would be the same as the one shown in Figure 9.28c but without the internal sources.

Anderson [4] shows that Equation 9.263 can be simplified as

$$\begin{bmatrix} \mathbf{V}_{a1} \\ \mathbf{V}_{a'1} \end{bmatrix} = \begin{bmatrix} \mathbf{V}_{s1} \\ \mathbf{V}_{s2} \end{bmatrix} - \begin{bmatrix} (\mathbf{Z}_{11-1} - \mathbf{Z}_{12-1}) \mathbf{I}_{a1} \\ -(\mathbf{Z}_{22-1} - \mathbf{Z}_{12-1}) \mathbf{I}_{a1} \end{bmatrix} \tag{9.267}$$

due to the fact that $\mathbf{I}_{a1}$ leaves the network at fault point F and enters at fault point F' due to external connection. This facilitates the voltage $\mathbf{V}_{a1}$ to be expressed in terms of the equivalent impedance $\mathbf{Z}_{s1}$ and the current $\mathbf{I}_{a1}$ to be expressed as it has been done for the shunt faults, where

$$\mathbf{V}_{a1} = \mathbf{V}_F - \mathbf{Z}_1\mathbf{I}_{a1} \tag{9.268}$$

Therefore, it can be concluded that the port of the positive-sequence network is completely uncoupled and that the resulting uncoupled positive-sequence network can be shown as in Figure 9.28d. The voltages $\mathbf{V}_{a1}$ and $\mathbf{V}_{a'1}$ can be found from Equation 9.263

$$\begin{bmatrix} \mathbf{V}_{a1} \\ \mathbf{V}_{a'1} \end{bmatrix} = \frac{1}{\Delta_y} \begin{bmatrix} \left(\mathbf{Y}_{12-1}\mathbf{I}_{s2} - \mathbf{Y}_{22-1}\mathbf{I}_{s1}\right) - \left(\mathbf{Y}_{12-1} + \mathbf{Y}_{22-1}\right)\mathbf{I}_{a1} \\ \left(\mathbf{Y}_{12-1}\mathbf{I}_{s1} - \mathbf{Y}_{11-1}\mathbf{I}_{s2}\right) + \left(\mathbf{Y}_{12-1} + \mathbf{Y}_{11-1}\right)\mathbf{I}_{a1} \end{bmatrix} \tag{9.269}$$

where

$$\Delta_y = \det \begin{bmatrix} \mathbf{Y}_{11-1} & \mathbf{Y}_{12-1} \\ \mathbf{Y}_{21-1} & \mathbf{Y}_{22-1} \end{bmatrix} \tag{9.270}$$

or

$$\Delta_y = \mathbf{Y}_{11-1}\mathbf{Y}_{22-1} - \mathbf{Y}_{12-1}^2 \tag{9.271}$$

Example 9.14

Consider the system shown in Figure 9.29 and assume that there is a series fault at fault point A, which is located at the middle of the transmission line TL_{AB}, as shown in the figure, and determine the following:

(a) Admittance matrix associated with positive-sequence network
(b) Two-port Thévenin equivalent of positive-sequence network
(c) Two-port Thévenin equivalent of negative-sequence network

Solution

Figure 9.30 shows the steps that are necessary to determine the positive- and negative-sequence network equivalents. Figure 9.30a shows the impedance diagram of the system for

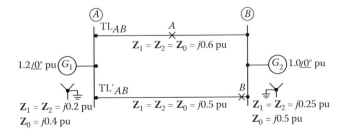

FIGURE 9.29 System diagram for Example 9.29.

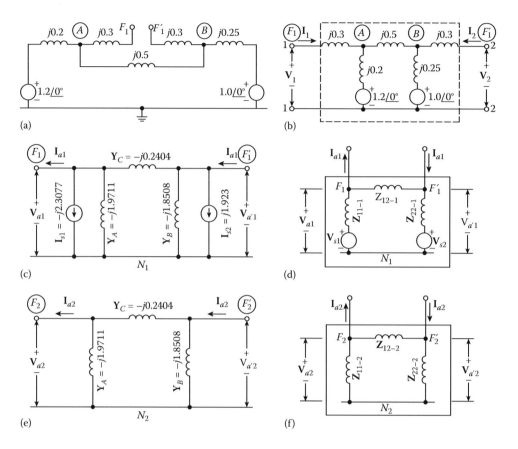

FIGURE 9.30 Steps in determining positive- and negative-sequence network equivalents for Example 9.14: (a) system diagram, (b) resulting two-port equivalent with input and output currents and voltages, (c) two-port Thévenin equivalent of positive-sequence network, (d) resulting coupled positive-sequence network, (e) two-port Thévenin equivalent of negative-sequence network, (f) resulting coupled negative-sequence network.

the positive sequence. Figure 9.30b shows the resulting two-port equivalent with input and output currents and voltages.

(a) To determine the elements of the admittance matrix **Y**, it is necessary to remove the internal voltage sources, shown in Figure 9.30b, by short-circuiting them. Then, with $V_2 = 0$ (i.e., by short-circuiting the terminals of the second port), apply $V_1 = 1.0\angle 0°$ pu and determine the parameters

$$Y_{11} = \left.\frac{I_1}{V_1}\right|_{V_2=0} = I_1 = \frac{1.0\angle 0°}{0.4522\angle 90°} = -j2.2115 \text{ pu}$$

and

$$Y_{21} = \left.\frac{I_2}{V_1}\right|_{V_2=0} = I_2 = -0.1087 I_1 = j0.2404 \text{ pu}$$

Now, with V_1 and $V_2 = 1.0\angle 0°$ pu, determine

$$Y_{22} = \left.\frac{I_2}{V_2}\right|_{V_1=0} = I_2 = \frac{1.0\angle 0°}{0.4782\angle 90°} = -j2.0912 \text{ pu}$$

and

$$\mathbf{Y}_{12} = \mathbf{Y}_{21} = j0.2404 \text{ pu}$$

Hence,

$$\mathbf{Y} = \begin{bmatrix} \mathbf{Y}_{11-1} & \mathbf{Y}_{12-1} \\ \mathbf{Y}_{21-1} & \mathbf{Y}_{22-1} \end{bmatrix} = \begin{bmatrix} -j2.2115 & j0.2404 \\ j0.2404 & -2.0912 \end{bmatrix}$$

(b) In order to find the source currents $\mathbf{I}_{s1}$ and $\mathbf{I}_{s2}$, short-circuit both F and F' to neutral and use the superposition theorem so that

$$\mathbf{I}_{s1} = \mathbf{I}_{s1(1.2)} + \mathbf{I}_{s1(1.0)}$$
$$= 2.0193\angle 90° + 0.2884\angle 90° = 2.3077\angle 90° \text{ pu}$$

and

$$\mathbf{I}_{s2} = \mathbf{I}_{s2(1.2)} + \mathbf{I}_{s2(1.0)}$$
$$= 0.4326\angle 90° + 1.4904\angle 90° = 1.9230\angle 90° \text{ pu}$$

Figure 9.30c shows the resulting two-port Thévenin equivalent of the positive-sequence network. Figure 9.30d shows the corresponding coupled positive-sequence network.

(c) Figure 9.30e shows the resulting two-port Thévenin equivalent of the negative-sequence network. Notice that it is the same as the one for the positive-sequence network but without its current sources. Figure 9.30f shows the corresponding coupled negative-sequence network.

Example 9.15

Consider the solution of Example 9.14 and determine the following:

(a) Uncoupled positive-sequence network
(b) Uncoupled negative-sequence network

Solution

(a) From Example 9.14,

$$\mathbf{Y} = \begin{bmatrix} -j2.2115 & j0.2404 \\ j0.2404 & -2.0912 \end{bmatrix}$$

where

$$\Delta_y = -4.6247 - (-0.0578) = -4.5669$$

Since

$$\begin{bmatrix} \mathbf{V}_{a1} \\ \mathbf{V}_{a'1} \end{bmatrix} = \frac{1}{\Delta_y} \begin{bmatrix} (\mathbf{Y}_{12-1}\mathbf{I}_{s2} - \mathbf{Y}_{22-1}\mathbf{I}_{s1}) - (\mathbf{Y}_{12-1} + \mathbf{Y}_{22-1})\mathbf{I}_{a1} \\ (\mathbf{Y}_{12-1}\mathbf{I}_{s1} - \mathbf{Y}_{11-1}\mathbf{I}_{s2}) + (\mathbf{Y}_{12-1} + \mathbf{Y}_{11-1})\mathbf{I}_{a1} \end{bmatrix}$$

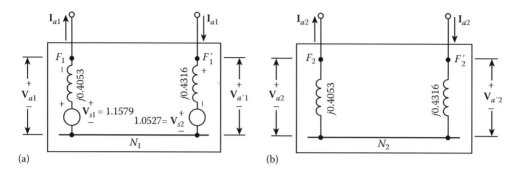

FIGURE 9.31 Uncoupled sequence networks: (a) positive-sequence network, (b) negative-sequence network.

where

$$\left(\mathbf{Y}_{12-1}\mathbf{I}_{s2} - \mathbf{Y}_{22-1}\mathbf{I}_{s1}\right) = j0.2404(j1.9230) - (-j2.0912)j2.3077$$
$$= -5.2882$$

$$\left(\mathbf{Y}_{12-1} + \mathbf{Y}_{22-1}\right)\mathbf{I}_{a1} = (j0.2404 - j2.0912)\mathbf{I}_{a1} = -j1.8508\mathbf{I}_{a1}$$

$$\left(\mathbf{Y}_{12-1}\mathbf{I}_{s1} - \mathbf{Y}_{11-1}\mathbf{I}_{s2}\right) = j0.2404(j2.3077) - (-j2.2115)j1.923$$
$$= 4.8075$$

$$\left(\mathbf{Y}_{12-1} + \mathbf{Y}_{11-1}\right)\mathbf{I}_{a1} = (j0.2404 - j2.2115)\mathbf{I}_{a1} = -j1.9711\mathbf{I}_{a1}$$

Therefore,

$$\begin{bmatrix} \mathbf{V}_{a1} \\ \mathbf{V}_{a'1} \end{bmatrix} = \frac{1}{-4.5669}\begin{bmatrix} (-5.2882) + j1.8508\mathbf{I}_{a1} \\ (-4.8075) - j1.9711\mathbf{I}_{a1} \end{bmatrix}$$
$$= \begin{bmatrix} 1.1579 - j0.4053\mathbf{I}_{a1} \\ 1.0527 - j0.4316\mathbf{I}_{a1} \end{bmatrix}$$

Figure 9.31a shows the corresponding uncoupled positive-sequence network.
(b) Figure 9.31b shows the corresponding uncoupled negative-sequence network.

9.15 SYSTEM GROUNDING

A *system neutral ground* is connected to ground from the neutral point or points of a system or rotating machine or transformer. Thus, a *grounded system* is a system that has at least one neutral point that is intentionally grounded, either solidly or through a current-limiting device. For example, most transformer neutrals of a transmission system are solidly grounded. But generator neutrals are usually grounded through some type of current-limiting device to limit the ground fault current. Figure 9.32 shows various neutral grounding methods used with generators and resulting zero-sequence networks. Hence, the methods of grounding the system neutral include the following:

1. Ungrounded
2. Solidly grounded
3. Resistance grounded
4. Reactance grounded
5. Peterson coil (PC) grounded

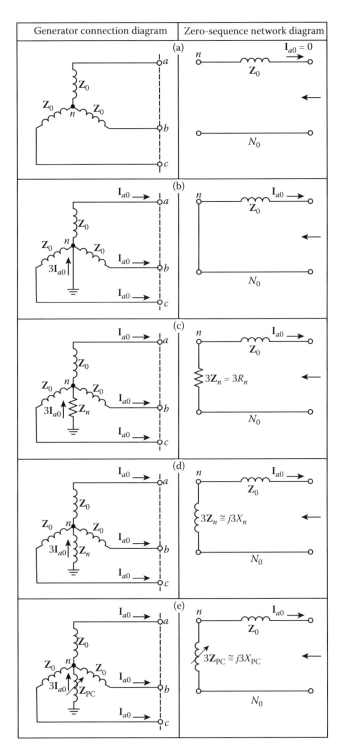

FIGURE 9.32 Various system (neutral) grounding methods used with generators and resulting zero-sequence network: (a) ungrounded, (b) solidly grounded, (c) resistance grounded, (d) reactance grounded, (e) grounded through PC.

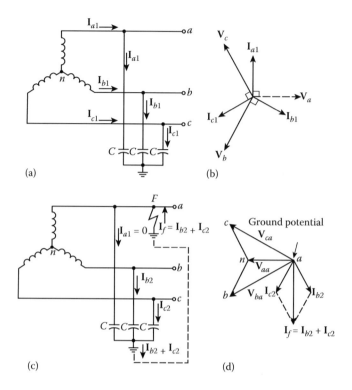

FIGURE 9.33 Representation of ungrounded system: (a) charging currents under normal condition, (b) phasor diagram under normal condition, (c) charging currents during SLG fault, (d) resulting phasor diagram.

The last four methods provide grounded neutrals, whereas the first provides an ungrounded (also called *isolated* or *free*) neutral system.

In ungrounded system, there is no intentional connection between the neutral point and neutral points of the system and the ground, as shown in Figure 9.33a. The line conductors have distributed capacitances between one another (not shown in the figure) and to ground due to capacitive coupling.

Under balanced conditions (assuming a perfectly transposed line), each conductor has the same capacitance to ground. Thus, the charging current of each phase is the same in Figure 9.33b. Hence, the potential of the neutral is the same as the ground potential, as illustrated in Figure 9.34a. The charging currents $\mathbf{I}_{a1}$, $\mathbf{I}_{b1}$, and $\mathbf{I}_{c1}$ lead their respective phase voltages by 90°. Thus,

$$\left|\mathbf{I}_{a1}\right| = \left|\mathbf{I}_{b1}\right| = \left|\mathbf{I}_{c1}\right| = \frac{\mathbf{V}_{\text{L-N}}}{X_c} \tag{9.272}$$

where X_c is the capacitive reactance of the line to ground. These phasor currents are in balance, as shown in Figure 9.33a.

Now assume that there is a line-to-ground fault involving phase a, as shown in Figure 9.33c. As a result of this SLG fault, the potential of phase a becomes equal to the ground potential, and hence, no charging current flows in this phase. Therefore, the neutral point shifts from ground potential position to the position shown in Figure 9.33d. It is also illustrated in Figure 9.34. A charging current of three times the normal per-phase charging current flows in the faulted phase because the phase voltage of each of the two healthy phases increases by three times its normal phase voltage. Therefore,

$$\mathbf{I}_f = 3\mathbf{I}_{b1} = 3\mathbf{I}_{c1} \tag{9.273}$$

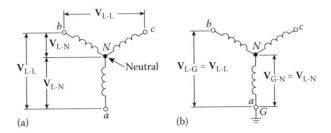

FIGURE 9.34 Voltage diagrams of ungrounded system: (a) before SLG fault, (b) after SLG fault.

The insulation of all apparatus connected to the lines is subjected to this HV. If it exists for a very short periods of time, the insulation may be adequate to withstand it. But, it will eventually cause the failure of insulation due to cumulative weakening action. For operating the protective devices, it is crucial that the magnitude of the current applied should be sufficient to operate them.

However, in the event of an SLG fault on an ungrounded neutral system, the resultant capacitive current is usually not large enough to actuate the protective devices. Furthermore, a current of such magnitude (over 4 or 5 A) flowing through the fault might be sufficient to maintain an arc in the ionized part of the fault. It is possible that such a current may exist even after the SLG fault is cleared.

The phenomenon of persistent arc is called the *arcing ground*. Under such conditions, the system capacity will be charged and discharged in cyclic order, due to which high-frequency oscillations are superimposed on the system. These high-frequency oscillations produce surge voltages as high as six times the normal value that may damage the insulation at any point of the system.*

The neutral grounding is effective in reducing such transient voltage buildup from such intermittent ground faults by reducing neutral displacement from ground potential and the destructiveness of any high-frequency voltage oscillations following each arc initiation or restrike. *Because of these problems with ungrounded neutral systems, in most of the modern HV systems, the neutral is grounded.*

The advantages of neutral grounding include the following:

1. Voltages of phases are restricted to the line-to-ground voltages since the neutral point is not shifted in this system.
2. The ground relays can be used to protect against the ground faults.
3. The HVs caused by arcing grounds or transient SLG faults are eliminated.
4. The overvoltages caused by lightning are easily eliminated contrary to the case of the isolated neutral systems.
5. The induced static charges do not cause any disturbance since they are conducted to ground immediately.
6. It provides a reliable system.
7. It provides a reduction in operating and maintenance expenses.

A power system is solidly (i.e., directly) grounded when a generator, power transformer, or grounding transformer neutral is connected directly to the ground, as shown in Figure 9.35a. When there is an SLG fault on any phase (e.g., phase *a*), the line-to-ground voltage of that phase becomes zero. However, the remaining two phases will still have the same voltages as before, since the neutral point remains unshifted, as shown in Figure 9.35b. Note that in this system, in addition to the charging currents, the power source also feeds the fault current $\mathbf{I}_f$. To keep the system stable, solid grounding is usually used where the circuit impedance is high enough so that the fault current can be kept within limits.

---

* The condition necessary for producing these overvoltages requires that the dielectric strength of the arc path build up at a higher rate, after extinction of the arc, than at the preceding extinction.

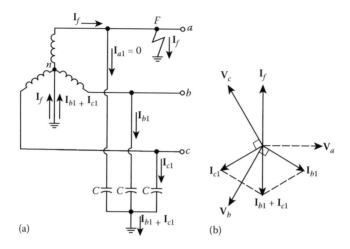

FIGURE 9.35 Representation of SLG fault on solidly grounded system: (a) solidly grounded system, (b) phasor diagram.

The comparison of the magnitude of the SLG fault current with the system three-phase current determines how solidly the system should be grounded. The higher the ground fault current in relation to the three-phase current, the more solidly the system is grounded. Most equipment rated 230 kV and above is designed to operate only on an effectively grounded system.*

As a rule of thumb, an *effectively grounded system* is one in which the ratio of the coefficient of grounding does not exceed 0.80. Here, the *coefficient of grounding* is defined as the ratio of the maximum sustained line-to-ground voltage during faults to the maximum operating line-to-line voltage. At higher voltage levels, insulation is more expensive, and therefore, more economy can be achieved from the insulation reduction. However, *solid grounding of a generator* without external impedance may cause the SLG fault current from the generator to exceed the maximum three-phase fault current the generator can deliver and to exceed the short-circuit current for which its windings are braces. Thus, generators are usually grounded through a resistance, reactance, or PC to limit the fault current to a value that is less than three-phase fault currents.

In a *resistance-grounded system*, the system neutral is connected to ground through one or more resistors. A system that is properly grounded by resistance is not subject to destructive transient overvoltages. Resistance grounding reduces the arcing hazards and permits ground fault protection.

In a *reactance-grounded system*, the system neutral is connected to ground through a reactor. Since the ground fault current that may flow in a reactance-grounded system is a function of the neutral reactance, the magnitude of the reactance in the neutral circuit determines how *solidly* the system is grounded. In fact, whether a system is solidly grounded or reactance grounded depends on the ratio of zero-sequence reactance X_0 to positive-sequence reactance X_1. Hence, a system is reactance grounded, if the ratio X_0/X_1 is greater than 3.0. Otherwise, if the ratio is less than 3.0, the system is solidly grounded. The system neutral grounding using PCs will be reviewed in Section 9.16.

The best way to obtain the system neutral for grounding purposes is to use source transformers or generators with wye-connected windings. The neutral is then readily available.

If the system neutral is not available for some reason, for example, when an existing system is delta connected, the grounding can be done using zigzag grounding transformer with no secondary winding or a wye–delta grounding transformer. In this case, the delta side must be closed to provide a path for zero-sequence current. The wye winding must be of the same voltage rating as the circuit that is to be grounded. On the other hand, the delta voltage rating can be selected at any standard voltage level.

---

* A system is defined as *effectively grounded* when $R_0 \ll X_1$ and $X_0 \ll 3X_1$, and such relationships exist at any point in the system for any condition of operation and for any amount of generator capacity.

9.16   ELIMINATION OF SLG FAULT CURRENT BY USING PETERSON COILS

In the event that the reactance of a neutral reactor is increased until it is equal to the system capacitance to ground, the system zero-sequence network is *in parallel resonance for SLG faults*. As a result, a fault current flows through the neutral reactor to ground. A current of approximately equal magnitude and about $180°$ out of phase with the reactor current flows through the system capacitance to ground. These two currents neutralize each other, except for a small resistance component, as they flow through the fault. Such a reactor is called a *ground fault neutralizer, arc suppression coil*, or *PC*. It is basically an iron core reactor that is adjustable by means of taps on the winding.

The *resonant grounding* is an effective means to clear both transient, due to lightning, small animals, or tree branches, and sustained SLG faults. Other advantages of PCs include extinguishing arcs and reduction of voltage dips due to SLG faults. The disadvantages of PCs include the need for retuning after any network modification or line-switching operation, the need for the lines to be transposed, and the increase in corona and RI under DLG fault conditions.

Example 9.16

Consider the subtransmission system shown in Figure 9.36. Assume that loads are connected to buses 2 and 3 and are supplied from bus1 through 69 kV lines of TL_{12}, TL_{13}, and TL_{23}. The line lengths are 5, 10, and 5 mi for lines TL_{12}, TL_{13}, and TL_{23}, respectively. The lines are transposed and made of three 500 kcmil, 30/7-strand ACSR conductors, and there are no ground wires. The GMD between the three conductors and their images (i.e., H_{aa}) is 81.5 ft. The self-GMD of OH conductors as a composite group (i.e., D_{aa}) is 1.658 ft. In order to reduce the SLG faults, a PC is to be installed between the neutral of the wye-connected secondary of the supply transformer T_1 and ground. The transformer T_1 has a leakage reactance of 5% based on its 25 MVA rating. Determine the following:

(a) The total zero-sequence capacitance and susceptance per phase of the system at 60 Hz.
(b) Draw the zero-sequence network of the system.
(c) The continuous-current rating of the PC.
(d) The required reactance value for the PC.
(e) The inductance value of the PC.
(f) The continuous kVA rating for the PC.
(g) The continuous-voltage rating for the PC.

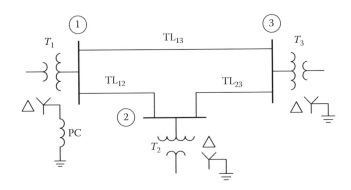

FIGURE 9.36   Subtransmission system for Example 9.16.

Solution

(a) $C_0 = \dfrac{29.842}{\ln(H_{aa}/D_{aa})} = \dfrac{29.842}{\ln(81.5/1.658)} = 7.6616 \text{ nF/mi}$

Therefore,

$$b_0 = \omega C_0 = 2.8884 \text{ μS/mi}$$

and for the total system,

$$B_0 = b_0 l = 2.8884 \times 20 = 57.7671 \text{ μS}$$

The total zero-sequence reactance is

$$\sum X_{c0} = \frac{1}{B_0} = \frac{10^6}{57.7671} = 17,310.8915 \text{ } \Omega$$

and the total zero-sequence capacitance of the system is

$$\sum C_0 = \frac{B_0}{\omega} = \frac{57.7671 \times 10^{-6}}{377} = 0.1532 \text{ μF}$$

(b) The resulting zero-sequence network is shown in Figure 9.37.
(c) Since the leakage reactance of transformer T_1 is

$$X_1 = X_2 = X_0 = 0.05 \text{ pu}$$

or since

$$Z_B = \frac{kV_B^2}{MVA_B} = \frac{69^2}{25} = 190.44 \text{ } \Omega$$

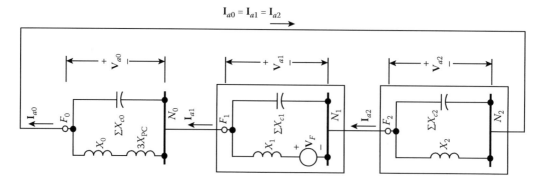

FIGURE 9.37   Interconnection of sequence networks for Example 9.16.

In order to have a zero SLG current,

$$\mathbf{I}_{a0} = \mathbf{I}_{a1} = \mathbf{I}_{a2} = 0$$

Thus, it is required that

$$\mathbf{V}_{a0} = -\mathbf{V}_f$$

where

$$\mathbf{V}_f = \frac{69 \times 10^3}{\sqrt{3}} = 39{,}837.17 \text{ V}$$

Since $\sum X_{c1} \gg X_1$ and $\sum X_{c2} \gg X_2$, the zero-sequence current component flowing through the PC can be expressed as

$$\mathbf{I}_{a0(PC)} = \frac{-\mathbf{V}_{a0}}{j(X_0 + 3X_{PC})} = \frac{\mathbf{V}_F}{j(X_0 + 3X_{PC})}$$

or

$$\mathbf{I}_{a0(PC)} = \frac{39{,}837.17\angle 0°}{j17{,}310.8915} = -j2.3013 \text{ A}$$

Therefore, the continuous-current rating for the PC is

$$\mathbf{I}_{PC} = 3\mathbf{I}_{a0(PC)} = 6.9038 \text{ A}$$

(d) Since

$$3X_{PC} + X_0 = 17{,}310.8915 \ \Omega$$

where

$$X_0 = 9.522 \ \Omega$$

therefore,

$$3X_{PC} = 17{,}310.8915 - 9.522 = 17{,}301.3695 \ \Omega$$

and thus, the required reactance value for the PC is

$$X_{PC} = \frac{17{,}301.3695 \ \Omega}{3} = 5767.1232 \ \Omega$$

(e) Hence, its inductance is

$$L_{PC} = \frac{X_{PC}}{\omega} = \frac{5767.1232}{377} = 15.2928\,H$$

(f) Its continuous kVA rating is

$$S_{PC} = I_{PC}^2 X_{PC} = (6.9030)^2 (5767.1232) = 274.88\,kVA$$

(g) The voltage across the PC is

$$V_{PC} = I_{PC} X_{PC} = (6.9030)(5767.1232) = 39,815.07\,V$$

which is approximately equal to the line-to-neutral voltage.

9.17 SIX-PHASE SYSTEMS

The six-phase transmission lines are proposed due to their ability to increase power transfer over existing lines and reduce electrical environmental impacts. For example, in six-phase transmission lines, voltage gradients of the conductors are lower, which in turn reduces both audible noise and electrostatic effects without requiring additional insulation.

In multiphase transmission lines, if the line-to-ground voltage is fixed, then the line-to-line voltage decreases as the number of phases increases. Consequently, this enables the line-to-line insulation distance to be reduced.

In such systems, the symmetrical components analysis can also be used to determine the unbalance factors that are caused by the unsymmetrical tower-top configurations.

9.17.1 APPLICATION OF SYMMETRICAL COMPONENTS

A set of unbalanced six-phase currents (or voltages) can be decomposed into six sets of balanced currents (or voltages) that are called the *symmetrical components*. Figure 9.38 shows the balanced voltage-sequence sets of a six-phase system [17].

The first set, that is, the first-order positive-sequence components, are equal in magnitude and have a 60° phase shift. They are arranged in *abcdef* phase sequence. The remaining sets are the first-order negative sequence, the second-order positive sequence, the second-order negative sequence, the odd sequence, and finally the zero-sequence components.

After denoting the phase sequence as *abcdef*, their sequence components can be expressed as

$$\left.\begin{array}{l}
V_a = V_{a0^+} + V_{a1^+} + V_{a2^+} + V_{a0^-} + V_{a2^-} + V_{a1^-} \\
V_b = V_{b0^+} + V_{b1^+} + V_{b2^+} + V_{b0^-} + V_{b2^-} + V_{b1^-} \\
V_c = V_{c0^+} + V_{c1^+} + V_{c2^+} + V_{c0^-} + V_{c2^-} + V_{c1^-} \\
V_d = V_{d0^+} + V_{d1^+} + V_{d2^+} + V_{d0^-} + V_{d2^-} + V_{d1^-} \\
V_e = V_{e0^+} + V_{e1^+} + V_{e2^+} + V_{e0^-} + V_{e2^-} + V_{e1^-} \\
V_f = V_{f0^+} + V_{f1^+} + V_{f2^+} + V_{f0^-} + V_{f2^-} + V_{f1^-}
\end{array}\right\} \tag{9.274}$$

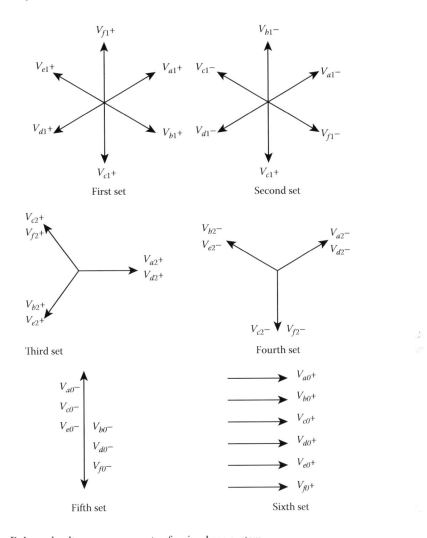

FIGURE 9.38 Balanced voltage-sequence sets of a six-phase system.

9.17.2 TRANSFORMATIONS

By taking phase a as the reference phase as usual, the set of voltages given in Equation 9.274 can be expressed in matrix form as

$$
\begin{bmatrix} V_a \\ V_b \\ V_c \\ V_d \\ V_e \\ V_f \end{bmatrix} = \begin{bmatrix} 1 & 1 & 1 & 1 & 1 & 1 \\ 1 & b^5 & b^4 & b^3 & b^2 & b \\ 1 & b^4 & b^2 & 1 & b^4 & b^2 \\ 1 & b^3 & 1 & b^3 & 1 & b^3 \\ 1 & b^2 & b^4 & 1 & b^2 & b^4 \\ 1 & b & b^2 & b^3 & b^4 & b^5 \end{bmatrix} \begin{bmatrix} V_{a0^+} \\ V_{a1^+} \\ V_{a2^+} \\ V_{a0^-} \\ V_{a2^-} \\ V_{a1^-} \end{bmatrix}
$$

(9.275)

or in shorthand matrix notation,

$$\left[\mathbf{V}_\phi\right] = \left[\mathbf{T}_6\right]\left[\mathbf{V}_s\right] \tag{9.276}$$

where
  $\left[\mathbf{V}_\phi\right]$ is the matrix of unbalanced phase voltages
  $\left[\mathbf{V}_s\right]$ is the matrix of balanced sequence voltages
  $\left[\mathbf{T}_6\right]$ is the six-phase symmetrical transformation matrix

Similar to the definition of the **a** operator in three-phase systems, it is possible to define a six-phase operator **b** as

$$\mathbf{b} = 1.0\angle 60° \tag{9.277}$$

or

$$\mathbf{b} = \exp\left(\frac{j\pi}{3}\right) = 0.5 + j0.866 \tag{9.278}$$

It can be shown that

$$\mathbf{b} = -\mathbf{a}^2$$

$$= -1\left(1.0\angle 120°\right)^2 = -\left(1.0\angle 240°\right)$$

$$= 1.0\angle 60° \tag{9.279}$$

The relation between the sequence components and the unbalanced phase voltages can be expressed as

$$\left[\mathbf{V}_s\right] = \left[\mathbf{T}_6\right]^{-1}\left[\mathbf{V}_\phi\right] \tag{9.280}$$

Similar equations can be written for the phase currents and their sequence components as

$$\left[\mathbf{I}_\phi\right] = \left[\mathbf{T}_6\right]\left[\mathbf{I}_s\right] \tag{9.281}$$

and

$$\left[\mathbf{I}_s\right] = \left[\mathbf{T}_6\right]^{-1}\left[\mathbf{I}_\phi\right] \tag{9.282}$$

The sequence impedance matrix $\left[\mathbf{Z}_s\right]$ can be determined from the phase impedance matrix $\left[\mathbf{Z}_\phi\right]$ by applying KVL. Hence,

$$\left[\mathbf{V}_\phi\right] = \left[\mathbf{Z}_\phi\right]\left[\mathbf{I}_\phi\right] \tag{9.283}$$

and

$$\left[\mathbf{V}_s\right] = \left[\mathbf{Z}_s\right]\left[\mathbf{I}_s\right] \tag{9.284}$$

where

$\left[\mathbf{Z}_\phi\right]$ is the phase impedance matrix of the line in 6×6

$\left[\mathbf{Z}_s\right]$ is the sequence impedance matrix of the line in 6×6

After multiplying both sides of Equation 9.284 by $\left[\mathbf{Z}_s\right]^{-1}$,

$$\left[\mathbf{I}_s\right] = \left[\mathbf{Z}_s\right]^{-1}\left[\mathbf{V}_s\right]$$

$$= \left[\mathbf{Y}_s\right]\left[\mathbf{V}_s\right] \tag{9.285}$$

where $\left[\mathbf{Y}_s\right]$ is the sequence admittance matrix.

Since the unbalanced factors are to be determined after having only the first-order positive-sequence voltage applied, Equation 9.285 can be reexpressed as

$$\begin{bmatrix} I_{a0^+} \\ I_{a1^+} \\ I_{a2^+} \\ I_{a0^-} \\ I_{a2^-} \\ I_{a1^-} \end{bmatrix} = \begin{bmatrix} Y_{0^+0^+} & Y_{0^+0^+} & Y_{0^+0^+} & Y_{0^+0^-} & Y_{0^+0^-} & Y_{0^+0^-} \\ Y_{0^+0^+} & Y_{0^+0^+} & Y_{0^+0^+} & Y_{0^+0^-} & Y_{0^+0^-} & Y_{0^+0^-} \\ Y_{0^+0^+} & Y_{0^+0^+} & Y_{0^+0^+} & Y_{0^+0^-} & Y_{0^+0^-} & Y_{0^+0^-} \\ Y_{0^-0^+} & Y_{0^-0^+} & Y_{0^-0^+} & Y_{0^-0^-} & Y_{0^-0^-} & Y_{0^-0^-} \\ Y_{0^-0^+} & Y_{0^-0^+} & Y_{0^-0^+} & Y_{0^-0^-} & Y_{0^-0^-} & Y_{0^-0^-} \\ Y_{0^-0^+} & Y_{0^-0^+} & Y_{0^-0^+} & Y_{0^-0^-} & Y_{0^-0^-} & Y_{0^-0^-} \end{bmatrix} \begin{bmatrix} 0 \\ V_{a1^+} \\ 0 \\ 0 \\ 0 \\ 0 \end{bmatrix} \tag{9.286}$$

9.17.3 Electromagnetic Unbalance Factors

For a six-phase transmission line, there are five electromagnetic sequence unbalanced factors. They are called *zero, second-order positive, odd, second-order negative,* and *first-order negative sequence factors.* Each of them is computed as the ratio of the corresponding current to the first-order positive-sequence current. For example, zero-sequence unbalanced factor is

$$\mathbf{m}_{0^+} = \frac{I_{a0^+}}{I_{a1^+}} \tag{9.287a}$$

or

$$\mathbf{m}_{0^+} = \frac{\left(y_{0^+1^+}\right)\left(V_{a1^+}\right)}{\left(y_{1^+1^+}\right)\left(V_{a1^+}\right)} = \frac{y_{0^+1^+}}{y_{1^+1^+}} \tag{9.287b}$$

The second-order positive unbalance factor is

$$\mathbf{m}_{2^+} = \frac{I_{a2^+}}{I_{a1^+}} \tag{9.288a}$$

or

$$\mathbf{m}_{2^+} = \frac{\left(y_{2^+1^+}\right)\left(V_{a1^+}\right)}{\left(y_{1^+1^+}\right)\left(V_{a1^+}\right)} = \frac{y_{2^+1^+}}{y_{1^+1^+}} \tag{9.288b}$$

The odd unbalance factor is

$$\mathbf{m}_{0^-} = \frac{I_{a0^-}}{I_{a1^+}} \tag{9.289a}$$

or

$$\mathbf{m}_{0^-} = \frac{\left(y_{0^-1^+}\right)\left(V_{a1^+}\right)}{\left(y_{1^+1^+}\right)\left(V_{a1^+}\right)} = \frac{y_{0^-1^+}}{y_{1^+1^+}} \tag{9.289b}$$

The second-order negative unbalance factor is

$$\mathbf{m}_{2^-} = \frac{I_{a2^-}}{I_{a1^+}} \tag{9.290a}$$

or

$$\mathbf{m}_{2^-} = \frac{\left(y_{2^-1^+}\right)\left(V_{a1^+}\right)}{\left(y_{1^+1^+}\right)\left(V_{a1^+}\right)} = \frac{y_{2^-1^+}}{y_{1^+1^+}} \tag{9.290b}$$

The first-order negative unbalance factor is

$$\mathbf{m}_{1^-} = \frac{I_{a1^-}}{I_{a1^+}} \tag{9.291a}$$

or

$$\mathbf{m}_{1^-} = \frac{\left(y_{1^-1^+}\right)\left(V_{a1^+}\right)}{\left(y_{1^+1^+}\right)\left(V_{a1^+}\right)} = \frac{y_{1^-1^+}}{y_{1^+1^+}} \tag{9.291b}$$

As a result of the unsymmetrical configuration, circulating residual (i.e., zero sequence) currents will flow in the HV system with solidly grounded neutrals. Such currents affect the proper operation of very sensitive elements in ground relays. In addition to the zero-sequence unbalance, negative-sequence charging currents are also produced. They are caused by the capacitive unbalances that will cause the currents flow through the lines and windings of the transformers and rotating machines in the system, causing additional power losses in the rotating machines and transformers.

9.17.4 Transposition on the Six-Phase Lines

The six-phase transmission lines can be transposed in *complete transposition, cyclic transposition,* and *reciprocal transposition.* In a complete transposition, every conductor assumes every possible position with respect to every other conductor over an equal length. Thus, the resultant impedance matrix for a *complete transposition* can be expressed as

$$
\left[\mathbf{Z}_\phi\right] = \begin{bmatrix}
Z_s & Z_m & Z_m & Z_m & Z_m & Z_m \\
Z_m & Z_s & Z_m & Z_m & Z_m & Z_m \\
Z_m & Z_m & Z_s & Z_m & Z_m & Z_m \\
Z_m & Z_m & Z_m & Z_s & Z_m & Z_m \\
Z_m & Z_m & Z_m & Z_m & Z_s & Z_m \\
Z_m & Z_m & Z_m & Z_m & Z_m & Z_s
\end{bmatrix}
\tag{9.292}
$$

In a six-phase transmission line, it is difficult to achieve a complete transposition. Also, it is not of interest due to the differences in the line-to-line voltages. Therefore, it is more efficient to implement cyclic transposition or reciprocal cyclic transposition. The impedance matrix for a cyclically transposed line can be expressed as

$$
\left[\mathbf{Z}_\phi\right] = \begin{bmatrix}
Z_s & Z_{m1} & Z_{m2} & Z_{m3} & Z_{m4} & Z_{m5} \\
Z_{m5} & Z_s & Z_{m1} & Z_{m2} & Z_{m3} & Z_{m4} \\
Z_{m4} & Z_{m5} & Z_s & Z_{m1} & Z_{m2} & Z_{m3} \\
Z_{m3} & Z_{m4} & Z_{m5} & Z_s & Z_{m1} & Z_{m2} \\
Z_{m2} & Z_{m3} & Z_{m4} & Z_{m5} & Z_s & Z_{m1} \\
Z_{m1} & Z_{m2} & Z_{m3} & Z_{m4} & Z_{m5} & Z_s
\end{bmatrix}
\tag{9.293}
$$

Similarly, the impedance matrix for a reciprocal cyclically transposed line can be given as

$$
\left[\mathbf{Z}_\phi\right] = \begin{bmatrix}
Z_s & Z_{m1} & Z_{m2} & Z_{m3} & Z_{m2} & Z_{m1} \\
Z_{m1} & Z_s & Z_{m1} & Z_{m2} & Z_{m3} & Z_{m2} \\
Z_{m2} & Z_{m1} & Z_s & Z_{m1} & Z_{m2} & Z_{m3} \\
Z_{m3} & Z_{m2} & Z_{m1} & Z_s & Z_{m1} & Z_{m2} \\
Z_{m2} & Z_{m3} & Z_{m2} & Z_{m1} & Z_s & Z_{m1} \\
Z_{m1} & Z_{m2} & Z_{m3} & Z_{m2} & Z_{m1} & Z_s
\end{bmatrix}
\tag{9.294}
$$

where
Z_s is the self-impedance
Z_m is the mutual impedance

9.17.5 Phase Arrangements

The values of the electromagnetic and electrostatic unbalances will change by changing the phase conductors. However, there is a phase configuration that has the minimum amount of electromagnetic unbalances. The circulating current unbalances can become very large under some phasing arrangements.

9.17.6 Overhead Ground Wires

OH ground wires are installed in order to protect the transmission lines against lightning. However, the OH ground wires affect both the self- and mutual impedances. The resistances of the self- and mutual impedances increase slightly, while their reactances decrease significantly. The OH ground wires can increase or decrease some or all of the unbalances depending on the type and size of the configuration. Kron reduction can be used to compare the equivalent impedance matrix for the transmission lines.

9.17.7 Double-Circuit Transmission Lines

The voltage equation of a double-circuit line is given by

$$\left[\frac{\sum \mathbf{V}_{ckt1}}{\sum \mathbf{V}_{ckt2}}\right] = \left[\begin{array}{c|c} \mathbf{Z}_{ckt1} & \mathbf{Z}_{ckt1\ ckt2} \\ \hline \mathbf{Z}_{ckt2\ ckt1} & \mathbf{Z}_{ckt2} \end{array}\right]\left[\frac{\mathbf{I}_{ckt1}}{\mathbf{I}_{ckt2}}\right] \tag{9.295}$$

where $\sum \mathbf{V}_{ckt1}$ and $\sum \mathbf{V}_{ckt2}$ and $\mathbf{I}_{ckt1}$ and $\mathbf{I}_{ckt2}$ are the phase voltages and currents, respectively. Each of them is a column vector of size 6×1. Each $\left[\mathbf{Z}\right]$ impedance matrix has dimensions of 6×6. The aforementioned matrix is solved for the currents, in order to express the unbalance factors in terms of sequence currents. Hence,

$$\left[\frac{\mathbf{I}_{ckt1}}{\mathbf{I}_{ckt2}}\right] = \left[\mathbf{Y}_{line}\right]\left[\frac{\sum \mathbf{V}_{ckt1}}{\sum \mathbf{V}_{ckt2}}\right] \tag{9.296}$$

where $\left[\mathbf{Y}_{line}\right]$ is the admittance matrix of the line having a size 12×12.

In order to determine the sequence admittance matrix of the line, the appropriate transformation matrix needs to be defined as

$$\left[\mathbf{T}_{12}\right] = \left[\begin{array}{c|c} \mathbf{T}_6 & \mathbf{0} \\ \hline \mathbf{0} & \mathbf{T}_6 \end{array}\right] \tag{9.297}$$

Premultiplying Equation 9.296 by the transformation matrix $\left[\mathbf{T}_{12}\right]$ and postmultiplying by $\left[\mathbf{T}_{12}\right]^{-1}$ and also inserting the unity matrix of $\left[\mathbf{T}_{12}\right]^{-1}\left[\mathbf{T}_{12}\right] = \left[\mathbf{U}\right]$ into the right-hand side of the equation,

$$\left[\frac{\mathbf{I}_{seq1}}{\mathbf{I}_{seq2}}\right] = \left[\mathbf{T}_{12}\right]\left[\mathbf{Y}_{line}\right]\left[\mathbf{T}_{12}\right]^{-1}\left[\frac{\sum \mathbf{V}_{seq1}}{\sum \mathbf{V}_{seq2}}\right] \tag{9.298}$$

where $\sum \mathbf{V}_{seq1}, \sum \mathbf{V}_{seq2}, \mathbf{I}_{seq1}$, and $\mathbf{I}_{seq2}$ are the sequence voltage drops and currents for the first and second circuits, respectively. The sequence admittance matrix is

$$\left[\mathbf{Y}_{seq}\right] = \left[\mathbf{T}_{12}\right]\left[\mathbf{Y}_{line}\right]\left[\mathbf{T}_{12}\right]^{-1} \tag{9.299}$$

The unbalance factors are to be determined with only the first-order positive-sequence voltage applied. There are two different unbalances, that is, the *net-through* and the *net-circulating* unbalances. The sequence matrix is found by expanding the previous equation to the full 12×12 matrix as

$$
\begin{bmatrix}
I_{a0^+} \\ I_{a1^+} \\ I_{a2^+} \\ I_{a0^-} \\ I_{a2^-} \\ I_{a1^-} \\ \hline
I_{a0^+} \\ I_{a1^+} \\ I_{a2^+} \\ I_{a0^-} \\ I_{a2^-} \\ I_{a1^-}
\end{bmatrix}
=
\left[
\begin{array}{cccccc|cccccc}
y_{0^+0^+} & y_{0^+1^+} & y_{0^+2^+} & y_{0^+0^-} & y_{0^+2^-} & y_{0^+1^-} & y_{0^+0'^+} & y_{0^+1'^+} & y_{0^+2'^+} & y_{0^+0'^-} & y_{0^+2'^-} & y_{0^+1'^-} \\
y_{1^+0^+} & y_{1^+1^+} & y_{1^+2^+} & y_{1^+0^-} & y_{1^+2^-} & y_{1^+1^-} & y_{1^+0'^+} & y_{1^+1'^+} & y_{0^+2'^+} & y_{1^+0'^-} & y_{1^+2'^-} & y_{1^+1'^-} \\
y_{2^+0^+} & y_{2^+1^+} & y_{2^+2^+} & y_{2^+0^-} & y_{2^+2^-} & y_{2^+1^-} & y_{2^+0'^+} & y_{2^+1'^+} & y_{0^+2'^+} & y_{2^+0'^-} & y_{2^+2'^-} & y_{2^+1'^-} \\
y_{0^-0^+} & y_{0^-1^+} & y_{0^-2^+} & y_{0^-0^-} & y_{0^-2^-} & y_{0^-1^-} & y_{0^-0'^+} & y_{0^-1'^+} & y_{0^-2'^+} & y_{0^-0'^-} & y_{0^-2'^-} & y_{0^-1'^-} \\
y_{2^-0^+} & y_{2^-1^+} & y_{2^-2^+} & y_{2^-0^-} & y_{2^-2^-} & y_{2^-1^-} & y_{2^-0'^+} & y_{2^-1'^+} & y_{0^-2'^+} & y_{2^-0'^-} & y_{2^-2'^-} & y_{2^-1'^-} \\
y_{1^-0^+} & y_{1^-1^+} & y_{1^-2^+} & y_{1^-0^-} & y_{1^-2^-} & y_{1^-1^-} & y_{1^-0'^+} & y_{1^-1'^+} & y_{0^-2'^+} & y_{1^-0'^-} & y_{1^-2'^-} & y_{1^-1'^-} \\ \hline
y_{0'^+0^+} & y_{0'^+1^+} & y_{0'^+2^+} & y_{0'^+0^-} & y_{0'^+2^-} & y_{0'^+1^-} & y_{0'^+0'^+} & y_{0'^+1'^+} & y_{0'^+2'^+} & y_{0'^+0'^-} & y_{0'^+2'^-} & y_{0'^+1'^-} \\
y_{1'^+0^+} & y_{1'^+1^+} & y_{1'^+2^+} & y_{1'^+0^-} & y_{1'^+2^-} & y_{1'^+1^-} & y_{1'^+0'^+} & y_{1'^+1'^+} & y_{1'^+2'^+} & y_{1'^+0'^-} & y_{1'^+2'^-} & y_{1'^+1'^-} \\
y_{2'^+0^+} & y_{2'^+1^+} & y_{2'^+2^+} & y_{2'^+0^-} & y_{2'^+2^-} & y_{2'^+1^-} & y_{2'^+0'^+} & y_{2'^+1'^+} & y_{2'^+2'^+} & y_{2'^+0'^-} & y_{2'^+2'^-} & y_{2'^+1'^-} \\
y_{0'^-0^+} & y_{0'^-1^+} & y_{0'^-2^+} & y_{0'^-0^-} & y_{0'^-2^-} & y_{0'^-1^-} & y_{0'^-0'^+} & y_{0'^-1'^+} & y_{0'^-2'^+} & y_{0'^-0'^-} & y_{0'^-2'^-} & y_{0'^-1'^-} \\
y_{2'^-0^+} & y_{2'^-1^+} & y_{2'^-2^+} & y_{2'^-0^-} & y_{2'^-2^-} & y_{2'^-1^-} & y_{2'^-0'^+} & y_{2'^-1'^+} & y_{2'^-2'^+} & y_{2'^-0'^-} & y_{2'^-2'^-} & y_{2'^-1'^-} \\
y_{1'^-0^+} & y_{1'^-1^+} & y_{1'^-2^+} & y_{1'^-0^-} & y_{1'^-2^-} & y_{1'^-1^-} & y_{1'^-0'^+} & y_{1'^-1'^+} & y_{1'^-2'^+} & y_{1'^-0'^-} & y_{1'^-2'^-} & y_{1'^-1'^-}
\end{array}
\right]
\begin{bmatrix}
0 \\ \sum V_{a1^+} \\ 0 \\ 0 \\ 0 \\ 0 \\ \hline
0 \\ \sum V_{a1^+} \\ 0 \\ 0 \\ 0 \\ 0
\end{bmatrix}
\tag{9.300}
$$

The *net-through unbalance factors* are defined as

$$
\mathbf{m}_{0^+ t} \triangleq \frac{I_{a0^+} + I_{a'0^+}}{I_{a1^+} + I_{a'1^+}}
$$

$$
= \frac{\left(y_{0^+1^+} + y_{0^+1'^+} + y_{0'^+1^+} + y_{0'^+1'^+} \right) \sum V_{a1+}}{\left(y_{1^+1^+} + y_{1^+1'^+} + y_{1'^+1^+} + y_{1'^+1'^+} \right) \sum V_{a1+}}
$$

$$
= \frac{y_{0^+1^+} + y_{0^+1'^+} + y_{0'^+1^+} + y_{0'^+1'^+}}{y_k}
\tag{9.301}
$$

where $y_k = y_{1^+1^+} + y_{1^+1'^+} + y_{1'^+1^+} + y_{1'^+1'^+}$

$$
\mathbf{m}_{2^+ t} = \frac{y_{2^+1^+} + y_{2^+1'^+} + y_{2'^+1^+} + y_{2'^+1'^+}}{y_k}
\tag{9.302}
$$

$$
\mathbf{m}_{0^- t} = \frac{y_{0^-1^+} + y_{0^-1'^+} + y_{2^-1^+} + y_{2^-1'^+}}{y_k}
\tag{9.303}
$$

$$
\mathbf{m}_{2^- t} = \frac{y_{2^-1^+} + y_{2^-1'^+} + y_{2'^-1^+} + y_{2'^-1'^+}}{y_k}
\tag{9.304}
$$

$$
\mathbf{m}_{1^- t} = \frac{y_{1^-1^+} + y_{1^-1'^+} + y_{1'^-1^+} + y_{1'^-1'^+}}{y_k}
\tag{9.305}
$$

The *net-circulating unbalances* are defined as

$$\mathbf{m}_{0^+c} \triangleq \frac{I_{a0^+} + I_{a'0^+}}{I_{a1^+} + I_{a'1^+}}$$

$$= \frac{y_{0^+1^+} + y_{0^+1'^+} - y_{0'1^+} - y_{0'1'^+}}{y_k} \tag{9.306}$$

$$\mathbf{m}_{2^+c} = \frac{y_{2^+1^+} + y_{2^+1'^+} - y_{2'+1^+} - y_{2'+1'^+}}{y_k} \tag{9.307}$$

$$\mathbf{m}_{0^-c} = \frac{y_{0^-1^+} + y_{0^-1'^+} - y_{0'-1^+} - y_{0'-1'^+}}{y_k} \tag{9.308}$$

$$\mathbf{m}_{2^-c} = \frac{y_{2^-1^+} + y_{2^-1'^+} - y_{2'-1^+} - y_{2'-1'^+}}{y_k} \tag{9.309}$$

$$\mathbf{m}_{1^-c} = \frac{y_{1^-1^+} + y_{1^-1'^+} - y_{1'-1^+} - y_{1'-1'^+}}{y_k} \tag{9.310}$$

PROBLEMS

9.1 Determine the symmetrical components for the phase currents of

$$\mathbf{I}_a = 125\angle 20°, \quad \mathbf{I}_b = 175\angle -100°, \quad \text{and} \quad \mathbf{I}_c = 95\angle 155° \, \text{A}.$$

9.2 Assume that the unbalanced phase currents are $\mathbf{I}_a = 100\angle 180°$, $\mathbf{I}_b = 100\angle 0°$, and $\mathbf{I}_c = 10\angle 20° \, \text{A}$.
  (a) Determine the symmetrical components.
  (b) Draw a phasor diagram showing I_{a0}, I_{a1}, I_{a2}, I_{b0}, I_{b1}, I_{b2}, I_{c0}, I_{c1}, and 1_{c2} (i.e., the positive-, negative-, and zero-sequence currents for each phase).
  (c) Draw the unbalanced phase current phasors in the phasor diagram of part (b).
9.3 Assume that $\mathbf{V}_{a1} = 180\angle 0°$, $\mathbf{V}_{a2} = 100\angle 100°$, and $\mathbf{V}_{a0} = 250\angle -40° \, \text{V}$.
  (a) Draw a phasor diagram showing all the nine symmetrical components.
  (b) Find the phase voltages $\left[\mathbf{V}_{abc} \right]$ using the equation

$$\left[\mathbf{V}_{abc} \right] = \left[\mathbf{A} \right] \left[\mathbf{V}_{012} \right]$$

  (c) Find the phase voltages $\left[\mathbf{V}_{abc} \right]$ graphically and check the results against the ones found in part (b).
9.4 Repeat Example 9.2 assuming that the phase voltages and currents are given as

$$\left[\mathbf{V}_{abc} \right] = \begin{bmatrix} 100\angle 0° \\ 100\angle 60° \\ 100\angle -60° \end{bmatrix} \quad \text{and} \quad \left[\mathbf{I}_{abc} \right] = \begin{bmatrix} 10\angle -30° \\ 10\angle 30° \\ 10\angle -90° \end{bmatrix}$$

9.5 Determine the symmetrical components for the phase currents of $\mathbf{I}_a = 100\angle 20°$, $\mathbf{I}_b = 50\angle -20°$, and $\mathbf{I}_c = 150\angle 180° \, \text{A}$. Draw a phasor diagram showing all the nine symmetrical components.

9.6 Assume that $\mathbf{I}_{a0} = 50 - j86.6$, $\mathbf{I}_{a1} = 200\angle0°$, and $\mathbf{I}_a = 400\angle0°$ A. Determine the following:
 (a) $\mathbf{I}_{a2}$
 (b) $\mathbf{I}_b$
 (c) $\mathbf{I}_c$

9.7 Determine the symmetrical components for the phase currents of $\mathbf{I}_a = 200\angle0°$, $\mathbf{I}_b = 175\angle-90°$, and $\mathbf{I}_c = 100\angle90°$ A.

9.8 Use the symmetrical components for the phase voltages and verify the following line-to-line voltage equations:
 (a) $\mathbf{V}_{ab} = \sqrt{3}\left(V_{a1}\angle30° + V_{a2}\angle-30°\right)$
 (b) $\mathbf{V}_{bc} = \sqrt{3}\left(V_{a1}\angle-90° + V_{a2}\angle90°\right)$
 (c) $\mathbf{V}_{ca} = \sqrt{3}\left(V_{a1}\angle150° + V_{a2}\angle-150°\right)$

9.9 Consider Example 9.3 and assume that the voltage applied at the sending end of the line is 69 $\angle0°$ kV. Determine the phase current matrix from Equation 9.35.

9.10 Consider a three-phase horizontal line configuration and assume that the phase spacings are $D_{ab} = 30$ ft, $D_{bc} = 30$ ft, and $D_{ca} = 60$ ft. The line conductors are made of 500 kcmil, 37-strand copper conductors. Assume that the 100-mi-long untransposed transmission line operates at 50°C, 60 Hz. If the earth has an average resistivity, determine the following:
 (a) Self-impedances of line conductors in ohms per mile
 (b) Mutual impedances of line conductors in ohms per mile
 (c) Phase impedance matrix of line in ohms

9.11 Consider a 50-mi-long completely transposed transmission line operating at 25°C, 50 Hz, having 500 kcmil ACSR conductors. The three-phase conductors have a triangular configuration with spacings of $D_{ab} = 6$ ft, $D_{bc} = 10$ ft, and $D_{ca} = 8$ ft. If the earth is considered to be dry earth, determine the following:
 (a) Zero-sequence impedance of line
 (b) Positive-sequence impedance of line
 (c) Negative-sequence impedance of line

9.12 Consider a three-phase, vertical pole-top conductor configuration. Assume that the phase spacings are $D_{ab} = 72$ in., $D_{bc} = 72$ in., and $D_{ca} = 144$ in. The line conductors are made of 795 kcmil, 30/19-strand ACSR. If the line is 100 mi long and not transposed, determine the following:
 (a) Phase impedance matrix of line
 (b) Phase admittance matrix of line
 (c) Sequence impedance matrix of line
 (d) Sequence admittance matrix of line

9.13 Repeat Problem 9.12 assuming that the phase spacings are $D_{ab} = 144$ in., $D_{bc} = 144$ in., and $D_{ca} = 288$ in.

9.14 Repeat Problem 9.12 assuming that the conductor is 795 kcmil, 61% conductivity, 37-strand, hard-drawn aluminum.

9.15 Repeat Problem 9.13 assuming that the conductor is 750 kcmil, 97.3% conductivity, 37-strand, hard-drawn copper conductor.

9.16 Consider the line configuration shown in Figure 9.5. Assume that the 115 kV line is transposed and its conductors are made up of 500 kcmil, 30/7-strand ACSR conductors. Ignore the OH ground wire but consider the heights of the conductors and determine the zero-sequence capacitance of the line in nanofarads per mile and nanofarads per kilometer.

9.17 Solve Problem 9.16 taking into account the OH ground wire. Assume that the OH ground wire is made of 3/8 in. E.B.B. steel conductor.

9.18 Repeat Example 9.6 without ignoring the OH ground wire. Assume that the OH ground wire is made of 3/8 in. E.B.B. steel conductor.

9.19 Consider the line configuration shown in Figure 9.5. Assume that the 115 kV line is transposed and its conductors are made of 500 kcmil, 30/7-strand ACSR conductors. Ignore the effects of conductor heights and OH ground wire and determine the following:
  (a) Positive- and negative-sequence capacitances to ground of line in nanofarads per mile
  (b) The 60 Hz susceptance of line in microsiemens per mile
  (c) Charging kilovolt-amperes per phase per mile of line
  (d) Three-phase charging kilovolt-amperes per mile of line

9.20 Repeat Problem 9.19 without ignoring the effects of conductor heights.

9.21 Consider the untransposed line shown in Figure P9.21. Assume that the 50-mi-long line has an OH ground wire of 3/0 ACSR and that the phase conductors are of 556.5 kcmil, 30/7-strand ACSR. Use a frequency of 60 Hz, an ambient temperature of 50°C, and average earth resistivity and determine the following:
  (a) Phase impedance matrix of line
  (b) Sequence impedance matrix of line
  (c) Sequence admittance matrix of line
  (d) Electrostatic zero- and negative-sequence unbalance factors of line

9.22 Repeat Problem 9.21 assuming that there are two OH ground wires, as shown in Figure P9.22.

9.23 Consider the power system given in Example 9.7 and assume that transformers T_1 and T_3 are connected as delta/wye-grounded and T_2 and T_4 are connected as wye-grounded/delta, respectively. Assume that there is a fault on bus 3 and do the following:
  (a) Draw the corresponding zero-sequence network.
  (b) Reduce the zero-sequence network to its Thévenin equivalent looking in at bus 3.

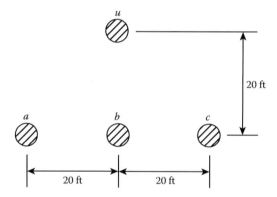

FIGURE P9.21   System for Problem 9.21.

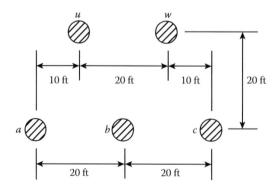

FIGURE P9.22   System for Problem 9.22.

9.24 Consider the power system given in Example 9.7 and assume that all four transformers are connected as wye-grounded/wye-grounded. Assume there is a fault on bus 3 and do the following:

(a) Draw the corresponding zero-sequence network.

(b) Reduce the zero-sequence network to its Thévenin equivalent looking in at bus 3.

9.25 Consider the power system given in Problem 9.36. Use 25 MVA as the megavolt-ampere base and draw the positive-, negative-, and zero-sequence networks (but do not reduce them). Assume that the two three-phase transformer bank connections are

(a) Both wye-grounded

(b) Delta/wye-grounded for transformer T_1 and wye-grounded/delta for transformer T_2

(c) Wye-grounded/wye for transformer T_1 and delta/wye for transformer T_2

9.26 Assume that a three-phase, 45 MVA, 34.5/115 kV transformer bank of three single-phase transformers, with nameplate impedances of 7.5%, is connected wye/delta with the HV side delta. Determine the zero-sequence equivalent circuit (in per-unit values) under the following conditions:

(a) If neutral is ungrounded

(b) If neutral is solidly grounded

(c) If neutral is grounded through 10 Ω resistor

(d) If neutral is grounded through 4000 µF capacitor

9.27 Consider the system shown in Figure P9.27. Assume that the following data are given based on 20 MVA and the line-to-line base voltages as shown in Figure P9.27.

Generator G_1: $X_1 = 0.25$ pu, $X_2 = 0.15$ pu, $X_0 = 0.05$ pu.

Generator G_2: $X_2 = 0.90$ pu, $X_2 = 0.60$ pu, $X_0 = 0.05$ pu.

Transformer T_1: $X_1 = X_2 = X_0 = 0.10$ pu.

Transformer T_2: $X_1 = X_2 = 0.10$ pu, $X_0 = \infty$.

Transformer T_3: $X_1 = X_2 = X_0 = 0.50$ pu.

Transformer T_4: $X_1 = X_2 = 0.30$ pu, $X_0 = \infty$.

Transmission line TL_{23}: $X, = X_2 = 0.15$ pu, $X_0 = 0.50$ pu.

Transmission line TL_{35}: $X_1 = X_2 = 0.30$ pu, $X_0 = 1.00$ pu.

Transmission line TL_{57}: $X_1 = X_2 = 0.30$ pu, $X_0 = 1.00$ pu.

(a) Draw the corresponding positive-sequence network.

(b) Draw the corresponding negative-sequence network.

(c) Draw the corresponding zero-sequence network.

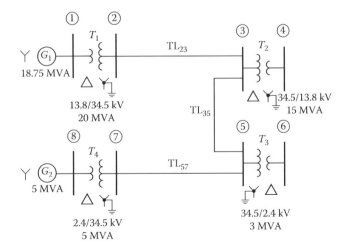

FIGURE P9.27   System for Problem 9.27.

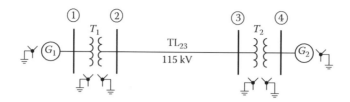

FIGURE P9.28 System for Problem 9.28.

9.28 Consider the system showing in Figure P9.28 and the following data:

Generator G_1: 15 kV, 50 MVA, $X_1 = X_2 = 0.10$ pu and $X_0 = 0.05$ pu based on its own ratings.

Generator G_1: 15 kV, 20 MVA, $X_1 = X_2 = 0.20$ pu and $X_0 = 0.07$ pu based on its own ratings.

Transformer T_1: 15/115 kV, 30 MVA, $X_1 = X_2 = X_0 = 0.06$ pu based on its own ratings.

Transformer T_2: 115/15 kV, 25 MVA, $X_1 = X_2 = X_0 = 0.07$ pu based on its own ratings.

Transmission line TL_{23}: $X_1 = X_2 = 0.03$ pu and $X_0 = 0.10$ pu based on its own ratings.

Assume an SLG fault at bus 4 and determine the fault current in per units and amperes. Use 50 MVA as the megavolt-ampere base and assume that Z_f is $j0.1$ pu based on 50 MVA.

9.29 Consider the system given in Problem 9.28 and assume that there is a line-to-line fault at bus 3 involving phases b and c. Determine the fault currents for both phases in per units and amperes.

9.30 Consider the system given in Problem 9.28 and assume that there is a DLG fault at bus 2, involving phases b and c. Assume that Z_f is $j0.1$ pu and Z_g is $j0.2$ pu (where Z_g is the neutral-to-ground impedance) both based on 50 VA.

9.31 Consider the system shown in Figure P9.31 and assume that the generator is loaded and running at the rated voltage with the CB open at bus 3. Assume that the reactance values of the generator are given as $X_d'' = X_1 = X_2 = 0.14$ pu and $X_0 = 0.08$ pu based on its ratings. The transformer impedances are $Z_1 = Z_2 = Z_0 = j0.05$ pu based on its ratings. The transmission line TL23 has $Z_1 = Z_2 = j0.04$ pu and $Z_0 = j0.10$ pu. Assume that the fault point is located on bus 1. Select 25 MVA as the megavolt-ampere base and 8.5 and 138 kV as the LV and HV bases, respectively, and determine the following:

(a) Subtransient fault current for three-phase fault in per units and amperes

(b) The SLG fault (Also find the ratio of this SLG fault current to the three-phase fault current found in part [a].)

(c) Line-to-line fault (Also find the ratio of this line-to-line fault current to previously calculated three-phase fault current.)

(d) DLG fault

9.32 Repeat Problem 9.31 assuming that the fault is located on bus 2.

9.33 Repeat Problem 9.31 assuming that the fault is located on bus 3.

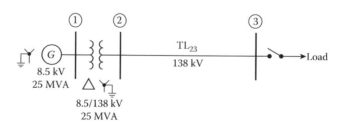

FIGURE P9.31 System for Problem 9.31.

9.34 Consider the system shown in Figure P9.34a. Assume that loads, line capacitance, and transformer-magnetizing currents are neglected and that the following data are given based on 20 MVA and the line-to-line voltages as shown in Figure P9.34a. Do not neglect the resistance of the transmission line TL_{23}. The prefault positive-sequence voltage at bus 3 is $\mathbf{V}_{an} = 1.0\angle0°$ pu, as shown in Figure P9.34b.

Generator: $X_1 = 0.20$ pu, $X_2 = 0.10$ pu, $X_0 = 0.05$ pu.

Transformer T_1: $X_1 = X_2 = 0.05$ pu, $X_0 = X_1$ (looking into HV side).

Transformer T_2: $X_1 = X_2 = 0.05$ pu, $X_0 = \infty$ (looking into HV side).

Transmission line: $\mathbf{Z}_1 = \mathbf{Z}_2 = 0.2 + j0.2$ pu, $\mathbf{Z}_0 = 0.6 + j0.6$ pu.

Assume that there is a bolted (i.e., with zero fault impedance) line-to-line fault on phases b and c at bus 3 and determine the following:

(a) Fault current I_{bf} in per units and amperes

(b) Phase voltages V_a, V_b, and V_c at bus 2 in per units and kilovolts

(c) Line-to-line voltages V_{ab}, V_{bc}, and V_{ca} at bus 2 in kilovolts

(d) Generator line currents I_a, I_b, and I_c

Given: Per-unit positive-sequence currents on the LV side of the transformer bank lag positive-sequence currents on the HV side by 30° and similarly for negative-sequence currents excepting that the LV currents lead the HV by 30°.

9.35 Consider Figure P9.35 and assume that the generator ratings are 2.40/4.16Y kV, 15 MW (3ϕ), 18.75 MVA (3ϕ), 80% power factor, two poles, 3600 rpm. Generator reactances are $X_1 = X_2 = 0.10$ pu and $X_0 = 0.05$ pu, all based on generator ratings. Note that the given value of X_1 is subtransient reactance X'', one of several different positive-sequence reactances of a synchronous machine. The subtransient reactance corresponds to the initial symmetrical fault current (the transient dc component not included) that occurs before demagnetizing armature magnetomotive force begins to weaken the net field excitation. If manufactured in accordance with US standards, the coils of a synchronous generator will withstand the mechanical forces that accompany a three-phase fault current, but not more. Assume that this generator is to supply a four-wire, wye-connected distribution. Therefore, the neutral grounding reactor X_n should have the smallest possible reactance.

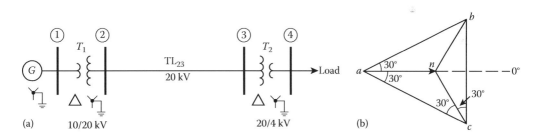

FIGURE P9.34   System for Problem 9.34.

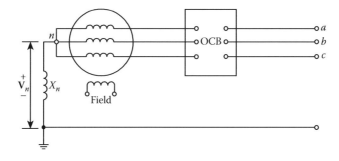

FIGURE P9.35   System for Problem 9.35.

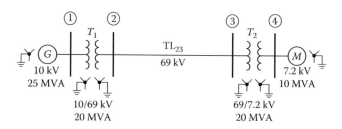

FIGURE P9.36   System for Problem 9.36.

Consider both SLG and DLG faults. Assume the prefault positive-sequence internal voltage of phase a is 2500 $\angle 0°$ or 1.042 0° 1.042 $\angle 0°$pu and determine the following:

(a) Specify X_n in ohms and in per units.

(b) Specify the minimum allowable momentary symmetrical current rating of the reactor in amperes.

(c) Find the initial symmetrical voltage across the reactor, $\mathbf{V}_n$, when a bolted SLG fault occurs on the oil circuit breaker (OCB) terminal in volts.

9.36 Consider the system shown in Figure P9.36 and the following data:

Generator G: $X_1 = X_2 = 0.10$ pu and $X_0 = 0.05$ pu based on its ratings.

Motor: $X_1 = X_2 = 0.10$ pu and $X_0 = 0.05$ pu based on its ratings.

Transformer T_1: $X_1 = X_2 = X_0 = 0.05$ pu based on its ratings.

Transformer T_2: $X_1 = X_2 = X_0 = 0.10$ pu based on its ratings.

Transmission line TL$_{23}$: $X_1 = X_2 = X_0 = 0.09$ pu based on 25 MVA.

Assume that bus 2 is faulted and determine the faulted phase currents.

(a) Determine the three-phase fault.

(b) Determine the line-to-ground fault involving phase a.

(c) Use the results of part (a) and calculate the line-to-neutral phase voltages at the fault point.

9.37 Consider the system given in Problem 9.36 and assume a line-to-line fault, involving phases b and c, at bus 2, and determine the faulted phase currents.

9.38 Consider the system shown in Figure P9.38 and assume that the associated data are given in Table P9.38 and are based on a 100 MVA base and referred to nominal system voltages.

Assume that there is a three-phase fault at bus 6. Ignore the prefault currents and determine the following:

(a) Fault current in per units at faulted bus 6

(b) Fault current in per units in transmission line TL$_{25}$

9.39 Use the results of Problem 9.38 and calculate the line-to-neutral phase voltages at the faulted bus 6.

9.40 Repeat Problem 9.38 assuming a line-to-ground fault, with $\mathbf{Z}_f = 0$ pu, at bus 6.

9.41 Use results of Problem 9.40 and calculate the line-to-neutral phase voltages at the following buses:

(a) Bus 6

(b) Bus 2

9.42 Repeat Problem 9.38 assuming a line-to-line fault at bus 6.

9.43 Repeat Problem 9.38 assuming a DLG fault, with $\mathbf{Z}_f = 0$ and $\mathbf{Z}_g = 0$, at bus 6.

9.44 Consider the system described in Example 9.7 and assume that there is an SLG fault, involving phase a, at the indicated bus. Show the interconnection of the resulting reduced equivalent sequence networks. Determine sequence and phase currents and sequence and phase voltages:

(a) Fault is at bus 1.

(b) Fault is at bus 2.

(c) Fault is at bus 4.

(d) Fault is at bus 5.

(e) Fault is at bus 6.

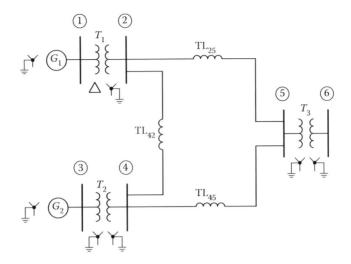

FIGURE P9.38   System for Problem 9.38.

TABLE P9.38
Data for Problem 9.38

Network Component	X_1 (pu)	X_2 (pu)	X_3 (pu)
G_1	0.35	0.35	0.09
G_2	0.35	0.35	0.09
T_1	0.10	0.10	0.10
T_2	0.10	0.10	0.10
T_3	0.05	0.05	0.05
TL_{42}	0.45	0.45	1.80
TL_{25}	0.35	0,45	1 15
TL_{45}	0.35	0.35	1.15

9.45 Repeat Problem 9.44 assuming a fault impedance of 5 Ω.

9.46 Repeat Problem 9.45 assuming a line-to-line fault involving phases b and c but without $\mathbf{Z}_f = 5$ Ω.

9.47 Repeat Problem 9.46 assuming a fault impedance of 5 Ω.

9.48 Repeat Problem 9.44 assuming a DLG fault involving phases b and c.

9.49 Repeat Problem 9.48 assuming a fault through a fault impedance $\mathbf{Z}_f$ of 5 Ω on each phase and then to ground G through impedance $\mathbf{Z}_g$ of 10 Ω.

9.50 Repeat Problem 9.44 assuming a three-phase fault.

9.51 Repeat Problem 9.50 assuming a fault impedance $\mathbf{Z}_f$ of 5 Ω on each phase.

9.52 Consider the system shown in Figure P9.52 and data given in Table P9.52. Assume there is a fault at bus 2. After drawing the corresponding sequence networks, reduce them to their Thévenin equivalents looking in at bus 2:
   (a) Positive-sequence network
   (b) Negative-sequence network
   (c) Zero-sequence network

9.53 Use the solution of Problem 9.52 and calculate the fault currents for the following faults, and draw the corresponding interconnected sequence networks:
   (a) SLG fault at bus 2 assuming faulted phase is phase a
   (b) DLG fault at bus 2 involving phases b and c
   (c) Three-phase fault at bus 2

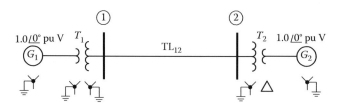

FIGURE P9.52 System for Problem 9.52.

TABLE P9.52
Table for Problem 9.52

Network Component MVA	Base (pu)	X_1 (pu)	X_2 (pu)	X_0 (pu)
G_1	100	0.2	0.15	0.05
G_2	100	0.3	0.2	0.05
T_1	100	0.2	0.2	0.2
T_2	100	0.15	0.15	0.15
TL_{12}	100	0.6	0.6	0.9

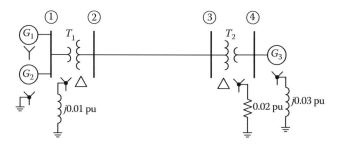

FIGURE P9.54 System for Problem 9.54.

9.54 Consider the system shown in Figure P9.54 and data given in Table P9.54. Assume that there is an SLG fault at bus 3. Determine the following:
(a) Thévenin equivalent positive-sequence impedance.
(b) Thévenin equivalent negative-sequence impedance.
(c) Thévenin equivalent zero-sequence impedance.
(d) Positive-, negative-, and zero-sequence currents.
(e) Phase currents in per units and amperes.
(f) Positive-, negative-, and zero-sequence voltages.
(g) Phase voltages in per units and kilovolts.
(h) Line-to-line voltages in per units and kilovolts.
(i) Draw a voltage phasor diagram using before-the-fault line-to-neutral and line-to-line voltage values.
(j) Draw a voltage phasor diagram using the resultant after-the-fault line-to-neutral and line-to-line voltage values.

9.55 Consider the system shown in Figure P9.55 and assume that the following data on the same base are given:
Generator G_1: $X_1 = 0.15$ pu, $X_2 = 0.10$ pu, $X_0 = 0.05$ pu.
Generator G_2: $X_1 = 0.30$ pu, $X_2 = 0.20$ pu, $X_0 = 0.10$ pu.
Transformer T_1: $X_1 = X_2 = X_0 = 0.10$ pu.

TABLE P9.54

Table for Problem 9.54

Network Component	MVA Rating	Voltage Rating (kV)	X_1 (pu)	X_2 (pu)	X_0 (pu)
G_1	100	13.8	0.15	0.15	0.05
G_2	100	13.8	0.15	0.15	0.05
G_3	100	13.8	0.15	0.15	0.05
T_1	100	13.8/115	0.20	0.20	0.20
T_2	100	115/13.8	0.18	0.18	0.18
TL_{23}	100	115	0.30	0.30	0.90

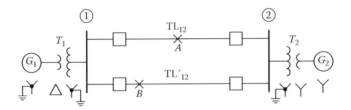

FIGURE P9.55 System for Problem 9.55.

Transformer T_2: $X_1 = X_2 = X_0 = 0.15$ pu.
Transmission line TL_{12}: $X_1 = X_2 = 0.30$ pu, $X_0 = 0.60$ pu.
Transmission line TL_{12}: $X_1 = X_2 = 0.30$ pu, $X_0 = 0.60$ pu.
Assume that fault point A is located at the middle of the top transmission line, as shown in the figure, and determine the fault current(s) in per units for the following faults:
(a) SLG fault (involving phase a)
(b) DLG fault (involving phases b and c)
(c) Three-phase fault

9.56 Repeat Problem 9.55 assuming that the fault point is B and is located at the beginning of the bottom line.

9.57 Consider the system shown in Figure P9.57 and assume that the following data on the same base are given:
Generator G_1: $X_1 = 0.15$ pu, $X_2 = 0.10$ pu, $X_0 = 0.05$ pu.
Generator G_2: $X_1 = 0.15$ pu, $X_2 = 0.10$ pu, $X_0 = 0.05$ pu.
Transformer T_1: $X_1 = X_2 = X_0 = 0.10$ pu.
Transformer T_2: $X_1 = X_2 = X_0 = 0.15$ pu.
Transmission lines: $X_1 = X_2 = 0.30$ pu, $X_0 = 0.60$ (all three are identical).
Assume that fault point A is located at the middle of the bottom line, as shown in the figure, and determine the fault current(s) in per units for the following faults:
(a) SLG fault (involving phase a)
(b) SLG fault (involving phases b and c)
(c) DLG fault (involving phases b and c)
(d) Three-phase fault

9.58 Repeat Problem 9.57 assuming that the faulted point is B and is located at the end of the bottom line.

9.59 Consider the system shown in Figure P9.59 and its data given in Table P9.59. Assume that there is an SLG fault involving phase a at fault point F.
(a) Draw the corresponding equivalent positive-sequence network.
(b) Draw the corresponding equivalent negative-sequence network.
(c) Draw the corresponding equivalent zero-sequence network.

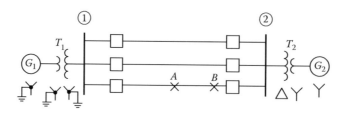

FIGURE P9.57   System for Problem 9.57.

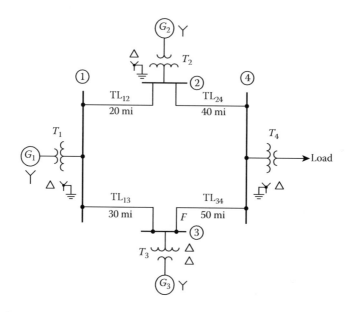

FIGURE P9.59   System for Problem 9.59.

TABLE P9.59
Table for Problem 9.59

Network Component	Base MVA	Base kV$_{(L-L)}$	X_1 (pu)	X_2 (pu)	X_3 (pu)
G_1	100	230	0–15	0 15	
G_2	100	230	0.20	0.20	
G_3	100	230	0.25	0.25	
T_1	100	230	0.10	0.10	0.10
T_2	100	230	0.09	0.09	0.09
T_3	100	230	0.08	0.08	0.08
T_4	100	230	0.11	0.11	0.11
TL_{12}	100	230	0.10	0.10	0.36
TL_{13}	100	230	0.20	0.20	0.60
TL_{24}	100	230	0.35	0.35	1.05
TL_{34}	100	230	0.40	0.40	1.20

9.60 Use the results of Problem 9.59 and determine the interior sequence currents flowing in each of the four transmission lines:
   (a) Positive-sequence currents
   (b) Negative-sequence currents
   (c) Zero-sequence currents

9.61 Use the results of Problem 9.60 and determine the interior phase currents in each of the four transmission lines:
   (a) Phase *a* currents
   (b) Phase *b* currents
   (c) Phase *c* currents

9.62 Use the results of Problems 9.60 and 9.61 and draw a three-line diagram of the given system. Show the phase and sequence currents on it.
   (a) Determine the SLG fault current.
   (b) Is the fault current equal to the sum of the zero-sequence currents (i.e., $\mathbf{I}_{f(\mathrm{SLG})} = \sum 3\mathbf{I}_{a0}$)?

REFERENCES

1. Fortescue, C. L. Method of symmetrical coordinates applied to the solution of polyphase networks, *Trans. Am. Inst. Electr. Eng.* 37, 1918, 1027–1140.
2. Carson, J. R. Wave propagation in overhead wires with ground return, *Bell Syst. Tech. J.* 5, 1926, 539–554.
3. Gross, E. T. B. and Hesse, M. H. Electromagnetic unbalance of untransposed lines, *Trans. Am. Inst. Electr. Eng.* 72 (Pt. 3), 1953, 1323–1336.
4. Anderson, P. M. *Analysis of Faulted Power Systems*, Iowa State University Press, Ames, IA, 1973.
5. Westinghouse Electric Corporation. *Electrical Transmission and Distribution Reference Book*, WEC, East Pittsburgh, PA, 1964.
6. Clarke, E. *Circuit Analysis of A-C Power Systems*, vol. 2, General Electric Co., Schenectady, NY, 1960.
7. Gönen, T. *Modern Power System Analysis*, Wiley, New York, 1987.
8. Clarke, E. *Circuit Analysis of A-C Power Systems*, vol. 1, General Electric Co., Schenectady, NY, 1960.
9. Atabekov, G. I. *The Relay Protection of High Voltage Networks*, Pergamon Press, New York, 1960.
10. Anderson, P. M. Analysis of simultaneous faults by two-port network theory, *IEEE Trans. Power Appar. Syst.* PAS-90(5), 1971, 2199–2205.
11. Beeman, D., ed. *Industrial Power System Handbook*, McGraw-Hill, New York, 1955.
12. North, J. R. et al. Discussions on some engineering features on Peterson coils and their application, *Trans. Am. Inst. Electr. Eng.* 57, 1938, 289–291.
13. Tomlinson, H. R. Ground-fault neutralizer grounding of unit-connected generators, *Trans. Am. Inst. Electr. Eng.* 72(8), 1953, 953–961.
14. Wagner, C. F. and Evans, R. D. *Symmetrical Components*, McGraw-Hill, New York, 1933.
15. Gönen, T., Nowikowski, J., and Brooks, C. L. Electrostatic unbalances of transmission lines with 'N' overhead ground wires, part I, *Proc. Model. Simul. Conf.* 17 (Pt. 2), 1986, 459–464.
16. Gönen, T., Nowikowski, J., and Brooks, C. L. Electrostatic unbalances of transmission lines with 'N' overhead ground wires, part I, *Proc. Model. Simul. Conf.* 17 (Pt. 2), 1986, 465–470.
17. Gönen, T. and M. S. Haj-Mohamadi. Electromagnetic unbalances of six-phase transmission lines, *Electr. Power Energ. Syst.* 11(2), April 1989, 78–84.
18. Gönen, T. *Electric Power Distribution System Engineering*, CRC Press, Boca Raton, FL, 2008.

GENERAL REFERENCES

Brown, H. E. *Solution of Large Networks by Matrix Methods*, Wiley, New York, 1975.
Calabrese, G. O. *Symmetrical Components Applied to Electric Power Network*, Ronald Press, New York, 1959.
Chen, M. S. and Dillon, W. E. Power system modeling, *Proc. IEEE* 62(7), 1974, 901–915.
Clarke, E. Simultaneous faults on three-phase systems, *Trans. Am. Inst. Electr. Eng.* 50, 1931, 919–941.
Clem, J. E. Reactance of transmission lines with ground return, *Trans. Am. Inst. Electr. Eng.* 50, 1931, 901–918.
Dawalibi, F. and Niles, G. B. Measurements and computations of fault current distribution of overhead transmission lines, *IEEE Trans. Power Appar. Syst.* PAS-103(3), 1984, 553–560.

Duesterhoeft, W. C., Schutz, M. W., Jr., and Clarke, E. Determination of instantaneous currents and voltages by means of alpha, beta, and zero components, *Trans. Am. Inst. Electr. Eng.* 70 (Pt. 3), 1951, 1248–1255.

Elgerd, O. I. *Electric Energy Systems Theory: An Introduction*, McGraw-Hill, New York, 1971.

Ferguson, W. H. Symmetrical component network connections for the solution of phase interchange faults, *Trans. Am. Inst. Electr. Eng.* 78 (Pt. 3), 1959, 948–950.

Garin, A. N. Zero-phase-sequence characteristics of transformers, parts I and 11, *Gen. Electr. Rev.* 43, 1940, 131–136, 174–170.

Gönen, T. *Electric Power Distribution System Engineering*, McGraw-Hill, New York, 1986.

Gross, C. A. *Power System Analysis*, Wiley, New York, 1979.

Guile, A. E. and Paterson, W. *Electrical Power Systems*, vol. 1, Pergamon Press, New York, 1978.

Harder, E. L. Sequence network connections for unbalanced load and fault conditions, *Electr. J.* 34(12), 1937, 481–488.

Hobson, J. E. and Whitehead, D. L. Symmetrical components, in *Electrical Transmission and Distribution Reference Book*, Chapter 2, WEC, East Pittsburgh, PA, 1964.

Kron, G. *Tensor Analysis of Networks*, Wiley, New York, 1939.

Lyle, A. G. *Major Faults on Power Systems*, Chapman & Hall, London, U.K., 1952.

Lyon, W. V. *Applications of the Method of Symmetrical Components*, McGraw-Hill, New York, 1937.

Mortlock, J. R., Davies, M. W. H., and Jackson, W. *Power System Analysis*, Chapman & Hall, London, U.K., 1952.

Neuenswander, J. R. *Modern Power Systems*, International Textbook Co., New York, 1971.

Roper, R. *Kurzschlussstrime in Drehstromnetzen*, 5th Ger. edn. (translated as *Short-Circuit Currents in Three-Phase Networks*), Siemens Aktienges, Munich, Germany, 1972.

Rildenberg, R. *Transient Performance of Electric Power Systems-Phenomena in Lumped Networks*, 1st edn., McGraw-Hill, New York, 1950.

Stevenson, W. D., Jr. *Elements of Power System Analysis*, 4th edn., McGraw-Hill, New York, 1982.

Stigant, S. A. *Mathematical and Geometrical Techniques for Symmetrical Component Fault Studies*, MacDonald & Co., London, U.K., 1965.

Wagner, C. F. and Evans, R. D. *Symmetrical Components*, McGraw-Hill, New York, 1941.

Weedy, B. M. *Electric Power Systems*, 3rd edn., Wiley, New York, 1979.

10 Protective Equipment and Transmission System Protection

Experience is the name everyone gives to their mistake.

Oscar Wilde

10.1 INTRODUCTION

The proper operation of a transmission system depends on protective equipment to detect fault conditions and disconnect malfunctioning equipment. The protective equipment must protect people and power system apparatus from malfunctions, whether the malfunction is the result of an equipment failure, accidents, weather, or misoperations by the personnel involved. The most important protective equipment for transmission system are CBs, disconnect switches, and relays to sense fault conditions.

10.2 INTERRUPTION OF FAULT CURRENT

The main function of interrupting equipment such as CBs is to stop the flow of current. During the process of interruption, an arc is created that must be extinguished. The arc is caused by any gas that is located between separating contacts and subject to the electrical field. The gas ionizes, becomes an arc, and starts to support current flow through it. The higher the voltage that the contacts are breaking, the more severe the arcing is. Inductive loads makes arc even more severe. Most industrial loads and faulted lines are inductive.

There are two methods to extinguish an arc. The first method involves lengthening the arc until it is long and thin, which causes the arc resistance to increase. This increase in resistance causes the arc current to decrease and the temperature of the arc to drop and eventually results in not having enough energy in the arc to keep it ionized. The second method involves the opening of the arc in a medium that can absorb energy from the arc causing it to cool and quench.

DC arcs are more difficult to break than ac arcs because ac goes through a current zero every half cycle, which dc does not. Hence, in an ac CB, the advantage of current zero is taken and then dielectric strength is injected between the contacts of the CB faster than the recovery voltage building up.

Note that after ac zero, the arc may establish itself beyond the first current zero, if the medium between the contacts is still ionized. Furthermore, even if the arc does not reestablish itself immediately due to the medium being ionized, the voltage rise across the contacts may cause the arc to reestablish in the event that the contacts are not sufficiently apart.

As illustrated in Figure 10.1c, during a short circuit, the current lags the system voltage by upwards of 90°, depending on the relative values of R and X. At the instant the fault current goes through zero, the system voltage may be nearly at maximum. It is at this instant that the arc goes out temporarily. But, the voltage across the breaker suddenly shoots from this low value toward full system voltage. The inductance and capacitance in the circuit, however, cause the voltage to

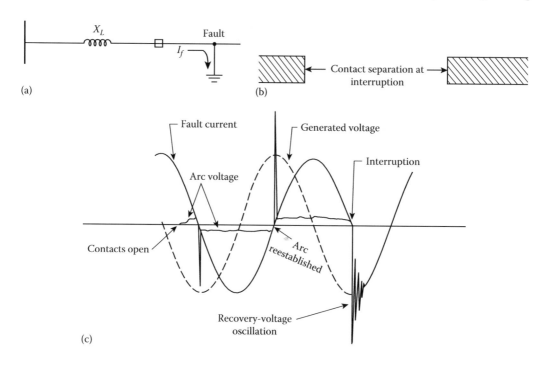

FIGURE 10.1 Interruption of short-circuit current: (a) equipment circuit, (b) contact separation, and (c) current and voltage waveforms.

overshoot to a value that is as far above the system voltage as it was below it at the beginning. Hence, the transient voltage across the breaker may be nearly double the steady-state system voltage.

Furthermore, if the sudden increase in the arc resistance, as the current approaches zero, should cause the current to reach zero prematurely, that would cause another transient and produce more voltage due to the greater rate of change of current in the inductive circuit. These voltages are called the *recovery voltages* and they appear across the breaker. The rate at which the voltage builds up is known as the *rate of rise of recovery voltage*. The arc that is established in the first ¼ cycle is called a *reignition*, and the arc that is reestablished after the first ¼ cycle is called a *restrike*.

In a plain-break CB, the earlier cycle may be repeated several times. Eventually though, arc extinction becomes permanent and circuit interruption is complete. The high *X/R* ratio of the circuit causes the arc to be more difficult to break.

A special problem occurs in interrupting the leading current of a capacitor or an unloaded transmission line. Here, at the first current zero of a leading current arc, interruption takes place very easily. This is due to the fact that the capacitor retains the instantaneous voltage of the source at the instant of current zero, and for several hundred microseconds thereafter, the voltage across the breaker is low.

Hence, interruption seems to be accomplished at the first current zero of arc despite the fact that contact separation is very small. A ¼ cycle later, however, the system voltage reverses, and another ¼ cycle after that, approximately a double voltage, appears across the breaker. If the CB withstands this voltage without restriking, then the interruption is complete. At high currents, the arc produces an increased amount of hotter gas. Hence, the short arc gap cannot withstand a double voltage, and this voltage causes a restrike during the ½ cycle immediately after the first interruption.

In the event that the restrike takes place just ½ cycle after the first interruption, the capacitor has a charge whose polarity is opposite to that of the system voltage. Thus, the current flow is limited by the inductance of the circuit. Because of the capacitance, the voltage overshoots its mark by the initial difference. As a result, the voltage can reach $-3E$ at exact moment that the transient current passes through zero.

Therefore, it is harder to switch off capacitors and open-circuited transmission lines than to open the same amount of lagging current. Doing so produces HVs. However, modern CBs have additional design features that help in the interruption of leading current.

Also, note that the arc energy transferred to the medium between the contacts causes the medium to reach temperatures as high as 30,000 K and high pressures very quickly. The resulting expansion of the medium is almost explosive. Hence, the combination of high mechanical arc forces can cause the ground to shake around a large CB when it operates. This fact has to be taken into account in the substation ground preparations.

10.3 HIGH-VOLTAGE CIRCUIT BREAKERS

According to IEEE Std. C.37.100-1992, "a circuit breaker is mechanical switching device capable of making, carrying, and breaking currents under normal circuit conditions and also making, carrying, and breaking for a specified time, and breaking currents under specified abnormal conditions such as a short circuit."

In general, CBs are categorized based on their interrupting medium used. The types of CBs are magnetic, vacuum, air blast, oil, and SF_6 gas.

In the United States, the air magnetic CBs are no longer being installed, and the old ones are being replaced by vacuum or SF_6 CBs.

Vacuum types are used in switchgear applications up to 38 kV class and below. Vacuum CBs use an interrupter that is a small cylinder enclosing the moving contacts under a hard vacuum. In a vacuum CB operation, when the contacts part, an arc is formed from contact separation. The resultant arc products are immediately forced to and deposited on a metallic shield surrounding the contacts. Since there is nothing to sustain the arc, it is instantly extinguished. These CBs are extensively used for metal-clad switchgear, as said before, up to 38 kV class.

Also, air blast breakers, which were used at 345 kV or above applications, are no longer manufactured. They are replaced by SF_6 CBs. Furthermore, oil CBs were very popular in the electric power utility industry in the past. Today, they are also being increasingly replaced by the SF_6 CBs in the old and new installations.

The oil CBs were used to be designed as a single-tank or three-tank apparatus for 69 kV or below. Otherwise, they had three tank designs for 115 kV and above applications. The disadvantages of the oil CBs were large space requirements, their significant foundation requirements due to their immense weights and impact loads taking place during their operations, and rightfully never ending environmental concerns and regulations. Two types of designs exist for the oil CBs, namely, *dead tank* (or bulk oil) design, which is the type used in the United States, or *live tank* (or minimum oil) design.

SF_6 gas CBs use sulfur hexafluoride (SF_6) gas as an interrupting and insulating medium. SF_6 is proven to be an excellent arc-quenching and insulating medium for CBs. It is a very stable compound, inert, nonflammable, nontoxic, and odorless. SF_6 gas CBs are of either the dead tank design for outdoor installations or live tank (or modular design) for outdoor installations, and increasingly, dead tank breakers are integrated in SF_6-insulated substations for indoor or outdoor installations.

All SF_6 CBs are designed as either the piston (*puffer*) or the dual-pressure (two-tank) system. In single puffer mechanisms, the interrupter is designed to compress the gas during the opening stroke and use the compressed gas as a transfer mechanism to cool the arc and also use the pressure to elongate the arc through a grid (i.e., *arc chutes*), causing the arc to be extinguished when the current passes through zero.

Puffer-type designs are simpler than two-tank designs since all of the SF_6 is at one pressure, 75 psi, which does not liquefy until the temperature drops to 30°C. Two-tank designs have a high-pressure tank in which the interrupter is located and a low-pressure reserve tank. When there is a fault, the high-pressure tank is vented to the low-pressure tank, thus creating turbulence to assist the interruption of the arc. The low-pressure SF_6 is then compressed and returned to the high-pressure tank. The high-pressure tank must be warmed at low temperature to keep the high-pressure SF_6 from liquefying.

In other designs, the arc heats the SF_6 gas and the resulting pressure is used for elongating and interrupting the arc. Some older dual-pressure SF_6 CBs used a pump to provide the high-pressure SF_6 gas for arc interruption.

In order to prevent liquefaction of SF_6 gas at low temperatures, many CBs are equipped with electric heating systems. This is due to the fact that the dielectric strength and interrupting performance of SF_6 gas are reduced significantly at lower pressures, normally as a result of lower ambient temperatures. Because of this, for cold temperature applications (ambient temperature as cold as $-40°C$), dead tank gas CBs are commonly supplied with tank heaters to keep the gas in vapor form rather than allowing it to liquefy. A liquefied SF_6 significantly derates the breaker's capability. For any colder temperature applications (ambient temperatures between $-40°C$ and $-50°C$), the SF_6 used is normally mixed with another gas, typically either nitrogen (N_2) or carbon tetrafluoride (CF_4), to prevent the liquefaction of the SF_6 gas.

The advantages of SF_6 gas CBs are the following:

1. SF_6 gas CBs have a high degree of reliability.
2. The compact design of SF_6 gas CBs substantially reduces space requirements and building installation costs.
3. SF_6 gas CBs can handle all known switching phenomena.
4. SF_6 gas CBs perfectly can adapt to environmental requirements since they have completely enclosed gas system that eliminates any exhaust during switching operations.
5. SF_6 gas CBs require very little maintenance.
6. The lower- and medium-current ratings of SF_6 gas CBs are very economically satisfied by the modular design.
7. Contact separation in SF_6 gas CBs is minimum due to dielectric strength provided by the high-pressure SF_6.
8. SF_6 gas CBs have low arcing time due to the very high rate of recovery of the dielectric.
9. In SF_6 gas CBs, arc reignition is minimized due to the chemical properties of SF_6.

In general, the only disadvantage of the SF_6 CBs is their relatively high costs, which have been somewhat coming down in recent years.

The SF_6 CBs are available as live tank, dead tank, or grounded tank designs. The *live tank* means the interruption happens in an enclosure that is at line potential. Such SF_6 CB has an interrupter chamber that is mounted on insulators and is at line potential. An interrupter with such a modular design can be connected in series to operate at higher-voltage levels.

The *dead tank* means that interruption takes place in a grounded enclosure and CTs are located on both sides of the break (i.e., interrupter contacts). In such CBs, the interruption maintenance takes place at ground level and its seismic withstand is better than CBs with the live tank designs. However, they require more insulating gas in order to provide the proper amount of insulation between the interrupter and the grounded tank enclosure. The modular dead tank CB has been especially developed for integration of SF_6-insulated substation systems.

The *grounded tank* means that interruption happens in an enclosure that is partially at line potential and partially at ground potential. The evolution of the grounded tank CB design is the result of installing a live tank CB interrupter into a dead tank CB design.

SF_6 CBs are available for all voltages ranging from 144 to 765 kV or even above, continuous currents up to 8000 A, and symmetrical interrupting ratings up to 63 kA at 765 kV and 80 kA at 230 kV. Figure 10.2 shows three-pole-operated 245 kV SF_6 dead tank CB fitted with 80 kA interrupters. Figure 10.3 shows single-pole-operated 138 kV SF_6 live tank CBs.

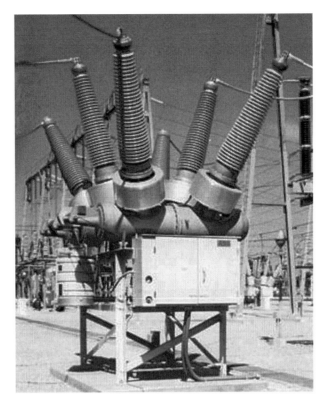

FIGURE 10.2 Three-pole-operated 245 kV SF$_6$ dead tank CB fitted with 80 kA interrupters. (Courtesy of ABB Corporation, Munich, Germany.)

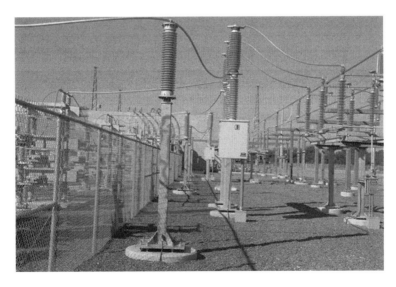

FIGURE 10.3 Single-pole-operated 138 kV SF$_6$ live tank CBs. (Courtesy of ABB Corporation, Munich, Germany.)

However, the pupper types have little lower interrupting capacities (about 50 kA) than dead tank types because their operating mechanisms are too massive when they are built for the same interrupting capacities.

Modern EHV breakers have an average span of about two cycles from the time the relays energize the trip coil to complete interruption of the fault. Clearing times of this order are necessary in many instances to maintain stability when a fault takes place on the system. Faults that last for nine or more cycles generally cause instability.

Some CBs have high-speed automatic reclosing capability. This is due to the fact that in a power system, most faults are temporary and self-clearing. Thus, if a circuit is deenergized for a short time, it is possible that whatever caused the fault has disintegrated and the associated ionized arc in the fault has dissipated.

If such reclosing CBs are used in EHV systems, it is a standard practice to reduce them only once in about 15–50 cycles, based on operating voltage after the CB interrupts the fault. If the fault still persists and the EHV CB recloses into it, the CB reinterrupts the fault current and then *locks out*, requiring operator resetting. Because of the transient stability considerations, repeated reclosing operations are not a standard practice in EHV systems. They are used in distribution systems up to 46 kV voltage levels.

10.4 CIRCUIT BREAKER SELECTION

A CB is selected based on the following factors:

1. The voltage class being considered (nominal rms voltage [class] level)
2. The continuous load current that the CB must carry under normal or emergency conditions
3. The short-circuit current that the breaker must interrupt
4. The speed of short-circuit interruption

The continuous load current can be found from substation loading data or from system load-flow studies. In general, the maximum load of a CB is limited to nameplate rating. However, it is possible to overload a CB under certain conditions. Basically, short-circuit data normally determine the CB selection, given an operating voltage. It is based on nominal three-phase MVA duty or on the basis of rated short-circuit current.

Each CB at the substation gets the extra short-circuit duty as additional circuits are added to a substation. Because of this, it is often required to base the selection of the CBs on future instead of present requirements. As a result of this procedure, the required symmetrical short-circuit ratings of the modern-day CBs have increased to as high as 80 kA.

In general, the faster the CB interrupts a fault, the better it is for the system. Fast interruptions reduce the possibility of extensive damage. Also, the primary reason for having faster CBs on transmission systems is improved transient stability. Because of this, some applications dictate independent pole operation. Independent pole operation provides that even during a breaker malfunction, a three-phase fault will be restricted to a single-pole fault until backup clearing takes place. This is due to the fact that in a breaker without independent pole operation, all three poles operate as one, and the malfunction of any pole prevents all poles from clearing the fault. Hence, a three-phase fault remains as a three-phase fault until backup clearing takes place. This may further cause the stability margin to be reduced. Finally, the selection of CBs is also based on economics, the type of breakers available in the voltage class being considered, and the advantages and disadvantages of competing interruption methods.

The CBs have an operating range that is designated as K factor and is given in IEEE Std. C37.06. For example, for a 72.5 kV CB, the voltage range is 1.21, meaning that the breaker is capable of its full interrupting rating down to a voltage of 60 kV. Interrupting time is defined usually in cycles, and it is usually two cycles for modern CBs used in transmission systems. Interrupting time is defined as the maximum possible delay between energizing the trip circuit at rated control voltage and the interruption of the circuit by the main contacts of all three poles.

The modern CBs usually operate in two cycles of 60 Hz. With fast-acting CBs, the actual current to be interrupted is increased by the dc component of the fault current, and the initial symmetrical rms current value is increased by a specific factor depending on the speed of the CB. For example, if the CB opening time is 8, 2, or 2 cycles, then the corresponding multiplying factor is 1.0, 1.2, or 1.4, respectively. The interrupting capacity (i.e., *rating*) of a CB is found from

$$S_{\text{interrupting}} = \sqrt{3}\left(V_{\text{prefault}}\right)\left(I''_{\text{rms}}\right)\zeta \times 10^{-6}\,\text{MVA} \tag{10.1}$$

where

V_{prefault} is the prefault line voltage at the point of fault in V
I''_{rms} is the initial symmetrical rms current (also called *subtransient current*) in A
ζ is the multiplying factor according to CB speed

However, it is important to note that only the ac component of the fault current is included in the earlier equation. This current is also called the *subtransient current*. Also, note that the *fault* MVA is often referred as the *fault level*.

The asymmetrical current wave decays gradually to a symmetrical current. The rate of such decay of the dc component is determined by the *X/R* or *L/R* of the system supplying the current. The time constant for dc component decay can be determined from

$$T_{\text{dc}} = \text{Circuit}\left(\frac{L}{R}\right) = \text{s}$$

or

$$T_{\text{dc}} = \frac{\text{Circuit}\left(L/R\right)}{2\pi}\,\text{cycles} \tag{10.2}$$

The maximum possible value of the dc current component is

$$I_{f(\text{dc}),\text{max}} = \sqrt{2}I''_f \tag{10.3}$$

The total maximum instantaneous current is

$$I''_{\text{max}} = 2I_{f(\text{dc}),\text{max}} \tag{10.4}$$

or

$$I''_{\text{max}} = 2\sqrt{2}I''_f \tag{10.5}$$

The momentary duty (or rating) of a CB also includes this dc component of the fault current. It can be expressed as

$$S_{\text{momentary}} = \sqrt{3}\left(V_{\text{prefault}}\right)\left(I''_{\text{rms}}\right)\times 1.6 \times 10^{-6}\,\text{MVA} \tag{10.6}$$

or

$$S_{\text{momentary}} = \sqrt{3}\left(V_{\text{prefault}}\right)\left(I_{\text{momentary}}\right) \times 10^{-6}\,\text{MVA} \tag{10.7}$$

The rms momentary current is the total rms current that includes both the ac and dc components and can be found from

$$I_{\text{momentary}} = 1.6 I_{f,\text{rms}} \tag{10.8}$$

and it is used for CBs of 115 kV and above. The CB must be able to withstand this rms current during the first half cycle after the fault occurs. If the $I_{f,\text{max}}$ is measured in peak amperes, then the peak momentary current is expressed as

$$I_{\text{momentary}} = 2.7 I_{f,\text{rms}} \tag{10.9}$$

A simplified procedure for determining the symmetrical fault current is known as the *E/X method* and is described in Section 5.3.1 of ANSI C37.010. This method [1,2] gives results approximating those obtained by more rigorous methods. In using this method, it is necessary first to make an *E/X* calculation. The method then corrects this calculation to take into account both ac and dc decay components of the fault current, depending on circuit parameters.

Example 10.1

Consider the power system shown in Figure 10.4 and assume that the generator is unloaded and running at the rated voltage with the CB open at bus 3. The reactance values of the generator are $X_1 = X_2 = X_d'' = 0.14$ pu and $X_0 = 0.08$ pu based on its ratings. The transformer impedances are $Z_1 = Z_2 = Z_0 = j0.10$ pu based on its ratings. The transmission line TL_{23} has the symmetrical component impedances of $Z_1 = Z_2 = j0.03$ pu and $Z_0 = j0.09$ pu. Select 25 MVA as the MVA base and 13.8 and 138 kV as the LV and HV bases. If the fault point is located on bus 1, find the subtransient fault current for a three-phase fault in per units and amperes.

Solution

The subtransient fault current for a three-phase fault located at bus 1 is

$$I_f'' = \frac{E_g}{X''} = \frac{1.0\angle0°}{j0.14} = -j7.143\,\text{pu}$$

The current base for the LV side is

$$I_{B(\text{LV})} = \frac{S_B}{\sqrt{3}V_{B(\text{L}-\text{V})}} = \frac{25{,}000\,\text{kVA}}{\sqrt{3}\left(13.8\,\text{kV}\right)} = 1{,}045.92\,\text{A}$$

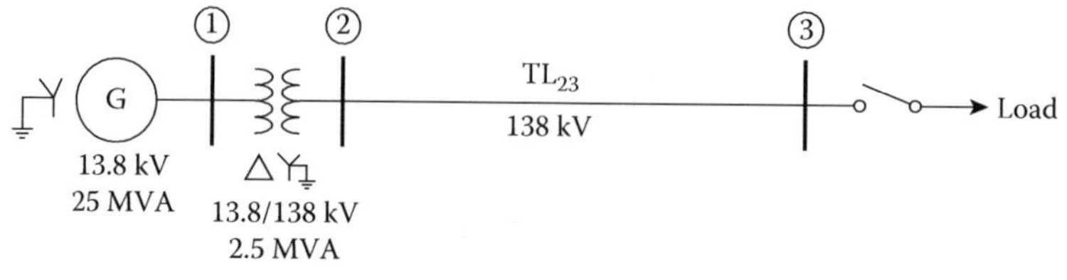

FIGURE 10.4 Transmission system for Example 10.1.

Hence, the magnitude of the fault current is

$$|I_f''| = (7.143 \text{ pu})(11{,}045.92 \text{ A}) \cong 7{,}471 \text{ A}$$

Example 10.2

Use the results of Example 10.1 and determine the following:

(a) Maximum possible value of dc current component
(b) Total maximum instantaneous current
(c) Momentary current
(d) Interrupting rating of a two-cycle CB, if it is located at bus 1
(e) Momentary duty of a two-cycle breaker, if it is located at bus 1

Solution

(a) Considering the peak-to-peak amplitude shown in Figure 10.5, the maximum possible value of dc component of the fault current is

$$I_{f(dc),max} = \sqrt{2}I_f''$$
$$= \sqrt{2}(7.143 \text{ pu}) \cong 10.1 \text{ pu}$$

(b) The total maximum instantaneous value of the fault current is

$$I_{max}'' = 2I_{f(dc),max}$$
$$= 2\left(\sqrt{2}I_f''\right) = 20.2 \text{ pu}$$

(c) The total rms momentary current is

$$I_{momentary} = 1.6I_{f,rms}$$
$$= 1.6(7.143 \text{ pu}) = 11.43 \text{ pu}$$

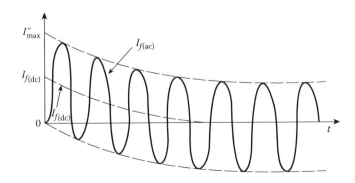

FIGURE 10.5 Asymmetrical fault current I_f with its symmetrical current component $I_{f(ac)}$ and its dc current component $I_{f(dc)}$.

(d) The interrupting rating of a two-cycle CB that is located at bus 1 is

$$S_{\text{interrupting}} = \sqrt{3}\left(V_{\text{prefault}}\right)\left(I''_f\right)\zeta \times 10^{-6}\ \text{MVA}$$

$$= \sqrt{3}\left(13{,}800\,\text{V}\right)\left(7{,}471\,\text{A}\right)\left(1.4\right)\times 10^{-6} \cong 250\ \text{MVA}$$

(e) The momentary duty of the CB is

$$S_{\text{momentary}} = \sqrt{3}\left(V_{\text{prefault}}\right)\left(I''_f\right)1.6\times 10^{-6}\ \text{MVA}$$

$$= \sqrt{3}\left(13{,}800\,\text{V}\right)\left(7{,}471\,\text{A}\right)\left(1.6\right)\times 10^{-6} \cong 285.7\ \text{MVA}$$

10.5 DISCONNECT SWITCHES

Based on its function, a *disconnect switch* is the simplest switch. It can be operated only when the CB is open, in no-load condition. It cannot open normal load current. They are used primarily for isolation of equipment such as buses or other live apparatus. For example, they are used to disconnect or connect transformers, CBs, other pieces of equipment, and short length of HV conductors, only after current through them has been interrupted by opening a CB or load-break switch.

They allow disconnecting the faulted circuit or apparatus for repair while the rest of the circuit is put back into service and provide for personnel safety while the malfunction is being repaired. However, they can open very small charging currents to unload on apparatus. The low-current arc is broken by swinging the moving arm in a 90° arc to provide a long air gap. (For example, an air gap of approximately 11 ft is required at 230 kV. Because of this, they cannot open a fault.) At their specific ratings, they are designed to carry normal load currents at their specific ratings and remain closed for momentary current flow such as fault currents. They are classified as station, transmission, and distribution disconnecting switches.

Disconnecting switches rated up through 3000 A are available. They can be of manual or automatic switching types. In station locations, manual switching is preferred. They are classified based on their voltage, continuous current rating, and function. They can be in single phase–single pole and three phase–three pole.

Transmission disconnect switches are generally used as load management tools. Increasing needs for transmission lines and decreasing availability of ROW make automatic switching of transmission load highly desirable. These load management activities are usually done during *dead time* by switching the proper disconnects automatically through sending loss of voltage. Such systems built up to 161 kV, 1200 A.

10.6 LOAD-BREAK SWITCHES

A load-break (disconnect) switch can interrupt normal load currents, but not large fault currents. They provide the desired capability of switching without CBs. A wall switch is the most common load-break switch. Generally, these interrupters are not continuous in duty in terms of carrying load. They have limited interrupting capability and are primarily used for line, transformers, capacitor, and reactor switching.

Load-break switches for medium and high voltages use interrupters built into the switch to break the load current before the switch disconnecting arms swing open. Some newer HV load-break switches that are equipped with SF_6 interrupters can break significant fault current and obey protective relay trip signals. Most load-break switches employ motors to open and close the switch blades, but the interrupters are operated by strong spring pressure.

10.7 SWITCHGEAR

Switchgear is a general term covering switching and interrupting devices, also assemblies of those devices with control, metering, protective, and regulatory equipment with the associated interconnections and supporting structures. Switchgears are used in industrial, commercial, and utility installations. They are used 34.5 kV and ratings of the heavy-duty range up to some 6000 A continuous current.

They can be either metal-clad switchgear, metal-enclosed switchgear, or isolated-phase metal-enclosed switchgear. In the metal-clad switchgear, there are usually factory-assembled electrical equipment that are required to control an individual circuit, including bus, CB, disconnecting devices, current and voltage transformers, controls, instruments, and relays. They are used for low- and medium-capacity circuits, for indoor and outdoor installations at 345 kV and lower voltages.

In the metal-enclosed switchgear, the aforementioned individual components are in separate metal housings and the CBs are of the stationary type.

In the isolated-phase metal-enclosed switchgear, each phase is enclosed in a separate metal housing. It is the most practical, the safest, and the most economical design in terms of preventing phase-to-phase faults. Switchgear can be used to perform the following two functions:

1. *Under normal conditions*: It is used to carry out a number of routine switching operations.
2. *Under abnormal conditions*: It is used to automatically disconnect the part of the system in trouble to prevent excessive damage and to restrict the trouble to the smallest possible segment of the system.

The routine switching operations include the following:

1. Disconnecting and isolating any piece of equipment for replacement or maintenance
2. Disconnecting a generator from the system when it is no longer required to serve the loads
3. Isolating regulators using switchgears
4. Bypassing CBs using switchgears
5. Reversing of various operations using switchgears

In the most inclusive definition, *directly connected switchgear* definition covers the following devices as well, including CBs, disconnecting switches or disconnecting devices, fuses, instrument transformers, buses, and connections between all these components and supporting structures, insulators, or housings.

Other switchgear devices may be located at some distance from the circuit with which they are identified. They include the indicators (e.g., annunciators, signal lamps, or instruments, control switches, meters, protective and control relays, generator voltage relays, and the panels on which they are mounted).

10.8 PURPOSE OF TRANSMISSION LINE PROTECTION

The purpose using protective relaying is to minimize service interruptions and limit damage to equipment when failure takes place. In order to achieve such protection, protective relays quickly detect the existence of abnormal system conditions by monitoring appropriate system quantities, decide which minimum number of CBs should be opened, and energize trip circuits of those breakers. The reasons for quick isolation are as follows:

1. To minimize the duration and seriousness of the effective element interference with the normal operation of power system
2. To minimize and prevent damage to the defective element (thus, reducing the time and cost of repairs and allowing faster restoration of the element to service)
3. To maximize the power that can be transferred on power systems (high-speed clearing of faults can often provide a means for achieving higher power transfers and by that means delay investment in additional transmission facilities)

10.9 DESIGN CRITERIA FOR TRANSMISSION LINE PROTECTION

The design criteria for transmission line protection are as follows:

1. *Reliability*: It is a measure of the degree that the protective system will function properly in terms of both dependability (i.e., *performing correctly when required*) and security (i.e., *avoiding unnecessary operation*).
2. *Selectivity (or discrimination)*: The quality whereby a protective system distinguishes between those conditions for which it is intended to operate and those for which it must not operate. In other words, the selectivity of a protective system is its ability to recognize a fault and trip a minimum number of CBs to clear the fault. A well-designed protective system should provide maximum continuity of service with minimum system disconnection.
3. *Speed*: It is the ability of the protective system to disconnect a faulty system element as quickly as possible with minimum fault time and equipment damage. Therefore, a protective relay must operate at the required speed. It should neither be too slow, which may result in damage to the equipment, nor should it be too fast, which may result in undesired operation during transient faults. The speed of operation also has direct effect on the general stability of the power system. The shorter the time for which a fault is allowed to persist on the system, the more load can be transferred between given points on the power system without loss of synchronism. Figure 10.6 shows the curves that

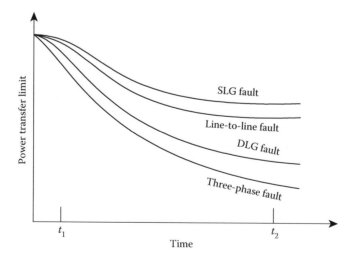

FIGURE 10.6 Typical values of power that can be transmitted as function of fault clearance time.

represent the power that can be transferred as a function of fault-clearing time for various types of faults. Obviously, a fast fault-clearing time t_1 permits a higher power transfer than longer clearing time t_2. Currently, the fault-clearing times of bulk power systems are in the t_1 region (about three cycles on a 60 Hz base), and thus, power transfers are almost at a maximum. Also, it can be observed that the most severe fault is the three-phase fault, and the least severe fault is the line-to-ground fault in terms of transmission of power.

4. *Simplicity*: It is the sign of a good design in terms of minimum equipment and circuitry. However, the simplest protective system may not always be the most economical one even though it may be the most reliable owing to fewer elements that can malfunction.

5. *Economics*: It dictates to achieve the maximum protection possible at minimum cost. It is possible to design a very reliable protective system but at a very high cost. Therefore, high reliability should not be pursued as an end in itself, regardless of cost, but should rather be balanced against economy, taking all factors into account.

Protection is not needed when the system is operating normally. It is only needed when the system is not operating normally. Therefore, in that sense, protection is a form of insurance against any failures of the system. Its premium is its capital and maintenance costs, and its return is the possible prevention of loss of stability and the minimization of any possible damages. The cost of protection is generally extremely small compared with the cost of equipment protected. The art of protective relaying is constantly changing and advancing. However, the basic principles of relay operation and application remain the same. Thus, the purpose of this chapter is to review these fundamental principles and then show their applications to the protection of particular system elements. However, the emphasis will be on the transmission system.

The most commonly occurring faults on transmission lines are short circuits. However, lightning is still the most common cause of faults on OH transmission lines. Single-phase faults contribute 75%–90% of all faults. In contrast, multiphase-to-ground faults are 5%–15% of all faults, while multiphase faults with no ground connection are the rarest 5%–10%. Other rare causes of faults are temporary contact with foreign objects, swinging of wires caused by strong winds, and insulator breakings.

10.10 ZONES OF PROTECTION

A power system is divided into various primary protective zones, as shown in Figure 10.7. The dashed lines indicate a separate zone of protection around each system element (e.g., generator, transformer, bus, transmission line) for which a given relay or protective system is responsible. The zone includes both the system element and the CBs that connect the element to the system. As shown in the figure, in order to be adequately protected with minimum interruptions, a power system can be divided into protective zones for (1) generators (or generator–transformer), (2) transformers, (3) buses, (4) transmission lines, and (5) loads, motors, etc.

Each protective zone has its own protective relays for detecting the existence of a fault in that zone and its own CBs for disconnecting that zone from the rest of the system. In that sense, a *protective zone* can be defined as the portion of a power system protected by a given protective system or a part of that protective system.

The boundary of a zone of protection is dictated by the CTs that supply the input to the relays. In a given power system, a CT provides the ability to detect a fault within its zone; the CB provides the ability to isolate the fault by disconnecting all of the power apparatus inside its protective zone. In the event that the CT is not an integral part of the CB, the CYs still define the zone of protection, but a communication channel has to be employed to implement the tripping function.

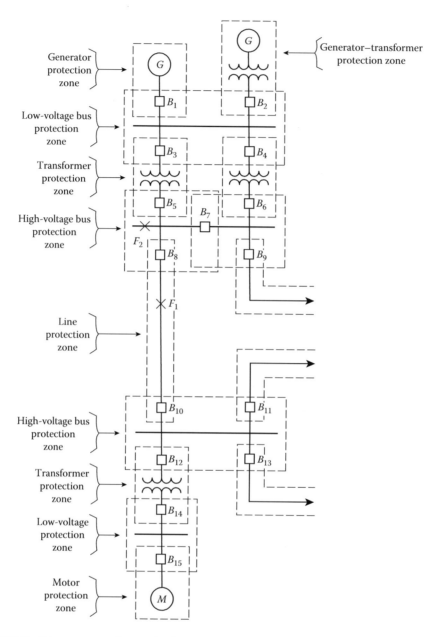

FIGURE 10.7 Primary zones of protection in a power system.

10.11 PRIMARY AND BACKUP PROTECTION

As illustrated in Figure 10.7, the primary zones are arranged in a manner so that they overlap around CBs. The purpose of the overlap is to eliminate the possibility of *blind spots* or unprotected areas. A fault in an overlap area will cause tripping of all CBs in two primary zones.

Primary protection: Operation of the protection must be fast, reliable, and sensitive. A fast speed of response and high reliability are crucial to limit the damage that could be caused by a fault. Furthermore, the protection must be selective so that only the faulty element is removed. Reliability is achieved by having high-quality apparatus and by using two different protection schemes for each element: the *primary protection* and the *backup protection*. The main protection system for a given zone of protection is called the *primary protection system*.* It operates the least amount of equipment from service.

Backup protection: Backup protection is provided for possible failure in the primary protection and for possible CB failures. The causes for such failure are (1) ac current or voltage supply failures to relays due to failures in CRs or VTs or wiring, (2) failure of auxiliary devices, (3) loss of dc control supply, and (4) relay failure. On the other hand, those causes that may cause the circuit greater failure may include (1) open or short-circuit trip coil, (2) loss of dc supply, (3) failure of main contacts to interrupt, and (4) mechanical failure of tripping mechanism.

Backup relays are slower than the primary relays and may remove more of the system elements than is necessary to clear a fault. The main protection should operate based on different physical principles than its backup. Also, any backup scheme must provide both relay backup as well as breaker backup.

It is important that the backup protection should be arranged so that the cause of primary protection failure will not also be the cause of backup protection failure.

Furthermore, the backup protection must not operate until primary protection had a chance to operate. Because of this, there is a time delay associated with the backup protection.

Remote backup: If the main protection of a neighboring element is used as the backup protection of the given element, then it is called *remote backup*. In other words, the backup relays are physically located in a separate location and are completely independent of the relays and CBs that are backing up. Because of this, there are no common failures that can affect both sets of relays. For EHV systems, it is not unusual to have two station batteries and separate circuitry so that the primary protection is electrically isolated from the backup protection.

Consider the protection scheme that is illustrated in Figure 10.8. In a remote backup scheme, time delays at bus 1 provide backup protection for transmission line TL_{34}. When there is a fault on transmission line TL_{34}, if there is a protection failure or CB failure at bus 3, the remote relays located at bus 1 will trip their CBs to isolate the fault. That means that the relays and CB at bus 1 provide relay and CB backup for breaker 3. By the same token, the relays and CB at bus 4 provide backup for breaker 2. Also, both 1 and 4 provide backup protection for the bus at the substation.

Now, consider the protection scheme shown in Figure 10.9. Note that the additional generation and transmission lines will feed the faults, on transmission lines TL_{12} and TL_{34}. Because of this, the remote backup relays located at 1 and 2 will have difficulty in seeing faults on adjacent transmission lines, especially the faults that are located near the remote buses. Hence, the infeed of fault current at the middle substation makes a fault seem farther away to the remote relays. In fact, the greater the infeed, the farther away the fault will appear. In such case, a local type of backup is employed.

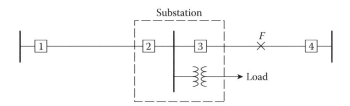

FIGURE 10.8 Illustration of remote backup protection.

---

* Note that on EHV transmission systems, it is common to duplicate the primary protection systems in case a component in one primary protection chain fails to operate as a result of a relay failure. Also, relays from a different manufacturer or relays based on different operational principles can be used to prevent common-mode failures. However, their operating time and the tripping logic are kept the same.

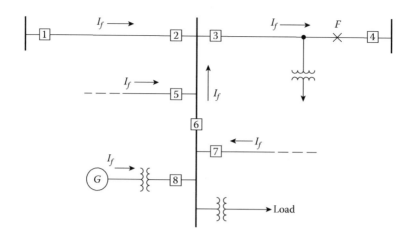

FIGURE 10.9 Illustration of remote backup protection with intermediate feed.

Local backup: If backup protection is placed in the same substation bay as the main protection, then it is called *local backup*. These relays are installed in the same substation and use some of the same elements as the primary protection. In other words, faults are cleared locally in the same substation where the failure has taken place. This type of backup provides both relay and CB failure backup, as illustrated in Figure 10.10.

Consider Figure 10.9 and assume that a local backup scheme is used at CB 3. In the event of a fault taking place on transmission line TL_{34} close to CB 3, the primary and backup distance relays at 3 will operate in high speed to clear the fault. In case CB 3 fails to clear the fault, the bus time can be set to operate to trip CB 2, 5, and 6 in about 0.15–0.20 s.

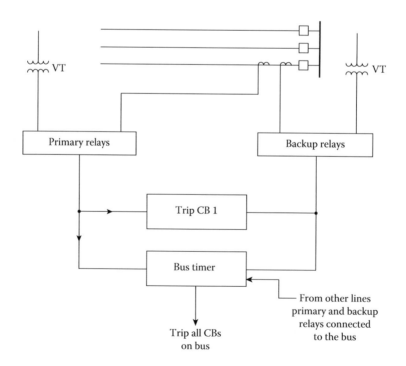

FIGURE 10.10 Local backup protection.

10.12 RECLOSING

The majority (80%–90%) of the faults on OH distribution lines are transient in nature. They are mainly caused by flashovers between phase conductors or between one or more of the phase conductors and earthed neutral and the ground caused by lightning or by wind. The wind may cause the conductors to move together to flashover or may cause a temporary tree contact that result in a fault. The remaining 10%–20% of faults are either semitransient or permanent.

Thus, the transient faults can be dealt with by deenergizing the line until the arc or arcs are extinguished, and then it can be energized again after a certain time period, which is called the *dead time*. The whole procedure is known as the *automatic line reclosing* or simply *autoreclosing*. It should be clear that such reclosing procedure substantially improves the continuity of energy supply and the service. However, if the fault is permanent, the reenergized line will be open again by its protection. The benefits of using high-speed reclosure are as follows:

1. It prevents and/or limits conductor damage.
2. It minimizes the effects of a line outage on critical loads.
3. It maintains the integrity of the system by returning the line back to the service.
4. It allows greater loading of the transmission system.
5. It improves the system stability.

Reclosing can be one single attempt (one shot) or several attempts at various time intervals (multiple shots). The first attempt of automatic reclosing can be either *instantaneous* or with *time delay*. There may be two or three such attempts, but usually, only a single-shot reclosure is used in HV transmission networks. The high-speed reclosing permits only enough time (usually 15–40 cycles) for the arc of a fault to dissipate. On the other hand, time-delayed reclosings have a delay time of 1 or more seconds. If the reclosure is not successful, the recloser relay moves to a lockout position so that no further automatic operation is possible.

The late Blackburn [3] suggested that in a three-phase circuit, the deenergized time for the fault arc to deionize and not restrike is

$$t = \frac{V_{kV}}{34.5} + 10.5 \text{ cycles} \tag{10.10}$$

This applies only for the case of having all three phases open. For single-pole trip–reclose operation, the required deionization times are longer since the energy from unopened phases supplies the arc.

In the United States, it is a common practice to trip all three phases for all faults and then reclose the three phases simultaneously. However, in Europe, it is not uncommon to trip only the faulted phase in the event of having a single line-to-ground fault. But in such situation, the voltage and current in the healthy phases tend to maintain the fault arc even after the faulted phase is deenergized. This event is known as the *secondary arc*. It may require compensating reactors to remedy the situation [5].

In general, it is the common practice to reclose automatically transmission lines that are remote from the generating station after they have been tripped for a fault. Usually, a single high-speed reclosing will be attempted only after the simultaneous, high-speed tripping of all line breakers by the primary pilot-relaying system. In the event of a persisting fault, the line relays will trip the line out again, and usually, no more automatic reclosing will be attempted after that attempt. If all attempts to close the line automatically fail, then a system operator may try to close the line manually after a certain time interval. If even the manual reclosing attempt fails, it becomes evident that the line is experiencing a permanent fault. Thus, it is taken out of service until it is repaired properly.

There is a potential danger for closing instantaneous reclosing on lines at or near generating stations since such reclosing may cause damage to the long turbine shafts of the turbine–generator units. This is due to the fact that the voltages on the two sides of the CB are at different angles. Thus, such reclosing causes a sudden shock and movement of the rotor and to transient oscillations and stresses.

According to Blackburn [3], reclosing on multiterminal lines is more complex. This is especially true, if more than five terminals have synchronous voltage sources. This may require reclosing one or two terminals instantaneously but reclosing others after proper voltage or synchro-clock. In the case that the transmission line has load taps, when the same line is used for both transmission and distribution purposes, reclosing of the source terminals can be used to service to the tap loads.

Transmission lines that end in a transfer bank without having a CB between them, or transmission lines having shunt reactors, should not be reclosed automatically. In such situations, a delay in reclosing is needed to be sure that there is no problem in either the transformer or the reactor.

Based on the past experiences, one can conclude that successful high-speed reclosure can be achieved 80%–90% of the time. However, the high-speed reclosing cannot be used in all cases. For example, a reclosure into a persistent fault may result in system instability. Furthermore, high-speed reclosure after tripping for phase faults is not advised on transmission lines leaving a generating station, since it has the possibility of generator shaft torque damage and should be closely examined before using it.

Rustebakke [4] suggested that such effects can be minimized by the following:

1. Delaying reclosure for a minimum of 10 s.
2. Employing selective reclosing, that is, reclosing only on single phase-to-ground faults.
3. Employing sequential reclosing. (In other words, reclose first at the remote end of the line and block reclosing at the generating station if the fault still exists.) Use this approach if the line is long and/or if there is no generating station at the remote end.

The lines used to send power between stations dictate high-speed reclosing on both terminals to restore service. Such high-speed reclosing is limited to the lines (that are made of sufficient parallel lines in the network) that are protected by pilot protection since it requires that the source voltages are in synchronism (i.e., in phase) with each other during the open-line period.

According to Blackburn [3], it is better to use the following methodologies when pilot protection is not used:

1. Use single-pole pilot trip and reclose as the method.
2. First use pilot relay protection for simultaneous line tripping. Reclose one end instantaneously and then close the other end after checking that the line and bus voltages are in synch or within the preset angle difference. Synchronizing relays can be used for this purpose.
3. If the pilot protection does not exist, then reclose with the following:
   a. Live line, dead bus
   b. Dead line, live bus, and/or dead bus
   c. Live line, live bus with synchronism checking

Note that since faults are often temporary in nature, the stability is often never reached. Hence, the instantaneous reclosing of both ends of lines simultaneously is practiced for line of 115 kV and above. Usually, this is attempted only one time. Further attempts require voltage check and/or the use of synchronism check apparatus. Such reclosing operation is used only for OH lines but not for transmission lines built in cables since they are not reclosed. The lines that have both the OH and cable sections require separate protection for the OH and cable protection for the OH and cable segments. In such applications, the reclosing is allowed only for the OH line faults.

10.13 TYPICAL RELAYS USED ON TRANSMISSION LINES

As defined previously, a protective relay is a device designed to initiate isolation of a part of electric system, or to operate an alarm signal, in the case of a fault or other abnormal condition. Basically, a protective relay consists of an operating element and a set of contacts. The operating element receives input from the instrument transformers in the form of currents, voltages, or a combination of currents and voltages (e.g., impedance and power). The relay may respond to (1) a change in the magnitude of the input quantity, (2) the phase angle between two quantities, (3) the sum (or difference) between two quantities, or (4) the ratio of the quantities. In any case, the relay performs a measuring (or comparison) operation based on the input and translates the result into a motion of contacts. Hence, for example, the output state of an electromechanical relay is either *trip* (with its contacts closed) or *block* or *block to trip* (with its contacts open). When they close, the contacts either actuate a warning signal or complete the trip circuit of a CB, which in turn isolates the faulty part by interrupting the flow of current into that part.

In general, protective relays can be classified by their constructions, functions, or applications. By construction, they can be either electromechanical or solid state (or *static*) types. In general, the electromechanical relays are robust, inexpensive, and relatively immune to the harsh environment of a substation. However, they require regular maintenance by skilled personnel. Furthermore, their design is somewhat limited in terms of available characteristics, tap settings, and burden capability.

On the other hand, solid-state relays have been primarily used in areas where the application of conventional methods is difficult or impossible (e.g., HV transmission line protection by phase comparison). The relays using transistors for phase or amplitude comparison can be made smaller, cheaper, faster, and more reliable than electromechanical relays. They can be made shockproof and require very little maintenance. Furthermore, their great sensitivity allows smaller CTs to be used and more sophisticated characteristics to be obtained. Contrary to the electromechanical relays, the solid-state relays provide switching action, without any physical motion of any contacts, by changing its state from nonconducting to conducting or vice versa. The electromechanical relays can be classified as magnetic attraction, magnetic induction, d'Arsonval, and thermal units. Most widely used types of magnetic attraction relays include plunger (solenoid), clapper, and polar.

The typical relays that are used for transmission line protection are (1) overcurrent relays, (2) distance relays, and (3) pilot relays.

10.13.1 Overcurrent Relays

The use of overcurrent relays is the simplest and cheapest type of line protection. Three types of overcurrent relays are used: inverse time delay overcurrent (TDOC) relays, instantaneous overcurrent relays, and directional overcurrent relays.

In general, overcurrent relays are difficult to implement where coordination, selectivity, and speed are important. They usually require changes to their settings as the system configuration changes. Also, they cannot discriminate between load and fault currents. Hence, when they are implemented only for phase fault protection, they are only useful when the minimum fault current exceeds the full load current. However, they can effectively be used on subtransmission systems and radial distribution systems. This is due to the fact that faults on these systems usually do not affect system stability and therefore high-speed protection is not needed.

10.13.1.1 Inverse Time Delay Overcurrent Relays

The main use of TDOC relays is on a radial system where they are used for both phase and ground protection. Basic complements of such relays are two phase and one ground relays. This can protect the line for all combinations of phase and ground faults using the minimum number of relays. According to Horowitz [5], adding a third phase relay can provide complete backup protection, having two relays for every type of fault, and is the preferred practice. These relays are usually applied on subtransmission lines and industrial systems due to the low cost involved.

10.13.1.2 Instantaneous Overcurrent Relays

Since the closer the fault is to the source, the greater the fault current magnitude but the longer the tripping time, the TDOC relay cannot be used all by itself. As illustrated in Figure 10.11, the addition of an instantaneous overcurrent relay makes such system of protection possible. However, there must be considerable reduction in fault current as the fault moves from the relay toward the far end of the line. In this manner, the instantaneous relay can be made to see almost up to, but not including, the next bus. The relay will not operate for faults beyond the end of the line but still provide high-speed protection for most of the line.

10.13.1.3 Directional Overcurrent Relays

When it is important to limit tripping for faults in only one direction in multiple-source circuits, the use of directional overcurrent relays becomes necessary. The overcurrent relaying is made directional to provide relay coordination between all the relays that can *see* a given fault. Otherwise, the coordination is often too difficult if not impossible.

The directional relays require two inputs that are the operating current and a *reference* (or *polarizing*) quantity that does not change with fault location. For phase relays, the polarizing quantity is the system voltage at the relay location. For ground directional reference, the zero-sequence

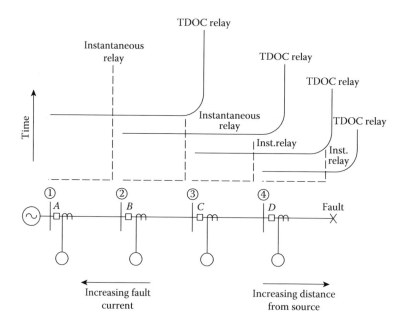

FIGURE 10.11 Application of instantaneous overcurrent relays.

voltage $(3V_{a0})$ is used. However, it is often that the current in the neutral of a wye-connected/delta power transformer is used as a directional reference instead.

10.13.2 DISTANCE RELAYS

The most common method of detecting faults on transmission lines is by impedance measurement. It is accomplished by relay units that respond to a ratio of voltage to current and, therefore, to impedance or a component of impedance. Since impedance is a measure of distance along a transmission line, between the relay location and the fault location, these relays are called *distance relays*. As the power systems become more complex and the fault currents vary with changes in generation and system configuration, directional overcurrent relays become difficult to implement and to set for all contingencies.

In comparison to directional overcurrent relays, the distance relay setting is constant for a wide variety of changes outside of the protected transmission line. The discrimination is obtained by limiting relay operation to a certain range of impedance. Hence, the operating limits of distance relays are usually given in terms of impedance or in terms of impedance components, resistance, and reactance. There are three basic distance relay characteristics, namely, impedance relay, admittance relay, and reactance relay. Each relay is distinguished by its application and its operational characteristic.

10.13.2.1 Impedance Relay

As shown in Figure 10.12, the impedance relay has a circular triggering characteristic centered at the origin of the R–X diagram. It is nondirectional, as shown in Figure 10.12a, and is used mainly as a fault detector. However, it is possible to have an impedance relay with a directional element, as shown in Figure 10.12b. Hence, a directional relay is commonly used to monitor the impedance relay.

10.13.2.2 Admittance Relay

It is the most commonly used distance relay. Its characteristic passes through the origin of the R–X diagram and is therefore directional. It is also used as the tripping relay in pilot schemes and as the backup relay in step distance schemes. Its characteristic is circular for the electromechanical relay, as shown in Figure 10.13. However, for the solid-state relays, it can be shaped according to the transmission line impedance, as shown in Figure 10.14.

10.13.2.3 Reactance Relay

The reactance relay is has straight-line characteristic that responds only to the reactance of the protected area, as shown in Figure 10.15a. It is nondirectional and is used to supplement the admittance (mho)

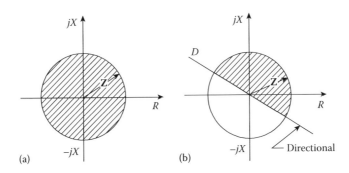

FIGURE 10.12   Impedance relays: (a) without directional element and (b) with directional element.

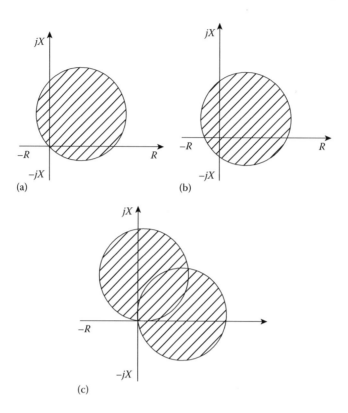

FIGURE 10.13 Electromechanical admittance (i.e., mho) relays: (a) regular admittance relay, (b) offset admittance relay, and (c) expanded admittance relay.

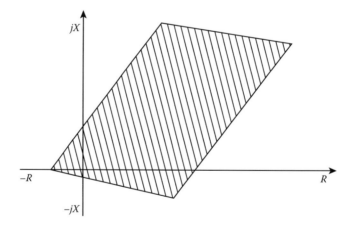

FIGURE 10.14 Solid-state admittance relay.

relay as a tripping relay to make the overall protection independent of resistance. It is especially used for short lines where the arc resistance of the fault is the same order of magnitude as the line length [5].

Consider a three-zone step distance relaying scheme shown in Figure 10.16. Assume that it provides instantaneous protection over 80%–90% of the protected line section (zone 1) and that time-delayed protection over the remainder of the line (zone 2) plus backup protection over the adjacent line section. Note that zone 3 also provides backup protection for sections of adjacent lines.

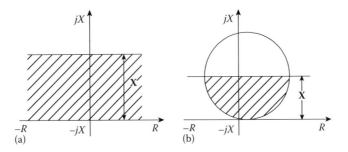

FIGURE 10.15   Reactance relays: (a) without mho characteristic and (b) with mho characteristic.

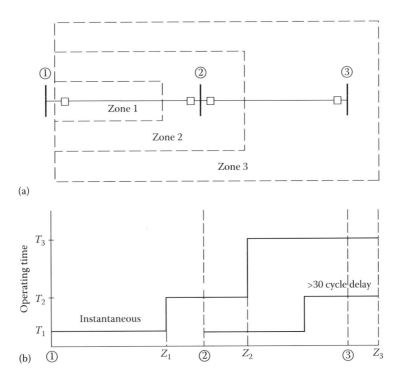

FIGURE 10.16   Three-zone step distance relaying: (a) to protect 100% of a line and (b) to provide backup of the neighboring line.

Example 10.3

Consider the one-line diagram of a 345 kV transmission line shown in Figure 10.17a. The equivalent systems behind buses A and B are represented by the equivalent system impedances in series with constant bus voltages, respectively. Assume that power flow direction is from bus A to bus B. Consider the directional distance relay located at A whose forward direction is in the direction from bus A to bus B. Assume that zone-type distance relays have two units, namely, three phase and phase to phase. Hence, for three-phase faults, the mho characteristic is directional and only operates for faults in the forward direction on line AB. For line-to-line faults (i.e., a–b, b–c, and c–a), the phase-to-phase unit operates. Also assume that all double line-to-ground faults are

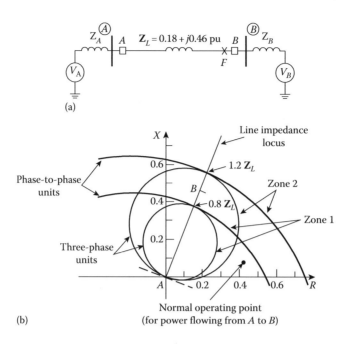

FIGURE 10.17 Typical application of distance relays for protection of transmission line: (a) system one-line diagram and (b) distance relays of A looking toward B.

protected by an overlap of the two distance units. All other line-to-ground faults are protected by ground distance relays and are not included in this example. Consider only zone 1 and 2 protection for the distance relay location at bus A and do the following:

(a) Draw the locus of the line impedance $\mathbf{Z}_L$ on the $R–X$ diagram.
(b) Draw the two-zone mho characteristics on the $R–X$ diagram for the three-phase units.
(c) Draw the two-zone characteristics on the $R–X$ diagram for the phase-to-phase units.
(d) Indicate the approximate vicinity for possible location of the normal operation point for power flow from bus A to bus B.

Solution

The solution is shown in Figure 10.17b.

Example 10.4

Assume that Figure 10.17a is a one-line diagram of a 138 kV subtransmission line with a line impedance of $0.2 + j0.7$ pu. Consider the directional distance (mho) relay located at A whose forward direction is in the direction from bus A to bus B. There is a line-to-line fault at the fault point F, which is located at 0.7 pu distance away from bus A. The magnitude of the fault current is 1.2 pu. Assume that the line spacing of 10.3 ft is equal to the arc length. The bus quantities for power, voltage, current, and impedance are given as 100 MVA, 138 kV, 418.4 A, and 190.4 Ω, respectively. Consider only zones 1 and 2 protection and determine the following:

(a) Value of arc resistance at fault point in ohms and per units
(b) Value of line impedance including the arc resistance
(c) Line impedance angle without and with arc resistance
(d) Graphically, whether or not relay will clear fault instantaneously

Solution

(a) Since the current in the arc is 1.2 pu or $I = 1.2 \times 418.4\ \text{A} = 502.08\ \text{A}$, the arc resistance can be found from the following equation as

$$R_{arc} = \frac{8750I}{I^{1.4}} = \frac{8750 \times 10.3}{502.08^{1.4}} = 14.92\,\Omega \quad \text{or} \quad 0.0784\ \text{pu}$$

(b) The impedance seen by the relay is

$$\mathbf{Z}_L + R_{arc} = (0.2 + j0.7)0.7 + 0.0784 = 0.2184 + j0.49\ \text{pu}$$

(c) The line impedance angle without the arc resistance is

$$\tan^{-1}\left(\frac{0.49}{0.14}\right) = 74.05°$$

and with the arc resistance is

$$\tan^{-1}\left(\frac{0.49}{0.2184}\right) = 65.98°$$

(d) Figure 10.18 shows that even after the addition of the arc resistance, the fault point F moved to point F', which is still within zone 1. Thus, the fault will be cleared instantaneously.

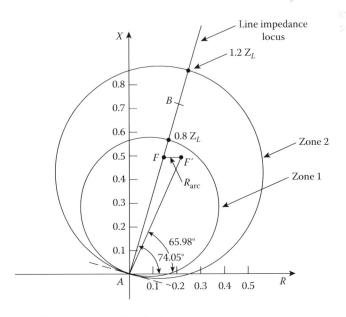

FIGURE 10.18 Graphical determination of fault clearance.

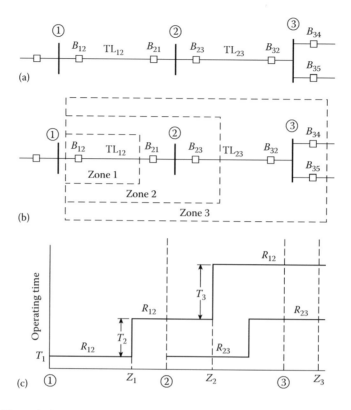

FIGURE 10.19 Transmission system for Example 10.5: (a) one line diagram of the system, (b) zones of protection, and (c) backup protection.

Example 10.5

Consider a transmission line TL_{12} protected by directional relays R_{12} and R_{21}, as shown in Figure 10.19a. Determine the following:

(a) Zones of protection for relay R_{12}
(b) Coordination of distance relays R_{12} and R_{21} in terms of operating time versus impedance

Solution

(a) The zone of protection for relay R_{12} is shown in Figure 10.19b.
(b) The coordination of the distance relays R_{12} and R_{21} in terms of operating time versus impedance is illustrated in Figure 10.19c. Note that zone 3 provides backup protection for the neighboring protection system.

Example 10.6

Consider the 230 kV transmission system shown in Figure 10.19a. Assume that the positive-sequence impedances of the lines TL_{12} and TL_{23} are $2 + j20$ and $2.5 + j25\ \Omega$, respectively. If the maximum peak load supplied by the line TL_{12} is 100 MVA with a lagging power factor of 0.9, design in a three-zone distance relaying system for the R_{12} impedance relay by determining the following:

(a) Maximum load current
(b) CT ratio
(c) VT ratio
(d) Impedance measured by relay

(e) Load impedance based on secondary ohms
(f) Zone 1 setting of relay R_{12}
(g) Zone 2 setting of relay R_{12}
(h) Zone 3 setting of relay R_{12}

Solution

(a) The maximum load current is

$$I_{max} = \frac{100 \times 10^6}{\sqrt{3}\left(230 \times 10^3\right)} = 251.02 \text{ A}$$

(b) Thus, the CT ratio is 250:5, which gives about 5 A in the secondary winding under the maximum loading.
(c) Since the system voltage to neutral is $(230/\sqrt{3}) = 132.79$ kV and selecting a secondary voltage of 69 V line to neutral, the VT ratio is calculated as

$$\frac{132.79 \times 10^3}{69} = \frac{1924.5}{1}$$

(d) The impedance measured by the relay is

$$\frac{V_\phi/1924.5}{I_\phi/50} = 0.026 \, Z_{line}$$

Hence, the impedances of lines TL_{12} and TL_{23} as seen by the relay are approximately 0.052 + $j0.5196$ and 0.065 + $j0.6495$ Ω, respectively.
(e) The load impedance based on secondary ohms is

$$\mathbf{Z}_{load} = \frac{69}{251.02\left(5/250\right)}\left(0.9 + j0.4359\right) = 12.37 + j5.99 \ \Omega \text{ (secondary)}$$

(f) The zone 1 setting of relay R_{12} is

$$\mathbf{Z}_r = 0.80\left(0.052 + j0.5196\right) = 0.0416 + j0.4157 \ \Omega \text{ (secondary)}$$

(g) The zone 2 setting of relay R_{12} is

$$\mathbf{Z}_r = 1.20\left(0.052 + j0.5196\right) = 0.0624 + j0.6235 \ \Omega \text{ (secondary)}$$

(h) Since the zone 3 setting must reach beyond the longest line connected to bus 2, it is

$$\mathbf{Z}_r = 0.052 + j0.5196 + 1.20\left(0.065 + j0.6495\right)$$

$$= 0.130 + j1.299 \ \Omega \text{ (secondary)}$$

Example 10.7

Assume that the R_{12} relay of Example 10.6 is a mho relay and that the relay characteristic angle may be either 30° or 45°. If the 30° characteristic angle is used, the relay ohmic settings can be determined by dividing the required zone reach impedance, in secondary ohms, by $\cos(\theta - 30°)$, where θ is the line angle. Use the 30° characteristic angle and determine the following:

(a) Zone 1 setting of mho relay R_{12}
(b) Zone 2 setting of mho relay R_{12}
(c) Zone 3 setting of mho relay R_{12}

Solution

(a) From Example 10.6, the required zone 1 setting was

$$\mathbf{Z}_r = 0.0416 + j0.4157 = 0.4178\angle 84.3° \ \Omega \text{ (secondary)}$$

Thus,

$$\text{Mho relay zone 1 setting} = \frac{0.4178}{\cos(84.3° - 30°)} = 0.7157 \ \Omega \text{ (secondary)}$$

(b) The required zone 2 setting was

$$\mathbf{Z}_r = 0.0624 + j0.6235 = 0.6266\angle 84.3° \ \Omega \text{ (secondary)}$$

Hence,

$$\text{Mho relay zone 2 setting} = \frac{0.6266}{\cos(84.3° - 30°)} = 1.0734 \ \Omega \text{ (secondary)}$$

(c) The required zone 3 setting was

$$\mathbf{Z}_r = 0.130 + j1.299 = 1.3055\angle 84.3° \ \Omega \text{ (secondary)}$$

Thus,

$$\text{Mho relay zone 3 setting} = \frac{1.3055}{\cos(84.3° - 30°)} = 2.2364 \ \Omega \text{ (secondary)}$$

that is, 312.5% of zone 1 setting.

10.13.3 Pilot Relaying

Pilot relaying, in a sense, is a means of remote controlling the CBs. Here, the term *pilot* implies that there is some type of channel (or medium) that interconnects the ends of a transmission line over which information on currents and voltages, from each end of the line to the other, can be transmitted.

Such systems use high-speed protective relays at the line terminals in order to ascertain in as short a time as possible whether a fault is within the protected line or external to it. If the fault is internal to the protected line, all terminals are tripped in high speed. If the fault is external to the protected line, tripping is blocked (i.e., prevented). The location of the fault is pointed out either by the presence or the absence of a pilot signal.

The advantages of such high-speed simultaneous clearing of faults at all line terminals by opening CBs include (1) minimum damage to the equipment, (2) minimum (transient) stability problems, and (3) automatic reclosing.

Pilot relaying, being a modified form of differential relaying, is the best protection that can be provided for transmission lines. It is inherently selective, suitable for high-speed operation, and capable of good sensitivity. It is usually used to provide primary protection for a line. Backup protection may be provided by a separate set of relays (*step distance relaying*) or the relays used in the channels available for protective relaying include the following:

1. *Separate wire circuits*: They are called *pilot wires*, operating at power system frequency, audio frequency tones, or in dc. They can be made of telephone lines either privately owned or leased. Refer to Figure 10.20.
2. *Power line carriers*: They use the protected transmission line itself to provide the channel medium for transmission signals at frequencies of 30–300 kHz. These are the most widely used *pilots* for protective relaying. The carrier transmitter receivers are connected to the transmission line by coupling capacitor devices that are also used for line voltage measurement. Line traps tuned to the carrier frequency are located at the line terminals, as shown in Figure 10.21. They prevent an external fault behind the relays from shorting out the channel by showing high impedance to the carrier frequency and a low impedance to the power frequency. The RF choke acts as low impedance to 60 Hz power frequency but as high impedance to the carrier frequency. Thus, it protects the apparatus from HV at the power frequency and, simultaneously, limits the attenuation of the carrier frequency.

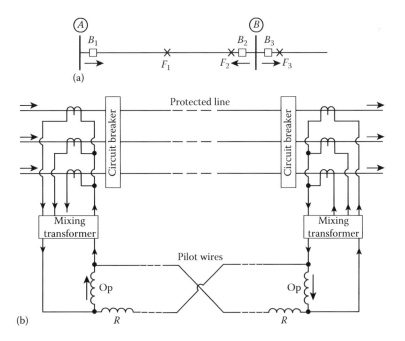

FIGURE 10.20 Line protection by pilot relaying: (a) example application and (b) one form of pilot wire relaying application.

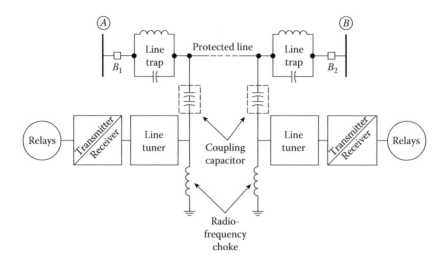

FIGURE 10.21 One-line diagram of power line carrier for pilot-relaying system.

3. *Microwave channel*: It uses beamed radio signals, usually in the range of 2–12 GHz, between line-of-sight antennas located at the terminals. This channel can also simultaneously be used for other functions. A continuous tone of one frequency, called the *guard frequency*, is transmitted under normal (or *no-fault*) conditions. When there is an internal fault, the audio tone transmitter is keyed by the protective relaying scheme so that its output is shifted from the guard frequency to a trip frequency.

Pilot-relaying systems use either comparison or directional comparison to detect faults. In the phase comparison, the phase position of the power system frequency current at the terminals is compared. Amplitude modulation is used in a phase comparison system. The phase of the modulation signal waveform is not affected by the signal attenuation.

Identical equipments at each end of the line are modulated in phase during an internal fault and in antiphase when a through-fault current flows (due to an external fault). Hence, current flow through the line to external faults is considered 180° out of phase, and tripping is blocked. If the currents are relatively in phase, an internal fault is indicated, and the line is tripped. Thus, modulation is of the all-or-nothing type, producing half-cycle pulses of carrier signals interspersed with half periods of zero signals, as shown in Figure 10.22.

Note that during an external fault, the out-of-phase modulation results in transmission of the carrier signal to the line alternatively from each end. Thus, transmission from one end fills in the signals from the other and vice versa, providing a continuous signal on the line. The presence of the signal is used to block the tripping function. On the other hand, when there is an internal fault, the resulting signal on the line has half-period gaps during which the tripping function, initiated by the relay, is completed.

A pilot-relaying system can also use directional comparison to detect faults. In this case, the fault-detecting relays compare the direction of power flow at the line terminals. Power flow into the line at the terminals points out an internal fault, and the line is tripped. If power flows into the line at one end and out at the other, the fault is considered external, and tripping is not allowed. Consider the line shown in Figure 10.20a.

Assume that directional relays are used and high-speed protection is provided for the entire line (instead of the middle 60%) by pilot relaying. Thus, both faults F_1 and F_2 are detected as internal faults by the relays located at B_1 and B_2, respectively, and are therefore cleared at a high speed.

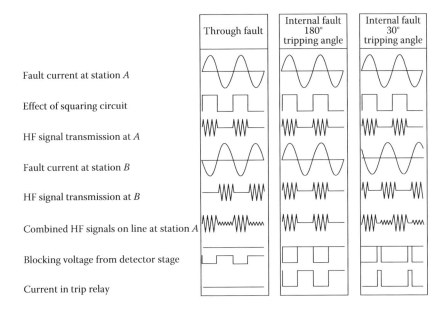

FIGURE 10.22 Carrier current phase comparison: key to operation.

Note that both relays see the fault current flowing in the forward direction. Thus, when this information is impressed on the signal by modulation and transmitted to the remote ends over a pilot channel, it is confirmed that the fault is indeed on the protected line.

Now assume that there is fault at F_3. The relay at B_2 sees it as an external fault and the relays at B_1 and B_3 see it as an internal fault. Upon receiving this directional information at B_1, that relay will be able to block tripping for the fault at F_3.

10.14 COMPUTER APPLICATIONS IN PROTECTIVE RELAYING

Computers have been widely used in the electric power engineering field since 1950s. The applications include a variety of off-line or online tasks. Examples of off-line tasks include fault studies, load-flow (power flow) studies, transient stability computations, unit commitment, and relay setting and coordination studies.

Examples of one-line tasks are economic generation scheduling and dispatching, load frequency control, SCADA, sequence-of-event monitoring, sectionalizing, and load management. The applications to computers in protective relaying have been primarily in relay settings and coordination studies and computer relaying.

A relay is essentially an analog computer. It receives inputs, processes them electromechanically or electronically to develop a torque or a logic input, and makes a decision resulting in a contact closure or output signal.

At the beginning, computer relays were used to take over existing protection functions, for example, transmission line and transformer or bus protection. Eventually, microprocessors were used in some relays to make the relay decision based on digitized analog signals. On the other hand, other relays continue to make the relaying decisions based on analog functions as well as provide for the necessary logic and auxiliary functions based on digital techniques. Also, a digital relay has the ability to diagnose itself. Furthermore, the today's relay has the ability to adapt itself in real time to changing system conditions.

10.14.1 Computer Applications in Relay Settings and Coordination

Today, there are various commercially available computer programs that are being used in the power industry to set and coordinate protective equipment. Advantages of using such programs include (1) sparing the relay engineer from routine, tedious, and time-consuming work, (2) facilitating system-wide studies, (3) providing consistent relaying practices throughout the system, and (4) providing complete and updated results of changes in system protection.

In 1960, the Westinghouse Electric Corporation developed its well-known protective device coordination program. It is one of the most comprehensive and complete programs for applying, setting, and checking the coordination of various types of protective relays, fuses, and reclosers. The user must specify the input data for the *data check study* block in terms of both device type and setting for each relay, fuse, or recloser. The program then evaluates the effectiveness of these devices and settings within the existing system and, if necessary, recommends alternative protective devices.

However, in the *coordination study* block, the user specifies the protective device with no settings or permits the program to select a device. The program then establishes settings within the ranges specified or it selects a device and settings. The settings and/or devices are chosen to optimize coordination.

The *final coordination study* shows how the system will behave with the revised settings, which can then be issued by the relay engineer [8]. Of course, no computer program can replace the relay engineer. Such a program is simply a tool to aid the engineer by indicating possible problems in the design and their solutions. The engineer has to use his *engineering judgment*, past experience, and skill in determining the best protection of the system.

10.14.2 Computer Relaying

Computer hardware technology has considerably advanced since the early 1960s. Newer generations of mini- and microcomputers tend to make digital computer relaying a viable alternative to the traditional relaying systems. Indeed, it appears that a simultaneous change is taking place in traditional relaying systems, which are using solid-state analog and digital subsystems as their building blocks. However, there are still electromechanical relays that are still in use extensively and especially in the old systems. The use of the digital computers for protection of power system equipment, however, is of relatively recent origin. The first serious proposals appeared in the late 1960s. For example, in 1966, Last and Stalewski [8] suggested that digital computers can be used in an online mode for protection of power systems. Since then, many authors have developed digital computer techniques for protection of line, transformers, and generators. Significantly, contributions have been made in the area of line protection. However, protection of transformers and generators using digital computers had somewhat received less attention for a while. In 1969, the feasibility of protecting a substation by a digital computer was investigated by Rockefeller [11]. He examined protection of all types of station equipment into one unified system. Researchers suggested the use of microcomputers in power system substations for control, data acquisition, and protection against faults and other abnormal operating conditions. This has become known as computer relaying and several papers and even books have been written on various techniques of performing or existing relaying characteristics. At first, a few field installations had been made to demonstrate computer relaying techniques and to show that computers can survive in the harsh substation environment. However, today, many utility companies have installations or plans for future implementations of computers as SCADA remotes. These substation control computers receive data from the transmit data to the central dispatch control computer.

It is interesting to note that at the beginning, most of the papers written on computer relaying have been under the auspices of universities. These tend to focus on algorithms and softwares or on models that can be tested on multipurpose minicomputers or on special-purpose circuits and hardware that are laboratory oriented. For example, a great deal of research has been undertaken at the University of Missouri at Columbia, since 1968, to develop a computer relaying system that would permit the computer to perform relaying as well as other substation functions [12–15].

However, the *real-world* test installations had been the result of cooperation between utilities and manufacturers and are mainly concerned with line protection using an impedance algorithm [16]. For example, in 1977, Westinghouse installed the PRODAR 70 computer in the Pacific Gas and Electric Company's Tesla Substation for protection of Bellota 230 kV line. Also, in 1971, a computer relaying project was initiated by the American Electric Power and later joined by IBM Service Corporation. The purpose of the project was to install an IBM System 7 in a substation to perform protective relaying and few data-logging functions [10]. General Electric initiated a joint project with Philadelphia Electric Company to install computer relaying equipment on a 500 kV line. Recently, Pacific Gas and Electric Company implemented substation automation techniques, based on the computer applications, at its substations in a great scale [26]. Therefore, it can be said that when the minicomputer becomes available, the industry realized the potential of the relatively low-cost computer and tried various applications. However, the extremely high costs of software programs to implement specific functions have played an inhibitive role. With the advent of micro-computers, the hardware costs can be further reduced. This permits software simplification since a microprocessor can be dedicated to a specific function.

PROBLEMS

10.1 Consider Example 10.1 and assume that the three-phase fault is located at bus 2 and determine the subtransient fault current in per units and amperes.

10.2 Consider Example 10.1 and assume that the three-phase fault is located at bus 3 and determine the subtransient fault current in per units and amperes.

10.3 First, solve Problem 10.1, and then based on its results, determine the following:
  (a) Maximum possible value of dc current component
  (b) Total maximum instantaneous current
  (c) Momentary current
  (d) Interrupting rating of a two-cycle CB located at bus 2
  (e) Momentary rating of a two-cycle CB located at bus 2

10.4 First, solve Problem 10.2, and then based on its results, determine the following:
  (a) Maximum possible value of dc current component
  (b) Total maximum instantaneous current
  (c) Momentary current
  (d) Interrupting rating of a two-cycle CB located at bus 3
  (e) Momentary rating of a two-cycle CB located at bus 3

10.5 Consider the system shown in Figure P10.5 and do the following:
  (a) Sketch the zones of protection.
  (b) Describe the backup protection necessary for a fault at fault point F_1.
  (c) Repeat part (b) for a fault at F_2.
  (d) Repeat part (b) for a fault at F_3.

10.6 Consider the system shown in Figure P10.6 and do the following:
  (a) Sketch the zones of protection.
  (b) Describe the backup protection necessary for a fault at fault point F_1.
  (c) Repeat part (b) for a fault at F_2.
  (d) Repeat part (b) for a fault at F_3.

10.7 Consider the system, with overlapped primary protective zones, shown in Figure P10.7 and assume that there is a fault at fault point F. Describe the necessary primary and backup protection with their possible implications.

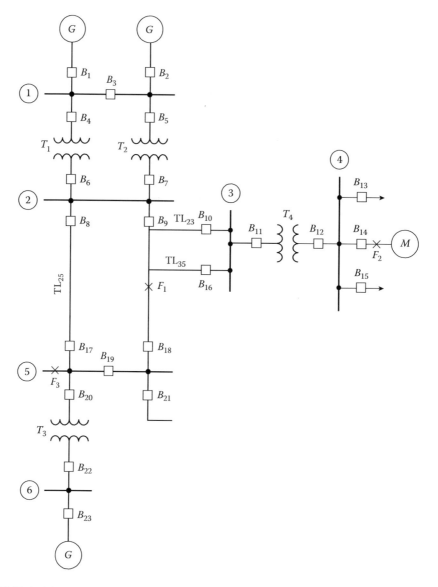

FIGURE P10.5 Transmission system for Problem 10.5.

10.8 Consider the system shown in Figure P10.8 and determine the locations of the necessary backup relays in the event of having a fault at the following locations:
  (a) Fault point F_1
  (b) Fault point F_2

10.9 Repeat Example 10.3 for the directional distance relay located at B whose forward direction is in the direction from bus B to bus A. Assume that the power flow direction is from bus B to bus A.

10.10 Repeat Example 10.4 assuming that the fault point F is located at 0.78 pu distance away from bus A.

10.11 Repeat Example 10.4 assuming that the arc resistance is increased by a 75 mph wind and that the zone 2 relay unit operates at a time delay of 18 cycles.

10.12 Repeat Example 10.6 assuming that the transmission system is being operated at 138 kV line to line and at a maximum peak load of 50 MVA at a lagging power factor of 0.85.

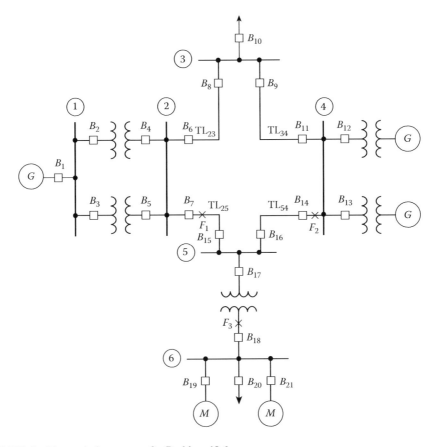

FIGURE P10.6   Transmission system for Problem 10.6.

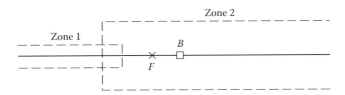

FIGURE P10.7   Protected system for Problem 10.7.

10.13 Repeat Example 10.7 using the results of Problem 10.12 and a 45° mho relay characteristic.

10.14 Consider the 345 kV transmission system shown in Figure P10.14. Assume that all three lines are identical with positive-sequence impedance of $0.02 + j0.2$ pu and that the megavoltampere base is 200 MVA. Assume also that all six line breakers are commanded by directional impedance distance relays and consider only three-phase faults. Set the settings of zone 1, zone 2, and zone 3 for 80%, 120%, and 250%, respectively. Determine the following:

(a)   Relay settings for all zones in per units.

(b)   Relay setting for all zones in ohms, if the VTs are rated $345 \times 10^3 / \sqrt{3} : 69\,\text{V}$ and the CTs are rated 400:5 A.

(c)   If there is a fault at fault point F located on the line TL_{35} at a 0.15 pu distance away from bus 3, explain the resulting relay operations.

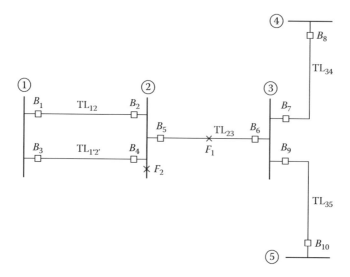

FIGURE P10.8 System for Problem P10.8.

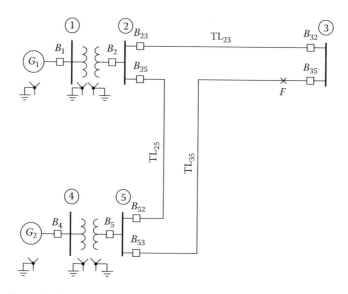

FIGURE P10.14 Transmission system for Problem P10.14.

10.15 Consider the transmission line shown in Figure P10.15. Assume that the line is compensated by SCs in order to improve stability limits and voltage regulation and to maximize the load-carrying capability of the system. Assume that the SCs are located at the terminals due to economics and that X_{CC} is equal to X_{CD}. If the line is protected by directional mho-type distance relays located at B and C, determine the following:

(a) Determine whether the SCs present any problem for the relays. If so, what are they?

(b) Sketch the possible locus of the line impedance on the R–X diagram.

(c) Sketch the operating characteristics of the distance relay located at B and set the relay to protect the line BC.

(d) Sketch the operating characteristics of the distance relay located at B and set the relay to protect the line BA.

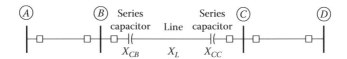

FIGURE P10.15 Transmission system for Problem P10.15.

REFERENCES

1. American National Standards Institute. IEEE standard application guide for ac high-voltage circuit breakers on a symmetrical current basis, ANSI C37.010-1972 (IEEE Stand. 320-1972), ANSI, New York, 1972.

2. Gönen, T. *A Practical Guide for Calculation of Short-Circuit Currents and Selection of High-Voltage Circuit Breakers*, Black & Veatch Company, Overland Park, KS, 1977.

3. Blackburn, J. L. *Protective Relaying: Principles and Applications*, Marcel Dekker, New York, 1987.

4. Rustebakke, H. M. *Electric Utility Systems and Practices*, 4th edn., Wiley, New York, 1983.

5. Horowitz, S. H. Transmission line protection, in *Power System Stability and Control*, L.L. Grigsby, ed., CRC Press, Boca Raton, FL, 2007.

6. GEC Measurements Ltd. *Protective Relays Application Guide*, 2nd edn., GEC Measurements Ltd., Stafford, England, 1975.

7. Westinghouse Electric Corporation. *Applied Protective Relaying*, Relay-Instrument Division, Newark, NJ, 1976.

8. Last, F. H. and Stalewski, A. Protective gear as a part of automatic power system control, *IEE Conf. Publ.* 16(Part I), 1966, 337–343.

9. Horowitz, S. H., ed. *Protective Relaying for Power Systems*, IEEE Press, New York, 1980.

10. Phadke, A. G., Ibrahim, M. A., and Hlibka, T. A digital computer system for EHV substations: Analysis and field tests, *IEEE Power Eng. Soc. Summer Meet.*, 1975, paper no. F75 543-9.

11. Rockefeller, G. D. Fault protection with a digital computer, *IEEE Trans. Power Apparatus Syst.* PAS-88, 1969, 438–462.

12. Boonyubol, C. Power transmission system fault simulation analysis and location, PhD dissertation, University of Missouri-Columbia, Columbia, MO, 1968.

13. Walker, L. N., Ott, A. D., and Tudor, J. R. Implementation of high frequency transient fault detector, *IEEE Power Eng. Soc. Winter Meet.*, 1970, paper no. 70CP 140-PWR.

14. Walker, L. N., Ott, A. D., and Tudor, J. R. Simulated power transmission substation, *SWIEEECO Rec.*, tech. pap., 1970, pp. 153–162.

15. Walker, L. N. Analysis, design, and simulation of a power transmission substation control system, PhD dissertation, University of Missouri-Columbia, Columbia, MO, 1970.

16. Gönen, T. *Modern Power System Analysis*, Wiley, New York, 1988.

17. General Electric Company. SLC 1000 transmission line protection, appl. manual GET-6749, General Electric Co., Schenectady, NY, 1984.

18. Westinghouse Electric Corporation. *Electrical Transmission and Distribution Reference Book*, WEC, East Pittsburgh, PA, 1964.

19. Atabekov, G. I. *The Relay Protection of High Voltage Networks*, Pergamon Press, New York, 1960.

20. Mason, C. R. *The Art and Science of Protective Relaying*, Wiley, New York, 1956.

21. Neher, J. H. A computerized method of determining the performance of distance relays, *Trans. Am. Inst. Electr. Eng.* 56, 1937, 833–844.

22. Hope, G. S. and Umamaheswaran, V. S. Sampling for computer protection of transmission lines, *IEEE Trans. Power Apparatus Syst.* PAS-93(5), 1974, 1524–1534.

23. Mann, B. J. and Morrison, I. F. Digital calculation of impedance for transmission line protection, *IEEE Trans. Power Apparatus Syst.* PAS-91(3), 1972, 1266–1272.

24. Sykes, J. A. and Morrison, I. F. A proposed method of harmonic–restrain differential protection of transformers by digital computer, *IEEE Trans. Power Apparatus Syst.* PAS-91(3), 1972, 1266–1272.

25. Gönen, T. *Electric Power Distribution System Engineering*, 2nd edn., CRC Press, Boca Raton, FL, 2008.

26. Bricker, S., Rubin, L., and Gönen, T. Substation automation techniques and advantages, *IEEE Comput. Appl. Power* 14(3), 2001, 31–37.

11 Transmission System Reliability

To fail to plan is to plan to fail.

A. E. Gascoigne, 1985

Now that I'm almost up the ladder,
I should, no doubt, be feeling gladder.
It is quite fine, the view and such,
If just it didn't shake so much.

Richard Armour

11.1 BASIC DEFINITIONS

The following definitions of terms for reporting and analyzing outages of power system facilities and interruptions are taken from Ref. [1] and included here by permission of the IEEE.

Outage. It describes the state of a component when it is not available to perform its intended function due to some event *directly associated* with that component. An outage may or may not cause an interruption of service to consumers depending on system configuration.

Forced outage. It is an outage that results from emergency conditions directly associated with a component requiring that component to be taken out of service immediately, either automatically or as soon as switching operations can be performed, or an outage caused by improper operation of equipment or human error.

Scheduled outage. It is an outage that results when a component is deliberately taken out of service at a selected time, usually for purposes of construction, preventive maintenance, or repair. The key test to determine if an outage should be classified as forced or scheduled is as follows: if it is possible to defer the outage when such deferment is desirable, the outage is a scheduled outage; otherwise, the outage is a forced outage. Deferring an outage may be desirable, for example, to prevent overload of facilities or an interruption of service to consumers.

Transient forced outage. It is a component outage whose cause is immediately self-clearing so that the affected component can be restored to service either automatically or as soon as a switch or a CB can be reclosed or a fuse replaced. An example of a transient forced outage is a lightning flashover that does not permanently disable the flashed component.

Persistent forced outage. It is a component outage whose cause is not immediately self-clearing but must be corrected by eliminating the hazard or by repairing or replacing the affected component before it can be returned to service. An example of a persistent forced outage is a lightning flashover that shatters an insulator, thereby disabling the component until repair or replacement can be made.

Interruption. It is the loss of service to one or more consumers or other facilities and is the result of one or more component outages, depending on system configuration.

Forced interruption. It is an interruption caused by a forced outage.

Scheduled interruption. It is an interruption caused by a scheduled outage.

Momentary interruption. It has a duration limited to the period required to restore service by automatic or supervisory controlled switching operations or by manual switching at locations where an operator is immediately available. Such switching operations are typically completed in a few minutes.

11.2 NATIONAL ELECTRIC RELIABILITY COUNCIL

The NERC was established by the electric utility industry in 1968 and incorporated in 1975. The purpose of the council is to increase the reliability and adequacy of bulk power supply of the electric utility systems in North America. It is a forum of nine regional reliability councils and covers essentially all of the power systems of the United States and the Canadian power systems in the provinces of Ontario, British Columbia, Manitoba, and New Brunswick, as shown in Figure 11.1. The figure shows the total number of bulk power outages reported and the ratio of the number of bulk outages to electric sales for each regional electric reliability council area.

Note that the terms *reliability* and *adequacy* define two separate but interdependent concepts. *Reliability* describes the security of the system and the avoidance of the power outages, whereas *adequacy* refers to having sufficient system capacity to supply the electric energy requirements of the customers.

The term *power pool* defines usually a formal organization established by two or more utilities for the purpose of increased economy, security, or reliability in power system planning or operations. Each pool arrangement is unique due to the different needs and system design of the individual member utilities that are included in the pool. The level of joint planning and operations in power pools can vary from very flexible arrangements for bulk power transfers to coordinated planning and operations to completely integrated operations. In the integrated operation–type pools, decisions are made centrally by the pool, and the benefits are allocated to the member utilities. There are approximately 30 power pools at the present time, both formal and informal [2].

Figure 11.2 shows the number of interruptions, load reduction incidents, and load involved per year for the years from 1971 to 1979 (based on the US Department of Energy reports; as are data for Figures 11.2 through 11.6). The number of customers affected per bulk power outage per year is shown in Figure 11.3. The generic causes of bulk power outages can be classified as weather, electric system components, electric system operation, and miscellaneous factors. Figure 11.4 shows bulk power outages by generic cause by year for the years from 1970 to 1979. The generic cause of bulk power outages for each utility subsystem, that is, generation, transmission, and distribution, is shown in Figure 11.5, whereas Figure 11.6 shows bulk power outages by utility subsystem. Note that the transmission system is involved in 60%–80% of all bulk power outages.

11.3 INDEX OF RELIABILITY

The index of reliability is a convenient performance measure that has been used in the past to provide an indication of positive system performance. It is defined as the ratio of the total customer hours per year minus the total customer hours interrupted per year to total customer hours per year. Therefore,

$$\text{Index of reliability} = \frac{(\text{Total customer - hours per year}) - \text{Total customer - hours interrupted per year}}{(\text{Total customer - hours per year})}$$

$$(11.1)$$

Table 11.1 gives the index of reliability for all reporting US power utility industries for the years from 1956 to 1967 and from 1974 to 1978. The data for the years from 1956 to 1967 have been taken from a 1968 Edison Electric Institute (EEI) Survey on service reliability. The data include distribution system interruptions as well as bulk power system interruptions. Whereas the data for the years from 1974 to 1978 have been taken from the National Electric Reliability Study [3] and include

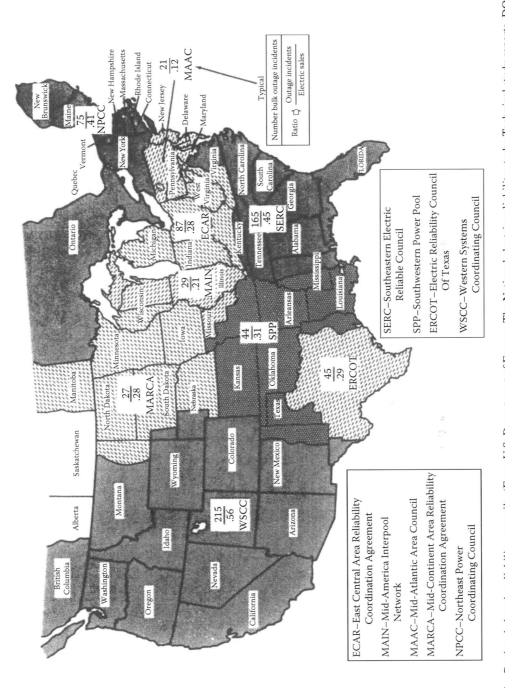

FIGURE 11.1 Regional electric reliability councils. (From U.S. Department of Energy, The National electric reliability study: Technical study reports, DOE/EP-0005, Office of Emergency Operations, USDOE, Washington, DC, 1981.)

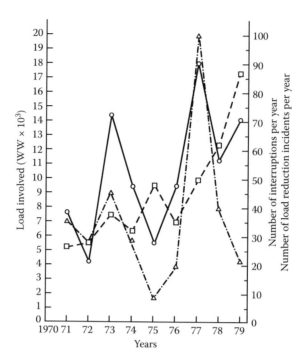

FIGURE 11.2 Bulk power system interruption data, 1971–1979. (From U.S. Department of Energy, The National electric reliability study: Technical study reports, DOE/EP-0005, Office of Emergency Operations, USDOE, Washington, DC, 1981.): o————o, load involved (×10³ MW); □————□, interruptions per year; △·············△, load reduction incidents per year.

only bulk power system interruptions. In either case, the reliability performance of the bulk power systems appears consistently high in the United States.

It is usually understood that the bulk power system includes basic generation plants and the transmission system that permits transportation of power from these plants to primary load centers.

11.4 SECTION 209 OF PURPA OF 1978

Figure 11.7 shows Section 209 of the Public Utility Regulatory Policies Act (PURPA) of 1978. The legislation requires study of numerous reliability-related questions, for example, appropriate levels of reliability; procedures to minimize public disruption during an outage; appropriate generation, transmission, and distribution mix; or appropriate electric utility reliability standards. The basic objectives of the legislation have been summarized in the 1981 National Electric Reliability Study [3] as follows:

1. Providing answers to the following three issues:
   a. The level of reliability appropriate to serve adequately the needs of electric consumers, taking into account cost-effectiveness and the need for energy conservation
   b. The various methods that could be used in order to achieve such a level of reliability and the cost-effectiveness of such methods
   c. The various procedures that might be used in case of an emergency outage to minimize the public disruption and economic loss that might result from such an outage and the cost of such procedures
2. Recommending industry and/or government goals or policies needed to maintain or improve reliability if necessary

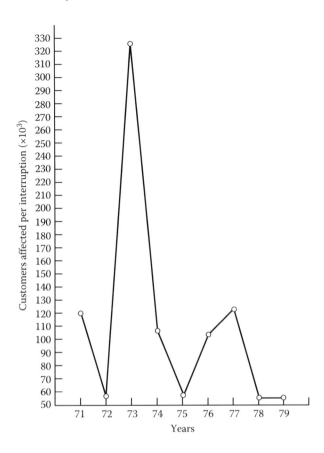

FIGURE 11.3 Number of customers, in thousands, affected per bulk power interruption, 1971–1979. (From U.S. Department of Energy, The National electric reliability study: Technical study reports, DOE/EP-0005, Office of Emergency Operations, USDOE, Washington, DC, 1981.)

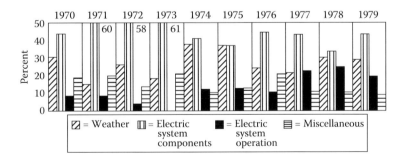

FIGURE 11.4 Bulk power outages by cause, 1970–1979. (From U.S. Department of Energy, The National electric reliability study: Technical study reports, DOE/EP-0005, Office of Emergency Operations, USDOE, Washington, DC, 1981.)

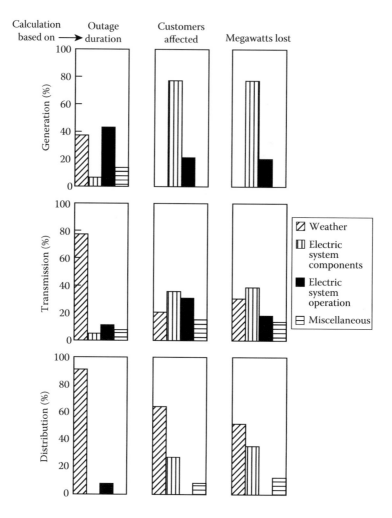

FIGURE 11.5 Bulk power outages by subsystem by cause. (From U.S. Department of Energy, The National electric reliability study: Technical study reports, DOE/EP-0005, Office of Emergency Operations, USDOE, Washington, DC, 1981.)

The objectives of Section 209 are consistent with the overall objectives stipulated in the National Energy Act to encourage conservation of energy supplied by electric utilities, optimize the efficient use of facilities and resources by electric utilities, and provide equitable rates to consumers of electric power.

However, in general, there is no one level of reliability that is suitable for all utilities. Furthermore, even the level of reliability that is suitable for a single utility can change over a period of time. The National Electric Reliability Study [4,5] points out the following:

1. Roughly 75% of all reported transmission outages causing customer interruptions resulting from problems related to components, maintenance, or operation and coordination, with the remaining 25% arising from events outside the control of the utility.
2. Roughly 20% of the interruptions that could have been avoided were caused by inadequate transmission system operation. High percentage of failures related to operations indicated that there are definite possibilities for improved transmission reliability performance with existing facilities by improving the adequacy of supporting systems such as communications and control.

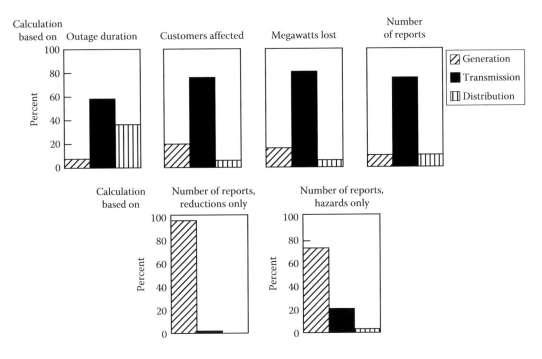

FIGURE 11.6 Bulk power outages by generic subsystem. (From U.S. Department of Energy, The National electric reliability study: Technical study reports, DOE/EP-0005, Office of Emergency Operations, USDOE, Washington, DC, 1981.)

TABLE 11.1
Service Reliability in the United States

Year	Index of Reliability
1956	99.8801
1957	99.9852
1959	99.9824
1959	99.9849
1960	99.9812
1961	99.9848
1962	99.9858
1963	99.9860
1964	99.9829
1965	99.9754
1966	99.9883
1967	99.9845
1974	99.9984[a]
1975	99.9987[a]
1976	99.9980[a]
1977	99.9968[a]
1978	99.9983[a]

[a] Includes only bulk power system outages.

SEC. 209.   RELIABILITY.

   (a) STUDY.——(1) The Secretary, in consultation with the Commission, shall conduct a study with respect to—

       (A) the level of reliability appropriate to adequately serve the
needs of electric consumers, taking into account cost effectiveness
and the need for energy conservation,

       (B) the various methods which could be used in order to achieve
such level of reliability and the cost effectiveness of such methods,
and

       (C) the various procedures that might be used in case of an
emergency outage to minimize the public disruption and economic
loss that might be caused by such an outage and the cost effectiveness of such procedures.

Such study shall be completed and submitted to the President and the
Congress not later than 18 months after the date of the enactment of
this Act. Before such submittal the Secretary shall provide an opportunity for public comment on the results of such study.

   (2) The study under paragraph (1) shall include consideration of
the following:

       (A) the cost effectiveness of investments in each of the com-
ponents involved in providing adequate and reliable electric
service, including generation, transmission, and distribution
facilities, and devices available to the electric consumer;

       (B) the environmental and other effects of the investments con-
sidered under subparagraph (A);

       (C) various types of electric utility systems in terms of gen-
eration, transmission, distribution and customer mix, the extent
to which differences in reliability levels may be desirable, and the
cost-effectiveness of the various methods which could be used to
decrease the number and severity of any outages among the
various types of systems;

       (D) alternatives to adding new generation facilities to achieve
such desired levels of reliability (including conservation);

       (E) the cost-effectiveness of adding a number of small, decen-
tralized conventional and nonconventional generating units
rather than a small number of large generating units with a similar total megawatt capacity for achieving the desired level of
reliability; and

       (F) any standards for electric utility reliability used by, or
suggested for use by, the electric utility industry in terms of
cost-effectiveness in achieving the desired level of reliability,
including equipment standards, standards for operating procedures and training of personnel, and standards relating the
number and severity of outages to periods of time.

   (b) EXAMINATION OF RELIABILITY ISSUES BY RELIABILITY COUN-
CILS.——The Secretary, in consultation with the Commission, may, from
time to time, request the reliability councils established under section
202(a) of the Federal Power Act or other appropriate persons
(including Federal agencies) to examine and report to him concerning
any electric utility reliability issue. The Secretary shall report to the
Congress (in its annual report or in the report required under subsec-
tion (a) if appropriate) the results of any examination under the
preceding sentence.

   (c) DEPARTMENT OF ENERGY RECOMMENDATIONS.——The Secretary,
in consultation with the Commission, and after opportunity for public
comment, may recommend industry standards for reliability to the
electric utility industry, including standards with respect to equipment, operating procedures and training of personnel, and standards
relating to the level or levels of reliability appropriate to adequately
and reliably serve the needs of electric consumers. The Secretary shall
include in his annual report—

       (1) any recommendations made under this subsection or any
recommendations respecting electric utility reliability problems
under any other provision of law, and

       (2) a description of actions taken by electric utilities with
respect to such recommendations.

Margin notes:
16 USC 824a-z.

Report to
President and
Congress.

Report to
Congress.

16 USC 824a.

EXHIBIT 1

FIGURE 11.7   Summary of PURPA.

3. The most major interruptions initiated by inadequate transmission operation are the results of protection and relaying problems that are not adequately addressed by current reliability evaluation techniques.
4. The level of transmission utility may be inadequate from a regional perspective.
5. The size and complexity of the transmission system make it very difficult to calculate meaningful transmission reliability measures.

11.5 BASIC PROBABILITY THEORY

There are various reliability indices that can be employed in measuring the reliability of a given system and/or comparing the reliabilities of various possible system designs. These reliability indices are defined in Section 6.4. The reliability indices may involve values that are probabilistic in nature (e.g., probability of an event occurring or not occurring), mean time between failures, etc. Thus, these values are random variables that may change randomly in time.

The probability theory can be defined as the theory based on an equally likely set of events or as relative frequencies. The relative frequency of the occurrence of an event in a large number of repetitions of situations where the event may occur is defined as the probability of the event. A set of outcomes is called an event. An event is said to occur if any one of its outcomes occurs. A series of events is said to be random if one event has no predictable effect on the next. The probability of an event E_i is a number between 0 and 1:

$$0 \leq P(E_i) \leq 1 \quad \forall_i \tag{11.2}$$

where $\forall_i$ means *for all i*. If the event cannot occur, its probability is 0. On the other hand, if it must occur (its occurrence is certain), its probability is 1. Otherwise, its probability is somewhere in between 0 and 1.

Assume that a chance experiment (an equation whose outcome cannot be predicted in advance) is to be performed and that there may be various possible outcomes that can occur when the experiment is performed. If an event A occurs with m of these outcomes, then the probability of the event A occurring is

$$p = P(A) = \frac{m}{n} \tag{11.3}$$

where
p is the probability of event A (also called its success), $= P(A)$
n is the total number of outcomes possible

For example, if the event occurs, on the average, in 4 out of every 10 trials, then the probability of its occurrence is 0.4. Similarly, the probability of nonoccurrence of the event is

$$q = P(\text{not } A) = P(\bar{A}) = \frac{n-m}{n} = 1 - \frac{m}{n} = 1 - p = 1 - P(A) \tag{11.4}$$

where q is the probability of nonoccurrence of event (also called its failure), $= p(\bar{A})$.

For example, the probability of nonoccurrence of the event in the previous example is 0.6. Therefore, the probability of an event A is equal to the sum of the probabilities of the sample points in A. Note that

$$p + q = 1 \tag{11.5}$$

or

$$P(A) + P(\overline{A}) = 1 \tag{11.6}$$

or, in a general expression,

$$\sum_{S} P(E_i) = 1 \tag{11.7}$$

where
   S is the sample space
   $P(E_i)$ is the probability of event E_i

11.5.1 SET THEORY

The discussion of probability is greatly facilitated if it can be presented in the terms of set theory. Thus, some very elementary definitions and operations of set theory will be presented in this section. A set is a well-defined collection of distinct elements. An *element* of a set is any one of its members. A set may have a finite or infinite number of elements or no elements at all. If $x_1, x_2, x_3, \ldots, x_n$ are elements of set A, it is denoted as

$$A = \{x_1, x_2, x_3, \ldots, x_n\}$$

If set A is a set and x is an element of A, the set membership is indicated as $x \in A$ and is read as x *belongs to A*. On the other hand, if x is not an element of A, this fact is indicated as $x \notin A$.

If $x \in A$ implies $x \in B$, then it can be said that A *is a subset of B* (A is contained in or equal to B), and this fact is indicated by writing $A \subseteq B$, which is read as A *is a subset of B*. In other words, $A \subseteq B$ if every element of A is also an element of B. An equivalent notation, $B \supseteq A$, is read as B *contains or equals A*.

The relationships that exist among sets can be more easily defined if a *Venn diagram*, that is, a *Euler diagram*, is utilized. The Venn diagram displays the entire sample space S as a rectangular area. Here, the sample space defines the entirety of the set of elements under consideration. (It is also called the *universal set* [or *universe*] and is denoted by U.) For example, Figure 11.8 shows a Venn diagram that illustrates the set–subset relationship. Note that $B \subseteq S$, $A \subseteq S$, and $A \subseteq B$.

If every element in A is also an element of B and if every element in B is also an element of A, then A equals B (i.e., if $A \subseteq B$ and $B \subseteq A$, then $A = B$). Alternatively, $A = B$ if $A \subseteq B$ and $A \supseteq B$. If A is a subset of B and $A \neq B$, then A is a proper subset of B. If A is any set, then A is a subset itself. A set that contains no elements is said to be *empty* and is called the *null set*. If A is any set, then $\varnothing \subseteq A$.

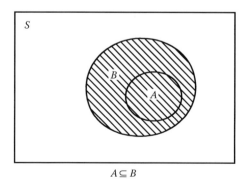

$A \subseteq B$

FIGURE 11.8   Set–subset relationship.

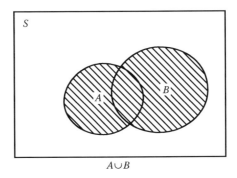

$A \cup B$

FIGURE 11.9   Union, $A \cup B$.

It is possible to form new sets from given sets. For instance, given two sets A and B, the *union* of A and B is the set of all elements that (1) are in A or (2) are in B or (3) are in both A and B. The word union is symbolized by $\cup$ so that A union B (the union of A and B) is written $A \cup B$. Figure 11.9 illustrates the concept of union in which the shaded area represents the union of A and B, symbolized by $A \cup B$ or, in some applications, by $A + B$. Here, the crucial word to remember about the concept of union is *or*. The criterion for including any element in the union of A and B is whether that element is contained in A or B or both A and B. Therefore, mathematically, $A \cup B$ is the set $\{x \in A \text{ or } x \in B\}$. For example, if A includes $\{1, 2, 3, 4, 5\}$ and B includes $\{3, 4, 5, 6, 7, 8\}$, then $A \cup B = \{1, 2, 3, 4, 5, 6, 7, 8\}$. Note that numbers contained in both A and B are not represented twice in $A \cup B$, that is, $A \cup B$ is not equal to $(1, 2, 3, 4, 5, 3, 4, 5, 6, 7, 8)$. Of course, there can be more than two sets in a given sample space, for example, A, B, and C, whose union can be expressed as $A \cup B \cup C$.

Given two sets A and B, the *intersection* of A and B contains all elements that are in both A and B but not in A or B alone. The symbol for intersection is $\cap$, and A intersection B is written $A \cap B$. Therefore, mathematically speaking, $A \cap B$ is the set $\{x \in S \mid x \in A \text{ and } x \in B\}$. Here, $A \cap B$ is read A *intersects* B. Figure 11.10a illustrates the intersection of A and B in which $A \cap B$ is the shaded portion of the diagram. For example, if $A = \{1, 2, 3, 4, 5\}$ and $B = \{3, 4, 5, 6, 7, 8\}$, then $A \cap B = \{3, 4, 5\}$. Here, the emphasis is on the word *and* because in order for an element to be a member of the intersection of A and B ($A \cap B$), it must be contained in both A *and* B. The intersection represents the *common* portion of two sets or the elements shared by two sets. Naturally, there can be more than two sets in a given sample space, for example, three sets, which would be expressed as $A \cap B \cap C$.

Assume that $A \cap B$ contains no elements (i.e., $A \cap B = \varnothing$); then A and B share no common elements, that is, no element in A is also in B and no element in B is also in A. If $A \cap B = \varnothing$, then A and B are called *disjoint sets*, or *mutually exclusive sets*, due to the fact that there is no common element to *join* them together. Figure 11.10b illustrates this concept. For instance, if $A = \{1, 2, 3, 4, 5\}$ and $B = \{6, 7, 8, 9, 10\}$, then $A \cap B = \varnothing$ or $A \cap B = \{\}$, where $\varnothing$ is said to be *empty* and is called *the null set*.

Another example of disjoint sets is A and $\bar{A}$. Here, the set $\bar{A}$ contains all elements that are not in the set A and is called the *complement* of A. Therefore, $\bar{A} = S - \bar{A}$ or $A \cup \bar{A} = S$, and $A \cap \bar{A} = 0$. For any set A, A and $\bar{A}$ are disjoint. Thus, mathematically speaking, the *complement* of A is the set $\{x \in S \mid x \notin A\}$. For example, if $S = \{1, 2, 3, 4, 5, 6, 7, 8, 9, 10\}$ and $A = \{1, 2, 3, 4, 5\}$, then $A = \{6, 7, 8, 9, 10\}$. Figure 11.11 illustrates the concept of complement.

Figure 11.12 shows the *difference* set $A - B$, which includes only those elements of A that are not also in B. It is crucial to be aware of the fact that $(A - B) + B = A + B$, not just A.*

---

* Because of this misleading result, the notation + should be avoided as much as possible.

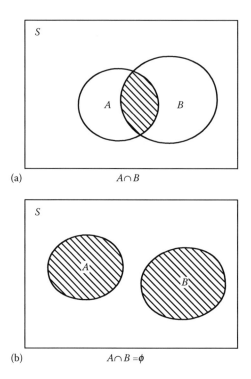

FIGURE 11.10   (a) Intersection, $A \cap B$; (b) two disjoint sets, $A \cap B = \varnothing$.

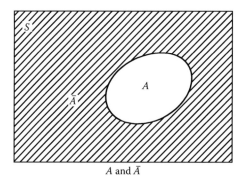

FIGURE 11.11   Complement set, $\bar{A}$.

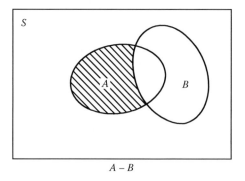

FIGURE 11.12   Difference, $A - B$.

11.5.2 PROBABILITY AND SET THEORY

It is possible to explain the probability theory in terms of set theory. In probability theory, any operation whose outcome cannot be predicted with certainty is called an *experiment*. The experiments that appear most often in examples to describe the concept of probability are flipping coins, rolling dice, selecting balls from an urn, and dealing cards from a deck. The set of all possible outcomes or results of an experiment is called the *sample space* and is denoted by *S*. For example, if a single die is rolled one time, then the experiment is the roll of the die. A sample space for this experiment could be

$$S = (1, 2, 3, 4, 5, 6)$$

where each of the integers 1–6 is meant to represent the face having that many spots being upper-most when the die stops rolling.

Each individual possible outcome is represented in the sample space by one *sample point* and is denoted by *A*. Therefore, the totality of sample points is the *sample space*. An *event* is a subset of the sample space. An event occurs if any one of its elements is the outcome of the experiment. The sample space used in the aforementioned example was

$$S = (1, 2, 3, 4, 5, 6)$$

Therefore, each of the sets

$$A = \{1\}$$

$$B = \{1, 3, 5)$$

$$C = \{2, 4, 6\}$$

$$D = \{4, 5, 6\}$$

$$E = (1, 3, 4, 6)$$

is an event (these are not the only events since they are not the only subsets of *S*). These are all different events since no two of these subsets are equal. If an actual experiment of rolling the die is performed and the resulting outcome is 4, then events *C*, *D*, and *E* are said to have occurred since each of these has 4 as an element. Events *A* and *B* did not occur since $4 \notin A$ and $4 \notin B$.

The theory of probability is concerned with consistent ways of assigning numbers of events (subsets of the sample space *S*), which are called the *probabilities of occurrence* of these events. Alternatively, assume that a weight w_i is assigned to each point p_i of the sample space in a way such that

$$w_i \geq 0 \quad \forall_i$$

and

$$w_1 + w_2 + w_3 + \cdots = \sum_i w_i = 1$$

Then the *probability that event A will occur* is the sum of the weights of the sample points that are in *A* and is denoted by *P(A)*. Succinctly put, a probability function is a real-valued set function defined on the class of all subsets of the sample space S; the value that is associated with a subset A is denoted by $P(A)$. The probability of an event is always nonnegative and can never exceed 1. The probabilities of the certain event and the impossible events are 1 and 0, respectively. The assignment of probabilities must satisfy the following three rules (which are called the *axioms of probability**) so that the set function may be called a *probability function*:

$$P(S) = 1 \tag{11.8}$$

$$P(A) \geq 0 \quad \text{for all} \quad A \subset S \tag{11.9}$$

$$P(A_1 \cup A_2 \cup \cdots) = P(A_1) + P(A_2) + \cdots \quad \text{if} \quad A_i \cap A_j = \varnothing \quad \forall_{i \neq j} \tag{11.10}$$

Equation 11.9 can alternatively be represented as

$$0 \leq P(A) \leq 1 \tag{11.11}$$

which implies that the probability of an event is always nonnegative and can never exceed 1. Equation 11.10 implies that if A and B are *disjoint* (*mutually exclusive*) events in S, as shown in Figure 11.10, then

$$P(A + B) = P(A) + P(B) \tag{11.12}$$

where $A + B$ is the event A or B, that is, the occurrence of one of them excludes the occurrence of the other. Note that the union of A and B ($A \cup B$) is defined to be the event containing all sample points in A or B or both. Therefore, it is usually expressed as A or B rather than $A + B$. Here, the events A and B may be said to be *disjoint* if they cannot both happen at the same time. The sample space represents a single trial of the experiment, and A and B are disjoint if they cannot both occur if one trial. For example, for rolling a pair of dice, the sample space consists of the 36 outcomes. If A is the event that the total is 4, then it includes three outcomes:

$$A = \{2\text{--}2, 1\text{--}3, 3\text{--}1\}$$

Similarly, if B is the event that the total is 3, it contains two outcomes:

$$B = \{1\text{--}2, 2\text{--}1\}$$

Then A or B is the event that the total is either 4 or 3:

$$A \text{ or } B = \{2\text{--}2, 1\text{--}3, 3\text{--}1, 1\text{--}2, 2\text{--}1\}$$

Therefore, it can be shown that

$$P(A \cup B) = P(A + B) = P(A \text{ or } B)$$

$$= P(A) + P(B)$$

$$= \frac{3}{36} + \frac{2}{36} = \frac{5}{36}$$

---

* Note that they are postulated and cannot be proved. However, the calculus of probability can be based on them.

Note that the dice cannot total both 4 and 3 at once, but none of these stops them from totaling 4 on one trial and 3 on another trial.

In general, it can be expressed that the probability of a union, as shown in Figure 11.8, is equal to

$$P(A \cup B) = P(A) + P(B) - P(AB) \tag{11.13}$$

or

$$P(A \cup B) = P(A) + P(B) - P(A \cap B) \tag{11.14}$$

If A and B are mutually exclusive,

$$P(AB) = 0 \tag{11.15}$$

and therefore,

$$P(A \cup B) = P(A) + P(B) \tag{11.16}$$

In other words, two events A and B are said to be *mutually exclusive* if the event AB contains no sample points. Note that Equation 11.13 can be reexpressed as

$$P(A \text{ or } B) = P(A) + P(B) - P(A \text{ and } B) \tag{11.17}$$

Equations 11.13 and 11.16 are referred to as the *additive law of probability*. For example, assume that a card is drawn at random from a deck and that A is the event of drawing a spade and B is the event of drawing a face card. Thus, A *and* B are the events that the card is both a spade and a face card. The number of outcomes in A is 13, the number in B is 12, and the number in A *and* B is 3. Therefore, the probability of drawing a spade or a face card is

$$P(A \text{ or } B) = \frac{13}{52} + \frac{12}{52} - \frac{3}{52} = \frac{22}{52}$$

The complement of an event A is the *opposite* event, the one that occurs exactly when A does not. Therefore, the complement of an event A is the collection of all sample points in S and not in A. The complement of A is denoted by the symbol $\bar{A}$. Since

$$\sum_S P(E_i) = 1 \tag{11.7}$$

then

$$P(A) + P(\bar{A}) \triangleq 1 \tag{11.6}$$

Therefore,

$$P(A) = 1 - P(\bar{A}) \tag{11.18}$$

or

$$P(\bar{A}) = 1 - P(A) \tag{11.19}$$

The *conditional probability* of an event B given another event A is denoted by $P(B|A)$ and is defined by

$$P(B|A) = \frac{P(A \cap B)}{P(A)} \quad \text{if } P(A) \neq 0 \tag{11.20}$$

or

$$P(B|A) = \frac{P(A \text{ and } B)}{P(A)} \quad \text{if } P(A) \neq 0 \tag{11.21}$$

or

$$P(B|A) = \frac{P(AB)}{P(A)} \quad \text{if } P(A) \neq 0 \tag{11.22}$$

Likewise,

$$P(A|B) = \frac{P(A \cap B)}{P(B)} \quad \text{if } P(B) \neq 0 \tag{11.23}$$

is called *the conditional probability of event A given event B*, where $A \cap B$ represents the event consisting of all points in the sample space S common to both A and B. In Equation 11.20, should one of the individual probabilities be zero, the corresponding conditional probability is undefined. The vertical bar in the parenthesis of $(B|A)$ is read *given*, and the events appearing to the right of the line are the events that are known to have occurred. Note that multiplying both sides of Equation 11.20 by $P(A)$ gives

$$P(A \cap B) = P(A)P(B|A) \tag{11.24}$$

or

$$P(A \text{ and } B) = P(A)P(B|A) \tag{11.25}$$

For example, assume that two cards are drawn at random without replacement from a bridge deck and that A is the event of the first card being red and B is the event of the second card being red. Then the probability of both cards being red is

$$P(\text{both cards red}) = P(A)P(B|A)$$

$$= 2 \times \frac{25}{51} = 0.2451$$

Two events A and B are said to be *independent* if either

$$P(A|B) = P(A) \tag{11.26}$$

or

$$P(B|A) = P(B) \tag{11.27}$$

Otherwise, the events are said to be *dependent*. If the events A and B are independent, then

$$P(B|A) = \frac{P(A \cap B)}{P(A)} = P(B) \tag{11.28}$$

Note that the probability of the *intersection AB* is

$$P(A \cap B) = P(AB)$$

$$= P(A)P(B|A) \tag{11.29}$$

$$= P(B)P(A|B) \tag{11.30}$$

If A and B are *independent*,

$$P(A \cap B) = P(AB)$$

$$= P(A)P(B) \tag{11.31}$$

Equations 11.29 through 11.31 are referred to as the *multiplicative law of probability*. An example for the independent events is the rolling of two dice where the outcome of rolling one die is independent of the roll of the second one. For instance, assume that a fair die is tossed twice; since the two tosses are made independently of each other, the probability of getting a pair of 4s is

$$P(\text{pair of 4s}) = P(\text{four spots on first toss})\,P(\text{four spots on second toss})$$

$$= \frac{1}{6} \times \frac{1}{6} = \frac{1}{36}$$

Assume that B is an event and $\bar{B}$ is its complement. If A is another event that occurs if and only if B or $\bar{B}$ occurs, then the probability is

$$P(B|A) = \frac{P(B)P(A|B)}{P(B)P(A|B) + P(\bar{B})P(A|\bar{B})} \tag{11.32}$$

This formula constitutes *Bayes's rule* or *Bayes's law* or *Bayes's theorem*. Given the prior probability $P(B)$ (and $P(\bar{B}) = 1 - P(B)$) and the respective probabilities $P(A|B)$ and $P(\bar{A}|B)$, one can use Bayes's law to calculate the *posterior* (after-the-fact) probability $P(B|A)$. In a sense, Bayes's law is updating or revising the prior probability $P(B)$ by incorporating the observed information contained within event A into the model.

11.6 COMBINATIONAL ANALYSIS

The probability problems often require the enumeration of the possible ways that events can occur. The combinational analysis methods make this cumbersome operation easier. If one thing can occur in n different ways and another thing can occur in m different ways, then both things can occur together or in succession in $m \times n$ different ways. For instance, if a couple of dice are rolled simultaneously, since one of them rolls in $n = 6$ ways and the other one rolls in $m = 6$ ways, then together they all roll in $n \times m = 36$ ways.

If n is a positive integer, then n factorial, denoted by $n!$, is defined as

$$n! = 1 \times 2 \times 3 \times \cdots \times (n - 1) \times n \tag{11.33}$$

For instance,

$$5! = 1 \times 2 \times 3 \times 4 \times 5 = 120$$

where

$$0! \triangleq 1$$

The number of ways of selecting and arranging r objects taken from n distinct objects is called a *permutation of n things taken r at a time*, denoted by $P_{(n,r)}$, $_nP_r$, or $P_{n,r}$, and is defined as

$$_nP_r \triangleq \frac{n!}{(n-r)!}$$

$$= n(n-1)(n-2)\cdots(n-r+1) \tag{11.34}$$

For example, the total number of possible permutations of the letters A, B, and C taken two at a time can be determined as

$$_3P_2 = \frac{3!}{(3-2)!}$$

$$= \frac{3!}{1!} = 6$$

which are *AB, BA, AC, CA, BC,* and *CB.*

The number of *combinations* of n distinct objects taken r at a time (the number of subsets of size r), denoted by $C_{(n,r)}$, $_nC_r$, $C_{n,r}$ or $\binom{n}{r}$, is defined as

$$_nC_r \triangleq \frac{n!}{r!(n-r)!}$$

$$= \frac{_nP_r}{r!}$$

$$= \frac{n(n-1)\cdots(n-r+1)}{r!} \tag{11.35}$$

For instance, the number of combinations of 5-card hands that can be dealt from a 52-card deck can be determined as

$$_{52}C_5 = \binom{52}{5}$$

$$= \frac{52!}{5!(52-5)!} = 2,598,960$$

11.7 PROBABILITY DISTRIBUTIONS

If a given set has the values of $x_1, x_2,\ldots, x_n$ and we have the probabilities $P(x_1)$, $P(x_2),\ldots, P(x_n)$ that $x_1, x_2,\ldots, x_n$ will occur, then this group of individual probabilities is referred to as a *density distribution*. By cumulating these individual probabilities of a discrete set of values $x_1, x_2,\ldots, x_n$, a *cumulative probability distribution* can be obtained. Because the variable x can assume certain values with given probabilities, it is often called a *discrete random variable* (or sometimes a *stochastic variable*). Random variables play an extremely important role in probability theory. Therefore, since random variables can be discrete or continuous, the resultant probability distributions can either be discrete or continuous. The following are some examples of discrete and continuous probability distributions.

The *binomial distribution* is a discrete distribution. It is also called the *Bernoulli distribution*. For example, if p is the probability that an event will occur (sometimes it is identified as the *probability of success*) in any single trial and $q = 1 - p$ is the probability that it will fail to occur (*probability of failure*), then the probability that the event will occur exactly x times in n trials is given by the expression

$$P(x = k) = {}_nC_k\, p^k q^{n-k}$$

$$= \frac{n!}{k!(n-k)!} p^k q^{n-k} \tag{11.36}$$

Note that this distribution is a function of the two parameters, p and n. The probability distribution of this random variable x is shown in Figure 11.13. An interesting interpretation of the binomial distribution is obtained when $n = 1$, that is,

$$P(x = 0) = 1 - P \quad \text{and} \quad P(x = 1) = P$$

Such a random variable is said to have a *Bernoulli distribution*. Thus, if a random variable takes on two values, say, 0 or 1, with probability $1 - p$ or p, respectively, it is defined as a *Bernoulli random variable*. The upturned face of a flipped coin is such an example. A binomial distribution has a mean value of $\mu = np$, a variance value of

$$\sigma^2 = npq \tag{11.37}$$

and a standard deviation of

$$\sigma = (npq)^{1/2} \tag{11.38}$$

The *Poisson distribution* is a discrete probability distribution, and it is a special case of the binomial distribution where n is large and p is small but the mean $\lambda = \mu = np$ is of moderate magnitude. Thus, a random variable x is said to have a Poisson distribution if its probability distribution can be written as

$$P\left(x = k\right) = \frac{\lambda^k e^{-\lambda}}{k!} \tag{11.39}$$

where
$k = 0, 1, 2,\ldots$
$e = 2.71823$
λ is a positive constant

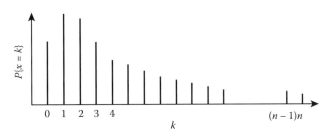

FIGURE 11.13 Binomial probability distribution with fixed n and p.

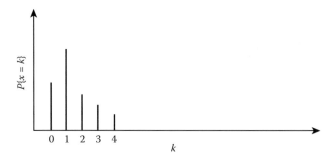

FIGURE 11.14   Poisson probability distribution.

An example of the probability distribution of a Poisson random variable is shown in Figure 11.14. A Poisson distribution has a mean value of $\mu = \lambda$, a variance value of $\sigma^2 = \lambda$, and a standard deviation of $\sigma = \sqrt{\lambda}$.

One of the most important and used distributions is the *normal distribution*. It is a continuous probability distribution, and it is also called *normal curve* or *Gaussian distribution* and is given by

$$Y = \frac{1}{\sigma \sum \sqrt{2\pi}} e^{-1/2(x-\mu)^2/\sigma^2}$$ (11.40)

where
  μ is the mean
  σ is the standard deviation
  $\pi = 3.14159$
  Y is the ordinate, that is, height of given curve corresponding to assigned value of x

A graph of a typical normal density function is given in Figure 11.15. Here, the total area bounded by the curve and x axis is 1. Therefore, the area under the curve between the ordinates $x = a$ and $x = b$ represents the probability that x lies between a and b, denoted by $P(a < x < b)$. Also see Figure 11.16. From Figures 11.15 and 11.16, it is obvious that a normal distribution curve is a symmetric curve. Here, the parameter σ is a measure of the relative width and maximum height of the curve, and the shape of the curve becomes higher and thinner as σ is reduced. Here, σ can be any real positive number. If the variable X is expressed in terms of standard units,

$$Z = \frac{X - \mu}{\sigma}$$ (11.41)

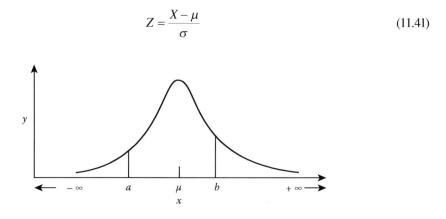

FIGURE 11.15   Normal probability distribution.

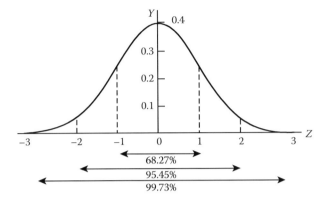

FIGURE 11.16　Standardized normal curve.

the distribution equation (11.40) becomes

$$Y = \frac{1}{\sqrt{2\pi}} e^{-1/2\left(z^2\right)}$$
(11.42)

where Z is normally distributed with a mean of 0 and variance of 1. Figure 11.16 shows a typical standardized normal curve. It shows the areas included between $Z = -1$ and $Z = +1$, $Z = -2$, $Z = +2$, and $Z = -3$ and $Z = +3$, which are equal to 68.27%, 95.45%, and 99.73%, respectively, of the total area, which is 1. A normal distribution has a mean value of μ, a variance value of σ^2, and a standard value of σ.

The *exponential distribution* is also a continuous probability distribution. It is often used in physical reliability problems. For example, the reliability $R(t)$ is usually given as a function of time and gives the number of identical components in a system surviving at time t and divided by the original number of components:

$$R(t) = \frac{N_s(t)}{N_0}$$
(11.43)

where
　　$N_s(t)$ is the number of components surviving at time t
　　N_0 is the number of original components at time t_0

It can be shown that if the failure rate is constant,

$$R(t) = e^{-\lambda t}$$
(11.44)

Therefore, the exponential distribution is given by

$$f(t) = \lambda e^{-\lambda t}$$
(11.45)

The exponential distribution is a special case of the gamma distribution and is shown in Figure 11.17.

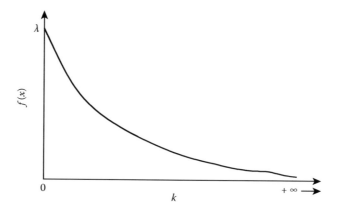

FIGURE 11.17   Exponential distribution.

11.8   BASIC RELIABILITY CONCEPTS

The probability of failure of a given component (or system) can be expressed as a function of time as

$$P(T \le t) = F(t) \quad t \le 0 \tag{11.46}$$

where
   T is the random variable representing failure time
   $F(t)$ is the probability that component will fail by time t

Therefore, the failure distribution function, $F(t)$, is also defined as the *unreliability function*. Thus, the *reliability function* can be expressed as

$$R(t) = 1 - F(t)$$
$$= P(T > t) \tag{11.47}$$

Hence, the probability that the component will survive at time t is defined as the *reliability function* $R(t)$. Note that

$$R(t) = 1 - F(t)$$
$$= 1 - \int_{0}^{t} f(t)\,dt$$
$$= \int_{0}^{\infty} f(t)\,dt \tag{11.48}$$

where

$$F(t) = \int_{0}^{\infty} f(t)\,dt \tag{11.49}$$

provided that the time to failure, random variable T, has a density function $f(t)$. Therefore, it is possible to express the probability of failure of a given system in a specific time interval (t_1, t_2) in terms of either the unreliability function as

$$\int_{t_1}^{t_2} f(t)\,dt = \int_{-\infty}^{t_2} f(t)\,dt - \int_{-\infty}^{t_1} f(t)\,dt$$

$$= F(T_2) - F(T_1) \tag{11.50}$$

or in terms of the *reliability function* as

$$\int_{t_1}^{t_2} f(t)\,dt = \int_{t1}^{\infty} f(t)\,dt - \int_{t_2}^{\infty} f(t)\,dt$$

$$= R(t_1) - R(t_2) \tag{11.51}$$

The *hazard rate* or *failure rate* is defined as the rate at which failures occur in a given time interval (t_1, t_2). In other words, it is the probability that a failure per-unit time occurs in the time interval provided that a failure has not occurred before the time t, that is, at the beginning of the time interval. Thus, the hazard rate can be expressed as

$$h(t) = \frac{R(t_1) - R(t_2)}{(t_2 - t_1)R(t_1)} \tag{11.52}$$

Alternatively, by redefining the time interval as

$$\Delta t = t_2 - t_1 \tag{11.53}$$

so that

$$t_1 = t \quad \text{and} \quad t_2 = t + \Delta t$$

the hazard rate can be expressed as

$$h(t) = \lim_{\Delta t \to 0} \frac{P\{\text{component of age } t \text{ will fail in } \Delta t \mid \text{it has survived up to } t\}}{\Delta t}$$

or

$$h(t) = \lim_{\Delta t \to 0} \frac{R(t) - R(t + \Delta t)}{\Delta t\, R(t)}$$

$$= \frac{1}{R(t)}\left[-\frac{d}{dt} R(t) \right]$$

$$= \frac{f(t)}{R(t)} \tag{11.54}$$

where $f(t)$ = probability density function

$$= -\frac{dR(t)}{dt} \tag{11.55}$$

By substituting Equation 11.48 into Equation 11.54,

$$h(t) = \frac{f(t)}{1 - F(t)} \tag{11.56}$$

Thus,

$$h(t)dt = \frac{dF(t)}{1 - F(t)} \tag{11.57}$$

or

$$\int_0^t h(t)dt = -\ln\left[1 - F(t)\right]\Big|_0^t$$

Therefore,

$$\ln\frac{1 - F(t)}{1 - F(0)} = -\int_0^t h(t)dt \tag{11.58}$$

or

$$1 - F(t) = \exp\left[-\int_0^t h(t)dt\right] \tag{11.59}$$

By substituting Equation 11.59 into Equation 11.56,

$$f(t) = h(t)\exp\left[-\int_0^t h(t)dt\right] \tag{11.60}$$

Furthermore, by substituting Equation 11.48 into Equation 11.59,

$$R(t) = \exp\left[-\int_0^t h(t)dt\right] \tag{11.61}$$

or

$$R(t) = \exp\left(-\int_0^t h(t)dt\right) \tag{11.62}$$

Let

$$\lambda(t) = h(t)$$

Therefore,

$$R(t) = \exp\left(-\int_0^t \lambda(t)dt\right) \tag{11.63}$$

which is called the *general reliability function*. Note that the failure $\lambda(t)$ is a transition rate associated with the number of transitions that a component makes between normal operating state and failure state. It is the rate at which failures happen and is a function of the number of failures in a given period of time during which failures can happen and the number of components exposed to failure. Therefore, it can be defined as

$$\lambda(t) = \frac{\text{Number of failures per unit exposure time}}{\text{Number of components exposed to failure}}$$

Alternatively, if the hazard rate can be assumed to be independent of time, that is,

$$h(t) = \lambda \quad \text{failures/unit time}$$

the failure density function can be expressed as

$$f(t) = \lambda e^{-\lambda t} \tag{11.64}$$

Thus, the *reliability function* can be expressed as

$$R(t) = e^{-\lambda t} \tag{11.65}$$

A typical hazard function can be represented as the *bathtub curve*, which can be segmented into three separate sections, as shown in Figure 11.18. The first segment represents the *break-in period* or *debugging period*, in which the failures occur due to design or manufacturing errors. The second segment represents the *useful life period* or *normal operating period*, in which the failure rates are relatively constant and are called *random failures*. The third represents the *wear-out period*, in which the failure rate increases due to the aging process of the component.

Further, it can be shown that

$$\int_0^t f(t)dt + \int_t^\infty f(t)dt = \int_0^\infty f(t)dt \triangleq 1 \tag{11.66}$$

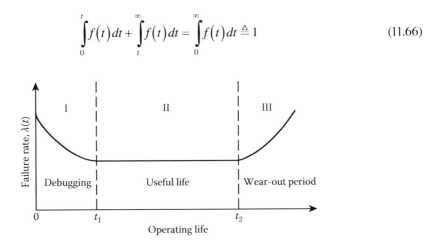

FIGURE 11.18 Bathtub hazard function.

from which

$$\int_0^t f(t)\,dt = 1 - \int_t^\infty f(t)\,dt \tag{11.67}$$

where

$$R(t) = \int_0^\infty f(t)\,dt$$

and

$$R(t) + Q(t) \triangleq 1 \tag{11.68}$$

Therefore, the *unreliability* can be defined as

$$
\begin{aligned}
Q(t) &= 1 - R(t) \\
&= 1 - \int_t^\infty f(t)\,dt \\
&= \int_0^t f(t)\,dt
\end{aligned} \tag{11.69}
$$

The relationship between reliability and unreliability has been illustrated graphically in Figure 11.19.

The *expected life* of a component is the expected time during which the component will survive and perform successfully. It can be expressed as

$$E(T) = \int_0^\infty R(t)\,dt \tag{11.70}$$

or

$$E(T) = \int_0^\infty \left\{ \exp\left[-\int_0^t \lambda(t)\,dt \right] \right\} dt \tag{11.71}$$

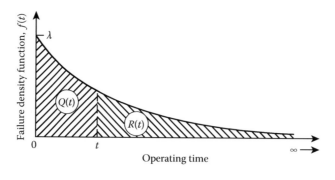

FIGURE 11.19 Relationship between reliability and unreliability.

or if the failure rate is constant,

$$E(T) = \int_{0}^{\infty} e^{-\lambda t} dt$$

$$= \frac{1}{\lambda} \tag{11.72}$$

If the component is not renewed through maintenance and repairs but simply replaced by a good component, the expected life can also be called the *mean time to failure* and is denoted as

$$\text{MTTF} = \bar{m} = \frac{1}{\lambda} \tag{11.73}$$

where λ is the constant failure rate.

On the other hand, if the component is renewed, through maintenance and repairs, the expected life can also be called the *mean time between failures* and is denoted as

$$\text{MTBF} = \bar{T} = \bar{m} + \bar{r} \tag{11.74}$$

where

t is the mean cycle time
$\bar{m}$ is the mean time to failure
$\bar{r}$ is the mean time to repair (MTTR), $= 1/\mu$
μ is the mean repair rate

Assume that a system can be represented by a two-state model so that the system is either in the *up* (or *in*) *state* or the *down* (or *out*) *state* at a given time. Thus, the mean time to failure of the system can be estimated as

$$\text{MTTF} = \bar{m} = \frac{\sum_{i=1}^{n} m_i}{n} \tag{11.75}$$

where

m_i is the observed time to failure for the ith cycle
n is the total number of cycles

In the same way, the estimate for the MTTR can be expressed as

$$\text{MTTR} = \bar{r} = \frac{\sum_{i=1}^{n} r_i}{n} \tag{11.76}$$

where

r_i is the observed time to repair the ith cycle
n is the total number of cycles

Thus, Equation 11.74 can be reexpressed as

$$\text{MTBF} = \text{MTTF} + \text{MTTR} \tag{11.77}$$

Alternatively, Equation 11.74 can be reexpressed as

$$\bar{T} = \frac{1}{\lambda} + \frac{1}{\mu} \tag{11.78}$$

or

$$\bar{T} = \frac{\lambda + \mu}{\lambda\mu} \tag{11.79}$$

Here, the average time that is necessary for the component to finish one cycle of operation (i.e., *failure*, *repair*, and *restart*) is called the *mean cycle time*. The reciprocal of the mean cycle time is called the *mean failure frequency* and is denoted

$$\bar{f} = \frac{1}{\bar{T}} \tag{11.80}$$

or

$$\bar{f} = \frac{\lambda\mu}{\lambda + \mu} \tag{11.81}$$

Alternatively, since in the two-state model the component is either *up* (*available for service*) or *down* (*unavailable for service*),

$$A + U = 1 \tag{11.82}$$

or

$$A + \bar{A} = 1 \tag{11.83}$$

where
   A is the availability of component, that is, fraction of time component is up
   U is the unavailability of component, that is, fraction of time component is down, $= \bar{A}$

Thus, as time t goes to infinity, the *availability* can be expressed as

$$A \triangleq \frac{\bar{m}}{\bar{T}} \tag{11.84}$$

or

$$A = \frac{\text{MTTF}}{\text{MTBT}} \tag{11.85}$$

or substituting Equation 11.77 into Equation 11.85,

$$A = \frac{\text{MTTF}}{\text{MTTF} + \text{MTTR}} \tag{11.86}$$

or

$$A = \frac{\bar{m}}{\bar{m} + \bar{r}} \tag{11.87}$$

or

$$A = \frac{\mu}{\lambda + \mu} \tag{11.88}$$

Therefore, the *unavailability* can be expressed as

$$U \triangleq 1 - A \tag{11.89}$$

or

$$U = \frac{\bar{r}}{\bar{T}} \tag{11.90}$$

or

$$U = \frac{\bar{r}}{\bar{r} + \bar{m}} \tag{11.91}$$

or

$$U = \frac{\lambda}{\lambda + \mu} \tag{11.92}$$

11.8.1 Series Systems

The definition of a series system can be given as a set of components that must all operate for system success in terms of reliability or only one requires to fail for system failure. A block diagram for a series system that has two independent components connected in series is shown in Figure 11.20a. Thus, in order to have the system perform its designated function, both components must perform successfully. Thus, a series system is a nonredundant system. Therefore, the system reliability can be expressed as the probability of system success as

$$R_{sys} = P[E_1 \cap E_2] \tag{11.93}$$

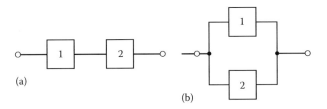

FIGURE 11.20 Block diagrams of system with two components: (a) connected in series and (b) connected in parallel.

or

$$R_{\text{sys}} = P(E_1)P(E_2) \tag{11.94}$$

assuming that the components are independent. Thus,

$$R_{\text{sys}} = R_1 \times R_2 \tag{11.95}$$

or

$$R_{\text{sys}} = \prod_{i=1}^{2} R_i \tag{11.96}$$

where
E_1 is the event that component i operates successfully
R_i is the reliability of component i, $= P(E_i)$
R_{sys} is the reliability of system

Therefore, the system reliability of a series system with n independent components can be expressed as

$$R_{\text{sys}} = P[E_1 \cap E_2 \cap \cdots \cap E_n] \tag{11.97}$$

or

$$R_{\text{sys}} = P(E_1)P(E_2)\cdots P(E_n) \tag{11.98}$$

or

$$R_{\text{sys}} = R_1 \times R_2 \times \cdots \times R_n \tag{11.99}$$

or

$$R_{\text{sys}} = \prod_{i=1}^{n} R_i \tag{11.100}$$

Thus, Equation 11.100 is called the *product rule* or the *chain rule* of reliability. Note that the reliability of a series system will always be less than or equal to the least reliable component, that is,

$$R_{\text{sys}} \leq \min_{i}\{R_i\} \tag{11.101}$$

The reliability of a series system decreases as the number of components increases due to the product rule. It is the function of the number of series components and the component reliability level. Alternatively, the *unreliability* (or failure) of the series system can be expressed as

$$Q_{\text{sys}} = 1 - R_{\text{sys}} \tag{11.102}$$

or

$$Q_{\text{sys}} = 1 - \prod_{i=1}^{n} R_i \tag{11.103}$$

Note that the product rule that is given in Equation 11.100 is applicable to both time-independent and time-dependent probabilities. In case of time-dependent probabilities, if the component reliability can be represented by a (negative) exponential distribution with a failure rate of λ_i, the system reliability can be expressed as

$$R_{sys}(t) = \prod_{i=1}^{n} \exp(-\lambda_i t) \tag{11.104}$$

or

$$R_{sys}(t) = \exp\left(-\sum_{i=1}^{n} \lambda_i t\right) \tag{11.105}$$

or

$$R_{sys}(t) = \exp(-\lambda_e t) \tag{11.106}$$

where λ_e is the equivalent failure rate of system

$$= \sum_{i=1}^{n} \lambda_i \tag{11.107}$$

Alternatively, if the probability of a component failure is q and is the same for all n components of a series system,

$$R_{sys} = (1-q)^n \tag{11.108}$$

or according to the binomial theorem,

$$R_{sys} = 1 + n(q)^1 + \frac{n(n-1)}{2}(-q)^2 + \cdots + (-q)^n \tag{11.109}$$

where
q is the probability of component failure
n is the total number of components connected in series

If the probability of component failure (q) is small, the system reliability approximately is

$$R_{sys} \cong 1 - nq \tag{11.110}$$

but if the q's are different for each component, the system reliability approximately is

$$R_{sys} \cong 1 - \sum_{i=1}^{n} q_i \tag{11.111}$$

11.8.2 PARALLEL SYSTEMS

The definition of a parallel system can be given as a set of components for which only one is required to operate for system success in terms of reliability or all must fail for system failure. Thus, a parallel system is a fully *redundant* system. A block diagram for a parallel system that has two independent components connected in parallel is shown in Figure 11.20b. Since both components must fail simultaneously to cause system reliability, the system unreliability can be expressed as

$$Q_{sys} = P[\bar{E}_1 \cap \bar{E}_2] \tag{11.112}$$

or

$$Q_{sys} = P(\bar{E}_1)P(\bar{E}_2) \tag{11.113}$$

assuming that the components are independent. Therefore,

$$Q_{sys} = Q_1 \times Q_2 \tag{11.114}$$

or

$$Q_{sys} = \prod_{i=1}^{2} Q_i \tag{11.115}$$

or

$$Q_{sys} = \prod_{i=1}^{2} (1 - R_i) \tag{11.116}$$

where
  $\bar{E}_i$ is the event that component i fails
  Q_i is the unreliability of component i, $= P(\bar{E}_i)$
  Q_{sys} is the unreliability of system

Then, the system reliability can be expressed as

$$R_{sys} = 1 - Q_{sys} \tag{11.117}$$

or

$$R_{sys} = 1 - \prod_{i=1}^{2} (1 - R_i) \tag{11.118}$$

Therefore, the system reliability of a parallel system with n independent component can be expressed as

$$Q_{sys} = P[\bar{E}_1 \cap \bar{E}_2 \cap \cdots \cap \bar{E}_n] \tag{11.119}$$

or

$$Q_{sys} = P(\bar{E}_1) \cap P(\bar{E}_2) \cap \cdots \cap P(\bar{E}_n) \tag{11.120}$$

or

$$Q_{\text{sys}} = Q_1 \times Q_2 \times \cdots \times Q_n = \prod_{i=1}^{n} Q_i \tag{11.121}$$

Thus, the system reliability can be expressed as

$$
\begin{aligned}
R_{\text{sys}} &= 1 - Q_{\text{sys}} \\
&= 1 - \left[Q_1 \times Q_2 \times \cdots \times Q_n \right] \\
&= 1 - \left[(1 - R_1) \times (1 - R_2) \times \cdots \times (1 - R_n) \right] \\
&= 1 - \prod_{i=1}^{n} Q_i \\
&= 1 - \prod_{i=1}^{n} (1 - R_i)
\end{aligned}
\tag{11.122}
$$

Note that the unreliability of a partial system decreases as the number of parallel components increases. Alternatively, the reliability of a parallel system increases as the number of parallel components increases. Note that Equation 11.122 is applicable to both time-independent and time-dependent probabilities. In the case of time-dependent probabilities, if the component unreliability can be represented by an exponential distribution with a failure rate of λ_i, the system unreliability can be expressed as

$$Q_{\text{sys}}(t) = \prod_{i=1}^{n} \left(1 - e^{-\lambda_i t} \right) \tag{11.123}$$

11.8.3 COMBINED SERIES–PARALLEL SYSTEMS

Simple combinations of series–parallel systems can be analyzed by using a *reduction technique* (similar to the network reduction technique). The reduction technique is simply sequential reduction of the given mixed configuration by combining proper series and parallel branches until a single equivalent element is left. For example, assume that a mixed series–parallel system has m parallel branches and that each branch involved has n components connected in series. Such a system may also be called a *parallel–series system* and has a high-level redundancy. The equivalent reliability of the system can be given as

$$R_{\text{sys}} = 1 - (1 - R^n)^m \tag{11.124}$$

where
R_{sys} is the equivalent reliability of system
R^n is the equivalent reliability of branch
R is the reliability of component
n is the total number of components connected in series in branch
m is the total number of paths

On the other hand, assume that a mixed series–parallel system has n series units (or banks) with m parallel components in each. Such a system may also be called a *series–parallel system*. The equivalent reliability of the system can be given as

$$R_{sys} = [1 - (1 - R)^m]^n \qquad (11.125)$$

where
   $1 - (1 - R)^m$ is the equivalent reliability of parallel unit (bank)
   R is the reliability of component
   m is the total number of components in parallel unit
   n is the total number of units

Note that the series–parallel configuration gives higher system reliability than the parallel–series configuration.

11.9   SYSTEMS WITH REPAIRABLE COMPONENTS

The series and parallel systems presented in Section 11.8 are based on the assumption that the components of the systems are not repairable. However, a more realistic approach would be to assume that the components are independent and repairable.

11.9.1   REPAIRABLE COMPONENTS IN SERIES

Consider a series system with two components, as shown in Figure 11.20a, and assume that the components are independent and repairable. Thus, the *availability* or *the steady-state probability of success* (i.e., *operation*) of the system is

$$A_{sys} = A_1 \times A_2 \qquad (11.126)$$

where
   A_{sys} is the availability of system
   A_1 is the availability of component 1
   A_2 is the availability of component 2

Since

$$A_1 = \frac{\bar{m}_1}{\bar{m}_1 + \bar{r}_1} \qquad (11.127)$$

and

$$A_2 = \frac{\bar{m}_2}{\bar{m}_2 + \bar{r}_2} \qquad (11.128)$$

the availability of the system can be expressed as

$$A_{sys} = \frac{\bar{m}_1}{\bar{m}_1 + \bar{r}_1} \times \frac{\bar{m}_2}{\bar{m}_2 + \bar{r}_2} \qquad (11.129)$$

or

$$A_{sys} = \frac{\bar{m}_{sys}}{\bar{m}_{sys} + \bar{r}_{sys}} \tag{11.130}$$

where
$\bar{m}_1$ is the mean time to failure of component 1
$\bar{m}_2$ is the mean time to failure of component 2
$\bar{m}_{sys}$ is the mean time to failure of system
$\bar{r}_1$ is the MTTR of component 1
$\bar{r}_2$ is the MTTR of component 2
$\bar{r}_{sys}$ is the MTTR of system

The average frequency of the system failure is the sum of the average frequency of component 1 failing, given that component 2 is operable, plus the average frequency of component 2 failing while component 1 is operable. Thus, the average frequency of the system failure is

$$\bar{f}_{sys} = A_2 \bar{f}_1 + A_1 \bar{f}_2 \tag{11.131}$$

where
$\bar{f}_i$ is the average frequency of failure of component i
$\bar{A}_i$ is the availability of component i

However,

$$\bar{f}_i = \frac{1}{\bar{m}_i + \bar{r}_i} \tag{11.132}$$

and

$$A_i = \frac{\bar{m}_i}{\bar{m}_i + \bar{r}_i} \tag{11.133}$$

Therefore,

$$\bar{f}_{sys} = \frac{1}{\bar{m}_1 + \bar{r}_1} \times \frac{\bar{m}_2}{\bar{m}_2 + \bar{r}_2} + \frac{1}{\bar{m}_2 + \bar{r}_2} \times \frac{\bar{m}_1}{\bar{m}_1 + \bar{r}_1} \tag{11.134}$$

From Equation 11.130,

$$A_{sys} = \bar{m}_{sys} \bar{f}_{sys} \tag{11.135}$$

The mean time to failure for the series system with two components is

$$\bar{m}_{sys} = \frac{1}{1/\bar{m}_1 + 1/\bar{m}_2} \tag{11.136}$$

Similarly, the mean time to failure of a series with n components is

$$\bar{m}_{sys} = \frac{1}{1/\bar{m}_1 + 1/\bar{m}_2 + \cdots + 1/\bar{m}_n} \tag{11.137}$$

However, the reciprocal of the mean time to failure is defined as the failure rate. Thus, the failure rate for the two-component series system is

$$\lambda_{sys} = \lambda_1 + \lambda_2 \tag{11.138}$$

and for the n-component system, it is

$$\lambda_{sys} = \lambda_1 + \lambda_2 + \cdots + \lambda_n \tag{11.139}$$

Similarly, the MTTR for the two-component series system can be expressed as

$$\bar{r}_{sys} = \frac{\lambda_1 \bar{r}_1 + \lambda_2 \bar{r}_2 + (\lambda_1 \bar{r}_1)(\lambda_2 \bar{r}_2)}{\lambda_{sys}} \tag{11.140}$$

or approximately,

$$\bar{r}_{sys} \cong \frac{\lambda_1 \bar{r}_1 + \lambda_2 \bar{r}_2}{\lambda_{sys}} \tag{11.141}$$

Thus, for an n-component series system, it is

$$\bar{r}_{sys} \cong \frac{\lambda_1 \bar{r}_1 + \lambda_2 \bar{r}_2 + \cdots + \lambda_n \bar{r}_n}{\lambda_{sys}} \tag{11.142}$$

or

$$\bar{r}_{sys} \cong \frac{\lambda_1 \bar{r}_1 + \lambda_2 \bar{r}_2 + \cdots + \lambda_n \bar{r}_n}{\lambda_1 + \lambda_2 + \cdots + \lambda_n} \tag{11.143}$$

The average total outage duration of the series system can be found as

$$U_{sys} = \frac{\bar{r}_{sys}}{\bar{r}_{sys} + 1/\lambda_{sys}}$$

$$\cong \lambda_{sys} \bar{r}_{sys} \tag{11.144}$$

so that for the two-component series system, it is

$$U_{sys} \cong \lambda_1 \bar{r}_1 + \lambda_2 \bar{r}_2 \tag{11.145}$$

and for an n-component series system, it is

$$U_{sys} \cong \sum_{i=1}^{n} \lambda_i \bar{r}_i \tag{11.146}$$

11.9.2 Repairable Components in Parallel

Consider a parallel system with two components, as shown in Figure 11.20b, and assume that the components are independent and repairable. The unavailability or the steady-state probability of failure of the system is

$$U_{sys} = U_1 \times U_2 \tag{11.147}$$

where
  U_1 is the unavailability of component 1
  U_2 is the unavailability of component 2

However,

$$U_1 = 1 - A_1$$

$$= \frac{\lambda_1 \bar{r}_1}{1 + \lambda_1 \bar{r}_1} \tag{11.148}$$

and

$$U_2 = 1 - A_2$$

$$= \frac{\lambda_2 \bar{r}_2}{1 + \lambda_2 \bar{r}_2} \tag{11.149}$$

Therefore, the system unreliability is

$$U_{sys} = \frac{\lambda_1 \bar{r}_1}{1 + \lambda_1 \bar{r}_1} \times \frac{\lambda_2 \bar{r}_2}{1 + \lambda_2 \bar{r}_2} \tag{11.150}$$

or

$$U_{sys} \cong \lambda_1 \times \lambda_2 \times \bar{r}_1 \times \bar{r}_2 \tag{11.151}$$

which gives the approximate average total outage duration of the parallel system.
  The average frequency of the system failure can be expressed as

$$f_{sys} = U_2 \bar{f}_1 + U_1 \bar{f}_2 \tag{11.152}$$

where
  $\bar{f}_i$ is the average frequency of failure of component i
  U_i is the unavailability of component i

Since

$$\bar{f}_1 = \frac{\lambda_1}{1 + \lambda_1 \bar{r}_1} \tag{11.153}$$

and

$$\bar{f}_2 = \frac{\lambda_2}{1 + \lambda_2 \bar{r}_2} \tag{11.154}$$

the average frequency of the system failure is

$$\bar{f}_{\text{sys}} = \frac{\lambda_1 \lambda_2 \left(\bar{r}_1 + \bar{r}_2 \right)}{\left(1 + \lambda_1 \bar{r}_1 \right) \left(1 + \lambda_2 \bar{r}_2 \right)} \tag{11.155}$$

The system unavailability is

$$U_{\text{sys}} \triangleq \frac{\bar{r}_{\text{sys}}}{T_{\text{sys}}} \tag{11.156}$$

or

$$U_{\text{sys}} = \bar{r}_{\text{sys}} \times \bar{f}_{\text{sys}} \tag{11.157}$$

so that

$$\bar{r}_{\text{sys}} = \frac{U_{\text{sys}}}{\bar{f}_{\text{sys}}} \tag{11.158}$$

Then, substituting Equations 11.150 and 11.155 into Equation 11.158, the *average repair time* (or *downtime*) of the two-component parallel system can be found as

$$\bar{r}_{\text{sys}} = \frac{\bar{r}_1 \times \bar{r}_2}{\bar{r}_1 + \bar{r}_2} \tag{11.159}$$

or

$$\frac{1}{\bar{r}_{\text{sys}}} = \frac{1}{\bar{r}_1} + \frac{1}{\bar{r}_2} \tag{11.160}$$

Similarly, the system unavailability can be given as

$$U_{\text{sys}} \triangleq \frac{\bar{r}_{\text{sys}}}{\bar{r}_{\text{sys}} + \bar{m}_{\text{sys}}} \tag{11.161}$$

then

$$\bar{m}_{\text{sys}} = \frac{\bar{r}_{\text{sys}} \left(1 - U_{\text{sys}} \right)}{U_{\text{sys}}} \tag{11.162}$$

so that the *average time to failure* (or *operation time* or *uptime*) of the parallel system can be found as

$$\bar{m}_{\text{sys}} = \frac{1 + \lambda_1 \bar{r}_1 + \lambda_2 \bar{r}_2}{\lambda_1 \lambda_2 \left(\bar{r}_1 + \bar{r}_2 \right)} \tag{11.163}$$

Since the failure rate of the parallel system is

$$\lambda_{\text{sys}} \triangleq \frac{1}{\bar{m}_{\text{sys}}} \tag{11.164}$$

then

$$\lambda_{\text{sys}} = \frac{\lambda_1 \lambda_2 \left(\bar{r}_1 + \bar{r}_2 \right)}{1 + \lambda_1 \bar{r}_1 + \lambda_2 \bar{r}_2} \tag{11.165}$$

Contrary to the series system, the equations derived for the two-component parallel system cannot be easily extended to a general *n*-component system. In certain parallel systems, it is possible to combine two components at a time. However, it is more recommendable to calculate the probabilities of the system by using the binomial distribution or conditional probabilities.

11.10 RELIABILITY EVALUATION OF COMPLEX SYSTEMS

Many systems cannot be classified as simple series–parallel structures. These non-series–parallel structures exhibit complex system characteristics. They can be evaluated by using the conditional probability method and minimal-cut-set method.

11.10.1 CONDITIONAL PROBABILITY METHOD

In this method [8,9], a proper component of the given complex system (say, C_i) is first short-circuited (i.e., *substituted by a component that never fails*) and then open-circuited (i.e., *assumed to be a failure*). The resulting series–parallel subsystems are reunited based on the conditional probability concept discussed in Section 11.5.2. Therefore, the probability of system success (i.e., *the system reliability*) can be expressed as

$$R_{\text{sys}} = P(\text{system operates} \mid C_i \text{ operates})P(C_i)$$
$$+ P(\text{system operates} \mid C_i \text{ fails})P(C_i) \tag{11.166}$$

Similarly, the probability of system failure (i.e., *system unreliability*) can be expressed as

$$Q_{\text{sys}} = P(\text{system fails} \mid C_i \text{ operates})P(C_i)$$
$$+ P(\text{system fails} \mid C_i \text{ fails})P(C_i) \tag{11.167}$$

As an example, consider the bridge-type network shown in Figure 11.21a. Here, the system success dictates that at least one of the paths (made up of components C_1C_3, C_2C_4, $C_1C_5C_4$, and $C_2C_5C_3$) is good, and therefore, the system operates. Thus, the best choice for component C_i is component 5 (i.e., C_5). Figure 11.21b and c show the modified networks with component 5 short-circuited and open-circuited, respectively. Therefore, from Equation 11.162, the system reliability can be expressed as

$$R_{\text{sys}} = P(\text{system operates } C_5 \text{ operates})P(C_5)$$
$$+ P(\text{system operates} \mid C_5 \text{ fails})P(C_5) \tag{11.168}$$

or, alternatively,

$$R_{\text{sys}} = R_{\text{sys}}(\text{if } C_5 \text{ operates})R_5 + R_{\text{sys}}(\text{if } C_5 \text{ fails})Q_5$$

where
$R_{\text{sys}}(\text{if } C_5 \text{ operates}) = (1 - Q_1Q_2)(1 - Q_3Q_4)$
$R_{\text{sys}}(\text{if } C_5 \text{ fails}) = 1 - (1 - R_1R_3)(1 - R_2R_4)$

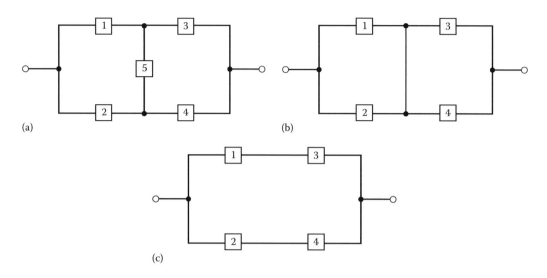

FIGURE 11.21 Reliability block diagrams: (a) bridge-type network, (b) modified network with component 5 shorted, and (c) modified network with component 5 opened.

Therefore,

$$R_{sys} = [(1 - Q_1Q_2)(1 - Q_3Q_4)]R_5 + [1 - (1 - R_1R_3)(1 - R_2R_4)]Q_5 \qquad (11.169)$$

If the components are identical, the system reliability becomes

$$R_{sys} = [1 - 2Q^2 + Q^4]R + [1 - (1 - 2R^2 + R^4)]Q$$
$$= [1 - 2(1 - R)^2 + (1 - R)^4]R + [1 - (1 - 2R^2 + R^4)](1 - R)$$
$$= 2R^2 + 2R^3 - 5R^4 + 2R^5 \qquad (11.170)$$

Similarly, the system unreliability can be calculated from Equation 11.167.

11.10.2 MINIMAL-CUT-SET METHOD

A *tie set* is a set of edges (representing components) that constitute a path from input to output. If the components operate, the system operates properly. If no node is passed through more than once when tracing the tie set, such a tie set is called the *minimal tie set*. In other words, if any one of the components of a given minimal tie set is removed, the remaining set is no longer a tie set. A cut set is a set of edges that, when removed, divides the block diagram into the input and output subblocks. That is, if the components of a given cut set fail, the system fails. If a given cut set cannot be divided into a subset that can be another cut set, it is called the *minimal cut set*. Hence, if all components of a minimal cut set fail, the system fails.

As an example, consider the bridge-type network given in Figure 11.22a. The minimal tie sets are made up of components C_1C_3, C_2C_4, $C_1C_5C_4$, and $C_2C_5C_3$, as shown in Figure 11.22b. Therefore, it can be shown that

$$S = (C_1 \cap C_3) \cup (C_2 \cap C_4) \cup (C_1 \cap C_5 \cap C_4) \cup (C_2 \cap C_5 \cap C_3) \qquad (11.171)$$

Similarly, the minimal cut sets are made up of components C_1C_2, C_3C_4, $C_1C_5C_4$, and $C_2C_5C_3$, as shown Figure 11.22c. Thus, it can be expressed that

$$\bar{S} = (\bar{C}_1 \cap \bar{C}_2) \cup (\bar{C}_3 \cap \bar{C}_4) \cup (\bar{C}_1 \cap \bar{C}_5 \cap \bar{C}_4) \cup (\bar{C}_2 \cap \bar{C}_5 \cap \bar{C}_3) \qquad (11.172)$$

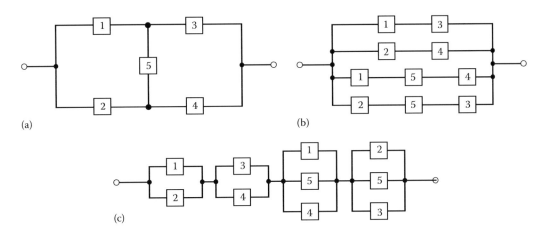

FIGURE 11.22 Reliability block diagrams showing bridge arrangement and its equivalents: (a) bridge-type network, (b) equivalent minimal-tie diagram, and (c) equivalent minimal-cut diagram.

As illustrated in Figure 11.22, a given nonseries–parallel structures' logic diagram can be converted to series–parallel diagrams using either minimal-tie-set or minimal-cut-set methods [9–12].

Using the minimum-cut-set method, the unreliability of the system can be expressed as

$$Q_{sys} = P(E_1 \cup E_2 \cup E_3 \cup E_4)$$
$$= P(E_1) + P(E_2) + P(E_3) + P(E_4) - P(E_1 \cap E_2) - P(E_1 \cap E_3)$$
$$- P(E_1 \cap E_4)P(E_2 \cap E_3) - P(E_2 \cap E_4) - P(E_3 \cap E_4)$$
$$+ P(E_1 \cap E_2 \cap E_3) + P(E_1 \cap E_2 \cap E_4) + P(E_1 \cap E_3 \cap E_4)$$
$$+ P(E_2 \cap E_3 \cap E_4) - P(E_1 \cap E_2 \cap E_3 \cap E_4) \tag{11.173}$$

where
$$P(E_1) = \bar{C}_1 \cap \bar{C}_2$$
$$P(E_2) = \bar{C}_3 \cap \bar{C}_4$$
$$P(E_3) = \bar{C}_1 \cap \bar{C}_5 \cap \bar{C}_4$$
$$P(E_4) = C_2 \cap \bar{C}_5 \cap \bar{C}_3$$

Note that Equation 11.173 is an exact one. However, usually, an approximation is made, and the system unreliability can be expressed as

$$Q_{sys} \cong P(E_1) + P(E_2) + P(E_3) + P(E_4) \tag{11.174}$$

which sets the upper limit to system unreliability. It can be reexpressed as

$$Q_{sys} \cong Q_1 Q_2 + Q_3 Q_4 + Q_1 Q_5 Q_4 + Q_2 Q_5 Q_3 \tag{11.175}$$

If the components are identical, the system unreliability becomes

$$Q_{sys} = 2Q^2 + 2Q_3^2 \tag{11.176}$$

11.11 MARKOV PROCESSES

A *stochastic process* can be defined as a family of random variables, $\{X(t), t \in T\}$, defined over some index set or parameter space T. For each t contained in the index set T, $X(t)$ is a random variable. The T is sometimes also defined as the *time range*, and $X(t)$ represents the observation at time t. The stochastic process is called a *discrete-parameter* or *continuous-parameter process* based on the nature of the time range. For example, if T is an infinite sequence, that is, $T = \{0, \pm 1, \pm 2, \ldots\}$ or $T = (0, 1, 2, \ldots)$, the stochastic process $\{X(t), t \in T\}$ is said to be a *discrete-parameter process* defined on the index set T. On the other hand, if T is an interval or algebraic combination of intervals, that is, $T = \{t: -\infty < T < +\infty\}$ or $T = (t: 0 \le t < +\infty\}$, the stochastic process $\{X(t), t \in T)$ is a continuous-parameter process defined on the index set T.

In reliability studies, the variable t denotes time, and $X(t)$ represents the state of the system at time t. The states at a given time t_n actually represent the mutually exclusive outcomes of the system at that time (i.e., operating, failed, in maintenance). All the possible states of a system are defined as the *state space*. The state space and the transitions between the states are illustrated in a state space diagram.

A stochastic process for which the occurrence of a future state depends only on the immediately prior state is defined as the *Markov process*. The Markovian process is characterized by a lack of memory. A discrete-parameter stochastic process, $\{X(t); t = 0, 1, 2\ldots\}$, or a continuous-parameter stochastic process, $\{X(t); t \ge 0\}$, is a Markov process if it has the following *Markovian property*:

$$P\{X(t_n) \le x_n | X(t_1) = x_1, \ldots, X(t_{n-1}) = x_{n-1}\}$$

$$= P\{X(t_n) \le x_n | X(T_n - 1) = x_n - 1\} \tag{11.177}$$

for any set of n time points $t_1 < t_2 \cdots < t_n$ in the index set of the process and any real numbers $x_1, x_2, \ldots, x_n$. In nonmathematical language, one can say that, given the *present* condition of the process, the *future* is independent of the *past*. The probability of

$$P_{x_{n-1}, x_n} = P\left\{X(t_n) = x_n | X(t_{n-1}) = x_{n-1}\right\} \tag{11.178}$$

is called the *transition probability* and represents the *conditional probability* of the system being in x_n at t_n, given it was x_{n-1} at t_{n-1}. It is also defined as a *one-step* transition probability as it represents the system between t_{n-1} and t_n.

A *Markov chain* can be defined by a sequence of discrete-valued random variables $\{X(t_n)\}$, where t_n is discrete valued or continuous. It is possible to define the Markov chain as the *Markov process* with a discrete state space. Define

$$p_{ij} = P\left\{X(t_n) = j | X(t_{n-1}) = i\right\} \tag{11.179}$$

as the *one-step transition probability* of going from state i at t_{n-1} to state j at t_n and assume that these probabilities do not change over time. The term used to describe this assumption is *stationarity*; if the transition probability depends only on the time difference, the Markov chain is defined to be *stationary in time*. A Markov chain is completely defined by its transition probabilities of going from state i to state j, given in matrix form as

$$[P] = \begin{bmatrix} p_{00} & p_{01} & p_{02} & \cdots & p_{0n} \\ p_{10} & p_{01} & p_{02} & \cdots & p_{0n} \\ p_{20} & p_{01} & p_{02} & \cdots & p_{0n} \\ p_{30} & p_{01} & p_{02} & \cdots & p_{0n} \\ \vdots & \vdots & \vdots & \vdots & \vdots \\ p_{n0} & p_{01} & p_{02} & \cdots & p_{0n} \end{bmatrix} \tag{11.180}$$

The matrix P is called a *one-step transition matrix* (or *stochastic matrix*) since all the transition probabilities p_{ij}'s are fixed and independent of time. The matrix P is also called just the *transition matrix* when there is no possibility of confusion. Since the p_{ij}'s are conditional, they must satisfy the conditions

$$\sum_{j}^{n} p_{ij} = 1 \quad \forall_{i} \tag{11.181}$$

and

$$p_{ij} \geq 0 \quad \forall_{ij} \tag{11.182}$$

where $i = 0, 1, 2, ..., n, j = 0, 1, 2, ..., n$. If the number of transitions (or states) are not too large, the information in a given transition matrix P can be represented by a transition diagram. For example, a given system has two states: (1) state 1, which represents the *system being up*, and (2) state 2, which represents the *system being down*. Then the associated transition probabilities can be defined as

p_{11} = probability of being in state 1 at time t given that it was in state 1 at time zero
p_{12} = probability of being in state 2 at time t given that it was in state 1 at time zero
p_{21} = probability of being in state 1 at time t given that it was in state 2 at time zero
p_{22} = probability of being in state 2 at time t given that it was in state 2 at time zero

Hence, the transition matrix can be expressed as

$$\begin{bmatrix} P \end{bmatrix} = \begin{bmatrix} p_{11} & p_{12} \\ p_{21} & p_{22} \end{bmatrix}$$

and its transition diagram can be drawn as in Figure 11.23.

By definition, the one-step transition probabilities are

$$p_{ij} = p_{ij}^{(1)} = P\{X(t_1) = j | X(t_0) = i\} \tag{11.183}$$

Therefore, the n-step transition probabilities can be defined by induction as

$$p_{ij}^{(n)} = P\{X(t_n) = j | X(t_0) = i\} \tag{11.184}$$

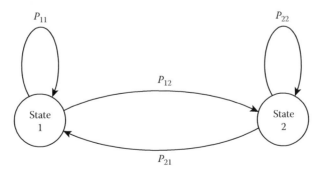

FIGURE 11.23   Transition diagram for two-state system.

In other words, $p_{ij}^{(n)}$ is the probability (*absolute probability*) that the process is in state j at time t_n given that it was in state i at time t_0. It can be observed from this definition that $p_{ij}^{(0)}$ must be 1 if $i = j$ and 0 otherwise.

The Chapman–Kolmogorov equations provide a method for determining these n-step transition probabilities. In general form, these equations are given as

$$p_{ij}^{(n)} = \sum_k P_{ik}^{(n-m)} p_{kj}^m \quad \forall_{ij} \tag{11.185}$$

for any m between zero and n. Note that this equation can be represented in matrix form by

$$P^{(n)} = P^{(n-m)} P^{(m)} \tag{11.186}$$

The elements of a higher-order transition matrix $\left(\text{e.g.,} \left\| p_{ij}^{(n)} \right\| \right)$ can be obtained directly by matrix multiplication. Hence,

$$\left\| p_{ij}^{(n)} \right\| = P^{(n-m)} P^{(m)} = P^{(n)} = P^n \tag{11.187}$$

Note that a special case of Equation 11.185 is

$$p_{ij}^{(n)} = \sum_k P_{ik}^{(n-1)} p_{kj} \quad \forall_{ij} \tag{11.188}$$

and therefore, the special cases of Equations 11.186 and 11.187 are

$$P^{(n)} = P^{(n-1)} P \tag{11.189}$$

and

$$\left\| p_{ij}^{(n)} \right\| = P^{(n-1)} P = P^{(n)} = P^n \tag{11.190}$$

respectively.

The unconditional probabilities such as

$$p_{ij}^n = P\left\{ X(t_n) = j \right\} \tag{11.191}$$

are called the *absolute probabilities* or *state probabilities*. In order to determine the state probabilities, the initial conditions must be known. Therefore,

$$
\begin{aligned}
p_j^{(n)} &= P\left\{ X(T_n) = j \right\} \\
&= P \sum_i \{ X(t_n) = j \,|\, X(t_0) = i \} P\{ X(t_0) = i \} \\
&= \sum_i P_i^{(0)} P_{ij}^{(n)}
\end{aligned}
\tag{11.192}
$$

Note that Equation 11.192 can be represented in matrix form by

$$p^{(n)} = p^{(0)}p^{(n)} \tag{11.193}$$

where
$p(n)$ is the vector of state probabilities at time t_0
$p(0)$ is the vector of initial state probabilities at time t_0
$p(n)$ is the n-step transition matrix

The state probabilities or absolute probabilities are defined in vector form as

$$p^{(n)} = \begin{bmatrix} p_1^{(n)} & p_2^{(n)} & p_3^{(n)} & \cdots & p_k^{(n)} \end{bmatrix} \tag{11.194}$$

and

$$p^{(0)} = \begin{bmatrix} p_1^{(0)} & p_2^{(0)} & p_3^{(0)} & \cdots & p_k^{(0)} \end{bmatrix} \tag{11.195}$$

The long-run absolute probabilities are independent of the initial state probabilities, that is, $p^{(0)}$. The resulting probabilities are called the *steady-state probabilities* and are defined as the set of π_i, where

$$\pi_j = \lim_{n \to \infty} p^{(n)} = \lim_{n \to \infty} P\{X(t_n) = j\} \tag{11.196}$$

In general, the initial state tends to be less important to the n-step transition probability as n increases, such that

$$\lim_{n \to \infty} P\{X(t_n) = j \mid X(t_0) = i\} = \lim_{n \to \infty} P\{X(t_n) = j\} = \Pi_i \tag{11.197}$$

so that one can get unconditional steady-state probability distribution from the n-step transition probabilities by taking n to infinity without taking the initial states into account.

Therefore,

$$p^{(n)} = p^{(n-1)}P \tag{11.198}$$

or

$$\lim_{n \to \infty} p^{(n)} = \lim_{n \to \infty} p^{(n-1)}P \tag{11.199}$$

and thus,

$$[\Pi] = [\Pi][P] \tag{11.200}$$

where

$$[\Pi] = \begin{bmatrix} \Pi_1 & \Pi_2 & \Pi_3 & \cdots & \Pi_k \\ \Pi_1 & \Pi_2 & \Pi_3 & \cdots & \Pi_k \\ \Pi_1 & \Pi_2 & \Pi_3 & \cdots & \Pi_k \\ \cdot & \cdot & \cdot & & \cdot \\ \cdot & \cdot & \cdot & & \cdot \\ \cdot & \cdot & \cdot & & \cdot \\ \Pi_1 & \Pi_2 & \Pi_3 & \cdots & \Pi_k \end{bmatrix} \qquad (11.201)$$

Note that the matrix Π has identical rows so that each row is a row vector of

$$[\Pi] = \begin{bmatrix} \Pi_1 & \Pi_2 & \Pi_3 & \cdots & \Pi_k \end{bmatrix} \qquad (11.202)$$

Since the transpose of a row vector Π is a column vector Π^t, Equation 11.200 can also be expressed as

$$\Pi^t = p^{(t)} \Pi^{(t)} \qquad (11.203)$$

which is a set of linear equations.

In order to be able to solve equation sets (11.200) or (11.203) for individual Π_i's, one additional equation is required. This equation is called the *normalizing equation* and can be expressed as

$$\sum_{\text{all } i} \Pi_i = 1 \qquad (11.204)$$

11.12 TRANSMISSION SYSTEM RELIABILITY METHODS

In recent years, transmission system reliability has gained considerable attention. Numerous methods have been developed for the quantitative evaluation of transmission system reliability. Some of the developed methods are included in this section.

11.12.1 AVERAGE INTERRUPTION RATE METHOD

This method has been introduced by Todd [13] in his paper published in 1964. The method determines the probability of forced outage of a specified minimum duration to calculate the customer interruption rate and the number of interruptions expected to exceed the given duration. Here, the *forced outage rate** is defined as the ratio of the total component outage time to the total component exposure time. In other words, the forced outage rate p is the probability of component outage presence and can be calculated from

$$p = \frac{\text{Sum of days on which outage of specified minimum duration occurred}}{\text{Sum of unit days}} \qquad (11.205)$$

The method is simple and can easily be applied to systems with series–parallel connected components. It is based on the assumption of complete redundancy in parallel components and the continuity of supply to the load points. The expected number of days in a year that the specified outage for

---

* The terms *outage rate* and *failure rate* mean the very same thing. Here, they are used interchangeably.

a given load point will happen is called the *average annual customer interruption rate* (AACIR). The systems that have a combination of series and parallel configurations can be included using the network reduction method.

Another alternative is to use the minimal-cut-set procedure. Todd [13] gives a practical example for the application of the average interruption rate method. It is usually assumed that all outages occur simultaneously.

11.12.2 FREQUENCY AND DURATION METHOD

In general, the failure rate of a given transmission line is a function of a fluctuating environment characterized by normal and severe (e.g., storms, ice, or sleet) weather conditions. It is possible that the failure rate during the severe weather conditions may become several orders of magnitude larger than the rate during the normal weather conditions. Also, it is possible for redundant systems to have multiple failures during the severe weather conditions. This phenomenon of overlapping forced outages during the periods of high environmental stress is known as *failure bunching*.

A method has been introduced by Gaver et al. [14] in their classical paper to take into account the changing environmental conditions. The proposed two-state weather model assumes that the weather fluctuates between normal and stormy periods. It again deals with series and parallel systems, as the first method. The method is based on the assumption that the component failure times, repair times, storm durations, and normal weather durations can be represented by exponential probability distributions. It is also based on the assumption of complete redundancy in parallel components and the continuity of supply to the load points. Unfortunately, the method results in an approximation as the number of parallel elements that are combined increases. In order to increase the computational efficiency of the method, a computer program has been developed [15]. The method gives two separate sets of equations for series and parallel systems. The parameters used are

λ_i = normal weather component failure rate of component i in failures per year of normal weather
λ'_i = stormy weather component failure rate of component i in failures per year of stormy weather
λ''_i = component maintenance outage rate of component i in outages per year
r_i = expected repair time for all forced outages of component i in years
r''_i = component maintenance repair rate of component i (i.e., expected downtime for maintenance outages) in years
N = expected duration of normal weather period in years
S = expected duration of stormy weather period in years

11.12.2.1 Series Systems

The *approximate* overall (normal and stormy weather) annual forced outage rate λ_f of component i can be expressed as

$$\lambda_{f,i} = \frac{N}{N+S}\lambda_i + \frac{S}{N+S}\lambda'_i \text{ outages/year} \tag{11.206}$$

The *overall* annual forced outage rate (i.e., failure rate) for an *n*-component series system is

$$\lambda_{f,e} = \sum_{i=1}^{n}\lambda_{f,i} \text{ outages/year} \tag{11.207}$$

Similarly, the *annual maintenance outage rate* for an *n*-component series system can be given as

$$\lambda''_e = \sum_{i=1}^{n}\lambda''_i \text{ outages/year} \tag{11.208}$$

If the series system is in parallel with other components, it is required to calculate the normal and stormy weather failure rates for the *equivalent component e* as

$$\lambda_e = \sum_{i=1}^{n} \lambda_i \text{ outages/year of normal weather} \tag{11.209}$$

and

$$\lambda'_e = \sum_{i=1}^{n} \lambda'_i \text{ outages/year of stormy weather} \tag{11.210}$$

Expected outage duration *due to forced outage* can be calculated from

$$r_{f,e} = \frac{\sum_{i=1}^{n} \lambda_{f,i} \times r_i}{\lambda_{f,e}} \text{ year} \tag{11.211}$$

Similarly, the expected outage duration *due to maintenance outages* can be calculated from

$$r''_{f,e} = \frac{\sum_{i=1}^{n} \lambda''_{f,i} \times r''_i}{\lambda''_{f,e}} \text{ year} \tag{11.212}$$

Therefore, the *total annual outage rate* can be expressed as

$$\lambda_{\text{sys}} = \lambda_{f,e} + \lambda''_e \text{ outages/year} \tag{11.213}$$

The *expected outage duration* (i.e., *restoration time*) can be expressed as

$$r_{\text{sys}} = \frac{\lambda_{f,e} \times r_{f,e} + \lambda''_e \times r''_e}{\lambda_{\text{sys}}} \text{ year} \tag{11.214}$$

or

$$r_{\text{sys}} = \frac{\lambda_{f,e} \times r_{f,e} + \lambda''_e \times r''_e}{\lambda_{\text{sys}}} \times 8760 \text{ year} \tag{11.215}$$

The total outage time per year can be expressed as

$$U_{\text{sys}} = \frac{r_{\text{sys}}}{r_{\text{sys}} + 1/\lambda_{\text{sys}}} \text{ year/year} \tag{11.216}$$

or

$$U_{\text{sys}} \cong A_{\text{sys}} \times r_{\text{sys}} \text{ year/year} \tag{11.217}$$

or

$$U_{sys} \cong A_{sys} \times r_{sys} \times 8760 \text{ h/year} \tag{11.218}$$

Note that Gaver et al. [14] included maintenance outages as a random parameter as given in the previous equations. However, Billinton [8] suggested to exclude them since it is questionable whether maintenance can be described as a random outage behavior.

11.12.2.2 Parallel Systems

In this method, the components are considered in pairs (two at a time) and are reduced to an equivalent component for some further combination based on the network reduction technique. However, unfortunately, this procedure increases the approximation involved in calculations as the number of parallel elements increases. Therefore, the approximate overall annual failure rate due to normal and stormy weather forced outages for a two-component parallel system can be expressed as

$$\lambda_{sys} = \frac{N}{N+S} \left[\lambda_1 \lambda_2 (r_1 + r_2) + \frac{S}{N} (\lambda_1 \lambda_2' r_1 + \lambda_2 \lambda_1' r_2) \right]$$

$$+ \frac{S}{N+S} \left[\lambda_1' \lambda_2 r_1 + \lambda_2' \lambda_1 r_2 + 2S\lambda_1' \lambda_2' \right] \text{ outages/year} \tag{11.219}$$

In the event that maintenance is to be included in the evaluation, a maintenance failure rate component, given by Equation 11.220, should be added to the right side of Equation 11.219. Here, it is assumed that the maintenance outages occur at random only during normal weather conditions. The maintenance failure rate can be calculated from

$$\lambda_e'' = \lambda_1'' \lambda_2 r_1'' + \lambda_2'' \lambda_1 r_2'' \text{ outages/year} \tag{11.220}$$

where
λ_i'' is the component maintenance outage rate in outages per year
r_i'' is the component maintenance repair rate in years

In the event that the parallel system operates in parallel with other components, normal and stormy weather outage rates and the expected outage duration for the equivalent component representing the parallel system for further combinations can be expressed as

$$\lambda_e = \lambda_1 \lambda_2 (r_1 + r_2) + \frac{S}{N} (\lambda_1' \lambda_2 r_1 + \lambda_1' \lambda_1 r_2) \text{ outages/year of normal weather} \tag{11.221}$$

$$\lambda_e' = \lambda_1 \lambda_2' r_1 + \lambda_2 \lambda_1' r_2 + 2S\lambda_1' \lambda_2' \text{ outages/year of stormy weather} \tag{11.222}$$

$$r_e = \frac{r_1 r_2}{r_1 + r_2} \text{ year} \tag{11.223}$$

Similarly, the equivalent failure rate of a two-component parallel system as a result of component forced-outage overlapping-component maintenance outage periods can be expressed as

$$\lambda_{m,e}'' = \lambda_1'' \lambda_2 r_1'' + \lambda_2'' \lambda_1 r_2'' \text{ outages/year} \tag{11.224}$$

Therefore, the expected downtime of the two-component system due to component forced-outages overlapping-component maintenance outage can be expressed as

$$r''_{m,e} = \frac{\lambda''_1 \lambda_2 r''_1}{\lambda''_1 \lambda_2 r''_1 + \lambda''_2 \lambda_1 r''_2} \times \frac{r_2 \times r''_1}{r_2 + r''_1} + \frac{\lambda''_2 \lambda_1 r''_2}{\lambda''_1 \lambda_2 r''_1 + \lambda''_2 \lambda_1 r''_2} \times \frac{r_1 \times r''_2}{r_1 + r''_2} \text{ year} \qquad (11.225)$$

or substituting Equation 6.224 into Equation 6.225,

$$r''_{m,e} = \frac{\lambda''_1 \lambda_2 r''_1}{\lambda''_{m,e}} \times \frac{r_2 \times r''_1}{r_2 + r''_1} + \frac{\lambda''_2 \lambda_1 r''_2}{\lambda''_{m,e}} \times \frac{r_1 \times r''_2}{r_1 + r''_2} \text{ year} \qquad (11.226)$$

Note that in the event that the stormy–normal weather approach cannot be applied and overall annual failure rates are used, the expected number of failures for a parallel system made up of two components can be expressed as [8]

$$\lambda_{f,e} = \lambda_1 \lambda_2 (r_1 + r_2) \text{ outages/year} \qquad (11.227)$$

The approximate value of the expected downtime duration can be expressed as

$$U_{\text{sys}} \cong \lambda_{f,e} \times r_T \text{ year/year} \qquad (11.228)$$

where r_T is the expected downtime duration due to overlapping forced outages

$$= \frac{r_1 \times r_2}{r_1 + r_2} \qquad (11.229)$$

Therefore, substituting Equation 11.229 into Equation 11.228, the expected downtime duration can be reexpressed as

$$U_{\text{sys}} \cong \frac{r_1 \times r_2}{r_1 + r_2} \times \lambda_{f,e} \text{ year/year} \qquad (11.230)$$

The previous equations give the failure rates due to permanent (or sustained) outages. Billinton and Grover [16] derived equations to take into account the temporary outages. For example, the equivalent temporary failure rate of a two-component parallel system due to component temporary outages overlapping-component permanent outages can be expressed as

$$\lambda_{t,e} = \lambda_{1T} \lambda_2 r_2 + \lambda_{2T} \lambda_1 r_1 \text{ outages/year} \qquad (11.231)$$

where λ_{iT} is the temporary outage rate of component i in outages per year.

In the event that the two components are identical, the system temporary outage rate can be expressed as

$$\lambda_{t,e} = 2\lambda_T \lambda r \text{ outages/year} \qquad (11.232)$$

Similarly, the equivalent temporary failure rate of a two-component parallel system due to component temporary outages overlapping-component maintenance outages can be expressed as

$$\lambda''_{t,e} = \lambda_{1T} \lambda''_2 r''_2 + \lambda_{2T} \lambda''_1 r''_1 \text{ outages/year} \qquad (11.233)$$

If the two components are identical,

$$\lambda''_{t,e} = 2\lambda_T \lambda'' r'' \text{ outages/year} \tag{11.234}$$

Therefore, the total temporary outage rate due to component temporary outages overlapping-component permanent and maintenance outage can be given as

$$\lambda_{T,e} = \lambda_{t,e} + \lambda''_{t,e} \text{ outages/year} \tag{11.235}$$

The previous equivalent temporary outage equations can be modified to take into account the failure bunching due to adverse weather [16].

11.12.3 MARKOV APPLICATION METHOD

In 1964, Desieno and Stine [17] have briefly introduced the application of Markov processes. They have mentioned the fact that within the limits of the assumptions made with regard to distributions involved, the Markov approach is theoretically the most accurate approach. Billinton and Bollinger [18] illustrated the application of the Markov method to series–parallel components operating in the two-state fluctuating weather environment. They have effectively demonstrated that the transitional probability matrix has all the probabilities of a transition from any one state to any of the other states. For example, in order to determine the limiting probabilities, the number of simultaneous equations that are necessary to be solved is 2×2^n for an n-component system in a two-state fluctuating weather environment. This number increases rapidly as the number of components increase.

In this method, it is assumed that the weather durations are distributed exponentially and that the system involved is operating in a two-state fluctuating weather environment (i.e., normal and stormy weather). In addition, the system can be represented as being either in the *up state* (the *system is operating*) or in the *down state* (the *system has failed*). Therefore, a state space diagram can be developed for each component, as shown in Figure 11.24. Thus, the required differential equations can be written directly from the state space diagram and can be expressed in matrix form as

$$\begin{bmatrix} P'_0(t) \\ P'_1(t) \\ P'_2(t) \\ P'_3(t) \end{bmatrix} = \begin{bmatrix} -(\lambda+n) & m & \mu & 0 \\ n & -(m+\lambda') & 0 & \mu' \\ \lambda & 0 & -(\mu+n) & m \\ 0 & \lambda' & n & -(\mu'+m) \end{bmatrix} \begin{bmatrix} P_0(t) \\ P_1(t) \\ P_2(t) \\ P_3(t) \end{bmatrix} \tag{11.236}$$

where
   λ is the normal weather failure rate of component
   μ is the normal weather repair rate of component
   λ' is the stormy weather failure rate of component
   μ' is the stormy weather repair rate of component

Also,

$$n = \frac{1}{N}$$

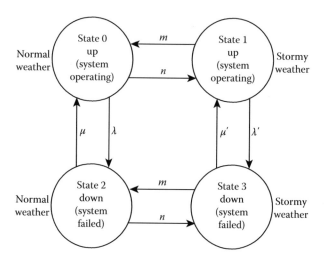

FIGURE 11.24 State space diagram for single component operating in two-weather environment.

and

$$m = \frac{1}{S}$$

where

N is the expected duration of normal weather period

S is the expected duration of stormy weather period

The long-term or steady-state probabilities of being in various states can be found by equating the differential matrix to zero so that

$$-(\lambda + n)P_0 + mP_1 + \mu P_2 = 0 \tag{11.237}$$

$$nP_0 - (m + \lambda') P_1 + \mu' P_3 = 0 \tag{11.238}$$

$$\lambda P_0 - (\mu + n)P_2 + mP_3 = 0 \tag{11.239}$$

$$\lambda' P_1 + nP_2 - (\mu' + m)P_3 = 0 \tag{11.240}$$

Also, of course, the sum of the steady-state probabilities of being in different states is equal to 1, that is,

$$P_0 + P_1 + P_2 + P_3 = 0 \tag{11.241}$$

From Equations 11.237 through 11.241, the steady-state probabilities can be determined. For the given system, the probability of the system being in the up state is the sum of probabilities of being in the states 0 and 1. Therefore,

$$P(\text{up}) = P_0 + P_1 \tag{11.242}$$

Similarly, the probability of the system being in the down state can be found as

$$P(\text{down}) = P_2 + P_3 \tag{11.243}$$

Based on the assumptions that the repair rate is independent of environment (i.e., $\mu = \mu'$), the probabilities of the system being in the up state and the down state can be expressed as [8]

$$P(\text{up}) = \frac{\mu}{m+n} \times \frac{(m+n)^2 + m(\mu + \lambda') + n(\mu + \lambda)}{(\mu + \lambda)(\mu + \lambda') + m(\mu + \lambda) + n(\mu + \lambda')} \qquad (11.244)$$

and

$$P(\text{down}) = \frac{1}{m+n} \times \frac{n\lambda'(n + \mu) + m\lambda(m + \mu) + nm(\lambda + \lambda') + \lambda\lambda'(m+n)}{(\mu + \lambda)(\mu + \lambda') + m(\mu + \lambda) + n(\mu + \lambda')} \qquad (11.245)$$

In the event that no repairs are done during the stormy weather (i.e., $\mu' = 0$), then, for example, the probability of being in the down state becomes

$$P(\text{down}) = \frac{1}{m+n} \times \frac{m(\lambda m + \lambda' n) + n(\lambda' \mu + \lambda m + \lambda' n)}{m + n(\mu + \lambda)(\mu + \lambda') + m(\mu + \lambda) + n(\mu + \lambda')} \qquad (11.246)$$

Note that the frequency of being in a given state can be found by multiplying the steady-state probability of being in that state by the rate of departure from that state. The average duration of a state can be found from the reciprocal of the rate of departure from that state [19].

In the event that only normal weather needs to be considered, then $\lambda = 0$, $m = 1$, and $n = 0$. Therefore,

$$P(\text{up}) = \frac{\mu}{\lambda + \mu} \qquad (11.247)$$

and

$$P(\text{down}) = \frac{\lambda}{\lambda + \mu} \qquad (11.248)$$

which are previously given in Equations 11.88 and 11.92, respectively.

Since in this case the absorbing states are states 2 and 3, Billinton [8] shows that the mean time to failure can be expressed as

$$\text{MTTF} = \frac{m + \lambda' + n}{\lambda m + \lambda' n + \lambda\lambda'} \qquad (11.249)$$

In the event that only normal weather needs to be considered, then $\lambda' = 0$, $m = 1$, and $n = 0$. Therefore,

$$\text{MITF} = \frac{1}{\lambda} \qquad (11.250)$$

which is previously given as Equation 11.73. The average failure rate can be found from Equation 11.249 as

$$\lambda_{av} = \frac{1}{\text{MITF}}$$

and

$$\lambda_{av} = \frac{\lambda m + \lambda' n + \lambda \lambda'}{m + \lambda' + n} \tag{11.251}$$

In the event that $\lambda\lambda' \ll \lambda m + n$ and $\lambda' \ll m + n$, from Equation 11.251, the approximate average failure rate can be expressed as

$$\lambda_{av} = \frac{\lambda m}{m + n} + \frac{\lambda' n}{m + n} \tag{11.252}$$

or

$$\lambda_{av} = \frac{N}{N + S}\lambda + \frac{S}{N + S}\lambda' \tag{11.253}$$

which is previously given as Equation 11.206.

11.12.4 Common-Cause Forced Outages of Transmission Lines

The task force of the IEEE-PES subcommittee on the application of probability methods [20] defines a common-cause or common-mode outage as an event having a single external cause with multiple failure effects where the effects are not consequences of each other (nor consequences of common protection system response). Most often, the common-cause outages are encountered among the transmission circuits that are located on the same ROW. In general, such outages involve common external causes such as storms, hurricanes, lightning, floods, lines broken by planes, and towers hit by cars. Other examples of common-cause failures may include systematic human error, changes in the characteristics of the system, and changes in the environment. The importance of including common-cause outages in the modeling of redundant transmission systems has been recognized recently [21–24]. In all the models developed, it is assumed that the component state residence times are distributed exponentially. Recently, the validity of this assumption has been questioned by Singh and Ebrahimian [25]. They suggest to use a nonexponential distribution (i.e., an Erlangian distribution) for the repair time on the reliability indices. Based on this assumption, they developed a non-Markovian model for common-mode failures in transmission systems.

PROBLEMS

11.1 A coin is tossed three times. On each result, head or tail is observed. Determine the following:
  (a) Sample space
  (b) Venn diagram
  (c) Tree diagram
11.2 A university has two scholarships, in the amounts of $400 and $1000, to award. If three freshmen, three sophomores, and three juniors are eligible, determine the sample space in terms of class rank by using the following:
  (a) Venn diagram
  (b) Tree diagram
11.3 Consider Problem 11.2 and use a Venn diagram and a tree diagram to represent each of the following events:
  (a) A = the presentation of the $400 scholarship to a freshman
  (b) B = the presentation of the $1000 scholarship to a sophomore
  (c) C = the presentation of both scholarships to a junior

11.4 If one card is drawn at random from a bridge deck, there are 52 possible outcomes, and each should occur with the same relative frequency. If the events are defined as (a) red card, (b) spade, (c) red card or spade, and (d) face card (king, queen, or jack), determine the following probabilities:
(a) $P(A)$
(b) $P(B)$
(c) $P(C)$
(d) $P(D)$

11.5 Assume that one card is drawn at random from a bridge deck and the following events are defined: A, spade; B, honor card (ace, king, queen, jack, or 10); and C, black card. Then
$A \cap B$: spade honor card
$A \cap C$: spade
$B \cap C$: black honor card

Determine the following:

(a) $P(A \cup B) = P(\text{spade or honor card})$
(b) $P(A \cup C)$
(c) $P(B \cup C)$

11.6 When dealing a 13-card hand from a bridge deck, determine the probability that the hand contains at least two spades.

11.7 If A is the event of drawing a king from a deck of cards and B is the event of drawing an ace, determine the probability of drawing either a king or an ace in a single draw.

11.8 If A is the event of drawing a spade from a deck of cards and B is the event of drawing an ace, determine the probability of drawing either an ace or a spade or both.

11.9 Verify, using set theory, that the probability of a null set is zero for a given sample space, that is,

$$P(\emptyset) = 0 \text{ for any } S$$

11.10 Verify Equation 11.19 using set theory.

11.11 By using set theory, verify that $P(A \cap B) = P(B) - P(A \cap B)$.

11.12 By using set theory, verify that $P(A \cup B) = P(A) + P(B) - P(A \cap B)$.

11.13 Assume that two balls are selected at random without replacement from an urn that contains four white and eight black balls. Determine the following:
(a) Probability that both balls are white
(b) Probability that the second ball is white

11.14 Assume that the personnel office of the NP&NL Utility Company has collected the following statistics of its 100 engineers:

Age	Bachelor's Degree Only	Master's Degree	Total
Under 30	45	5	50
30–40	10	15	25
Over 40	20	5	25
Total	75	25	100

If one engineer is selected at random from the company, determine the following:
(a) Probability that he or she has only a bachelor's degree
(b) Probability that he has a master's degree, given that he is over 40
(c) Probability that he is under 30, given that he has only a bachelor's degree

11.15 Assume that the NL&NP Utility Company has 40 distribution transformers, of which 6 are defective, in its riverside warehouse. Determine the probability of finding exactly two defective transformers in a group of five chosen randomly.

11.16 Determine the probability of getting exactly three heads out of eight tosses of a fair coin.

11.17 Assume that the expected life of a component can be given as $E(T) = \int_0^\infty tf(t)dt$ and derive Equation 11.70.

11.18 Verify Equation 11.90.

11.19 Consider Equation 11.86 and assume that the total number of components involved in the system is very large and that the mean time to failure is very much larger than the MTTR. Show that

$$A = 1 \cong \frac{\text{MTTR}}{\text{MTTF}}$$

11.20 Assume that 10 identical components are going to be connected in series in a given system and that the minimum acceptable system reliability is required to be 0.98. Determine the approximate value of the component reliability.

11.21 Assume that five components are going to be connected in series in a given system and that the individual component reliabilities are given as 0.90, 0.92, 0.94, 0.96, and 0.98. Determine the approximate value of the system reliability.

11.22 Assume that two components are connected in parallel and that the probabilities involved are time-dependent exponentials. If λ_1 and λ_2 are the failure rates of components 1 and 2, respectively, verify that the system reliability can be expressed as

$$R_{\text{sys}}(t) = e^{-\lambda_1 t} + e^{-\lambda_2 t} - e^{-(\lambda_1 + \lambda_2)t}$$

11.23 Consider the various combinations of the reliability block diagrams shown in Figure P11.23. Assume that each component has a reliability of 0.95. Determine the equivalent system reliability of each configuration.

11.24 Determine the equivalent reliability of the system shown in Figure P11.24, assuming that each component has the indicated reliability.

11.25 Determine the equivalent reliability of each of the system configurations shown in Figure P11.25, assuming that each component has the indicated reliability.

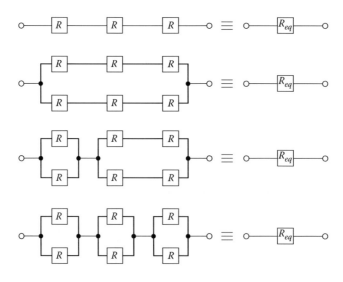

FIGURE P11.23 System configurations for Problem P11.23.

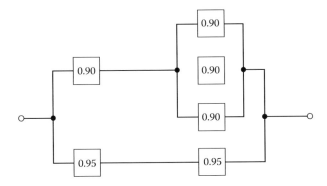

FIGURE P11.24 System configuration for Problem P11.24.

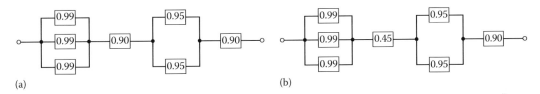

(a) (b)

FIGURE P11.25 System configurations for Problem P11.25.

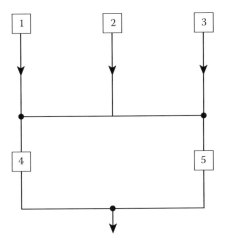

FIGURE P11.27 System configuration for Problem P11.27.

11.26 Assume that the components of the bridge-type network shown in Figure 11.20a are identical with a component reliability of 0.95. Determine the system reliability.

11.27 Assume that in the block diagram shown in Figure P11.27 two parallel paths (i.e., 14 and 25) operate to assure system supply if at least one of the paths is good. However, since neither 1 nor 2 is sufficiently reliable, a third element, 3, is added to supply either 4 or 5. Use the conditional probability method (or Bayes's theorem) and determine the system reliability.

11.28 Assume that the block diagram given in Problem 11.27 has been modified, as shown in Figure P11.28. Use the conditional probability method (or Bayes's theorem) and determine the system reliability.

11.29 Assume that the components of the bridge-type network given in Problem 11.26 are identical with a component reliability of 0.95. Determine the system unreliability using the following:
(a) Equation 11.170
(b) Equation 11.176

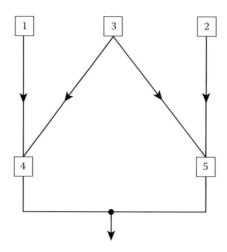

FIGURE P11.28   System configuration for Problem P11.28.

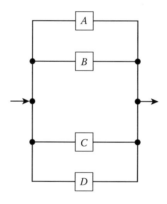

FIGURE P11.30   System configuration for Problem P11.30.

11.30 For the network block diagram shown in Figure P11.30 (which represents four subtransmission systems supplying a load), use the conditional probability method (or Bayes's theorem) and determine system reliability when three out of four subtransmission lines are required for system success.

11.31 For the network block diagram shown in Figure P11.31, use the conditional probability method (or Bayes's theorem) and determine system reliability. Assume that the successful operation of the system requires that at least one of the paths (i.e., 12, 32, or 45) is good and operating.

11.32 Assume that the components given in Problem 11.31 are all identical:
   (a) Determine the system reliability.
   (b) Calculate the system reliability if the component reliability is 0.99.

11.33 Repeat Problem 11.30 using the binomial theorem.

11.34 Consider the transmission system network configuration shown in Figure P11.34. Assume that the annual failure rates for line sections 1, 2, and 3 are given as 0.4, 0.3, and 0.6 failures per year, respectively. Use the average interruption rate method:
   (a) Determine the probability of an outage occurring on each of the lines 1, 2, and 3.
   (b) Determine the probability of an outage occurring for load bus B and the associated AACIR.
   (c) Repeat part (b) for load bus C.

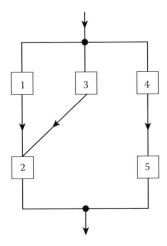

FIGURE P11.31 System configuration for Problem P11.31.

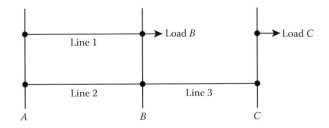

FIGURE P11.34 F System configuration for Problem P11.34.

11.35 Consider Problem 11.34 and assume that an additional line has been connected between buses B and C with an annual failure rate of 0.5 failure per year, as shown in the Figure P11.35. Use the average interruption rate method:
(a) Determine the probability of an outage occurring on line 4.
(b) Determine the probability of an outage occurring for load bus B and the associated AACIR.
(c) Repeat part (b) for load bus C.

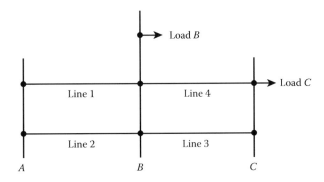

FIGURE P11.35 System configuration for Problem P11.25.

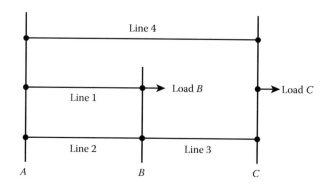

FIGURE P11.36   System configuration for Problem P11.36.

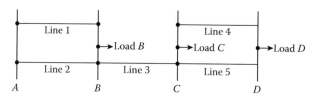

FIGURE P11.37   System configuration for Problem P11.37.

11.36 Consider Problem 11.34 and assume that an additional line has been connected between buses *A* and *C* with an annual failure rate of 0.7 failures per year, as shown in Figure P11.36. Use the average interruption rate method:

   (a) Determine the probability of an outage occurring on line 4.

   (b) Determine the probability of an outage occurring for load bus *B* and the associated AACIR.

   (c) Repeat part (b) for load bus *C*.

11.37 Consider Problem 11.34 and assume that an additional bus, bus *D*, has been added, as shown in Figure P11.37, and that the annual failure rates of the connecting lines 4 and 5 are given as 0.1 and 0.2, respectively. Use the average interruption rate method:

   (a) Determine the probability of an outage occurring for load bus *B* and the associated AACIR.

   (b) Repeat part (a) for load bus *C*.

   (c) Repeat part (a) for load bus *D*.

11.38 Consider the 50 mi long, 138 kV line shown in Figure P11.38, and assume that the outage rate for the 138 kV line is 0.0065 failures per mile per year and that the annual failure rates for the 138 kV CBs, 69 kV CBs, 138/69 kV transformer, and 69 kV bus are given as 0.00857, 0.00612, 0.0891, and 0.0111, respectively. Use the average interruption rate method, and determine the probability of an outage occurring for the 69 kV load bus and the associated AACIR. Assume that the 138 kV bus is 100% reliable.

11.39 Consider Problem 11.38 and assume that an identical line (with identical component failure rates) has been connected in parallel with the first line, as shown in Figure P11.39. Use the average interruption rate method and determine the following:

   (a) Probability of outage occurring for 69 kV load bus

   (b) Associated AACIR

   (c) Number of interruptions observed in the past 10 years

11.40 Consider the transmission system shown in Figure P11.40a. Assume that the annual failure rates for components 1 and 2 are given as 0.5 and 0.6 failures for normal weather and 15 and 18 failures for stormy weather, respectively. Assume that annual component

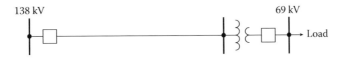

FIGURE P11.38 System configuration for Problem P11.38.

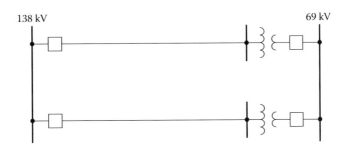

FIGURE P11.39 System configuration for Problem P11.39.

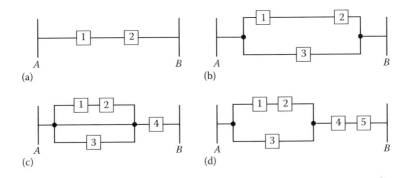

FIGURE P11.40 System configurations for Problem P11.40.

maintenance outage rates and expected repair times for all forced outages for each of the components are given as 2 outages and 8 h, respectively. Expected downtimes for maintenance outages for each of the components are 8 h. The expected durations of normal and stormy weather periods are 3 and 195 h, respectively. Assume that bus *A* is a 100% reliable source bus and that bus *B* is the load bus. Use the frequency and duration method and determine the following:

(a) Overall annual forced outage rates for each component
(b) Overall annual forced outage rate for series system
(c) Annual maintenance outage rate of series system
(d) Expected outage duration due to forced outage for system
(e) Expected outage duration due to maintenance outages for system
(f) Total annual outage rate for system
(g) Expected restoration time, in hours, for system

11.41 Assume that the two components given in Problem 11.40 are connected in parallel with respect to each other. Use the frequency and duration method and determine the overall annual failure rate due to normal and stormy weather forced outages for the system.

11.42 Consider Problem 11.40 and determine the average total outage time per year in hours.

11.43 Consider Problem 11.40 and assume that an additional component has been connected in parallel with respect to the previous components, as shown in Figure P11.40b. Use the results of Problem 11.40 and determine the overall annual failure rate due to normal and stormy weather forced outages for the new system. Assume that the following data have been given for the third component:

$$\lambda_3 = 0.4 \text{ failure/year of normal weather}$$

$$\lambda_3' = 20 \text{ failures/year of stormy weather}$$

$$\lambda_3'' = 2 \text{ maintenance outages/year}$$

$$r_3 = 10 \text{ h}$$

$$r_3' = 12 \text{ h}$$

$$r_3'' = 8 \text{ h}$$

11.44 Consider Problem 11.43 and assume that an additional component has been connected in series with respect to the previous system, as shown in Figure P11.40c. Use the results of Problem 11.43 and determine the overall annual failure rate due to normal and stormy weather forced outages for the new system. Assume that components 3 and 4 are identical.

11.45 Consider Problem 11.44 and assume that an additional component has been connected in series with respect to the previous system, as shown in Figure P11.40d. Use the results of Problem 11.44 and determine the overall annual failure rate due to normal and stormy weather forced outages for the new system. Assume that components 3, 4, and 5 are identical.

11.46 Assume that the following permanent outage data have been given for the subtransmission system shown in Figure P11.39.

System Component	Outage Rate (Outages/Year)	Average Repair Time (h)
138 kV breakers	0.0058	66
138 kV line	0.627	10
138/69 kV transformer	0.0119	360
69 kV breakers	0.0045	44
69 kV bus	0.0111	5

Assume that the 138 kV bus is 100% reliable and determine the following:
(a) Total failure rate for one parallel line
(b) Total MTTR for one parallel line
(c) Total failure rate for system
(d) Total MTTR for system
(e) Total failure time due to overlapping-component permanent failures

11.47 Consider Problem 11.46 and assume that the following maintenance outage data have been given for the system.

System Component	Outage Rate (Outages/Year)	Average Repair Time (h)
138 kV breakers	2	10
138 kV line	4	9
138/69 kV transformer	2	9
69 kV bus	1.5	5

Determine the following:

(a) Maintenance outage rate for one parallel line

(b) Expected maintenance outage duration for one parallel line

(c) Outage rate due to component permanent outages overlapping-component maintenance outages

(d) Expected outage duration due to component permanent outages overlapping-component maintenance outages

(e) Overall annual permanent outage rate

(f) Overall expected outage duration

(g) Overall average total outage time per year

11.48 Consider Problem 11.46 and assume that the following temporary forced outage data have been given for the system.

System Component	Outage Rate (Outages/Year)	Average Repair Time (h)
138 kV line	3.069	7
138/69 kV transformer	0.0048	90
69 kV bus	0.0164	7

Determine the following:

(a) Temporary outage rate for one parallel line

(b) Expected temporary outage duration for one parallel line

(c) System outage rate due to component temporary outages overlapping-component permanent outages

(d) Overlapping restoration time due to temporary outage

11.49 Consider Problem 11.48 and determine the following:

(a) Temporary outage rate due to component temporary outages overlapping-component maintenance outages

(b) Overlapping restoration time in part (a)

(c) Total temporary outage rate due to component temporary outages overlapping-component permanent and maintenance outages

(d) Restoration time for temporary outages

(e) Overall temporary outage rate

REFERENCES

1. IEEE Committee Report. Proposed definitions of terms for reporting and analyzing outages of electrical transmission and distribution facilities and interruptions, *IEEE Trans*. PAS-87(5), 1968, 1318–1323.

2. U.S. Department of Energy. The National power grid study: Technical study reports, vol. 2, DPE/ERA-0056-02, Economic Regulatory Administration, Office of Utility Systems, Washington, DC, 1979.

3. U.S. Department of Energy. The National electric reliability study: Technical study reports, DOE/EP-0005, Office of Emergency Operations, USDOE, Washington, DC, 1981.

4. U.S. Department of Energy. The National electric reliability study: Executive summary, DOE/EP-0003, Office of Emergency Operations, USDOE, Washington, DC, 1981.

5. U.S. Department of Energy. The National electric reliability study: Final report, DOE/EP-0004, Office of Emergency Operations, USDOE, Washington, DC, 1981.

6. Gönen, T. *Electric Power Distribution System Engineering*, McGraw-Hill, New York, 1986.

7. Billinton, R., Ringler, R. J., and Wood, A. J. *Power System Reliability Calculations*, MIT Press, Cambridge, MA, 1973.

8. Billinton, R. *Power System Reliability Evaluation*, Gordon & Breach, New York, 1970.

9. Endrenyi, J. *Reliability Modeling in Electric Power Systems*, Wiley, New York, 1978.

10. Allan, R. N., Billinton, R., and de Oliveira, M. F. An efficient algorithm for deducing the minimal cut and reliability indices of a general network configuration, *IEEE Trans. Reliab.* R-25, 1976, 226–233.

11. Allan, R. N. Basic concepts in reliability evaluation, in *Power System Reliability Evaluation*, IEEE Tutorial Course, Publ. No. 82 EHO 195-8-PWR, IEEE, New York, 1982.

12. Shooman, M. L. *Probabilistic Reliability: An Engineering Approach*, McGraw-Hill, New York, 1968.

13. Todd, Z. G. A probability method for transmission and distribution outage calculations, *IEEE Trans. Power Apparatus Syst.* PAS-84, 1964, 695–701.

14. Gaver, D. P., Montmeat, F. E., and Patton, A. D. Power system reliability. I. Measures of reliability and methods of calculation, *IEEE Power Eng. Soc. Winter Power Meet.*, 1964, paper no. 64-90; also in *IEEE Trans. Power Apparatus Syst.* PAS-84, 1964, 727–737.

15. Montmeat, F. E., Patton, A. D., Zemkoski, J., and Cumming, D. J., Power system reliability II-applications and a computer program, *IEEE Trans. Power Apparatus Syst.* PAS-84, 1965, 636–643.

16. Billinton, R. and Grover, M. S. Reliability evaluation in transmission and distribution systems, *Proc. Inst. Electr. Eng.* 122(5), 1975, 517–523.

17. Desieno, C. F. and Stine, L. L. A probability method for determining the reliability of electric power systems, *IEEE Trans. Power Apparatus Syst.* PAS-83, 1964, 174–191.

18. Billinton, R. and Bollinger, K. E. Transmission system reliability evaluation using Markov processes, *IEEE Trans. Power Apparatus Syst.* PAS-87, 1968, 538–547.

19. Hall, J. D., Ringlee, R. J., and Wood, A. J. Frequency and duration methods for power system reliability calculations, part I—Generation system model, *IEEE Trans. Power Apparatus Syst.* PAS-S7, 1968, 1787–1796.

20. IEEE Committee Report. Common mode forced outages of overhead transmission lines, *IEEE Trans. Power Apparatus Syst.* PAS-95(3), 1976, 859–863.

21. Billinton, R., Medicherla, T. K. P., and Sachdev, M. S. Application of common-cause outage models in composite system reliability evaluation, *IEEE Trans. Power Apparatus Syst.* PAS-100(7), 1981, 3648–3657.

22. Billinton, R., Medicherla, T. K. P., and Sachdev, M. S. Application of common-cause outage models in composite system reliability evaluation, *IEEE Power Eng. Soc. Summer Meet.*, 1979, paper no. A 79 461–5.

23. Allan, R. N., Dialynas, E. N., and Homer, I. R. Modeling common mode failures in the reliability evaluation of power system networks, *IEEE Power Eng. Soc. Winter Power Meet.*, 1979, paper no. A 79 040-7.

24. Billinton, R. and Kumar, Y. Transmission line reliability models including common mode and adverse weather effects, *IEEE Power Eng. Soc. Winter Meet.*, 1980, paper no. A80 080-2.

25. Singh, C. and Ebrahimian, M. R. Non-Markovian models for common mode failures in transmission systems, *IEEE Trans. Power Apparatus Syst.* PAS-101(6), 1982, 1545–1550.

GENERAL REFERENCES

Albrecht, P. F. Evaluating system reliability, *IEEE Spectr.* 59, 1978, 43–47.

Bhavaraju, M. P. and Billinton, R. Transmission planning using a reliability criterion. Part II. Transmission planning. *IEEE Trans. Power Apparatus Syst.* PAS-90(1), 1971, 70–78.

Bhavaraju, M. P. and Billinton, R. Transmission system reliability methods, *IEEE Power Eng. Soc. Winter Power Meet.*, 1971, paper no. 71 TP 91-PWR.

Billinton, R. and Bhavaraju, M. P. Transmission planning using a reliability criterion, Part I. A reliability criterion, *IEEE Trans. Power Apparatus Syst.* PAS-89(1), 28–34.

Billinton, R. and Grover, M. S. Reliability assessment of transmission and distribution schemes, *IEEE Trans. Power Apparatus Syst.* PAS-94(3), 1975, 724–732.

Billinton, R. and Grover, M. S. Quantitative evaluation of permanent outages in distribution systems, *IEEE Trans. Power Apparatus Syst.* PAS-94, 1975, 733–741.

Billinton, R. and Lee, S. Y. Unavailability analysis of an underwater cable system, *IEEE Trans. Power Apparatus Syst.* PAS-96(1), 1977, 27–31.

Billinton, R. and Medicherla, T. K. P. Station originated multiple outages in the reliability analysis of a composite generation and transmission system, *IEEE Trans. Power Apparatus Syst.* PAS-100(8), 1981, 3870–3878.

Chemical Engineering in Australia. *Instruction Manual for Reporting Component Forced Outages of Transmission Equipment*, CEA, Sydney, New South Wales, Australia, 1978.

Christiaanse, W. R. A new technique for reliability calculations, *IEEE Trans. Power Apparatus Syst.* PAS-89(8), 1970, 1836–1847.

Christiaanse, W. R. Reliability calculations including the effects of overloads and maintenance, *IEEE Power Eng. Soc. Winter Power Meet.*, 1971, paper no. TP 119-PWR.

Economic Regulatory Administration. Reports on outages, load reductions, and other emergency situations on the bulk electric system, U.S. Department of Energy, Washington, DC, 1970–1979.

Electric Power Research Institute. Reliability indexes for power systems, EPRI Rep. EL-1773, EPRI, Palo Alto, CA, 1981.

Electric Power Research Institute. Bulk transmission system component outage data base, EPRI Rep. EL-1797, EPRI, Palo Alto, CA, 1981.

Esser, W. F., Wasilew, S. G., and Egly, D. T. Computer programs for reliability, *Proc. Power Ind. Comput. Appl. Conf.* 1967, 513–518.

Ford, D. V. The British electricity boards national fault and interruption reporting scheme—Objectives, development and operating experience, *IEEE Winter Power Meet.*, 1972, paper no. T 72 082-1.

Garver, L. L. and Van Horne, P. R. Reliability analysis of transmission plans, *Electr. Forum* 5(1), 1979, 5–10.

IEEE Committee Report. Bibliography on the application of probability methods in power system reliability evaluation, *IEEE Trans. Power Apparatus Syst.* PAS-91, 1972, 649–660.

IEEE Committee Report. Bibliography on the application of probability methods in power system reliability evaluation, *IEEE Trans. Power Apparatus Syst.* PAS-97, 1978, 2235–2242.

IEEE Task Force Report. IEEE reliability test system, *IEEE Trans. Power Apparatus Syst.* PAS-98(6), 2047–2054.

IEEE Working Group Report. List of transmission and distribution components for use in outage reporting and reliability calculations, *IEEE Trans. Power Apparatus Syst.* PAS-95(4), 1976, 1210–1215.

IEEE Working Group Report. Reliability indices for use in bulk power supply adequacy evaluation, *IEEE Trans. Power Apparatus Syst.* PAS-98(4), 1978, 1097–1103.

Landren, G. L. and Anderson, S. W. Data base for EHV transmission reliability, *IEEE Trans. Power Apparatus Syst.* PAS-100(4), 1981, 2046–2058.

Noferi, P. L. and Paris, L. Quantitative evaluation of power system reliability in planning studies, *IEEE Trans. Power Apparatus Syst.* PAS-91(2), 1972, 611–618.

Noferi, V. I., Paris, T., and Salvaderi, T. Monte Carlo methods for power system reliability evaluations in transmission or generation planning, *Proceedings of Annual Reliability Maintainability Symposium*, Washington, DC, 1975, pp. 111–119.

PJM Transmission Reliability Task Force. Bulk power area reliability evaluation considering probabilistic transfer capability, *IEEE Trans. Power Apparatus Syst.* PAS-101(9), 1982, 3551–3562.

Ringlee, R. J. and Goode, S. D. On procedures for reliability evaluations of transmission systems, *IEEE Trans. Power Apparatus Syst.* PAS-89(4), 1970, 527–536.

Sharaf, T. A. M. and Berg, G. J. Reliability optimization for transmission expansion planning, *IEEE Trans. Power Apparatus Syst.* PAS-101(7), 1982, 2243–2248.

Singh, C. Markov cut-set approach for the reliability evaluation of transmission and distribution system, *IEEE Trans. Power Apparatus Syst.* PAS-100(6), 1981, 2719–2725.

Singh, C. and Billinton, R. A new method to determine the failure frequency of a complex system, *Microelectron. Reliab.* 12, 1974, 459–465.

Stanton, K. E. Reliability analysis for power system applications, *IEEE Trans. Power Apparatus Syst.* PAS-88(4), 1969, 431–437.

Van Horne, P. R. and Schoenberger, C. N. Trap: An innovative approach to analyzing the reliability of transmission paths, *IEEE Trans. Power Apparatus Syst.* PAS-101(1), 1982, 11–16.

Vemuri, S. An annotated bibliography power system reliability literature: 1972–1977, *IEEE Power Eng. Soc. Summer Meet.*, 1978, paper no. A 78 548-0.

Wang, L. The effects of scheduled outages in transmission system reliability evaluation, *IEEE Trans. Power Apparatus Syst.* PAS-97(6), 1978, 2346–2353.

Section II

Mechanical Design and Analysis

12 Construction of Overhead Lines

Much learning does not teach understanding.

Heraclitus

12.1 INTRODUCTION

OH construction* is only 15%–60% as costly as underground and is therefore more economical. The first consideration in the design of an OH line, of course, is its electrical characteristics. As explained in the previous chapters, the electrical design of the line must be sufficient for the required power to be transmitted without excessive voltage drop and/or energy losses, and the line insulation must be adequate to cope with the system voltage. The mechanical factors influencing the design must then be considered. For example, the poles supporting the conductors must have sufficient mechanical strength to withstand all expected loads. Another example is that the material chosen for the conductors must be strong enough to withstand the forces to which it is subjected.

The conductors and poles must have sufficient strength with a predetermined safety factor to withstand the loads due to the line itself and stresses imposed by ice and wind loads. Thus, the OH line should provide satisfactory service over a long period of time without the necessity for too much maintenance. Ultimate economy is provided by a good construction since excessive maintenance or especially short life can easily more than overbalance a saving in the first cost.

The OH line must have a proper strength to withstand the stresses imposed on its component parts by the line itself. These include stresses set up by the tension in conductors at dead-end points, compression stresses due to guy tension, transverse loads due to angles in the line, vertical stresses due to the weight of conductors, and the vertical component of conductor tension. The tension in the conductors should be adjusted so that it is well within the permissible load of the material. This will mean in practice that one must allow for an appreciable amount of sag.

The poles must have sufficient height and be so located, taking into account the topography of the land, as to provide adequate ground clearances at both maximum loading and maximum temperature condition. The conductor ground clearance for railroad tracks and wire line crossings, as well as from buildings and other objects, must meet the requirements of the NESC.†

A proper mechanical design is one of the essentials in providing good service to customers. A large majority of service interruptions can be traced to physical failures on the distribution system, broken wires, broken poles, damaged insulation, damaged equipment, etc. Many of these service interruptions are more or less unavoidable. But their numbers can be reduced if the design and construction of the various physical parts can withstand, with reasonable safety factors, not only normal conditions but also some probable abnormal conditions.

---

* In this chapter, the emphasis has been placed on the LV and HV OH lines, including OH distribution lines.

† It is important to note that the material in this book, especially in this and following chapters, illustrates only some selected requirements of the NESC. It is not advocated that the material in this book be used as the sole basis for line design in practice. Any line design must satisfy all applicable laws, ordinances, commission rules and orders, etc. While every precaution has been taken in the preparation of this book, the author and the publisher assume no responsibility for errors or omissions. Neither is any liability assumed for damages resulting from the use of information contained herein.

The OH line must be designed from the mechanical point of view to withstand the worst probable, but not the worst possible, conditions. For example, the cost of an OH line that would withstand a severe hurricane would be tremendous, and thus from the economical point of view, it may be justifiable to run the risk of failure under such conditions.

Example 12.1

The No Power & No Light (NP&NL) utility company provides service by an OH line to a small number of farms at a remote area at the outskirts of Ghost City. The past experiences with the line indicate that frequent repairs of the line are needed as a result of lightning, windstorms, and snow. Each repair, on the average, costs the company $1500. The probability of damage to the line in a given year is as follows:

Number of times repair required	0	1	2	3
Probability of exactly that number of repairs	0.4	0.3	0.2	0.1

The distribution engineer of the NP&NL company estimates that relocating and rebuilding of the line could reduce the probabilities to the following:

Number of times repair required	0	1
Probability of exactly that number of repairs	0.9	0.1

Assuming a useful life of 25 years, zero salvage value, and a carrying charge rate of 20% and that operating costs other than those for repairs are unaffected by the proposed change, find how much the NP&NL company could afford to pay for relocating and rebuilding the line.

Solution

Let B be the affordable cost of relocating the line. At the break-even point, the present equivalent of savings should be equal to the present equivalent of the added costs as a result of relocating the line. Therefore,*

$$B = \$1500[3(0.1) + 2(0.2) + 1(0.3) + 0(0.4) - 1(0.1) - 0(0.9)](P/A)_{25}^{20\%}$$

$$= \$1500[0.9](4.948)$$

$$= \$6679.8$$

Since the actual relocating and rebuilding of the line would cost much more than the amount found, the distribution engineer decides to keep the status quo.

12.2 FACTORS AFFECTING MECHANICAL DESIGN OF OVERHEAD LINES

In general, the factors affecting a *mechanical design* of the OH lines are as follows:

1. Character of line route
2. ROW
3. Mechanical loading
4. Required clearances
5. Type of supporting structures
6. Grade of construction
7. Conductors
8. Type of insulators
9. Joint use by other utilities

---

* $(P/A)_n^{i\%}$ is the present worth of a uniform series, and it is the reciprocal of the capital recovery factor. It is also called the *discount factor*. For a given interest rate and number of years, its value can be found from interest tables or it can be calculated from $(P/A)_n^{i\%} = [(1 + i)^n - 1]/i(1 + i)^n$.

12.3 CHARACTER OF LINE ROUTE

The routes of OH transmission lines are usually selected across the country on private ROW in order to obtain the most direct route and proper space for towers as well as to avoid buildings, roads, highways, and LV lines. Lower-voltage OH distribution lines are run along streets and highways, as much as possible, in order to reach customers more easily and to make the lines accessible for maintenance. In urban and suburban areas, poles are spaced 100 to about 150 ft apart to provide convenient points for service attachments or service drops and to keep the service lengths to a minimum. Usually, poles are set from half to one foot inside the curb when along streets.

Transmission lines may have spans of several hundred feet. The general character of the country in which the OH line is to be located affects the design primarily in terms of selecting the conductor and type of supporting structures. The line location task requires judgment, experience, and skill not only in minimizing the costs of ROW and construction but also in providing convenience in maintenance and eliminating some possible operational bottlenecks that might occur in the future. In general, the factors affecting the length of a span are as follows:

1. Character of route
2. Proper clearance between conductors
3. Excessive tensions under maximum load
4. Structures adequate to carry additional loads

It is usually not recommended, especially in mountainous country or in heavily populated areas, to choose a direct route or try to locate the line on long tangents.

12.4 RIGHT-OF-WAY

It is important to have all ROW and easements for a given line secured before final plans, designs, and specifications for construction. Higher-voltage transmission lines on private ROW are usually built with long spans, and the type of terrain covered by the line has an impact on the selection of the construction type.

Existing ROW should be utilized whenever possible, especially for augmented transmission systems, and in many cases, this is done with less environmental disruption than would occur with the acquisition of a new ROW. Advance planning and scheduling of road, pipeline, telephone, and electrical transmission is imperative for the future.

In general, rather than purchasing the ROW in fee, a permanent easement is obtained in which the owner or owners permit the necessary rights to construct and operate the line but keep ownership and use of the land. The easement secured must stipulate the following:

1. Permission to build all supporting structures
2. Permission for a means of access to each supporting structure
3. Permission to clear all trees and brush over a width of at least 10 ft larger than the spread of the conductors in order to allow sufficient working space for construction
4. Permission to remove all trees, which might violate the minimum required clearance to the conductors if they were to fall
5. Permission to remove all trees, which might violate the minimum required clearance to conductors if the conductor were to swing out under maximum wind
6. Permission to remove all obstacles, for example, buildings, lumber piles, and haystacks, which might cause a fire

As a rule, trees that may interfere with conductors should be trimmed or removed. Normal tree growth, the combined movement of trees and conductors under adverse conditions, voltage, and sagging of a conductor at elevated temperatures are among the factors to be considered in determining the extent of trimming required. Where trimming or removal is not practical, especially in distribution lines, the conductor should be separated from the tree with suitable insulating materials or devices to prevent conductor damage by abrasion and grounding of the circuit through the tree.

12.5 MECHANICAL LOADING

12.5.1 DEFINITIONS OF STRESSES

The term *mechanical loading* refers to the external conditions that produce mechanical stresses in the line conductors and supports, that is, poles or towers. Mechanical loading also includes the weight of the conductors and structures themselves. Structures are subject to vertical and horizontal loads. Vertical loading includes the dead weight of equipment such as crossarms, insulators, conductors, transformers, etc. It also includes ice and snow clinging on the structures and the conductors.

Poles supporting OH conductors and other equipment are subjected to strains from the tension with which they are strung. When a force is applied against an object, it produces stress within the object. There are five kinds of stress:

1. *Tensile stress.* Caused by the forces acting in opposite directions, away from the body and along the same straight line, to elongate, or stretch, the body beyond its normal length, as shown in Figure 12.1. For example, a conductor strung between two poles or a guy wire, under tension, is subjected to tensile stress.
2. *Compressive stress.* The opposite of the tensile stress. Caused by the forces acting toward the body to shorten the body, as shown in Figure 12.2. For example, a distribution transformer hung on a pole subjects the pole to a compressive stress.
3. *Shearing stress.* Caused by the forces, not in the same straight line, that tend to cut the body in two, as shown in Figure 12.3. For example, bolts attaching a crossarm to a pole are subjected to a shearing stress between the crossarm and the pole.
4. *Bending stress.* Caused by the forces acting along a body. For example, a pole supporting a corner in the line, and not guyed, is subject to a bending stress.
5. *Twisting stress* or *torque.* Caused by line tensions that are not equal on the two sides of a pole. For example, a pole may be subjected to a twisting stress when a conductor breaks between supports.

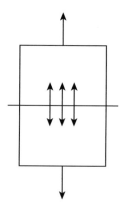

FIGURE 12.1   Tension.

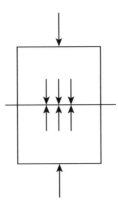

FIGURE 12.2   Compression.

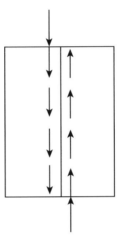

FIGURE 12.3   Shear.

12.5.2 ELASTICITY AND ULTIMATE STRENGTH

Elasticity is the property of a material that enables it to recover its original shape and size after being stressed. The ratio of normal stress (in pounds per square inch) to strain (in inches per inch) is called *Young's modulus* or the *modulus of elasticity*. It is constant for a given material up to the proportional limit, as shown in Figure 12.4. Up to a certain limit, stress applied to a material causes deformation, which disappears when the stress is removed.

Every material has a stress limit, and stress beyond this point causes a certain amount of permanent deformation. This limit is the *elastic limit* of the material. When the stress is less than the elastic limit of the material, the deformation is directly proportional to the unit stress. When the stress exceeds the elastic limit, the material still resists the stress but has lost certain of its original characteristics. The deformation increases until failure occurs.

The stress that causes failure or rupture is the *ultimate stress* of the material. For some materials, for example, glass, the elastic limit and the ultimate strength are very nearly the same. However, most materials show the deformation or yield point of elastic limit at a lower value than the breaking or ultimate strength.

In the design of mechanical structures, there are a number of variables and possibilities that make the exact determination of stresses and strengths difficult. The maximum stress at which a structure is designed to operate normally is the allowable or working stress. The ratio of working

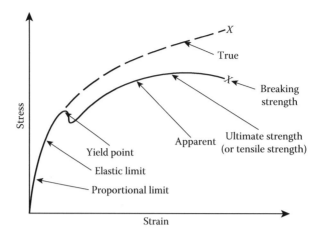

FIGURE 12.4 Stress–strain diagram.

stress to the ultimate strength of the material is the *design safety factor*. It is usual practice to design for the assumed loading conditions and to use this safety factor, or constant, to make reasonable provision for unusual and unforeseen conditions and hazards to which the structure may be subjected. Furthermore, these safety factors make allowance for the difference between elastic limit and ultimate strength and make allowance for variations from average quality.

The NESC and/or the local rules and regulations provide the *minimum required safety factors*. Where the NESC or the local regulations are not in effect, to specify safety factors that must be applied under various conditions, the design engineer must use his or her own engineering judgment in choosing such safety factors as will best meet the existing conditions.

12.5.3 NESC LOADINGS

In general, the map shown in Figure 12.5 is taken as a basis for determining the thickness of ice, wind velocity, and temperature for a given OH line in any region of the country. In the design of an important OH line, the past records of the local weather bureau should be studied.

When the local conditions are found to be different from the general conditions in the surrounding area indicated on this map, the line should be designed and constructed to meet such conditions. For example, certain districts are more subject to sleet storms than others even in the same general locality.

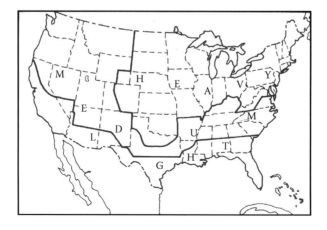

FIGURE 12.5 NESC's mechanical loading map for OH lines.

In general, sleet storms are most frequent in the moderate climates, since precipitation takes place more often at freezing temperatures. In large cities, sleet formation is much less likely to occur than in rural areas. Also, the exposure of lines to wind is extremely different since hills, buildings, trees, etc., make a fair amount of shields against the full pressure that a wind might cause in open country.

It is possible to have very heavy ice formation without much wind or very strong winds in warm weather with no ice formation. The NESC defines three conditions of loading, namely, heavy, medium, and light, and divides the country into three areas in which these loadings are possibly taking place.

12.5.4 Wind Pressure

The method of calculating wind pressure on cylindrical surfaces, for example, conductors and wood poles, was developed by H. W. Buck and is given by Buck's formula [1]

$$p = 0.00256V^2 \text{ lb/ft}^2 \tag{12.1}$$

where V is the actual wind velocity in miles per hour. It is, in general, accepted in span calculations.

The pressure on flat surfaces, for example, crossarms and towers, normal to the direction of the wind can be calculated by using the following formula developed by C. F. Marvin:

$$p = 0.004 \left(\frac{B}{30} \right) V^2 \text{ lb/ft}^2 \tag{12.2}$$

where
  B is the barometric pressure in millimeters of mercury
  V is the actual wind velocity in miles per hour

This equation can be written as

$$p = 0.004V^2 \text{ lb/ft}^2 \tag{12.3}$$

since $B/30$ is, in general, equal to unity.

When using the data for Vs given by the US Weather Bureau, the necessary correction factors should also be obtained since the observed values are taken at elevations considerably different than those on which conductors are usually hung. For the minimum required wind pressures by the NESC, see Chapter 13.

In still air, the conductor is subject to its own weight only, and if the temperature is high at the same time, the resulting sag gives a low tension. Thus, the combination of still air with high temperature gives the easiest conditions. The worst conditions are a combination of low temperature, which lessens the sag of the line, and accumulations of ice or snow, which increase the weight per-unit length and consequently the effect of the wind blowing against the conductor. This topic is discussed in greater detail in Chapter 13.

12.6 REQUIRED CLEARANCES

In general, the following clearances need to be considered: ground, tracks, buildings, trees, conductors and structures of another line, other conductors on the same structure, the structure itself, guy wires and other equipment on the structure, and the edge of the ROW. The NESC gives the

TABLE 12.1

Clearance of Conductors Passing by But Not Attached to Buildings (ft)

Clearance of Buildings	Communication Conductors, etc.	Open-Supply Conductors with Phase-to-Ground Voltages			
		0–750 V	750 V–8.7 kV	8.7–15 kV	15–50 kV
Horizontal					
To walls and projections	3	5	5	8	10
To unguarded windows	3	5	5	8	10
To balconies, etc.	3	5	5	8	10
Vertical					
Above or below roofs, etc. (accessible to pedestrians)	3	10	10	10	12
Above or below balconies and roofs (accessible to pedestrians)	8	15	15	15	17
Above roofs (accessible to vehicular traffic)	18	18	20	20	22
Chimneys, antennas, etc.					
Horizontal	3	5	5	8	10
Vertical, above or below	3	5	8	8	10

minimum required clearances. Space does not permit the tabulation here of clearances for all these conditions for all voltages used for OH lines. However, some information is summarized in the following sections.

12.6.1 HORIZONTAL CLEARANCES

Briefly, the location of poles must be chosen to provide sufficient clearance from driveways, fire hydrants, street traffic, railroad tracks, buildings, fire escapes, etc. Table 12.1 gives the clearance of conductors passing by but not attached to building and other installations except bridges. The given clearances are taken from the NESC, 1984 edition.

Conductors of one line should be not less than 4 ft from those of another and conflicting line. If conductors pass near the pole of another OH line, provided that they are not attached, they should not interfere with the climbing space.

12.6.2 VERTICAL CLEARANCES

Table 12.2, taken from the NESC, 1984 edition, presents vertical clearances. The given values are applicable to crossings where span lengths do not exceed 175 ft in heavy-loading districts, 250 ft in medium-loading districts, or 350 ft in light-loading districts. The given clearances are based on a temperature of 60°F with no wind and voltages not over 50 kV to ground. For longer spans and higher voltages, larger clearances are required, depending upon sag and tension in the span.

12.6.3 CLEARANCES AT WIRE CROSSINGS

Crossings should be made on a common crossing structure where practical. If not practical, the clearance between any two wires, conductors, or cables crossing each other and carried on different supports should be not less than the values given in Table 12.3 in order to prevent the possibility of accidental contact under varying wind, temperature, and ice loading.

TABLE 12.2

Minimum Vertical Clearances of Conductors above Ground or Rails (ft)

Location Type	Communication Conductors, Guys, Messengers, etc.	Open-Supply Conductors with Phase-to-Ground Voltages			Trolley Conductors with Phase-to-Ground Voltages	
		0–750 V	750 V–15 kV	15–50 kV	0–750 V	Over 750 V
When crossing above railroads	27	27	28	30	22	22
Streets, alleys, and roadways	18	18	20	22	18	20
Private driveways	10	15	20	22	18	20
Walks for pedestrians only	15	15	15	17	16	18
When conductors are along streets or alleys	18	18	20	22	18	20
Roads in rural districts	14	15	18	20	18	20

TABLE 12.3

Crossing Clearances of Wires Carried on Different Supports (ft)

Nature of Wires Crossed Over	Communication Conductors	Services, Supply Cables 0–750 V	Open-Supply Conductors with Phase-to-Ground Voltages		
			0–750 V	750 V–8.7 kV	8.7–50 kV
Communication wires	2	2	4	4	6
Aerial-supply cables	4	2	2	2	4
Open-supply wires (0–750 V)	4	2	2	2	4
Open-supply wires (750 V–8.7 kV)	4	4	2	2	4
Open-supply wires (8.7–50 kV)	6	6	4	4	4
Trolley conductors	4	4	4	6	6
Guys, lightning protection wires	2	2	2	4	4

The given clearances apply at 60°F with no wind and for spans not exceeding 175, 250, or 350 ft, in heavy-, medium-, and light-loading districts, respectively. For longer spans and higher voltages, greater clearances are required, depending on sag and tension in the span.

12.6.4 Horizontal Separation of Conductors from Each Other

The NESC requires that for supply conductors of the same circuit, at voltages up to 8.7 kV, the minimum horizontal clearances between the conductors should be 12 in. and for higher voltages should be 12 in. plus 0.4 in. per kilovolt over 8.7 kV.

It is required that for supply conductors of different circuits, at voltages up to 8.7 kV, the minimum horizontal clearances between the conductors should be 12 in.; for voltages between 8.7 and 50 kV, the clearances should be 12 in. plus 0.4 in. per kilovolt over 8.7 kV; and for voltages between 50 and 814 kV, the clearances should be 28.5 in. plus 0.4 in. per kilovolt over 50 kV.

TABLE 12.4

Horizontal Clearances at Supports between Line Conductors Smaller than No. 2 AWG Based on Sags

Voltage between Conductors (kV)	Sag (in.)							But Not Less than
	36	48	72	96	120	180	240	
	Horizontal Clearance (in.)							
2.4	14.7	20.5	28.7	35.0	40.3	51.2	60.1	12.0
4.16	15.3	21.1	29.3	35.6	40.9	51.8	60.7	12.0
12.47	17.7	23.5	31.7	38.0	43.3	54.2	63.1	13.5
13.2	18.0	23.8	32.0	38.3	43.6	54.5	63.4	13.8
13.8	18.1	23.9	32.1	38.4	43.7	54.6	63.5	14.0
14.4	18.3	24.1	32.3	38.6	43.9	54.8	63.7	14.3
24.94	21.5	27.3	35.5	41.8	47.1	58.0	66.9	18.5
34.5	24.4	30.2	38.4	44.7	50.0	60.9	69.8	22.4
46	27.8	33.6	41.8	48.1	53.4	64.3	73.2	26.9

Source: American National Standards Institute, *National Electrical Safety Code*, 1984 edn., IEEE, New York, 1984.

The minimum required horizontal clearances by the NESC for line conductors smaller than No. 2 AWG can be calculated by using the following formula:

$$\text{Minimum clearance} = 0.3 \text{ in.}/\text{kV} + 7\left(\frac{1}{3}S - 8\right)^{1/2} \tag{12.4}$$

where S is the apparent sag of the conductor in inches.

Table 12.4 gives the minimum horizontal clearances between the conductors up to 46 kV.

The minimum required horizontal clearances by the NESC for line conductors of No. 2 AWG or larger can be calculated by using the following formula:

$$\text{Minimum clearance} = 0.3 \text{ in.}/\text{kV} + 8\left(\frac{1}{12}S\right)^{1/2} \tag{12.5}$$

where S is the apparent sag of the conductor in inches.

Table 12.5 gives the minimum horizontal clearances between the conductors up to 46 kV.

In addition to those clearance requirements included here, the NESC provides other minimum requirements such as for climbing space through lower wires on a pole to gain access to wires on upper arms or for vertical separation of crossarms. For further information, see the current edition of the National Electrical Safety Code and local rules and regulations.

12.7 TYPE OF SUPPORTING STRUCTURES

12.7.1 POLE TYPES

There are basically four different pole types: (1) wood poles, (2) concrete poles, (3) steel poles, and (4) aluminum poles. In general, wood poles are preferred over others for OH distribution lines because of the abundance of the material, ease of handling, and cost. Concrete poles reinforced with

TABLE 12.5

Horizontal Clearance at Supports between Line Conductor No. 2 AWG or Larger Based on Sags

Voltage between Conductors (kV)	Sag (in.)							But Not Less than
	36	48	72	96	120	180	240	
	Horizontal Clearance (in.)							
2.4	14.6	16.7	20.2	23.3	26.0	31.7	36.5	12.0
4.16	15.1	17.3	20.8	23.8	26.5	32.2	37.0	12.0
12.47	17.6	19.7	23.6	26.3	29.0	34.7	39.5	13.5
13.2	17.8	20.0	23.5	26.5	29.2	34.9	39.7	13.8
13.8	18.0	23.7	26.7	29.4	35.1	39.9	14.0	
14.4	18.2	20.3	3.8	26.9	29.6	35.3	40.1	14.3
24.94	21.3	23.5	27.0	30.0	32.8	38.4	43.2	18.5
34.5	24.2	26.2	29.9	32.9	35.6	41.3	46.1	22.4
46	27.7	29.8	33.3	36.4	39.1	44.8	49.6	26.9

Source: American National Standards Institute, *National Electrical Safety Code*, 1984 edn., IEEE, New York, 1984.

steel have been used for street lighting because of their neat appearances. Steel poles have been used to support trolley OHs and street and parkway lighting. Both concrete and steel poles have been used to a limited extent for distribution. Aluminum poles are used basically for parkway lighting.

The life of wood poles is materially extended by impregnation with wood preservatives. Wood that has been properly treated for the environment in which it will be used will resist decay and maintain its mechanical strength for many years. A minimum life expectancy of 35 years has been accepted by the wood industry [3]. Cedar, pine, and fir are best suited by their proportions and properties for use as distribution poles.

Besides their usage in distribution systems, wood structures have been utilized for many years as a means of supporting single- and double-circuit transmission lines at voltages of 115–230 kV and single circuit of 345 kV. As a result of developing technology, wood structures have recently been designed for applications up to 765 kV and tested for 500 kV [3].

Wood structure design is based on an assigned or calculated ultimate stress for the species used. The inherent flexibility of wood adds a certain degree of cushion when severe loadings are imposed. This property provides wood construction the ability to absorb shock loads and longitudinal load capability not found in rigid structures.

Figure 12.6 shows some typical single-column wood structure designs used in distribution systems. Figure 12.7 shows typical single-column structure designs. Single wood column designs have been used for double-circuit lines through 230 kV and appear feasible for 345 kV. Structures using two columns, as shown in Figure 12.8, provide the basis for conventional H-frame designs with variations. Wood crossarms are normally used, although metal arms are sometimes specified. Double-circuit structures have been built using two columns for voltages through 230 kV and appear feasible for double circuits of 345 kV.

In distribution systems, single poles are widely used to support three transformer banks and their fused disconnects and surge arresters. A-frame poles are used where greater strength is required, and H-frame poles are used where it is necessary to support switching equipment and/or a transformer as well as the line.

The poles must have sufficient height and be so located as to provide adequate ground clearance at either maximum loading or maximum temperature condition. The conductor ground clearance for

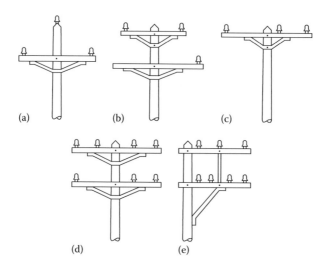

FIGURE 12.6 Typical single-pole designs used in distribution systems: (a) pole top, (b) two arms, (c) single arm, (d) line arms, and (e) side arms.

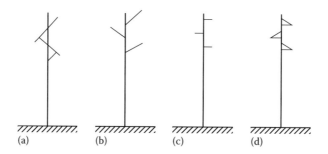

FIGURE 12.7 Typical single-column designs: (a) wishbone design, (b) unbraced upswept arms, (c) horizontal line post, and (d) braced horizontal arms.

railroad tracks and wire line crossings, as well as from buildings and other subjects, must meet the requirements of the NESC and other local rules and regulations. In essence, the height of a pole required for a particular location is determined by the following factors:

1. Length of vertical pole space required for wires and equipment
2. Clearance required above ground or obstructions for wires and equipment
3. Sag of conductors
4. Depth of pole to be set in ground

In distribution systems, the most commonly used pole is the 35 ft pole, and poles shorter than 30 ft are generally not used. The 30ft pole may be used in alleys and on rear lot lines. The larger sizes are, of course, used for providing clearance over obstructions, for heavier leads, etc.

The size (i.e., class), or diameter, of the pole is determined by the strength required to endure the mechanical loading imposed upon it. The critical point of strength for an unguyed pole at or near the ground line, therefore, the circumference of the pole at this point, determines the resisting moment of the pole when bending as a cantilever. However, if a pole is guyed, the diameter of the pole at the point of attachment of the guy is the measure of its strength. The resisting moment at the point

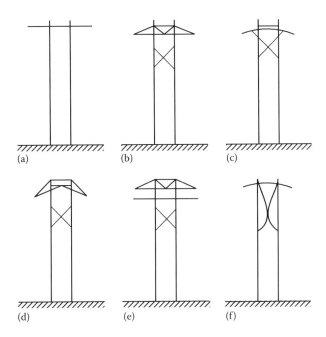

FIGURE 12.8 Typical two-column designs: (a) unbraced H-frame, (b) H-frame with wood (solid or laminated) crossarm, (c) H-frame with curved laminated crossarm, (d) K-frame, (e) double-circuit H-frame, and (f) Dreyfus design.

of guy attachment must be sufficient to endure the bending stresses caused at that point. Also, the top of the pole must be of adequate circumference to permit the attachment of crossarms without excessively weakening the pole near the top.

The wood poles are divided into several classes according to top circumference and the circumference 6 ft from the butt end for each nominal length. The word *class* refers to the dimensional classifications set up by the American Standards Association. The classes are numbered from 1 to 10. Class 1 provides the largest ground circumference and class 7 the smallest. Classes 8 to 10 specify minimum top circumferences only.

All poles in a given class, regardless of length, have approximately the same strength against load applied horizontally at the top. Table 12.6 gives the standard pole dimensions for yellow pine, chestnut, and western cedar. In order to identify any particular wood pole, its class, pole length, and wood type should be given.

12.7.2 Soil Types and Pole Setting

A stable pole must have sufficient setting depth. Table 12.7 provides minimum depth of pole settings. However, the distribution engineer chooses the depth of settings as the situation dictates. For example, corner poles should have about 6 in. deeper settings. Of course, the stability or rigidity of the pole depends not only on the depth of setting but also on the type of earth, moisture content of soil, size of pole butt, and setting technique used. Figure 12.9 shows some of the pole butt and setting techniques used. Figure 12.9 shows some of the setting techniques.

Earth can be classified into eight different groups, as given in Table 12.8, for the purpose of settings. Table 12.8 also gives the resistance S, as percentage of pole ultimate resisting moments, that the earth around the pole base shows to displacement for various earth types [4]. The values given in the table are somewhat arbitrary, and based on the assumptions that the pole setting is standard, the hole diameter is minimum, and the backfilling is properly tamped.

TABLE 12.6
Standard Wood Pole Dimensions

Class		1	2	3	4		6	7
Minimum Top Circumference (in.)		27	25	23	21	19	17	15
Minimum Top Diameter (in.)		8.6	8.0	7.3	6.7	6.1	5.4	4.8
Pole Length (ft)	**Wood Type[a]**	**Minimum Circumference at Ground Level (in.)**						
25	P	34.5	32.5	30.0	28.0	26.0	24.0	22.0
	C	37.0	34.5	32.5	30.0	28.0	25.5	24.0
	W	38.0	35.5	33.0	30.5	28.5	26.0	24.5
30	P	37.5	35.0	32.5	30.0	28.0	26.0	24.0
	C	40.0	37.5	35.0	32.5	30.0	28.0	26.0
	W	41.0	38.5	35.5	33.0	30.5	28.5	26.5
35	P	40.0	37.5	35.0	32.0	30.0	27.5	25.5
	C	42.5	40.0	37.5	34.5	32.0	30.0	27.5
	W	43.5	41.0	38.0	35.5	32.5	30.5	28.0
40	P	42.0	39.5	37.0	34.0	31.5	29.0	27.0
	C	45.0	42.5	39.5	36.5	34.0	31.5	29.5
	W	46.0	43.5	40.5	37.5	34.5	32.0	30.0
45	P	44.0	41.5	38.5	36.0	33.0	30.5	28.5
	C	47.5	44.5	41.5	38.5	36.0	33.0	31.0
	W	48.5	45.5	42.5	39.5	36.5	33.5	31.5
50	P	46.0	43.0	40.0	37.5	34.5	32.0	29.5
	C	49.5	46.5	43.5	40.0	37.5	34.5	32.0
	W	50.5	47.5	44.5	41.0	38.0	35.0	32.5
55	P	47.5	44.5	41.5	39.0	36.0	33.5	
	C	51.5	48.5	45.0	42.0	39.0	36.0	
	W	52.5	49.5	46.0	42.5	39.5	36.5	
60	P	49.5	46.0	43.0	40.0	37.0	34.5	
	C	53.5	50.0	46.5	43.0	40.0	37.5	
	W	54.5	51.0	47.5	44.0	41.0	38.5	
65	P	51.0	47.5	44.5	41.5	38.5		
	C	55.0	51.5	48.0	45.0	42.0		
	W	56.0	52.5	49.0	45.5	42.5		
70	P	52.5	49.0	46.0	42.5	39.5		
	C	56.5	53.0	48.5	45.5	43.5		
	W	57.5	54.0	50.5	47.0	45.0		
75	P	54.0	50.5	47.0	44.0			
	C	59.0	54.0	50.0	47.0			
	W	59.5	55.5	52.0	48.5			

[a] Yellow pine, chestnut, and western cedar are denoted as P, C, and W, respectively.

TABLE 12.7
Minimum Required Setting Depths

Pole size (ft)	30	35	40	45	50	55	60	70
Setting depth (ft)	5	5.5	6	6.5	6.5	7	7	7.5

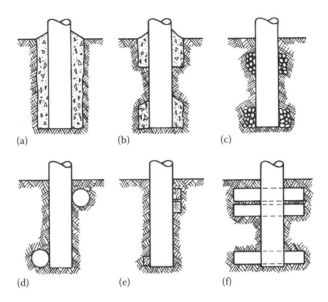

FIGURE 12.9 Setting techniques: (a) full-concrete setting, (b) concrete setting, (c) crushed stone setting, (d) plain earth setting, (e) heel-and-breast concrete blocks setting, and (f) bolted-timber setting.

TABLE 12.8
Various Earth Resistance to Displacement

Class	Earth Type	Percentage of Pole Resisting Moment, S_e
1	Hard rock	50
2	Shale, sandstone, or soft rock	50
3	Hard, dry hardpan	50
4	Crumbly, damp	40
5	Firm, moist	35
6	Plastic, wet	30
7	Loose, dry of loose, wet	25
8	Swamps, marshes	20

Source: Hubbard, A. and Watkins, W., *Electr. World*, 128, 94, 1947.

12.8 MECHANICAL CALCULATIONS

12.8.1 INTRODUCTION

In general, the forces acting on a given supporting structure, for example, the pole, are as follows:

1. Vertical forces due to the weight of the pole, conductors, and ice clinging to conductors
2. Vertical forces due to downward pull of guys
3. Lateral horizontal forces due to wind across line pole, conductors, ice, etc.
4. Longitudinal horizontal forces due to unbalanced pull of conductors
5. Torsional forces due to unbalanced pull of conductors

Any given pole is strong for vertical forces but weak for horizontal forces, and any given crossarm is weak for the torsional forces. In order to achieve a good line design, the horizontal and torsional forces should be reduced to a minimum by balancing the stresses, and the remains of unbalanced horizontal stresses should be transformed into vertical stresses on the pole by the use of guys. Hence, the strength of a wood pole must be sufficient to withstand transverse forces, such as wind pressure, on the pole and conductors, unbalanced pull on conductors when they are broken, and side pull on curves and corners where guys cannot be used. These forces place the fiber of the wood under tension, and the load a pole can carry is determined by the inherent strength of its wood fiber under tension and the moments of forces.

However, the calculations for the strength of a given pole, at best, give only approximate results since there will usually be a slight movement of the pole at the ground level. Therefore, the calculated fiber stress can be different than the actual value. In order to find the length of an unguyed span for a given height, kind, and class of pole, the bending moment of the pole at the ground level, which is usually the point of failure, is calculated. It is assumed that the pole is set in firm soil. The minimum radial thicknesses of ice and the wind pressures to be used in calculating loadings for the specified wind loading under light-, medium-, and heavy-loading conditions are given by the NESC.

There are two bending moments of wind affecting the pole:

1. The bending moment due to wind on the conductors
2. The bending moment due to wind on the pole itself

12.8.2 Bending Moment due to Wind on Conductors

The bending moment is equal to the force applied times its distance in inches (at right angles to its direction) from the point, that is, its moment arm, whose strength is being considered (see Figure 12.10). Therefore, the total bending moment due to wind on the conductors is

$$M_{tc} = \sum_{i=1}^{m}\sum_{j=1}^{n} m_i \times n_{ij} \times PL_{avg} \times h_{ij} \ \ \text{lb}\cdot\text{ft} \tag{12.6}$$

where
  M is the total bending moment due to wind on conductors in pound feet
  m is the number of crossarms on pole
  n is the number of conductors on each crossarm
  P is the transversal and horizontal wind force (i.e., load) exerted on line in pounds per feet
  L_{avg} is the average span in feet
  h_{ij} is the height of conductor j on crossarm i in feet

The amount of transversal and horizontal wind load exerted on the conductors depends on whether or not the conductors are covered with ice. This topic is discussed in greater detail in Section 13.5.

In Figure 12.11, L_{avg} represents the average horizontal span, and it is equal to one-half the length of the two adjacent spans L_1 and L_2. Here, the L_{avg} can be calculated as

$$L_{avg} = \frac{L_1 + L_2}{2} \quad \text{when} \ L_1 \neq L_2 \tag{12.7}$$

or

$$L_{avg} = L_1 = L_2 = L \quad \text{when} \ L_1 = L_2$$

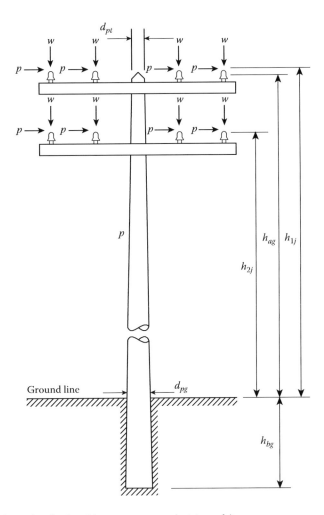

FIGURE 12.10   Schematic of pole with two crossarms (not to scale).

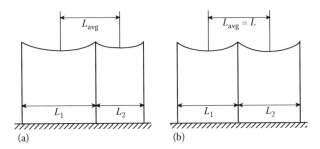

FIGURE 12.11   Pole-loading diagrams: (a) when two adjacent spans are not equal to each other and (b) when two adjacent spans are equal to each other.

12.8.3   Bending Moment due to the Wind on the Poles

The bending moment due to the wind on the pole (see Figure 12.10), which is usually a maximum at the ground level of an unguyed pole, is

$$M_{gp} = \frac{p \times h_{ag}^2}{72} \left(d_{pg} + 2d_{pt} \right) \ \text{lb} \cdot \text{ft} \tag{12.8}$$

or

$$M_{gp} = \frac{p \times h_{ag}^2}{72} \left(c_{pg} + 2c_{pt} \right) \ \text{lb} \cdot \text{ft} \tag{12.9}$$

where
M_{gp} is the bending moment due to wind on pole in pound feet
h_{ag} is the height of pole above ground in feet
d_{pg} is the diameter of pole at ground line in inches
d_{pt} is the diameter of pole at pole top in inches
p is the wind pressure in pounds per square feet
c_{pg} is the circumference of pole at ground line in inches
c_{pt} is the circumference of pole at pole top in inches

The internal resisting moment of the wood pole, when the maximum stress is at the ground line, is

$$M = \frac{1}{3790} S \times c_{pg}^3 \ \text{lb} \cdot \text{ft} \tag{12.10}$$

or

$$M = 2.6385 \times 10^{-4} S \times c_{pg}^3 \ \text{lb} \cdot \text{ft} \tag{12.11}$$

where the maximum stress is aboveground line,

$$M = 2.6385 \times 10^{-4} S \times c_1^2 \left(c_{pg} - c_1 \right) \ \text{lb} \cdot \text{ft} \tag{12.12}$$

where
M is the bending moment at ground line in pound feet
c_{pg} is the circumference of pole at ground line in inches
c_1 is the circumference of pole at point of maximum stress
S is the allowable maximum fiber stress in pounds per square inch

where

$$S = \frac{\text{ultimate fiber strength of pole}}{\text{safety factor}} \tag{12.13}$$

TABLE 12.9
Resisting Moments of Wood Poles

Pole Circumference at Ground (in.)	Pound Feet at One-Half Ultimate Fiber Stress Ratings of (lb/in.^{2})						
	8,400	**8,000**	**7,400**	**6,600**	**6,000**	**5,600**	**4,000**
28	24,300	23,150	21,400	19,150	17,350	16,250	11,550
30	29,900	28,500	26,350	23,500	21,350	19,950	14,250
32	36,300	34,600	32,000	28,500	25,950	24,200	17,300
34	43,600	41,500	38,400	34,200	31,150	29,000	20,750
36	51,750	49,300	45,600	40,700	36,950	34,450	24,650
38	60,750	57,850	53,500	47,800	43,400	40,550	28,900
40	70,950	67,550	62,500	55,700	50,650	47,250	33,800
42	82,200	78,250	72,400	64,400	58,700	54,700	39,150
44	94,450	89,950	83,200	74,100	67,450	62,900	44,950
46	107,950	102,800	95,100	84,600	77,100	71,900	51,400
48	122,600	116,750	108,000	96,200	87,550	81,700	58,350
50	138,600	132,000	122,100	108,700	99,000	92,300	66,000
52	155,850	148,400	137,300	122,400	111,300	103,900	74,200

Source: Fink, D.G. and Carroll, J.M., eds., *Standard Handbook for Electrical Engineers*, 10th edn., McGraw-Hill, New York, 1969. With permission.

The minimum safety factors required, according to the grades of construction, are given by the NESC. Table 12.9 provides the resisting moments of wood poles, given circumference of the pole at the ground line, and ultimate fiber stress rating of the pole [4].

The condition that a given pole will not break is

$$M > M_{tc} + M_{gp}$$

Fiber stress should not be more than 15% than at the breaking point for normal unbalanced forces, for example, forces affecting an unguyed corner pole. For wind pressures and an unbalanced force of broken conductors that are abnormal and do not persist, the stress is usually used at about 50% of that at breaking point.

Equation 12.11 is based on the assumption that the ground line is the weakest point of the pole. This is not so correct, especially for northern cedar or other wood poles tapering 1 in. in 5–6 ft of length and being approximately a truncated cone in shape. For a bending loading, that is, force applied at one end, such a cone is weakest at the point where the diameter is 3/2 or 1.5 the diameter at the point (near the small end) where the result and load or force is applied.

For example, a pole with a 10 in. diameter at the crossarm is weakest where it is 15 in. in diameter. If a northern cedar pole has a taper of 1 in. in 6 ft of length, the weakest point would be $6 \times (15 - 10) = 30$ ft below the crossarms.

However, in practice, the weakest section of the pole is taken at ground line since the pole at that point tends to become weaker than any point above ground as a result of its greater moisture content and its greater tendency to decay as the pole ages.

Since pole-top transformers impose not only vertical but also transversal loading on poles, the wood poles used to carry transformers greater than 25 kVA are usually selected having a pole-top diameter of 1 in. or larger than would be required elsewhere. Usually, a transformer of 300 kVA or greater is installed on a platform supported by two wood poles placed 10–15 ft apart.

Example 12.2

Assume a 35 ft pole set 6 ft in ground, with a 28 in. circumference at the pole top and a 40 in. circumference at ground level. Also assume a wind velocity of 40 mi/h and an average span of 120 ft. The conductor used is 4/0 copper of 0.81 in. diameter. There are eight conductors on the line, as shown in Figure 12.10. Calculate the following:

(a) Total pressure of wind on pole
(b) Total pressure of wind on conductors

Solution

(a) Using Equation 12.1,

$$p = 0.00256V^2$$

$$= 0.00256 \times 40^2$$

$$= 4.096 \text{ lb/ft}^2$$

The projected area of the pole is

$$S_{pni} = \left(\frac{d_{pg} + d_{pt}}{2} \right) h_{ag} \times 12 \text{ in.}^2 \tag{12.14}$$

where
  d_{pg} is the diameter of pole at ground line in inches
  d_{pt} is the diameter of pole at pole top in inches
  h_{ag} is the height of pole above ground in feet

Therefore,

$$S_{pni} = \frac{1}{2}(12.7 + 8.9) \times 29 \times 12$$

$$= 3758.4 \text{ in.}^2$$

or

$$= 3758.4 \text{ in.}^2 \times 0.0069444 \text{ ft}^2/\text{in.}^2$$

$$\cong 26.1 \text{ ft}^2$$

Hence, the total pressure of the wind on the pole is

$$P = S_{pni} \times p$$

$$= 26.1 \times 4.096$$

$$= 106.9 \text{ lb} \tag{12.15}$$

(b) The diameter of the conductor is 0.810 in. Therefore, the projected area of the conductor, a 120 ft span, is

$$S_{pni} = 0.810 \text{ in} \times 120 \text{ ft} \times 12 \text{ in./ft}$$

$$= 1166.4 \text{ in.}^2$$

or

$$= 1166 \text{ in.}^2 \times 0.006944 \text{ ft}^2/\text{in.}^2$$

$$= 8.1 \text{ ft}^2$$

Thus, the total pressure of the wind on the conductors is

$$P = S_{pni} \times p$$

$$= 8 \times 8.1 \text{ ft}^2 \times 4.096 \text{ lb/ft}^2$$

$$= 265.4 \text{ lb} \tag{12.16}$$

Example 12.3

A section of an OH line needs to be built on 45 ft wood poles set 6.5 ft deep in the ground. Each pole will carry two crossarms, and each crossarm has four conductors, as shown in Figure 12.10. The top crossarm will be 1 ft below the pole top, and the lower crossarm will be 3 ft below the pole top. The conductors located on the top crossarm and on the lower crossarm have transverse wind loads of 0.6861 and 0.4769 lb/ft of conductor, respectively. The rated ultimate strength of the wood pole is 8000 lb/in.^{2} and a safety factor of 2. Assume that the transverse wind load on the wood poles will not exceed 9clb/ft^2. Calculate the minimum required pole circumference at the ground line if the average span is 250 ft.

Solution

First, let us find the moment arms:

For the top arm, $h_{1j} = 45 - 6.5 - 1 = 37.5$ ft
For the lower arm, $h_{2j} = 45 - 6.5 - 3 = 35.5$ ft

By using Equation 12.6, the total bending moment due to wind on the conductors is

$$M_{tc} = \sum_{i=1}^{2}\sum_{j=1}^{4} m_i \times n_{ij} \times PL_{avg} \times h_{ij} \text{ lb} \cdot \text{ft}$$

For the top arm,

$$M_{tc} = 1 \times 4 \times 0.6861 \times 250 \times 37.5 = 25{,}729 \text{ lb} \cdot \text{ft}$$

For the lower arm,

$$M_{tc} = 1 \times 4 \times 0.4769 \times 250 \times 35.5 \cong 16{,}930 \text{ lb} \cdot \text{ft}$$

Then, for both crossarms together,

$$M_{tc} = 25{,}729 + 16{,}930 = 42{,}659 \text{ lb} \cdot \text{ft}$$

Using Equation 12.11, the internal resisting moment of the pole is

$$M = 2.6385 \times 10^{-4} \times S \times c^3$$

where

$$M = 42{,}659 \text{ lb} \cdot \text{ft}$$

$$S = \frac{8000}{2} = 400 \text{ psi}$$

Therefore,

$$c_{pg}^3 = \frac{M}{2.6385 \times 10^{-4} \times S}$$

$$= \frac{42{,}659}{2.6385 \times 10^{-4} \times 4000}$$

$$\cong 40{,}419.8$$

Hence,

$$c_{pg} = 34.3 \text{ in.}$$

Assume that, from the proper tables, the minimum pole-top circumference for the kind of pole corresponding to an ultimate fiber stress of 8000 psi is found to be 22 in. Therefore, the bending moment due to wind on the pole, using Equation 12.9, is

$$M_{gp} = \frac{p \times h_{ag}^2}{72} \left(c_{pg} + 2c_{pt} \right)$$

$$= \frac{9 \times (38.5)^2}{72\pi} (34.3 + 2 \times 22)$$

$$\cong 4618 \text{ lb} \cdot \text{ft}$$

Therefore, the total bending moment due to wind on conductors and pole is

$$M_T = M_{tc} + M_{gp}$$

$$= 42{,}659 + 4{,}618$$

$$= 47{,}277 \text{ lb} \cdot \text{ft}$$

Using Equation 12.11,

$$c_{pg}^3 = \frac{42{,}277}{2.6485 \times 10^{-4} \times 400}$$

$$\cong 44{,}795$$

or the required minimum circumference of the pole at the ground line is

$$c = 35.5 \text{ in.}$$

Therefore, the nearest standard size pole, which has a ground line circumference larger than 35.5 in., has to be used. Instead of using Equation 12.11 to find the required minimum circumference of the pole at ground level, one can find it directly from Table 12.9 as 36 in., which is a standard size.

12.8.4 Stress due to the Angle in the Line

If there is an angle in the line, an additional stress is imposed upon the supporting structure at the angle point because of the tensions in the conductors. Figure 12.12 shows a plan view of a diagram of the forces acting on an angle pole.

If the conductors in the adjacent spans have equal tensions of T and the angle of departure of the line is α, the resultant side pull force on the pole is T_r. This force can be calculated by using the following formula:

$$T_r = 2 \times n \times T_1 \times \sin\frac{\alpha}{2} \text{ lb} \tag{12.17}$$

where
    T_r is the resultant side pull force due to angle in line in pounds
    n is the number of conductors on pole
    T_1 is the maximum tension in conductors in pounds
    α is the angle departure of line in degrees

When this force is large enough, the bending stress may become greater than the allowable working stress or even the ultimate fiber strength of the pole. Because of this, it must be balanced by the guy wire.

If the conductor tensions in the adjacent spans are not equal, then the resultant side pull force is

$$T_1 = \sqrt{T_1^2 + T_2^2 - 2T_1 \times T_2 \cos\alpha} \text{ lb} \tag{12.18}$$

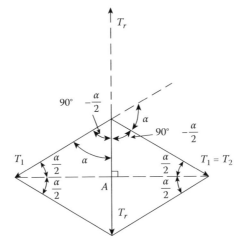

FIGURE 12.12 Plan view of angle pole and diagram of forces.

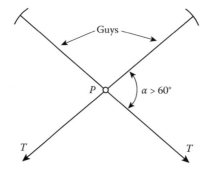

FIGURE 12.13 Installment of two guys when angle of departure of line is larger than 60°.

and the angle γ between the resultant and the span in which the tension T_1 is obtained from can be determined from

$$\cos\gamma = \frac{T_r^2 + T_1^2 - T_2^2}{2T_rT_1} \tag{12.19}$$

where γ is the angle between direction of resultant and direction of either span, that is, $90° - \alpha/2$.

If the angle departure of the line is less than 60°, the resultant side pull force is less than the maximum tension of the conductors in the adjacent spans. Therefore, one single guy installed in the opposite direction of the resultant side pull force, as shown in Figure 12.13, will be sufficient.

However, if the angle departure of the line is larger than 60°, the resultant side pull force is larger than the maximum tension of the conductors in the adjacent spans. In order to stop a tendency to displace the pole if the angle does not exactly bisect the line angle and not use a guy of extreme strength, install two guys each located in the opposite direction of the line, as shown in Figure 12.13.

12.8.5 Strength Determination of an Angle Pole

In order to determine whether a given pole, which will be used as an angle pole in the line, has the required strength to meet the NESC requirements, the following equation is used [5]:

$$M = \frac{M_{gp} + M_{tc}}{S_1} \times 100 + \frac{M_r}{S_2} \times 100 \ \text{lb} \cdot \text{ft} \tag{12.20}$$

where
    M is the required internal resisting moment of pole in pound feet
    M_{gp} is the total bending moment due to wind on pole in pound feet
    M_{tc} is the total bending moment due to wind on conductors in pound feet
    M_r is the bending moment due to tensions in conductors in pound feet
    S_1 is the permissible stress in pole for transverse loading, in percentage of ultimate fiber strength
    S_2 is the permissible stress in pole, for longitudinal loading at dead ends, in percentage of ultimate fiber strength

Here,

$$M_r = T_r \times h \ \text{lb} \cdot \text{ft} \tag{12.21}$$

or

$$M_r = 2n \times h \times T \times \sin\frac{\alpha}{2} \ \text{lb}\cdot\text{ft} \tag{12.22}$$

which has to be calculated for every conductor and added together. Theoretically, if M is larger than the ultimate resisting moment of the pole, use guy; otherwise, do not. However, in practice, if the pole does not have a proper rigid setting, there is still a need for the guy.

12.8.6 PERMISSIBLE MAXIMUM ANGLE WITHOUT GUYS

It is almost impossible to build an OH line of any considerable length, especially transmission lines, without several angles, which may vary in magnitude from only a few degrees to 90° or more. The earth settings, depending on earth type, may allow a certain amount of pole stresses, which are caused by angles in the line, to be in excess of the permissible fiber stress of a given wood pole. If the conductor tensions in the adjacent spans are equal, the allowable maximum angle, without any side guying, in a given line can be found from the following equation:

$$M_{tc} + M_{gp} + 2n \times h \times T \times \sin\frac{\alpha}{2} = \left(\frac{S_e}{100}\right)M \tag{12.23}$$

where
  M_{tc} is the total bending moment due to wind on conductors in pound feet
  M_{gp} is the bending moment due to wind on pole in pound feet
  T is the maximum tension of conductors in adjacent spans in pounds
  h_{ag} is the height of pole above ground in feet
  α is the angle of departure of line
  S_e is the earth resistance to displacement, in percentage of pole internal resisting moment
  M is the required internal resisting moment of pole in pound feet

If a given angle in the line is larger than the allowable maximum angle obtained from Equation 9.23 or if the earth resistance to displacement is not large enough, then a guy or guys need to be used.

12.8.7 GUYING

Whenever a pole is not strong enough to endure the bending stresses imposed on it by unbalanced forces, it should be guyed. For example, at the pole where the direction of a line changes, the tension of the conductor should be supported by guying to other poles, to a ground anchor, or to a

The strength of a guy should be large enough to take the entire horizontal stress in the direction in which it acts, the pole acting only as a strut taking only the vertical component of guy tension. Special structures such as A-frames and push braces are sometimes used instead of guys in some applications; but the most common technique is to install guys or steel wire or other high-strength material to take the stress. Figure 12.14 illustrates various guying techniques. Figure 12.15 shows a plan and elevation views of a guy installation at an angle. Figure 12.16 shows a dead-end guy installation.

Guys are firmly attached to poles by wrapping the end of the guy wire twice or more around the pole and clamping the free end to the main section of the guy, usually, by means of one or more guy clamps. However, nowadays, the guy is usually attached to the pole by a thimble-eye or by a guy eyebolt and a stubbing washer, as shown in Figure 12.17.

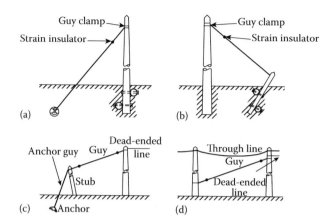

FIGURE 12.14　Various guying techniques: (a) anchor guy, (b) stub guy, (c) pole-to-stub-to-anchor guy, and (d) pole-to-pole guy.

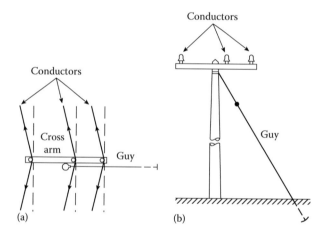

FIGURE 12.15　Guy installation at an angle: (a) plan and (b) elevation.

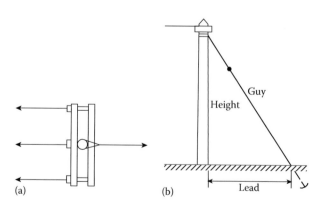

FIGURE 12.16　Dead-end guy installation: (a) plan and (b) elevation.

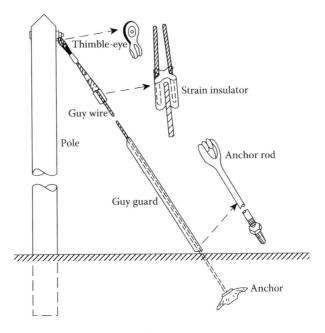

FIGURE 12.17 Components of anchor guy installation.

The attachment point of a guy should be as close as possible to the point where the resultant side pull force is imposed upon the supporting structure. If there are several crossarms mounted on the pole at different elevations, then the load at those elevations has to be converted to an equivalent load applied at the level where the guy is attached.

Usually, one or two strain insulators* are installed in guys to prohibit the lower part from becoming electrically energized by contact of the upper part with conductors or by leakage. Figure 12.17 shows the basic components of an anchor wire guy, which include the guy wire, clamps, the anchor, and a strain insulator. The guy wire is usually copperweld, galvanized, or bethanized steel.

Burring logs, which were called deadmen, in the ground to anchor the guy wire, as shown in Figure 12.14c, have been abandoned since the soil conditions often deteriorated the wood. Instead, in the present practice, metal anchors are used in any type of ground from swamp to solid rock.

12.8.8 CALCULATION OF GUY TENSION

Consider the dead-end pole supported by a guy wire, as shown in Figure 12.18. Assume that the line conductors are carried by the pole at two different heights. The resultant side pull is counterbalanced by the tension in the guy wire. This tension T_g can be resolved into two components, T_h and T_v. The summation of the bending moments created by T_1 and T_2 loads at heights h_1 and h_2, respectively, must be balanced by the bending moment created by T_h:

$$T_h \times h_g = T_r \times h_g \tag{12.24}$$

or

$$T_h \times h_g = T_1 \times h_1 + T_2 \times h_2 \tag{12.25}$$

---

* However, there is also the widespread use of uninsulated, grounded guys on multigrounded neutral distribution systems.

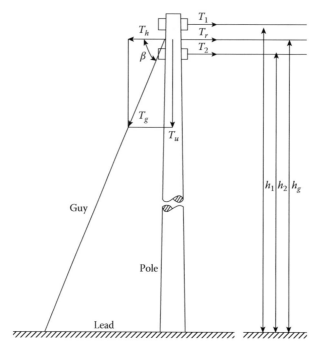

FIGURE 12.18 Guy-loading diagram.

Therefore, the horizontal component of the tension in the guy wire is

$$T_h = \frac{1}{h_g}\left(T_1 \times h_1 + T_2 \times h_2\right)$$

(12.26)

where
   T_h is the horizontal component of guy wire tension in pounds
   T_1 is the horizontal load at height h_1 in pounds
   T_2 is the horizontal load at height h_2 in pounds
   h_g is the height of attachment point of guy in feet
   h_1 is the height of horizontal load T_1 in feet
   h_2 is the height of horizontal load T_2 in feet

From Figure 12.18,

$$\tan \beta = \frac{h_g}{L}$$

(12.27)

or

$$\beta = \arctan\left(\frac{h_g}{L}\right)$$

(12.28)

where L is the lead of the guy in feet. Then, the tension in the guy wire is

$$T_g = \frac{T_h}{\cos \beta}$$

(12.29)

or

$$T_g = T_h \times \sec \beta \tag{12.30}$$

Also,

$$T_g = T_r \sqrt{1 + \left(\frac{h_g}{L}\right)^2} \tag{12.31}$$

since

$$T_r = T_h \quad \text{and} \quad \sec \beta = \sqrt{1 + \left(\frac{h_g}{L}\right)^2}$$

Further,

$$\tan \beta = \frac{h_g}{L} \tag{12.32}$$

or

$$\tan \beta = \frac{T_v}{T_h} \tag{12.33}$$

and the vertical component of the tension in the guy wire is

$$T_v = T_h \times \tan \beta \tag{12.34}$$

or

$$T_v = T_h \left(\frac{h_g}{L}\right) \tag{12.35}$$

Therefore, the total vertical load on the pole is

$$W_v = \frac{T_h \times h_g}{L} + W_e + W_p \text{ lb} \tag{12.36}$$

where
W_v is the total vertical load on pole in pounds
W_p is the weight of pole in pounds
W_e is the weight of equipment, hardware, and conductors on the pole in pounds

As the angle β decreases, the tension T_g in the guy wire and its vertical component T_v also decreases, despite the fact that the horizontal component of the guy wire tension T_h stays the same. Therefore, in practice, the tangent of the angle β should be held minimum.

If the attachment point of a given guy is too far from the center of the horizontal loads T_1 and T_2, the stress in the pole at that point may become important. Thus, the bending moment of the pole at the point of attachment becomes

$$M = T_1(h_1 - h_g) + T_2(h_2 - h_g) \text{ lb} \cdot \text{ft} \tag{12.37}$$

It should be kept less than the required minimum pole resisting moment.

Example 12.4

A dead-end pole is supported by a guy wire, as shown in Figure 12.18. The bending moments are created by 3000 and 2500 lb at heights of 37.5 and 35.5 ft, respectively. The guy is attached to a pole at the height of 36.5 ft. The lead of the guy is lift. Calculate the following:

(a) Horizontal component of tension in guy wire
(b) Angle β
(c) Vertical component of tension in guy wire
(d) Tension in guy wire

Solution

(a) Using Equation 12.26,

$$T_h = \frac{T_1 \times h_1 + T_2 \times h_2}{h_g}$$

$$= \frac{3000 \times 37.5 + 2500 \times 35.5}{36.5}$$

$$\cong 5513.7 \ \text{lb}$$

(b) Using Equation 12.28,

$$\beta = \arctan\left(\frac{h_g}{L}\right)$$

$$= \arctan\left(\frac{36.5}{15}\right)$$

$$\cong 67.6°$$

(c) Using Equation 12.34,

$$T_v = T_h \tan\beta$$

$$= 5513.7 \tan 67.6°$$

$$\cong 13{,}416.67 \ \text{lb}$$

(d) Using Equation 12.29,

$$T_g = \frac{T_h}{\cos\beta}$$

$$= \frac{5513.7}{\cos 67.6°}$$

$$\cong 14{,}505.4 \ \text{lb}$$

or from

$$T_g = \sqrt{T_h^2 + T_v^2}$$

$$= \sqrt{5513.7^2 + 13{,}416.67^2}$$

$$\cong 14{,}505.4 \ \text{lb}$$

12.9 GRADE OF CONSTRUCTION

The criterion used for the strength of requirements of a line is called the *grade of construction*. The grades of construction are specified on the basis of the required strengths for safety. The NESC designates the grades for supply and communication lines by the letters B, C, D, E, and N. Grade B is the highest and requires the greatest strength. Grade D is specified only for communication lines, and it is higher than grade N.

The grade used depends on the type of circuit, the voltage, and the surroundings of the line. For example, a power line of any voltage crossing over a main track of a railroad requires grade B construction, but under certain other conditions may be as low as grade N. In addition to the NESC requirements, there are also local rules and regulations for the grades of construction.

12.10 LINE CONDUCTORS

Copper and aluminum are the metals most frequently used as conductors in distribution systems. The selection criteria include conductivity, cost, mechanical strength, and weight. According to these selection criteria, copper conductor is the best and aluminum conductor is the second best conductor in terms of conductivity and availability. Aluminum has the advantage of about 70% less weight for a given size, but its conductivity is only about 61% that of annealed copper. Its breaking strength is about 43% that of hard-drawn copper. In general, aluminum conductor is rated as equivalent to a copper conductor two AWG sizes smaller, which has almost identical resistance.

The factors affecting voltage drop, power loss, and mechanical strength to prevent excessive sag are important in selecting the type of conductor for OH lines. In order to obtain proper ground clearance without excessively increasing the height of poles, for rural OH distribution lines with lower load densities and longer spans, conductors of high tensile strength are usually preferable. However, for urban underground distribution, serving high-load density areas, current-carrying capacity and voltage drop are more important in selecting the conductor type.

The relatively small diameter of copper conductors, solid or stranded, in comparison with their current-carrying capacity, allows a minimum of projected area to wind and ice loads. This provides a greater safety factor for the poles and demands only a minimum of guying against transverse loading.

However, because of its comparatively low ratio of strength to weight, copper conductors necessarily require greater sag for a given span length when compared with copperweld or ASCR conductors. Because of this greater sag, higher poles or shorter spans have been used to provide adequate ground clearance at maximum temperature conditions.

Copper wires or cables are made in three standard degrees of hardness: (1) hard drawn, (2) medium hard drawn, and (3) soft drawn. Hard-drawn copper has the greatest tensile strength and is used for OH lines with span lengths of 200 ft or more. Medium- to hard-drawn copper has less tensile strength and is used for common types of local distribution OH lines with shorter span lengths. Soft-drawn copper has the least tensile strength and is used almost only for underground cables because of its greater flexibility. Maximum transmission capacity for a given power loss and voltage drop is the largest for hard-drawn copper conductors. Hard-drawn wire is cold-drawn to size from a stock copper bar. This cold-drawing process increases the tensile strength of the copper, hardens it, and slightly decreases its conductivity.

If a hard-drawn copper wire is heated at the proper temperature for a specific time period, its small tensile strength decreases, and the wire becomes softer and more ductile and is said to be annealed. Medium- to hard-drawn copper is annealed after being cold-drawn to size and then cold-drawn to size and strength, whereas soft-drawn copper wire is cold-drawn to size and then annealed.

Aluminum stranded around a steel core sized to give the required strength is especially used in rural OH lines. It is called *aluminum cable steel-reinforced* and is commonly designated as ACSR.

The development of high-strength aluminum alloys has led to such alternative cables as ACAR and AAAC, which also combine conductivity with tensile strength.

Because of their high resistance, steel conductors are rarely used in distribution lines. But a high-strength steel strand covered with a thin sheet of copper welded on, known as *copperweld*, or with a thin sheet of aluminum welded on, known as *alumoweld*, has conductivity of about 40% that of copper and is used.

When a conductor of high conductivity and high tensile strength is required, copper strands combined with the copperweld strands form a conductor called *copperweld copper*. Another composite conductor is made out of hard-drawn aluminum strands combined with the alumoweld strands. Some guy cables are made out of copperweld or alumoweld since they are more durable than galvanized steel cables.

In general, the size of conductors used for an OH line is determined by the electric power to be transmitted and permissible voltage drop. The requirements for mechanical strength, however, place a minimum on the conductor size that is practical to use. The NESC specifies the minimum conductor sizes that are permissible to use.

12.11 INSULATOR TYPES

The OH line insulators are classified as (1) pin-type insulators, (2) suspension insulators, and (3) strain insulators. Pin-type insulators are used for LV and medium-voltage distribution lines. Suspension insulators are used for all voltage lines. Strain insulators are used in guys and for dead-ending LV lines.

Usually, pin-type or post-type insulators are used on the OH lines with not more than 70 kV. Above 70 kV, suspension insulators are used for dead-ending lines of any voltage, although small conductors of LV distribution lines are often dead-ended on double-arm construction using pin-type insulators.

Suspension insulators are also used for tangent and angle construction for practically all voltage lines. Suspension insulators are manufactured either with clevis-and-pin connections or with ball-and-socket connections. Both connection types are commonly used.

Pin insulators are generally mounted on pins bolted directly to the crossarms of the pole or tower. Pin insulators mounted on metal crossarms should be provided with metal pins that have sufficient length above the crossarm to ensure that flashover will take place on the pin rather than the crossarm. The method of attaching suspension insulator strings varies. In one of the attachment methods, a U-bolt is fastened on the underside of the crossarm to which the insulator hardware is attached. This would provide flexibility both longitudinally and transversely. In another method, in the form of a bent plate or angle, it is fastened to the underside of the crossarm with a sufficient hole to receive a hook or shackle at the top of the insulator string.

The minimum weight that should be allowed on a supporting structure may be obtained by calculating the transverse angle to which a suspension insulator string may swing without lessening the clearance from the conductor to the structure too much and by requiring that the ratio of vertical weight to horizontal wind load be maintained such as not to permit the insulator to swing beyond this angle. The maximum wind is assumed at a temperature of 60°F. However, the wind pressure in pounds per square feet to be applied in sag calculations is somewhat arbitrary, and it depends on local conditions.

The required minimum angle of conductor swing to be used in calculations, where nearness to other circuits is involved, is 30° according to the NESC. Usually, a clearance corresponding to about 75% of the flashover value of the insulator is sufficient. A suspension insulator swings in the direction of the resultant of the vertical and horizontal forces affecting the insulator swing. For further information, see Chapter 13.

Figure 12.19 shows a vee arrangement (V-strings) of suspension insulator strings carrying four bundled conductors per phase. Figure 12.19 shows a vee arrangement of suspension insulator strings

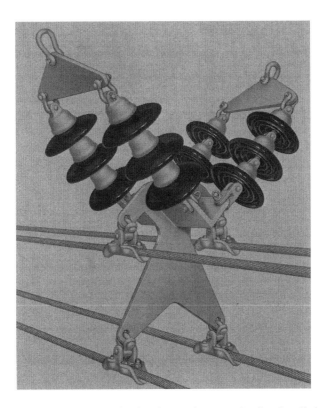

FIGURE 12.19 Vee arrangement of suspension insulator strings carrying four bundled conductors per phase. (Courtesy of Ohio Brass Company, Wadsworth, OH.)

carrying four bundled conductors per phase at 500 kV being installed. From a contamination point of view, the V-strings are more effective than vertical strings because of a *self-cleaning* possibility. Both sides of each insulator V-strings are exposed to the rain, allowing contaminants to be shed more effectively.

12.12 JOINT USE BY OTHER UTILITIES

There are advantages in the use of joint poles. However, when supporting structures of the OH lines are used jointly by other utilities, such as telephone or other communication systems, additional factors are introduced into the problem of line design beside those needing consideration in the case of power lines alone. For example, often a higher grade of construction is necessary, and consideration must be given the required separations between the conductors and equipment of the two utilities.

The cost of providing the pole is borne jointly by the companies that share in its ownership. In general, the allocation of the expense is made in proportion to the space assigned to owners. The cost of the clearance between higher-voltage and lower-voltage power circuits is usually charged to the higher-voltage circuits. However, the required clearance space, between power and communication circuits or between the lowest attachment and ground, is disregarded in determining percentage ownership. It is also possible that poles are used jointly under a lease agreement in which case the lessee has only the right to occupy a designated space.

In general, conductors are placed in such an order so that the higher-voltage conductors are at the higher levels. As a result of this, the highest-voltage circuits are near the pole top, and communication circuits are at a lower level, as shown in Figure 12.20.

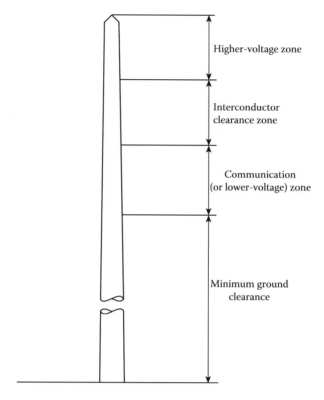

FIGURE 12.20 Allotment of pole space.

12.13 CONDUCTOR VIBRATION

The failure of conductors under tensions that are much below maximum design stresses has been caused by fatigue due to very fast vertical vibrations of the conductor (from 15 to possibly 100 Hz) caused by steady nonturbulent winds blowing across the line. In general, the mechanical vibrations in OH conductors and GWs are of six types:

1. *Aeolian vibration.* It is a resonant oscillation caused by vortex shedding from the leeward side of a conductor in a steady wind. Its amplitudes are of approximately one conductor diameter, with frequencies of oscillation on the order of 2–150 Hz. If uncorrected, these vibrations can cause chafing and fatigue failures of conductor strands, typically at oscillation nodes such as splices and suspension points. It causes wires to hum in the wind and the *whistle of wind* in the rigging of ships. Aeolian vibrations can be controlled by adding energy-dissipating vibration dampers (usually Stockbridge), which are attached to the conductor. Such dampers are a compound pendulum type of arrangement that detunes the vibrating conductor and absorbs enough of the energy to stop or greatly lessen vibration. Aeolian vibration can also be prevented by the use of armor rod and/or reduced conductor tensions and by the use of self-damped conductors that have recently been developed as another control alternative.

2. *Swinging of conductors caused by changes in wind pressure.* This type of vibration is not harmful provided there is enough clearance left between conductors to prevent flashover.

3. *Galloping* (or *dancing*). It is usually created by a nonuniform airfoil surface formed around the conductor by ice. It can be very severe, is of a very low frequency, and is extremely

difficult to control since the shapes of the ice and the wind velocity combine to result in a critical stability condition. Therefore, winds from 15 mph upward can create violent conductor motion with amplitudes measuring up to two times the amount of conductor sag. Cases have occurred where this galloping has displaced the phase conductor all the way up to the GWs, causing multiple trip outs. It has also resulted in damage to conductors, spacers, and towers. Although galloping produces severe motions, it is almost always limited to areas of icing and is dependent on terrain and wind exposure. It is more common in regions (e.g., Nebraska, Iowa) where steady, moderate-velocity winds (19–35 mph) occur. Luckily, it occurs very infrequently.

4. *Conductor ice loading and shedding.* Conductor icing and the subsequent shedding of ice loads can cause large vertical conductor motions (i.e., jumping). The worst jumping takes place when ice melts from the center span of a section after it has fallen from the other spans. Serious jumping also occurs when ice slips down the conductor toward midspan. The conductor jumping can be controlled by fitting special insulator assemblies at the suspension points and by increasing the mass per-unit length of line at midspan. Vertical motion of the conductor due to ice shedding is dependent on span length, tension, conductor size, ice thickness, and the amount of ice shed at any one time. EPRI [6] suggests the following criteria for ice shedding on 138 kV lines:

   a. Assume a maximum sag error of 6 in.
   b. Assume the upper conductor has an ice load equal to 50% of the criterion for unequal static ice load (usually 0.5×1 in. or 0.5 in.). Ice is assumed to weigh 57 lb/ft^3.
   c. Assume that the lower conductor, previously with the same ice load as cited earlier, has already shed 25%.
   d. Assume that the remaining 75% of the ice on lower conductor is shed at one time.
   e. Provide sufficient initial separation to ensure that the minimum clearance during the subsequent jump is 16 in., adequate for 60 Hz withstand.

5. *Subconductor vibration.* It is only possible on bundled conductor arrangements. On a bundled conductor, the windward conductor has a wake that spreads out its leeward side. One or more of the leeward conductors is riding in a wake that has a shear flow and different velocities of wind cross over the top and bottom of the conductor. Depending on the conductor position, this can result in either negative or positive lift. There is also a decreased drag on the leeward conductor compared with the windward conductor, tending to displace the conductors horizontally with respect to each other. Therefore, for example, in a horizontally twin-bundled conductor system, the windward conductor is exposed to the wind velocity, while the leeward conductor is exposed to the wake of the wind. The interaction of resonant forces due to the wind and mechanical coupling by spacers may cause an elliptical motion of the system. Amplitude may be in the range of 2–5 ft for winds 20 mph or greater. Subconductor vibration occurs at lower frequency (2–4 Hz) than aeolian vibration and is more difficult to control. It may lead to the ultimate breaking of spacers and, in some cases, destruction of suspension points at the insulators. In general, it can be controlled by the use of vibration dampers, the spacing of subconductors as far apart as practical, orienting the subconductors so that they are at advantageous points in the wind wake, and more frequent use of spacers within each span.

6. *Corona vibration.* It usually takes place in wet weather when water drops clinging to the underside of the conductor are forced off by an expulsion action due to the electrostatic field forces at the bottom of the conductor. Therefore, vibrational displacements of a few inches can appear between vibration nodes on any span. Corona vibration has relatively low amplitude and does not occur often; however, it may be important on the UHV lines.

With the exception of the corona vibration, the aforementioned vibration problems can also be controlled by the use of self-damped conductors that have recently been developed. For example, since two factors can cause conductor motion, namely, conductor shape and weather, Kaiser

Aluminum engineers deduced that wind-induced motion can be controlled by changing the shape of the conductor. It is obvious that a round conductor presents the same profile to the wind along its entire length between structures. Therefore, it was reasoned that a twisted double conductor would present a continually changing profile to the wind, thus preventing the buildup of resonant vibrations.

Hence, under ice buildup conditions, the ice-coated figure 8 shape and constantly changing profile of the T_2 conductor would act as a spoiler rather than as the airfoil shape associated with violent conductor galloping. A T_2 conductor is made up of two round aluminum conductors twisted at the factory to make one complete $360°$ revolution gradually over approximately every 9 ft of length. Its profile is like a figure 8. This configuration results in a continually changing orientation of major and minor axes.

This ever-changing profile to the wind interferes with the wind forces that create conductor motion. Because of its profile, the T_2 conductor has a lower operating temperature than the standard round conductor of equal aluminum circular mil area. Lower operating temperature means lower operating resistance, less sag, less loss in strength, and less creep. Figure 12.21 illustrates the installation of T_2 conductors. Figure 12.22 shows a corner tower carrying T_2 conductors.

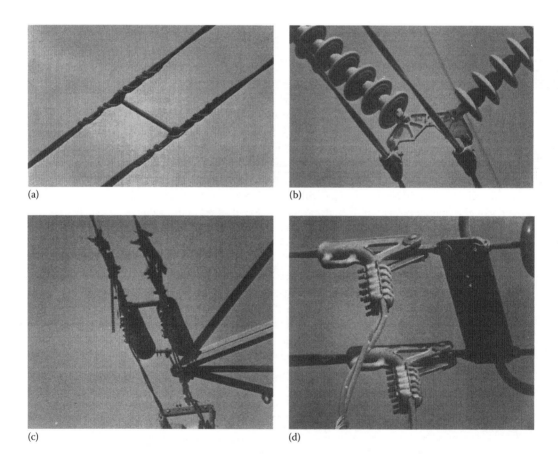

(a) (b)

(c) (d)

FIGURE 12.21 Installation of T_2 conductors: (a) clipping crew installing suspension clamp, (b) typical 345 kV two-conductor suspension clamp and yoke plate arrangement, (c) rigged used to dead-end T_2 conductor, and (d) strain clamp dead ends. (Courtesy of Kaiser Aluminum, Foothill Ranch, CA.)

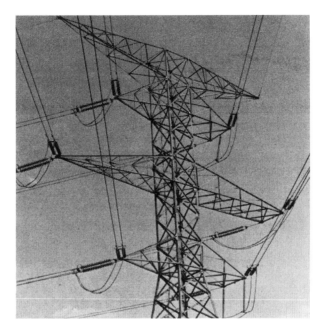

FIGURE 12.22 View of corner tower carrying T_2 conductors. (Courtesy of Kaiser Aluminum, Foothill Ranch, CA.)

12.14 CONDUCTOR MOTION CAUSED BY FAULT CURRENTS

Two parallel and current-carrying conductors are under a force of attraction or repulsion, depending on current direction. The magnitude of the force on each conductor can be expressed as

$$F \propto \frac{I^2}{d} \tag{12.38}$$

where
   I is the current in each conductor
   d is the distance (spacing) between conductors

In the event the current flow in each conductor is in the same direction, the resulting force will cause attraction. Otherwise, the force will cause repulsion. During short circuits, these forces may be great enough to cause significant conductor movement, especially where conductors are closely spaced (e.g., in EHV or UHV conductor bundles). Such conductor movement depends on the fault current magnitude and the fault duration and therefore the interruption time of the CB involved.

A line-to-line fault will cause current in the two affected phases to flow in opposite directions. The two conductors will then be repelled and, on interruption of the fault current, will swing together. If the fault is on an adjacent line section, the motion may be serious since it might cause interruption on the unfaulted section. Therefore, such conductor movement should be taken into account in determining the phase-to-phase spacing or in establishing the need for insulating spacers.

PROBLEMS

12.1 A 3/0 OH conductor is subjected to a tension of 2000 lb. Find the unit tensile stress of the following conductors:
(a) Copper with seven strands
(b) ACSR
(c) Copperweld copper, 3/0 E

12.2 A heavy transformer hung on a wood crossarm attached to a wood pole by a steel bolt sets up a shearing stress in the bolt between the crossarm and the pole. Calculate the shearing stress in the bolt. Assume that the transformer weighs 400 lb and a 3/4 in. bolt, having a cross-sectional area of 0.302 in.^{2}, fastens the crossarm to the pole.

12.3 A western cedar pole carries two crossarms, one of which is subjected to a normal transverse force of 450 lb at a height of 34 ft and the other 225 lb at 32 ft. Assume that the pole tapers 3 in. in circumference for each 8 ft of length and has an ultimate fiber stress rating of 5600 psi. Calculate the following:
(a) Minimum required pole diameter at ground line
(b) Relevant pole-top diameter of pole
(c) Permissible bending moment during storms

12.4 Repeat Problem 12.3 if the pole used is a northern white cedar with an ultimate fiber stress rating of 3600 psi.

12.5 A 46 ft pole with 24 in. circumference at the pole top and 50 in. circumference at the ground line. Use a wind velocity of 60 mph and an average span of 250 ft. The pole carries two crossarms, and each crossarm carries three conductors. The top crossarm is 1 ft below the pole top, and the lower crossarm is 2 ft below the top crossarm. Use hard-drawn copper conductors of 250 kcmil with 12 strands and 4/0 with 7 strands for the top and lower conductors, respectively. Assume that 6.5 ft of the pole is below the ground and find the following:
(a) Total pressure due to wind on pole
(b) Total pressure due to wind on conductors
(c) Total pressure due to wind on pole and conductors

12.6 The conductors in the adjacent spans have equal tensions of 400 lb and the angle of departure of the line is 46°. The pole, which carries the conductors of the adjacent spans, has a crossarm with four conductors. Calculate the additional stress imposed upon the supporting pole due to the angle in the line.

12.7 If the conductors in the adjacent spans of Problem 12.6 have different tensions of 400 and 300 lb for T_1 and T_2 and the angle of departure of the line is 46° as before, calculate the following:
(a) Resultant side pull force
(b) Angle γ

12.8 Repeat Problem 12.6 assuming the angle of departure of the line is 80°.

12.9 Consider Problem 12.5. Assume that the conductors in the adjacent spans have different tensions of 300 and 350 lb and the angle of departure of the line is 40°. Also assume that the permissible stress in pole is 50% and 60% of ultimate fiber strength for transverse loading and longitudinal loading, respectively. Find the required internal resisting moment of the pole in pound feet.

12.10 Find the allowable maximum angle of departure of the line, without any side guying, for the angle pole of Problem 12.9 if the pole is to be set in firm soil.

12.11 Repeat Example 12.4 if the bending moments are created by 4000 and 3000 lb at heights of 45 and 40 ft, respectively. The guy is attached to the pole at the heights of 45 ft. The lead of the guy is 20 ft.

12.12 Consider Figure 12.12 and assume that $T_2 \neq T_1$ and verify Equation 12.19.

REFERENCES

1. DeWeese, F. C. *Transmission Lines: Design, Construction and Performance*, McGraw-Hill, New York, 1945.
2. American National Standards Institute. *National Electrical Safety Code*, 1984 edn., IEEE, New York, 1984.
3. Pender, H. and Del Mar, W. A., eds. *Electrical Engineers' Handbook: Electric Power*, 4th edn., Wiley, New York, 1962.
4. Hubbard, A. and Watkins, W. Good anchoring a inexpensive guy insurance against storms, *Electr. World* 128, 1947, 94–96.
5. Fink, D. G. and Carroll, J. M., eds. *Standard Handbook for Electrical Engineers*, 10th edn., McGraw-Hill, New York, 1969.
6. Electric Power Research Institute. *Transmission Line Reference Book: 115–138 kV Compact Line Design*, EPRI, Palo Alto, CA, 1978.

GENERAL REFERENCES

American Society of Chemical Engineers. *Guide for Design of Steel Transmission Towers*, ASCE-Manuals Rep. Eng. Prac. no. 52., ASCE, New York, 1971.

Dwight, H. B. *Electrical Elements of Power Transmission Lines*, MacMillan, New York, 1954.

Edison Electric Institute. *EHV Transmission Line Reference Book*, EEI, New York, 1968.

Electric Power Research Institute. *Transmission Line Reference Book: 345 kV and Above*, 2nd edn., EPRI, Palo Alto, CA, 1982.

Freeman, P. J. *Electric Power Transmission & Distribution*, George G. Harrap & Co., London, U.K., 1977.

Gönen, T. *Electric Power Distribution System Engineering*, 2nd edn., CRC Press, Boca Raton, FL, 2008.

Guile, A. E. and Paterson, W. *Electrical Power Systems*, 2nd edn., Pergamon Press, New York, 1977.

Mallik, U. G. *Solution of Problems in Electrical Power*, Pitman, London, U.K., 1968.

Powel, C. A. *Principles of Electric Utility Engineering*, MIT Press, Cambridge, MA, 1955.

Rapson, E. T. A. *Electrical Transmission and Distribution*, Oxford University Press, London, U.K., 1933.

Seelye, H. P. *Electrical Distribution Engineering*, McGraw-Hill, New York, 1930.

Siemens Aktienges. *Electrical Engineering Handbook*, Berlin, Germany, 1976.

Skrotzki, B. G. A., ed. *Electric Transmission and Distribution*, McGraw-Hill, New York, 1954.

Taylor, E. O., and Boal, G. A., eds. *Electric Power Distribution: 415 V-33 kV*, Arnold, London, U.K., 1966.

Woodruff, L. F. *Principles of Electric Power Transmission*, 2nd edn., Wiley, New York, 1938.

13 Sag and Tension Analysis

There is no great genius without a mixture of madness.

Aristotle

13.1 INTRODUCTION

Conductor sag and tension analysis is an important consideration in OH distribution line design as well as in OH transmission line design. The quality and continuity of electric service supplied over a line (regardless of whether it is a distribution, a subtransmission, or a transmission line) depend largely on whether the conductors have been properly installed. Thus, the designing engineer must determine in advance the amount of sag and tension to be given to the wires or cables of a particular line at a given temperature. In order to specify the tension to be used in stringing the line conductors, the values of sag and tension for winter and summer conditions must be known. Tension in the conductors contributes to the mechanical load on structures at angles in the line and at dead ends. Excessive tension may cause mechanical failure of the conductor itself.

The factors affecting the sag of a conductor strung between supports are

1. Conductor load per unit length
2. Span, that is, distance between supports
3. Temperature
4. Conductor tension

In order to determine the conductor load properly, the factors that need to be taken into account are

1. Weight of conductor itself
2. Weight of ice or snow clinging to wire
3. Wind blowing against wire

The maximum effective weight of the conductor is the vector sum of the vertical weight and the horizontal wind pressure. It is very important to include the most adverse condition. The wind is considered to be blowing at right angles to the line and to act against the projected area of the conductor, including the projected area of ice or snow that may be clinging to it.

Economic design dictates that conductor sag should be minimum to refrain from extra pole height, to provide sufficient clearance above ground level, and to avoid providing excessive horizontal spacing between conductors to prevent them swinging together in midspan.

Conductor tension pulls the conductor up and decreases its sag. At the same time, tension elongates the conductor, from elastic stretching, which tends to relieve tension and increase sag. The elastic property of metallic wire is measured by its modulus of elasticity. The modulus of elasticity of a material equals the stress per unit of area divided by the deformation per unit of length. That is, since

$$\alpha = \frac{T}{A} \text{ psi} \tag{13.1}$$

where
  σ is the stress per unit area in pounds per square inches
  T is the conductor tension in pounds
  A is the actual metal cross section of conductor in square inches, in.^{2} = cmil/1,273,000

the resultant elongation e of the conductor due to the tension is

$$e = \frac{\text{Stress}}{\text{Modulus of elasticity}}$$

If the modulus of elasticity is low, the elongation is high, and vice versa. Thus, a small change in conductor length has a comparatively large effect on conductor sag and tension.

Sags and stresses in conductors are dependent on the initial tension put on them when they are clamped in place and are due to the weight of the conductors themselves, to ice or sleet clinging to them, and to wind pressure.

The stress in the conductor is the parameter on which everything else is based. But the stress itself is determined by the sag in the conductor as it hangs between adjacent poles or towers. Since the stress depends on sag, any span can be used provided the poles or towers are high enough and strong enough. The matter is merely one of extending the catenary in both directions. But the cost of poles or towers sharply increases with height and loading. Thus, the problem becomes the balancing of a larger number of lighter and shorter poles or towers against a smaller number of heavier and taller ones.

13.2 EFFECT OF CHANGE IN TEMPERATURE

Sags and stresses vary with temperature on account of the thermal expansion and contraction of the conductors. A temperature rise increases conductor length, with resulting increase in sag and decrease in tension. A temperature drop causes reverse effects. The change in length per unit of conductor length per degree Fahrenheit of temperature change is the temperature coefficient of linear expansion. The maximum stress occurs at the lowest temperature, when the line has contracted and is also possibly covered with ice and sleet:

1. If the conductor is *unstressed* or the conductor stress is *constant* while the temperature changes, the change in length of the conductor is

$$\Delta l = l_0 \alpha \Delta t \tag{13.2}$$

  where

$$\Delta t = t_1 - t_0 \quad \Delta l = l_1 - l_0$$

  where
    t_0 is the initial temperature
    l_0 is the conductor length at initial temperature t_0
    l_1 is the conductor length at t_1
    α is the coefficient of linear expansion of conductor per degree Fahrenheit
    Δt is the change in temperature
    Δl is the change in conductor length in feet

2. If the temperature is *constant* while the conductor stress changes (i.e., loading), the change in length of the conductor is

$$\Delta l = l_0 \left(\frac{\Delta T}{MA} \right) \tag{13.3}$$

where

$$\Delta T = T_1 - T_0$$

where

T_0 is the conductor initial tension in pounds
ΔT is the change in conductor tension in pounds
M is the modulus of elasticity of conductor in pound inches
A is the actual metal cross section of conductor in square inches

13.3 LINE SAG AND TENSION CALCULATIONS

A conductor suspended freely from two supports, which are at the same level and spaced L unit length apart, as shown in Figure 10.1, takes the form of a catenary curve providing the conductor is perfectly flexible and its weight is uniformly distributed along its length. If the conductor is tightly stretched (i.e., when sag d is very small in comparison to span L), the resultant curve can be considered a parabola. If the conductor's sag is less than 6% of its span length, the error in sag computed by the parabolic equations is less than 0.5%. If the conductor's sag is less than 10% of the span, the error is about 2%.

In distribution systems, determining accurate values of sag is not so important as it is in transmission systems. Nevertheless, even in the distribution lines, if the conductor is strung with too low tension, the resultant sag will be excessive, with the likelihood of wires swinging together and short-circuited. The usual tendency, however, is to pull the conductor too tight, which causes the conductor to be overstressed and stretched when the heaviest loading takes place and the normal sag after this loading becomes excessive. Then the excessive sag needs to be pulled out of the conductor, a process that also causes the conductor to be overstressed on the heaviest loading. This process of overstressing and pulling up may cause the conductors, especially the smaller ones, to be broken. This can be eliminated by measuring the line tension more accurately [2].

13.3.1 Supports at the Same Level

13.3.1.1 Catenary Method

Figure 13.1 shows a span of conductor with two supports at the same level and separated by a horizontal distance L. Let 0 be the lowest point on the catenary curve and 1 be the length of the conductor between two supports. Let w be the weight of the conductor per unit length, T be the tension of the conductor at any point P in the direction of the curve, and H be the tension at origin 0. Further, let s be the length of the curve between points 0 and P, so that the weight of the portion s is ws.

Tension T can be resolved into two components, T_x the horizontal component and T_y the vertical component. Then, for equilibrium,

$$T_x = H \quad \text{and} \quad T_y = ws$$

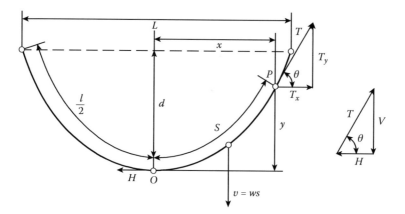

FIGURE 13.1 Conductor suspended between supports at the same elevation.

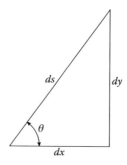

FIGURE 13.2 Triangle.

Thus, the portion OP of the conductor is in equilibrium under the tension T at P, the weight ws acting vertically downward, and the horizontal tension H.

In the triangle shown in Figure 13.2, ds represents a very short portion of the conductor, in the region of point P. When s is increased by ds, the corresponding x and y are increased by dx and dy, respectively. Hence,

$$\tan\theta = \frac{dy}{dx} = \frac{ws}{H}$$

since

$$\left(\frac{ds}{dx}\right)^2 = 1 + \left(\frac{dy}{dx}\right)^2$$

then

$$\left(\frac{ds}{dx}\right)^2 = 1 + \left(\frac{ws}{H}\right)^2$$

Therefore,

$$dx = \frac{ds}{\sqrt{1 + \left(ws/H\right)^2}}$$

Integrating both sides gives

$$x = \int \frac{1}{\sqrt{1 + (ws/H)^2}} \, ds$$

Therefore,

$$x = \frac{H}{w} \sinh^{-1}\left(\frac{ws}{H}\right) + K$$

where K is the constant of integration. When $x = 0$, $s = 0$, and $K = 0$,

$$s = \frac{H}{w} \sinh\left(\frac{wx}{H}\right) \tag{13.4}$$

When $x = \frac{1}{2}L$,

$$s = \frac{l}{2} = \frac{H}{w} \sinh\left(\frac{wL}{2H}\right) \tag{13.5}$$

Therefore,

$$l = \frac{2H}{w} \sinh\left(\frac{wL}{2H}\right) \tag{13.6}$$

or

$$l = \frac{2H}{w}\left[\frac{1}{1!}\left(\frac{wL}{2H}\right) + \frac{1}{3!}\left(\frac{wL}{2H}\right)^3 + \cdots\right] \tag{13.7}$$

or approximately

$$l \cong L\left(1 + \frac{w^2 L^2}{24H^2}\right) \tag{13.8}$$

From Equations 13.3 and 13.4,

$$\frac{dy}{dx} = \frac{ws}{H} = \sinh\left(\frac{wx}{H}\right)$$

or

$$dy = \sinh\left(\frac{wx}{H}\right) dx$$

Integrating both sides,

$$y = \int \sinh\left(\frac{wx}{H}\right) dx$$

or

$$y = \left(\frac{H}{w}\right) \cos\left(\frac{wx}{H}\right) + K_1 \tag{13.9}$$

If the lowest point of the curve is taken as the origin, when $x = 0$, $y = 0$, then $K_1 = -H/w$, since, by the series, $\cosh 0 = 1$. Therefore,

$$y = \frac{H}{w}\left(\cosh \frac{wx}{H} - 1\right) \tag{13.10}$$

is the equation of the curve that is called a *catenary*. Equation 13.10 can also be written as

$$y = \frac{H}{w}\left[1 + \frac{1}{2!}\left(\frac{wx}{H}\right)^2 + \cdots - 1\right] \tag{13.11}$$

or in approximate form

$$y \cong \frac{wx^2}{2H} \tag{13.12}$$

The total tension in the conductor at any point x is

$$T = H\sqrt{1 + \left(\frac{dy}{dx}\right)^2}$$

or

$$T = H \cos\left(\frac{wx}{H}\right) \tag{13.13}$$

whereas the total tension in the conductor at the support is

$$T = H \cos\left(\frac{wL}{2H}\right) \tag{13.14}$$

or

$$T = H\left[1 + \frac{1}{2!}\left(\frac{wL}{2H}\right)^2 + \frac{1}{4!}\left(\frac{wL}{2H}\right)^4 + \cdots\right] \tag{13.15}$$

The *sag*, or *deflection*, of the conductor for a span of length L between supports on the same level is

$$d = \frac{H}{w}\left(\cosh\left(\frac{wL}{2H}\right) - 1\right) \tag{13.16}$$

or

$$d = \frac{L}{2}\left[\frac{1}{2}\left(\frac{wL}{2H}\right) + \frac{1}{4!}\left(\frac{wL}{2H}\right)^3 + \frac{1}{6!}\left(\frac{wL}{2H}\right)^5 + \cdots\right] \tag{13.17}$$

The NESC gives the minimum (required) clearance height for the line above ground, and if to this is added the sag, the minimum height of the insulator support points can be found.

In Figure 13.3, it can be observed that c is the ordinate of the lowest point of the curve with respect to the directrix and y is the ordinate of the point of tangency with respect to the directrix. The form of the curve depends on the slope of the conductor at a support. In turn, the slope itself is the factor to determine the conductor tension. As previously mentioned, the tension T can be resolved into two components, T_x and T_y, where

$$T_y = \frac{1}{2}w$$

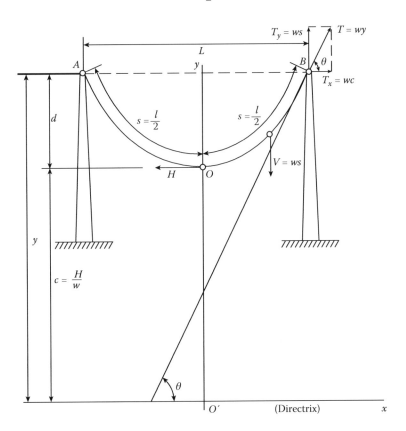

FIGURE 13.3 Parameters of catenary.

or if $s = \dfrac{1}{2}l$,

$$T_y = ws \tag{13.18}$$

$$T_x = wc \tag{13.19}$$

where T_x can be defined as the mass of some unknown length c of the conductor and T_y and T can also be defined similarly. Then for equilibrium,

$$T_x = H \quad \text{and} \quad T_y = V$$

where

H is the horizontal tension in conductor at origin 0
V is the weight of wire per foot of span times distance from point of maximum sag to support

Thus, from the triangle of forces,

$$T^2 = H^2 + V^2$$

so that

$$T = \sqrt{H^2 + V^2} \tag{13.20}$$

or

$$T = \sqrt{(wc)^2 + (ws)^2}$$

from which

$$T = w\sqrt{c^2 + s^2} \tag{13.21}$$

Equation 13.4 can be written as

$$s = c\left(\sinh \frac{x}{c}\right) \tag{13.22}$$

since $c = H/w$. Also, Equation 13.9 can be written as

$$y = c\left(\cosh \frac{x}{c}\right) + K_1 \tag{13.23}$$

where x is half of the span length ($L/2$). From Figure 13.3, when $x = 0$, Equation 13.23 becomes

$$c = c(\cosh 0) + K_1$$

Thus, $K_1 = 0$, and therefore,

$$y = c\left(\cosh\frac{x}{c}\right) \tag{13.24}$$

If both sides of Equations 13.22 and 13.24 are squared,

$$s^2 = c^2\left(\sinh^2\frac{x}{c}\right) \tag{13.25}$$

and

$$y^2 = c^2\left(\cosh^2\frac{x}{c}\right) \tag{13.26}$$

Subtracting Equation 13.26 from Equation 13.25,

$$y^2 - s^2 = c^2\left(\cosh^2\frac{x}{c} - \sinh^2\frac{x}{c}\right)$$

or

$$y^2 - s^2 = c^2 \tag{13.27}$$

since

$$\cosh^2\frac{x}{c} - \sinh^2\frac{x}{c} = 0$$

From Equation 13.27,

$$y = \sqrt{c^2 + s^2} \tag{13.28}$$

By substituting Equation 13.28 into Equation 13.21,

$$T_{\max} = wy \tag{13.29}$$

Also,

$$T_{\max} = w\sqrt{c^2 + s^2} \tag{13.30}$$

According to Equation 13.29, the maximum tension T occurs at the supports where the conductor is at an angle to the horizontal whose tangent is V/H, or s/c, since

$$V = ws \quad \text{and} \quad H = wc$$

At supports,

$$y = c + d \tag{13.31}$$

Thus, Equation 13.28 can be written as

$$c + d = \sqrt{c^2 + s^2}$$

from which

$$c = \frac{s^2 - d^2}{2d} \tag{13.32}$$

Also, Equation 13.29 can be written as

$$T_{max} = w(c + d) \tag{13.33}$$

Substituting Equation 13.32 into Equation 13.33,

$$T_{max} = \frac{w}{2d}\left(s^2 + d^2\right) \tag{13.34}$$

which gives the maximum value of the conductor tension.

A line tangent to the conductor is horizontal at the points of maximum sag and has the greatest angle from the horizontal at the supports. Since the supports are the same level, the weight of the conductor in one-half span on each side is supported at each pole. At midspan, or point of maximum sag, the vertical component of tension equals zero. Thus, the minimum tension occurs at the point of maximum sag. The tension at this point (the point at which $y = c$) acts in a horizontal direction and equals the horizontal component of total tension. Therefore,

$$T_{min} = H$$

or since $H = wc$,

$$T_{min} = wc \tag{13.35}$$

or

$$T_{min} = \frac{w}{2d}\left(s^2 - d^2\right) \tag{13.36}$$

Also from Figure 13.3,

$$y = \frac{1}{2}c\left(e^{x/c} + e^{-x/c}\right) \tag{13.37}$$

or

$$y = c\left(\cosh\frac{x}{c}\right) \tag{13.38}$$

where

$$C = \frac{H}{w}$$

Also,

$$d = y - c \quad \text{or} \quad c = y - d \qquad (13.39)$$

The conductor length is

$$l = 2s$$

or

$$l = 2\left[\frac{1}{2}c\left(e^{x/c} - e^{-x/c}\right)\right] \qquad (13.40)$$

or

$$l = 2c\left(\sinh\frac{x}{c}\right) \qquad (13.41)$$

Another useful equation can be developed by substituting $c = H/w$ into Equation 13.33:

$$T_{max} = H + wd \qquad (13.42)$$

or

$$T_{max} = T_{min} + wd \qquad (13.43)$$

since

$$T_{min} = H$$

13.3.1.2 Parabolic Method

In the case of short spans with small sags, the curve can be considered as a parabola. When the horizontal tension is the same, the radius of curvature at the lowest point of the conductor is the same for both the parabola and the catenary, but the outlines of the two curves are different at all points between the lowest point of the curve and the point of support. As the span length and sag are increased, the difference in outline of the two curves becomes more significant. Changes in the loading will produce different changes in the length of the two curves to make the sags different.

Since the sag by the parabola solution is smaller than the sag by the catenary solution for the same horizontal tension, the angle θ will be smaller. Thus, the vertical component of tension is smaller for the parabola solution than for the catenary. This difference increases along the curve toward the support, becoming maximum at the supports. However, for the sake of simplicity, the following assumptions are made:

1. The tension is considered uniform throughout the span, the slight excess of tension at the supports over that in the middle being neglected.
2. The change in length of the conductor due to elastic stretch or temperature expansion is taken as equal to the change of length of a conductor equal in length to the horizontal distance between the points of supports.

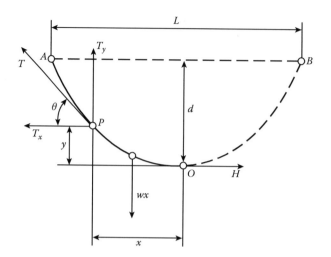

FIGURE 13.4   Parameters of parabola.

In Figure 13.4, let P be any point on the parabolic curve such that arc OP is equal to x. The portion OP of the conductor is in equilibrium under the action of T, H, and wx. As previously done, the tension T can be resolved into two components, T_x and T_y. Then, for equilibrium,

$$T_x = H \quad \text{and} \quad T_y = wx$$

Taking moments about P,

$$\text{Moments clockwise} = \text{Moments anticlockwise}$$

or

$$H_y = wx\,\frac{x}{2}$$

from which

$$y = \frac{wx^2}{2H} \tag{13.44}$$

Distribution lines usually have comparatively short spans with small sag. The difference between the maximum tension T and the horizontal tension H is relatively small because of short spans and small sags. Under such conditions, a slight error will result if T is substituted for H in the equation for sag. Therefore,

$$y = \frac{wx^2}{2T} \tag{13.45}$$

When $x = \dfrac{1}{2}L$, y is equal to sag or deflection d; therefore, the sag is

$$d = \frac{wL^2}{8T} \tag{13.46}$$

It is interesting to note that if the terms $(wL/2H)^3$ and $(wL/2H)^4$ are omitted in Equation 13.17, as is appropriate for spans of only a few hundred feet, the very same Equation 13.46 can be obtained.

After replacing T with H in Equation 13.46, if it is combined with Equation 13.8, the following equation can be derived for the conductor length (i.e., the perimeter of the conductor in the span):

$$l = L\left(1 + \frac{8d^2}{3L^2}\right)$$
(13.47)

Example 13.1

A subtransmission line conductor has been suspended freely from two towers and has taken the form of a catenary that has $c = 1600$ ft. The span between the two towers is 500 ft, and the weight of the conductor is 4122 lb/mi. Calculate the following:

(a) Length of conductor by using Equations 13.6 and 13.8
(b) Sag
(c) Maximum and minimum values of conductor tension using catenary method
(d) Approximate value of tension by using parabolic method

Solution

(a) Using Equation 13.6,

$$l = \frac{2H}{w}\sinh\frac{wL}{2H}$$

or

$$l = 2c\left(\sinh\frac{L}{2c}\right)$$

since

$$c = \frac{H}{w}$$

Therefore,

$$l = 2 \times 1600 \ \sinh\frac{500}{2 \times 1600}$$

$$= 3200 \ \sinh 0.15625$$

$$= 502.032 \text{ ft}$$

Using Equation 13.8,

$$l = L\left(1 + \frac{w^2L^2}{24H^2}\right)$$

or

$$l = L\left(1 + \frac{L^2}{24c^2}\right)$$
$$= 500\left(1 + \frac{500^2}{24 \times 1600^2}\right)$$
$$= 502.0345 \text{ ft}$$

(b) Using Equation 13.16,

$$d = \frac{H}{w}\left(\cosh\frac{wL}{2H} - 1\right)$$

or

$$d = c\left(\cosh\frac{L}{2c} - 1\right)$$

since

$$c = \frac{H}{w}$$

Therefore,

$$d = 1600\left(\cosh\frac{500}{2 \times 1600} - 1\right)$$
$$= 1600(\cosh 0.15625 - 1)$$
$$\cong 19.6 \text{ ft}$$

(c) Using Equation 13.33,

$$T_{max} = w(c + d)$$
$$= \frac{4122}{5280}(1600 + 19.6)$$
$$\cong 1264.4 \text{ lb}$$

Using Equation 13.35,

$$T_{min} = wc$$
$$= \frac{4122}{5280} \times 1600$$
$$\cong 1249.1 \text{ lb}$$

(d) From Equation 13.46,

$$T \cong \frac{wL^2}{8d}$$
$$\cong \frac{(4122/5280) \times 500^2}{8 \times 19.6}$$
$$\cong 1244.7 \text{ lb}$$

13.3.2 SUPPORTS AT DIFFERENT LEVELS: UNSYMMETRICAL SPANS

Consider a span L between two supports, as shown in Figure 13.5, whose elevations differ by a distance h. Let the horizontal distance from the lowest point of the curve to the lower and the higher supports be x_1 and x_2, respectively.

By using Equation 13.46, that is,

$$y = \frac{wx^2}{2T}$$

d_1 and d_2 sags can be found as

$$d_1 = \frac{wx_1^2}{2T} \tag{13.48}$$

and

$$d_2 = \frac{wx_2^2}{2T} \tag{13.49}$$

Therefore,

$$h = d_2 - d_1 \tag{13.50}$$

or

$$h = \frac{w}{2T}\left(x_2^2 - x_1^2\right) \tag{13.51}$$

or

$$h = \frac{wL}{2T}\left(x_2 - x_1\right) \tag{13.52}$$

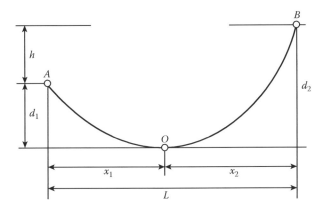

FIGURE 13.5 Supports at different levels.

Since

$$L = x_1 + x_2 \tag{13.53}$$

Therefore,

$$\frac{2Th}{wL} = x_2 - x_1 \tag{13.54}$$

By adding Equations 13.53 and 13.54,

$$2x_2 = L + \frac{2Th}{wL}$$

or

$$x_2 = \frac{L}{2} + \frac{Th}{wL} \tag{13.55}$$

Also by subtracting Equation 13.54 from Equation 13.53,

$$2x_1 = L - \frac{2Th}{wL}$$

or

$$x_1 = \frac{L}{2} - \frac{Th}{wL} \tag{13.56}$$

In Equation 13.56,

$$\text{If } \frac{L}{2} > \frac{Th}{wL}, \quad \text{then } x_1 \text{ is positive.}$$

$$\text{If } \frac{L}{2} = \frac{Th}{wL}, \quad \text{then } x_1 \text{ is zero.}$$

$$\text{If } \frac{L}{2} < \frac{Th}{wL}, \quad \text{then } x_1 \text{ is negative.}$$

If x_1 is negative, the lowest point (the point 0) of the imaginary curve lies outside the actual span, as shown in Figure 13.6.

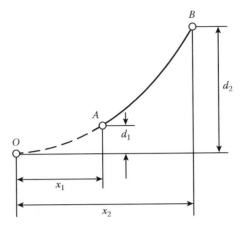

FIGURE 13.6 Case of negative x_1.

13.4 SPANS OF UNEQUAL LENGTH: RULING SPAN

When a line consists of spans of unequal length, each span should theoretically be tensioned according to its own length. However, this is not possible with suspension insulators since the insulator strings would swing so as to equalize the tension in each span. It is impractical to dead-end and erect each span separately. However, it is possible to assume a uniform tension between dead-end supports by defining an equivalent span, which is called a *ruling span*,* and basing all the calculations on this equivalent span.

If the actual spans are known, the ruling span can be calculated from the equation

$$L_e = \sqrt{\frac{L_1^3 + L_2^3 + L_3^3 + \cdots + L_n^3}{L_1 + L_2 + L_3 + \cdots + L_n}} \tag{13.57}$$

where
L_e is the ruling span or equivalent span
L_i is the each individual span in line

Generally, an exact value of the ruling span is not necessary. An approximate ruling span can be calculated as

$$L_e = L_{avg} + \frac{2}{3}\left(L_{max} - L_{avg}\right) \tag{13.58}$$

where
L_{avg} is the average span in line
L_{max} is the maximum span in line

The line tension T can be estimated using this equivalent span length, and then the sag for each actual span can be calculated from

$$d = \frac{wL^2}{8T} \tag{13.59}$$

---

* Mostly used for distribution lines.

13.5   EFFECTS OF ICE AND WIND LOADING

The span design consists in determining the sag at which the line is constructed so that heavy winds, accumulations of ice or snow, and excessive temperature changes will not stress the conductor beyond its elastic limit, cause a serious permanent stretch, or result in fatigue failures from continued vibrations. In other words, the lines will be erected under warmer and nearly still-air conditions and yet must comply with the worst conditions.

13.5.1   Effect of Ice

In mountainous geographic areas, the thickness of ice formed on the conductor becomes very significant. Depending on the circumstances, it might be as much as several times the diameter of the conductor. Ice accumulations on the conductor affect the design of the line (1) by increasing the dead weight per foot of the line and (2) by increasing the projected surface of the line subject to wind pressure.

Even though the more likely configuration of a conductor with a coating of ice is as shown in Figure 13.7, for the sake of simplicity, it can be assumed that the ice coating, of thickness t_i inches, is uniform over the surface of a conductor, as shown in Figure 13.8.

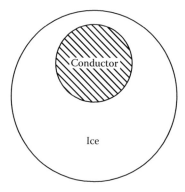

FIGURE 13.7   Probable configuration of ice-covered conductor cross-sectional area.

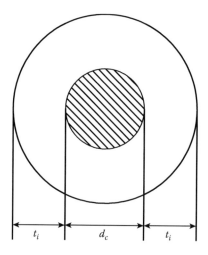

FIGURE 13.8   Assumed configuration of ice-covered conductor cross-sectional area.

Then the cross-sectional area of the ice is

$$A_i = \frac{\pi}{4}\left[\left(d_c + 2t_i\right)^2 - d_c^2\right]$$

or

$$A_i = \pi t_i \left(d_c + t_i\right) \text{ in.}^2 \tag{13.60}$$

or

$$A_i = \frac{\pi t_i}{144}\left(d_c + t_i\right) \text{ ft}^2 \tag{13.61}$$

where

d_c is the diameter of conductor in inches

t_i is the radial thickness of ice coating in inches

If the ice load is assumed to be uniform throughout the length of the conductor, the volume of ice per foot is

$$V_i = \frac{\pi}{144} \times \frac{1}{1} t_i \left(d_c + t_i\right) \text{ ft}^3/\text{ft} \tag{13.62}$$

The weight of the ice is 57 lb/ft³, so that the weight of ice per foot is

$$w_i = \frac{57}{144} \pi t_i \left(d_c + t_i\right)$$

or approximately

$$w_i = 1.25 t_i \left(d_c + t_i\right) \text{ lb/ft} \tag{13.63}$$

Therefore, the total vertical load on the conductor per unit length is

$$w_T = w + w_i \tag{13.64}$$

where

w_T is the total vertical load on conductor per unit length

w is the weight of conductor per unit length

w_i is the weight of ice per unit length

13.5.2 Effect of Wind

It is customary to assume that the wind blows uniformly and horizontally across the projected area of the conductor covered with no ice and ice, respectively.

The projected area per unit length of the conductor with no ice is

$$S_{ni} = A_{ni} \times l \tag{13.65}$$

where
  S_{ni} is the projected area of conductor covered with no ice in square feet per unit length
  A_{ni} is the cross-sectional area of conductor covered with no ice in square feet
  l is the length of conductor in unit length

For a 1 ft length of conductor with no ice,

$$S_{ni} = \frac{1}{12} d_c \times l \tag{13.66}$$

whereas with ice, it is

$$S_{wi} = A_{wi} \times l \tag{13.67}$$

where
  S_{wi} is the projected area of conductor covered with ice in square feet per unit length
  A_{wi} is the cross-sectional area of conductor covered with ice in square feet
  l is the length of conductor in unit length

For a 1 ft length of conductor,

$$S_{wi} = \frac{d_c + 2t_i}{12} l \text{ ft}^3/\text{ft} \tag{13.68}$$

Therefore, the horizontal force exerted on the line as a result of the wind pressure with no ice (Figure 13.9) is

$$P = S_{ni} \times p \text{ lb/unit length} \tag{13.69}$$

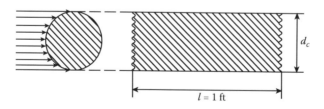

FIGURE 13.9 Force of wind on conductor covered with no ice.

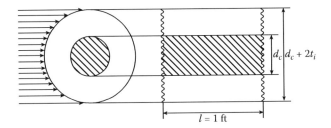

FIGURE 13.10   Force of wind on conductor covered with ice.

For a 1 ft length of conductor,

$$P = \frac{1}{12} d_c \times p \text{ lb/ft}$$ (13.70)

where
    P is the horizontal wind force (i.e., load) exerted on line in pounds per feet
    p is the wind pressure in pounds per square feet

whereas with ice (Figure 13.10), it is

$$P = S_{wi} \times p \text{ lb/unit length}$$ (13.71)

For a 1 ft length of conductor,

$$P = \frac{d_c + 2t_i}{12} p \text{ lb/ft}$$ (13.72)

Therefore, the effective load acting on the conductor is

$$w_e = \sqrt{P^2 + (w + wi)^2} \text{ lb/ft}$$ (13.73)

acting at an angle θ to the vertical, as shown in Figure 13.11.

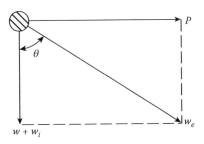

FIGURE 13.11   The effective load acting on the conductor.

By replacing w by w_e in the previously derived equations for tension and sag of the line in still air, these equations can be applied to a wind- and ice-loaded line. For example, the sag equation (13.46) becomes

$$d = \frac{w_e L^2}{8T} \text{ ft} \tag{13.74}$$

Example 13.2

A stress-crossing OH subtransmission line has a span of 500 ft over the stream. The line is located in a heavy-loading district in which the horizontal wind pressure is 4 lb/ft^2 and the radial thickness of the ice is 0.50 in. Use an ACSR conductor of 795 kcmil having an outside diameter of 1.093 in., a weight of 5,399 lb/mi, and an ultimate strength of 28,500 1b. Also use a safety factor of 2 and 57 lb/ft^3 for the weight of ice. Using the parabolic method, calculate the following:

(a) Weight of ice in pounds per feet
(b) Total vertical load on conductor in pounds per feet
(c) Horizontal wind force exerted on line in pounds per feet
(d) Effective load acting on conductor in pounds per feet
(e) Sag in feet
(f) Vertical sag in feet

Solution

(a) Using Equation 13.63,

$$w_i = 1.25 t_i \left(d_c + t_i \right)$$

$$= 1.25 \times 0.50 \left(1.093 + 0.50 \right)$$

$$\cong 0.9956 \text{ lb}$$

(b) Using Equation 13.64,

$$w_T = w + w_i$$

The weight of the conductor is

$$w = 5399 \text{ lb/mi}$$

or

$$w = \frac{5399}{5280} \cong 1.0225 \text{ lb/ft}$$

Therefore,

$$w_T = 1.0225 + 0.9956$$

$$= 2.0181 \text{ lb/ft}$$

(c) From Equation 13.72,

$$P = \frac{d_c + 2t_i}{12} p$$

$$= 1.093 + 2 \times \frac{0.50}{12} \times 4$$

$$= 0.6977 \text{ lb/ft}$$

(d) Using Equation 13.73 and Figure 13.11,

$$w_e = \sqrt{P^2 + (w + w_i)^2}$$

$$= \sqrt{0.6977^2 + 2.0181^2}$$

$$= 2.1353 \text{ lb/ft}$$

as shown in Figure 13.12.

(e) $T = \dfrac{28,500}{2} = 14,250 \text{ lb}$

From Equation 13.74,

$$d = \frac{w_e L^2}{8T}$$

$$= \frac{2.1353 \times 500^2}{8 \times 14,250}$$

$$= 4.68 \text{ ft}$$

(f) Vertical sag $= d \times \cos\theta$

$$= 4.68 \times \frac{2.0181}{2.1353}$$

$$= 4.42 \text{ ft}$$

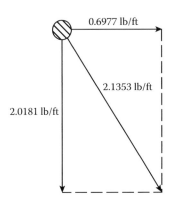

FIGURE 13.12 Effective load acting on the conductor.

13.6 NATIONAL ELECTRIC SAFETY CODE

More than 60% of the states in the United States use the NESC as either an official state code or a guide [1]. Therefore, the design of the OH lines should comply with NESC rules and regulations.

The following information has been based on the 1984 edition of the NESC [1]. Figure 13.13 shows the general loading map of the United States with respect to loading of OH lines. Table 13.1 gives the corresponding normal ice and wind loads for each of the loading districts. However, the NESC recognizes the possible variations in the ice and wind loads due to regional differences.

Table 13.1 shows the minimum radial thickness of ice and the wind pressures to be used in determining loadings. Here, ice is assumed to weigh 57 lb/ft³.

Figure 13.14 shows the NESC wind map of the United States. It shows the minimum horizontal wind pressures to be used for determining loads on tall structures. If any portion of a structure of supported facilities is located in excess of 60 ft above ground, these wind pressures are applied to the entire structure and supported facilities without ice covering. Note the fact that wind velocity usually increases with height. Hence, the given wind pressures have to be increased accordingly.

The total load on a conductor or messenger is the sum of vertical loading and horizontal loading components calculated at the temperature specified in Table 13.2, to which resultant has been added the constant given in Table 13.1. In all cases, therefore, the conductor or messenger tension is determined from this total loading.

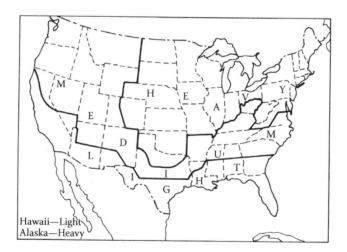

FIGURE 13.13   NESC's general loading map of the United States with respect to loading of OH lines.

TABLE 13.1
Ice and Wind Loads for Specified Districts
according to NESC

	Loading Districts		
	Heavy	**Medium**	**Light**
Radial thickness of ice, in.	0.50	0.25	0
Horizontal wind pressure, lb/ft	4	4	9

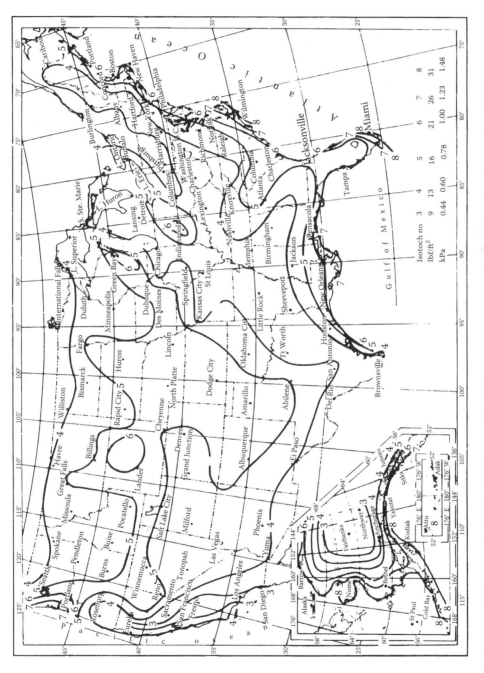

FIGURE 13.14 Extreme wind pressure in lbf/ft² at 30 ft above ground, 50-year mean recurrence interval (based on fastest mile of wind).

TABLE 13.2
Temperatures and Constants as Specified by NESC

| | Loading Districts | | | |
	Heavy	Medium	Light	Extreme Wind Loading
Temperature, °F	0	+15	+30	+60
Constant to be added to resultant in pounds per foot for all conductors	0.30	0.20	0.05	0.0

13.7 LINE LOCATION

The routing of a transmission line or a rural distribution line requires thorough investigation and study with several different routings explored to assure that the most desirable and practical route is selected, taking into consideration not only cost of construction, cost of easements, and cost of clearing but also environmental and maintenance requirements. Therefore, the line location is a matter of judgment and requires sound evaluation of divergent requirements. In practice, the ground is rarely level, and the poles are actually located to conform to the irregularities of the ground. The irregularities of the ground are ordinarily advantageous and allow slightly longer spans on the average than could be obtained with the same height of structures on level ground.

13.7.1 PROFILE AND PLAN OF RIGHT-OF-WAY

The basic purpose of the profile and the final plan of the ROW of a given line is to ensure correct design and economical construction. They are permanent drawings, as they are the key construction drawings, ROW record, and permanent property record. Accurate collection of field data and translation of such data to plan and profile drawings are of utmost importance since errors in this work will defeat the purposes of the drawings and cancel out the accuracy of structure spotting with a template.

In general, profiles are plotted on standard ruled profile section paper to a vertical scale of 40 ft to the inch and a horizontal scale of 400 ft to the inch. This scaling arrangement provides a most compact drawing with sufficient accuracy for most conditions. For some lines, three profiles may be desirable, one along the center of the line and one on each side, that is, at each edge of ROW. The two side profiles indicate the amount and direction of the slope of the ground across the line that must be allowed for in determining ground clearance.

A plan of the secured ROW is also required for determining the construction at angles in the line and the clearances from the conductor to the edge of the ROW when the conductor is deflected by the wind.

The planning engineer selects a tentative line route, making use of aerial photographs and the following maps: geological survey, county soil, county plat, road, post office routes, the US Forest Service, Bureau of Indian Affairs, aerial strip, and any other maps that may be available. These maps contain detailed topography from which a tentative paper location can be made. Also, aerial reconnaissance may be desirable over hilly and mountainous country. However, nowadays, typically the Google Earth is used for these purposes, as illustrated in Figure 13.15.

Based on this tentative line route, a more detailed survey needs to be prepared to show the proposed HV line and the angle positions, together with the obstructions mentioned. The angles in the line must be more accurately positioned by the surveyor according to site conditions. The surveyor measures the angles of deviation of the line at each angle or control point (marked by hub stakes, with tack points of alignment) and measures the straight-line distance between them. He has to take levels, entering

FIGURE 13.15 Selection of line route using Google Earth.

them in a level book, along the measuring chain at intervals depending on the gradient of the land at the point concerned. Other methods of survey are as follows:

1. *Slight grading*: It is cheaper and much faster if it is done by an experienced surveyor. However, of course, it is not economic if each pole ends up being much longer than it needs to be. Thus, it may be used only for level ground.
2. *Tacheometric survey*: It is done by using a theodolite if the ground is hilly and the measuring chain is not used.
3. *Aerial survey*: It may be useful for very long HV transmission lines, but it is hardly applicable to ordinary rural distribution.

13.7.2 TEMPLATES FOR LOCATING STRUCTURES

The location of structures on the profile with a template is essential for both correct design and economy. The sag template is a convenient device used in the design of a transmission line to determine graphically on plan and profile drawings the location and height of structures. It is cut from a transparent plastic material approximately 0.72 mm in thickness. It has the same horizontal and vertical scales as used for the profile and plan of the ROW. With reasonable competence and some experience, this method can be relied upon to provide the following:

1. Maintenance of proper clearance from conductor to ground and to crossing conductors
2. Economic layout
3. Minimum possibility of errors in design and layout
4. Proper grading of structures
5. Prevention of excessive insulator swing or uplift at structures
6. Exactly the correct quantity of material purchased and delivered to the proper site

A sag template is cut as a parabola on the maximum sag, usually at 120°F, of the ruling span, and is extended by calculating the sag as proportional to square of the span for spans both shorter and longer than the ruling span. Since the curvature of the catenary or parabola in which the conductor hangs depends only on the tension and loading and not on the length of the span or on the difference in elevation of the points of support, all spans having the same tension and loading can be drawn from a single template, irrespective of their lengths or of the differences in elevation of the support points. However, when the elevations of the support points are not the same, the lowest point of the curve is shifted from the middle of the span toward the lower support, but the axis of the curve remains vertical.

The sag template has three curves on it: one for ground clearance with maximum sag, one for uplift at times of minimum sag, and one for maximum side swing. Therefore, the required curves are as follows:

1. *Hot curve*: It is drawn for 120°F, no ice, no wind, final sag curve. It is used to locate position of structure and to check clearance, insulator swing, and structure height on the plotted profile.
2. *Cold curve*: It is drawn for minimum temperature (0°F), no ice, no wind, minimum initial sag curve. It is used to check for uplift and insulator swing.
3. *Normal curve*: It is drawn for 60°F, no ice, no wind, final sag curve. It is used to check normal clearances and insulator swing.

Uplift conditions for the OH conductors must be avoided. It can be checked by the cold curve. Conductors of underbuilt lines may be of different sizes. The hot curve of the lowest conductor should be used for checking ground clearance. Cold curves are required for each size of conductor to check for uplift or insulator swing.

A sag template drawing, as shown in Figure 13.16, is prepared for each line as a guide in cutting the template. A new template has to be prepared for each line where there is any variation in conductor size, conductor configuration, assumed loading conditions, design tension, ruling span, or voltage because a change in any one of these factors will change the characteristics of the template. The sags in Table 13.3 are determined as follows [3]:

1. Read applicable ruling span sag from sag and tension chart furnished by conductor manufacturer.
2. Calculate the other sag by using the formula

$$d = \frac{L^2 d_e}{L_e^2}$$

where
      d is the sag of other span in feet
      d_e is the sag of ruling span in feet
      L is the length of other span in feet
      L_e is the length of ruling span in feet

3. Apply catenary sag correction to long spans having large sags.

Table 13.3 gives sags for preparing a template for 4/0 ACSR conductor with 4210 lb design tension and 600 ft ruling span and for heavy-loading conditions. The template allows 1 ft greater clearances than the ones required by the NESC to allow minor shifts in structure location.

As shown in Figure 13.16, the intersection of the template with ground line determines the location of the structure. The vertical distance between this intersection and the lowest conductor curve gives the basic height of the pole. In order to achieve this, the ground clearance curve should be tangent to the ground profile. The vertical axis aids in holding the template vertical when spotting structures.

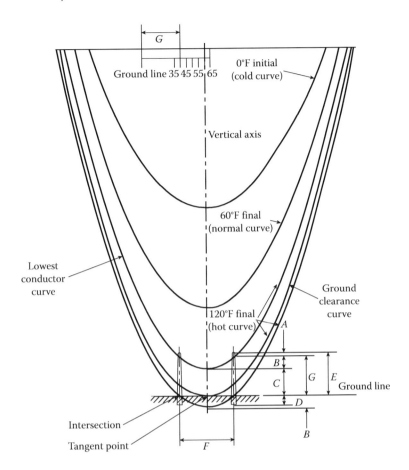

FIGURE 13.16 Sag template based on values given in Table 13.3: *A*, dimension from top of pole to point of attachment of lowest conductor; *B*, sag in level ground; *C*, ground clearance; *D*, setting depth of pole; *E*, length of pole; *F*, level ground span; *G*, dimension from ground to point of attachment of lowest conductor.

Ice and snow on the conductors may cause weights several times that of the 0.5 in. ice loading, and conductors have been known to sag to within reach of the ground. Such occurrences are not considered in line design, and when they happen, the line is taken out of service until the ice or snow falls. Checks made afterward have nearly always shown no permanent deformation.

The template must be used subject to a *creep* correction when aluminum conductors are involved. The creep is a constant nonelastic conductor stretch that continues for the life of the line. It causes a continuous slow increase in the sag of the line that must be estimated and allowed for. The manufacturers of aluminum conductors provide creep-estimating curves. The remedy is to check all close clearance points on the profile with a template made with no creep allowance and to choose higher structure at these points if the addition of extra creep sag encroaches on the required clearances.

The lowest point of the sag, on step and inclined spans, may fall beyond the lower support. This indicates that the conductor in the uphill span exerts a negative or upward pull on the lower structure, that is, the pole or tower. The amount of this upward pull is equal to the weight of the conductor from the structure to the low point in the sag. If the upward pull of the uphill span is greater than the downward load of the next adjacent span, actual uplift is caused, and the conductor tends to swing clear of the structure.

Therefore, the designer should not allow sudden changes in elevation of the structures.

In the design of lines with suspension insulators, each structure must carry a considerable weight of the conductor, and the uplift condition should not even be approached. The minimum weight that each structure must carry can be determined by finding the transverse angle to which the insulator

TABLE 13.3

Sags for Preparing Spotting Template

Condition Tension, lb Span (ft)	0°F Initial 2150 Sag (ft)	60°F Final 1174 Sag (ft)	120°F Final 981 Sag (ft)
200	0.68	1.24	1.49
400	2.71	4.98	5.96
600	6.11	11.2	13.4
800	10.9	19.9	23.8
1000	16.9	31.1	37.2
1200	24.4	44.8	53.6
1400	33.2	60.9	73.2[a]
1600	43.4	79.8[a]	95.7[a]
1800	55.0	101.2[a]	121.3[a]
2000	67.9	125.0[a]	150.0[a]
2200	82.1	151.51	181.7[a]
2400	98.0	180.4[a]	216.6[a]
2600	115.0	212.0[a]	254.7[a]
2800	133.5	246.3[a]	296.0[a]
3000	153.3	283.2[a]	340.6[a]

[a] Corrected by catenary method; a maximum of 1.64%.

string may swing without reducing the clearance from the conductor to the structure too greatly and by maintaining the ratio of vertical weight to horizontal wind load such that the insulator is not permitted to swing beyond this angle. Usually, the maximum wind is assumed at 60°F.

The insulator swings in the direction of the resultant of the vertical and horizontal forces acting on the insulator string. The minimum angle of conductor swing to be used in computations, where proximity to other circuits is involved, is 30° according to sixth edition of the NESC. In general, a clearance corresponding to approximately 75% of the flashover value of the insulator is appropriate.

13.7.3 SUPPORTING STRUCTURES

The structure heights, locations, and types can be determined by use of plan and profile sheets. It requires both engineering and economics. The following design factors should be considered:

1. Conductor sag and tension limitations
2. Clearance involved
3. Separation distances between conductors
4. Uplift or insulator swing
5. Loading of conductors
6. Height and strength of structures
7. Soil conditions
8. Control, or angle, points
9. Operation and maintenance problems

In order to spot or locate structures, the template is held tangent to the profile, and the ground clearance curve is held tangent to the profile. The edge of the template intersects the ground profile

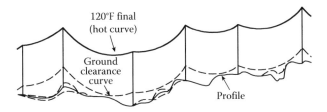

FIGURE 13.17 Locating structures by templates.

at points where structures of the basic height should be set. Here, the ground clearance curve represents the actual position of the lowest conductor. The procedure that is illustrated in Figure 13.16 for a level span is the same for any given type of terrain.

Once the height and the location of the structure is determined, the template should be shifted so that the clearance curve barely touches tangent to the profile, and the point where the edge of the template intersects the profile determines the location of the next structure of basic height. The point may be marked by drawing an arc along the edge of the template where it intersects the profile. The template should then be shifted and adjusted so that with the opposite edge of the template held on the point previously located, the clearance curve will again barely touch the profile. As is done before, an arc should be drawn to mark the location of the next structure of basic height, and the process is repeated to locate each structure of the line, as shown in Figure 13.17. Figure 13.18 shows an application using a computer program to locate each structure of the line.

After all structures are located, the structures and lowest conductor's arc should be drawn in. When line angles, broken terrain, and crossings are encountered, it may be necessary to cut and try several different arrangements of structure heights, increased clearances, and locations to determine the best arrangement. In addition to maintaining clearances, uplift must be avoided on lines with pin-type insulators, and excessive insulator swings must be avoided on lines with suspension-type insulators. On the lines with pin-type insulators, there is no danger of uplift if the low-temperature initial curve does not pass above the point of conductor support on the two adjacent structures.

13.8 CONSTRUCTION TECHNIQUES

Construction of transmission line in the rugged mountainous terrain requires access to the proposed route and transmission tower locations (PIs). The access roads to and along the ROW need to be carefully selected and surveyed before the construction of these roads are started to take into account the width, grade, and surface conditions. It also has to be determined which segments or site could not be accessed with conventional access roads and will need to be accessed by air (helicopter). Selected photographs shown in Figures 13.19 through 13.22 are provided for general information about transmission line construction in various terrains.

It is also essential that applicable national local government permits and approvals be secured before the access road and transmission work commences. Special care must be taken in identifying and listing any sites and routes that require special environmental care. A restoration plan should also be prepared prior to commencing with construction work complete with aerial or site photographs.

The actual construction will follow standard construction and mitigation best practices that were developed from past project experience. These best practices address ROW clearing, staging, erecting transmission line structures, and stringing transmission lines. Construction and mitigation practices to minimize impacts will be developed based on the proposed schedule for activities, permit requirements, prohibitions, maintenance guidelines, inspection procedures, terrain, and other practices. In some cases, these activities, such as schedules, are modified to minimize impacts to sensitive environments.

Transmission line structures are generally designed for installation at existing grades. Typically, structure sites with 10% or less slope will not be graded or leveled. At sites with more than 10% slope, working areas graded level or fill will be brought in for working pads.

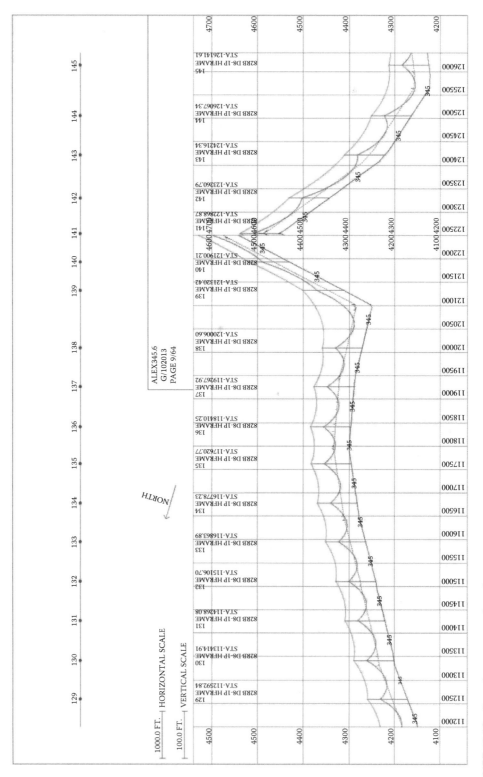

FIGURE 13.18 Locating structures by using a computer program.

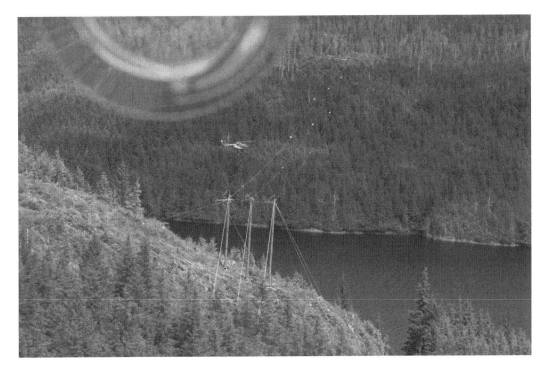

FIGURE 13.19 A river crossing of an HV transmission line.

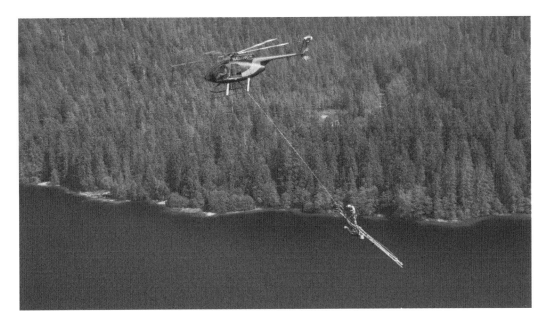

FIGURE 13.20 A helicopter carrying an incomplete pole to its location across a river.

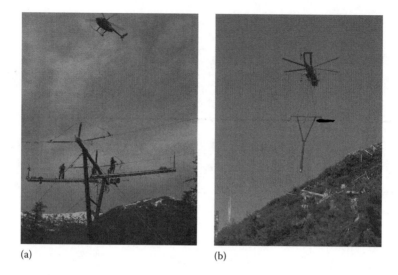

(a)   (b)

FIGURE 13.21 (a) Pole-top construction at the location and (b) a helicopter carrying an incomplete pole to its location.

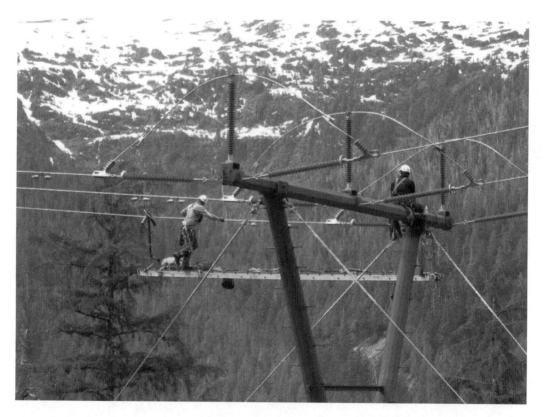

FIGURE 13.22 A crew is working on pole-top construction.

Staging areas will be established for the project and involve delivering the equipment and materials necessary to construct the new transmission line facilities. The materials will be stored at staging areas until they are needed for construction.

Temporary lay-down areas may be required for additional storage space during construction. These areas will be selected for their location, access, security, and ability to efficiently and safely warehouse supplies. The areas are chosen to minimize excavation and grading. The temporary lay-down areas outside of the transmission line ROW will be obtained from affected landowners through rental agreements.

Access to the transmission line ROW corridor is made directly from existing roads or trails that run parallel or perpendicular to the transmission line ROW. In some situations, private field roads or trails are used. Permission from the property owner is obtained prior to accessing the transmission line route. Where necessary to accommodate the heavy equipment used in construction (including cranes, cement trucks, and hole drilling equipment), existing access roads may be upgraded or new roads may be constructed. New access roads may also be constructed when no current access is available or the existing access is inadequate to cross roadway ditches.

When it is time to install the poles, they are generally moved from the staging areas and delivered to the staked location. The structures are typically placed within the transmission line ROW until the structure is set. Insulators and other hardware are attached while the pole is on the ground. The pole is then lifted, placed, and secured using a crane.

Medium-angle, heavy-angle, or dead-end structures will have concrete foundations. In those cases, holes are drilled in preparation for concrete. Drilled pier foundations may vary from 5 to 7 ft in diameter for the 400 kV transmission line and bolted to it. Concrete trucks are required to bring concrete from a local concrete batch plant.

Preparation for construction begins with the development of access points from existing roads. Clearing of all woody vegetation and brush within the 130-ft-wide ROW would be required to facilitate the safe and efficient construction, operation, and maintenance of the transmission line. A reasonably level access path is required to provide for safe passage of construction equipment. At structure locations, a stable working surface free of tripping hazards is required for framing and erecting structures and for the installation of concrete foundations if required.

Vegetation would be cut at or slightly above the ground surface. Rootstock would be left in place to stabilize existing soils and to regenerate vegetation after construction. With the approval of the landowner or land manager, stumps of tall-growing species would be treated with an approved herbicide to discourage regrowth. Merchantable timber is typically cut to standard log lengths and stacked along the ROW edge. Vegetation clearing debris (trees, brush, and slash) may be cut and scattered, placed in windrow piles, chipped, or burned, depending on location. In some special circumstances, this material may be collected for use as fuel.

To minimize the potential for tire and chassis damage to construction equipment and to maintain a safe, level access path and structure installation area, incidental stump removal would occur. Stumps that interfere with the placement of mats or movement of construction equipment would be ground down to a point at or slightly below ground level. If temporary removal or relocation of fences were necessary, the installation of temporary or permanent gates would be coordinated with the property owner(s).

Environmentally sensitive areas or areas susceptible to soil erosion would require special construction techniques. These techniques may include the use of low ground pressure equipment, timber mats, terracing, water bars, bale checks, rock checks, or temporary mulching and seeding of disturbed areas exposed during long periods of construction inactivity. Permanent erosion control measures may include permanent seeding, mulching, erosion control mats, or other measures depending on site conditions. Temporary bio-roll, silt fence, sedimentation ponds, and other measures may be utilized to prevent sediment from running off into wetlands or other surface waters.

The wire stringing process starts in a setup area prepared to accommodate the stringing equipment and materials, normally located midspan on the centerline of the ROW. The rope machine, new conductor wire trailers, and tensioner are located at the wire stringing setup area. This phase of construction occurs after the structures have been erected and fitted with stringing blocks (also called dollies or sheaves) and with single-leader *p-line* ropes that reach the ground. Stringing blocks are a type of pulley that attach to the insulator assembly and temporarily support a pulling rope or p-line and a wire rope or *hard line*, which in turn supports the conductor before it is permanently *clipped in*. The process starts as the construction crew pulls the p-lines toward the first structure beyond the setup area. The p-lines are normally pulled down the ROW with a small wide-track bombardier or other small equipment.

At each structure, the ropes are detached from the bombardier and attached to the single-leader p-line to lift the ropes up into the dollies. Then the ropes are reattached to the bombardier and driven to the next structure for the same process. After the p-line has been strung through all the structures for all phases within the stringing interval, the pulling ropes are attached to a hard line and pulled, one at a time, back through the dollies to the beginning of the interval. A hard-line setup is located at the opposite end of the interval from the wire stringing setup area. Each hard line is then attached to the conductor wire with an attachment called a *sock*, which is pulled back through the dollies to the end of the interval. Crew members travel along the access route in a pickup truck, following the *sock* as it is being pulled to make sure it does not get hung up in the dollies.

One at a time, the conductor wires are then pulled to the appropriate tension and clipped into place utilizing permanent suspension hardware. Wire stringing and hard-line setup areas are normally located in upland areas during spring, summer, or fall conditions.

If construction is performed during winter when frozen conditions provide a stable working surface, setups may be located in wetland areas. If setups in wetlands are required when surface conditions are not stable, extensive use of timber matting is required.

PROBLEMS

13.1 A single span of an OH line is 250 ft in length, having the supporting poles at the same level. The maximum tension in the conductor is 855 lb. The weight of the conductor is 0.125 lb/ft. Calculate the sag:
(a) Using the catenary method
(b) Using the parabolic method

13.2 An OH line conductor has taken the form of a catenary of $y = c \cosh(x/c)$, where c is 925 ft. The span between the poles is 235 ft, and the weight of the conductor is 0.139 lb/ft. Calculate the following:
(a) Length of conductor by using Equations 13.24 and 13.27
(b) Sag
(c) Maximum tension of conductor
(d) Minimum tension of conductor

13.3 An OH line over a hillside is supported from two towers, as shown in Figure P13.3, at levels of 28.1 and 49.6 ft above a horizontal datum line. The span is 350 ft. The copper conductor of the line has a breaking strength of 15,140 lb and a weight of 5,706 lb/mi. Use the parabolic method:
(a) Calculate the location of the lowest point of the curve.
(b) Calculate sags d_1 and d_2.
(c) Which of the sags should be considered as the principal sag?

13.4 An OH line conductor is supported at a water crossing from two towers, the heights of the supports being 30 and 34.2 m, respectively, above water level, with a horizontal span of 325 m. The conductor weighs 8.42 N/m, and its tension is not to exceed 4.44×10^4 N. Calculate the following:
(a) Clearance between lowest point of conductor and water
(b) Horizontal distance of this point from lower support

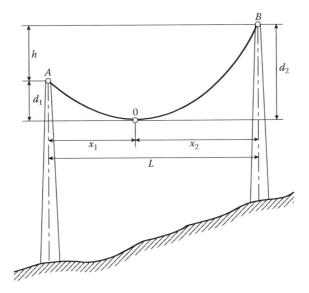

FIGURE P13.3 Figure for Problem P13.3.

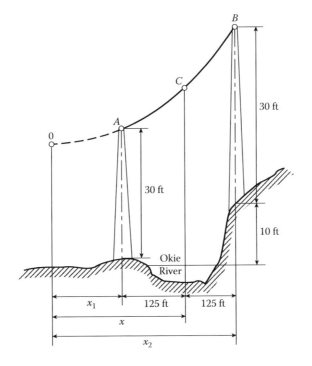

FIGURE P13.5 Figure for Problem P13.5.

13.5 A river-crossing OH line is supported from two poles at heights of 30 and 40 ft above the water level, as shown in Figure P13.5. The conductor of the line is a 1/0 copper conductor. Use a safety factor of 2. Calculate the clearance between the water level and the conductor at a point midway between the poles.

13.6 The ACSR conductors of an OH line have 1.63 cm overall diameter and are supported by suspension insulator strings of 1.02 m long. The permissible tension is 2.50×10^4 N, the conductor weighs 5.35 N/m, and the ice weighs 8920 N/m^3. Find the height of the lowest crossarm above ground level if the minimum clearance between conductor and ground is 6.9 m when there is an ice load 1.27 cm thick and a horizontal wind pressure of 461 N/m^2 on span lengths of 195 m.

13.7 Find the minimum permissible sag for a span of 225 m using a copper conductor with 1.2 cm diameter and allowing a maximum conductor tension of 2200 kg/cm^2. The horizontal wind pressure is 6 g/cm^2, and the specific gravity of copper is 8.9.

13.8 Calculate the sag in a 90 yd span of a 0.035 in.^{2} OH line when covered with ice to a radial thickness of 5/8 in., in a wind that exerts a pressure of 9 lb/ft^2. Assume the breaking load as 1620 lb and the weight of the conductor as 0.1 lb/ft. Allow a safety factor of 2.

REFERENCES

1. American National Standards Institute. *National Electrical Safety Code*, 1984 edn., IEEE, New York, 1984.
2. Electric Power Research Institute. *Transmission Line Reference Book: 115–138 kV Compact Line Design*, EPRI, Palo Alto, CA, 1978.
3. Rural Electrification Administration. *Transmission Line Manual*, REA Bull. No. 62-1, U.S. Department of Agriculture, U.S. Government Printing Office, Washington, DC, 1972.

GENERAL REFERENCES

American Society of Chemical Engineers. *Guide for Design of Steel Transmission Towers*, ASCE-Manuals Rep. Eng. Pract. No. 52, ASCE, New York, 1971.
DeWeese, F. C. *Transmission Lines: Design, Construction and Performance*, McGraw-Hill, New York, 1945.
Dwight, H. B. *Electrical Elements of Power Transmission Lines*, MacMillan, New York, 1954.
Edison Electric Institute. *EHV Transmission Line Reference Book*, EEI, New York, 1968.
Electric Power Research Institute. *Transmission Line Reference Book: 345 kV and Above*, 2nd edn., EPRI, Palo Alto, CA, 1982.
Fink, D. G. and Carroll, J. M., eds. *Standard Handbook for Electrical Engineers*, 10th edn., McGraw-Hill, New York, 1969.
Freeman, P. J. *Electric Power Transmission & Distribution*, George G. Harrap & Co., London, U.K., 1977.
Gönen, T. *Electric Power Distribution System Engineering*, 2nd edn., CRC Press, Boca Raton, FL, 2008.
Guile, A. E. and Paterson, W. *Electrical Power Systems*, 2nd edn., Pergamon Press, New York, 1977.
Mallik, U. G. *Solution of Problems in Electrical Power*, Pitman, London, U.K., 1968.
Pender, H. and Del Mar, W. A., eds. *Electrical Engineers' Handbook: Electric Power*, 4th edn., Wiley, New York, 1962.
Powel, C. A. *Principles of Electric Utility Engineering*, MIT Press, Cambridge, MA, 1955.
Rapson, E. T. A. *Electrical Transmission and Distribution*, Oxford University Press, London, U.K., 1933.
Seelye, H. P. *Electrical Distribution Engineering*, McGraw-Hill, New York, 1930.
Siemens Aktienges. *Electrical Engineering Handbook*, Berlin, Germany, 1976.
Skrotzki, B. G. A., ed. *Electric Transmission and Distribution*, McGraw-Hill, New York, 1954.
Taylor, E. O. and Boal, G. A., eds. *Electric Power Distribution: 413–33 kV*, Arnold, London, U.K., 1966.
Woodruff, L. F. *Principles of Electric Power Transmission*, 2nd edn., Wiley, New York, 1938.

Appendix A: Impedance Tables for Overhead Lines, Transformers, and Underground Cables

TABLE A.1
Characteristics of Copper Conductors, Hard Drawn, 97.3% Conductivity

Size of Conductor (Circular Mils)	AWG or B&S	Number of Strands	Diameter of Individual Strands (in.)	Outside Diameter (in.)	Breaking Strength (lb)	Weight (lb/mi)	Approx. Current-Carrying Capacity[a] (A)	Geometric Mean Radius at 60 Cycles (ft)
1,000,000	...	37	0.1644	1.151	43,830	16,300	1300	0.0368
900,000	...	37	0.1560	1.092	39,610	14,670	1220	0.0349
800,000	...	37	0.1470	1.029	35,120	13,040	1130	0.0329
750,000	...	37	0.1424	0.997	33,400	12,230	1090	0.0319
700,000	...	37	0.1375	0.963	31,170	11,410	1040	0.0306
500,000	...	37	0.1273	0.891	27,020	9,781	940	0.0285
500,000	...	37	0.1162	0.814	22,610	8,161	840	0.0260
500,000	...	19	0.1622	0.811	21,590	8,161	840	0.0256
450,000	...	19	0.1539	0.770	19,750	7,336	780	0.0243
400,000	...	19	0.1451	0.726	17,560	6,521	730	0.0229
350,000	...	19	0.1357	0.679	16,890	5,706	670	0.0214
350,000	...	12	0.1708	0.710	16,140	5,706	670	0.0225
300,000	...	19	0.1257	0.629	13,510	4,891	610	0.01987
300,000	...	12	0.1581	0.657	13,170	4,891	610	0.0208
250,000	...	19	0.1147	0.574	11,360	4,076	540	0.01813
250,000	...	12	0.1443	0.600	11,130	4,076	540	0.01902
211,600	4/0	19	0.1055	0.528	9,617	3,450	480	0.01668
211,600	4/0	12	0.1328	0.552	9,483	3,450	490	0.01750
211,600	4/0	7	0.1739	0.522	9,154	3,450	480	0.01579
167,800	3/0	12	0.1183	0.492	7,556	2,736	420	0.01569
167,800	3/0	7	0.1548	0.464	7,366	2,736	420	0.01404
133,100	2/0	7	0.1379	0.414	5,926	2,170	360	0.01252
106,500	1/0	7	0.1228	0.368	4,752	1,720	310	0.01113
83,690	1	7	0.1093	0.328	3,804	1,364	270	0.00992
63,690	1	3	0.1670	0.360	3,620	1,351	270	0.01016
66,370	2	7	0.0974	0.292	3,045	1,082	230	0.00883
66,370	2	3	0.1487	0.320	2,913	1,071	240	0.00903
66,370	2	1	...	0.258	3,003	1,061	220	0.00836
52,630	3	7	0.0867	0.260	2,433	858	200	0.00787
52,630	3	3	0.1325	0.286	2,359	850	200	0.00805
52,630	3	1	...	0.229	2,439	841	190	0.00745
41,740	4	3	0.1180	0.254	1,879	674	180	0.00717
41,740	4	1	...	0.204	1,970	667	170	0.00663
33,100	5	3	0.1050	0.226	1,605	534	180	0.00638
33,100	5	1	...	0.1819	1,591	529	140	0.00590
26,250	6	3	0.0935	0.201	1,205	424	130	0.00568
26,250	6	1	...	0.1620	1,280	420	120	0.00526
20,820	7	1	...	0.1443	1,030	333	110	0.00468
16,510	8	1	...	0.1286	826	264	90	0.00417

Sources: Westinghouse Electric Corporation, *Electric Utility Engineering Reference Book—Distribution Systems*, Westinghouse Electric Corporation, East Pittsburgh, PA, 1965; Gönen, T., *Electric Power Distribution System Engineering*, CRC Press.

[a] For conductor at 75°C, air at 25°C, wind 1.4 mi/h (2 ft/s), frequency = 60 cycles.

r_a Resistance (Ω/Conductor/mi)								X_a Inductive Reactance (Ω/Conductor/mi) at 1 ft Spacing			X'_a Shunt Capacitive Reactance (MΩ mi/Conductor) at 1 ft Spacing		
25°C (77°F)				50°C (122°F)									
DC	25 Cycles	50 Cycles	60 Cycles	DC	25 Cycles	50 Cycles	60 Cycles	25 Cycles	50 Cycles	60 Cycles	25 Cycles	50 Cycles	60 Cycles
0.0585	0.0594	0.0620	0.0634	0.0640	0.0648	0.0672	0.0685	0.1666	0.333	0.400	0.216	0.1081	0.0901
0.0650	0.0658	0.0682	0.0695	0.0711	0.0718	0.0740	0.0752	0.1693	0.339	0.406	0.220	0.1100	0.0916
0.0731	0.0739	0.0760	0.0772	0.0800	0.0808	0.0826	0.0837	0.1722	0.344	0.413	0.224	0.1121	0.0934
0.0780	0.0787	0.0807	0.6818	0.0853	0.0859	0.0878	0.0888	0.1739	0.348	0.417	10.225	0.1132	0.0943
0.0836	0.0842	0.0661	0.0671	0.0914	0.0920	0.0937	0.0947	0.1789	0.352	0.422	0.229	0.1145	0.0954
0.0975	0.0981	0.0997	0.1006	0.1066	0.1071	0.1086	0.1095	0.1799	0.360	0.432	0.235	0.1173	0.0977
0.1170	0.1175	0.1188	0.1196	0.1280	0.1283	0.1296	0.1303	0.1845	0.369	0.443	0.241	0.1206	0.1004
0.1170	0.1175	0.1188	0.1196	0.1280	0.1283	0.1296	0.1303	0.1853	0.371	0.445	0.241	0.1206	0.1006
0.1300	0.1304	0.1316	0.1323	0.1422	0.1426	0.1437	0.1443	0.1879	0.376	0.451	0.245	0.1224	0.1020
0.1462	0.1466	0.1477	0.1484	0.1600	0.1603	0.1613	0.1519	0.1909	0.382	0.458	0.249	0.1245	0.1038
0.1671	0.1675	0.1684	0.1690	0.1828	0.1831	0.1840	0.1845	0.1943	0.389	0.466	0.254	0.1269	0.1058
0.1671	0.1675	0.1684	0.1690	0.1828	0.1831	0.1840	0.1845	0.1918	0.384	0.460	0.251	0.1253	0.1044
0.1950	0.1953	0.1961	0.1966	0.213	0.214	0.214	0.215	0.1982	0.396	0.476	0.259	0.1296	0.1060
0.1950	0.1953	0.1961	0.1966	0.213	0.214	0.214	0.215	0.1957	0.392	0.470	0.256	0.1281	0.1068
0.234	0.234	0.235	0.236	0.256	0.256	0.257	0.257	0.203	0.406	0.487	0.266	0.1329	0.1108
0.234	0.234	0.235	0.236	0.256	0.256	0.257	0.257	0.200	0.401	0.481	0.263	0.1313	0.1094
0.276	0.277	0.277	0.278	0.302	0.303	0.303	0.303	0.207	0.414	0.497	0.272	0.1359	0.1132
0.276	0.277	0.277	0.278	0.302	0.303	0.303	0.303	0.208	0.409	0.491	0.269	0.1343	0.1119
0.276	0.277	0.277	0.278	0.302	0.303	0.303	0.303	0.210	0.420	0.603	0.273	0.1363	0.1136
0.349	0.349	0.349	0.350	0.381	0.381	0.382	0.382	0.210	0.421	0.606	0.277	0.1384	0.1153
0.349	0.349	0.349	0.350	0.381	0.381	0.382	0.382	0.216	0.431	0.518	0.281	0.1405	0.1171
0.440	0.440	0.440	0.440	0.481	0.481	0.481	0.481	0.222	0.443	0.532	0.289	0.1445	0.1205
0.555	0.555	0.555	0.555	0.606	0.607	0.607	0.607	0.227	0.455	0.546	0.298	0.1488	0.1240
0.599	0.699	0.699	0.699	0.766				0.233	0.467	0.560	0.306	0.1528	0.1274
0.692	0.692	0.692	0.692	0.757				0.232	0.464	0.557	0.299	0.1495	0.1246
0.881	0.882	0.882	0.882	0.964				0.239	0.478	0.574	0.314	0.1570	0.1308
0.873				0.956				0.238	0.476	0.571	0.307	0.1637	0.1281
0.884				0.946				0.242	0.484	0.581	0.323	0.1614	0.1346
1.112				1.216				0.245	0.490	0.588	0.322	0.1611	0.1343
1.101				1.204				0.244	0.488	0.585	0.316	0.1578	0.1315
1.090		Same as dc		1.192		Same as dc		0.248	0.496	0.595	0.331	0.1656	0.1380
1.388				1.518				0.250	0.499	0.599	0.324	0.1619	0.1349
1.374				1.503				0.264	0.507	0.609	0.339	0.1697	0.1416
1.750				1.914				0.256	0.511	0.613	0.332	0.1661	0.1384
1.733				1.895				0.260	0.519	0.623	0.348	0.1738	0.1449
2.21				2.41				0.262	0.523	0.628	0.341	0.1703	0.1419
2.18				2.39				0.265	0.531	0.637	0.356	0.1779	0.1483
2.75				3.01				0.271	0.542	0.651	0.364	0.1821	0.1517
3.47				3.80				0.277	0.564	0.665	0.372	0.1862	0.1652

TABLE A.2

Characteristics of Alcoa Aluminum Conductors, Hard Drawn, 61% Conductivity

Size of Conductor (Circular Mils or AWG)	No. of Strands	Diameter of Individual Strands (in.)	Outside Diameter (in.)	Ultimate Strength (lb)	Weight (lb/mi)	GMR at 60 Cycles (ft)	Approx. Current-Carrying Capacity[a] (A)
6	7	0.0612	0.184	528	130	0.00556	100
4	7	0.0772	0.232	826	207	0.00700	134
3	7	0.0867	0.260	1,022	261	0.00787	155
2	7	0.0974	0.292	1,266	329	0.00883	180
1	7	0.1094	0.328	1,537	414	0.00992	209
1/0	7	0.1228	0.368	1,865	523	0.01113	242
1/0	19	0.0745	0.373	2,090	523	0.01177	244
2/0	7	0.1379	0.414	2,350	659	0.01251	282
2/0	19	0.0837	0.419	2,586	659	0.01321	283
3/0	7	0.1548	0.464	2,845	832	0.01404	327
3/0	19	0.0940	0.470	3,200	832	0.01483	328
4/0	7	0.1739	0.522	3,590	1049	0.01577	380
4/0	19	0.1055	0.528	3,890	1049	0.01666	381
250,000	37	0.0822	0.575	4,860	1239	0.01841	425
266,800	7	0.1953	0.586	4,525	1322	0.01771	441
266,800	37	0.0849	0.594	5,180	1322	0.01902	443
300,000	19	0.1257	0.629	5,300	1487	0.01983	478
300,000	37	0.0900	0.630	5,830	1487	0.02017	478
336,400	19	0.1331	0.666	5,940	1667	0.02100	514
336,400	37	0.0954	0.668	6,400	1667	0.02135	514
350,000	37	0.0973	0.681	6,680	1735	0.02178	528
397,500	19	0.1447	0.724	6,880	1967	0.02283	575
477,000	19	0.1585	0.793	8,090	2364	0.02501	646
500,000	19	0.1623	0.812	8,475	2478	0.02560	664
500,000	37	0.1162	0.813	9,010	2478	0.02603	664
556,500	19	0.1711	0.856	9,440	2758	0.02701	710
636,000	37	0.1311	0.918	11,240	3152	0.02936	776
715,500	37	0.1391	0.974	12,640	3546	0.03114	817
750,000	37	0.1424	0.997	12,980	3717	0.03188	864
750,000	61	0.1109	0.998	13,510	3717	0.03211	864
795,000	37	0.1466	1.026	13,770	3940	0.03283	897
874,500	37	0.1538	1.077	14,830	4334	0.03443	949
954,000	37	0.1606	1.024	16,180	4728	0.03596	1000
1,000,000	61	0.1280	1.152	17,670	4956	0.03707	1030
1,000,000	91	0.1048	1.153	18,380	4956	0.03720	1030
1,033,500	37	0.1672	1.170	18,260	5122	0.03743	1050
1,113,000	61	0.1351	1.216	19,660	5517	0.03910	1110
1,192,500	61	0.1398	1.258	21,000	5908	0.04048	1160
1,192,500	91	0.1145	1.259	21,400	5908	0.04062	1160
1,272,000	61	0.1444	1.300	22,000	6299	0.04180	1210
1,351,500	61	0.1489	1.340	23,400	6700	0.04309	1250
1,431,000	61	0.1532	1.379	24,300	7091	0.04434	1300
1,510,500	61	0.1574	1.417	25,600	7487	0.04556	1320
1,590,000	61	0.1615	1.454	27,000	7883	0.04674	1380
1,590,000	91	0.1322	1.454	28,100	7883	0.04691	1380

Sources: Westinghouse Electric Corporation, *Electric Utility Engineering Reference Book—Distribution Systems,* Westinghouse Electric Corporation, East Pittsburgh, PA, 1965; Gönen, T., *Electric Power Distribution System Engineering,* CRC Press.

[a] For conductor at 75°C, wind 1.4 mi/h (2 ft/s), frequency = 60 cycles.

| r_a Resistance (Ω/Conductor/mi) | | | | | | | | X_a Inductive Reactance (Ω/Conductor/mi) at 1 ft Spacing | | | X'_a Shunt Capacitive Reactance (MΩ mi/Conductor) at 1 ft Spacing | | |
| 25°C (77°F) | | | | 50°C (122°F) | | | | | | | | | |
DC	25 Cycles	50 Cycles	60 Cycles	DC	25 Cycles	50 Cycles	60 Cycles	25 Cycles	50 Cycles	60 Cycles	25 Cycles	50 Cycles	60 Cycles
3.56	3.56	3.56	3.56	3.91	3.91	3.91	3.91	0.2626	0.5251	0.6301	0.3468	0.1734	0.1445
2.24	2.24	2.24	2.24	2.46	2.46	2.46	2.46	0.2509	0.5017	0.6201	0.3302	0.1651	0.1376
1.77	1.77	1.77	1.77	1.95	1.95	1.95	1.95	0.2450	0.4899	0.5879	0.3221	0.1610	0.1342
1.41	1.41	1.41	1.41	1.55	1.55	1.55	1.55	0.2391	0.4782	0.5739	0.3139	0.1570	0.1308
1.12	1.12	1.12	1.12	1.23	1.23	1.23	1.23	0.2333	0.4665	0.5598	0.3055	0.1528	0.1273
0.885	0.8851	0.8853	0.885	0.973	0.9731	0.9732	0.973	0.2264	0.4528	0.5434	0.2976	0.1488	0.1240
0.885	0.8851	0.8853	0.885	0.973	0.9731	0.9732	0.973	0.2246	0.4492	0.5391	0.2964	0.1482	0.1235
0.702	0.7021	0.7024	0.702	0.771	0.7711	0.7713	0.771	0.2216	0.4431	0.5317	0.2890	0.1445	0.1204
0.702	0.7021	0.7024	0.702	0.771	0.7711	0.7713	0.771	0.2188	0.4376	0.5251	0.2882	0.1441	0.1201
0.557	0.5571	0.5574	0.558	0.612	0.6121	0.6124	0.613	0.2157	0.4314	0.5177	0.2810	0.1405	0.1171
0.557	0.5571	0.5574	0.558	0.612	0.6121	0.6124	0.613	0.2129	0.4258	0.5110	0.2801	0.1400	0.1167
0.441	0.4411	0.4415	0.442	0.485	0.4851	0.4855	0.486	0.2099	0.4196	0.5036	0.2726	0.1363	0.1136
0.441	0.4411	0.4415	0.442	0.485	0.4851	0.4855	0.486	0.2071	0.4141	0.4969	0.2717	0.1358	0.1132
0.374	0.3741	0.3746	0.375	0.411	0.4111	0.4115	0.412	0.2020	0.4040	0.4848	0.2657	0.1328	0.1107
0.350	0.3502	0.3506	0.351	0.385	0.3852	0.3855	0.386	0.2040	0.4079	0.4895	0.2642	0.1321	0.1101
0.350	0.3502	0.3506	0.351	0.385	0.3852	0.3855	0.386	0.2004	0.4007	0.4809	0.2633	0.1316	0.1097
0.311	0.3112	0.3117	0.312	0.342	0.3422	0.3426	0.343	0.1983	0.3965	0.4758	0.2592	0.1296	0.1080
0.311	0.3112	0.3117	0.312	0.342	0.3422	0.3426	0.343	0.1974	0.3947	0.4737	0.2592	0.1296	0.1080
0.278	0.2782	0.2788	0.279	0.306	0.3062	0.3067	0.307	0.1953	0.3907	0.4688	0.2551	0.1276	0.1063
0.278	0.2782	0.2788	0.279	0.306	0.3062	0.3067	0.307	0.1945	0.3890	0.4668	0.2549	0.1274	0.1062
0.267	0.2672	0.2678	0.268	0.294	0.2942	0.2947	0.295	0.1935	0.3870	0.4644	0.2537	0.1268	0.1057
0.235	0.2352	0.2359	0.236	0.258	0.2582	0.2589	0.259	0.1911	0.3822	0.4587	0.2491	0.1246	0.1038
0.196	0.1963	0.1971	0.198	0.215	0.2153	0.2160	0.216	0.1865	0.3730	0.4476	0.2429	0.1214	0.1012
0.187	0.1873	0.1882	0.189	0.206	0.2062	0.2070	0.208	0.1853	0.3707	0.4448	0.2412	0.1206	0.1005
0.187	0.1873	0.1882	0.189	0.206	0.2062	0.2070	0.208	0.1845	0.3689	0.4427	0.2410	0.1205	0.1004
0.168	0.1683	0.1693	0.170	0.185	0.1853	0.1862	0.187	0.1826	0.3652	0.4383	0.2374	0.1187	0.0989
0.147	0.1474	0.1484	0.149	0.162	0.1623	0.1633	0.164	0.1785	0.3569	0.4283	0.2323	0.1162	0.0968
0.137	0.1314	0.1326	0.133	0.144	0.1444	0.1455	0.146	0.1754	0.3508	0.4210	0.2282	0.1141	0.0951
0.125	0.1254	0.1267	0.127	0.137	0.1374	0.1385	0.139	0.1743	0.3485	0.4182	0.2266	0.1133	0.0944
0.125	0.1254	0.1267	0.127	0.137	0.1374	0.1385	0.139	0.1739	0.3477	0.4173	0.2263	0.1132	0.0943
0.117	0.1175	0.1188	0.120	0.129	0.1294	0.1306	0.131	0.1728	0.3455	0.4146	0.2244	0.1122	0.0935
0.107	0.1075	0.1089	0.110	0.118	0.1185	0.1198	0.121	0.1703	0.3407	0.4088	0.2210	0.1105	0.0921
0.0979	0.0985	0.1002	0.100	0.108	0.1085	0.1100	0.111	0.1682	0.3363	0.4036	0.2179	0.1090	0.0908
0.0934	0.0940	0.0956	0.0966	0.103	0.1035	0.1050	0.106	0.1666	0.3332	0.3998	0.2162	0.1081	0.0901
0.0934	0.0940	0.0956	0.0966	0.103	0.1035	0.1050	0.106	0.1664	0.3328	0.3994	0.2160	0.1080	0.0900
0.0904	0.0910	0.0927	0.0936	0.0994	0.0999	0.1015	0.102	0.1661	0.3322	0.3987	0.2150	0.1075	0.0895
0.0839	0.0845	0.0864	0.0874	0.0922	0.0928	0.0945	0.0954	0.1639	0.3278	0.3934	0.2124	0.1062	0.0885
0.0783	0.0790	0.0810	0.0821	0.0860	0.0866	0.0884	0.0895	0.1622	0.3243	0.3892	0.2100	0.1050	0.0875
0.0783	0.0790	0.0810	0.0821	0.0860	0.0866	0.0884	0.0895	0.1620	0.3240	0.3888	0.2098	0.1049	0.0874
0.0734	0.0741	0.0762	0.0774	0.0806	0.0813	0.0832	0.0843	0.1606	0.3211	0.3853	0.2076	0.1038	0.0865
0.0691	0.0699	0.0721	0.0733	0.0760	0.0767	0.0787	0.0798	0.1590	0.3180	0.3816	0.2054	0.1027	0.0856
0.0653	0.0661	0.0685	0.0697	0.0718	0.0725	0.0747	0.0759	0.1576	0.3152	0.3782	0.2033	0.1016	0.0847
0.0618	0.0627	0.0651	0.0665	0.0679	0.0687	0.0710	0.0722	0.1562	0.3123	0.3748	0.2014	0.1007	0.0839
0.0597	0.0596	0.0622	0.0636	0.0645	0.0653	0.0677	0.0690	0.1549	0.3098	0.3718	0.1997	0.0998	0.0832
0.0587	0.0596	0.0622	0.0636	0.0645	0.0653	0.0677	0.0690	0.1547	0.3094	0.3713	0.1997	0.0998	0.0832

TABLE A.3
Characteristics of Aluminum Cable, Steel Reinforced (Aluminum Company of America)

Aluminum (Circular Mils or AWG)	Aluminum Strands	Layers	Strand Dia. (in.)	Steel Strands	Strand Dia. (in.)	Outside Diameter (in.)	Copper (Equivalent[a] Circular Mils or AWG)	Ultimate Strength (lb)	Weight (lb/mi)	GMR at 60 Cycles (ft)	Approx. Current-Carrying Capacity[b] (A)	Resistance 25°C (77°F) DC	Resistance 25°C (77°F) 25 Cycles
1,590,000	54	3	0.1716	19	0.1030	1.545	1,000,000	56,000	10,777	0.0520	1380	0.0587	0.0588
1,510,500	54	3	0.1673	19	0.1004	1.506	950,000	53,200	10,237	0.0507	1340	0.0618	0.0619
1,431,000	54	3	0.1628	19	0.0977	1.465	900,000	50,400	9,699	0.0493	1300	0.0652	0.0653
1,351,000	54	3	0.1582	19	0.0949	1.424	850,000	47,600	9,160	0.0479	1250	0.0691	0.0692
1,272,000	54	3	0.1535	19	0.0921	1.382	800,000	44,800	8,621	0.0465	1200	0.0734	0.0735
1,192,500	54	3	0.1486	19	0.0892	1.338	750,000	43,100	8,082	0.0450	1160	0.0783	0.0784
1,113,000	54	3	0.1436	19	0.0862	1.293	700,000	40,200	7,544	0.0435	1110	0.0839	0.0840
1,033,500	54	3	0.1384	7	0.1384	1.246	650,000	37,100	7,019	0.0420	1060	0.0903	0.0905
954,000	54	3	0.1329	7	0.1329	1.196	600,000	34,200	6,479	0.0403	1010	0.0979	0.0980
900,000	54	3	0.1291	7	0.1291	1.162	566,000	32,300	6,112	0.0391	970	0.104	0.104
874,500	54	3	0.1273	7	0.1273	1.146	550,000	31,400	5,940	0.0386	950	0.107	0.107
795,000	54	3	0.1214	7	0.1214	1.093	500,000	28,500	5,399	0.0368	900	0.117	0.118
795,000	26	2	0.1749	7	0.1360	1.108	500,000	31,200	5,770	0.0375	900	0.117	0.117
795,000	30	2	0.1628	19	0.0977	1.140	500,000	38,400	6,517	0.0393	910	0.117	0.117
715,500	54	3	0.1151	7	0.1151	1.036	450,000	26,300	4,859	0.0349	830	0.131	0.131
715,500	26	2	0.1659	7	0.1290	1.051	450,000	28,100	5,193	0.0355	840	0.131	0.131
715,500	30	2	0.1544	19	0.0926	1.081	450,000	34,600	5,865	0.0372	840	0.131	0.131
666,600	54	3	0.1111	7	0.1111	1.000	419,000	24,500	4,527	0.0337	800	0.140	0.140
636,000	54	3	0.1085	7	0.1085	0.977	400,000	23,600	4,319	0.0329	770	0.147	0.147
636,000	26	2	0.1564	7	0.1216	0.990	400,000	25,000	4,616	0.0335	780	0.147	0.147
636,000	30	2	0.1456	19	0.0874	1.019	400,000	31,500	5,213	0.0351	780	0.147	0.147
605,000	54	3	0.1059	7	0.1059	0.953	380,500	22,500	4,109	0.0321	750	0.154	0.155
605,000	26	2	0.1525	7	0.1186	0.966	380,500	24,100	4,391	0.0327	760	0.154	0.154
556,500	26	2	0.1463	7	0.1138	0.927	350,000	22,400	4,039	0.0313	730	0.168	0.168
556,500	30	2	0.1362	7	0.1362	0.953	350,000	27,200	4,588	0.0328	730	0.168	0.168
500,000	30	2	0.1291	7	0.1291	0.904	314,500	24,400	4,122	0.0311	690	0.187	0.187
477,000	26	2	0.1355	7	0.1054	0.858	300,000	19,430	3,462	0.0290	670	0.196	0.196
477,000	30	2	0.1261	7	0.1261	0.883	300,000	23,300	3,933	0.0304	670	0.196	0.196
397,500	26	2	0.1236	7	0.0961	0.783	250,000	16,190	2,885	0.0265	590	0.235	
397,500	30	2	0.1151	7	0.1151	0.806	250,000	19,980	3,277	0.0278	600	0.235	Same
336,400	26	2	0.1138	7	0.0885	0.721	4/0	14,050	2,442	0.0244	530	0.278	
336,400	30	2	0.1059	7	0.1059	0.741	4/0	17,040	2,774	0.0255	530	0.278	
300,000	26	2	0.1074	7	0.0835	0.680	188,700	12,650	2,178	0.0230	490	0.311	
300,000	30	2	0.1000	7	0.1000	0.700	188,700	15,430	2,473	0.0241	500	0.311	
266,800	26	2	0.1013	7	0.0788	0.642	3/0	11,250	1,936	0.0217	460	0.350	
										For current approx. 75% capacity[c]			
266,800	6	1	0.2109	7	0.0703	0.633	3/0	9,645	1,802	0.00684	460	0.351	0.351
4/0	6	1	0.1878	1	0.1878	0.563	2/0	8,420	1,542	0.00814	340	0.441	0.442
3/0	6	1	0.1672	1	0.1672	0.502	1/0	6,675	1,223	0.00600	300	0.556	0.557
2/0	6	1	0.1490	1	0.1490	0.447	1	5,345	970	0.00510	270	0.702	0.702
1/0	6	1	0.1327	1	0.1327	0.398	2	4,280	769	0.00446	230	0.885	0.885
1	6	1	0.1182	1	0.1182	0.355	3	3,480	610	0.00418	200	1.12	1.12
2	6	1	0.1052	1	0.1052	0.316	4	2,790	484	0.00418	180	1.41	1.41
2	7	1	0.0974	1	0.1299	0.325	4	3,525	566	0.00504	180	1.41	1.41
3	6	1	0.0937	1	0.0937	0.281	5	2,250	384	0.00430	160	1.78	1.78
4	6	1	0.0834	1	0.0834	0.250	6	1,830	304	0.00437	140	2.24	2.24
4	7	1	0.0772	1	0.1029	0.257	6	2,288	356	0.00452	140	2.24	2.24
5	6	1	0.0743	1	0.0743	0.223	7	1,460	241	0.00416	120	2.82	2.82
6	6	1	0.0661	1	0.0661	0.198	8	1,170	191	0.00394	100	3.56	3.56

Sources: Gönen, T., *Electric Power Distribution System Engineering*, CRC Press.

[a] Based on copper 97%, aluminum 61% conductivity.

[b] For conductor at 75°C, air at 25°C, wind 1.4 mi/h (2 ft/s), frequency = 60 cycles.

[c] Current approx. 75% capacity is 75% of the approx. current-carrying capacity in amperes and is approximately the current that will produce 50°C conductor temp. (25°C rise) with 25°C air temp., wind 1.4 mi/h.

| Ohms per Conductor per Mile | | | | | | X_a | | | X'_a | | |
| Small Currents | | 50°C (122°F) Current Approx. 75% Capacity^c | | | | X_a Inductive Reactance Ohms per Conductor per Mile at 1 ft Spacing All Currents | | | x'_a Shunt Capacitive Reactance MΩ mi/ Conductor at 1 ft Spacing | | |
50 Cycles	60 Cycles	DC	25 Cycles	50 Cycles	60 Cycles	25 Cycles	50 Cycles	60 Cycles	25 Cycles	50 Cycles	60 Cycles
0.0590	0.0591	0.0646	0.0656	0.0675	0.0684	0.1495	0.299	0.359	0.1953	0.0977	0.0814
0.0621	0.0622	0.0680	0.0690	0.0710	0.0720	0.1508	0.302	0.362	0.1971	0.0986	0.0821
0.0655	0.0656	0.0718	0.0729	0.0749	0.0760	0.1522	0.304	0.365	0.1991	0.0996	0.0830
0.0694	0.0695	0.0761	0.0771	0.0792	0.0803	0.1536	0.307	0.369	0.201	0.1006	0.0838
0.0737	0.0738	0.0808	0.0819	0.0840	0.0851	0.1551	0.310	0.372	0.203	0.1016	0.0847
0.0786	0.0788	0.0862	0.0872	0.0894	0.0906	0.1568	0.314	0.376	0.206	0.1028	0.0857
0.0842	0.0844	0.0924	0.0935	0.0957	0.0969	0.1585	0.317	0.380	0.208	0.1040	0.0867
0.0907	0.0908	0.0994	0.1005	0.1025	0.1035	0.1603	0.321	0.385	0.211	0.1053	0.0878
0.0981	0.0982	0.1078	0.1088	0.1118	0.1128	0.1624	0.325	0.390	0.214	0.1068	0.0890
0.104	0.104	0.1145	0.1155	0.1175	0.1185	0.1639	0.328	0.393	0.216	0.1078	0.0898
0.107	0.108	0.1178	0.1188	0.1218	0.1228	0.1646	0.329	0.395	0.217	0.1083	0.0903
0.118	0.119	0.1288	0.1308	0.1358	0.1378	0.1670	0.334	0.401	0.220	0.1100	0.0917
0.117	0.117	0.1288	0.1288	0.1288	0.1288	0.1660	0.332	0.399	0.219	0.1095	0.0912
0.117	0.117	0.1288	0.1288	0.1288	0.1288	0.1637	0.327	0.393	0.217	0.1085	0.0904
0.131	0.132	0.1442	0.1452	0.1472	0.1482	0.1697	0.339	0.407	0.224	0.1119	0.0932
0.131	0.131	0.1442	0.1442	0.1442	0.1442	0.1687	0.337	0.405	0.223	0.1114	0.0928
0.131	0.131	0.1442	0.1442	0.1442	0.1442	0.1664	0.333	0.399	0.221	0.1104	0.0920
0.141	0.141	0.1541	0.1571	0.1591	0.1601	0.1715	0.343	0.412	0.226	0.1132	0.0943
0.148	0.148	0.1618	0.1638	0.1678	0.1688	0.1726	0.345	0.414	0.228	0.1140	0.0950
0.147	0.147	0.1618	0.1618	0.1618	0.1618	0.1718	0.344	0.412	0.227	0.1135	0.0946
0.147	0.147	0.1618	0.1618	0.1618	0.1618	0.1693	0.339	0.406	0.225	0.1125	0.0937
0.155	0.155	0.1695	0.1715	0.1755	0.1775	0.1739	0.348	0.417	0.230	0.1149	0.0957
0.154	0.154	0.1700	0.1720	0.1720	0.1720	0.1730	0.346	0.415	0.229	0.1144	0.0953
0.168	0.168	0.1849	0.1859	0.1859	0.1859	0.1751	0.350	0.420	0.232	0.1159	0.0965
0.168	0.168	0.1849	0.1859	0.1859	0.1859	0.1728	0.346	0.415	0.230	0.1149	0.0957
0.187	0.187	0.206				0.1754	0.351	0.421	0.234	0.1167	0.0973
0.196	0.196	0.216				0.1790	0.358	0.430	0.237	0.1186	0.0988
0.196	0.196	0.216				0.1766	0.353	0.424	0.235	0.1176	0.0980
		0.259				0.1836	0.367	0.441	0.244	0.1219	0.1015
As dc		0.259		Same as dc		0.1812	0.362	0.435	0.242	0.1208	0.1006
		0.306				0.1872	0.376	0.451	0.250	0.1248	0.1039
		0.306				0.1855	0.371	0.445	0.248	0.1238	0.1032
		0.342				0.1908	0.382	0.458	0.254	0.1269	0.1057
		0.342				0.1883	0.377	0.452	0.252	0.1258	0.1049
		0.385				0.1936	0.387	0.465	0.258	0.1289	0.1074

Single-Layer Conductors

| | | | | | | Small Currents | | | Current Approx. 75% Capacity^c | | | | | |
50 Cycles	60 Cycles	DC	25 Cycles	50 Cycles	60 Cycles	25 Cycles	50 Cycles	60 Cycles	25 Cycles	50 Cycles	60 Cycles	25 Cycles	50 Cycles	60 Cycles
0.351	0.352	0.386	0.430	0.510	0.552	0.194	0.388	0.466	0.252	0.504	0.605	0.259	0.1294	0.1079
0.444	0.445	0.485	0.514	0.567	0.592	0.218	0.437	0.524	0.242	0.484	0.581	0.267	0.1336	0.1113
0.559	0.560	0.612	0.642	0.697	0.723	0.225	0.450	0.540	0.259	0.517	0.621	0.275	0.1377	0.1147
0.704	0.706	0.773	0.806	0.866	0.895	0.231	0.462	0.554	0.267	0.534	0.641	0.284	0.1418	0.1182
0.887	0.888	0.974	1.01	1.08	1.12	0.237	0.473	0.568	0.273	0.547	0.656	0.292	0.1460	0.1216
1.12	1.12	1.23	1.27	1.34	1.38	0.242	0.483	0.580	0.277	0.554	0.665	0.300	0.1500	0.1250
1.41	1.41	1.55	1.59	1.66	1.69	0.247	0.493	0.592	0.277	0.554	0.665	0.308	0.1542	0.1285
1.41	1.41	1.55	1.59	1.62	1.65	0.247	0.493	0.592	0.267	0.535	0.642	0.306	0.1532	0.1276
1.78	1.78	1.95	1.95	2.04	2.07	0.252	0.503	0.604	0.275	0.551	0.661	0.317	0.1583	0.1320
2.24	2.24	2.47	2.50	2.54	2.57	0.257	0.514	0.611	0.274	0.549	0.659	0.325	0.1627	0.1355
2.24	2.24	2.47	2.50	2.53	2.55	0.257	0.515	0.618	0.273	0.545	0.655	0.323	0.1615	0.1346
2.82	2.82	3.10	3.12	3.16	3.18	0.262	0.525	0.630	0.279	0.557	0.665	0.333	0.1666	0.1388
3.56	3.56	3.92	3.94	3.97	3.98	0.268	0.536	0.643	0.281	0.561	0.673	0.342	0.1708	0.1423

TABLE A.4

Characteristics of *"Expanded"* Aluminum Cable, Steel Reinforced[a]
(Aluminum Company of America)

| | Aluminum | | | Steel | | Filler Section | | | | | | | | | |
| | | | | | | Aluminum | | Paper | | | | | | | |
Aluminum (Circular Mils or AWG)	Strands	Layers	Strand Dia. (in.)	Strand	Strand Dia. (in.)	Strands	Strand Dia. (in.)	Strands	Layers	Outside Dia. (in.)	Copper (Equivalent Circular Mils or AWG)	Ultimate Strength (lb)	Weight (lb/mi)	GMR at 60 Cycles (ft)	Approx. Current-Carrying Capacity (A)
850,000	54	2	0.1255	19	0.0834	4	0.1182	23	2	1.38	534,000	35,371	7,200		
1,150,000	54	2	0.1409	19	0.0921	4	0.1353	24	2	1.55	724,000	41,900	9,070	(1)	(1)
1,338,000	66	2	0.1350	19	0.100	4	0.184	18	2	1.75	840,000	49,278	11,340		

Source: Gönen, T., *Electric Power Distribution System Engineering*, CRC Press.

[a] Electrical characteristics not available until laboratory measurements are completed.

r_a Resistance Ohms per Conductor per Mile								X_a Inductive Reactance Ohms per Conductor per Mile at 1 ft Spacing All Currents			X_a' Shunt Capacitive Reactance (MΩ mi/ Conductor) at 1 ft Spacing		
25°C (77°F) Small Currents				50°C (122°F) Current Approx. 75% Capacity[a]									
DC	25 Cycles	50 Cycles	60 Cycles	DC	25 Cycles	50 Cycles	60 Cycles	25 Cycles	50 Cycles	60 Cycles	25 Cycles	50 Cycles	60 Cycles
(a)				(a)				(a)	(a)	(a)	(a)	(a)	(a)

TABLE A.5

Characteristics of Copperweld Copper Conductors

Nominal Designation	Size of Conductor		Outside Diameter (in.)	Copper (Equivalent Circular Mils or AWG)	Rated Breaking Load (lb)	Weight (lb/mi)	GMR at 60 Cycles (ft)	Approx. Current-Carrying Capacity at 60 Cycles (A)[a]
	Number and Diameter of Wires							
	Copperweld	Copper						
350 E	7 × .1576″	12 × .1576″	0.788	350,000	32,420	7409	0.0220	660
350 EK	4 × .1470″	15 × .1470″	0.735	350,000	23,850	6536	0.0245	680
350 V	3 × .1751″	9 × .1893″	0.754	350,000	23,480	6578	0.0226	650
300 E	7 × .1459″	12 × .1459″	0.729	300,000	27,770	6351	−0.0204	500
300 EK	4 × .1361″	15 × .1361″	0.680	300,000	20,960	5602	0.0227	610
300 V	3 × .1621″	9 × .1752″	0.698	300,000	20,730	5639	0.0208	590
250 E	7 × .1332″	12 × .1332″	0.666	250,000	23,920	5292	0.01859	540
250 EK	4 × .1242″	15 × .1242″	0.621	250,000	17,840	4669	0.0207	540
250 V	3 × .1480″	9 × .1600″	0.637	250,000	17,420	4699	0.01911	530
4/0 E	7 × .1225″	12 × .1225″	0.613	4/0	20,730	4479	0.01711	480
4/0 G	2 × .1944″	5 × .1944″	0.583	4/0	1,540	4168	0.01409	460
4/0 EK	4 × .1143″	15 × .1143″	0.571	4/0	15,370	3951	0.01903	490
4/0 V	3 × .1361″	9 × .1472″	0.586	4/0	15,000	3977	0.01758	470
4/0 F	1 × .1833″	6 × .1833″	0.550	4/0	12,290	3750	0.01558″	470
3/0 E	7 × .1091″	12 × .1091″	0.545	3/0	16,800	3522	0.01521	420
3/0 J	3 × .1851″	4 × .1851″	0.555	3/0	16,170	3732	0.01158	410
310 G	2 × .1731″	2 × .1731″	0.519	3/0	12,860	3305	0.01254	400
3/0 EK	4 × .1018″	4 × .1018″	0.509	3/0	12,370	3134	0.01697	420
3/0 V	3 × .1311″	9 × .1311″	0.522	3/0	12,220	3154	0.01566	410
3/0 F	1 × .1632″	6 × .1632″	0.490	3/0	9,980	2974	0.01388	410
2/0 K	4 × .1780″	3 × .1780″	0.534	2/0	17,600	3411	0.00912	360
2/0 J	3 × .1648″	4 × .1648″	0.494	2/0	13,430	2960	0.01029	350
2/0 G	2 × .1542″	6 × .1542″	0.463	2/0	10,510	2622	0.01119	350
2/0 V	3 × .1080″	9 × .1167″	0.465	2/0	9,846	2502	0.01395	360
2/0 F	1 × .1454″	6 × .1454″	0.436	2/0	8,094	2359	0.01235	350
1/0 K	4 × .1585″	3 × .1585″	0.475	1/0	14,490	2703	0.00812	310
1/0 J	3 × .1467″	4 × .1467″	0.440	1/0	10,970	2346	0.00917	310
1/0 G	2 × .1373″	5 × .1373″	0.412	1/0	8,563	2078	0.00995	310
1/0 F	1 × .1294″	6 × .1294″	0.388	1/0	6,536	1870	0.01099	310
1 N	5 × .1546″	2 × .1546″	0.464	1	15,410	2541	0.00638	280
1 K	4 × .1412″	3 × .1412″	0.423	1	11,900	2144	0.00723	270
1 J	3 × .1307″	4 × .1307″	0.392	1	9,000	1881	0.00817	270
1 G	2 × .1222″	5 × .1222″	0.367	1	6,956	1649	0.00887	260
1 F	1 × .1153″	6 × .1153″	0.346	1	5,266	1483	0.00980	270
2 P	6 × .1540″	1 × .1540″	0.452	2	16,870	2487	0.00501	250
2 N	5 × .1377″	2 × .1377″	0.413	2	12,880	2015	0.00568	240
2 K	4 × .1257″	3 × .1257″	0.377	2	9,730	1701	0.00644	240
2 J	3 × .1164″	4 × .1164″	0.349	2	7,322	1476	0.00727	230
2 A	1 × .1699″	2 × .1699″	0.366	2	5,876	1356	0.00763	240
2 G	2 × .1089	5 × .1089″	0.327	2	5,626	1307	0.00790	230
2 F	1 × .1026″	6 × .1026″	0.308	2	4,233	1176	0.00873	230

r_a Resistance (Ω/Conductor/mi)								X_a Inductive Reactance (Ω/Conductor/mi) 1 ft Spacing Average Currents			X'_a Capacitive Reactance (MΩ mi/Conductor) 1 ft Spacing		
At 25°C (77°F) Small Currents				At 50°C (122°F) Current Approx. 75% of Capacity[b]									
DC	25 Cycles	50 Cycles	60 Cycles	DC	25 Cycles	50 Cycles	60 Cycles	25 Cycles	50 Cycles	60 Cycles	25 Cycles	50 Cycles	60 Cycles
0.1658	0.1728	0.1789	0.1812	0.1812	0.1915	0.201	0.204	0.1929	0.386	0.463	0.243	0.1216	0.1014
0.1658	0.1682	0.1700	0.1705	0.1812	0.1845	0.1873	0.1882	0.1875	0.375	0.450	0.248	0.1241	0.1034
0.1655	0.1725	0.1800	0.1828	0.1809	0.1910	0.202	0.206	0.1915	0.383	0.460	0.246	0.1232	0.1027
0.1934	0.200	0.207	0.209	0.211	0.222	0.232	0.235	0.1969	0.394	0.473	0.249	0.1244	0.1037
0.1934	0.1958	0.1976	0.198	0.211	0.215	0.218	0.219	0.1914	0.383	0.460	0.254	0.1269	0.1057
0.1930	0.200	0.208	0.210	0.211	0.222	0.233	0.237	0.1954	0.391	0.469	0.252	0.1259	0.1050
0.232	0.239	0.245	0.248	0.254	0.265	0.275	0.279	0.202	0.403	0.484	0.255	0.1276	0.1604
0.232	0.235	0.236	0.237	0.254	0.258	0.261	0.261	0.1960	0.392	0.471	0.260	0.1301	0.1084
0.232	0.239	0.246	0.249	0.253	0.264	0.276	0.281	0.200	0.400	0.480	0.258	0.1292	0.1077
0.274	0.281	0.287	0.290	0.300	0.312	0.323	0.326	0.206	0.411	0.493	0.261	0.1306	0.1088
0.273	0.284	0.294	0.298	0.299	0.318	0.336	0.342	0.215	0.431	0.517	0.265	0.1324	0.1103
0.274	0.277	0.278	0.279	0.300	0.304	0.307	0.308	0.200	0.401	0.481	0.266	0.1331	0.1109
0.274	0.281	0.288	0.291	0.299	0.311	0.323	0.328	0.204	0.409	0.490	0.264	0.1322	0.1101
0.273	0.280	0.285	0.287	0.299	0.309	0.318	0.322	0.210	0.421	0.505	0.269	0.1344	0.1220
0.346	0.353	0.359	0.361	0.378	0.391	0.402	0.407	0.212	0.423	0.608	0.270	0.1348	0.1123
0.344	0.356	0.367	0.372	0.377	0.398	0.419	0.428	0.225	0.451	0.541	0.268	0.1341	0.1118
0.344	0.355	0.365	0.369	0.377	0.397	0.416	0.423	0.221	0.443	0.531	0.273	0.1365	0.1137
0.346	0.348	0.350	0.351	0.378	0.382	0.386	0.386	0.206	0.412	0.495	0.274	0.1372	0.1143
0.345	0.352	0.360	0.362	0.377	0.390	0.403	0.408	0.210	0.420	0.504	0.273	0.1363	0.1136
0.344	0.351	0.366	0.358	0.377	0.388	0.397	0.401	0.216	0.432	0.519	0.277	0.1385	0.1155
0.434	0.447	0.459	0.466	0.475	0.499	0.524	0.535	0.237	0.476	0.570	0.271	0.1355	0.1129
0.434	0.446	0.457	0.462	0.475	0.498	0.520	0.530	0.231	0.463	0.555	0.277	0.1383	0.1152
0.434	0.445	0.456	0.459	0.475	0.497	0.518	0.526	0.227	0.454	0.545	0.281	0.1406	0.1171
0.435	0.442	0.450	0.452	0.476	0.489	0.504	0.509	0.216	0.432	0.518	0.281	0.1404	0.1170
0.434	0.441	0.446	0.448	0.475	0.487	0.497	0.501	0.222	0.444	0.533	0.285	0.1427	0.1189
0.548	0.560	0.573	0.579	0.599	0.625	0.652	0.664	0.243	0.487	0.584	0.279	0.1397	0.1164
0.548	0.559	0.570	0.576	0.699	0.624	0.648	0.659	0.237	0.474	0.589	0.285	0.1423	0.1188
0.548	0.559	0.568	0.573	0.699	0.623	0.645	0.654	0.233	0.466	0.559	0.289	0.1447	0.1206
0.548	0.554	0.559	0.562	0.599	0.612	0.622	0.627	0.228	0.456	0.547	0.294	0.1469	0.1224
0.691	0.705	0.719	0.726	0.755	0.787	0.818	0.832	0.256	0.512	0.614	0.281	0.1405	0.1171
0.691	0.704	0.716	0.722	0.755	0.784	0.813	0.825	0.249	0.498	0.598	0.288	0.1438	0.1198
0.691	0.703	0.714	0.719	0.755	0.783	0.808	0.820	0.243	0.486	0.583	0.293	0.1465	0.1221
0.691	0.702	0.712	0.716	0.755	0.781	0.805	0.815	0.239	0.478	0.573	0.298	0.1488	0.1240
0.691	0.698	0.704	0.705	0.755	0.769	0.781	0.786	0.234	0.468	0.561	0.302	0.1509	0.1258
0.871	0.886	0.901	0.909	0.952	0.988	1.024	1.040	0.268	0.536	0.643	0.281	0.1406	0.1172
0.871	0.885	0.899	0.906	0.952	0.986	1.020	1.035	0.261	0.523	0.627	0.289	0.1445	0.1208
0.871	0.884	0.896	0.902	0.952	0.983	1.014	1.028	0.255	0.510	0.612	0.296	0.1479	0.1232
0.871	0.883	0.894	0.899	0.952	0.982	1.010	1.022	0.249	0.498	0.598	0.301	0.1506	0.1255
0.869	0.875	0.880	0.882	0.950	0.962	0.973	0.979	0.247	0.493	0.592	0.298	0.1489	0.1241
0.871	0.882	0.892	0.896	0.952	0.980	1.006	1.016	0.246	0.489	0.587	0.306	0.1529	0.1276
0.871	0.878	0.884	0.885	0.952	0.967	0.979	0.986	0.230	0.479	0.576	0.310	0.1551	0.1292

(*continued*)

TABLE A.5 (continued)

Characteristics of Copperweld Copper Conductors

	Size of Conductor							Approx.
	Number and Diameter of Wires			Copper (Equivalent			GMR at	Current-Carrying Capacity
Nominal Designation	Copperweld	Copper	Outside Diameter (in.)	Circular Mils or AWG)	Rated Breaking Load (lb)	Weight (lb/mi)	60 Cycles (ft)	at 60 Cycles (A)[a]
3 P	6 × .1371″	1 × .1371″	0.411	3	13,910	1973	0.00445	220
3 N	5 × .1226″	2 × .1226″	0.368	3	10,390	1598	0.00506	210
3 K	4 × .1120″	3 × .1120″	0.336	3	7,910	1349	0.00674	210
3 J	3 × .1036″	4 × .1036″	0.311	3	5,956	1171	0.00648	200
3 A	1 × .1513″	2 × .1513″	0.326	3	4,810	1075	0.00679	210
4 P	6 × .1221″	1 × .1221″	0.366	4	11,420	1584	0.00397	190
4 N	5 × .1092″	2 × .1092″	0.328	4	8,460	1267	0.00451	180
4 D	2 × .1615″	1 × .1615″	0.348	4	7,340	1191	0.00586	190
4 A	1 × .1347″	2 × .1347″	0.290	4	3,938	853	0.00604	180
5 P	6 × .1087″	1 × .1087″	0.326	5	9,311	1240	0.00353	160
5 D	2 × .1438″	1 × .1438″	0.310	5	6,035	944	0.00504	160
5 A	1 × .1200″	2 × .1200″	0.258	5	3,193	675	0.00538	160
6 D	2 × .1281″	1 × .1281″	0.276	6	4,942	749	0.00449	140
6 A	1 × .1068″	2 × .1068″	0.230	6	2,585	536	0.00479	140
6 C	1 × .1046″	2 × .1046″	0.225	6	2,143	514	0.00469	130
7 D	2 × .1141″	1 × .1141″	0.246	7	4,022	594	0.00400	120
7 A	1 × .1266″	2 × .0895″	0.223	7	2,754	495	0.00441	120
8 D	2 × .1016″	1 × .1016″	0.219	8	3,256	471	0.00356	110
8 A	1 × .1127″	2 × .0797″	0.199	8	2,233	392	0.00394	100
8 C	1 × .0808″	2 × .0834″	0.179	8	1,362	320	0.00373	100
9½ D	2 × .0808″	1 × .0808″	0.174	9½	1,743	298	0.00283	85

Sources: Westinghouse Electric Corporation, *Electric Utility Engineering Reference Book—Distribution Systems*, Westinghouse Electric Corporation, East Pittsburgh, PA, 1965; Gönen, T., *Electric Power Distribution System Engineering*, CRC Press.

[a] Based on a conductor temperature of 75°C and an ambient of 25°C wind 1.4 mi/h (2 ft/s), (frequency = 60 cycles, average tarnished surface).

[b] Resistances at 50°C total temperature, based on an ambient of 25°C plus 25°C rise due to heating effect of current. The approximate magnitude of the current necessary to produce the 25°C rise is 75% of the *approximate current-carrying capacity 60 cycles.*

r_a Resistance (Ω/Conductor/mi)								X_a Inductive Reactance (Ω/Conductor/mi) 1 ft Spacing Average Currents			X'_a Capacitive Reactance (MΩ mi/Conductor) 1 ft Spacing		
At 25°C (77°F) Small Currents				At 50°C (122°F) Current Approx. 75% of Capacity[b]									
DC	25 Cycles	50 Cycles	60 Cycles	DC	25 Cycles	50 Cycles	60 Cycles	25 Cycles	50 Cycles	60 Cycles	25 Cycles	50 Cycles	60 Cycles
1.098	1.113	1.127	1.136	1.200	1.239	1.273	1.296	0.274	0.647	0.657	0.290	0.1448	0.1207
1.098	1.112	1.126	1.133	1.200	1.237	1.273	1.289	0.267	0.634	0.641	0.298	0.1487	0.1239
1.098	1.111	1.123	1.129	1.200	1.233	1.267	1.281	0.261	0.622	0.626	0.304	0.1520	0.1266
1.098	1.110	1.121	1.126	1.200	1.232	1.262	1.275	0.255	0.609	0.611	0.309	0.1547	0.1289
1.096	1.102	1.107	1.109	1.198	1.211	1.226	1.229	0.252	0.606	0.606	0.306	0.1531	0.1275
1.385	1.400	1.414	1.423	1.514	1.555	1.598	1.616	0.280	0.559	0.671	0.298	0.1489	0.1241
1.385	1.399	1.413	1.420	1.514	1.554	1.593	1.610	0.273	0.546	0.655	0.306	0.1528	0.1274
1.382	1.389	1.396	1.399	1.511	1.529	1.544	1.542	0.262	0.523	0.628	0.301	0.1507	0.1256
1.382	1.388	1.393	1.395	1.511	1.525	1.540	1.545	0.258	0.517	0.620	0.316	0.1572	0.1310
1.747	1.762	1.776	1.785	1.909	1.954	2.00	2.02	0.285	0.571	0.685	0.306	0.1531	0.1275
1.742	1.749	1.756	1.759	1.905	1.924	1.941	1.939	0.268	0.535	0.642	0.310	0.1548	0.1290
1.742	1.748	1.753	1.755	1.905	1.920	1.938	1.941	0.264	0.528	0.634	0.323	0.1514	0.1245
2.20	2.21	2.21	2.22	2.40	2.42	2.44	2.44	0.273	0.547	0.555	0.318	0.1590	0.1325
2.20	2.20	2.21	2.21	2.40	2.42	2.44	2.44	0.270	0.540	0.648	0.331	0.1655	0.1379
2.20	2.20	2.21	2.21	2.40	2.42	2.44	2.44	0.271	0.542	0.651	0.333	0.1663	0.1384
2.77	2.78	2.79	2.79	3.03	3.06	3.07	3.07	0.279	0.558	0.670	0.326	0.1831	0.1359
2.77	2.78	2.78	2.78	3.03	3.06	3.07	3.07	0.274	0.548	0.658	0.333	0.1665	0.1388
3.49	3.50	3.51	3.51	3.82	3.84	3.86	3.86	0.285	0.570	0.684	0.334	0.1872	0.1392
3.49	3.50	3.51	3.51	3.82	3.84	3.86	3.87	0.280	0.560	0.672	0.341	0.1706	0.1422
3.49	3.50	3.51	3.51	3.82	3.84	3.86	3.86	0.283	0.565	0.679	0.349	0.1744	0.1453
4.91	4.92	4.92	4.93	5.37	5.39	5.42	5.42	0.297	0.593	0.712	0.351	0.1754	0.1462

TABLE A.6
Characteristics of Copperweld Conductors

Nominal Conductor Size	Number and Size of Wires	Outside Diameter (in.)	Area of Conductor (Circular Mils)	Rated Breaking Load (lb) Strength		Weight (lb/mi)	GMR at 60 Cycles and Average Currents (ft)	Approx. Current-Carrying Capacity[a] (A) at 60 Cycles
				High	Extra High			
30% Conductivity								
7/8[a]	19 No. 5	0.910	628,900	55,570	66,910	9344	0.00758	620
18/16[a]	19 No. 6	0.810	498,800	45,830	55,530	7410	0.00675	540
23/32[a]	19 No. 7	0.721	395,500	37,740	45,850	5877	0.00501	470
21/32[a]	19 No. 8	0.642	313,700	31,040	37,690	4560	0.00535	410
9/16[a]	19 No. 9	0.572	248,800	25,500	30,610	3698	0.00477	350
5/8[a]	7 No. 4	0.613	292,200	24,780	29,430	4324	0.00511	410
9/16[a]	7 No. 5	0.546	231,700	20,470	24,650	3429	0.00455	350
1/2[a]	7 No. 6	0.485	183,800	16,890	20,460	2719	0.00405	310
7/16[a]	7 No. 7	0.433	145,700	13,910	15,890	2157	0.00351	270
3/8[a]	7 No. 8	0.385	115,600	11,440	13,890	1710	0.00321	230
11/32[a]	7 No. 9	0.343	91,650	9,393	11,280	1356	0.00286	200
9/16[a]	7 No. 10	0.306	72,680	7,758	9,196	1076	0.00255	170
3 No. 5	3 No. 5	0.392	99,310	9,262	11,860	1467	0.00457	220
3 No. 6	3 No. 6	0.349	78,750	7,639	9,754	1163	0.00407	190
3 No. 7	3 No. 7	0.311	62,450	6,291	7,922	922.4	0.00363	160
3 No. 8	3 No. 8	0.277	49,530	5,174	6,282	731.5	0.00323	140
3 No. 9	3 No. 9	0.247	39,280	4,250	6,129	580.1	0.00288	120
3 No. 10	3 No. 10	0.220	31,150	3,509	4,160	460.0	0.00257	110
40% Conductivity								
7/6[a]	19 No.5	0.910	628,900	50,240	...	9344	0.01175	690
18/16[a]	19 No. 6	0.810	498,800	41,600	...	7410	0.01046	610
23/32[a]	19 No. 7	0.721	395,500	34,390	...	5877	0.00931	530
21/32[a]	19 No. 8	0.642	313,700	28,380	...	4660	0.00829	470
9/16[a]	19 No. 9	0.572	248,800	23,390	...	3696	0.00739	410
5/8[a]	7 No. 4	0.613	292,200	22,310	...	4324	0.00792	470
9/16[a]	7 No. 5	0.546	231,700	18,510	...	3429	0.00705	410
1/2[a]	7 No. 6	0.486	183,800	15,330	...	2719	0.00628	350
7/16[a]	7 No. 7	0.433	145,700	12,670	...	2157	0.00559	310
3/8[a]	7 No. 8	0.385	115,600	10,460	...	1710	0.00497	270
11/32[a]	7 No. 9	0.343	91,650	8,616	...	1356	0.00443	230
8/16[a]	7 No. 10	0.306	72,680	7,121	...	1076	0.00395	200
3 No. 5	3 No. 5	0.392	99,310	8,373	...	1467	0.00621	250
3 No.6	3 No.6	0.349	78,750	6,934	...	1163	0.00553	220
3 No. 7	3 No. 7	0.311	62,450	5,732	...	922.4	0.00492	190
3 No. 8	3 No. 8	0.277	49,530	4,730	...	731.5	0.00439	160
3 No. 9	3 No. 9	0.247	39,280	3,898	...	580.1	0.00391	140
3 No. 10	3 No. 10	1.220	31,150	3,221	...	460.0	0.00348	120
3 No. 12	3 No. 12	0.174	19,590	2,236	...	289.3	0.00276	90

Sources: Westinghouse Electric Corporation, *Electric Utility Engineering Reference Book—Distribution Systems,* Westinghouse Electric Corporation, East Pittsburgh, PA, 1965; Gönen, T., *Electric Power Distribution System Engineering,* CRC Press.

[a] Based on conductor temperature of 125°C and an ambient of 25°C.

[b] Resistance at 75°C total temperature, based on an ambient of 25°C plus 50°C rise due to heating effect of current. The approximate magnitude of current necessary to produce the 50°C rise is 75% of the *approximate current-carrying capacity at 60 cycles.*

r_a Resistance (Ω/Conductor/mi) at 25°C (77°F) Small Currents				r_a Resistance (Ω/Conductor/mi) at 75°C (157°F) Current Approx. 75% of Capacity[b]				X_a Inductive Reactance (Ω/Conductor/mi) 1 ft Spacing Average Currents			X'_a Capacity Reactance (MΩ·mi/Conductor) 1 ft Spacing		
DC	25 Cycles	50 Cycles	60 Cycles	DC	25 Cycles	50 Cycles	60 Cycles	25 Cycles	50 Cycles	60 Cycles	25 Cycles	50 Cycles	60 Cycles
0.306	0.316	0.328	0.331	0.363	0.419	0.476	0.499	0.261	0.493	0.592	0.233	0.1165	0.0971
0.386	0.396	0.406	0.411	0.458	0.518	0.580	0.605	0.267	0.505	0.605	0.241	0.1206	0.1006
0.486	0.495	0.506	0.511	0.577	0.643	0.710	0.737	0.273	0.517	0.621	0.250	0.1248	0.1040
0.613	0.623	0.633	0.638	0.728	0.799	0.872	0.902	0.279	0.529	0.635	0.258	0.1289	0.1074
0.773	0.783	0.793	0.798	0.917	0.995	1.076	1.106	0.285	0.541	0.649	0.266	0.1330	0.1109
0.656	0.664	0.672	0.676	0.778	0.824	0.870	0.887	0.281	0.533	0.640	0.261	0.1306	0.1088
0.827	0.836	0.843	0.847	0.981	1.030	1.080	1.090	0.287	0.545	0.654	0.269	0.1347	0.1122
1.042	1.050	1.058	1.062	1.237	1.290	1.343	1.354	0.293	0.557	0.668	0.278	0.1388	0.1157
1.315	1.323	1.331	1.335	1.550	1.617	1.675	1.897	0.299	0.569	0.683	0.286	0.1420	0.1191
1.658	1.656	1.574	1.578	1.957	2.03	2.09	2.12	0.305	0.581	0.597	0.294	0.1471	0.1226
2.09	2.10	2.11	2.11	2.48	2.55	2.81	2.64	0.311	0.592	0.711	0.303	0.1512	0.1260
2.64	2.64	2.65	2.66	3.13	3.20	3.27	3.30	0.316	0.804	0.725	0.311	0.1553	0.1294
1.926	1.931	1.936	1.938	2.29	2.31	2.34	2.35	0.289	0.545	0.654	0.293	0.1465	0.1221
2.43	2.43	2.44	2.44	2.88	2.91	2.94	2.95	0.295	0.556	0.688	0.301	0.1506	0.1255
3.06	3.07	3.07	3.07	3.63	3.66	3.70	3.71	0.301	0.568	0.682	0.310	0.1547	0.1289
3.86	3.87	3.87	3.87	4.58	4.61	4.65	4.66	0.307	0.580	0.695	0.318	0.1589	0.1324
4.87	4.87	4.88	4.88	5.78	5.81	5.85	5.86	0.313	0591	0.710	0.326	0.1629	0.1358
6.14	6.14	6.15	6.15	7.28	7.32	7.36	7.38	0.319	0.603	0.724	0.334	0.1671	0.1392
0.229	0.239	0.249	0.254	0.272	0.321	0.371	0.391	0.236	0.449	0.539	0.233	0.1165	0.0971
0.289	0.299	0.309	0.314	0.343	0.395	0.450	0.472	0.241	0.461	0.553	0.241	0.1206	0.1005
0.365	0.375	0.385	0.390	0.433	0.490	0.549	0.573	0.247	0.473	0.567	0.250	0.1248	0.1040
0.460	0.470	0.480	0.485	0.546	0.608	0.672	0.698	0.253	0.485	0.582	0.258	0.1289	0.1074
0.580	0.590	0.800	0.605	0.688	0.756	0.826	0.753	0.259	0.496	0.595	0.266	0.1330	0.1109
0.492	0.500	0.508	0.512	0.584	0.824	0.664	0.680	0.255	0.489	0.587	0.261	0.1306	0.1088
0.620	0.628	0.636	0.640	0.736	0.780	0.843	0.840	0.261	0.501	0.601	0.269	0.1347	0.1122
0.782	0.790	0.798	0.802	0.928	0.975	1.021	1.040	0.267	0.513	0.615	0.278	0.1388	0.1167
0.986	0.994	1.002	1.006	1.170	1.220	1.271	1.291	0.273	0.524	0.629	0.286	0.1429	0.1191
1.244	1.252	1.260	1.264	1.476	1.530	1.584	1.606	0.279	0.536	0.644	0.294	0.1471	0.1226
1.568	1.576	1.584	1.588	1.851	1.919	1.978	2.00	0.285	0.548	0.658	0.303	0.1512	0.1260
1.978	1.986	1.994	1.998	2.35	2.41	2.47	2.50	0.291	0.559	0.671	0.311	0.1553	0.1294
1.445	1.450	1.455	1.457	1.714	1.738	1.762	1.772	0.269	0.514	0.617	0.293	0.1485	0.1221
1.821	1.826	1.831	1.833	2.16	2.19	2.21	2.22	0.275	0.526	0.631	0.301	0.1506	0.1255
2.30	2.30	2.31	2.31	2.73	2.75	2.78	2.79	0.281	0.537	0.645	0.310	0.1547	0.1289
2.90	2.90	2.91	2.91	3.44	3.47	3.50	3.51	0.286	0.549	0.659	0.318	0.1589	0.1324
3.65	3.66	3.66	3.66	4.33	4.37	4.40	4.41	0.292	0.561	0.673	0.326	0.1629	0.1358
4.61	4.61	4.62	4.62	5.46	5.50	5.53	5.55	0.297	0.572	0.687	0.334	0.1671	0.1392
7.32	7.33	7.33	7.34	8.69	8.73	8.77	8.78	0.310	0.596	0.715	0.361	0.1754	0.1462

TABLE A.7
Electrical Characteristics of Overhead Ground Wires

Part A: Alumoweld Strand

| Strand (AWG) | Resistance (Ω/mi) | | | | 60 Hz Reactance for 1 ft Radius | | 60 Hz GMR (ft) |
| | Small Currents | | 75% of Cap. | | | | |
	25°C OC	25°C 60 Hz	75°C OC	75°C 60 Hz	Inductive (Ω/mi)	Capacitive (MΩ mi)	
7 No. 5	1.217	1.240	1.432	1.669	0.707	0.1122	0.002958
7 No. 6	1.507	1.536	1.773	2.010	0.721	0.1157	0.002633
7 No. 7	1.900	1.937	2.240	2.470	0.735	0.1191	0.002345
7 No. 8	2.400	2.440	2.820	3.060	0.749	0.1226	0.002085
7 No. 9	3.020	3.080	3.560	3.800	0.763	0.1260	0.001858
7 No. 10	3.810	3.880	4.480	4.730	0.777	0.1294	0.001658
3 No. 5	2.780	2.780	3.270	3.560	0.707	0.1221	0.002940
3 No. 6	3.510	3.510	4.130	4.410	0.721	0.1255	0.002618
3 No. 7	4.420	4.420	5.210	5.470	0.735	0.1289	0.002333
3 No. 8	5.580	5.580	6.570	6.820	0.749	0.1324	0.002078
3 No. 9	7.040	7.040	8.280	8.520	0.763	0.1358	0.001853
3 No. 10	8.870	8.870	10.440	10.670	0.777	0.1392	0.001650

Part B: Single-Layer ACSR

| Code | 25°C DC | Resistance (Ω/mi) 60 Hz, 75°C | | | 60 Hz Reactance for 1 ft Radius Inductive (Ω/mi) at 75°C | | | Capacitive (MΩ mi) |
		I = 0 A	I = 100 A	I = 200 A	I = 0 A	I = 100 A	I = 200 A	
Brahma	0.394	0.470	0.510	0.565	0.500	0.520	0.545	0.1043
Cochin	0.400	0.480	0.520	0.590	0.505	0.515	0.550	0.1065
Dorking	0.443	0.535	0.575	0.650	0.515	0.530	0.565	0.1079
Dotterel	0.479	0.565	0.620	0.705	0.515	0.530	0.575	0.1091
Guinea	0.531	0.630	0.685	0.780	0.520	0.545	0.590	0.1106
Leghorn	0.630	0.760	0.810	0.930	0.530	0.550	0.605	0.1131
Minorca	0.765	0.915	0.980	1.130	0.540	0.570	0.640	0.1160
Petrel	0.830	1.000	1.065	1.220	0.550	0.580	0.655	0.1172
Grouse	1.080	1.295	1.420	1.520	0.570	0.640	0.675	0.1240

Part C: Steel Conductors

| Grade (7 Strand) | Diameter (in.) | Resistance (Ω/mi) at 60 Hz | | | 60 Hz Reactance for 1 ft Radius Inductive (Ω/mi) | | | Capacitive (MΩ mi) |
		I = 0 A	I = 30 A	I = 60 A	I = 0 A	I = 30 A	I = 60 A	
Ordinary	1/4	9.5	11.4	11.3	1.3970	3.7431	3.4379	0.1354
Ordinary	9/32	7.1	9.2	9.0	1.2027	3.0734	2.5146	0.1319
Ordinary	5/16	5.4	7.5	7.8	0.8382	2.5146	2.0409	0.1288
Ordinary	3/8	4.3	6.5	6.6	0.8382	2.2352	1.9687	0.1234
Ordinary	1/2	2.3	4.3	5.0	0.7049	1.6893	1.4236	0.1148
E.B.	1/4	8.0	12.0	10.1	1.2027	4.4704	3.1565	0.1354
E.B.	9/32	6.0	10.0	8.7	1.1305	3.7783	2.6255	0.1319
E.B.	5/16	4.9	8.0	7.0	0.9843	2.9401	2.5146	0.1288
E.B.	3/8	3.7	7.0	6.3	0.8382	2.5997	2.4303	0.1234
E.B.	1/2	2.1	4.9	5.0	0.7049	1.8715	1.7616	0.1148
E.B.B.	1/4	7.0	12.8	10.9	1.6764	5.1401	3.9482	0.1354
E.B.B.	9/32	5.4	10.9	8.7	1.1305	4.4833	3.7783	0.1319
E.B.B.	5/16	4.0	9.0	6.8	0.9843	3.6322	3.0734	0.1288
E.B.B.	3/8	3.5	7.9	6.0	0.8382	3.1168	2.7940	0.1234
E.B.B.	1/2	2.0	5.7	4.7	0.7049	2.3461	2.2352	0.1148

Sources: Reprinted from Anderson, P.M., *Analysis of Faulted Power Systems*, The Iowa State University Press, Ames, IA, Copyright 1973. With permission; Gonen, T., *Electric Power Distribution System Engineering*, CRC Press.

TABLE A.8

(a) Inductive Reactance Spacing Factor X_d, Ω/(Conductor·mi), at 60 Hz

ft	0.0	0.1	0.2	0.3	0.4	0.5	0.6	0.7	0.8	0.9
0		−0.2794	−0.1953	−0.1461	−0.1112	−0.0841	−0.0620	−0.0433	−0.0271	−0.0128
1	0.0	0.0116	0.0221	0.0318	0.0408	0.0492	0.0570	0.0644	0.0713	0.0779
2	0.0841	0.0900	0.0957	0.1011	0.1062	0.1112	0.1159	0.1205	0.1249	0.1292
3	0.1333	0.1373	0.1411	0.1449	0.1485	0.1520	0.1554	0.1588	0.1620	0.1651
4	0.1682	0.1712	0.1741	0.1770	0.1798	0.1825	0.1852	0.1878	0.1903	0.1928
5	0.1953	0.1977	0.2001	0.2024	0.2046	0.2069	0.2090	0.2112	0.2133	0.2154
6	0.2174	0.2194	0.2214	0.2233	0.2252	0.2271	0.2290	0.2308	0.2326	0.2344
7	0.2361	0.2378	0.2395	0.2412	0.2429	0.2445	0.2461	0.2477	0.2493	0.2508
8	0.2523	0.2538	0.2553	0.2568	0.2582	0.2597	0.2611	0.2625	0.2639	0.2653
9	0.2666	0.2680	0.2693	0.2706	0.2719	0.2732	0.2744	0.2757	0.2769	0.2782
10	0.2794	0.2806	0.2818	0.2830	0.2842	0.2853	0.2865	0.2876	0.2887	0.2899
11	0.2910	0.2921	0.2932	0.2942	0.2953	0.2964	0.2974	0.2985	0.2995	0.3005
12	0.3015	0.3025	0.3035	0.3045	0.3055	0.3065	0.3074	0.3084	0.3094	0.3103
13	0.3112	0.3122	0.3131	0.3140	0.3149	0.3158	0.3167	0.3176	0.3185	0.3194
14	0.3202	0.3211	0.3219	0.3228	0.3236	0.3245	0.3253	0.3261	0.3270	0.3278
15	0.3286	0.3294	0.3302	0.3310	0.3318	0.3326	0.3334	0.3341	0.3349	0.3357
16	0.3364	0.3372	0.3379	0.3387	0.3394	0.3402	0.3409	0.3416	0.3424	0.3431
17	0.3438	0.3445	0.3452	0.3459	0.3466	0.3473	0.3480	0.3487	0.3494	0.3500
18	0.3507	0.3514	0.3521	0.3527	0.3534	0.3540	0.3547	0.3554	0.3560	0.3566
19	0.3573	0.3579	0.3586	0.3592	0.3598	0.3604	0.3611	0.3617	0.3623	0.3629
20	0.3635	0.3641	0.3647	0.3653	0.3659	0.3665	0.3671	0.3677	0.3683	0.3688
21	0.3694	0.3700	0.3706	0.3711	0.3717	0.3723	0.3728	0.3734	0.3740	0.3745
22	0.3751	0.3756	0.3762	0.3767	0.3773	0.3778	0.3783	0.3789	0.3794	0.3799
23	0.3805	0.3810	0.3815	0.3820	0.3826	0.3831	0.3836	0.3841	0.3846	0.3851
24	0.3856	0.3861	0.3866	0.3871	0.3876	0.3881	0.3886	0.3891	0.3896	0.3901
25	0.3906	0.3911	0.3916	0.3920	0.3925	0.3930	0.3935	0.3939	0.3944	0.3949
26	0.3953	0.3958	0.3963	0.3967	0.3972	0.3977	0.3981	0.3986	0.3990	0.3995
27	0.3999	0.4004	0.4008	0.4013	0.4017	0.4021	0.4026	0.4030	0.4035	0.4039
28	0.4043	0.4048	0.4052	0.4056	0.4061	0.4065	0.4069	0.4073	0.4078	0.4082
29	0.4086	0.4090	0.4094	0.4098	0.4103	0.4107	0.4111	0.4115	0.4119	0.4123
30	0.4127	0.4131	0.4135	0.4139	0.4143	0.4147	0.4151	0.4155	0.4159	0.4163
31	0.4167	0.4171	0.4175	0.4179	0.4182	0.4186	0.4190	0.4194	0.4198	0.4202
32	0.4205	0.4209	0.4213	0.4217	0.4220	0.4224	0.4228	0.4232	0.4235	0.4239
33	0.4243	0.4246	0.4250	0.4254	0.4257	0.4261	0.4265	0.4268	0.4272	0.4275
34	0.4279	0.4283	0.4286	0.4290	0.4293	0.4297	0.4300	0.4304	0.4307	0.4311
35	0.4314	0.4318	0.4321	0.4324	0.4328	0.4331	0.4335	0.4338	0.4342	0.4345
36	0.4348	0.4352	0.4355	0.4358	0.4362	0.4365	0.4368	0.4372	0.4375	0.4378
37	0.4382	0.4385	0.4388	0.4391	0.4395	0.4398	0.4401	0.4404	0.4408	0.4411
38	0.4414	0.4417	0.4420	0.4423	0.4427	0.4430	0.4433	0.4436	0.4439	0.4442
39	0.4445	0.4449	0.4452	0.4455	0.4458	0.4461	0.4464	0.4467	0.4470	0.4473
40	0.4476	0.4479	0.4492	0.4485	0.4488	0.4491	0.4494	0.4497	0.4500	0.4503
41	0.4506	0.4509	0.4512	0.4515	0.4518	0.4521	0.4524	0.4527	0.4530	0.4532
42	0.4535	0.4538	0.4541	0.4544	0.4547	0.4550	0.4553	0.4555	0.4558	0.4561
43	0.4564	0.4567	0.4570	0.4572	0.4575	0.4578	0.4581	0.4584	0.4586	0.4589
44	0.4592	0.4595	0.4597	0.4600	0.4603	0.4606	0.4608	0.4611	0.4614	0.4616
45	0.4619	0.4622	0.4624	0.4627	0.4630	0.4632	0.4635	0.4638	0.4640	0.4643
46	0.4646	0.4648	0.4651	0.4654	0.4656	0.4659	0.4661	0.4664	0.4667	0.4669
47	0.4672	0.4674	0.4677	0.4680	0.4682	0.4685	0.4687	0.4690	0.4692	0.4695
48	0.4697	0.4700	0.4702	0.4705	0.4707	0.4710	0.4712	0.4715	0.4717	0.4720
49	0.4722	0.4725	0.4727	0.4730	0.4732	0.4735	0.4737	0.4740	0.4742	0.4744
50	0.4747	0.4749	0.4752	0.4754	0.4757	0.4759	0.4761	0.4764	0.4766	0.4769

(continued)

TABLE A.8 (continued)

(a) Inductive Reactance Spacing Factor X_d, Ω/(Conductor · mi), at 60 Hz

ft	0.0	0.1	0.2	0.3	0.4	0.5	0.6	0.7	0.8	0.9
51	0.4771	0.4773	0.4776	0.4778	0.4780	0.4783	0.4785	0.4787	0.4790	0.4792
52	0.4795	0.4797	0.4799	0.4801	0.4804	0.4806	0.4808	0.4811	0.4813	0.4815
53	0.4818	0.4820	0.4822	0.4824	0.4827	0.4829	0.4831	0.4834	0.4836	0.4838
54	0.4840	0.4843	0.4845	0.4847	0.4849	0.4851	0.4854	0.4856	0.4858	0.4860
55	0.4863	0.4865	0.4867	0.4869	0.4871	0.4874	0.4876	0.4878	0.4880	0.4882
56	0.4884	0.4887	0.4889	0.4891	0.4893	0.4895	0.4897	0.4900	0.4902	0.4904
57	0.4906	0.4908	0.4910	0.4912	0.4914	0.4917	0.4919	0.4921	0.4923	0.4925
58	0.4927	0.4929	0.4931	0.4933	0.4935	0.4937	0.4940	0.4942	0.4944	0.4946
59	0.4948	0.4950	0.4952	0.4954	0.4956	0.4958	0.4960	0.4962	0.4964	0.4966
60	0.4968	0.4970	0.4972	0.4974	0.4976	0.4978	0.4980	0.4982	0.4984	0.4986
61	0.4988	0.4990	0.4992	0.4994	0.4996	0.4998	0.5000	0.5002	0.5004	0.5006
62	0.5008	0.5010	0.5012	0.5014	0.5016	0.5018	0.5020	0.5022	0.5023	0.5025
63	0.5027	0.5029	0.5031	0.5033	0.5035	0.5037	0.5039	0.5041	0.5043	0.5045
64	0.5046	0.5048	0.5050	0.5052	0.5054	0.5056	0.5058	0.5060	0.5062	0.5063
65	0.5065	0.5067	0.5069	0.5071	0.5073	0.5075	0.5076	0.5078	0.5080	0.5082
66	0.5084	0.5086	0.5087	0.5089	0.5091	0.5093	0.5095	0.5097	0.5098	0.5100
67	0.5102	0.5104	0.5106	0.5107	0.5109	0.5111	0.5113	0.5115	0.5116	0.5118
68	0.5120	0.5122	0.5124	0.5125	0.5127	0.5129	0.5131	0.5132	0.5134	0.5136
69	0.5138	0.5139	0.5141	0.5143	0.5145	0.5147	0.5148	0.5150	0.5152	0.5153
70	0.5155	0.5157	0.5159	0.5160	0.5162	0.5164	0.5166	0.5167	0.5169	0.5171
71	0.5172	0.5174	0.5176	0.5178	0.5179	0.5181	0.5183	0.5184	0.5186	0.5188
72	0.5189	0.5191	0.5193	0.5194	0.5196	0.5198	0.5199	0.5201	0.5203	0.5204
73	0.5206	0.5208	0.5209	0.5211	0.5213	0.5214	0.5216	0.5218	0.5219	0.5221
74	0.5223	0.5224	0.5226	0.5228	0.5229	0.5231	0.5232	0.5234	0.5236	0.5237
75	0.5239	0.5241	0.5242	0.5244	0.5245	0.5247	0.5249	0.5250	0.5252	0.5253
76	0.5255	0.5257	0.5258	0.5260	0.5261	0.5263	0.5265	0.5266	0.5268	0.5269
77	0.5271	0.5272	0.5274	0.5276	0.5277	0.5279	0.5280	0.5282	0.5283	0.5285
78	0.5287	0.5288	0.5290	0.5291	0.5293	0.5294	0.5296	0.5297	0.5299	0.5300
79	0.5302	0.5304	0.5305	0.5307	0.5308	0.5310	0.5311	0.5313	0.5314	0.5316
80	0.5317	0.5319	0.5320	0.5322	0.5323	0.5325	0.5326	0.5328	0.5329	0.5331
81	0.5332	0.5334	0.5335	0.5337	0.5338	0.5340	0.5341	0.5343	0.5344	0.5346
82	0.5347	0.5349	0.5350	0.5352	0.5353	0.5355	0.5356	0.5358	0.5359	0.5360
83	0.5362	0.5363	0.5365	0.5366	0.5368	0.5369	0.5371	0.5372	0.5374	0.5375
84	0.5376	0.5378	0.5379	0.5381	0.5382	0.5384	0.5385	0.5387	0.5388	0.5389
85	0.5391	0.5392	0.5394	0.5395	0.5396	0.5398	0.5399	0.5401	0.5402	0.5404
86	0.5405	0.5406	0.5408	0.5409	0.5411	0.5412	0.5413	0.5415	0.5416	0.5418
87	0.5419	0.5420	0.5422	0.5423	0.5425	0.5426	0.5427	0.5429	0.5430	0.5432
88	0.5433	0.5434	0.5436	0.5437	0.5438	0.5440	0.5441	0.5442	0.5444	0.5445
89	0.5447	0.5448	0.5449	0.5451	0.5452	0.5453	0.5455	0.5456	0.5457	0.5459
90	0.5460	0.5461	0.5463	0.5464	0.5466	0.5467	0.5468	0.5470	0.5471	0.5472
91	0.5474	0.5475	0.5476	0.5478	0.5479	0.5480	0.5482	0.5483	0.5484	0.5486
92	0.5487	0.5488	0.5489	0.5491	0.5492	0.5493	0.5495	0.5496	0.5497	0.5499
93	0.5500	0.5501	0.5503	0.5504	0.5505	0.5506	0.5508	0.5509	0.5510	0.5512
94	0.5513	0.5514	0.5515	0.5517	0.5518	0.5519	0.5521	0.5522	0.5523	0.5524
95	0.5526	0.5527	0.5528	0.5530	0.5531	0.5532	0.5533	0.5535	0.5536	0.5537
96	0.5538	0.5540	0.5541	0.5542	0.5544	0.5545	0.5546	0.5547	0.5549	0.5550
97	0.5551	0.5552	0.5554	0.5555	0.5556	0.5557	0.5559	0.5560	0.5561	0.5562
98	0.5563	0.5565	0.5566	0.5567	0.5568	0.5570	0.5571	0.5572	0.5573	0.5575
99	0.5576	0.5577	0.5578	0.5579	0.5581	0.5582	0.5583	0.5584	0.5586	0.5587
100	0.5588	0.5589	0.5590	0.5592	0.5593	0.5594	0.5595	0.5596	0.5598	0.5599

TABLE A.8 (continued)

(b) Zero-Sequence Resistive and Inductive Factors r_e^*, x_e^*, Ω/(Conductor · mi)

	p ($\Omega \cdot$ m)	r_e, x_e ($f = 60$ Hz)
r_e	All	0.2860
	1	2.050
	5	2.343
	10	2.469
x_e	50	2.762
	100[†]	2.888[†]
	500	3.181
	1000	3.307
	5000	3.600
	10,000	3.726

Sources: Reprinted by permission from *Analysis of Faulted Power Systems* by Paul M. Anderson; © 1973 by The Iowa State University Press, Ames, Iowa 50010.

From Gonen, *Electric Power Distribution System Engineering*, CRC Press.

* From formulas:

$$r_e = 0.004764 f$$

$$x_e = 0.006985 f \log_{10} 4,665,600 \frac{r}{f}$$

where f = frequency and ρ = resistivity ($\Omega \cdot$ m).

[†] This is an average value which may be used in the absence of definite information.

Fundamental equations:

$$z_1 = z_2 = r_a + j(x_a + x_d)$$

$$z_0 = r_a + r_e + j(x_a + x_e - 2x_d)$$

where $x_d = wk \ln d$ and d = separation (ft).

TABLE A.9

(a) Shunt Capacitive Reactance Spacing Factor x'_d (MΩ/Conductor $\cdot$ mi), at 60 Hz

ft	0.0	0.1	0.2	0.3	0.4	0.5	0.6	0.7	0.8	0.9
0		−0.0683	−0.0477	−0.0357	−0.0272	−0.0206	−0.0152	−0.0106	−0.0066	−0.0031
1	0.0000	0.0028	0.0054	0.0078	0.0100	0.0120	0.0139	0.0157	0.0174	0.0190
2	0.0206	0.0220	0.0234	0.0247	0.0260	0.0272	0.0283	0.0295	0.0305	0.0316
3	0.0326	0.0336	0.0345	0.0354	0.0363	0.0372	0.0380	0.0388	0.0396	0.0404
4	0.0411	0.0419	0.0426	0.0433	0.0440	0.0446	0.0453	0.0459	0.0465	0.0471
5	0.0477	0.0483	0.0489	0.0495	0.0500	0.0506	0.0511	0.0516	0.0521	0.0527
6	0.0532	0.0536	0.0541	0.0546	0.0551	0.0555	0.0560	0.0564	0.0569	0.0573
7	0.0577	0.0581	0.0586	0.0590	0.0594	0.0598	0.0602	0.0606	0.0609	0.0613
8	0.0617	0.0621	0.0624	0.0628	0.0631	0.0635	0.0638	0.0642	0.0645	0.0649
9	0.0652	0.0655	0.0658	0.0662	0.0665	0.0668	0.0671	0.0674	0.0677	0.0680
10	0.0683	0.0686	0.0689	0.0692	0.0695	0.0698	0.0700	0.0703	0.0706	0.0709
11	0.0711	0.0714	0.0717	0.0719	0.0722	0.0725	0.0727	0.0730	0.0732	0.0735
12	0.0737	0.0740	0.0742	0.0745	0.0747	0.0749	0.0752	0.0754	0.0756	0.0759
13	0.0761	0.0763	0.0765	0.0768	0.0770	0.0772	0.0774	0.0776	0.0779	0.0781
14	0.0783	0.0785	0.0787	0.0789	0.0791	0.0793	0.0795	0.0797	0.0799	0.0801
15	0.0803	0.0805	0.0807	0.0809	0.0811	0.0813	0.0815	0.0817	0.0819	0.0821
16	0.0823	0.0824	0.0826	0.0828	0.0830	0.0832	0.0833	0.0835	0.0837	0.0839
17	0.0841	0.0842	0.0844	0.0846	0.0847	0.0849	0.0851	0.0852	0.0854	0.0856
18	0.0857	0.0859	0.0861	0.0862	0.0864	0.0866	0.0867	0.0869	0.0870	0.0872
19	0.0874	0.0875	0.0877	0.0878	0.0880	0.0881	0.0883	0.0884	0.0886	0.0887
20	0.0889	0.0890	0.0892	0.0893	0.0895	0.0896	0.0898	0.0899	0.0900	0.0902
21	0.0903	0.0905	0.0906	0.0907	0.0909	0.0910	0.0912	0.0913	0.0914	0.0916
22	0.0917	0.0918	0.0920	0.0921	0.0922	0.0924	0.0925	0.0926	0.0928	0.0929
23	0.0930	0.0931	0.0933	0.0934	0.0935	0.0937	0.0938	0.0939	0.0940	0.0942
24	0.0943	0.0944	0.0945	0.0947	0.0948	0.0949	0.0950	0.0951	0.0953	0.0954
25	0.0955	0.0956	0.0957	0.0958	0.0960	0.0961	0.0962	0.0963	0.0964	0.0965
26	0.0967	0.0968	0.0969	0.0970	0.0971	0.0972	0.0973	0.0974	0.0976	0.0977
27	0.0978	0.0979	0.0980	0.0981	0.0982	0.0983	0.0984	0.0985	0.0986	0.0987
28	0.0989	0.0990	0.0991	0.0992	0.0993	0.0994	0.0995	0.0996	0.0997	0.0998
29	0.0999	0.1000	0.1001	0.1002	0.1003	0.1004	0.1005	0.1006	0.1007	0.1008
30	0.1009	0.1010	0.1011	0.1012	0.1013	0.1014	0.1015	0.1016	0.1017	0.1018
31	0.1019	0.1020	0.1021	0.1022	0.1023	0.1023	0.1024	0.1025	0.1026	0.1027
32	0.1028	0.1029	0.1030	0.1031	0.1032	0.1033	0.1034	0.1035	0.1035	0.1036
33	0.1037	0.1038	0.1039	0.1040	0.1041	0.1042	0.1043	0.1044	0.1044	0.1045
34	0.1046	0.1047	0.1048	0.1049	0.1050	0.1050	0.1051	0.1052	0.1053	0.1054
35	0.1055	0.1056	0.1056	0.1057	0.1058	0.1059	0.1060	0.1061	0.1061	0.1062
36	0.1063	0.1064	0.1065	0.1066	0.1066	0.1067	0.1068	0.1069	0.1070	0.1070
37	0.1071	0.1072	0.1073	0.1074	0.1074	0.1075	0.1076	0.1077	0.1078	0.1078
38	0.1079	0.1080	0.1081	0.1081	0.1082	0.1083	0.1084	0.1085	0.1085	0.1086
39	0.1087	0.1088	0.1088	0.1089	0.1090	0.1091	0.1091	0.1092	0.1093	0.1094
40	0.1094	0.1095	0.1096	0.1097	0.1097	0.1098	0.1099	0.1100	0.1100	0.1101
41	0.1102	0.1102	0.1103	0.1104	0.1105	0.1105	0.1106	0.1107	0.1107	0.1108
42	0.1109	0.1110	0.1110	0.1111	0.1112	0.1112	0.1113	0.1114	0.1114	0.1115
43	0.1116	0.1117	0.1117	0.1118	0.1119	0.1119	0.1120	0.1121	0.1121	0.1122
44	0.1123	0.1123	0.1124	0.1125	0.1125	0.1126	0.1127	0.1127	0.1128	0.1129
45	0.1129	0.1130	0.1131	0.1131	0.1132	0.1133	0.1133	0.1134	0.1135	0.1135
46	0.1136	0.1136	0.1137	0.1138	0.1138	0.1139	0.1140	0.1140	0.1141	0.1142
47	0.1142	0.1143	0.1143	0.1144	0.1145	0.1145	0.1146	0.1147	0.1147	0.1148
48	0.1148	0.1149	0.1150	0.1150	0.1151	0.1152	0.1152	0.1153	0.1153	0.1154
49	0.1155	0.1155	0.1156	0.1156	0.1157	0.1158	0.1158	0.1159	0.1159	0.1160
50	0.1161	0.1161	0.1162	0.1162	0.1163	0.1164	0.1164	0.1165	0.1165	0.1166

TABLE A.9 (continued)

(a) Shunt Capacitive Reactance Spacing Factor x'_d (MΩ/Conductor $\cdot$ mi), at 60 Hz

ft	0.0	0.1	0.2	0.3	0.4	0.5	0.6	0.7	0.8	0.9
51	0.1166	0.1167	0.1168	0.1168	0.1169	0.1169	0.1170	0.1170	0.1171	0.1172
52	0.1172	0.1173	0.1173	0.1174	0.1174	0.1175	0.1176	0.1176	0.1177	0.1177
53	0.1178	0.1178	0.1179	0.1180	0.1180	0.1181	0.1181	0.1182	0.1182	0.1183
54	0.1183	0.1184	0.1184	0.1185	0.1186	0.1186	0.1187	0.1187	0.1188	0.1188
55	0.1189	0.1189	0.1190	0.1190	0.1191	0.1192	0.1192	0.1193	0.1193	0.1194
56	0.1194	0.1195	0.1195	0.1196	0.1196	0.1197	0.1197	0.1198	0.1198	0.1199
57	0.1199	0.1200	0.1200	0.1201	0.1202	0.1202	0.1203	0.1203	0.1204	0.1204
58	0.1205	0.1205	0.1206	0.1206	0.1207	0.1207	0.1208	0.1208	0.1209	0.1209
59	0.1210	0.1210	0.1211	0.1211	0.1212	0.1212	0.1213	0.1213	0.1214	0.1214
60	0.1215	0.1215	0.1216	0.1216	0.1217	0.1217	0.1218	0.1218	0.1219	0.1219
61	0.1220	0.1220	0.1221	0.1221	0.1221	0.1222	0.1222	0.1223	0.1223	0.1224
62	0.1224	0.1225	0.1225	0.1226	0.1226	0.1227	0.1227	0.1228	0.1228	0.1229
63	0.1229	0.1230	0.1230	0.1231	0.1231	0.1231	0.1232	0.1232	0.1233	0.1233
64	0.1234	0.1234	0.1235	0.1235	0.1236	0.1236	0.1237	0.1237	0.1237	01238
65	0.1238	0.1239	0.1239	0.1240	0.1240	0.1241	0.1241	0.1242	0.1242	0.1242
66	0.1243	0.1243	0.1244	0.1244	0.1245	0.1245	0.1246	0.1246	0.1247	0.1247
67	0.1247	0.1248	0.1248	0.1249	0.1249	0.1250	0.1250	0.1250	0.1251	0.1251
68	0.1252	0.1252	0.1253	0.1253	0.1254	0.1254	0.1254	0.1255	0.1255	0.1256
69	0.1256	0.1257	0.1257	0.1257	0.1258	0.1258	0.1259	0.1259	0.1260	0.1260
70	0.1260	0.1261	0.1261	0.1262	0.1262	0.1262	0.1263	0.1263	0.1264	0.1264
71	0.1265	0.1265	0.1265	0.1266	0.1266	0.1267	0.1267	0.1268	0.1268	0.1268
72	0.1269	0.1269	0.1270	0.1270	0.1270	0.1271	0.1271	0.1272	0.1272	0.1272
73	0.1273	0.1273	0.1274	0.1274	0.1274	0.1275	0.1275	0.1276	0.1276	0.1276
74	0.1277	0.1277	0.1278	0.1278	0.1278	0.1279	0.1279	0.1280	0.1280	.01280
75	0.1281	0.1281	0.1282	0.1282	0.1282	0.1283	0.1283	0.1284	0.1284	0.1284
76	0.1285	0.1285	0.1286	0.1286	0.1286	0.1287	0.1287	0.1288	0.1288	0.1288
77	0.1289	0.1289	0.1289	0.1290	0.1290	0.1291	0.1291	0.1291	0.1292	0.1292
78	0.1292	0.1293	0.1293	0.1294	0.1294	0.1294	0.1295	0.1295	0.1296	0.1296
79	0.1296	0.1297	0.1297	0.1297	0.1298	0.1298	0.1299	0.1299	0.1299	0.1300
80	0.1300	0.1300	0.1301	0.1301	0.1301	0.1302	0.1302	0.1303	0.1303	0.1303
81	0.1304	0.1304	0.1304	0.1305	0.1305	0.1306	0.1306	0.1306	0.1307	0.1307
82	0.1307	0.1308	0.1308	0.1308	0.1309	0.1309	0.1309	0.1310	0.1310	0.1311
83	0.1311	0.1311	0.1312	0.1312	0.1312	0.1313	0.1313	0.1313	0.1314	0.1314
84	0.1314	0.1315	0.1315	0.1316	0.1316	0.1316	0.1317	0.1317	0.1317	0.1318
85	0.1318	0.1318	0.1319	0.1319	0.1319	0.1320	0.1320	0.1320	0.1321	0.1321
86	0.1321	0.1322	0.1322	0.1322	0.1323	0.1323	0.1324	0.1324	0.1324	0.1325
87	0.1325	0.1325	0.1326	0.1326	0.1326	0.1327	0.1327	0.1327	0.1328	0.1328
88	0.1328	0.1329	0.1329	0.1329	0.1330	0.1330	0.1330	0.1331	0.1331	0.1331
89	0.1332	0.1332	0.1332	0.1333	0.1333	0.1333	0.1334	0.1334	0.1334	0.1335
90	0.1335	0.1335	0.1336	0.1336	0.1336	0.1337	0.1337	0.1337	0.1338	0.1338
91	0.1338	0.1339	0.1339	0.1339	0.1340	0.1340	0.1340	0.1340	0.1341	0.1341
92	0.1341	0.1342	0.1342	0.1342	0.1343	0.1343	0.1343	0.1344	0.1344	0.1344
93	0.1345	0.1345	0.1345	0.1346	0.1346	0.1346	0.1347	0.1347	0.1347	0.1348
94	0.1348	0.1348	0.1348	0.1349	0.1349	0.1349	0.1350	0.1350	0.1350	0.1351
95	0.1351	0.1351	0.1352	0.1352	0.1352	0.1353	0.1353	0.1353	0.1353	0.1354
96	0.1354	0.1354	0.1355	0.1355	0.1355	0.1356	0.1356	0.1356	0.1357	0.1357
97	0.1357	0.1357	0.1358	0.1358	0.1358	0.1359	0.1359	0.1359	0.1360	0.1360
98	0.1360	0.1361	0.1361	0.1361	0.1361	0.1362	0.1362	0.1362	0.1363	0.1363
99	0.1363	0.1364	0.1364	0.1364	0.1364	0.1365	0.1365	0.1365	0.1366	0.1366
100	0.1366	0.1366	0.1367	0.1367	0.1367	0.1368	0.1368	0.1368	0.1369	0.1369

(continued)

TABLE A.9 (continued)

(b) Zero-Sequence Shunt Capacitive Reactance Factor X'_0, MΩ/(Conductor · mi)

Conductor Height Aboveground (ft)	x'_0 ($f = 60$ Hz)
10	0.267
15	0.303
20	0.328
25	0.318
30	0.364
40	0.390
50	0.410
60	0.426
70	0.440
80	0.452
90	0.462
100	0.472

Sources: Reprinted from Anderson, P.M., *Analysis of Faulted Power Systems*, The Iowa State University Press, Ames, IA, Copyright 1973. With permission; Gönen, T., *Electric Power Distribution System Engineering*, CRC Press.

$$x'_0 = \frac{12.30}{f} \log_{10} 2h$$

where h = height aboveground and f = frequency.

Fundamental equations:

$x'_1 = x'_2 = x'_a = x'_d$.

$x'_0 = x'_a + x'_c - 2x'_d$.

where $x'_d = (1/\omega k') \ln d$ and d = separation (ft).

TABLE A.10
Standard Impedances for Power Transformers 10,000 kVA and below

Highest-Voltage Winding (BIL kV)	Low-Voltage Winding, BIL kV (For Intermediate BIL, Use Value for the Next Higher BIL Listed)	At kVA Base Equal to 55°C Rating of the Largest Capacity Winding Self-Cooled (OA), Self-Cooled Rating of Self-Cooled/Forced-Air-Cooled (OA/FA) Standard Impedance (%)	
		Ungrounded Neutral Operation	Grounded Neutral Operation
110 and below	45	5.75	
	60, 75, 95, 110	5.5	
150	45	5.75	
	60, 75, 95, 110	5.5	
200	45	6.25	
	60, 75, 95, 110	6.0	
	150	6.5	
250	45	6.75	
	60, 150	6.5	
	200	7.0	
350	200	7.0	
	250	7.5	
450	200	7.5	7.00
	250	8.0	7.50
	350	8.5	8.00
550	200	8.0	7.50
	350	9.0	8.25
	450	10.0	9.25
650	200	8.5	8.00
	350	9.5	8.50
	550	10.5	9.50
750	250	9.0	8.50
	450	10.0	9.50
	650	11.0	10.25

Sources: Westinghouse Electric Corporation, *Applied Protective Relaying*, Westinghouse Electric Corporation, Newark, NJ, 1970. With permission; Gönen, T., *Electric Power Distribution System Engineering*, CRC Press.
BIL, basic impulse insulation level.

TABLE A.11

Standard Impedance Limits for Power Transformers above 10,000 kVA

Highest-Voltage Winding (BIL KV)	Low-Voltage Winding, BIL KV (For Intermediate BIL, Use Value for Next Higher BIL Listed)	At kVA Base Equal to 55°C Rating of Largest Capacity Winding							
		Self-Cooled (OA), Self-Cooled Rating of Self-Cooled/Forced-Air-Cooled (OA/FA), Self-Cooled Rating of Self-Cooled/Forced-Air, Forced-Oil-Cooled (OA/FOA) Standard Impedance (%)				Forced-Oil-Cooled (FOA and FOW) Standard Impedance (%)			
		Ungrounded Neutral Operation		Grounded Neutral Operation		Ungrounded Neutral Operation		Grounded Neutral Operation	
		Min.	Max.	Min.	Max.	Min.	Max.	Min.	Max.
110 and below	110 and below	5.0	6.25			8.25	10.5		
150	110	5.0	6.25			8.25	10.5		
200	110	5.5	7.0			9.0	12.0		
	150	5.75	7.5			9.75	12.75		
250	150	5.75	7.5			9.5	12.75		
	200	6.25	8.5			10.5	14.25		
350	200	6.25	8.5			10.25	14.25		
250	6.75	9.5				11.25	15.75		
450	200	6.75	9.5	6.0	8.75	11.25	15.75	10.5	14.5
	250	7.25	10.75	6.75	9.5	12.0	17.25	11.25	16.0
	350	7.75	11.75	7.0	10.25	12.75	18.0	12.0	17.25
550	200	7.25	10.75	6.5	9.75	12.0	18.0	10.75	16.5
	350	8.25	13.0	7.25	10.75	13.25	21.0	12.0	18.0
	450	8.5	13.5	7.75	11.75	14.0	22.5	12.75	19.5

650	200	7.75	11.75	7.0	10.75	12.75	19.5	11.75	18.0
	350	8.5	13.5	7.75	12.0	14.0	22.5	12.75	19.5
	450	9.25	14.0	8.5	13.5	15.25	24.5	14.0	22.5
750	250	8.0	12.75	7.5	11.5	13.5	21.25	12.5	19.25
	450	9.0	13.75	8.25	13.0	15.0	24.0	13.75	21.5
	650	10.25	15.0	9.25	14.0	16.5	25.0	15.0	24.0
825	250	8.5	13.5	7.75	12.0	14.25	22.5	13.0	20.0
	450	9.5	14.25	8.75	13.5	15.75	24.0	14.5	22.25
	650	10.75	15.75	9.75	15.0	17.25	26.25	15.75	24.0
900	250			8.25	12.5			13.75	21.0
	450			9.25	14.0			15.25	23.5
	750			10.25	15.0			16.5	25.5
1050	250			8.75	13.5			14.75	22.0
	550			10.0	15.0			16.75	25.0
	825			11.0	16.5			18.25	27.5
1175	250			9.25	14.0			15.5	23.0
	550			10.5	15.75			17.5	25.5
	900			12.0	17.5			19.5	29.0
1300	250			9.75	14.5			16.25	24.0
	550			11.25	17.0			18.75	27.0
	1050			12.5	18.25			20.75	30.5

Sources: Westinghouse Electric Corporation, *Applied Protective Relaying*, Westinghouse Electric Corporation, Newark, NJ, 1970. With permission; Gönen, T., *Electric Power Distribution System Engineering*, CRC Press.

BIL, basic impulse insulation level.

TABLE A.12

60 Hz Characteristics of Three-Conductor Belted Paper-Insulated Cables

Voltage Class	Insulation Thickness (Mils)		Circular Mils or AWG (B&S)	Type of Conductor	Weight per 1000 ft	Diameter[d] or Sector Depth (in.)	Resistance[a] (Ω/mi)	GMR of One Conductor[b] (in.)
	Conductor	Belt						
1 kV	60	35	6	SR	1,500	0.184	2.50	0.067
	60	35	4	SR	1,910	0.232	1.58	0.084
	60	35	2	SR	2,390	0.292	0.987	0.106
	60	35	1	SR	2,820	0.332	0.786	0.126
	60	35	0	SR	3,210	0.373	0.622	0.142
	60	35	00	CS	3,160	0.323	0.495	0.151
	60	35	000	CS	3,650	0.364	0.392	0.171
	60	35	0000	CS	4,390	0.417	0.310	0.191
	60	35	250,000	CS	4,900	0.455	0.263	0.210
	60	35	300,000	CS	5,660	0.497	0.220	0.230
	60	35	350,000	CS	6,310	0.539	0.190	0.249
	60	35	400,000	CS	7,080	0.572	0.166	0.265
	60	35	500,000	CS	8,310	0.642	0.134	0.297
	65	40	600,000	CS	9,800	0.700	0.113	0.327
	65	40	750,000	CS	11,800	0.780	0.0901	0.366
3 kV	70	40	6	SR	1,680	0.184	2.50	0.067
	70	40	4	SR	2,030	0.232	1.58	0.084
	70	40	2	SR	2,600	0.292	0.987	0.106
	70	40	1	SR	2,930	0.332	0.786	0.126
	70	40	0	SR	3,440	0.373	0.622	0.142
	70	40	00	CS	3,300	0.323	0.495	0.151
	70	40	000	CS	3,890	0.364	0.392	0.171
	70	40	0000	CS	4,530	0.417	0.310	0.191
	70	40	250,000	CS	5,160	0.455	0.263	0.210
	70	40	300,000	CS	5,810	0.497	0.220	0.230
	70	40	350,000	CS	6,470	0.539	0.190	0.249
	70	40	400,000	CS	7,240	0.572	0.166	0.265
	70	40	500,000	CS	8,660	0.642	0.134	0.297
	75	40	600,000	CS	9,910	0.700	0.113	0.327
	75	40	750,000	CS	11,920	0.780	0.091	0.366
5 kV	105	55	6	SR	2,150	0.184	2.50	0.067
	100	55	4	SR	2,470	0.232	1.58	0.084
	95	50	2	SR	2,900	0.292	0.987	0.106
	90	45	1	SR	3,280	0.332	0.786	0.126
	90	45	0	SR	3,660	0.373	0.622	0.142
	85	45	00	CS	3,480	0.323	0.495	0.151
	85	45	000	CS	4,080	0.364	0.392	0.171
	85	45	0000	CS	4,720	0.417	0.310	0.191
	85	45	250,000	CS	5,370	0.455	0.263	0.210
	85	45	300,000	CS	6,050	0.497	0.220	0.230

Positive and Negative Sequences			Zero Sequence			Sheath	
Series Reactance (Ω/mi)	Shunt Capacitive Reactance[c]	GMR— Three Conductors	Series Resistance[d] (Ω/mi)	Series Resistance[d] (Ω/mi)	Shunt Capacitive Reactance[c] (Ω/mi)	Thickness (Mils)	Resistance (Ω/mi) at 50°C
0.185	6300	0.184	10.66	0.315	11,600	85	2.69
0.175	5400	0.218	8.39	0.293	10,200	90	2.27
0.165	4700	0.262	6.99	0.273	9,000	90	2.00
0.165	4300	0.295	6.07	0.256	8,400	95	1.76
0.152	4000	0.326	5.54	0.246	7,900	95	1.64
0.138	2800	0.290	5.96	0.250	5,400	95	1.82
0.134	2300	0.320	5.46	0.241	4,500	95	1.69
1.131	2000	0.355	4.72	0.237	4,000	100	1.47
0.129	1800	0.387	4.46	0.224	3,600	100	1.40
0.128	1700	0.415	3.97	0.221	3,400	105	1.25
0.126	1500	0.446	3.73	0.216	3,100	105	1.18
0.124	1500	0.467	3.41	0.214	2,900	110	1.08
0.123	1300	0.517	3.11	0.208	2,600	110	0.993
0.122	1200	0.567	2.74	0.197	2,400	115	0.877
0.121	1100	0.623	2.40	0.194	2,100	120	0.771
0.192	6700	0.192	9.67	0.322	12,500	90	2.39
0.181	5800	0.227	8.06	0.298	11,200	90	2.16
1.171	5100	0.271	6.39	0.278	9,800	95	1.80
0.181	4700	0.304	5.83	0.263	9,200	95	1.68
0.158	4400	0.335	5.06	0.256	8,600	100	1.48
0.142	3500	0.297	5.69	0.259	6,700	95	1.73
0.138	2700	0.329	5.28	0.246	5,100	95	1.63
0.135	2400	0.367	4.57	0.237	4,600	100	1.42
0.132	2100	0.396	4.07	0.231	4,200	105	1.27
0.130	1900	0.424	3.82	0.228	3,800	105	1.20
0.129	1800	0.455	3.61	0.219	3,700	105	1.14
0.128	1700	0.478	3.32	0.218	3,400	110	1.05
0.126	1500	0.527	2.89	0.214	3,000	115	0.918
0.125	1400	0.577	2.68	0.210	2,800	115	0.855
0.123	1300	0.633	2.37	0.204	2,500	120	0.758
0.215	8500	0.218	8.14	0.342	15,000	95	1.88
0.199	7600	0.250	6.86	0.317	13,600	95	1.76
0.184	6100	0.291	5.88	0.290	11,300	95	1.63
0.171	5400	0.321	5.23	0.270	10,200	100	1.48
0.165	5000	0.352	4.79	0.259	9,600	100	1.39
0.148	3600	0.312	5.42	0.263	9,300	95	1.64
0.143	3200	0.343	4.74	0.254	6,700	100	1.45
0.141	2800	0.380	4.33	0.245	8,300	100	1.34
0.138	2600	0.410	3.89	0.237	7,800	105	1.21
0.135	2400	0.438	3.67	0.231	7,400	105	1.15

(continued)

TABLE A.12 (continued)

60 Hz Characteristics of Three-Conductor Belted Paper-Insulated Cables

Voltage Class	Insulation Thickness (Mils) Conductor	Belt	Circular Mils or AWG (B&S)	Type of Conductor	Weight per 1000 ft	Diameter[d] or Sector Depth (in.)	Resistance[a] (Ω/mi)	GMR of One Conductor[b] (in.)
	85	45	350,000	CS	6,830	0.539	0.190	0.249
	85	45	400,000	CS	7,480	0.572	0.166	0.265
	85	45	500,000	CS	8,890	0.642	0.134	0.297
	85	45	600,000	CS	10,300	0.700	0.113	0.327
	85	45	750,000	CS	12,340	0.780	0.091	0.366
8 kV	130	65	6	SR	2,450	0.184	2.50	0.067
	125	65	4	SR	2,900	0.232	1.58	0.084
	115	60	2	SR	3,280	0.292	0.987	0.106
	110	55	1	SR	3,560	0.332	0.786	0.126
	110	55	0	SR	4,090	0.373	0.622	0.142
	105	55	00	CS	3,870	0.323	0.495	0.151
	105	55	000	CS	4,390	0.364	0.392	0.171
	105	55	0000	CS	5,150	0.417	0.310	0.191
	105	55	250,000	CS	5,830	0.455	0.263	0.210
	105	55	300,000	CS	6,500	0.497	0.220	0.230
	105	55	350,000	CS	7,160	0.539	0.190	0.249
	105	55	400,000	CS	7,980	0.572	0.166	0.265
	105	55	500,000	CS	9,430	0.642	0.134	0.297
	105	55	600,000	CS	10,680	0.700	0.113	0.327
	105	55	750,000	CS	12,740	0.780	0.091	0.366
15 kV	170	85	2	SR	4,350	0.292	0.987	0.106
	165	80	1	SR	4,640	0.332	0.786	0.126
	160	75	0	SR	4,990	0.373	0.622	0.142
	155	75	00	SR	5,600	0.419	0.495	0.159
	155	75	000	SR	6,230	0.470	0.392	0.178
	155	75	0000	SR	7,180	0.528	0.310	0.200
	155	75	250,000	SR	7,840	0.575	0.263	0.218
	155	75	300,000	CS	7,480	0.497	0.220	0.230
	155	75	350,000	CS	8,340	0.539	0.190	0.249
	155	75	400,000	CS	9,030	0.572	0.166	0.265
	155	75	500,000	CS	10,550	0.642	0.134	0.297
	155	75	600,000	CS	12,030	0.700	0.113	0.327
	155	75	750,000	CS	14,190	0.780	0.091	0.366

Sources: Westinghouse Electric Corporation, *Electrical Transmission and Distribution Reference Book*, Westinghouse Electric Corporation, East Pittsburgh, PA, 1964; Gönen, T., *Electric Power Distribution System Engineering*, CRC Press.

The following symbols are used to designate the cable types: SR, stranded round; CS, compact sector.

[a] AC resistance based on 100% conductivity at 65°C including 2% allowance for stranding.

[b] GMR of sector-shaped conductors is an approximate figure close enough for most practical applications.

[c] Dielectric constant = 3.7.

[d] Based on all return current in the sheath; none in ground.

[e] See Figure 7, p. 67, of Ref. [1].

Positive and Negative Sequences			Zero Sequence			Sheath	
Series Reactance (Ω/mi)	Shunt Capacitive Reactance[c]	GMR— Three Conductors	Series Resistance[d] (Ω/mi)	Series Resistance[d] (Ω/mi)	Shunt Capacitive Reactance[c] (Ω/mi)	Thickness (Mils)	Resistance (Ω/mi) at 50°C
0.133	2200	0.470	3.31	0.225	7,000	110	1.04
0.131	2000	0.493	3.17	0.221	6,700	110	1.00
0.129	1800	0.542	2.79	0.216	6,200	115	0.885
0.128	1600	0.587	2.51	0.210	5,800	120	0.798
0.125	1500	0.643	2.21	0.206	5,400	125	0.707
0.230	9600	0.236	7.57	0.353	16,300	95	1.69
0.212	8300	0269	6.08	0.329	14,500	100	1.50
0.193	6800	0.307	5.25	0.302	12,500	100	1.42
0.179	6100	0.338	4.90	0.280	11,400	100	1.37
0.174	5700	0.368	4.31	0.272	10,700	105	1.23
0.156	4300	0.330	4.79	0.273	8,300	100	1.43
0.151	3800	0.362	4.41	0.263	7,400	100	1.34
0.147	3500	0.399	3.88	0.254	6,600	105	1.19
0.144	3200	0.428	3.50	0.246	6,200	110	1.08
0.141	2900	0.458	3.31	0.239	5,600	110	1.03
0.139	2700	0.489	3.12	0.233	5,200	110	0.978
0.137	2500	0.513	2.86	0.230	4,900	115	0.899
0.135	2200	0.563	2.53	0.224	4,300	120	0.800
0.132	2000	0.606	2.39	0.218	3,900	120	0.758
0.129	1800	0.663	2.11	0.211	3,500	125	0.673
0.217	8600	0.349	4.20	0.323	15,000	110	1.07
0.202	7800	0.381	3.88	0.305	13,800	110	1.03
0.193	7100	0.409	3.62	0.288	12,800	110	1.00
0.185	6500	0.439	3.25	0.280	12,000	115	0.918
0.180	6000	0.476	2.99	0.272	11,300	115	0.867
0.174	5600	0.520	2.64	0.263	10,600	120	0.778
0.168	5300	0.555	2.50	0.256	10,200	120	0.744
0.155	5400	0.507	2.79	0.254	7,900	115	0.855
0.152	5100	0.536	2.54	0.250	7,200	120	0.784
0.149	4900	0.561	2.44	0.245	6,900	120	0.758
0.145	4600	0.611	2.26	0.239	6,200	125	0.690
0.142	4300	0.656	1.97	0.231	5,700	130	0.620
0.139	4000	0.712	1.77	0.226	5,100	135	0.558

TABLE A.13
60 Hz Characteristics of Three-Conductor Shielded Paper-Insulated Cables

Voltage Class	Insulation Thickness (Mils)	Circular Mils or AWG (B&S)	Type of Conductor[f]	Weight per 1000 ft	Diameter or Sector Depth[b] (in.)	Resistance (Ω/mi)[a]	GMR of One Conductor[c] (in.)
15 kV	205	4	SR	3,860	0.232	1.58	0.084
	190	2	SR	4,260	0.292	0.987	0.106
	185	1	SR	4,740	0.332	0.786	0.126
	180	0	SR	5,090	0.373	0.622	0.141
	175	00	CS	4,790	0.323	0.495	0.151
	175	000	CS	5,510	0.364	0.392	0.171
	175	0000	CS	6,180	0.417	0.310	0.191
	175	250,000	CS	6,910	0.455	0.263	0.210
	175	300,000	CS	7,610	0.497	0.220	0.230
	175	350,000	CS	8,480	0.539	0.190	0.249
	175	400,000	CS	9,170	0.572	0.166	0.265
	175	500,000	CS	10,710	0.642	0.134	0.297
	175	600,000	CS	12,230	0.700	0.113	0.327
	175	750,000	CS	14,380	0.780	0.091	0.366
23 kV	265	2	SR	5,590	0.292	0.987	0.106
	250	1	SR	5,860	0.332	0.786	0.126
	250	0	SR	6,440	0.373	0.622	0.141
	240	00	CS	6,060	0.323	0.495	0.151
	240	000	CS	6,620	0.364	0.392	0.171
	240	0000	CS	7,480	0.410	0.310	0.191
	240	250,000	CS	8,070	0.447	0.263	0.210
	240	300,000	CS	8,990	0.490	0.220	0.230
	240	350,000	CS	9,720	0.532	0.190	0.249
	240	400,000	CS	10,650	0.566	0.166	0.265
	240	500,000	CS	12,280	0.635	0.134	0.297
	240	600,000	CS	13,610	0.690	0.113	0.327
	240	750,000	CS	15,830	0.767	0.091	0.366
35 kV	355	0	SR	8,520	0.288	0.622	0.141
	345	00	SR	9,180	0.323	0.495	0.159
	345	000	SR	9,900	0.364	0.392	0.178
	345	0000	CS	9,830	0.410	0.310	0.191
	345	250,000	CS	10,470	0.447	0.263	0.210
	345	300,000	CS	11,290	0.490	0.220	0.230
	345	350,000	CS	12,280	0.532	0.190	0.249
	345	400,000	CS	13,030	0.566	0.166	0.265
	345	500,000	CS	14,760	0.635	0.134	0.297
	345	600,000	CS	16,420	0.690	0.113	0.327
	345	750,000	CS	18,860	0.767	0.091	0.366

Sources: Westinghouse Electric Corporation, *Electrical Transmission and Distribution Reference Book*, Westinghouse Electric Corporation, East Pittsburgh, PA, 1964; Gönen, T., *Electric Power Distribution System Engineering*, CRC Press.

[a] AC resistance based on 100% conductivity at 65°C including 2% allowance for stranding.

[b] GMR of sector-shaped conductors is an approximate figure close enough for most practical applications.

[c] Dielectric constant = 3.7.

[d] Based on all return current in the sheath; none in ground.

[e] See Figure 7, p. 67, of Ref. [1].

[f] The following symbols are used to designate the conductor types: SR, stranded round; CS, compact sector.

Positive and Negative Sequences		GMR—	Zero Sequence			Sheath	
Series Reactance (Ω/mi)	Shunt Capacitive Reactance (Ω/mi)	Three Conductors	Series Resistance (Ω/mi)[d]	Series Reactance (Ω/mi)[d]	Shunt Capacitive Reactance (Ω/Mils)[e]	Thickness (mi)	Resistance (Ω/mi) at 50°C
0.248	8200	0.328	5.15	0.325	8200	105	1.19
0.226	6700	0.365	4.44	0.298	6700	105	1.15
0.210	6000	0.398	3.91	0.285	6000	110	1.04
0.201	5400	0.425	3.65	0.275	5400	110	1.01
0.178	5200	0.397	3.95	0.268	5200	105	1.15
0.170	4800	0.432	3.48	0.256	4800	110	1.03
0.166	4400	0.468	3.24	0.249	4400	110	0.975
0.158	4100	0.498	2.95	0.243	4100	115	0.897
0.156	3800	0.530	2.80	0.237	3800	115	0.860
0.153	3600	0.561	2.53	0.233	3600	120	0.783
0.151	3400	0.585	2.45	0.228	3400	120	0.761
0.146	3100	0.636	2.19	0.222	3100	125	0.684
0.143	2900	0.681	1.98	0.215	2900	130	0.623
0.139	2600	0.737	1.78	0.211	2600	135	0.562
0.250	8300	0.418	3.60	0.317	8300	115	0.870
0.232	7500	0.450	3.26	0.298	7500	115	0.851
0.222	8800	0.477	2.99	0.290	6800	120	0.788
0.196	6600	0.446	3.16	0.285	6600	115	0.890
0.188	6000	0.480	2.95	0.285	6000	115	0.851
0.181	5600	0.515	2.64	0.268	5800	120	0.775
0.177	5200	0.545	2.50	0.261	5200	120	0.747
0.171	4900	0.579	2.29	0.252	4900	125	0.690
0.167	4600	0.610	2.10	0.249	4600	125	0.665
0.165	4400	0.633	2.03	0.240	4400	130	0.620
0.159	3900	0.687	1.82	0.237	3900	135	0.562
0.154	3700	0.730	1.73	0.230	3700	135	0.540
0.151	3400	0.787	1.56	0.225	3400	140	0.488
0.239	9900	0.523	2.40	0.330	9900	130	0.594
0.226	9100	0.548	2.17	0.322	9100	135	0.559
0.217	8500	0.585	2.01	0.312	8500	135	0.538
0.204	7200	0.594	2.00	0.290	7200	135	0.563
0.197	6800	0.628	1.90	0.280	6800	135	0.545
0.191	6400	0.663	1.80	0.273	6400	135	0.527
0.187	6000	0.693	1.66	0.270	6000	140	0.491
0.183	5700	0.721	1.61	0.265	5700	140	0.480
0.177	5200	0.773	1.46	0.257	5200	145	0.441
0.171	4900	0.819	1.35	0.248	4900	150	0.412
0.165	4500	0.879	1.22	0.243	4500	155	0.377

TABLE A.14

60 Hz Characteristics of Three-Conductor Oil-Filled Paper-Insulated Cables

Voltage Class	Insulation Thickness (Mils)	Circular Mils or AWG (B&S)	Type of Conductor[f]	Weight per 1000 ft	Diameter or Sector Depth[e] (in.)	Resistance (Ω/mi)[a]	GMR of One Conductor[b] (in.)
35 kV	190	00	CS	5,590	0.323	0.495	0.151
		000	CS	6,150	0.364	0.392	0.171
		0000	CS	6,860	0.417	0.310	0.191
		250,000	CS	7,680	0.455	0.263	0.210
		300,000	CS	9,090	0.497	0.220	0.230
		350,000	CS	9,180	0.539	0.190	0.249
		400,000	CS	9,900	0.572	0.166	0.265
		500,000	CS	11,550	0.642	0.134	0.297
		600,000	CS	12,900	0.700	0.113	0.327
		750,000	CS	15,660	0.780	0.091	0.366
46 kV	225	00	CS	6,360	0.323	0.495	0.151
		000	CS	6,940	0.364	0.392	0.171
		0000	CS	7,660	0.410	0.310	0.191
		250,000	CS	8,280	0.447	0.263	0.210
		300,000	CS	9,690	0.490	0.220	0.230
		350,000	CS	10,100	0.532	0.190	0.249
		400,000	CS	10,820	0.566	0.166	0.265
		500,000	CS	12,220	0.635	0.134	0.297
		600,000	CS	13,930	0.690	0.113	0.327
		750,000	CS	16,040	0.767	0.091	0.366
		1,000,000	CS				
69 kV	315	00	CR	8,240	0.370	0.495	0.147
		000	CS	8,830	0.364	0.392	0.171
		0000	CS	9,660	0.410	0.310	0.191
		250,000	CS	10,330	0.447	0.263	0.210
		300,000	CS	11,540	0.490	0.220	0.230
		350,000	CS	12,230	0.532	0.190	0.249
		400,000	CS	13,040	0.566	0.166	0.205
		500,000	CS	14,880	0.635	0.134	0.297
		600,000	CS	16,320	0.690	0.113	0.327
		750,000	CS	18,980	0.767	0.091	0.366
		1,000,000					

Sources: Westinghouse Electric Corporation, *Electrical Transmission and Distribution Reference Book*, Westinghouse Electric Corporation, East Pittsburgh, PA, 1964; Gönen, T., *Electric Power Distribution System Engineering*, CRC Press.

[a] AC resistance based on 100% conductivity at 65°C, including 2% allowance for stranding.

[b] GMR of sector-shaped conductors is an approximate figure close enough for most practical applications.

[c] Dielectric constant = 3.5.

[d] Based on all return current in sheath, none in ground.

[e] See Figure 7, p. 67, of Ref. [1].

[f] The following symbols are used to designate the cable types: CR, compact round; CS, compact sector.

Positive and Negative Sequences			Zero Sequence			Sheath	
Series Reactance (Ω/mi)	Shunt Capacitive Reactance[c] (Ω/mi)	GMR— Three Conductors	Series Resistance (Ω/mi)[d]	Series Reactance (Ω/mi)[d]	Shunt Capacitive Reactance (Ω/mi)[c]	Thickness (Mils)	Resistance (Ω/mi) at 50°V
0.185	6030	0.406	3.56	0.265	6030	115	1.02
0.178	5480	0.439	3.30	0.256	5480	115	0.970
0.172	4840	0.478	3.06	0.243	4840	115	0.918
0.168	4570	0.508	2.72	0.238	4570	125	0.820
0.164	4200	0.539	2.58	0.232	4200	125	0.788
0.160	3900	0.570	2.44	0.227	3900	125	0.752
0.157	3690	0.595	2.35	0.223	3690	125	0.729
0.153	3400	0.646	2.04	0.217	3400	135	0.636
0.150	3200	0.691	1.94	0.210	3200	135	0.608
0.148	3070	0.763	1.73	0.202	3070	140	0.548
0.195	6700	0.436	3.28	0.272	6700	115	0.928
0.188	6100	0.468	2.87	0.265	6100	125	0.826
0.180	5520	0.503	2.67	0.256	5520	125	0.788
0.177	5180	0.533	2.55	0.247	5180	125	0.761
0.172	4820	0.566	2.41	0.241	4820	125	0.729
0.168	4490	0.596	2.16	0.237	4400	135	0.658
0.165	4220	0.623	2.08	0.232	4220	135	0.639
0.160	3870	0.672	1.94	0.226	3870	135	0.603
0.156	3670	0.718	1.74	0.219	3670	140	0.542
0.151	3350	0.773	1.62	0.213	3350	140	0.510
0.234	8330	0.532	2.41	0.290	8330	135	0.639
0.208	7560	0.538	2.32	0.284	7560	135	0.642
0.200	6840	0.575	2.16	0.274	6840	135	0.618
0.195	6500	0.607	2.06	0.266	6500	135	0.597
0.190	6030	0.640	1.85	0.260	6030	140	0.543
0.185	5700	0.672	1.77	0.254	5700	140	0.527
0.181	5430	0.700	1.55	0.248	5430	140	0.513
0.176	5050	0.750	1.51	0.242	5050	150	0.460
0.171	4740	0.797	1.44	0.235	4740	150	0.442
0.165	4360	0.854	1.29	0.230	4360	155	0.399

TABLE A.15

60 Hz Characteristics of Single-Conductor Concentric-Strand Paper-Insulated Cables

						x_a	z_a	r_a	r_a		
Voltage Class	Insulation Thickness (Mils)	Circular Mils or AWG (B&S)	Weight per 1000 ft	Diameter of Conductor (in.)	GMR of One Conductor[a] (in.)	Reactance at 12 in. (Ω/Phase/mi)	Reactance of Sheath (Ω/Phase/mi)	Resistance of One Conductor (Ω/Phase/mi)[a]	Resistance of Sheath (Ω/Phase/mi) at 50°C	Shunt Capacitive Reactance[c] (Ω/Phase/mi)	Lead Sheath Thickness (Mils)
1 kV	60	6	560	0.184	0.067	0.628	0.489	2.50	6.20	4040	75
	60	4	670	0.232	0.084	0.602	0.475	1.58	5.56	3360	75
	60	2	880	0.292	0.106	0.573	0.458	0.987	4.55	2760	80
	60	1	990	0.332	0.126	0.552	0.450	0.786	4.25	2490	80
	60	0	1,110	0.373	0.141	0.539	0.442	0.622	3.61	2250	80
	60	00	1,270	0.418	0.159	0.524	0.434	0.495	3.34	2040	80
	60	000	1,510	0.470	0.178	0.512	0.425	0.392	3.23	1840	85
	60	0000	1,740	0.528	0.200	0.496	0.414	0.310	2.98	1650	85
	60	250,000	1,930	0.575	0.221	0.484	0.408	0.263	2.81	1530	85
	60	350,000	2,490	0.681	0.262	0.464	0.392	0.190	2.31	1300	90
	60	500,000	3,180	0.814	0.313	0.442	0.378	0.134	2.06	1090	90
	60	750,000	4,380	0.998	0.385	0.417	0.358	0.091	1.65	885	95
	60	1,000,000	5,560	1.152	0.445	0.400	0.344	0.070	1.40	800	100
	60	1,500,000	8,000	1.412	0.543	0.374	0.319	0.050	1.05	645	110
	60	2,000,000	10,190	1.632	0.633	0.356	0.305	0.041	0.894	555	115
3 kV	75	6	600	0.184	0.067	0.628	0.481	2.50	5.80	4810	75
	75	4	720	0.232	0.084	0.602	0.467	1.58	5.23	4020	75
	75	2	930	0.292	0.106	0.573	0.453	0.987	4.31	3300	80
	75	1	1,040	0.332	0.126	0.552	0.445	0.786	4.03	2990	80
	75	0	1,170	0.373	0.141	0.539	0.436	0.622	3.79	2670	80
	75	00	1,320	0.418	0.159	0.524	0.428	0.495	3.52	2450	80
	75	000	1,570	0.470	0.178	0.512	0.420	0.392	3.10	2210	85
	75	0000	1,800	0.528	0.200	0.496	0.412	0.310	2.87	2010	85
	75	250,000	1,990	0.575	0.221	0.484	0.403	0.263	2.70	1860	85
	75	350,000	2,550	0.681	0.262	0.464	0.389	0.190	2.27	1610	90
	75	500,000	3,340	0.814	0.313	0.442	0.375	0.134	1.89	1340	95
	75	750,000	4,570	0.998	0.385	0.417	0.352	0.091	1.53	1060	100
	75	1,000,000	5,640	1.152	0.445	0.400	0.341	0.070	1.37	980	100
	75	1,500,000	8,090	1.412	0.543	0.374	0.316	0.050	1.02	805	110
	75	2,000,000	10,300	1.632	0.633	0.356	0.302	0.041	0.877	685	115

						x_z	z_a	r_a	r_a		
Voltage Class	Insulation Thickness (Mils)	Circular Mils or AWG (B&S)	Weight per 1000 ft	Diameter of Conducto (in.)	GMR of One Conductor[a] (in.)	Reactance at 12 in. (Ω/Phase/mi)	Reactance of Sheath (Ω/Phase/mi)	Resistance of One Conductor (Ω/Phase/mi)[a]	Resistance of Sheath (Ω/Phase/mi) at 50°C	Shunt Capacitive Reactance[c] (Ω/Phase/mi)[b]	Lead Sheath Thickness (Mils)
15 kV	220	4	1340	0.232	0.084	0.602	0.412	1.58	2.91	8580	85
	215	2	1500	0.292	0.106	0.573	0.406	0.987	2.74	7270	85
	210	1	1610	0.332	0.126	0.552	0.400	0.786	2.64	6580	85
	200	0	1710	0.373	0.141	0.539	0.397	0.622	2.59	5880	85
	195	00	1940	0.418	0.159	0.524	0.391	0.495	2.32	5290	90
	185	000	2100	0.470	0.178	0.512	0.386	0.392	2.24	4680	90
	180	0000	2300	0.528	0.200	0.496	0.380	0.310	2.14	4200	90
	175	250,000	2500	0.575	0.221	0.484	0.377	0.263	2.06	3820	90
	175	350,000	3110	0.681	0.262	0.464	0.366	0.190	1.98	3340	95
	175	500,000	3940	0.814	0.313	0.442	0.352	0.134	1.51	2870	100
	175	750,000	5240	0.998	0.385	0.417	0.336	0.091	1.26	2420	105
	175	1,000,000	6350	1.152	0.445	0.400	0.325	0.070	1.15	2130	105
	175	1,500,000	8810	1.412	0.546	0.374	0.305	0.050	0.90	1790	115
	175	2,000,000	11,080	1.632	0.633	0.356	0.294	0.041	0.772	1570	120
23 kV	295	2	1920	0.292	0.106	0.573	0.383	0.987	2.16	8890	90
	285	1	2010	0.332	0.126	0.552	0.380	0.786	2.12	8050	90
	275	0	2120	0.373	0.141	0.539	0.377	0.622	2.08	7300	90
	265	00	2250	0.418	0.159	0.524	0.375	0.495	2.02	6580	90
	260	000	2530	0.470	0.178	0.512	0.370	0.392	1.85	6000	95
	250	0000	2740	0.528	0.200	0.496	0.366	0.310	1.78	5350	95
	245	250,000	2930	0.575	0.221	0.484	0.361	0.263	1.72	4950	95
	240	350,000	3550	0.681	0.262	0.464	0.352	0.190	1.51	4310	100
	240	500,000	4300	0.814	0.313	0.442	0.341	0.134	1.38	3720	100
	240	750,000	5630	0.998	0.385	0.417	0.325	0.091	1.15	3170	105
	240	1,000,000	6910	1.152	0.445	0.400	0.313	0.070	1.01	2800	110
	240	1,500,000	9460	1.412	0.546	0.374	0.296	0.050	0.806	2350	120
	240	2,000,000	11,790	1.632	0.633	0.356	0.285	0.041	0.697	2070	125

(*continued*)

TABLE A.15 (continued)
60 Hz Characteristics of Single-Conductor Concentric-Strand Paper-Insulated Cables

Voltage Class	Insulation Thickness (Mils)	Circular Mils or AWG (B&S)	Weight per 1000 ft	Diameter of Conductor (in.)	GMR of One Conductor[a] (in.)	x_a Reactance at 12 in. (Ω/Phase/mi)	z_a Reactance of Sheath (Ω/Phase/mi)	r_a Resistance of One Conductor (Ω/Phase/mi)[a]	r_a Resistance of Sheath (Ω/Phase/mi) at 50°C	Shunt Capacitive Reactance (Ω/Phase/mi)	Lead Sheath Thickness (Mils)
5 kV	120	6	740	0.184	0.067	0.628	0.456	2.50	4.47	6700	80
	115	4	890	0.232	0.084	0.573	0.447	1.58	4.17	5540	80
	110	2	1,040	0.292	0.106	0.573	0.439	0.987	3.85	4520	80
	110	1	1,160	0.332	0.126	0.552	0.431	0.786	3.62	4100	80
	105	0	1,270	0.373	0.141	0.539	0.425	0.622	3.47	3600	80
	100	00	1,520	0.418	0.159	0.524	0.420	0.495	3.09	3140	85
	100	000	1,710	0.470	0.178	0.512	0.412	0.392	2.91	2860	85
	95	0000	1,870	0.525	0.200	0.496	0.406	0.310	2.74	2480	85
	90	250,000	2,080	0.575	0.221	0.484	0.400	0.263	2.62	2180	85
	90	350,000	2,620	0.681	0.262	0.464	0.386	0.190	2.20	1890	90
	90	500,000	3,410	0.814	0.313	0.442	0.396	0.134	1.85	1610	95
	90	750,000	4,650	0.998	0.385	0.417	0.350	0.091	1.49	1360	100
	90	1,000,000	5,850	1.152	0.445	0.400	0.339	0.070	1.27	1140	105
	90	1,500,000	8,160	1.412	0.543	0.374	0.316	0.050	1.02	950	110
	90	2,000,000	10,370	1.632	0.663	0.356	0.302	0.041	0.870	820	115
8 kV	150	6	890	0.184	0.067	0.628	0.431	2.50	3.62	7780	80
	150	4	1,010	0.232	0.084	0.602	0.425	1.58	3.$2	6660	85
	140	2	1,150	0.292	0.106	0.573	0.417	0.987	3.06	5400	85
	140	1	1,330	0.332	0.126	0.552	0.411	0.786	2.91	4920	85
	135	0	1,450	0.373	0.141	0.539	0.408	0.622	2.83	4390	85
	130	00	1,590	0.418	0.159	0.524	0.403	0.495	2.70	3890	85
	125	000	1,760	0.470	0.178	0.512	0.397	0.392	2.59	3440	85
	120	0000	1,980	0.528	0.200	0.496	0.389	0.310	2.29	3020	90
	120	250,000	2,250	0.575	0.221	0.484	0.383	0.263	2.18	2790	90
	115	350,000	2,730	0.681	0.262	0.464	0.375	0.190	1.90	2350	95
	115	500,000	3,530	0.814	0.313	0.442	0.361	0.134	1.69	2010	95
	115	750,000	4,790	0.998	0.385	0.417	0.341	0.091	1.39	1670	100
	115	1,000,000	6,000	1.152	0.415	0.400	0.330	0.070	1.25	1470	105
	115	1,500,000	8,250	1.412	0.543	0.374	0.310	0.050	0.975	1210	110
	115	2,000,000	10,480	1.632	0.663	0.356	0.297	0.041	0.797	1055	120

Sources: Westinghouse Electric Corporation, *Electrical Transmission and Distribution Reference Book*, Westinghouse Electric Corporation, East Pittsburgh, PA, 1964; Gönen, T., *Electric Power Distribution System Engineering*, CRC Press.

[a] Conductors are standard concentric stranded, not compact round.

[b] AC resistance based on 100% conductivity at 65°C including 2% allowance for stranding.

[c] Dielectric constant = 3.7.

						x_z	z_a	r_a	r_a		
Voltage Class	Insulation Thickness (Mils)	Circular Mils or AWG (B&S)	Weight per 1000 ft	Diameter of Conductor (in.)	GMR of One Conductor[a] (in.)	Reactance at 12 in. (Ω/Phase/mi)	Reactance of Sheath (Ω/Phase/mi)	Resistance of One Conductor (Ω/Phase/mi)[a]	Resistance of Sheath (Ω/Phase/mi) at 50°C	Shunt Capacitive Reactance[c] (Ω/Phase/mi)[b]	Lead Sheath Thickness (Mils)
35 kV	395	0	2,900	0.373	0.141	0.539	0.352	0.622	1.51	9150	100
	385	00	3,040	0.418	0.159	0.524	0.350	0.495	1.48	8420	100
	370	000	3,190	0.470	0.178	0.512	0.347	0.392	1.46	7620	100
	355	0000	3,380	0.528	0.200	0.496	0.344	0.310	1.43	6870	100
	350	250,000	3,590	0.575	0.221	0.484	0.342	0.263	1.39	6410	100
	345	350,000	4,230	0.681	0.262	0.464	0.366	0.190	1.24	5640	105
	345	500,000	5,040	0.814	0.313	0.442	0.325	0.134	1.15	4940	105
	345	750,000	5,430	0.998	0.385	0.417	0.311	0.091	0.975	4250	110
	345	1,000,000	7,780	1.152	0.445	0.400	0.302	0.070	0.866	3780	115
	345	1,500,000	10,420	1.412	0.546	0.374	0.285	0.050	0.700	3210	125
	345	2,000,000	12,830	1.632	0.633	0.356	0.274	0.041	0.811	2830	130
46 kV	475	000	3,910	0.470	0.178	0.512	0.331	0.392	1.20	8890	105
	460	0000	4,080	0.528	0.200	0.496	0.329	0.310	1.19	8100	105
	450	250,000	4,290	0.575	0.221	0.484	0.326	0.263	1.16	7570	105
	445	350,000	4,990	0.681	0.262	0.464	0.319	0.190	1.05	6720	110
	445	500,000	5,820	0.814	0.313	0.442	0.310	0.134	0.930	5950	115
	445	750,000	7,450	0.998	0.385	0.417	0.298	0.091	0.807	5130	120
	445	1,000,000	8,680	1.152	0.445	0.400	0.290	0.070	0.752	4610	120
	445	1,500,000	11,420	1.412	0.546	0.374	0.275	0.050	0.615	3930	130
	445	2,000,000	13,910	1.632	0.633	0.356	0.264	0.041	0.543	3520	135
69 kV	650	350,000	6,720	0.681	0.262	0.464	0.292	0.190	0.773	8590	120
	650	500,000	7,810	0.814	0.313	0.442	0.284	0.134	0.695	7680	125
	650	750,000	9,420	0.998	0.385	0.417	0.275	0.091	0.615	6700	130
	650	1,000,000	10,940	1.152	0.445	0.400	0.267	0.070	0.557	6060	135
	650	1,500,000	13,680	1.412	0.546	0.374	0.258	0.050	0.488	5250	140
	650	2,000,000	16,320	1.632	0.633	0.356	0.246	0.041	0.437	4710	145

TABLE A.16

60 Hz Characteristics of Single-Conductor Oil-Filled (Hollow-Core) Paper-Insulated Cables

Inside Diameter of Spring Core = 0.5 in.

Voltage Class	Insulation Thickness (Mils)	Circular Mils or AWG (B&S)	Weight per 1000 ft	Diameter of Conductor (in.)	GMR of One Conductor[c] (in.)	X_a Reactance at 12 in. (Ω/Phase/mi)	X_a Reactance of Sheath (Ω/Phase/mi)	r_c Resistance of One Conductor (Ω/Phase/mi)[a]	R_a Resistance of Sheath (Ω/Phase/mi) at 50°C	Shunt Capacitive Reactance[c] (Ω/Phase/mi)[b]	Lead Sheath Thickness (Mils)
69 kV	315	00	3,980	0.736	0.345	0.431	0.333	0.495	1.182	5240	110
		000	4,090	0.768	0.356	0.427	0.331	0.392	1.157	5070	110
		0000	4,320	0.807	0.373	0.421	0.328	0.310	1.130	4900	110
		250,000	4,650	0.837	0.381	0.418	0.325	0.263	1.057	4790	115
		350,000	5,180	0.918	0.408	0.410	0.320	0.188	1.009	4470	115
		500,000	6,100	1.028	0.448	0.399	0.312	0.133	0.905	4070	120
		750,000	7,310	1.180	0.505	0.384	0.302	0.089	0.838	3620	120
		1,000,000	8,630	1.310	0.550	0.374	0.294	0.068	0.752	3380	125
		1 $$ 000	11,090	1.547	0.639	0.356	0.281	0.048	0.649	2920	130
		2,000,000	13,750	1.760	0.716	0.342	0.270	0.039	0.550	2570	140
115 kV	480	0000	5,720	0.807	0.373	0.421	0.305	0.310	0.805	6650	120
		250,000	5,930	0.837	0.381	0.418	0.303	0.263	0.793	6500	120
		350,000	6,390	0.918	0.408	0.410	0.298	0.188	0.730	6090	125
		500,000	7,480	1.028	0.448	0.399	0.291	0.133	0.692	5600	125
		750,000	8,950	1.180	0.505	0.381	0.283	0.089	0.625	5040	130
		1,000,000	10,350	1.310	0.550	0.374	0.276	0.068	0.568	4700	135
		1,500,000	12,960	1.547	0.639	0.356	0.265	0.048	0.500	4110	140
		2,000,000	15,530	1.760	0.716	0.342	0.255	0.039	0.447	3710	145
138 kV	560	0000	6,480	0.807	0.373	0.421	0.205	0.310	0.758	7410	125
		250,000	6,700	0.837	0.381	0.418	0.293	0.263	0.746	7240	125
		350,000	7,460	0.918	0.408	0.410	0.288	0.188	0.690	6820	130
		500,000	8,310	1.028	0.448	0.399	0.282	0.133	0.658	6260	130
		750,000	9,800	1.180	0.505	0.384	0.274	0.089	0.592	5680	135
		1,000,000	11,270	1.310	0.550	0.374	0.268	0.068	0.541	5240	140
		1,500,000	13,720	1.547	0.639	0.356	0.257	0.048	0.477	4670	145
		2,000,000	16,080	1.760	0.716	0.342	0.248	0.039	0.427	4170	150
161 kV	650	250,000	7,600	0.837	0.381	0.418	0.283	0.263	0.660	7980	130
		350,000	8,390	0.918	0.408	0.410	0.279	0.188	0.611	7520	135
		500,000	9,270	1.028	0.448	0.399	0.273	0.133	0.585	6980	135
		750,000	10,840	1.180	0.505	0.384	0.266	0.089	0.532	6320	140
		1,000,000	12,340	1.310	0.550	0.374	0.259	0.068	0.483	5880	145
		1,500,000	15,090	1.547	0.639	0.356	0.246	0.048	0.433	5190	150
		2,000,000	18,000	1.760	0.716	0.342	0.241	0.039	0.391	4710	155

Sources: Westinghouse Electric Corporation, *Electrical Transmission and Distribution Reference Book*, Westinghouse Electric Corporation, East Pittsburgh, PA, 1964; Gönen, T., *Electric Power Distribution System Engineering*, CRC Press.

[a] AC resistance based on 100% conductivity at 65°C including 2% allowance for stranding.

[b] Dielectric constant = 3.5.

[c] Calculated for circular tube.

Voltage Class	Insulation Thickness (Mils)	Circular Mils or AWG (B&S)	Weight per 1000 ft	Diameter of Conductor (in.)	GMR of One Conductor[c] (in.)	X_z Reactance at 12 in. (Ω/Phase/mi)	X_a Reactance of Sheath (Ω/Phase/mi)	r_c Resistance of One Conductor (Ω/Phase/mi)[a]	r_s Resistance of Sheath (Ω/Phase/mi) at 50°C	Shunt Capacitive Reactance (Ω/Phase/mi)[2]	Lead Sheath Thickness (Mils)
							Inside Diameter of Spring Core = 0.59 in.				
69 kV	315	000	4,860	0.924	0.439	0.399	0.320	0.392	1.007	4450	115
		0000	5,090	0.956	0.450	0.398	0.317	0.310	0.985	4350	115
		250,000	5,290	0.983	0.460	0.396	0.315	0.263	0.975	4230	115
		350,000	5,950	1.050	0.483	0.390	0.310	0.188	0.897	4000	120
		500,000	6,700	1.145	0.516	0.382	0.304	0.132	0.850	3700	120
		750,000	8,080	1.286	0.550	0.374	0.295	0.089	0.759	3410	125
		1,000,000	9,440	1.416	0.612	0.360	0.288	0.067	0.688	3140	130
		1,500,000	11,970	1.635	0.692	0.346	0.276	0.047	0.601	2750	135
		2,000,000	14,450	1.835	0.763	0.334	0.266	0.038	0.533	2510	140
115 kV	480	0000	6,590	0.956	0.450	0.398	0.295	0.310	0.760	5950	125
		250,000	6,800	0.983	0.460	0.396	0.294	0.263	0.752	5790	125
		350,000	7,340	1.050	0.483	0.390	0.290	0.188	0.729	5540	125
		500,000	8,320	1.145	0.516	0.382	0.284	0.132	0.669	5150	130
		750,000	9,790	1.286	0.550	0.374	0.277	0.089	0.606	4770	135
		1,000,000	11,060	1.416	0.612	0.360	0.270	0.067	0.573	4430	135
		1,500,000	13,900	1.635	0.692	0.346	0.260	0.047	0.490	3920	145
		2,000,000	16,610	1.835	0.763	0.334	0.251	0.038	0.440	3580	150
138 kV	560	0000	7,390	0.956	0.450	0.398	0.786	0.310	0.678	6590	130
		250,000	7,610	0.983	0.460	0.396	0.285	0.263	0.669	6480	130
		350,000	8,170	1.050	0.483	0.390	0.281	0.188	0.649	6180	130
		500,000	9,180	1.145	0.516	0.382	0.276	0.132	0.601	5790	135
		750,000	10,660	1.286	0.550	0.374	0.269	0.089	0.545	5320	140
		1,000,000	12,010	1.416	0.612	0.360	0.263	0.067	0.519	4940	140
		1,500,000	14,450	1.635	0.692	0.346	0.253	0.047	0.462	4460	145
		2,000,000	16,820	1.835	0.763	0.334	0.245	0.038	0.404	4060	155
161 kV	650	250,000	8,560	0.983	0.460	0.396	0.275	0.263	0.596	7210	135
		350,000	9,140	1.050	0.483	0.390	0.272	0.188	0.580	6860	135
		500,000	10,280	1.145	0.516	0.382	0.267	0.132	0.537	6430	140
		750,000	11,770	1.286	0.550	0.374	0.261	0.089	0.492	5980	145
		1,000,000	13,110	1.416	0.612	0.360	0.255	0.067	0.469	5540	145
		1,500,000	15,840	1.635	0.692	0.346	0.246	0.047	0.421	4980	150
		2,000,000	18,840	1.835	0.763	0.334	0.238	0.038	0.369	4600	160
230 kV	925	750,000	15,360	1.286	0.550	0.374	0.238	0.089	0.369	7610	160
		1,000,000	16,790	1.416	0.612	0.360	0.233	0.067	0.355	7140	160
		2,000,000	22,990	1.835	0.763	0.334	0.219	0.038	0.315	5960	170

TABLE A.17
Current-Carrying Capacity of Three-Conductor Belted Paper-Insulated Cables

Conductor Size AWG or MCM	Conductor Type[a]	Number of Equally Loaded Cables in Duct Bank							
		One				Three			
		30	50	75	100	30	50	75	100
		Amperes per Conductor[b]							
	4,500 V								
6	S	82	80	78	75	81	78	73	68
4	SR	109	106	103	98	108	102	96	89
2	SR	143	139	134	128	139	133	124	115
1	SR	164	161	153	146	159	152	141	130
0	CS	189	184	177	168	184	175	162	149
00	CS	218	211	203	192	211	201	185	170
000	CS	250	242	232	219	242	229	211	193
0000	CS	286	276	264	249	276	260	240	218
250	CS	316	305	291	273	305	288	263	239
300	CS	354	340	324	304	340	321	292	264
350	CS	392	376	357	334	375	353	320	288
400	CS	424	406	385	359	406	380	344	309
500	CS	487	465	439	408	465	433	390	348
600	CS	544	517	487	450	517	480	430	383
750	CS	618	581	550	505	585	541	482	427
		(1.07 at 10°C, 0.92 at 30°C, 0.83 at 40°C, 0.73 at 50°C)[c]				(1.07 at 10°C, 0.92 at 30°C, 0.83 at 40°C, 0.73 at 50°C)[c]			
	7,500 V								
6	S	81	80	77	74	79	76	72	67
4	SR	107	105	101	97	104	100	94	87
2	SR	140	137	132	126	136	131	122	113
1	SR	161	156	150	143	156	149	138	128
0	CS	186	180	174	165	180	172	156	146
00	CS	214	206	198	188	206	196	181	166
000	CS	243	236	226	214	236	224	206	188
0000	CS	280	270	258	243	270	255	235	214
250	CS	311	300	287	269	300	283	259	235
300	CS	349	336	320	300	335	316	288	260
350	CS	385	369	351	328	369	346	315	283
400	CS	417	399	378	353	398	373	338	303
500	CS	476	454	429	399	454	423	381	341
600	CS	534	508	479	443	507	471	422	376
750	CS	607	576	540	497	575	532	473	413
		(1.08 at 10°C, 0.92 at 30°C, 0.83 at 40°C, 0.72 at 50°C)[c]				(1.08 at 10°C, 0.92 at 30°C, 0.83 at 40°C, 0.72 at 50°C)[c]			

Number of Equally Loaded Cables in Duct Bank

Six Percent Load Factor				Nine				Twelve			
30	50	75	100	30	50	75	100	30	50	75	100
Amperes per Conductor[a]											
Copper Temperature, 85°C											
79	74	68	63	78	72	65	58	76	69	61	54
104	97	89	81	102	94	84	74	100	90	79	69
136	127	115	104	133	121	108	95	130	117	101	89
156	145	130	118	152	138	122	108	148	133	115	100
180	166	149	134	175	159	140	122	170	152	130	114
208	190	170	152	201	181	158	138	195	173	148	126
237	217	193	172	229	206	179	156	223	197	167	145
270	246	218	194	261	234	202	176	254	223	189	163
297	271	239	212	288	258	221	192	279	244	206	177
332	301	264	234	321	285	245	211	310	271	227	195
366	330	288	255	351	311	266	229	341	296	248	211
395	355	309	272	380	334	285	244	367	317	264	224
451	403	348	305	433	378	320	273	417	357	296	251
501	444	383	334	480	416	350	298	462	393	323	273
566	500	427	371	541	466	390	331	519	439	359	302
(1.07 at 10°C, 0.92 at 30°C, 0.83 at 40°C, 0.73 at 50°C)[c]				(1.07 at 10°C, 0.92 at 30°C, 0.83 at 40°C, 0.73 at 50°C)[c]				(1.07 at 10°C, 0.92 at 30°C, 0.83 at 40°C, 0.73 at 50°C)[c]			
Copper Temperature, 83°C											
78	74	67	62	77	71	64	57	75	69	60	53
103	96	87	79	100	92	82	73	98	89	77	68
134	125	113	102	130	119	105	93	127	114	99	87
153	142	128	115	149	136	120	105	145	130	112	98
177	163	148	131	172	155	136	120	167	149	128	111
202	186	166	148	196	177	155	135	191	169	145	125
230	211	188	168	223	200	174	152	217	192	163	141
264	241	213	190	255	229	198	172	247	218	184	159
293	266	235	208	282	252	217	188	273	240	202	174
326	296	259	230	315	279	240	207	304	265	223	190
359	323	282	249	345	305	261	224	333	289	242	206
388	348	303	267	371	317	279	239	360	309	257	220
440	392	340	298	422	369	312	267	406	348	288	245
491	436	375	327	469	408	343	291	451	384	315	267
555	489	418	363	529	455	381	323	507	428	350	295
(1.08 at 10°C, 0.92 at 30°C, 0.83 at 40°C, 0.72 at 50°C)[c]				(1.08 at 10°C, 0.92 at 30°C, 0.83 at 40°C, 0.72 at 50°C)[c]				(1.08 at 10°C, 0.92 at 30°C, 0.83 at 40°C, 0.72 at 50°C)[c]			

(*continued*)

TABLE A.17 (continued)

Current-Carrying Capacity of Three-Conductor Belted Paper-Insulated Cables

		Number of Equally Loaded Cables in Duct Bank							
		One				Three			
Conductor Size AWG or MCM	Conductor Type[a]	30	50	75	100	30	50	75	100
		Amperes per Conductor[b]							
	15,000 V								
6	S	78	77	74	71	76	74	69	64
4	SR	102	99	96	92	98	95	89	83
2	SR	132	129	125	119	129	123	115	106
1	SR	151	147	142	135	146	140	131	120
0	CS	175	170	163	155	169	161	150	138
00	CS	200	194	187	177	194	184	170	156
000	CS	230	223	214	202	222	211	195	178
0000	CS	266	257	245	232	253	242	222	202
250	CS	295	284	271	255	281	268	245	221
300	CS	330	317	301	283	316	297	271	245
350	CS	365	349	332	310	348	327	297	267
400	CS	394	377	357	333	375	352	319	286
500	CS	449	429	406	377	428	399	359	321
600	CS	502	479	450	417	476	443	396	352
750	CS	572	543	510	468	540	499	444	393
		(1.09 at 10°C, 0.90 at 30°C, 0.79 at 40°C, 0.67 at 50°C)[c]				(1.09 at 10°C, 0.90 at 30°C, 0.79 at 40°C, 0.67 at 50°C)[c]			

Sources: Westinghouse Electric Corporation, *Electrical Transmission and Distribution Reference Book*, Westinghouse Electric Corporation, East Pittsburgh, PA, 1964; Gönen, T., *Electric Power Distribution System Engineering*, CRC Press.

[a] The following symbols are used here to designate conductor types: S, solid copper; SR, standard round concentric stranded; CS, compact sector stranded.

[b] Current ratings are based on the following conditions:
  i. Ambient earth temperature = 20°C.
  ii. 60-cycle ac.
  iii. Ratings include dielectric loss and all induced ac losses.
  iv. One cable per duct; all cables equally loaded and in outside ducts only.

[c] Multiply tabulated currents by these factors when earth temperature is other than 20°C.

Number of Equally Loaded Cables in Duct Bank

Six Percent Load Factor				Nine				Twelve			
30	50	75	100	30	50	75	100	30	50	75	100

Amperes per Conductor[a]

Copper Temperature, 85°C

Six Percent Load Factor				Nine				Twelve			
75	70	64	59	73	68	61	54	72	65	57	50
97	91	83	75	95	87	78	69	93	85	73	64
126	117	106	96	123	112	99	88	120	108	93	82
144	133	120	109	140	128	112	99	136	122	107	92
166	153	137	123	161	146	128	112	156	139	120	104
189	175	156	139	183	166	145	127	178	158	135	117
217	199	177	158	210	189	165	143	203	180	153	132
249	228	201	179	240	215	187	158	233	205	173	149
276	251	220	196	266	239	204	177	257	225	189	163
307	278	244	215	295	264	225	194	285	248	208	178
339	305	266	235	324	289	245	211	313	271	227	193
365	327	285	251	349	307	262	224	336	290	241	206
414	396	319	280	396	346	293	250	379	326	269	229
459	409	351	306	438	380	319	273	420	358	294	249
520	458	391	341	494	425	356	302	471	399	326	275

(1.09 at 10°C, 0.90 at 30°C, 0.79 at 40°C, 0.66 at 50°C)[c]	(1.09 at 10°C, 0.90 at 30°C, 0.79 at 40°C, 0.66 at 50°C)[c]	(1.09 at 10°C, 0.90 at 30°C, 0.79 at 40°C, 0.66 at 50°C)[c]

TABLE A.18

Current-Carrying Capacity of Three-Conductor Shielded Paper-Insulated Cables

Conductor Size AWG or MCM	Conductor Type[a]	Number of Equally Loaded							
		One				Three			
		30	50	75	100	30	50	75	100
		Amperes per Conductor[b]							
	15,000 V	*Copper Temperature, 81°C*							
6	S	94	91	88	83	91	87	81	75
4	SR	123	120	115	107	119	114	104	95
2	SR	159	154	146	137	153	144	139	121
1	SR	179	174	166	156	172	163	149	136
0	CS	203	195	182	176	196	185	169	154
00	CS	234	224	215	202	225	212	193	175
000	CS	270	258	245	230	258	242	220	198
0000	CS	308	295	281	261	295	276	250	223
250	CS	341	327	310	290	325	305	276	246
300	CS	383	365	344	320	364	339	305	272
350	CS	417	397	375	346	397	369	330	293
400	CS	453	428	403	373	429	396	354	314
500	CS	513	487	450	418	483	446	399	350
600	CS	567	537	501	460	534	491	437	385
750	CS	643	606	562	514	602	551	485	426
		(1.08 at 10°C, 0.91 at 30°C, 0.82 at 40°C, 0.71 at 50°C)[b]				(1.08 at 10°C, 0.91 at 30°C, 0.82 at 40°C, 0.71 at 50°C)[b]			
	23,000 V	*Copper Temperature, 77°C*							
2	SR	156	150	143	134	149	141	130	117
1	SR	177	170	162	152	170	160	145	133
0	CS	200	192	183	172	192	182	166	149
00	CS	227	220	210	197	221	208	189	170
000	CS	262	251	238	223	254	238	216	193
0000	CS	301	289	271	251	291	273	246	219
250	CS	334	315	298	277	321	299	270	239
300	CS	373	349	328	306	354	329	297	263
350	CS	405	379	358	331	384	356	318	283
400	CS	434	409	386	356	412	379	340	302
500	CS	492	465	436	401	461	427	379	335
600	CS	543	516	484	440	512	470	414	366
750	CS	616	583	541	495	577	528	465	407
		(1.09 at 10°C, 0.90 at 30°C, 0.80 at 40°C, 0.67 at 50°C)[b]				(1.09 at 10°C, 0.90 at 30°C, 0.80 at 40°C, 0.67 at 50°C)[c]			
	34,500 V	*Copper Temperature, 70°C*							
0	CS	193	185	176	165	184	174	158	141
00	CS	219	209	199	187	208	197	178	160
000	CS	250	238	225	211	238	222	202	182
0000	CS	288	275	260	241	273	256	229	205
250	CS	316	302	285	266	301	280	253	224
300	CS	352	335	315	293	334	310	278	246
350	CS	384	364	342	318	363	336	301	267

Cables in Duct Bank

Six Percent Load Factor				Nine				Twelve			
30	50	75	100	30	50	75	100	30	50	75	100

Amperes per Conductor[b]

Copper Temperature, 81°C

89	83	74	66	87	78	69	60	84	75	64	56
116	108	95	85	113	102	89	77	109	96	83	75
149	136	120	107	144	129	112	97	139	123	104	90
168	153	136	121	162	145	125	109	158	138	117	100
190	173	154	137	183	164	141	122	178	156	131	112
218	198	174	156	211	187	162	139	203	177	148	127
249	225	198	174	241	212	182	157	232	202	168	144
285	257	224	196	275	241	205	176	265	227	189	162
315	283	245	215	303	265	224	193	291	250	207	177
351	313	271	236	337	293	246	211	322	276	227	194
383	340	293	255	366	318	267	227	350	301	245	208
413	366	313	273	394	340	285	242	376	320	262	222
467	410	350	303	444	381	318	269	419	358	292	247
513	450	384	330	488	416	346	293	465	390	317	269
576	502	423	365	545	464	383	323	519	432	348	293

(1.08 at 10°C, 0.91 at 30°C, 0.82 at 40°C, 0.71 at 50°C)[b]				(1.08 at 10°C, 0.91 at 30°C, 0.82 at 40°C, 0.71 at 50°C)[b]				(1.08 at 10°C, 0.91 at 30°C, 0.82 at 40°C, 0.71 at 50°C)[b]			

Copper Temperature, 77°C

145	132	117	105	140	125	107	84	134	119	100	86
164	149	132	117	159	140	121	105	154	133	112	97
186	169	147	132	178	158	136	118	173	149	126	109
212	193	168	149	202	181	156	134	196	172	144	123
242	220	191	169	230	206	175	150	222	195	162	139
278	250	215	190	264	233	197	169	255	221	182	157
308	275	236	207	290	258	216	184	279	242	199	170
341	302	259	227	320	283	232	202	309	266	217	186
369	327	280	243	347	305	255	217	335	285	233	199
396	348	298	260	374	325	273	232	359	303	247	211
443	391	333	288	424	363	302	257	400	336	275	230
489	428	365	313	464	396	329	279	441	367	299	248
550	479	402	347	520	439	364	306	490	408	329	276

(1.09 at 10°C, 0.90 at 30°C, 0.79 at 40°C, 0.67 at 50°C)[c]				(1.09 at 10°C, 0.90 at 30°C, 0.79 at 40°C, 0.66 at 50°C)[c]				(1.09 at 10°C, 0.90 at 30°C, 0.79 at 40°C, 0.65 at 50°C)[a]			

Copper Temperature, 70°C

178	161	140	124	171	149	129	111	164	142	119	103
202	182	158	140	194	170	145	126	185	161	134	115
229	206	179	158	220	193	165	141	209	182	152	128
263	234	203	179	251	219	186	160	238	205	170	144
289	258	222	196	276	240	202	174	262	222	187	157
320	284	244	213	304	264	221	190	288	244	203	171
346	308	264	229	329	285	238	204	311	263	217	184

(continued)

TABLE A.18 (continued)

Current-Carrying Capacity of Three-Conductor Shielded Paper-Insulated Cables

Conductor Size AWG or MCM	Conductor Type[a]	Number of Equally Loaded							
		One				Three			
		30	50	75	100	30	50	75	100
		Amperes per Conductor[b]							
400	CS	413	392	367	341	384	360	321	284
500	CS	468	442	414	381	436	402	358	317
600	CS	514	487	455	416	481	440	391	344
750	CS	584	548	510	466	541	496	435	383
		(1.10 at 10°C, 0.89 at 30°C, 0.76 at 40°C, 0.61 at 50°C)[c]				(1.10 at 10°C, 0.89 at 30°C, 0.76 at 40°C, 0.60 at 50°C)[b]			

Sources: Westinghouse Electric Corporation, *Electrical Transmission and Distribution Reference Book*, Westinghouse Electric Corporation, East Pittsburgh, PA, 1964; Gönen, T., *Electric Power Distribution System Engineering*, CRC Press.

[a] The following symbols are used here to designate conductor types: S, solid copper; SR, standard round concentric stranded; CS, compact sector stranded.

[b] Current ratings are based on the following conditions:
  i. Ambient earth temperature = 20°C.
  ii. 60-cycle ac.
  iii. Ratings include dielectric loss and all induced ac losses.
  iv. One cable per duct; all cables equally loaded and in outside ducts only.

[c] Multiply tabulated currents by these factors when earth temperature is other than 20°C.

TABLE A.19

Current-Carrying Capacity of Single-Conductor Solid Paper-Insulated Cables

Number of Equally Loaded Cables in Duct Bank

Conductor Size AWG or MCM	Three				Six Percent Load Factor			
	30	50	75	100	30	50	75	100
	Amperes per Conductor[a]							
	7,500 V				Copper Temperature, 85°C			
6	116	113	109	103	115	110	103	96
4	164	149	142	135	152	144	134	125
2	202	196	186	175	199	189	175	162
1	234	226	214	201	230	218	201	185
0	270	262	245	232	266	251	231	212
00	311	300	283	262	309	290	270	241
000	356	344	324	300	356	333	303	275
0000	412	395	371	345	408	380	347	314
250	456	438	409	379	449	418	379	344
300	512	491	459	423	499	464	420	380
350	561	537	500	460	546	507	457	403
400	607	580	540	496	593	548	493	445
500	692	660	611	561	679	626	560	504
600	772	735	679	621	757	696	621	557
700	846	804	741	677	827	758	674	604

Cables in Duct Bank

Six Percent Load Factor				Nine				Twelve			
30	50	75	100	30	50	75	100	30	50	75	100
					Amperes per Conductor[b]						
372	329	281	244	352	303	254	216	334	282	232	195
418	367	312	271	393	337	281	238	372	313	256	215
459	401	340	294	430	367	304	259	406	340	277	232
515	447	378	324	481	409	337	284	452	377	304	255

(1.10 at 10°C, 0.89 at 30°C, 0.76 at 40°C, 0.60 at 50°C)[1]

(1.10 at 10°C, 0.88 at 30°C, 0.75 at 40°C, 0.58 at 50°C)[3]

(1.10 at 10°C, 0.88 at 30°C, 0.74 at 40°C, 0.56 at 50°C)[3]

Nine				Twelve			
30	50	75	100	30	50	75	100
		Amperes per Conductor[a]					
		Copper Temperature, 85°C					
113	107	98	90	111	104	94	85
149	140	128	116	147	136	122	110
196	183	167	151	192	178	159	142
226	210	190	172	222	204	181	162
261	242	219	196	256	234	208	184
303	278	250	224	295	268	236	208
348	319	285	255	340	308	270	236
398	364	325	290	390	352	307	269
437	400	358	316	427	386	336	294
486	442	394	349	474	428	371	325
532	483	429	379	518	466	403	352
576	522	461	407	560	502	434	378
659	597	524	459	641	571	490	427
733	663	579	506	714	632	542	470
802	721	629	548	779	688	587	508

(continued)

TABLE A.19 (continued)
Current-Carrying Capacity of Single-Conductor Solid Paper-Insulated Cables

Number of Equally Loaded Cables in Duct Bank

Conductor Size AWG or MCM	Three				Six Percent Load Factor			
	30	50	75	100	30	50	75	100
				Amperes per Conductor[a]				
750	881	837	771	702	860	789	700	627
800	914	866	797	725	892	817	726	648
1000	1037	980	898	816	1012	922	815	725
1250	1176	1108	1012	914	1145	1039	914	809
1500	1300	1224	1110	1000	1268	1146	1000	884
1750	1420	1332	1204	1080	1382	1240	1078	949
2000	1546	1442	1300	1162	1500	1343	1162	1019

(1.07 at 10°C, 0.92 at 30°C, 0.83 at 40°C, 0.73 at 50°C)[b]   (1.07 at 10°C, 0.92 at 30°C, 0.83 at 40°C, 0.73 at 50°C)[b]

	15,000 V				Copper Temperature, 81°C			
6	113	110	105	100	112	107	100	93
4	149	145	138	131	147	140	131	117
2	195	190	180	170	193	183	170	157
1	226	218	208	195	222	211	195	179
0	256	248	234	220	252	239	220	203
00	297	287	271	254	295	278	253	232
000	344	330	312	290	341	320	293	267
0000	399	384	361	335	392	367	335	305
250	440	423	396	367	432	404	367	334
300	490	470	439	406	481	449	406	369
350	539	516	481	444	527	491	443	401
400	586	561	522	480	572	530	478	432
500	669	639	592	543	655	605	542	488
600	746	710	656	601	727	668	598	537
700	810	772	712	652	790	726	647	581
750	840	797	736	674	821	753	672	602
800	869	825	762	696	850	780	695	622
1000	991	939	864	785	968	882	782	697
1250	1130	1067	975	864	1102	1000	883	784
1500	1250	1176	1072	966	1220	1105	972	856
1750	1368	1282	1162	1044	1330	1198	1042	919
2000	1464	1368	1233	1106	1422	1274	1105	970

(1.08 at 10°C, 0.92 at 30°C, 0.82 at 40°C, 0.71 at 50°C)[b]   (1.08 at 10°C, 0.92 at 30°C, 0.82 at 40°C, 0.71 at 50°C)[b]

	23,000 V				Copper Temperature, 77°C			
2	186	181	172	162	184	175	162	150
1	214	207	197	186	211	200	185	171
0	247	239	227	213	244	230	213	196
00	283	273	258	242	278	263	243	221
000	326	314	296	277	320	302	276	252
0000	376	362	340	317	367	345	315	288
250	412	396	373	346	405	380	346	316
300	463	444	416	386	450	422	382	349

Nine				Twelve			
30	**50**	**75**	**100**	**30**	**50**	**75**	**100**
			Amperes per Conductor[a]				
835	750	651	568	810	714	609	526
865	776	674	588	840	740	630	544
980	874	758	657	950	832	705	606
1104	981	845	730	1068	941	784	673
1220	1078	922	794	1178	1032	855	731
1342	1166	992	851	1280	1103	919	783
1442	1260	1068	914	1385	1190	986	839
(1.07 at 10°C, 0.92 at 30°C, 0.83 at 40°C, 0.73 at 50°C)[b]				(1.07 at 10°C, 0.92 at 30°C, 0.83 at 40°C, 0.73 at 50°C)[b]			
			Copper Temperature, 81°C				
110	104	96	87	108	10L	92	83
144	136	125	114	142	132	119	107
189	177	161	146	186	172	154	137
218	204	185	167	214	197	175	157
247	230	209	188	242	223	198	177
287	265	239	214	283	257	226	202
333	306	274	245	327	296	260	230
383	352	315	280	374	340	298	263
422	387	345	306	412	372	325	286
470	429	382	338	457	413	359	316
514	468	416	367	501	450	391	342
556	506	447	395	542	485	419	366
636	577	507	445	618	551	474	412
705	637	557	488	685	608	521	452
766	691	604	528	744	659	564	488
795	716	625	547	772	684	584	505
823	741	646	565	800	707	604	522
933	832	724	631	903	794	675	581
1063	941	816	706	1026	898	759	650
1175	1037	892	772	1133	987	828	707
1278	1124	958	824	1230	1063	886	755
1360	1192	1013	889	1308	1125	935	795
(1.08 at 10°C, 0.92 at 30°C, 0.82 at 40°C, 0.71 at 50°C)[b]				(1.08 at 10°C, 0.92 at 30°C, 0.82 at 40°C, 0.71 at 50°C)[b]			
			Copper Temperature, 77°C				
180	169	154	140	178	164	147	132
206	193	176	159	203	187	167	150
239	222	197	182	234	216	192	171
275	253	225	205	267	245	217	193
315	290	259	233	307	280	247	220
360	332	297	265	351	320	281	250
396	365	326	290	386	351	307	272
438	404	360	319	428	389	340	301

(continued)

TABLE A.19 (continued)

Current-Carrying Capacity of Single-Conductor Solid Paper-Insulated Cables

Number of Equally Loaded Cables in Duct Bank

Conductor Size AWG or MCM	Three				Six Percent Load Factor			
	30	50	75	100	30	50	75	100
				Amperes per Conductor[a]				
350	508	488	466	422	493	461	418	380
400	548	525	491	454	536	498	451	409
500	627	600	559	514	615	570	514	464
600	695	663	616	566	684	632	568	511
700	765	729	675	620	744	689	617	554
750	797	759	702	643	779	717	641	574
800	826	786	726	665	808	743	663	595
1000	946	898	827	752	921	842	747	667
1250	1080	1020	935	848	1052	957	845	751
1500	1192	1122	1025	925	1162	1053	926	818
1750	1296	1215	1106	994	1256	1130	991	875
2000	1390	1302	1180	1058	1352	1213	1053	928
	(1.09 at 10°C, 0.90 at 30°C, 0.80 at 40°C, 0.68 at 50°C)[b]				(1.09 at 10°C, 0.90 at 30°C, 0.80 at 40°C, 0.68 at 50°C)[b]			
	34,500 V				**Copper Temperature, 70°C**			
0	227	221	209	197	225	213	197	182
00	260	251	239	224	255	242	224	205
000	299	290	273	256	295	278	256	235
0000	341	330	312	291	336	317	291	267
250	380	367	345	322	374	352	321	294
300	422	408	382	355	416	390	356	324
350	464	446	419	389	455	426	388	353
400	502	484	451	419	491	460	417	379
500	575	551	514	476	562	524	474	429
600	644	616	573	528	629	584	526	475
700	710	675	626	577	690	639	574	517
750	736	702	651	598	718	664	595	535
800	765	730	676	620	747	690	617	555
1000	875	832	766	701	852	783	698	624
1250	994	941	864	786	967	882	782	696
1500	1098	1036	949	859	1068	972	856	760
1750	1192	1123	1023	925	1156	1048	919	814
2000	1275	1197	1088	981	1234	1115	975	860
2500	1418	1324	1196	1072	1367	1225	1064	936
	(1.10 at 10°C, 0.89 at 30°C, 0.76 at 40°C, 0.61 at 50°C)[b]				(1.10 at 10°C, 0.89 at 30°C, 0.76 at 40°C, 0.61 at 50°C)[b]			
	46,000 V				**Copper Temperature, 65°C**			
000	279	270	256	240	274	259	230	221
0000	322	312	294	276	317	299	274	251
250	352	340	321	300	346	326	299	274
300	394	380	358	334	385	364	332	304
350	433	417	392	365	425	398	364	331
400	469	451	423	393	459	430	391	356

Nine				Twelve			
30	50	75	100	30	50	75	100

Amperes per Conductor[a]

Nine				Twelve			
481	442	393	347	468	424	369	326
521	478	423	373	507	458	398	349
597	546	480	423	580	521	450	392
663	603	529	466	645	577	496	431
725	656	574	503	703	627	538	467
754	681	596	527	732	650	558	483
782	706	617	540	759	674	576	500
889	797	692	603	860	759	646	580
1014	904	781	676	980	858	725	630
1118	993	855	736	1081	940	791	682
1206	1067	911	785	1162	1007	843	720
1293	1137	967	831	1240	1073	893	760

(1.09 at 10°C, 0.90 at 30°C, 0.80 at 40°C, 0.68 at 50°C)[b]

(1.09 at 10°C, 0.90 at 30°C, 0.80 at 40°C, 0.62 at 50°C)[b]

Copper Temperature, 70°C

Nine				Twelve			
220	205	187	169	215	199	177	158
249	234	211	190	245	226	200	179
288	268	242	217	282	259	230	204
328	304	274	246	321	293	259	230
364	337	303	270	356	324	286	253
405	374	334	298	395	359	315	278
443	408	364	324	432	392	343	302
478	440	390	347	466	421	368	323
547	500	442	392	532	479	416	364
610	556	491	433	593	532	459	401
669	608	535	470	649	580	500	435
696	631	554	486	675	602	518	450
723	654	574	503	700	624	535	465
823	741	646	564	796	706	601	520
930	833	722	628	898	790	670	577
1025	914	788	682	988	865	730	626
1109	984	845	730	1066	929	780	668
1182	1045	893	770	1135	985	824	704
1305	1144	973	834	1248	1075	893	760

(1.10 at 10°C, 0.89 at 30°C, 0.76 at 40°C, 0.60 at 50°C)[b]

(1.10 at 10°C, 0.89 at 30°C, 0.76 at 40°C, 0.60 at 50°C)[b]

Copper Temperature, 65°C

Nine				Twelve			
268	249	226	204	262	241	214	191
309	287	259	232	302	276	244	217
336	313	282	252	329	301	266	236
377	349	313	280	367	335	295	260
413	382	341	304	403	366	321	283
446	411	367	326	433	394	344	307

(*continued*)

TABLE A.19 (continued)
Current-Carrying Capacity of Single-Conductor Solid Paper-Insulated Cables

Number of Equally Loaded Cables in Duct Bank

Conductor Size AWG or MCM	Three				Six Percent Load Factor			
	30	50	75	100	30	50	75	100
				Amperes per Conductor[a]				
500	534	512	482	444	522	487	441	400
600	602	577	538	496	589	546	494	447
700	663	633	589	542	645	598	538	488
750	689	658	611	561	672	622	559	504
800	717	683	638	583	698	645	578	522
1000	816	776	718	657	794	731	653	585
1250	927	879	810	738	900	825	732	654
1500	1020	968	887	805	992	904	799	703
1750	1110	1047	959	867	1074	976	859	762
2000	1184	1115	1016	918	1144	1035	909	805
2500	1314	1232	1115	1002	1265	1138	994	875
	(1.11 at 10°C, 0.87 at 30°C, 0.73 at 40°C, 0.54 at 50°C)[b]				(1.11 at 10°C, 0.87 at 30°C, 0.72 at 40°C, 0.53 at 50°C)[b]			
	69,000 V				*Copper Temperature, 60°C*			
350	395	382	360	336	387	364	333	305
400	428	413	389	362	418	393	358	328
500	489	470	441	409	477	446	406	370
600	545	524	490	454	532	496	450	409
700	599	573	536	495	582	543	490	444
750	623	597	556	514	605	562	508	460
800	644	617	575	531	626	582	525	475
1000	736	702	652	599	713	660	592	533
1250	832	792	734	672	806	742	664	595
1500	918	872	804	733	886	814	724	647
1750	994	942	865	788	957	876	776	692
2000	1066	1008	924	840	1020	931	822	732
2500	1163	1096	1001	903	1115	1013	892	791
	(1.13 at 10°C, 0.85 at 30°C, 0.67 at 40°C, 0.42 at 50°C)[b]				(1.13 at 10°C, 0.85 at 30°C, 0.66 at 40°C, 0.42 at 50°C)[b]			

Sources: Westinghouse Electric Corporation, *Electrical Transmission and Distribution Reference Book*, Westinghouse Electric Corporation, East Pittsburgh, PA, 1964; Gönen, T., *Electric Power Distribution System Engineering*, CRC Press.

[a] Current ratings are based on the following conditions:
  i. Ambient earth temperature = 20°C.
  ii. 60-cycle ac.
  iii. Sheaths bonded and grounded at one point only (open-circuited sheaths).
  iv. Standard concentric-stranded conductors.
  v. Ratings include dielectric loss and skin effect.
  vi. One cable per duct; all cables equally loaded and in outside ducts only.
[b] Multiply tabulated values by these factors when earth temperature is other than 20°C.

Nine				Twelve			
30	50	75	100	30	50	75	100
Amperes per Conductor[a]							
506	464	412	365	492	444	386	339
570	520	460	406	553	497	430	377
626	569	502	441	605	542	468	408
650	590	520	457	629	562	485	422
674	612	538	472	652	582	501	436
766	691	604	528	740	657	562	487
865	777	675	589	834	736	626	541
951	850	735	638	914	802	679	585
1028	915	788	682	987	862	726	623
1094	970	833	718	1048	913	766	656
1205	1062	905	778	1151	996	830	708
(1.11 at 10°C, 0.87 at 30°C, 0.72 at 40°C, 0.52 at 50°C)[b]				(1.11 at 10°C, 0.87 at 30°C, 0.70 at 40°C, 0.51 at 50°C)[b]			
Copper Temperature, 60°C							
375	348	312	279	365	332	293	259
405	375	335	300	394	358	315	278
461	425	379	337	447	405	354	312
513	471	419	371	497	448	391	343
561	514	455	403	542	489	425	372
583	533	472	417	563	506	439	384
603	554	487	430	582	523	453	396
685	622	547	481	660	589	508	442
772	698	610	535	741	659	564	489
848	763	664	580	812	718	612	529
913	818	711	618	873	770	653	563
972	868	750	651	927	814	688	592
1060	942	811	700	1007	880	741	635
(1.13 at 10°C, 0.84 at 30°C, 0.65 at 40°C, 0.36 at 50°C)[b]				(1.14 at 10°C, 0.84 at 30°C, 0.64 at 40°C, 0.32 at 50°C)[b]			

TABLE A.20

60 Hz Characteristics of Self-Supporting Rubber-Insulated Neoprene-Jacketed Aerial Cable

Voltage Class	Conductor Size	Stranding	Insulation Thickness	Shielding	Jacket Thickness	Diameter	Messenger Used with Copper Conductors	Weight per 1000 ft; Messenger and Copper	Messenger Used with Aluminum Conductors
3 kV ungrounded neutral, 5 kV grounded neutral	6	7	$10/4$	No	¼	0.59	$3/4''$30%CCS	1020	$3/0''$30%CCS
	4	7	$10/4$	No	¼	0.67	$3/4''$30%CCS	1230	$3/0''$30%CCS
	2	7	$10/4$	No	¼	0.73	$3/4''$30%CCS	1630	$3/0''$30%CCS
	1	19	$10/4$	No	¼	0.77	$3/4''$30%CCS	1780	$3/0''$30%CCS
	1/0	19	$10/4$	No	¼	0.81	$3/4''$30%CCS	2070	$3/0''$30%CCS
	2/0	19	$10/4$	No	¼	0.85	$3/4''$30%CCS	2510	$3/0''$30%CCS
	3/0	19	$10/4$	No	¼	0.91	$3/4''$30%CCS	2890	$3/0''$30%CCS
	4/0	19	$10/4$	No	¼	0.99	$3/4''$30%CCS	3570	$3/0''$30%CCS
	250	37	$11/4$	No	¼	1.08	$3/2''$30%CCS	4080	$3/0''$30%CCS
	300	37	$11/4$	No	¼	1.13	$3/2''$30%CCS	4620	$3/0''$30%CCS
	350	37	$11/4$	No	¼	1.18	$3/2''$30%CCS	5290	$3/0''$30%CCS
	400	37	$11/4$	No	¼	1.23	$3/2''$30%CCS	5800	$3/0''$30%CCS
	500	37	$11/4$	No	¼	1.32	$3/2''$30%CCS	6860	$3/0''$30%CCS
5 kV ungrounded neutral	6	7	$11/4$	Yes	¼	0.74	$3/2''$30%CCS	1310	$3/2''$30%CCS
	4	7	$11/4$	Yes	¼	0.79	$3/2''$30%CCS	1540	$3/2''$30%CCS
	2	7	$11/4$	Yes	¼	0.88	$3/2''$30%CCS	1950	$3/2''$30%CCS
	1	19	$11/4$	Yes	¼	0.92	$3/2''$30%CCS	2180	$3/2''$30%CCS
	1/0	19	$11/4$	Yes	¼	0.96	$3/2''$30%CCS	2450	$3/2''$30%CCS
	2/0	19	$11/4$	Yes	¼	1.00	$3/2''$30%CCS	2910	$3/2''$30%CCS
	3/0	19	$11/4$	Yes	¼	1.06	$3/2''$30%CCS	3320	$3/2''$30%CCS
	4/0	19	$11/4$	Yes	¼	1.11	$3/2''$30%CCS	4030	$3/2''$30%CCS
	250	37	$11/4$	Yes	¼	1.20	$3/2''$30%CCS	4570	$3/2''$30%CCS
	300	37	$11/4$	Yes	¼	1.29	$3/2''$30%CCS	5260	$3/2''$30%CCS
	350	37	$11/4$	Yes	¼	1.34	$3/2''$30%CCS	5840	$3/2''$30%CCS
	400	37	$11/4$	Yes	¼	1.39	$3/2''$30%CCS	6380	$3/2''$30%CCS
	500	37	$11/4$	Yes	¼	1.47	$3/2''$30%CCS	7470	$3/2''$30%CCS

Weight per 1000 ft Messenger and Aluminum	Positive Sequence 60~ AC Ω/mi				Zero Sequence[c] 60~ AC Ω/mi				
	Resistance[a]		Reactance		Resistance[a]		Reactance Series Inductive		
	Copper	Aluminum	Series Inductive	Shunt Capacitive[b]	Copper	Aluminum	Copper	Aluminum	Shunt Capacitive[b]
854	2.52	4.13	0.258	...	3.592	5.082	3.712	3.712	...
958	1.58	2.58	0.246	...	2.632	3.572	3.662	3.662	
1100	1.00	1.64	0.229	...	2.025	2.605	3.615	3.615	...
1250	0.791	1.29	0.211	...	1.815	2.275	3.582	3.582	...
1390	0.635	1.03	0.207	...	1.644	2.015	3.555	3.555	...
1530	0.501	0.816	0.200	...	1.622	1.803	3.162	3.526	...
1690	0.402	0.644	0.194	...	1.517	1.637	3.135	3.499	...
1900	0.318	0.518	0.191	...	1.401	1.508	2.665	3.459	...
2160	0.269	0.437	0.189	...	1.351	1.430	2.635	3.429	...
2500	0.228	0.366	0.184	...	1.308	1.465	2.612	3.042	...
2780	0.197	0.316	0.180	...	1.277	1.415	2.591	3.021	...
3040	0.172	0.276	0.176	...	1.252	1.377	2.576	3.006	...
3650	0.141	0.223	0.172	...	1.219	1.290	2.543	2.543	...
1140	2.52	4.13	0.292	4970	...	...	...	...	...
1270	1.58	2.58	0.272	4320	...	...	...	...	...
1520	1.00	1.64	0.257	3630	...	...	...	...	...
1640	0.791	1.29	0.241	3330	...	...	...	...	...
1770	0.655	1.03	0.233	3080	...	...	...	...	...
1930	0.501	0.816	0.223	2830	...	...	...	...	...
2120	0.402	0.644	0.215	2580	...	...	...	...	...
2350	0.318	0.518	0.207	2380	...	...	...	...	...
2770	0.269	0.437	0.206	2380	...	...	...	...	...
3140	0.228	0.366	0.203	2280	...	...	...	...	...
3380	0.197	0.316	0.199	2090	...	...	...	...	...
3610	0.172	0.276	0.194	1890	...	...	...	...	...
4240	0.141	0.223	0.187	1740	...	...	...	...	...

(*continued*)

TABLE A.20 (continued)

60 Hz Characteristics of Self-Supporting Rubber-Insulated Neoprene-Jacketed Aerial Cable

Voltage Class	Conductor Size	Stranding	Insulation Thickness	Shielding	Jacket Thickness	Diameter	Messenger Used with Copper Conductors	Weight per 1000 ft; Messenger and Copper	Messenger Used with Aluminum Conductors
15 kV grounded neutral	6	19	$11/4$	Yes	¼	1.05	$3/2''$30%CCS	2090	$3/2''$30%CCS
	4	19	$11/4$	Yes	¼	1.10	$3/2''$30%CCS	2350	$3/2''$30%CCS
	2	19	$11/4$	Yes	¼	1.16	$3/2''$30%CCS	2860	$3/2''$30%CCS
	1	19	$11/4$	Yes	¼	1.20	$3/2''$30%CCS	3120	$3/2''$30%CCS
	1/0	19	$11/4$	Yes	¼	1.27	$3/2''$30%CCS	3560	$3/2''$30%CCS
	2/0	19	$11/4$	Yes	¼	1.32	$3/2''$30%CCS	4120	$3/2''$30%CCS
	3/0	19	$11/4$	Yes	¼	1.37	$3/2''$30%CCS	4580	$3/2''$30%CCS
	4/0	19	$11/4$	Yes	¼	1.43	$3/2''$30%CCS	5150	$3/2''$30%CCS
	250	37	$11/4$	Yes	¼	1.47	$3/2''$30%CCS	5590	$3/2''$30%CCS
	300	37	$11/4$	Yes	¼	1.53	$3/2''$30%CCS	6260	$3/2''$30%CCS
	350	37	$11/4$	Yes	¼	1.59	$3/2''$30%CCS	6870	$3/2''$30%CCS
	400	37	$11/4$	Yes	¼	1.63	$3/2''$30%CCS	7450	$3/2''$30%CCS
	500	37	$11/4$	Yes	¼	1.75	$3/2''$30%CCS	8970	$3/2''$30%CCS

Sources: Westinghouse Electric Corporation, *Electrical Transmission and Distribution Reference Book*, Westinghouse Electric Corporation, East Pittsburgh, PA, 1964; Gönen, T., *Electric Power Distribution System Engineering*, CRC Press.

[a] AC resistance based on 65°C with allowance for stranding, skin effect, and proximity effect.

[b] Dielectric constant assumed to be 6.0.

[c] Zero-sequence impedance based on return current both in the messenger and in 100 mΩ earth.

Weight per 1000 ft Messenger and Aluminum	Positive Sequence 60~ AC Ω/mi				Zero Sequence[c] 60~ AC Ω/mi				
	Resistance[a]		Reactance		Resistance[a]		Reactance Series Inductive		
	Copper	Aluminum	Series Inductive	Shunt Capacitive[b]	Copper	Aluminum	Copper	Aluminum	Shunt Capacitive[b]
1920	2.52	4.13	0.326	7150	3.846	5.346	3.396	3.396	7150
2080	1.58	2.58	0.302	6260	2.901	3.831	3.364	3.364	6260
2430	1.00	1.64	0.279	5460	2.459	3.039	2.851	2.851	5460
2580	0.791	1.29	0.268	5110	2.238	2.701	2.837	2.837	5110
2880	0.655	1.03	0.260	4720	2.052	2.426	2.825	2.825	4720
3070	0.501	0.816	0.249	4370	1.896	2.214	2.251	2.801	4370
3510	0.402	0.644	0.241	4120	1.782	2.008	2.240	2.240	4120
3790	0.318	0.518	0.231	3770	1.681	1.864	2.235	2.235	3770
3980	0.269	0.437	0.223	3570	1.630	1.782	2.227	2.227	3570
4330	0.228	0.366	0.217	3330	1.577	1.701	2.226	2.226	3330
4600	0.197	0.316	0.212	3130	1.536	1.640	2.226	2.226	3130
4860	0.172	0.276	0.208	2980	1.500	1.592	2.216	2.216	2980
5560	0.141	0.223	0.204	2830	1.454	1.524	2.198	2.198	2830

REFERENCES

1. Westinghouse Electric Corporation. *Electrical Transmission and Distribution Reference Book*, Westinghouse Electric Corporation, East Pittsburgh, PA, 1964.
2. Westinghouse Electric Corporation. *Electric Utility Engineering Reference Book—Distribution Systems*, vol. 3, Westinghouse Electric Corporation, East Pittsburgh, PA, 1965.
3. Anderson, P. M. *Analysis of Faulted Power Systems*, Iowa State University Press, Ames, IA, 1973.
4. Westinghouse Electric Corporation. *Applied Protective Relaying*, Westinghouse Electric Corporation, Newark, NJ, 1970.

Appendix B: Methods for Allocating Transmission-Line Fixed Charges among Joint Users

In general, interconnections can help to achieve the two fundamental objectives of power system operations, the economy of power production and the continuity of service. Therefore, interchanges between adjacent utilities are scheduled to take advantage of load diversity or available low-cost generating capacity, allowing lower overall operating costs and possible deferment of capital investment for new plants. Thus, interconnections provide the ability to use larger plants and relative flexibility in locating them and the ability to share spinning reserve capacity during emergencies for continuities of service. While sharing in the benefits of interconnected operation, each participating utility is expected to share its responsibilities.

B.1 THEORETICAL METHODS FOR ALLOCATING DEMAND COSTS

In general, the fixed charges of a transmission line include the return of investment, taxes, depreciation, insurance costs, and O&M costs. The methods* used in the past to allocate fixed charges (i.e., demand costs) are

1. Energy method
2. Peak responsibility method
3. Maximum-demand method
4. Greene's method
5. Eisenmenger's method
6. Phantom method
7. Weighted peak method

B.1.1 ENERGY METHOD

The energy method is the simplest and one of the most commonly used methods. It allocates the demand costs in proportion to the energy used by each class of consumer during a period of months or years [1,2]. It is a simple method due to the fact that the values of energy consumed by various consumer classes during the past periods are readily available from the records. However, it is not fair to all users involved since it does not take into account the cost of providing service that is largely dependent on short-time power demands rather than energy. If all customers had 100% load factor, the method would be perfectly fair to all consumers. Therefore, the method is usually not an appropriate one because demand costs are not basically proportional to the energy used but rather to the maximum demand of the class of consumers. With this method, the class with the large energy consumption would be overburdened.

---

* The methods presented are useful in rate design work as well as in the design of interconnection agreements.

B.1.2   PEAK RESPONSIBILITY METHOD

The peak responsibility method [3] allocates the demand costs in proportion to the demand made by each class of consumer on the system at the time of system maximum demand. It attempts to place the burden on those classes of consumers responsible for the large amount of investment required to serve the peak-load period. If a company serves classes of consumers whose peaks are coincident in forming the annual peak on the company's system, the peak responsibility method is fair and just. In the early days, when the principal load was lighting, this condition existed.

It is obviously unfair to charge one class of customers who happens to use energy at the time of the annual system peak with all of the demand costs and let the other customers use the equipment for nothing. This is not only unfair but it is impracticable. For example, a peak due to one class of customers may coincide with the system annual peak, and in the following year, the system peak may be caused by different classes.

B.1.3   MAXIMUM-DEMAND METHOD

The criticism of the peak responsibility method suggested that the demand costs may be more equitably allocated by the ratio of the maximum demand of the class under consideration to the summation of the maximum demands of all classes. However, the maximum-demand method [3] gives correct results only in certain isolated cases. If the customer's peaks coincide, it agrees with the peak responsibility. In cases where the customer's maximum demands are not coincident, there is no overlapping of curves, and when the load factors (average load/maximum load) of all customers are the same, this method is applicable, and the results are just and fair.

However, there are two important aspects that are neglected in the method. First, it ignores the important item of time that the peaks occur. Second, it entirely neglects the energy required by those classes. Therefore, it encourages long hour use of the individual demand because all consumers who have a load factor higher than the average are charged too little, and all who have a load factor lower than the average are charged too much.

B.1.4   GREENE'S METHOD

Greene's method [4] uses a combination of the maximum-demand and the energy methods. Part of the demand costs is a direct function of the maximum demands, and the remainder is a direct function of energy. The proper values can be obtained by solving the following equations:

$$Kx + Dy = C \tag{B.1}$$

$$8760x + y = \frac{C}{P} \tag{B.2}$$

where
x is the cost per kilowatt-hour of that portion of demand costs that functions with kilowatt-hour supplied consumers
y is the demand cost per kilowatt of the portion of demand costs that function with maximum demand of customers
D is the sum of consumers' maximum demands
P is the maximum coincident demand or peak responsibility of all consumers on sources of supply
K is the kilowatt-hours used by all consumers in a year
C is the kilowatt-hours in a year for 1 kW load operated at 100% power factor and 100% load factor (number of hours in a year)

Without any doubt, this is a fairer method than any one of the previously mentioned methods. It is a simple method. However, it neglects a very important parameter, the time at which the individual maximum demands occur, even though it does recognize the duration of such load.

B.1.5   EISENMENGER'S METHOD

Eisenmenger [5] made the most elaborate study of central station (i.e., power plant) load curves and their relative contribution to the demand costs of the system. He advocated the following simplified method of allocation. Eisenmenger's method is usually a more appropriate one than the three previous methods. This is due to the fact that it takes into consideration not only the on-peak but also the off-peak load of the various consumer classes and their duration.

If the proportionality factors of the classes of consumers sharing the annual demand costs are represented by F_{class} and the total demand costs are divided by their sum, the demand costs to be allocated to each class can be expressed as

$$\text{Demand costs allocated to class } i = \frac{F_{class\,i}}{\sum_{i=1}^{n} F_{class\,i}} \times (\text{Total demand costs}) \qquad \text{(B.3)}$$

From an elaborate graphical analysis of many load curves, the following empirical formula has been developed for determining F_{class} factors:

$$\begin{aligned}
F_{class} = &\; MD_{class} \times \frac{\%SP_{class}}{100} \\
&+ MD_{class} \times \left(1.0 - \frac{\%SP_{class}}{100}\right) \times \frac{\text{Peak hours}}{24} \\
&+ \left(MD_{class}OP\right) \times \frac{OP_{hours}}{24}
\end{aligned} \qquad \text{(B.4)}$$

This equation states that the proportionality factor of a class is equal to the sum of the following terms:

1. Maximum demand of class (MD_{class}) times percentage of station peak of class ($\%SP_{class}/100$)
2. Maximum demand of class times remainder percentage of station peak of class times ratio of hours per day to 24 h during which the class peak and station peak coincide
3. Maximum-demand off-peak (MD_{class} OP) of class times ratio of hours per day to 24 h during which the class peak and the station peak do not overlap

For off-peak consumers, this method gives correct results. However, it does not divide the demand costs correctly among those consumers who are on at the time of the station peak. In this method, every customer who is on at the time of station peak contributes to that peak. However, the favorable 100% load factor consumer has no peak in his or her individual demand curve. Therefore, the method burdens rather heavily this favorable class of consumer who has a steady load.

B.1.6   PHANTOM METHOD

If a public utility could operate steadily at its maximum demand for 24 h a day every day (i.e., at 100% load factor), its investment in equipment would be used most economically. The loss of any customer will affect the load factor, or efficiency of plant use, regardless of the fact that one might have twice the demand of the other. This was the conclusion of Hills [6] when he inserted that a fair and just division of cost will be on a kilowatt-hour basis, for every block of energy used is just as important and every other block of the same size as far as costs to the central station are concerned.

Thus, with a plant operating at 100% load factor, the demand costs divided by the number of kilowatt-hours generated and multiplied by the consumption of each customer at the generating plant will give the true demand costs that should be allocated to each customer. Therefore, under these conditions, the demand costs per kilowatt-hour can be expressed as

$$\text{Demand costs} = \frac{\text{Total annual demand costs}}{8760 \,(\text{max demand station})} \tag{B.5}$$

In actual practice, the load factor is usually not 100%. Here, the demand costs are divided among the groups of customers according to their kilowatt-hour consumption, charging this phantom customer in the same way as the real customers. Hence, now the problem is to divide the bill of this phantom customer, which would be required to operate the existing plant at 100% load factor, among the existing customers in an equitable manner.

Certainly, the customers who already have a 100% load factor are not responsible for the bill and neither are those customers who are off-peak, for they are doing their share toward reducing the size of this phantom. Those customers that cause the peak are responsible since they use more than their average demand during the period of that peak load. Furthermore, their degree of responsibility is limited to the excess demand during the period of the station peak load over the average demand.

In many cases, it may be that there is not only one station peak during the year, due to one set of conditions, but perhaps two or more peaks at other times due to different groups of customers or under different conditions. It often happens that the annual station peak is just as likely to occur because of one group of customers as because of another. This is a case where the phantom method can be applied with accuracy and ease.

B.1.7 Weighted Peak Method

In 1927, Knights [3], in an effort to correct some of the defects of Greene's [4], Eisenmenger's [5], and Hills' [6] methods in overcharging the off-peak customers, presented a new method called the *weighted peak method*. This method allocates the demand costs to the various classes of consumer according to the share of each class in the total weighted peak.

The weighted peak of any class of consumer is taken as equal to the demand of that class at the time of the plant peak plus a fraction of the difference between the maximum demand of that class of consumers and its demand at the time of the plant peak. This fraction that is added is the ratio of the plant demand at the time of the class maximum demand to the total peak demand.

B.2 METHODS FOR PLANNING FUTURE INVESTMENTS

In 1950, Watchorn [8] developed a method for determining capacity benefits resulting from an interconnection of generating systems and used this to justify the installation of transmission facilities as a substitute for generating capacity. Also, he described several possible bases for allocating such benefits. He pointed out that when only two systems are involved in an interconnection, the resulting capacity benefit should be divided equally between them.

However, in the event that more than two systems are involved, the benefit allocated to any of the participating systems should not be reduced by the addition of any new participants into the interconnection. He suggested what may be defined as the mutual benefit method of allocation, which recognizes that the benefit should be divided among the participating systems in proportion to the benefits for all combinations of two's among them. This method meets the two basic requirements so long as the installed capacity requirements are determined on the basis of consistent application of probability methods.

In 1957, Phillips [8] developed a method that he asserted to be more equitable to allocate saving from energy interchange in power pools where more than three companies are involved. He pointed out that it is a generally accepted principle throughout the United States that on interchange where only two parties are involved, the savings are divided equally between buyer and seller. The accounting involved in applying this theory is given by a simple equation for the billing rate, which is a function of energy interchange, replacement cost of purchasing company, and supplying cost of selling company.

When the magnitude of the interconnection grows to include three companies, the accounting is slightly more complicated, since for any specified period, either one company is buying and two are selling or two companies are buying and one is selling. Again, the total interchange can be broken down into separate two-party transactions, and no arbitrary method is involved for determining the distribution of energy. A similar equation for billing rate can be applied in the three-company interconnection.

When the magnitude of the power pool grows to four companies, it is no longer possible to say which company receives a given block of power except in those hours when only one company is buying or only one company is selling. He suggested that if more than one company is buying during a particular period, each buying company's replacement cost is compared with the weighted average of all the selling companies in order to determine the billing rate. Conversely, in any period, the selling cost of any selling company is compared with the weighted average of the replacement costs of all the buying companies for that specific period in order to determine the billing rate for that company.

It is very difficult to determine an equitable method of allocating the fixed charges of the interconnection facilities for power interchange among the various participants. Suggestions have been made that such fixed charges be divided annually among participating parties of the interconnection arrangement on the basis of the actual dollar benefits derived by the individual members from power interchange transactions. Watchorn [7] recommended that such allocation may well be on approximately the same basis as the allocation of the capacity benefits.

However, Bary (in his discussion in Phillips [8]) suggested that the disposition of fixed charges on interconnection facilities should be made at the time they enter into an interconnection agreement. Furthermore, he suggested that benefits should be allocated on an equitable basis with the amounts applicable to each participating system to remain fixed for a prolonged period and be subjected to modification only as a result of future changes in the scope or extent of the facilities involved in the interconnection or due to major changes in the components of fixed charges (i.e., return on investment, taxes, depreciation, insurance, and maintenance). He argued that the disposition of fixed charges should not be made automatically dependent on the actual day-to-day or year-to-year operational benefits of power interchanges.

Anthony [9] described the exchange of seasonal diversity capacity between Tennessee Valley Authority (TVA) and the South Central Electric Companies (SCECs). Basically, each SCEC was to own, operate, and maintain those EHV facilities required in its *service area*. Financing was to be handled on a group basis.

The annual cost of ownership, operation, and maintenance of individual company facilities was to be prorated to each company by an arbitrary formula based on the portion of such facilities installed by that company compared with the total EHV facilities installed by all SCECs and the percentage of participation by that company in diversity capacity exchange of TVA power.

Since the company in whose service area EHV facilities are installed is in a position to use the facilities for purposes other than the interchange of power with TVA, each company owning EHV facilities was to begin to absorb 5% of the annual charges of those EHV facilities in its service area. Each year thereafter, for a total of 19 years, the amount to be absorbed was to be increased by 5%. Consequently, at the end of the 19-year period, annual charges to be shared by the companies were projected to be 50% of the initial annual charges. Incremental losses occasioned by the receipt or delivery of power under the agreements were to be distributed in proportion to each company's participation in each power transfer.

Firestone et al. [10] extended the use of probability techniques for analyzing a system's generation reserve position and applied this method to the Central Area Power Coordination Group (CAPCO) system. A probabilistic capacity model is merged with a load model to develop the expected frequency distribution of daily capacity margins. The daily capacity margin is considered to be the difference between the load that exists during a daily peak period and the operable capacity at that time.

Operable capacity for this purpose is the normal rating of installed generating capacity, adjusted for various limitations, plus purchases of firm power from other utilities less outages, both planned and forced. Each of these capacity margins is associated with the probability of the corresponding capacity level.

The CAPCO group, like other power pools, required a mechanism for ensuring the equitable sharing of benefits and responsibilities arising from such an association. The fundamental basis of equity adopted by the CAPCO group was that each party should contribute to the group reserve in the same proportion as they expected to utilize it. Negative margins were quite useful as the measure of a system's need for help from outside the pool, whereas the positive margins were used as the measure of a system's ability to provide help to outside systems.

An energy quantity called *megawatt-days* was developed as a useful measurement here. *Positive megawatt-days* is equal to the sum of the products of each positive margin and its respective frequency. *Negative megawatt-days* is calculated in a similar manner, from the negative margin data.

By proper distribution of capacity responsibility, it is possible to make the relationship of each party's contribution to the group reserve (positive-megawatt-day value) to this potential use of the group reserve (negative-megawatt-day value) equal to that for each of the other parties. The capacity responsibility assigned represents the power in megawatts for which the individual party bears financial responsibility.

In 1967, Rincliffe [11] described the Pennsylvania–New Jersey–Maryland (PJM) policy for allocating the annual costs of the 500 kV transmission system to all pool members. The 500 kV transmission system, owned by six companies, was being constructed to bring power from the mine-mouth stations to the load centers and to provide high-capacity interpool tie lines.

The total cost of the transmission system was divided into an interarea tie function and a generation delivery function. The interarea function was allocated to all PJM members and associated systems in proportion to their sizes as measured by peak loads. The generation delivery function was allocated to the owners of the stations in proportion to ownership of the combined capacity of these stations.

The methods that have been described so far take into account the benefits of interconnection facilities from the savings to the participating systems due to power interchange transactions. However, Brandt [12] defined the benefits to be gained from transmission facilities in a more comprehensive way in an Edison Electric Institute's (EEI) committee report.

According to the report, the benefits that a company receives from an interconnection include distribution benefits, wheeling benefits, and pool benefits (i.e., the value associated with increased reliability of the pool).

Therefore, the possible bases for ownership of transmission lines, based on the methods mentioned earlier, can be summarized as follows:

1. Ownership may be divided equally among the members.
2. Ownership may be proportional to the installed capacity requirements of each company when operating separately.
3. Ownership may be proportional to the peak load of each for separate operation.
4. Ownership may be proportional to a combination of energy consumed, average load, and the difference between the maximum load and the average load of each company (excess demand).
5. Ownership may be proportional to the distribution and the reliability benefits each member company derives from using the transmission system.

The first ownership base is equitable in a very uncommon situation, that is, when the companies involved have nearly the same size and similar fundamental characteristics. However, the second and third ownership bases are not equitable as far as a transmission line is concerned because the line is not planned for construction on these bases. On the other hand, if the problem was one of adding generating units, these bases may be more equitable.

The fourth ownership base appears to be more equitable if one can find an appropriate way to formulate the concept. The phantom customer method of allocating fixed charges is suggested. It allocates the costs from both the energy and the power point of views. It may be an appropriate method for operating purpose on a day-to-day or month-to-month basis. However, the fifth ownership base appears to be more equitable and logical for planning purposes.

In the event that there are n member companies in a given power pool, based on energy and excess demand considerations, the fixed charges of path (i.e., tie line) j allocated to service area i can be expressed as [13]

$$F_{ij} = \frac{L_i}{\sum_{i=1}^{n} L_i} P_{aj} + \frac{\Delta P_{cj}}{\sum_{i=1}^{n} \Delta P_{cj}} \left(P_{pj} - P_{aj} \right) \tag{B.6}$$

where
F_{ij} is the fixed charge of path j allocated to service area i in megawatts
L_i is the total load of area i at pool average load level in megawatts
P_{aj} is the magnitude of real power flow in path j at pool average load level in megawatts
ΔP_{cj} is the incremental real power flow in path j due to any load condition designated as C (positive value only) in megawatts
P_{pj} is the magnitude of real power flow in path j at pool peak-load level in megawatts

Equation B.6 is based on the phantom method. Note that the first term of the equation represents the energy charge in megawatts, which is equivalent to the power flow in that particular line when the pool is operating at the average load level.

The second term of the equation represents the fixed charges in megawatts due to excess demand and is called the *phantom demand charge of the line*. The demand charge in megawatts is equivalent to the difference between the power flows in the line at the pool peak load level and at the pool average load level. The difference should have only a positive value in order to be significant. A negative value means that there is no excess demand at the time of pool peak.

The reliance on the transmission lines (tie lines) in a modern pool is more crucial than just providing help in an emergency. It applies whenever generating capacity is insufficient for any reason (e.g., during the refueling of a nuclear unit), and physical backup has now become as necessary to reliable operation as emergency assistance. This is the reason the reliability benefit should be included in the allocation. Therefore, the fifth ownership base appears to be more equitable than the other four bases for planning purposes. Thus, it can be used by the planning engineer to allocate fixed charges of jointly used transmission lines.

Therefore, in the event that there are n member companies in a given pool, based on distribution and reliability benefits, the fixed charges of path j allocated to service area i can be expressed as [13]

$$F_{ij} = \frac{1}{2} \left(\frac{R_{ij}}{\sum_{i=1}^{n} R_{ij}} + \frac{D_{ij}}{\sum_{i=1}^{n} D_{ij}} \right) F_j \tag{B.7}$$

where
F_{ij} is the fixed charges of path j allocated to area i in dollars
R_{ij} is the reliability benefit to area i from path j
D_{ij} is the distribution benefit to area i from path j in megawatts
F_j is the fixed charges of path j in dollars

Note that a 50–50 split of the fixed charges is assumed in Equation B.7. The base value to determine the per-unit quantity of the distribution benefit is the sum of the distribution benefits of that particular line to each separate area in the pool. Similarly, the base value to determine the per-unit quantity of the reliability benefit is the sum of the reliability benefits for the entire system:

$$\text{Basic reliability benefit} = \sum_{i=1}^{n} R_{ij} \tag{B.8}$$

Therefore, the fixed charge allocation of company i for the transmission line j can be expressed as [14]

$$F_{ij} = \frac{1}{2}\left(R_{ij} + D_{ij}\right)F_j \tag{B.9}$$

where
R_{ij} is the reliability benefit in per units
D_{ij} is the distribution benefit in per units

The distribution benefit of a transmission line to a power system is defined as the increment of real power flowing over that line when the total load of the power system is changed from one arbitrary load level to a higher arbitrary load level under economic production schedules from the dispatch control center under normal conditions, measured either in physical units (i.e., megawatts or kilowatts) or in per units on some appropriate base.

The per-unit distribution benefit of a line can be expressed in several ways, depending on how the base value is chosen. For example, if the base value may be chosen to be some arbitrary number (e.g., 100 MW), the per-unit distribution benefit of a line (i.e., per-unit ΔP_{line}) can be expressed as

$$D_{\text{line}} = \frac{\Delta P_{\text{line}}\ \text{MW}}{100\ \text{MW base}}\ \text{pu} \tag{B.10}$$

In the event that the base value is chosen to be the total change in area load in megawatts, it can be calculated as

$$D_{\text{line}} = \frac{\Delta P_{\text{line}}\ \text{MW}}{\Delta P_{\text{area}}\ \text{MW}}\ \text{pu} \tag{B.11}$$

Finally, if the base value is chosen to be the sum of the changes in every line flow (megawatts) in the area, the per-unit distribution benefit of a line can be expressed as

$$D_{\text{line}} = \frac{\Delta P_{\text{line}}\ \text{MW}}{\sum \Delta P\ \text{in all lines}}\ \text{pu} \tag{B.12}$$

Note that the base value may be chosen for each individual line separately to be the total sum of the distribution benefits of that particular line to each separate area in the pool. The increments of real power flowing over the line can be found from load-flow studies.

The reliability benefit of a transmission line to a power system is defined as an increment of the total probability of system failure, calculated at the load buses in the power system, with the line in service and with the line out of service. The total probability of system failure in the system is the sum of the probabilities of system failure to serve the load at each load bus in the system. The probabilities are calculated at each of the individual load buses in the power system. The conditional probability approach can be used to calculate the probability of system failure.

REFERENCES

1. Hills, H. W. Demand costs and their allocation, *Electr. World* 89, 1927, 198–203.
2. Harding, C. F. and Confield, D. T. *Business Administration for Engineers*, 1st edn., McGraw-Hill, New York, 1937.
3. Knight, A. S. Peak responsibility as a basis for allocating fixed costs, *Electr. World* 87, 1926, 495–496.
4. Greene, W. J. Determining demand charges, *Electr. World* 86, 1925, 947.
5. Eisenmenger, H. E. *Central Station Rates in Theory and Practices*, Fred J. Drake & Co., Chicago, IL, 1921.
6. Hills, H. W. Proposed allocation of demand costs, *Electr. World* 89, 1927, 249–252.
7. Watchorn, C. W. The determination and allocation of the capacity benefits resulting from interconnecting two or more generating systems, *AIEE Trans. Power Appar. Syst.* PAS-69, 1950, 1180–1186.
8. Phillips, H. W. An equitable method for the distribution of power pool savings, *AIEE Trans. Power Appar. Syst.* PAS-76, 1957, 103–105.
9. Anthony, C. W. SCEC-TVA seasonal capacity agreement supplements existing interconnections, *Electr. Light Power* 42, 1964, 30–33.
10. Firestone, L., Monteith, A. H., and Masters, W. D. The CAPCO Group probability technique for timing capacity additions and allocation of capacity responsibility, *IEEE Trans. Power Appar. Syst.* PAS-88, 1969, 1174–1182.
11. Rincliffe, R. G. Planning and operation of a large power pool. *IEEE Spectr.* (4), 1967, 91–96.
12. Brandt, R. Transmission problems in establishing a power pool, *Edison Electr. Inst. Interconnect. Agreements Comm.* 86, 1969, 12.
13. Bijayendrayodhin, I. Allocation of transmission line fixed charges among joint users according to the benefits, Unpublished PhD dissertation, Iowa State University, Ames, IA, 1971.

GENERAL REFERENCES

Federal Energy Regulatory Commission. *Power Pooling in the United States*, FERC-0049, FERC, Washington, DC, 1981.
Happ, H. H. The Interarea matrix: A tie line flow model for power pools, *IEEE Trans. Power Appar. Syst.* PAS-90, 1971, 36–45.
Mochon, H. H., Jr. Practices of the New England power exchange, *Proc. Am. Power Conf.* 34, 1972, 911–925.
U.S. Department of Energy. Power pooling: Issues and approaches, DOE/ERA/6385-1, USDOE, Washington, DC, 1980.

Appendix C: New Electrical Infrastructure Trends and Regulations in the United States

C.1 INTRODUCTION

The electrical infrastructure in the United States and other countries is undergoing major changes with steadily increasing demand for energy and introduction of renewable power generating resources. This trend is affecting the planning, development, and operation of power grid and associated infrastructure.

On the planning side, the builders and operators of cross-country transmission lines are increasingly affected by federal, regional, and local regulatory policies, which apply to siting, permitting, and security of new or existing transmission lines. On the technical side, the electrical grid—the transmission and distribution systems—is undergoing significant modernization with advanced technologies, such as *smart grid*, and real-time information collection systems.

On the security side of the current trend, the electrical infrastructure and transmission lines specifically have been gradually reinforced physically and via cybersecurity measures. These major trends are discussed in detail in this appendix.

C.1.1 REGULATORY TRENDS

The electrical infrastructure, which includes transmission lines, substations, and power generation plants, is regulated or monitored by two key federal government agencies in the United States. The FERC collects transmission information from investor-owned utilities and intrastate bulk lines. The Energy Information Administration (EIA) collects similar information from entities outside of FERC jurisdiction—IPPs, cooperatives, municipal systems, federal power, and Texas. EIA also collects data from generators under FERC jurisdiction. The DOE collects trade data with Canada and Mexico. The Department of Agriculture collects data from cooperatives having loans with the Rural Utilities Service.

The operation of transmission lines is regulated by the North American NERC, which operates under oversight of FERC. In addition to federal regulatory agencies, the transmission-line siting and permitting is regulated by numerous other state and local agencies in the state of California, including California Independent System Operator (CAISO) and California Public Utility Commission (CPUC).

The overall structures of the government agencies that oversee the transmission lines are shown in Figure C.1 and described in numerous government publications and professional article. The key areas of regulatory control for the transmission lines are as follows:

In addition to the technical aspects of transmission system analysis, this appendix addresses the planning and execution of the type of cross-country overhead transmission line in the current regulatory environment and smart-grid technology application. Although the regulations may vary from location and countries, the new trend in regulating and permitting transmission lines is becoming key elements in electrical infrastructure development in most of industrial regions.

The other aspect of transmission system growth is the *smart-grid* technologies application to facilitate load growth and infrastructure security. This appendix provides overview of these technologies and the trend in power grid security.

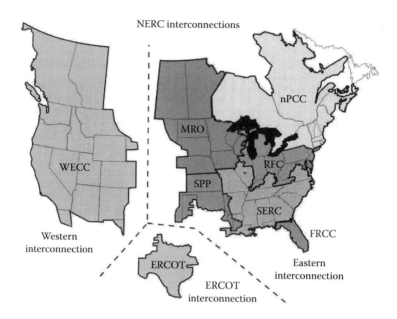

FIGURE C.1 Overall structures of the government agencies that oversee the transmission lines. *Note:* ERCOT, Electric Reliability Council of Texas; FRCC, Florida Reliability Coordinating Council; MRO, Midwest Reliability Organization; NPCC, Northwest Power Coordinating Council; RFC, Reliability First Corporation; SERC, Southeastern Electric Reliability Council; SPP, Southwest Power Pool, Inc.; WECC, Western Electricity Coordinating Council.

The final rule reflects FERC's extensive experience in licensing transmission and hydroelectric generation facilities and issuing certificates for interstate natural gas pipelines. It applies this knowledge and experience to the electric transmission construction permit program. The application process will assist the commission to determine if the proposed transmission facilities

- Are eligible for an electric transmission construction permit
- Are in the public interest
- Will reduce transmission congestion and protect and benefit consumers
- Are consistent with sound national energy policy and will enhance energy independence
- Maximize the use of existing facilities

This information as well as information necessary for FERC to complete a thorough environmental analysis is the basis of the information required by the application. FERC regulations require an extensive prefiling process to facilitate issue identification and resolution, to facilitate maximum participation from all stakeholders, and to provide all interested entities with timely and accurate project information to base their comments and recommendations. This process provides for openness and transparency throughout the permitting process.

This process provides for preparation of one National Environmental Policy Act (NEPA) document for all federal actions and the setting of binding intermediate milestones and ultimate deadlines (consistent with existing law) for actions by other agencies issuing permits under federal law. This process provides for numerous opportunities throughout the process for input from

- States
- Tribes
- Regional planning agencies

- Other permitting entities
- Land owners
- The public

Order No. 1000 is a Final Rule that reforms the commission's electric transmission planning and cost allocation requirements for public utility transmission providers. The rule builds on the reforms of Order No. 890 and corrects the remaining deficiencies with respect to transmission planning processes and cost allocation methods.

C.1.2 BACKGROUND

On June 17, 2010, FERC issued a notice of proposed rulemaking seeking comment on potential changes to its transmission planning and cost allocation requirements. Industry participants and other stakeholders provided extensive comment in response to the notice of proposed rulemaking. The commission received more than 180 initial comments and more than 65 reply comments.

C.1.3 PLANNING REFORMS

The rule establishes three requirements for transmission planning:

1. Each public utility transmission provider must participate in a regional transmission planning process that satisfies the transmission planning principles of Order No. 890 and produces a regional transmission plan.
2. Local and regional transmission planning processes must consider transmission needs driven by public policy requirements established by state or federal laws or regulations. Each public utility transmission provider must establish procedures to identify transmission needs driven by public policy requirements and evaluate proposed solutions to those transmission needs.
3. Public utility transmission providers in each pair of neighboring transmission planning regions must coordinate to determine if there are more efficient or cost-effective solutions to their mutual transmission needs.

C.1.4 COST ALLOCATION REFORMS

The rule establishes three requirements for transmission cost allocation:

1. Each public utility transmission provider must participate in a regional transmission planning process that has a regional cost allocation method for new transmission facilities selected in the regional transmission plan for purposes of cost allocation. The method must satisfy six regional cost allocation principles.
2. Public utility transmission providers in neighboring transmission planning regions must have a common interregional cost allocation method for new interregional transmission facilities that the regions determine to be efficient or cost-effective. The method must satisfy six similar interregional cost allocation principles.
3. Participant funding of new transmission facilities is permitted but is not allowed as the regional or interregional cost allocation method.

C.1.5 NONINCUMBENT DEVELOPER REFORMS

1. Public utility transmission providers must remove from commission-approved tariffs and agreements a federal right of first refusal for a transmission facility selected in a regional transmission plan for purposes of cost allocation, subject to three limitations:
   (a) This does not apply to a transmission facility that is not selected in a regional transmission plan for purposes of cost allocation.
   (b) This allows, but does not require, public utility transmission providers in a transmission planning region to use competitive bidding to solicit transmission projects or project developers.
   (c) Nothing in this requirement affects state or local laws or regulations regarding the construction of transmission facilities, including but not limited to authority over siting or permitting of transmission facilities.
2. The rule recognizes that incumbent transmission providers may rely on regional transmission facilities to satisfy their reliability needs or service obligations. The rule requires each public utility transmission provider to amend its tariff to require reevaluation of the regional transmission plan to determine if delays in the development of a transmission facility require evaluation of alternative solutions, including those proposed by the incumbent, to ensure incumbent transmission providers can meet reliability needs or service obligations.

C.1.6 COMPLIANCE

- Order No. 1000 takes effect 60 days from publication in the *Federal Register*.
- Each public utility transmission provider is required to make a compliance filing with the commission within 12 months of the effective date of the Final Rule.
- Compliance filings for interregional transmission coordination and interregional cost allocation are required within 18 months of the effective date.

C.2 SECURITY GUIDELINES OVERVIEW FOR THE ELECTRICITY SECTOR

The appendix of the proceedings of *1998–1999 National Conference of State Legislatures* states that these guidelines and their attachments describe general approaches, considerations, practices, and planning philosophies to be applied in protecting the electrical infrastructure systems. Specific program or implementation of security considerations must reflect an individual organization's assessment of its own needs, vulnerabilities, and consequences and its tolerance for risk.

Recognizing these guidelines does not represent any single or *cookbook* approach to electricity sector (ES) infrastructure protection. Presidential Decision Directive 63 (PDD-63), *Protecting America's Critical Infrastructures*, officially identifies *electricity* as a critical infrastructure.

Homeland Security Presidential Directive 3 (HSPD-3) dictates the following:

- A framework for cooperation within individual infrastructure sectors and with government for the vital mission of protecting critical infrastructures.
- The US DOE to be the lead agency for the energy sectors.
- Sector coordinator functions and responsibilities. The DOE has designated the North American NERC as the sector coordinator for the ES.

NERC, as the sector coordinator, has the responsibility to

- Assess sector vulnerabilities
- Develop a plan to reduce electric system vulnerabilities
- Propose a system for identifying and averting attacks

- Develop a plan to alert ES participants and appropriate government agencies that an attack is imminent or in progress
- Assist in reconstituting minimum essential electric system capabilities in the aftermath of an attack

The idea of protecting the electric system infrastructure is not new. The electrical grid is designed to ensure a reliable supply of electricity, even in the face of adverse conditions. Throughout its history, the industry has been able to restore service consistently and quickly after earthquakes, hurricanes, major floods, ice storms, and a variety of other natural and man-made disasters. Its experience in emergency management has prepared the industry to respond effectively to a *spectrum of threats* using its existing structure, resources, and plans.

This spectrum ranges from simple trespassing, to vandalism, to civil disturbances, to dedicated acts of terror and sabotage. Perpetrators include *insiders* and *outsiders* whose actions may be cyber or physical in nature. In this context, it may be appropriate to periodically reevaluate existing plans, procedures, and protocols to consider vulnerabilities to a full spectrum of threats, particularly the unique aspects associated with terrorism.

These guidelines are meant to support those efforts. They are advisory in nature. Each company must assess their usefulness within the context of its operating environment and subject to its own evaluation of its vulnerability and risk to its perceived spectrum of threats.

These guidelines apply to *critical* operating assets. Each company is free to define and identify those facilities and functions it believes to be critical, keeping in mind that the ability to mitigate the loss of a facility through redundancies may make that facility less critical than others.

Each security guideline for the ES is summarized as follows. Companies may wish to review their plans, practices, and procedures for these elements:

1. *Vulnerability and risk assessment*
   Helps identify those facilities that may be critical to overall operations, as well as their vulnerabilities. Consideration should be given to closely safeguarding such information and restricting it to only a few individuals with a *need to know.*
2. *Threat response capability*
   Ensures that company personnel at critical operating facilities understand how to respond to a spectrum of threats, both physical and cyber. Consideration should be given to NERC's *Threat Alert Levels and Response Guidelines.*
3. *Emergency management*
   Ensures that companies are prepared to respond to a spectrum of threats, both physical and cyber. Consideration should be given to reviewing, revising, and testing emergency plans on a regular basis.

   Plans might include training provisions for key responders to ensure they have the skills and knowledge to effectively carry out those plans. Maintaining comprehensive mutual assistance agreements at the local, state, and regional levels also supports response, repair, and restoration activities in the event a critical facility is disrupted. Liaison relationships with local FBI offices as well as with other local law enforcement agencies may be necessary.

   For purposes of these guidelines, a critical facility may be defined as any facility or combination of facilities, if severely damaged or destroyed, would have a significant impact on the ability to serve large quantities of customers for an extended period of time, would have a detrimental impact on the reliability or operability of the energy grid, or would cause significant risk to public health and safety.
4. *Continuity of business processes*
   Reduces the likelihood of prolonged interruptions and enhances prompt resumption of operations when interruptions occur. Consider flexible plans that address key areas such as

telecommunications, information technology, customer service centers, facilities security, operations, generation, power delivery, customer remittance, and payroll processes. It is useful to revise and test plans on a regular basis. It also is advisable to train personnel so they fully understand their roles with respect to the plans.

5. *Communications*

Ensure the effectiveness of threat response, emergency management, and business continuity plans. Consideration should be given to establishing liaison relationships with federal, state, county, and local law enforcement agencies in the area. Building the relationship might include providing tours of critical facilities for law enforcement agencies having jurisdiction in areas where those facilities are located and planning to identify possible response needs. Such liaisons may need to be periodically updated and tested.

Consideration also should be given to planning how personnel will respond to alarms, outages, or other issues at critical operating facilities. Robust communications systems such as radio, cellular phone, or similar communications devices are effective.

6. *Physical security*

Mitigates the threat from inside and outside the organization. A physical security program might include deterrence and prevention strategies. A systems approach is advisable, where detection, assessment, communication, and response are planned and supported by adequate policies, procedures, and resources.

7. *Information technology/cybersecurity*

Mitigates the threat from inside and outside the organization. Consideration should be given to computer network monitoring and intrusion detection, placing particular attention on EMS, SCADA, or other key operating systems. It is advisable that only authorized persons have access to those critical systems and only for valid purposes. Consideration also should be given to adequate firewall protection and periodic audits of the network and existing security protocols. Third-party penetration testing may be useful.

8. *Employment screening*

Mitigates the threat from inside the organization. Hiring standards and preemployment background investigations may help ensure the trustworthiness and reliability of personnel who have unescorted access to critical facilities, including contractors and vendors.

9. *Protecting potentially sensitive information*

Reduces the likelihood that information could be used by those intending to damage critical facilities, disrupt operations, or harm individuals. Consider creating a hierarchical confidentiality classification framework (e.g., public, market participant confidential, company confidential, and highly confidential) and the authorization requirements and conditions to permit disclosure.

Overall, training for new personnel and ongoing training for existing personnel on physical and cybersecurity policies, standards, and procedures are effective tools to mitigate threats. Finally, each company must consider and comply with all applicable laws.

C.2.1 Problem Statement

The United States faces numerous, complex energy security challenges in the twenty-first century. Central to those challenges is the national security requirement that the nation must continue to function even during catastrophic naturally occurring events, unintentional man-made calamities, and asymmetric physical or virtual threats or attacks perpetrated by nation-state or non-nation-state actors against assets, systems, or networks.

The nation's critical dependency on the commercial electric power grid to achieve its global mission is very well established. Since most of the bulk power infrastructure nodes and systems are commercially owned, identifying and remediating the vulnerabilities that characterize this dependent relationship require complex partnership arrangements with industry. In addition, the ES is critically dependent on the communications, transportation, water, and chemical sectors in terms of output and continuity—a fact that extends vulnerabilities to these sectors. ES risks and disruptions include those caused by inherent attributes of the infrastructure itself, as well as a variety of naturally occurring and man-made causes, whether deliberate or accidental in nature.

Frequently, electric power is primarily supplied by commercial service providers tied to the bulk power system, with on-site backup diesel generators used during short-duration commercial power disruptions. Diesel backup generators are typically not designed to support extended outages of the grid. Therefore, we need a new approach in partnership with the industry.

Additionally, the nation is in the midst of significant electric power grid upgrades, system expansions, integrating various renewable generation sources, and bringing on intelligent metering and control systems to increase efficiency and reduce demand management. Yet, the electric power grid remains vulnerable to physical and cyber attacks. Key nodes in the electrical network, such as the substations located in remote areas with little physical protection, are viable *targets* to criminals and terrorists. Key components in a substation consist of large transformers, circuit breakers, and the substation control house, which are all readily identifiable from outside of the chain-link fence protection and easily accessible once the protective fence is breached. Cyber intrusion can also damage transformers, transmission lines, electric breakers, and generators by causing electric overloads. Electric overloads will either destroy grid components or cause a reduction of equipment life expectancy.

The question is, what should *future grid* be in order to accommodate intelligent, for example, smart-grid technologies and maintain resilient power for the consumer, while decreasing the vulnerabilities to homeland security and defense missions?

- What are the best practices that are necessary to achieve these objectives?
- What national policies should the United States put in place that will get us from the *grid of 2010* to the *optimal grid of the future*?
- What technologies best serve to increase grid resilience?
- What can/should we do to increase mission efficiencies, increase grid reliance, reduce demand, and develop technologies or practices that can be leveraged to meet these national goals?
- What can/should the federal government do to increase mission efficiencies, increase grid reliance, reduce demand, and develop technologies or practices that can be leveraged to meet these national goals?
- What are the *best case* effects of a national grid policy and technology insertion to reduce vulnerabilities?
- Can our reliance on imported fuels be increased?
- Can our reliance on new technologies increase homeland security?
- Can our reliance on new technologies assist homeland defense and reduce vulnerabilities to defense missions worldwide?
- Can the federal government play a positive role in grid improvements? How?
- Can industry rise to increase grid resilience?
- What technologies best fit our current regulatory environment?
- What legal/regulatory changes must occur to make *future grid* possible?

C.2.2 Approach

The focus is on the anticipated impact of a renewable and clean energy future on energy production and distribution, specifically via the electric power grid. The fundamental approach is to identify an end state or *vision* of an optimal electric power grid and work backward to the present day. Working backward from the end state to the present state will identify milestones that must be met in order to get to the future state. We can then decide what policies are needed today that will take us to the end state. The end state is roughly defined as a production and distribution system with the following characteristics:

- *Energy independence*: 90% of the energy consumed by the United States is also produced by the United States.
- *Clean*: CO_2 emissions equal to or better than the Kyoto Protocols.
- *Resilient*: Energy production and distribution reliability is *five nines* reliable (no more than a few hours per year of outages), and cascade failures are containable (controlled islanding via load shedding).

There are multiple visions of what the future power grid might look like. Rather than postulate distinct *scenarios*, for our purposes, this paper uses the visions of the writers. In order for this paper to be useful in the future development of policy, we will build our collective vision through the series of questions posed in the previous section within the following steps.

Step 1: Vision of future grid
What is the optimal future grid? An incrementally robust grid? A collection of microgrids? Government Electric Power Inc.? The objective here is to define the aspects of the most resilient, most efficient grid possible. It is anticipated that this vision will encompass the incorporation of a two-way communication and a sophisticated computer and sensor control network for sensing and adjusting the flow of electrons throughout a national grid that has incorporated intermittent generation from wind, solar, natural gas, nuclear, etc., sources. New technologies will be incorporated as they become available, for example, *smart transformers*. The vision could also incorporate a variety of base power, intermittent power, and storage facilities focused on support of localized microgrids. New technologies are designed to address this new architecture and incorporate a variety of sources of power.

Step 2: Relevance to national security/defense
The vision of *future grid* will have a significant effect on national security and national defense policies. In the case of national defense, the Department of Defense has a continuing reliance on commercial and defense infrastructures to complete its worldwide missions. Achieving these many requirements depends on a reliable grid. National security, as expressed in our reliance on commercial ports under the purview of the US Coast Guard, has a similar dependence on a reliable and efficient grid. *Future grid* must serve the mission needs of the Departments of Defense and homeland security. What policies must be in place for *future grid* to enhance our national security and national defense?

Step 3: Enabling technologies
Achievement of *future grid* depends on expansion of existing technologies; the development of new technologies; integration of complex generation, transmission, and distribution systems; and new security protocols, standards, and systems. While some currently exist but require efficiency increases, for example, photovoltaic power generation and storage systems, and other technologies currently used only for laboratory experiments, for example, fusion power generation, it is essential that major technological advances are envisioned and achieved. What are these technologies?

Step 4: Enabling national security and national defense policies
In terms of the big picture, our recommendations aim to drive toward a *national energy policy* at the national level. What policies are necessary to build and protect the grid to assure that the grid enables and enhances the US Coast Guard missions to protect our ports, to assure that defense facilities have reliable power for their missions, and to integrate our public and private grid research and development?

Many ideas were discussed by the participants. These centered on a handful of critical elements:

- Transformers
- Storage
- Cap banks
- IT integration
- PMUs/RTUs
- Transmission policy
- Demand response
- Renewable energy
- Breeder technology

A follow-up meeting was recommended to develop recommendations to the White House.

REFERENCE

Congressional Research Service, Electric power transmission: Background and policy issues, Congressional Document No. R40511, Library of Congress, Washington, DC (also at www.loc.gov; accessed 2011).

Appendix D: Guide to the FERC: Electric Transmission Facilities Permit Process

This guide explains the FERC's permitting process for electric transmission facilities and addresses some of the basic concerns of interested entities and individuals that may be impacted by a proposed project.

This commission's Office of Energy Projects is available at 1-202-502-8700 to answer questions concerning the procedures involved. A website has been established for transmission-line siting at http://www.ferc.gov/idutrires/electric/indus-act/sitin.asp for further information.

D.1 PURPOSE

The purpose of this is to

1. Describe the scope of FERC's electric transmission-line siting authority
2. Describe FERC's prefiling and application filing processes for an electric transmission construction permit
3. Explain how to obtain accurate and timely information concerning a proposed electric transmission project that is located in a national interest electric transmission corridor (national corridor)
4. Explain how to participate in the FERC review process
5. Provide contact information should additional information be needed

D.2 INTRODUCTION

Electric transmission lines provide reliable electric power to homes, offices, and industry. Construction of electric transmission facilities has lagged in recent years, and additional transmission is required to ensure a reliable source of power.

In August 2005, Congress enacted the Energy Policy Act of 2005 (EPAct 2005). This act required the Secretary of Energy (secretary) to conduct a study of electric transmission congestion and release the study for public comment. In August 2006, the DOE published its first National Electric Transmission Congestion Study and released the study for public comment. In 2007, based on the findings of that study and after considering comments of stakeholders, the secretary designated two national corridors, one in the mid-Atlantic area and one covering Southern California and part of the Western Arizona. In April 2010, the DOE published its second National Electric Transmission Congestion Study. The 2009 study identified areas that are transmission constrained, but did not make recommendations concerning existing or new national corridor designations.

Most electric transmission projects will continue to be approved by the states in which they are proposed. However, under EPAct 2005, the commission has the authority to consider an application and to issue a permit to construct proposed facilities if a state either withholds approval for more than a year, does not have authority to site transmission facilities, or cannot consider interstate benefits of a proposed project located in a national corridor.

Before an application can be filed at FERC, a potential applicant (project sponsor or company) must participate in a prefiling process that is designed to encourage early participation from all interested entities and individuals during the review of a proposed project. During this process, the information necessary to file an application is compiled for review. Once the prefiling process has been successfully complied, the applicant may submit a permit application for further FERC review.

FERC staff will conduct an environmental analysis for consideration in the commission's determination whether to issue a permit to construct electric transmission facilities in national corridors. The purpose of the analysis is to identify and inform the public, other permitting agencies, and the FERC commoners about reasonable alternatives as required by the NEPA.

In order to issue a permit under Section 216 of the EPA, the commission must find that the proposed project

- Is eligible for a construction permit issued by the commission
- Is located in a national corridor designated by the DOE
- Will be used in interstate commerce
- Is in the public interest
- Will significantly reduce transmission congestion and protect and benefit consumers
- Is consistent with sound national energy policy and will enhance energy independence
- Will maximize the use of existing towers or structures to the extent reasonably and economically possible

D.3   STATE REVIEW

The project sponsor must file an applicant with that proposed facilities are located in a state that has authority to approve the siting of the facilities and to consider its interstate state. A sponsor must be engaged in the state process for at least 1 year prior to initiating prefiling with the commission. In all other instances, a sponsor may request to initiate prefiling whenever sufficient project-related information is available.

Where possible, FERC encourages potential applicants to complete ongoing state permit review processes. Where successful, this may allow projects to be constructed sooner.

D.4   INITIAL REVIEW

Prior to a company requesting the initiation of the prefiling process, company representatives are required to meet commission staff to explain the proposed project. These meetings provide the staff the opportunity to offer suggestions and comments related to the environmental, engineering, and safety features of the proposed project. Based on the input received, the project sponsor will be able to further define their proposed project. Once there is sufficient project definition, the sponsor may submit its request to initiate the prefiling process to the commission's director of the Office of Energy Projects (director).

D.5   PREFILING REVIEW PROCESS

If the director approves the request, the commission will issue a notice informing the public of the initiation of the prefiling process. As part of the prefiling process, a potential applicant is required to implement a project participation plan. The plan must identify specific tools and actions to facilitate stakeholder communication and the dissemination of public information to those who are interested in the proposed project.

During the prefiling process, communication staff will review the company's proposal and identify information needed for the preparation of a complete application. Staff activities may include conducting site visits, facilitating the identification and resolution of issues, coordinating with other agencies, and initiating the environmental review of the proposed project. By engaging the stakeholders early in the process and resolving relevant issues, the proposed project will become better defined, and the benefits and impact of the proposed project will be better understood. The work performed in the prefiling process will form the basis for the application that is subsequently filed with the commission.

D.6 APPLICATION PROCESS

An applicant may be filed only after the director has determined that all necessary information gathering is complete. After an application is filed, commission staff will conduct a comprehensive project review, including issuing an environmental document. All comments and recommendations from all affected entities and individuals will be compiled and carefully reviewed. Commission staff may conduct public meetings and technical conferences, as appropriate, to clarify project-related issues. After the issuance of a final environmental document, the commission will act on the request for construction permit. The commission must act within 1 year from the date the application is filed with the commission.

D.7 FREQUENTLY ASKED QUESTIONS

D.7.1 Getting Involved

D.7.1.1 How Will I First Hear about a Proposed Electric Transmission Facility?

You may first hear about the proposed project from a variety of sources. If you live in the vicinity of a proposed project, you may first learn of it through the state permit process. Once the commission's prefiling is initiated, you may learn of it through open-house meetings, newspaper notices, or direct mailing from FERC or the applicant.

D.7.1.2 How Can I Obtain Details about the Company's Application?

FERC's record on a project is publicly accessible and can be obtained from the FERC website at www.ferc.gov. The prefiling or application material may be reviewed or downloaded (free of charge) through the FERC website using the *eLibrary* link and the project's docket number. User assistance is available at 1-866-208-3676 (toll-free). In addition, information may be obtained from the applicant's project-specific website.

D.7.1.3 How Do I Make My Views Known?

You are encouraged to contact the transmission company directly with your questions, comments, or concerns. You may contact the company through the contact person listed in the notification you received or from the applicant's project-specific website.

There are also ways to make your views known directly to FERC. First, if you want FERC to consider your views on various environmental issues associated with the proposed project, you can do so by simply writing a letter. FERC affords you the opportunity to comment at various stages of the environmental review process, including public hearings. Details are available from the commission's Office of External Affairs at 1-866-208-3372 (toll-free). Check the FERC website for details on filing electronically at www. ferc.gov/docs-filing/efiling.asp. By filing comments, your views will be considered and addressed in the environmental documents or final order. Please include the docket number at the top of your letter.

Second, once an application is filed, you may become an intervenor and a party to the FERC proceeding. Instructions on how to do this are available from the commission's Office of External Affairs and the FERC website at www.ferc.gov/help.how-to/intervene.asp. As an intervenor, you will receive the applicant's filings and other commission's documents related to the case and materials filed by other interested parties. You will also be able to file the briefs and appear at hearings and be heard by the courts if you choose to appeal the commission's final ruling. However, along with these rights come responsibilities. For example, you may serve copies of your filings on all other parties. The secretary of the commission maintains a mailing list of all parties to the proceeding. Typically, you must file for intervenor status within 21 days of FERC's notice of the application in the Federal Register, although the commission may accept late intervention for a good cause. You may also file for intervenor status during the comment period for a draft environmental document.

Request for intervention is not accepted during the prefiling process. You must wait until an application is filed with the commission. As detailed earlier, ample opportunity is provided for filing requests to intervene after the application is filed.

D.7.1.4   Will the Commission Consider a State's Regulatory Record?

A state's regulatory record will be carefully considered by the commission and, to the extent practicable, will be used to expedite the commission's proceeding of a permit application. While the commission will accept any pertinent information developed in the state proceeding or elsewhere into the record, the commission is required to do an independent review of environmental impacts. The commission's ultimate determination on whether to issue a permit will be based on the entire record developed in the commission proceeding. The formal record will be used to determine if the proposed project meets the criteria in Section 216 of the FPA.

D.7.2   Project Location

D.7.2.1   How Is the Transmission-Line Route Selected?

The project sponsor identifies the project purpose and an initial proposed route or routes to achieve that purpose. During the prefiling process, the commission staff works with the project sponsor and all other interested entities to better define the route. During this process, the prospective applicant must study alternative routes or location to reduce project-related impacts; in addition, minor route variations are often evaluated to avoid or minimize certain impacts to property owners or sensitive environmental resources. The commission staff, the company, or other entities may suggest alternative and modifications to reduce project impacts.

D.7.2.2   Will the Commission Consider Alternatives Other than New Transmission Lines?

The commission requires the prospective applicant to address a variety of alternatives, including, where appropriate, alternatives other than new transmission lines. Under NEPA, the commission is required to analyze all reasonable alternatives, even if the alternative does not fall under the commission's jurisdiction. Thus, the commission may be required to look at a wide range of *nonwire* alternatives (e.g., local generation, demand-side management, and energy storage), in addition to transmission-line route alternatives, as part of the environmental review process.

D.7.2.3   How Does the Applicant Obtain an ROW?

The company negotiates an ROW easement and compensation for the easement with each landowner. Landowners may be paid for loss of certain uses of the land during and after construction, loss of any other resources, and any damage to property. If the commission approves the project and no agreement with the landowner is reached through negotiation, the company may acquire the easement under eminent domain (a right given to the company by statue to take private land for commission-authorized use) with a court determining just compensation under state law.

D.7.2.4   What Authorization Allows the Company to Use Eminent Domain?

If the commission issues a construction permit for a project and the necessary easements cannot be negotiated, an applicant is granted the right of eminent domain (Section 216[e] of DPA) and the procedure set forth under the Federal Rules of Civil Procedure (Rule 71 A). Under the conditions, the landowner would receive just compensation as determined by the courts. This right of eminent domain does not apply to federal or state land.

D.7.2.5   Who Pays Taxes on the ROW?

When an applicant has an easement across a portion of the land, the landowner typically pays on the ROW unless a local taxing authority grants relief.

D.7.2.6   How Large Is the ROW and How Is It Maintained?

The width of the ROW depends on the type and voltage of the transmission line. ROW widths of approximately 100–200 ft would be typical for the types of projects we expect to review for construction permits. The transmission company must adhere to the vegetative management standard required by the state and the North American NERC.

D.7.2.7   Must the Company Obey Local, County, and State Laws and Zoning Ordinances?

Yes, but if there is a conflict between these ordinances and what the commission requires, the commission requirement prevails.

D.7.2.8   In General, Will I Still Be Able to Use the ROW?

The easement agreement will specify restricted users on or across the ROW and any types of uses for which the company's permission must be sought. An easement acquired under eminent domain shall be used by the transmission company exclusively for the construction and modification of electric transmission facilities and will also specify restricted uses.

D.7.2.9   What If I Have Problems with Erosion or Other Issues during Restoration and/or Maintenance of the ROW?

The landowner should first contact the company to address and resolve the issue. If the landowner is not satisfied that the problem has adequately addressed, he or she can contact the commission's Dispute Resolution Service Helpline at 1-877-377-2237 (toll-free) or send an e-mail to ferc.adr@ferc.gov.

D.7.2.10   Must Companies Post Bonds to Guarantee Performance?

No, but the commission inspects the ROW during and after the construction prior to the facilities being place in service to ensure that the terms of its permit are met.

D.7.2.11   Can the Applicant Come on the Proposed Route without Landowner Permission?

State or local trespass laws prevail. Some states have laws that allow a company to get across to property for survey purposes (procedures vary by state). Once a permit is issued or an easement/survey agreement or court order is obtained, the company may come onto your land. Usually the company will notify the landowner in advance.

D.7.2.12   When Can Construction Begin?

Construction cannot commence until the commission issues a permit, the applicant accepts it, and the applicant receives all other necessary permits and authorizations. Once a permit has been issued, construction may start within a few weeks of the company having complied with any preconditions set by the commission. Authorization to commence construction will be issued when the applicant demonstrates compliance with the terms and conditions of the permit.

D.7.2.13   Why Would the Company Approach a Landowner before the Project Is Approved?

If you are a potential ROW landowner, the company may try to obtain easement agreements in advance of project approval. A company must conduct environmental studies during the prefiling process. For those studies to be completed as soon as possible, the company will try to obtain access from the individual landowners along the entire length of the proposed ROW. If commission approval is ultimately denied, or the route changes, the initial easement agreement with the landowner is usually void (depending on the wording of the ROW or access contract). Disputes over the wording of an easement agreement are subject to state law.

D.7.2.14   Can the Company Place Other Facilities Not Authorized by the Permit on a Landowner's Property? Can the Facilities and the Easement Be Used for Anything Other than Transmitting Electricity?

The permit issued by the commission would require that eminent domain only be used for the proposed facilities in the location described. If the company wishes to install additional facilities under commission jurisdiction, it must obtain additional approval from the commission. Other utilities may wish to use an adjacent or overlapping easement, but they would have to obtain approval from the landowner or from another permitting authority that can grant eminent domain (usually the state). Of course, the landowner may agree to other uses.

D.7.2.15   Can a Landowner Receive Service from the Facilities?

Not directly. The operation of interstate transmission facilities is incompatible with direct residential use, which is provided by local electric providers.

D.7.2.16   How Soon after Construction Will the Transmission Company Restore the Vegetation in Disturbed Areas?

Commission rules require the land be restored as soon as weather permits.

D.7.3   SAFETY ISSUES

D.7.3.1   Who Is Responsible for Safety?

Standards of construction and operation are governed by the ANSI, Inc., the NESC, NERC, FERC, and municipal regulators. While the commission has oversight in ensuring that the facilities are safely constructed, on the facility if operational, the transmission company is responsible for the safety of its facilities.

D.7.4   ENVIRONMENTAL ISSUES

D.7.4.1   What If Endangered Species, Wetlands, or Archeological Sites Are Identified along the Proposed Route?

The transmission company is required to prepare environmental repots, which address resources, fish, wildlife, vegetation, cultural resources, socioeconomics, geological resources, sols, land use, recreation, aesthetics, alternatives, reliability and safety, and design and engineering. The minimum filing requirements for these reports are described in Section 380.16 of our regulations.

D.7.4.2   What Environmental Documents Will Be Prepared by FERC?

FERC's environmental review will build on any previous environmental review process. The following provides some general guidance.

A notice of intent (NOI) to prepare an environmental assessment (EA) or an environmental impact statement (EIS) is issued for most major proposals. It is sent to federal, state, and local agencies; local media and libraries; environmental groups; Native American tribes; and affected landowners. For most major projects, the NOI will announce a schedule of public meetings along the proposed route. The NOI seeks comments from interested parties on the scope of the environmental document, and any comments must be submitted to the commission, normally within 30 days.

After the comment period, the commission staff begins to prepare an EA or a draft EIS outlining its findings and recommendations. For major proposals, further comments are sought and public meetings may be conducted during 45 days allotted for review of a draft EIS or 30 days in the case of an EA. These comments are considered and addressed in the final EIS or the final order granting or denying the permit.

ADDITIONAL INFORMATION

For additional information, contact
Federal Energy Regulatory Commission
Office of External Affairs
888 First Street NE, Washington, DC 20426
Toll-free: 1-866-208-3372
TTY: 202-502-3372
www.ferc.gov or customer@ferc.gov

Dispute Resolution Service Helpline
Toll-Free: 1-977-337-223
Local: 202-502-8702
ferc.adr@ferc.gov

For assistance with ferc.gov or eFiling, please contact
FERC Online Technical Support
Toll-free: 1-866-208-3676
Local: 202-502-6652
ferconlinesuppot@ferc.gov

For materials and copying assistance, please contact
Public Reference Room
Toll-free: 1-866-208-3676
Local: 202-502-8371
TTY: 202-502-8659
public.referenceroom@ferc.gov

Other related FERC documents you may find helpful are listed in the following. These are available on our website:

- *Handbook for Using Third-Party Contractors to Prepare Environmental Documents* (http://www.ferc.gov/indutiries/electric/indus-act/siting/third-party-handbook.pdf)
- *Guide to Electronic Information at FERC* (http://www.ferc.gov/for-citizens/citizen-guides.asp)
- *Guidance Manual for Environmental Report Preparation*
- *Guidelines for Reporting on Cultural Resources Investigations*
- *Interim Guidelines for Applicant-Prepared Draft Environmental Assessments*
- *Upland Erosion Control, Vegetation, and Maintenance Plan*
- *Wetland and Waterbody Construction and Mitigation Procedures* (http://www. ferc.gov/industries/gas/environ/guidelines.asp)

REFERENCE

Federal Energy Regulatory Commission. *Order 1000: Final Rule on Transmission Planning and Cost Allocation by Transmission Owning and Operating Public Utilities*, Washington, DC, July 21, 2011.

Appendix E: Standard Device Numbers Used in Protection Systems

Some of the frequently used device numbers are listed as follows. A complete list and definitions are given in ANSI/IEEE Standard C37.2-1079:

1. Master element, normally used for hand-operated devices
2. Time-delay starting or closing relay
3. Checking or interlocking relay
4. Master contactor
5. Stopping device
6. Starting CB
7. Anode CB
8. Control power disconnecting device
9. Reversing device
10. Unit sequence switch
12. Synchronous-speed device
14. Underspeed device
15. Speed- or frequency-matching device
17. Shunting or discharge switch
18. Accelerating or decelerating device
20. Electrically operated valve
21. Distance relay
23. Temperature control device
25. Synchronizing or synchronism-check device
26. Apparatus thermal device
27. Undervoltage relay
29. Isolating contactor
30. Annunciator relay
32. Directional power relay
37. Undercurrent or underpower relay
46. Reverse-phase or phase-balance relay
47. Phase-sequence voltage relay
48. Incomplete sequence relay
49. Machine or transformer thermal relay
50. Instantaneous overcurrent or rate-of-rise relay
51. AC time overcurrent relay
52. AC CB, mechanism-operated contacts are
    a. 52a, 52aa, open when breaker closed that is, when breaker contacts closed
    b. 52b, 52bb, operates just as mechanism motion starts; known as high-speed contacts
55. Power factor relay
57. Short-circuiting or grounding device
59. Overvoltage relay

60. Voltage or current balance relay
62. Time-delay stopping or opening relay
64. Ground detector relay
67. AC directional overcurrent relay
68. Blocking relay
69. Permissive control device
72. AC circuit breaker
74. Alarm relay
76. DC overcurrent relay
78. Phase-angle measuring or out-of-step protective relay
79. AC reclosing relay
80. Flow switch
81. Frequency relay
82. DC reclosing relay
83. Automatic selective control or transfer relay
84. Operating mechanism
85. Carrier or pilot-wire receiver relay
86. Lockout relay
87. Differential protective relay
89. Line switch
90. Regulating device
91. Voltage directional relay
92. Voltage and power directional relay
93. Field-changing contactor
94. Tripping or trip-free relay

Appendix F: Final Rule on Transmission Planning and Cost Allocation by Transmission Owning and Operating Public Utilities

FEDERAL ENERGY REGULATORY COMMISSION

Order No. 1000   **July 21, 2010**

Order No. 1000 is a Final Rule that reforms the Commission's electric transmission planning and cost allocation requirements for public utility transmission providers. The rule builds on the reforms of Order No. 890 and corrects remaining deficiencies with respect to transmission planning processes and cost allocation methods.

F.1 BACKGROUND

On June 17, 2010, the FERC issued a Notice of Proposed Rulemaking seeking comments on potential changes to its transmission planning and cost allocation requirements. Industry participants and other stakeholders provided extensive comments in response to the Notice of Proposed Rulemaking. The commission received more than 180 initial comments and more than 65 rely comments.

F.2 PLANNING REFORMS

The rule establishes three requirements for transmission planning:

1. Each public utility transmission provider must participate in a regional transmission planning process that satisfies the transmission planning principles of Order No. 890 and produces a regional transmission plan.
2. Local and regional transmission planning processes must consider transmission planning needs driven by public policy requirements established by state or federal laws or regulations. Each public utility transmission provider must establish procedures to identify transmission needs driven by public policy requirements and evaluate proposed solutions to those transmission needs.
3. Public utility transmission providers in each pair of neighboring transmission planning regions must coordinate to determine if there are more efficient or cost-effective solutions to their mutual transmission needs.

F.3 COST ALLOCATION REFORMS

The rule establishes three requirements for transmission cost allocation:

1. Each public utility transmission provider must participate in a regional transmission planning process that has a regional cost allocation method for new transmission facilities selected in the regional transmission plan for the purpose of cost allocation. The method must satisfy six regional cost allocation principles.
2. Public utility transmission providers in neighboring transmission planning regions must have a common interregional cost allocation method for new interregional facilities that the regions determine to be efficient and cost-effective. The method must satisfy six similar interregional cost allocation principles.
3. Participant funding of new transmission facilities is permitted, but is not allowed as the regional or interregional cost allocation method.

F.4 NONINCUMBENT DEVELOPER REFORMS

Public utility transmission providers must remove from commission-approved tariffs and agreements—a federal right of first refusal for a transmission facility selected in a regional plan for purpose of cost allocation, subject to four limitations:

1. This does not apply to a transmission facility that is not selected in a regional transmission plan for the purpose of cost allocation.
2. This does not apply to upgrades to transmission facilities, such as tower change outs or reconductoring.
3. This allows, but does not require, public utility transmission providers in a transmission planning region to use competitive bidding to solicit transmission projects or project developers.
4. Nothing in this requirement affects state or local laws or regulations over siting or permitting of transmission facilities.

The rule recognizes that incumbent transmission providers must rely on regional transmission providers to satisfy their reliability needs or service obligations. The rule requires each public utility transmission provider to amend their tariff to require reevaluation of the regional transmission plan to determine if delays in the development of a transmission facility require evaluation of alternative solutions, including those proposed by the incumbent, to ensure incumbent transmission providers meet reliability needs or service obligations.

F.5 COMPLIANCE

Order No. 1000 takes effect 60 days from publication in the Federal Register.

Each public utility transmission provider is required to make a compliance filing with the commission within 12 months of the effective date of the Final Rule.

Compliance filing for interregional transmission coordination and interregional cost allocation are required within 18 months of the effective date.

REFERENCE

Federal Energy Regulatory Commission. *A Guide to the FERC-Electric Transmission Facilities Permit Process*, FERC, Washington, DC, September, 2010.

Appendix G: Unit Conversions from the English System to SI System

The following are useful when converting from the English system to the SI system:

Length	1 in. = 2.54 cm = 0.0245 m
	1 ft = 30.5 cm = 0.305 m
	1 mile = 1609 m
Area	$1 \text{ mile}^2 = 2.59 \times 106 \text{ m}^2$
	$1 \text{ in.}^2 = 0.000645 \text{ m}^2$
	$1 \text{ in.}^2 = 6.45 \text{ cm}^2$
Volume	$1 \text{ ft}^3 = 0.0283 \text{ m}^3$
Linear speed	1 ft/s = 0.305 m/s = 30.3 cm/s
	1 mph = 0.447 m/s
	1 in./s = 0.0254 m/s = 2.54 cm/s
Rotational speed	1 rev/min = 0.105 rad/s = 6 deg/s
Force	1 lb = 4.45 N
Power	1 hp = 746 W = 0.746 kW
Torque	1 ft-lb = 1.356 N-m
Magnetic flux	$1 \text{ line} = 1 \text{ maxwell} = 10^{-8} \text{ Wb}$
	$1 \text{ kiloline} = 1000 \text{ maxwells} = 10^{-5} \text{ Wb}$
Magnetic flux density	$1 \text{ line/in.}^2 = 15.5 \times 10^{-6} \text{ T}$
	$100 \text{ kilolines/in.}^2 = 1.55 \text{ T} = 1.55 \text{ Wb/m}^2$
Magnetomotive force	1 A-turn = 1 A
Magnetic field intensity	1 A-turn/in. = 39.37 A/m

Appendix H: Unit Conversions from the SI System to English System

The following are useful when converting from the SI system to the English system:

Length	1 m = 100 cm = 39.37 in.
	1 m = 3.28 ft
	$1 \text{m} = 6.22 \times 10^{-4}$ mile
Area	$1 \text{m}^2 = 0.386 \times 10^{-6}$ mile
	1 m² = 1550 in.²
	1 cm² = 0.155 in.²
Volume	1 m³ = 35.3 ft³
Linear speed	1 m/s = 100 cm/s = 3.28 ft/s
	1 m/s = 2.237 mph
	1 m/s = 39.37 in./s
Rotational speed	1 rad/s = 9.55 rev/min = 57.3 deg/s
Force	1 N = 0.225 lb
Power	1 kW = 1000 W = 1.34 hp
Torque	1 N-m = 0.737 ft-lb
Magnetic flux	$1 \text{Wb} = 10^8$ lines $= 10^8$ maxwells
	$1 \text{Wb} = 10^5$ kilolines
Magnetic flux density	$1 \text{T} = 6.45 \times 10^4$ lines / in.²
	1 T = 1 Wb/m²
Magnetomotive force	1 A = 1 A-turn
Magnetic field intensity	1 A/m = 0.0254 A-turn/in.

Appendix I: Classroom Examples for Designing Transmission Lines by Using MATLAB®

I.1 CLASSROOM ASSIGNMENT #1

Problem 1 Assume that a 60 Hz three-phase transmission line is 178 mi long. The line is connected to a load of 200 MW at a lagging PF of 0.95 at 345 kV. Choose an appropriate ACSR conductor for the line so that the efficiency and voltage regulation of the line are equal or greater than 0.95% and equal or less than 5%. And the power loss of the line is less than 5%. Select an appropriate 345 kV EPRI tower among the towers that are given in Chapter 2, and determine the following by using MATLAB®:

(a) A, B, C, and D transmission-line constants
(b) Sending-end voltage
(c) Sending-end current
(d) Sending-end PF
(e) Sending-end power
(f) Power loss in line
(g) Transmission-line efficiency
(h) Percentage of voltage regulation
(i) Sending-end charging current at no load
(j) The amount of rise in the receiving-end voltage at no load, if sending-end voltage is held constant

Solution

```
clc
clear all

disp('')
disp(' xxxxxxxxxxxxxxxxxxxxxxxxxxxxxxxxxxxxxxxxxxxxxxxxxxxxxxxxxx')
disp(
disp(' TRANSMISSION LINE 178 miles Long FOR Project: EEE-500:')
disp(' From: Bishop, CA. to Kramer Junction along Hwy-395')
disp(' xxxxxxxxxxxxxxxxxxxxxxxxxxxxxxxxxxxxxxxxxxxxxxxxxxxxxxxxxx')
disp(' ')
disp('LoadPower, Pr = 200MW ')
disp('ACSR conductors are made up of 397,500-kcmil 26/7-strand')
disp('Distances between conductors are:')
disp('D12 = 27.2 ft. D23 = 27.23 ft. D13 = 54.4 ft.')
disp('')
TL = 178;        % transmission line length, mi
VrLL = 345*10^3; % line to line voltage, V
```

```
Pr = 200*10^6; % load power, Watts
pf = 0.95;     % power factor, pf
D12 = 27.2;    % ft
D23 = 27.2;    % ft
D13 = 54.4;    % ft
disp(' ')
disp('Characteristics of ACSR 397,500-kcmil 26/7-strand, Table A.3, A.8,
 and A.9')
disp('do = 0.783 outside diameter of conductor, inches')
do = 0.783;
disp('ra = 0.259 resistance, ohms/mi ')
ra = 0.259;
disp('')
disp('xa = 0.441 inductive reactance, ohms/mi')
xa = 0.441;
disp('')
disp('xaa = 0.1015 from Table A.3, shunt capacitive reactance,
 MegOhms*mi')
xaa = 0.1015;
disp('')
disp('xd = 0.4289 from Table A.8 based on calculated Deq, inductive
 reactance')
disp('spacing factor, MegOhms/mi')
xd = 0.4289;
disp('')
disp('xdd = 0.1049 from Table A.9 based on calculated Deq, shunt
 capacitive')
disp('reactance spacing factor, MegOhms/mi')
xdd = 0.1049;
disp(' ')
disp(' *** EQUATIONS: ***')
disp('equivalent spacing, Deq = (D12*D23*D13)^(1/3), feet')
Deq = (D12*D23*D13)^(1/3)
disp('VrLN = VrLL/(3)^(1/2), V')
VrLN = VrLL/(3)^(1/2)
disp('V')
disp('thetap = acosd(pf) power factor angle')
thetap = acosd(pf)
thetar = (pf+sind(thetap)*i) % rectangular form of pf angle
disp('Ir = Pr/(sqrt(3)*VrLL*pf) magnitude of the current, A')
Ir = Pr/(sqrt(3)*VrLL*pf)    % magnitude of the current
disp('A')
Irp = Ir/thetar              % Ir with phase angle
thetarangle = -1*(angle(thetar)*(180/pi))% lagging
disp('degrees lagging')
disp('')
raL = (ra*TL)
disp('ohms')
xaL = (xa*TL)
disp('ohms')
xaaL = (xaa/TL)
disp('ohms')
xdL = xd*TL
disp('ohms')
xddL = xdd/TL
disp('ohms')
```

```
disp('Xl = xaL+xdL ohms')
Xl = xaL+xdL
disp('ohms')
disp('Zl = raL+Xl*i ohms')
Zl = raL+Xl*i
disp('ohms')
disp('xcL = -1*(xaaL+xddL)*(10^6)*i ohms')
xcL = -1*(xaaL+xddL)*(10^6)*i
disp('ohms')
disp('Yl = 1/xcL Siemens')
Yl = 1/xcL
disp('Siemens')
disp('Yl magnitude is, Siemens')
Ylmag = abs(Yl)
disp('Siemens')
disp('PropK = propagation constant')
disp('')
disp('PropK = (Yl*Zl)^(1/2)')
PropK = (Yl*Zl)^(1/2)
disp('Zc = (Zl/Yl)^(1/2)')
Zc = (Zl/Yl)^(1/2)
disp('ohms')
disp('Yc = 1/Zc')
Yc = 1/Zc
disp('Siemens')
disp('')
disp('a. A B C D constants of the Trans-Line')
disp('A = cosh(PropK) ; where: PropK is the propagation constant')
disp('B = Zc*(sinh(PropK))')
disp('C = Yc*(sinh(PropK)) and D = A')
disp('')
A = cosh(PropK)
B = Zc*(sinh(PropK))
C = Yc*(sinh(PropK))
D = A
disp('')
disp('[ABCD] = Matrix constants ABCD')
[ABCD] = [A B;C D]
disp('')
disp('[VsLN ; Is] = [A B;C D]*[VrLN ; Irp]')
[VsLNIs] = [ABCD]*[VrLN;Irp]
disp('b. Sending end voltage')
VsLN = VsLNIs(1,1)
VsLNmag = abs(VsLN)
VsLNangle = angle(VsLN)*(180/pi) % angle in degrees
disp('')
disp('c. Sending end current')
disp('')
Is = VsLNIs(2,1)
Ismag = abs(Is)
Isangle = angle(Is)*(180/pi)     % angle in degrees
disp('')
disp('VsLL = (3)^(1/2)*(VsLN)')
VsLL = (3)^(1/2)*(VsLN)
VsLLmag = abs(VsLL)
VsLLangle = angle(VsLL)*(180/pi) % angle in degrees
```

```
disp('')
disp('d. Sending end power factor, spf')
disp('')
thets = VsLNangle-(Isangle)
spf = cosd(thets)
disp('lagging')
disp('')
disp('e. Sending end power, SEP Watts')
disp('')
disp('SEP = (3)^(1/2)*(VsLLmag*Ismag*spf)')
SEP = (3)^(1/2)*(VsLLmag*Ismag*spf)
disp('')
disp('f. Receiving end power, REP Watts')
disp('')
disp('')
REP = (3)^(1/2)*(VrLL*Ir*pf)
disp('REP = (3)^(1/2)*(VrLL*Ir*pf)')
disp('Therefore, PL = power loss = SEP-REP, Watts')
disp('')
disp('PL = SEP-REP')
PL = SEP-REP
disp('')
disp('g. Efficiency,% n = REP/SEP')
disp('')
n = (REP/SEP)*100
disp('%')
disp('')
disp('h.% Voltage regulation,% VR = ((((|VsLN|/|A|)-/VrLN/)/|VrLN|)*100')
disp('')
VR = (((VsLNmag/A)-VrLN)/VrLN)*100
disp('%')
disp('')
disp('i. Sending-end charging current at no load is,')
disp('Ic = 1/2*(Yl*VsLN), A')
Ic = 1/2*(Yl*VsLN)
disp('')
disp('Ic magnitude and angle')
Icmag = abs(Ic)
disp('')
Icangle = angle(Ic)*(180/pi) % angle in degrees
disp('j. Receiving-end voltage "rise" at no load VrLNr is')
disp('VrRLNr VsLN-Ic*Zl, V')
VrLNr = VsLN-Ic*Zl
disp('VrLNr magnitude and angle')
VRLNmag = abs(VrLNr)
VrLNrangle = angle(VrLNr)*(180/pi)
disp(' Therefore, the line_to_line voltage at the receiving end is,')
disp(' VrLLr = (3)^(1/2)* VrLNr, V ')
disp(' Converting VrLNr to VrLLr, there is a 30 degree phase shift')
disp(' Let: phase_shift = 30 degrees phase shift')
disp('')
phase_shift = 30;
ps = (cosd(phase_shift)+sind(phase_shift)*i);
VrLLr = (3)^(1/2)* VrLNr*ps
disp('VrLLr magnitude and angle')
VrLLrmag = abs(VrLLr);
VrLLrangle = angle(VrLLr)*(180/pi) % angle in degrees
```

xxxxxxxxxxxxxxxxxxxxxxxxxxxxxxxxxxxxxxxxxxxxxxxxxxxxxxxxxxxx
TRANSMISSION LINE 178 miles Long FOR Project: EEE-500:
From: Bishop, CA. to Kramer Junction along Hwy-395
xxxxxxxxxxxxxxxxxxxxxxxxxxxxxxxxxxxxxxxxxxxxxxxxxxxxxxxxxxxx

LoadPower, Pr = 200MW
ACSR conductors are made up of 397,500-kcmil 26/7-strand
Distances between conductors are:
D12 = 27.2 ft. D23 = 27.23 ft. D13 = 54.4 ft.

Characteristics of ACSR 397,500-kcmil 26/7-strand, Tables A.3, A.8, and A.9
do = 0.783 outside diameter of conductor, inches
ra = 0.259 resistance, ohms/mi
xa = 0.441 inductive reactance, ohms/mi
xa = 0.1015 from Table A.3, shunt capacitive reactance, MegOhms*mi
xd = 0.4289 from Table A.8 based on calculated Deq, inductive reactance spacing factor, MegOhms/mi
xdd = 0.1049 from Table A.9 based on calculated Deq, shunt capacitive reactance spacing factor, MegOhms/mi

*** EQUATIONS: ***
equivalent spacing, Deq = (D12*D23*D13)^(1/3), feet
Deq =
    34.2699
VrLN = VrLL/(3)^(1/2), V
VrLN =
    1.9919e+05
V
thetap = acosd(pf) power factor angle
thetap =
    18.1949
thetar =
    0.9500 + 0.3122i
Ir = Pr/(sqrt(3)*VrLL*pf) magnitude of the current, A
Ir =
    352.3114
A
Irp =
    3.3470e + 02 − 1.1001e + 02i
thetarangle =
    −18.1949
degrees lagging
raL =
    46.1020
ohms
xaL =
    78.4980
ohms

xaaL =
   5.7022e−04
ohms
xdL =
   76.3442
ohms
xddL =
   5.8933e−04
ohms
Xl = xaL+xdL ohms
Xl =
   154.8422
ohms
Zl = raL+Xl*i ohms
Zl =
   4.6102e+01 + 1.5484e+02i

ohms
xcL = −1*(xaaL+xddL)*(10^6)*i ohms
xcL =
   0 − 1.1596e + 03i
ohms
Yl = 1/xcL Siemens
Yl =
   0 + 8.6240e−04i
Siemens
Yl magnitude is, Siemens
Ylmag =
   8.6240e-04
Siemens
PropK = propagation constant
PropK = (Yl*Zl)^(1/2)
PropK =
   0.0538 + 0.3694i

Zc = (Zl/Yl)^(1/2)
Zc =
   4.2830e+02 − 6.2407e + 01i
ohms
Yc = 1/Zc
Yc =
   0.0023 + 0.0003i
Siemens
a. A B C D constants of the Trans-Line
A = cosh(PropK) ; where: PropK is the propagation constant
B = Zc*(sinh(PropK))
C = Yc*(sinh(PropK)) and D = A

A =
   0.9339 + 0.0194i
B =
   4.4070e+01 + 1.5172e+02i
C =
   −5.6387e−06 + 8.4333e−04i
D =
   0.9339 + 0.0194i
[ABCD] = Matrix constants ABCD
ABCD =
   1.0e+02 *
   0.0093 + 0.0002i 0.4407 + 1.5172i
   −0.0000 + 0.0000i 0.0093 + 0.0002i
[VsLN ; Is] = [A B;C D]*[VrLN ; Irp]
VsLNIs =
   1.0e+05 *
   2.1746 + 0.4980i
   0.0031 + 0.0007i

b. Sending end voltage
VsLN =
   2.1746e+05 + 4.9804e+04i
VsLNmag =
   2.2309e+05
VsLNangle =
   12.8996

c. Sending end current
Is =
   3.1359e+02 + 7.1747e+01i
Ismag =
   321.6928
Isangle =
   12.8870
VsLL = (3)^(1/2)*(VsLN)
VsLL =
   3.7665e+05 + 8.6262e+04i
VsLLmag =
   3.8641e+05
VsLLangle =
   12.8996

d. Sending end power factor, spf
thets =
   0.0126

spf =

   1.0000
lagging

e. Sending end power, SEP Watts
SEP = (3)^(1/2)*(VsLLmag*Ismag*spf)
SEP =

   2.1530e+08

f. Receiving end power, REP Watts
REP =

   200000000
REP = (3)^(1/2)*(VrLL*Ir*pf)
Therefore, PL = power loss = SEP-REP, Watts
PL = SEP-REP
PL =

   1.5301e + 07

g. Efficiency,% n = REP/SEP
n =

   92.8933
%

h.% Voltage regulation,% VR = ((((|VsLN|/|A|)−/VrLN/)/|VrLN|)*100
VR =

   19.8762 − 2.4953i
%

i. Sending-end charging current at no load is
Ic = 1/2*(Yl*VsLN), A
Ic =

   −21.4754 + 93.7697i
Ic magnitude and angle
Icmag =

   96.1974
Icangle =

   102.8996

j. Receiving-end voltage "rise" at no load VrLNr is
VrRLNr VsLN-Ic*Zl, V
VrLNr =

   2.3297e + 05 + 4.8806e + 04i
VrLNr magnitude and angle
VRLNmag =

   2.3803e + 05
VrLNrangle =

   11.8320

Therefore, the line_to_line voltage at the receiving end is
VrLLr = (3)^(1/2)* VrLNr, V
Converting VrLNr to VrLLr, there is a 30 degree phase shift
Let: phase_shift = 30 degrees phase shift
VrLLr =

   3.0719e+05 + 2.7497e + 05i
VrLLr magnitude and angle
VrLLrangle =

   41.8320
>>

I.2   CLASSROOM ASSIGNMENT #2

I.2.1   TRANSMISSION-LINE PARAMETERS

I.2.1.1   Input Data: Project Data

The input data used for calculations are summarized to perform a graduate project study for a long transmission line. This project study used EDSA DesignBase, which is a collection of practical equipment and commercially available data.

```
            Transmission Line Constants
            = = = = = = = = = = = = = = = = = = = = = = = = = = = =
Project Name:           Graduate Project
System Voltage:         345 kV, 3-Phase, 60 Hz
Length:                 168 miles (321.9 km)
Structures:             Tower # 3H2 (See Figure I.1)
Conductors:             397.5 kcmil 26/7 Strands ACSR ("Ibis")
Load:                   200 MW

            Physical Conditions
            = = = = = = = = = = = = = = = = = = = = = = =
Earth Resistivity          = 100.00 (ohm-meter)
Average Height Calculation = Method 1
Transposition              = Yes
Circuit Name               = C1
From                       = Bus 1
To                         = Bus 2

            Target Performance
            = = = = = = = = = = = = = = = = = = = = = = = = =
Voltage Regulation:        Less than 5%
Efficiency:                Greater than 95%

            Conductor Selection
            = = = = = = = = = = = = = = = = = = = = = = = = =
Conductors:         200 mm2 ACSR "Jaguar") - 400 kcmil A397.5 kcmil 26/7
Strands ACSR ("Ibis")
Conductor per Phase: Single (1 conductor per phase)
```

I.2.1.2   Conductor Data

The conductor selected for this study is type *Ibis* 397.5 kcmil ACSR conductor, which has the physical characteristics as shown in Table I.1, Conductor Data. Case 1 is based on the single conductor

TABLE I.1
Conductor Data

Code Word	Size (AWG or kcmil)	Stranding (Al/Stl)	Diameter (in.) Individual Wires Al	Diameter (in.) Individual Wires Stl	Diameter (in.) Steel Core	Diameter (in.) Complete Cable	Weight per 1000 ft. (lb) Al	Weight per 1000 ft. (lb) Stl	Weight per 1000 ft. (lb) Total	Content (%) Al	Content (%) Stl	Rated Strength (lb)	Resistance ohms/1000 ft. DC at 20°C	Resistance ohms/1000 ft. AC at 75°C	Allowable Ampacity + (amps)
Merlin	336.4	18/1	0.1367	0.1367	0.1367	0.684	315	49	365	86.43	13.57	8680	0.0510	0.0625	519
Linnet	336.4	26/7	0.1137	0.0885	0.2654	0.72	317	146	462	68.51	31.49	14100	0.0505	0.0618	529
Oriole	336.4	30/7	0.1059	0.1059	0.3177	0.741	318	209	526	60.35	39.65	17300	0.0502	0.0613	535
Chickadee	397.5	18/1	0.1486	0.1486	0.1486	0.743	373	58	431	86.43	13.57	9940	0.0432	0.0529	576
Brant	397.5	24/7	0.1287	0.0858	0.2574	0.772	374	137	511	73.21	26.79	14600	0.0430	0.0526	584
Ibis	397.5	26/7	0.1236	0.0962	0.2885	0.783	374	172	546	68.51	31.49	16300	0.0428	0.0523	587
Lark	397.5	30/7	0.1151	0.1151	0.3453	0.806	375	247	622	60.35	39.65	20300	0.0425	0.0519	594

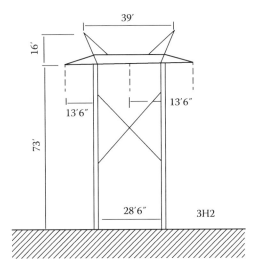

FIGURE I.1   The tower type no. 3H2 used in the project.

per phase configuration and Case 2 is based on bundle (two conductors per phase) arrangement. Data are taken from Table I.1. Figure I.1 shows the tower type that has been used in the project. Table I.2 gives conductor input data.

I.2.1.3   Study Results
Calculation results are summarized in Table I.3.

I.2.1.4   Power-Flow Calculations
Based on the results presented in the previous section, the DesignBase power-flow model is created. The model is depicted in Figure I.2. DesignBase files are attached to this report as well.

The summary of the input data is given as follows:

- *SendingEnd*—swing bus with a nominal voltage of 345 kV
- Feeder—line of *200 miles* with parameters as defined in Section 3
- *ReceivingEnd*—load of *200 MW* and 0 Mvar

Power-flow calculations are performed for the base case of 200 MW of loads and several loads up to 350 MW. Power-flow results are summarized in Table I.4 and their visualization is given in Figure I.3.

TABLE I.2

Conductor Input Data

No.	Phase Bdl.	Wrs	DC RES. (ohm/km)	Avg. Hight (m)	Horz. Pos. (m)	DIA. (cm)	TDR.	GMR (cm)	Voltage (kV)	Voltage (deg)	Bundle Sep Angle (cm)	Bundle Sep Angle (deg)	Phase Current (A)	Current Angle (deg)
1	A	2	0.13670	19.000	-8.460	1.930	0.50	n/a	345.0	0.0	40.0	0.0	415.000	0.0
2	B	2	0.13670	19.000	0.000	1.930	0.50	n/a	345.0	240.0	40.0	0.0	415.000	240.0
3	C	2	0.13670	19.000	8.460	1.930	0.50	n/a	345.0	120.0	40.0	0.0	415.000	120.0

Ground Wires

No.	Grnd Wire	SEG	DC RES (ohm/km)	Avg Hght (m)	Horz Pos (m)	DIA (cm)	TDR	GMR (cm)	Voltage (kV)	Voltage (deg)
1	G1	N	0.10000	27.900	5.940	1.300	0.50	n/a	0.0	0.0
2	G2	N	0.10000	27.900	-5.940	1.300	0.50	n/a	0.0	0.0

TABLE I.3
Impedance Calculation Results

```
Series-impedance matrix(Ohm/km):
9.6434E-02    0.5626    2.7128E-02    0.1784    2.6823E-02    0.1340
2.7128E-02    0.1784    9.6151E-02    0.5518    2.7128E-02    0.1784
2.6823E-02    0.1340    2.7128E-02    0.1784    9.6434E-02    0.5626

Shunt-admittance matrix(Mho/km)
0.000    3.6037E-06    0.000    -6.4865E-07    0.000    -2.2236E-07
0.000    -6.4865E-07    0.000    3.7393E-06    0.000    -6.4865E-07
0.000    -2.2236E-07    0.000    -6.4865E-07    0.000    3.6037E-06

Current Eigenvectors [Ti]:
0.6059    -7.1917E-03    0.7071    -9.3211E-16    -0.4009    -6.8038E-03
0.5160    1.6890E-02    -1.4131E-15    1.9970E-15    0.8238    -6.6220E-03
0.6059    -7.1917E-03    -0.7071    -9.3211E-16    -0.4009    -6.8038E-03

[Y'] Diag (Mho/km):
6.3521E-09    2.6490E-06    1.8773E-23    3.8261E-06    -6.3521E-09    4.4718E-06

[Z'] Diag (Ohm/km):
0.1479    0.8815    6.9611E-02    0.4286    6.9542E-02    0.3626

Eigenvalues of [Y].[Z]:
Mode 1: -.233407E-11    0.397259E-12
Mode 2: -.163989E-11    0.266340E-12
Mode 3: -.162189E-11    0.308674E-12

Modal propagation constants:
Mode 1: 0.129548E-06    0.153325E-05
Mode 2: 0.103653E-06    0.128477E-05
Mode 3: 0.120648E-06    0.127924E-05

Surge impedances (Ohm):
Mode 1: 578.928    -47.5171
Mode 2: 335.791    -27.0909
Mode 3: 286.030    -27.3861

Sequence Impedances Assuming Complete Transposition
Impedances for Circuit number 1:
```

	Resistance (ohm/km)	Reactance (ohm/km)	Susceptance (Micro-Siemens/km)
Positive Sequence	0.0693	0.3954	4.155
Zero Sequence	0.1504	0.8862	2.636

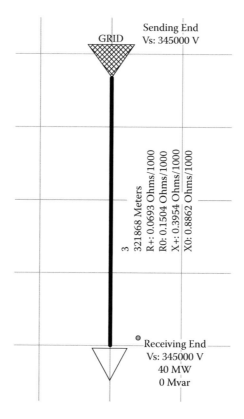

Sending End
Vs: 345000 V

GRID

3
321868 Meters
R+: 0.0693 Ohms/1000
R0: 0.1504 Ohms/1000
X+: 0.3954 Ohms/1000
X0: 0.8862 Ohms/1000

Receiving End
Vs: 345000 V
40 MW
0 Mvar

FIGURE I.2   Power-flow model.

TABLE I.4
Power-Flow Results

Load (MW)	Efficiency (%)	Regulation (%)	Losses (MW)	Voltage (PU)
200	95.74142	−2.20049	8.896	1.0225
250	94.76984	0.68466	13.797	0.9932
300	93.54945	4.65725	20.686	0.9555
350	91.92239	10.65619	30.756	0.9037

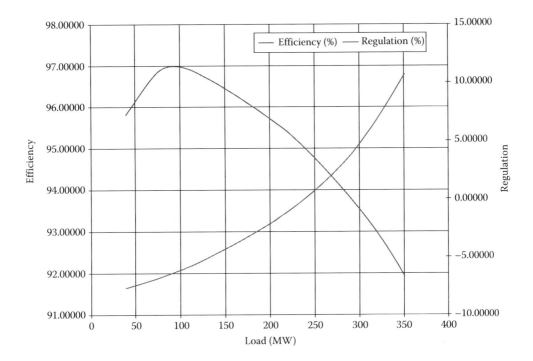

FIGURE I.3   Power-flow results.

Appendix J

Example J.1

Consider the system shown in Figure J.1 and the following data:

Generator G_1: 15 kV, 50 MVA, $X_1 = X_2 = 0.10$ pu and $X_0 = 0.05$ pu based on its own ratings.
Synchronous motor M: 15 kV, 20 MVA, $X_1 = X_2 = 0.20$ pu and $X_0 = 0.07$ pu based on its own ratings.
Transformer T_1: 15/115 kV, 30 MVA, $X_1 = X_2 = X_0 = 0.06$ pu based on its own ratings.
Transformer T_2: 115/15 kV, 25 MVA, $X_1 = X_2 = X_0 = 0.07$ pu based on its own ratings.
Transmission line TL_{23}: $X_1 = X_2 = 0.03$ pu and $X_0 = 0.10$ pu based on its own ratings.

Assume an SLG fault at bus 4 and determine the fault current in per units and amperes. Use 50 MVA as the megavolt-ampere base and assume that $\mathbf{Z}_f$ is $j0.1$ pu based on 50 MVA.

Solution

Assuming an SLG fault at bus 4 with a $\mathbf{Z}_f = j0.1$ pu on 50 MVA base, the given reactance has to be adjusted based on the new S_B. Hence, using

$$\mathbf{Z}_{\text{adjusted}} = X_{\text{pu(old)}} \times \left(\frac{S_{B(\text{new})}}{S_{B(\text{old})}} \right)$$

where in this example $S_{B(\text{new})} = 50$ MVA, for generator G_1,

$$\mathbf{Z}_1 = \mathbf{Z}_2 = j0.10 \times \left(\frac{50\,\text{MVA}}{50\,\text{MVA}} \right) = j0.10 \text{ pu}$$

$$\mathbf{Z}_0 = j0.05 \times \left(\frac{50\,\text{MVA}}{50\,\text{MVA}} \right) = j0.00 \text{ pu}$$

For transformer T_1,

$$\mathbf{Z}_1 = \mathbf{Z}_2 = \mathbf{Z}_0 = j0.06 \times \left(\frac{50\,\text{MVA}}{50\,\text{MVA}} \right) = j0.01 \text{ pu}$$

For transmission line TL_{23},

$$\mathbf{Z}_1 = \mathbf{Z}_2 = j0.03 \times \left(\frac{50\,\text{MVA}}{50\,\text{MVA}} \right) = j0.03 \text{ pu}$$

and

$$\mathbf{Z}_0 = j0.10 \times \left(\frac{50\,\text{MVA}}{50\,\text{MVA}} \right) = j0.10 \text{ pu}$$

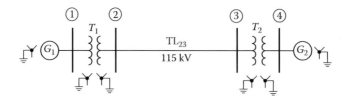

FIGURE J.1   System for Example J.1.

For transformer T_2,

$$\mathbf{Z}_1 = \mathbf{Z}_2 = \mathbf{Z}_0 = j0.07 \times \left(\frac{50 \text{ MVA}}{25 \text{ MVA}} \right) = j0.14 \text{ pu}$$

For synchronous motor M,

$$\mathbf{Z}_1 = \mathbf{Z}_2 = j0.20 \times \left(\frac{50 \text{ MVA}}{20 \text{ MVA}} \right) = j0.5 \text{ pu}$$

and

$$\mathbf{Z}_0 = j0.07 \times \left(\frac{50 \text{ MVA}}{20 \text{ MVA}} \right) = j0.175 \text{ pu}$$

Thus, the Thévenin impedance at the faulted bus 4 is

$$\mathbf{Z}_{1,th} = \frac{\left(\mathbf{Z}_{1,G_1} + \mathbf{Z}_{1,T_1} + \mathbf{Z}_{1,TL} + \mathbf{Z}_{1,T_2} \right)\left(\mathbf{Z}_{1,M} \right)}{\mathbf{Z}_{1,G_1} + \mathbf{Z}_{1,T_1} + \mathbf{Z}_{1,TL} + \mathbf{Z}_{1,T_2} + \mathbf{Z}_{1,M}}$$

$$= j\frac{(0.10 + 0.10 + 0.03 + 0.14)(0.5)}{(0.10 + 0.10 + 0.03 + 0.14 + 0.5)}$$

$$= j0.213 \text{ pu}$$

and since

$$\mathbf{Z}_{2,th} = \mathbf{Z}_{1,th} = j0.213 \text{ pu}$$

and

$$\mathbf{Z}_{0,th} = \frac{\left(\mathbf{Z}_{0,G} + \mathbf{Z}_{0,T_1} + \mathbf{Z}_{0,TL} + \mathbf{Z}_{0,M} \right)\left(\mathbf{Z}_{0,M} \right)}{\mathbf{Z}_{0,G} + \mathbf{Z}_{0,T_1} + \mathbf{Z}_{0,TL} + \mathbf{Z}_{0,T_2} + \mathbf{Z}_{0,M}}$$

$$= j\frac{(0.05 + 0.10 + 0.03 + 0.14)(0.175)}{(0.05 + 0.10 + 0.10 + 0.14 + 0.175)}$$

$$= j0.1208 \text{ pu}$$

Since the voltage at the faulted bus 4 before the fault has taken place is $1.0\angle 0°$ puV, then

$$\mathbf{I}_{af} = 3\mathbf{I}_{a1} = 3\left(\frac{\mathbf{V}_F}{(\mathbf{Z}_{0,th} + \mathbf{Z}_{1,th} + \mathbf{Z}_{2,th}) + 3\mathbf{Z}f}\right)$$

$$= \frac{3.0\angle 0°}{j0.1208 + j0.2126 + j0.2126 + 3(j0.1)}$$

$$\cong 3.555\angle -90° \text{ pu}$$

Since the current base at bus 4 is

$$I_B = \frac{S_{B(3\phi)}}{\sqrt{3} \times V_{L-L}}$$

$$= \frac{50 \times 10^6 \text{ VA}}{\sqrt{3} \times (15 \times 10^3 \text{ V})}$$

$$= 192.45 \text{ A}$$

the phase fault current in amps is

$$I_f = |\mathbf{I}_{af}| \times I_B$$

$$= (5.555 \text{ pu})(192.45 \text{ A})$$

$$\cong 684.16 \text{ A}$$

Example J.2

Consider the system given in Example J.1 and assume that there is a line-to-line fault at bus 3 involving phases b and c. Determine the fault currents for both phases in per units and amperes. Consider the system showing in Figure G.1 and the following data:

Generator G_1: 15 kV, 50 MVA, $X_1 = X_2 = 0.10$ pu and $X_0 = 0.05$ pu based on its own ratings.
Synchronous motor: 15 kV, 20 MVA, $X_1 = X_2 = 0.20$ pu and $X_0 = 0.07$ pu based on its own ratings.
Transformer T_1: 15/115 kV, 30 MVA, $X_1 = X_2 = X_0 = 0.06$ pu based on its own ratings.
Transformer T_2: 115/15 kV, 25 MVA, $X_1 = X_2 = X_0 = 0.07$ pu based on its own ratings.
Transmission line TL_{23}: $X_1 = X_2 = 0.03$ pu and $X_0 = 0.10$ pu based on its own ratings.

Assume an SLG fault at bus 3 and determine the fault current in per units and amperes. Use 50 MVA as the megavolt-ampere base and assume that $\mathbf{Z}_f$ is $j0.1$ pu based on 50 MVA.

Solution

Assuming a line-to-line fault at bus 3 with a $\mathbf{Z}_f = j0.1$ pu on 50 MVA base, the given reactance has already been adjusted based on the new $S_{B(new)} = 50$ MVA. Hence, for generator G_1,

$$\mathbf{Z}_1 = \mathbf{Z}_2 = j0.10 \text{ pu}$$

and

$$\mathbf{Z}_0 = j0.05 \text{ pu}$$

For transformer T_1,

$$\mathbf{Z}_1 = \mathbf{Z}_2 = \mathbf{Z}_0 = j0.01\,\text{pu}$$

For transmission line TL_{23},

$$\mathbf{Z}_1 = \mathbf{Z}_2 = j0.03\,\text{pu}$$

and

$$\mathbf{Z}_0 = j0.10\,\text{pu}$$

For transformer T_2,

$$\mathbf{Z}_1 = \mathbf{Z}_2 = \mathbf{Z}_0 = j0.14\,\text{pu}$$

For synchronous motor M,

$$\mathbf{Z}_1 = \mathbf{Z}_2 = j0.5\,\text{pu}$$

and

$$\mathbf{Z}_0 = j0.175\,\text{pu}$$

Thus, the Thévenin impedance at the faulted bus 3 is

$$
\begin{aligned}
\mathbf{Z}_{1,th} &= \frac{\left(\mathbf{Z}_{1,G_1} + \mathbf{Z}_{1,T_1} + \mathbf{Z}_{1,TL}\right)\left(\mathbf{Z}_{1,M} + \mathbf{Z}_{1,T_2}\right)}{\mathbf{Z}_{1,G_1} + \mathbf{Z}_{1,T_1} + \mathbf{Z}_{1,TL} + \mathbf{Z}_{1,T_2} + \mathbf{Z}_{1,M}} \\
&= j\frac{(0.10 + 0.10 + 0.03)(0.14 + 0.5)}{(0.10 + 0.10 + 0.03 + 0.14 + 0.5)} \\
&= j0.1692\ \text{pu}
\end{aligned}
$$

Since

$$\mathbf{Z}_{2,th} = \mathbf{Z}_{1,th} = j0.1692\ \text{pu}$$

and the voltage at the faulted bus 3 before the fault has taken place is $1.0\angle 0°\ \text{pu V}$,

$$
\begin{aligned}
\mathbf{I}_{a1} &= \left(\frac{\mathbf{V}_F}{\mathbf{Z}_{1,th} + \mathbf{Z}_{2,th}}\right) \\
&= \frac{1.0\angle 0°}{j0.1692 + j0.1692} \\
&= 2.9552\angle -90°\ \text{pu}
\end{aligned}
$$

Hence, faulted phase currents for phases b and c are

$$\mathbf{I}_{bf} = \sqrt{3}\mathbf{I}_{a1}\angle - 90°$$

$$= \sqrt{3}\left(-j2.9552\,\text{pu}\right)\angle - 90°$$

$$= -5.1186\,\text{pu}$$

where

$$\angle - 90° = -j$$

Since current base 3 is

$$I_B = \frac{S_{B(3\phi)}}{\sqrt{3}\times V_{L-L}}$$

$$= \frac{50\times 10^6\,\text{VA}}{\sqrt{3}\times\left(115\times 10^3\,\text{V}\right)}$$

$$= 251.02\,\text{A}$$

then the phase fault current in amperes is

$$I_{bf} = \left|\mathbf{I}_{bf}\right|\times I_B$$

$$= \left(5.1186\,\text{pu}\right)\left(251.02\,\text{A}\right)$$

$$= -1284.9\,\text{A}$$

and

$$\mathbf{I}_{cf} = -\mathbf{I}_{bf} = -\left(-5.1186\right) = 5.1186\,\text{pu}$$

$$\mathbf{I}_{cf} = -\mathbf{I}_{bf} = -\left(-1284.9\,\text{A}\right) = 1284.9\,\text{A}$$

Example J.3

Consider the system given in Example J.1 and assume that there is a DLG fault at bus 2, involving phases b and c. Assume that $\mathbf{Z}_f$ is $j0.1$ pu and $\mathbf{Z}_g$ is $j0.2$ pu (where $\mathbf{Z}_g$ is the neutral-to-ground impedance) both based on 50 VA. Consider the system shown in Figure J.1 and the following data:

Generator G_1: 15 kV, 50 MVA, $X_1 = X_2 = 0.10$ pu and $X_0 = 0.05$ pu based on its own ratings.
Synchronous motor: 15 kV, 20 MVA, $X_1 = X_2 = 0.20$ pu and $X_0 = 0.07$ pu based on its own ratings.
Transformer T_1: 15/115 kV, 30 MVA, $X_1 = X_2 = X_0 = 0.06$ pu based on its own ratings.
Transformer T_2: 115/15 kV, 25 MVA, $X_1 = X_2 = X_0 = 0.07$ pu based on its own ratings.
Transmission line TL$_{23}$: $X_1 = X_2 = 0.03$ pu and $X_0 = 0.10$ pu based on its own ratings.

Assume a DLG fault at bus 2, involving phases b and c, and determine the fault current in per units and amperes. Use 50 MVA as the megavolt-ampere base and assume that $\mathbf{Z}_f$ is $j0.1$ pu and $\mathbf{Z}_g$ is $j0.2$ pu (where $\mathbf{Z}_g$ is the neutral-to-ground impedance) both based on 50 MVA.

Solution

The Thévenin impedance at the faulted bus 2 is

$$\mathbf{Z}_{1,th} = \frac{\left(\mathbf{Z}_{1,G} + \mathbf{Z}_{1,T_1}\right)\left(\mathbf{Z}_{1,TL_{23}} + \mathbf{Z}_{1,T_2} + \mathbf{Z}_{1,M}\right)}{\mathbf{Z}_{1,G} + \mathbf{Z}_{1,T_1} + \mathbf{Z}_{1,TL_{23}} + \mathbf{Z}_{1,T_2} + \mathbf{Z}_{1,M}}$$

$$= j\frac{(0.10 + 0.10)(0.03 + 0.14 + 0.05)}{(0.10 + 0.10)(0.03 + 0.14 + 0.05)}$$

$$= j0.15402 \text{ pu}$$

Since

$$\mathbf{Z}_{2,th} = \mathbf{Z}_{1,th} = j0.15402 \text{ pu}$$

and

$$\mathbf{Z}_{0,th} = \frac{\left(\mathbf{Z}_{0,G} + \mathbf{Z}_{0,T_1}\right)\left(\mathbf{Z}_{0,TL_{23}} + \mathbf{Z}_{0,T_2} + \mathbf{Z}_{0,M}\right)}{\mathbf{Z}_{0,G} + \mathbf{Z}_{0,T_1} + \mathbf{Z}_{0,TL_{23}} + \mathbf{Z}_{0,T_2} + \mathbf{Z}_{0,M}}$$

$$= j\frac{(0.05 + 0.10)(0.10 + 0.14 + 0.175)}{(0.05 + 0.10)(0.10 + 0.14 + 0.175)}$$

$$= j0.11018 \text{ pu}$$

then

$$\mathbf{I}_{a1} = \frac{\mathbf{V}_F}{\mathbf{Z}_f + \mathbf{Z}_{1,th} + \dfrac{\left(\mathbf{Z}_{2,th} + \mathbf{Z}_f\right)\left(\mathbf{Z}_{0,TL_{23}} + \mathbf{Z}_f + 3\mathbf{Z}_g\right)}{\mathbf{Z}_{2,th} + \mathbf{Z}_{0,th} + 2\mathbf{Z}_f + 3\mathbf{Z}_g}}$$

$$= -j\frac{1.0\angle 0°}{0.1 + 0.154 + \dfrac{(0.154 + 0.1)(0.110 + 0.1 + 0.6)}{0.154 + 0.110 + 0.2 + 0.6}}$$

$$= -j2.2351 \text{ pu}$$

Here, by applying current division,

$$\mathbf{I}_{a0} = -\left(\frac{\mathbf{Z}_{2,th} + \mathbf{Z}_f}{\mathbf{Z}_{2,th} + \mathbf{Z}_{0,th} + 2\mathbf{Z}_f + 3\mathbf{Z}_g}\right)\mathbf{I}_{a1}$$

$$= -\left(\frac{(j0.254)(-j2.2354)}{j0.154 + j0.110 + j0.2 + j0.6}\right)(-j2.2351)$$

$$= j0.53351 \text{ pu}$$

and similarly,

$$\mathbf{I}_{a2} = -\left(\frac{\mathbf{Z}_{0,th} + \mathbf{Z}_f + 3\mathbf{Z}_g}{\mathbf{Z}_{2,th} + \mathbf{Z}_{0,th} + 2\mathbf{Z}_f + 3\mathbf{Z}_g}\right)\mathbf{I}_{a1}$$

$$= -\left(\frac{(j0.254)(-j2.2352)}{j0.154 + j0.110 + j0.2 + j0.6}\right)(-j2.2351)$$

$$= j1.70161 \text{ pu}$$

or

$$\mathbf{I}_{a2} = -\left(\mathbf{I}_{a1} + \mathbf{I}_{a0}\right)$$

$$= -\left(-j2.2351 + j0.53351\right)$$

$$\cong j1.70161 \text{ pu}$$

Hence, the ground current is

$$\mathbf{I}_{G} = 3\mathbf{I}_{a0}$$

$$= 3\left(-0.53351\angle -90°\right)$$

$$\cong 1.6005\angle -90° \text{ pu}$$

Or since

$$I_{B} = \frac{50,000 \text{ kVA}}{\sqrt{3}\left(115 \text{ kV}\right)}$$

$$= 251.02 \text{ A}$$

or

$$I_{G} = I_{G,\text{pu}} \times I_{B}$$

$$= \left|\left(1.6005\angle -90°\right)\right|\left(251.02\right)$$

$$= 401.77 \text{ A}$$

then the faulted phase current is

$$\mathbf{I}_{bf} = \mathbf{I}_{a0} + a^{2}\mathbf{I}_{a1} + a\mathbf{I}_{a2}$$

$$= \left(0.53351\angle -90°\right) + \left(1\angle 240°\right)\left(2.2351\angle -90°\right) + \left(1\angle 120°\right)\left(1.70161\angle -90°\right)$$

$$= 3.5017\angle 166.79° \text{ pu}$$

or

$$I_{bf} = \left|I_{bf,\text{pu}}\right| \times I_{B}$$

$$= 3.5017 \times 251.02$$

$$= 879.62 \text{ A}$$

and

$$\mathbf{I}_{cf} = \mathbf{I}_{a0} + a\mathbf{I}_{a1} + a^{2}\mathbf{I}_{a2}$$

$$= \left(0.53351\angle -90°\right) + \left(1\angle 120°\right)\left(2.2351\angle -90°\right) + \left(1\angle 240°\right)\left(1.70161\angle -90°\right)$$

$$= 3.5017\angle 13.21° \text{ pu}$$

or

$$I_{cf} = \left|I_{cf,\text{pu}}\right| \times I_{B}$$

$$= 3.5017 \times 251.02$$

$$= 879.62 \text{ A}$$

Example J.4

Consider the system shown in Figure J.4 and assume that the generator is loaded and running at the rated voltage with the CB open at bus 3. Assume that the reactance values of the generator are given as $X_d'' = X_1 = X_2 = 0.14$ pu and $X_0 = 0.08$ pu based on its ratings. The transformer impedances are $Z_1 = Z_2 = Z_0 = j0.05$ pu based on its ratings. The transmission line TL_{23} has $Z_1 = Z_2 = j0.04$ pu and $Z_0 = j0.10$ pu. Assume that the fault point is located on bus 1. Select 25 MVA as the megavolt-ampere base and 8.5 and 138 kV as the LV and HV voltage bases, respectively, and determine the following:

(a) Subtransient fault current for three-phase fault in per units and amperes.
(b) SLG fault. [Also find the ratio of this SLG fault current to the three-phase fault current found in part (a).]
(c) Line-to-line fault. (Also find the ratio of this line-to-line fault current to previously calculated three-phase fault current.)
(d) DLG fault.

Solution

(a) The subtransient fault current is

$$\mathbf{I}_{f,3\phi}'' = \frac{1.0\angle 0°}{\mathbf{Z}_1}$$

$$= \frac{1.0\angle 0°}{j0.14}$$

$$= 0.7143\angle -90° \text{ pu}$$

Since $\mathbf{I}_{f(L-L)}$ is about 86.6% of $\mathbf{I}_{f(3\phi)}$, then

$$\left|\mathbf{I}_{f(L-L)}\right| = \frac{\sqrt{3}}{2}\left|\mathbf{I}_{f(3\phi)}\right|$$

$$= \frac{\sqrt{3}}{2}\left|8.3333\right|$$

$$= 7.2169 \text{ A}$$

(b) The SLG fault current is

$$\mathbf{I}_{af} = \mathbf{I}_{a(L-G)} = 3\mathbf{I}_{a0} = \frac{3(1.0\angle 0°)}{\mathbf{Z}_0 + \mathbf{Z}_1 + \mathbf{Z}_2}$$

$$= \frac{3.0\angle 0°}{j(0.08 + 0.14 + 0.14)}$$

$$= -j8.3333 \text{ pu}$$

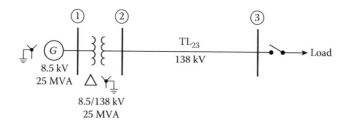

FIGURE J.4 System for Example J.4.

and

$$\frac{I_{f(\text{L-G})}}{I_{f(3\phi)}} = \frac{8.3333}{7.2169} = 1.1547$$

(c) Since $\mathbf{I}_{a0} = 0$ and $\mathbf{I}_{af} = 0$,

$$\mathbf{I}_{a1} = -\mathbf{I}_{a2} = \frac{1.0\angle 0}{\mathbf{Z}_1 + \mathbf{Z}_2}$$

$$= \frac{1.0\angle 0°}{j0.14 + j0.14}$$

$$= -j3.571 \text{ pu}$$

Therefore,

$$\mathbf{I}_{cf} = -\sqrt{3}\mathbf{I}_{a1}\angle -90°$$

$$= \sqrt{3}\,(3.571)\angle -90°$$

$$= -6.186 \text{ pu}$$

and

$$\mathbf{I}_{cf} = -\mathbf{I}_{bf}$$

$$= (6.186 \text{ pu})(1{,}698.089 \text{ A})$$

$$= 10{,}504.2 \text{ A}$$

and the ratio is

$$\frac{I_{f(\text{L-L})}}{I_{f(3\phi)}} = \frac{6.186}{7.143} = 0.866$$

Thus,

$$I_{f(\text{L-L})} = 86.6\% \text{ of } I_{f(3\phi)}$$

(d) In order to calculate the DLG fault current,

$$\mathbf{I}_{a1} = \frac{1.0\angle 0°}{\mathbf{Z}_1 + \dfrac{\mathbf{Z}_2 \times \mathbf{Z}_0}{\mathbf{Z}_2 + \mathbf{Z}_0}}$$

$$= \frac{1.0\angle 0°}{j0.14 + j\dfrac{0.14 \times 0.08}{0.14 + 0.08}}$$

$$= -j5.2381 \text{ pu}$$

where

$$\mathbf{V}_{a1} = 1.0\angle 0° - \mathbf{I}_{a1}\mathbf{Z}_{1,G}$$

$$= 1 - (-j5.2381)(j0.14)$$

$$= 0.26667 \text{ pu}$$

so that

$$\mathbf{I}_{a2} = -\frac{\mathbf{V}_{a1}}{\mathbf{Z}_2}$$

$$= -\frac{0.26667}{j0.14}$$

$$= j1.9048 \text{ pu}$$

and

$$\mathbf{I}_{a0} = -\frac{\mathbf{V}_{a1}}{\mathbf{Z}_0}$$

$$= -\frac{2.6667}{j0.08}$$

$$= j3.3333 \text{ pu}$$

also,

$$\mathbf{I}_{nf} = \text{neutral current at fault}$$

$$= 3\mathbf{I}_{a0}$$

$$= 3(j3.3333)$$

$$= j10.013 \text{ pu}$$

The faulted phase currents are

$$\mathbf{I}_{bf} = \mathbf{I}_{a0} + a^2\mathbf{I}_{a1} + a\mathbf{I}_{a2}$$

$$= j3.3333 + (1.0\angle 240°)(-j5.238) + (1.0\angle 120°)(j1.905)$$

$$\cong -6.1857 + j5.0001$$

$$\cong 7.954\angle 218.95° \text{ pu}$$

and

$$\mathbf{I}_{cf} = \mathbf{I}_{a0} + a\mathbf{I}_{a1} + a^2\mathbf{I}_{a2}$$

$$= j3.3333 + (1.0\angle 120°)(-j5.238) + (1.0\angle 240°)(j1.905)$$

$$\cong 6.1857 + j5.0001$$

$$\cong 7.954\angle 38.95° \text{ pu}$$

Hence,

$$I_{bf} = I_{cf} = \left| \mathbf{I}_{bf,pu} \right| I_B$$

$$= 7.954 \times 1698.089$$

$$= 13.501 \text{ A}$$

Example J.5

Repeat Example J.4 assuming that the fault is located on bus 2.

Solution

(a) The subtransient fault current is

$$\mathbf{I}''_{f,3\phi} = \frac{1.0\angle 0°}{\mathbf{Z}_{1,G} + \mathbf{Z}_{1,T_1}}$$

$$= \frac{1.0\angle 0°}{j0.14 + j0.05}$$

$$= \frac{1.0\angle 0°}{j0.19}$$

$$= 5.2632\angle -90° \text{ pu}$$

Since $\mathbf{I}_{f(L-L)}$ is about 86.6% of $\mathbf{I}_{f(3\phi)}$, then

$$\left|\mathbf{I}_{f(L-L)}\right| = \frac{\sqrt{3}}{2}\left|\mathbf{I}_{f(3\phi)}\right|$$

$$= \frac{\sqrt{3}}{2}\left|5.2632\right|$$

$$= 4.5580 \text{ A}$$

(c) The SLG fault current is

$$\mathbf{I}_{af} = \mathbf{I}_{a(L-G)} = 3\mathbf{I}_{a0} = \frac{3(1.0\angle 0°)}{\mathbf{Z}_0 + \mathbf{Z}_1 + \mathbf{Z}_2}$$

$$= \frac{3.0\angle 0°}{j(0.05 + 0.19 + 0.19)}$$

$$= -j6.9767 \text{ pu}$$

where

$$\mathbf{Z}_1 = \mathbf{Z}_{1,G} + \mathbf{Z}_{1,T_1} = j0.14 + j0.05 = j0.19 \text{ pu}$$

$$\mathbf{Z}_2 = \mathbf{Z}_{2,G} + \mathbf{Z}_{2,T_1} = j0.14 + j0.05 = j0.19 \text{ pu}$$

$$\mathbf{Z}_0 = \mathbf{Z}_{0,T_1} = j0.05 = j0.05 \text{ pu}$$

and

$$I_B = \frac{25 \times 10^6}{\sqrt{3}(138 \times 10^3)} 104.59 \text{ A}$$

Also,

$$\mathbf{I}_{af} = \left|\mathbf{I}_{af}\right| \times I_B$$

$$= \left|-j6.9767\right| \times (104.59 \text{ A})$$

$$= 729.71 \text{ A}$$

and

$$\frac{I_{f(\text{L-G})}}{I_{f(3\phi)}} = \frac{6.9767}{5.2632} = 1.3255$$

(c) Since $\mathbf{I}_{a0} = 0$ and $\mathbf{I}_{af} = 0$,

$$\mathbf{I}_{a1} = -\mathbf{I}_{a2} = \frac{1.0\angle 0°}{\mathbf{Z}_1 + \mathbf{Z}_2}$$

$$= \frac{1.0\angle 0°}{j0.19 + j0.19}$$

$$= -j2.6316 \text{ pu}$$

Therefore,

$$\mathbf{I}_{cf} = -\sqrt{3}\mathbf{I}_{a1}\angle - 90°$$

$$= \sqrt{3}\,(2.6316)\angle - 90°$$

$$= -4.558 \text{ pu}$$

And

$$\mathbf{I}_{cf} = -\mathbf{I}_{bf}$$

$$= (4.558 \text{ pu})(104.592 \text{ A})$$

$$= 476.73 \text{ A}$$

and the ratio is

$$\frac{I_{f(\text{L-L})}}{I_{f(3\phi)}} = \frac{4.558}{5.2632} = 0.866$$

thus,

$$I_{f(\text{L-L})} = 86.6\% \text{ of } I_{f(3\phi)}$$

(d) In order to calculate the DLG fault current,

$$\mathbf{I}_{a1} = \frac{1.0\angle 0°}{\mathbf{Z}_1 + \dfrac{\mathbf{Z}_2 \times \mathbf{Z}_0}{\mathbf{Z}_2 + \mathbf{Z}_0}}$$

$$= \frac{1.0\angle 0°}{j0.19 + j\dfrac{0.19 \times 0.08}{0.19 + 0.08}}$$

$$= -j4.3557 \text{ pu}$$

where

$$\mathbf{V}_{a1} = 1.0\angle 0° - \mathbf{I}_{a1}\mathbf{Z}_{1,G}$$

$$= 1 - (-j4.3557)(j0.19)$$

$$= 0.17241 \text{ pu}$$

so that

$$\mathbf{I}_{a2} = -\frac{\mathbf{V}_{a1}}{\mathbf{Z}_2}$$

$$= -\frac{0.17241}{j0.19}$$

$$= j1.90744 \text{ pu}$$

and

$$\mathbf{I}_{a0} = -\frac{\mathbf{V}_{a1}}{\mathbf{Z}_0}$$

$$= -\frac{0.17241}{j0.05}$$

$$= j3.4483 \text{ pu}$$

also,

$$\mathbf{I}_{nf} = \text{neutral current at fault}$$

$$= 3\mathbf{I}_{a0}$$

$$= 3(j3.4483)$$

$$= j10.345 \text{ pu}$$

The faulted phase currents are

$$\mathbf{I}_{bf} = \mathbf{I}_{a0} + a^2\mathbf{I}_{a1} + a\mathbf{I}_{a2}$$

$$= j3.4483 + (1.0\angle240°)(-j4.3557) + (1.0\angle120°)(j0.90744)$$

$$\cong -4.5579 + j5.1722$$

$$\cong 6.8939\angle228.6° \text{ pu}$$

and

$$\mathbf{I}_{cf} = \mathbf{I}_{a0} + a\mathbf{I}_{a1} + a^2\mathbf{I}_{a2}$$

$$= j3.483 + (1.0\angle120°)(-j4.3557) + (1.0\angle240°)(j0.90744)$$

$$\cong 4.186 + j5.1722$$

$$\cong 6.8939\angle48.6° \text{ pu}$$

hence,

$$I_{bf} = I_{cf} = \left|\mathbf{I}_{bf,pu}\right| I_B$$

$$= 6.8939 \times 104.59$$

$$= 721.03 \text{ A}$$

Example J.6

Repeat Example J.4 assuming that the fault is located on bus 3.

Solution

(a) The subtransient fault current is

$$\mathbf{I}''_{f,3\phi} = \frac{1.0\angle 0°}{\mathbf{Z}_{1,G} + \mathbf{Z}_{1,T_1} + \mathbf{Z}_{TL_{23}}}$$

$$= \frac{1.0\angle 0°}{j0.14 + j0.05 + j0.05}$$

$$= \frac{1.0\angle 0°}{j0.23}$$

$$= 4.918\angle -90° \text{ pu}$$

Since $\mathbf{I}_{f(L\text{-}L)}$ is about 86.6% of $\mathbf{I}_{f(3\phi)}$, then

$$\left|\mathbf{I}_{f(L\text{-}L)}\right| = \frac{\sqrt{3}}{2}\left|\mathbf{I}_{f(3\phi)}\right|$$

$$= \frac{\sqrt{3}}{2}\left|4.918\right|$$

$$= 4.259 \text{ A}$$

(b) The SLG fault current is

$$\mathbf{I}_{af} = \mathbf{I}_{a(L\text{-}G)} = 3\mathbf{I}_{a0} = \frac{3(1.0\angle 0°)}{\mathbf{Z}_0 + \mathbf{Z}_1 + \mathbf{Z}_2}$$

$$= \frac{3.0\angle 0°}{j(0.15 + 0.23 + 0.23)}$$

$$= -j4.918 \text{ pu}$$

where

$$\mathbf{Z}_1 = \mathbf{Z}_{1,G} + \mathbf{Z}_{1,TL_{23}} = j0.14 + j0.05 + j0.04 = j0.23 \text{ pu}$$

$$\mathbf{Z}_2 = \mathbf{Z}_{2,G} + \mathbf{Z}_{2,T_1} + \mathbf{Z}_{2,TL_{23}} = j0.14 + j0.05 + j0.04 = j0.23 \text{ pu}$$

$$\mathbf{Z}_0 = \mathbf{Z}_{0,T_1} + \mathbf{Z}_{0,TL_{23}} = j0.05 + j0.10 = j0.15 \text{ pu}$$

and

$$I_B = \frac{25 \times 10^6}{\sqrt{3}(138 \times 10^3)} 104.59 \text{ A}$$

Also,

$$\mathbf{I}_{af} = \left|\mathbf{I}_{af}\right| \times I_B$$

$$= \left|-j4.918\right| \times (104.59 \text{ A})$$

$$= 514.39 \text{ A}$$

and

$$\frac{I_{f(L\text{-}G)}}{I_{f(3\phi)}} = \frac{4.918}{4.3478} \cong 1.1311$$

(c) Since $I_{a0} = 0$ and $I_{af} = 0$ for line-to-line fault,

$$I_{a1} = -I_{a2} = \frac{1.0\angle 0°}{Z_1 + Z_2}$$

$$= \frac{1.0\angle 0°}{j0.23 + j0.23}$$

$$= -j2.1739 \text{ pu}$$

Therefore,

$$I_{bf} = -\sqrt{3}I_{a1}\angle -90°$$

$$= \sqrt{3}(2.1739)\angle -90°$$

$$= -3.7653 \text{ pu}$$

or

$$I_{bf} = \left|I_{bf,pu}\right| \times I_B$$

$$= \sqrt{2}(2.1739\angle -90°)$$

$$= -3.7653 \text{ pu}$$

and

$$I_{cf} = -I_{bf}$$

$$= (3.7653 \text{ pu})(104.592 \text{ A})$$

$$= 393.82 \text{ A}$$

and the ratio is

$$\frac{I_{f(L-L)}}{I_{f(3\phi)}} = \frac{3.7653}{4.3478} = 0.866$$

thus,

$$I_{f(L-L)} = 86.6\% \text{ of } I_{f(3\phi)}$$

(c) In order to calculate the DLG fault current,

$$I_{a1} = \frac{1.0\angle 0°}{Z_1 + \dfrac{Z_2 \times Z_0}{Z_2 + Z_0}}$$

$$= \frac{1.0\angle 0°}{j0.23 + j\dfrac{0.23 \times 0.15}{0.23 + 0.15}}$$

$$= -j3.1173 \text{ pu}$$

where

$$V_{a1} = 1.0\angle 0° - I_{a1}Z_{1,G}$$

$$= 1 - (-j3.1173)(j0.23)$$

$$= 0.28302 \text{ pu}$$

so that

$$\mathbf{I}_{a2} = -\frac{\mathbf{V}_{a1}}{\mathbf{Z}_2}$$

$$= -\frac{0.28302}{j0.23}$$

$$= j1.2305 \text{ pu}$$

and

$$\mathbf{I}_{a0} = -\frac{\mathbf{V}_{a1}}{\mathbf{Z}_0}$$

$$= -\frac{0.28302}{j0.15}$$

$$= j1.8868 \text{ pu}$$

also,

$$\mathbf{I}_{nf} = \text{neutral current at fault}$$

$$= 3\mathbf{I}_{a0}$$

$$= 3(j1.8868)$$

$$= j5.6604 \text{ pu}$$

The faulted phase currents are

$$\mathbf{I}_{bf} = \mathbf{I}_{a0} + a^2\mathbf{I}_{a1} + a\mathbf{I}_{a2}$$

$$= j1.8868 + (1.0\angle 240°)(-j3.1173) + (1.0\angle 120°)(j1.2305)$$

$$\cong -3.7652 + j2.2801$$

$$\cong 4.4018\angle 211.2° \text{ pu}$$

and

$$\mathbf{I}_{cf} = \mathbf{I}_{a0} + a\mathbf{I}_{a1} + a^2\mathbf{I}_{a2}$$

$$= j1.8868 + (1.0\angle 120°)(-j3.1173) + (1.0\angle 240°)(j1.2305)$$

$$\cong 3.7652 + j2.8302$$

$$\cong 4.7103\angle 36.93° \text{ pu}$$

hence,

$$I_{bf} = I_{cf} = \left|\mathbf{I}_{bf,\text{pu}}\right| I_B$$

$$= 4.7103 \times 104.59$$

$$= 492.66 \text{ A}$$

Example J.7

Consider the system shown in Figure J.7. Assume that loads, line capacitance, and transformer-magnetizing currents are neglected and that the following data are given based on 20 MVA and the line-to-line voltages as shown in Figure G.7. Do not neglect the resistance of the transmission line TL_{23}. The prefault positive-sequence voltage at bus 3 is $\mathbf{V}_{an} = 1.0\angle 0°$ pu, as shown in Figure J.7.

Generator: $X_1 = 0.20$ pu, $X_2 = 0.10$ pu, $X_0 = 0.05$ pu.
Transformer T_1: $X_1 = X_2 = 0.05$ pu, $X_0 = X_1$ (looking into the HV side).
Transformer T_2: $X_1 = X_2 = 0.05$ pu, $X_0 = \infty$ (looking into the HV side).
Transmission line: $Z_1 = Z_2 = 0.2 + j0.2$ pu, $Z_0 = 0.6 + j0.6$ pu.

Assume that there is a bolted (i.e., with zero fault impedance) line-to-line fault on phases b and c at bus 3 and determine the following:

(a) Fault current $\mathbf{I}_{bf}$ in per units and amperes
(b) Phase voltages $\mathbf{V}_a$, $\mathbf{V}_b$, and $\mathbf{V}_c$ at bus 2 in per units and kilovolts
(c) Line-to-line voltages $\mathbf{V}_{ab}$, $\mathbf{V}_{bc}$, and $\mathbf{V}_{ca}$ at bus 2 in kilovolts
(d) Generator line currents $\mathbf{I}_a$, $\mathbf{I}_b$, and $\mathbf{I}_c$

Given: Per-unit positive-sequence currents on the LV side of the delta–wye-connected transformer bank and lag positive-sequence currents on the HV side by 30° and similarly negative-sequence currents on the LV side of the transformer bank and lead positive-sequence currents on the HV side by 30°

Solution

When fault is located on bus 3,

$$I_B = \frac{20 \times 10^6}{\sqrt{3}\left(20 \times 10^3\right)}$$

$$= 577.35 \text{ A}$$

(a) Since there is a bolted line-to-line fault, $\mathbf{I}_{a0} = 0$, $\mathbf{I}_{af} = 0$, and $\mathbf{Z}_f = 0$, then

$$\mathbf{I}_{a1} = -\mathbf{I}_{a2} = \frac{1.0\angle 0°}{\mathbf{Z}_1 + \mathbf{Z}_2}$$

$$= \frac{1.0\angle 0°}{\left(0.2 + j0.45\right) + \left(0.2 + j0.35\right)}$$

$$= \frac{1.0\angle 0°}{\left(0.4 + j\right)0.80}$$

$$= 1.118\angle -63.43° \text{ pu}$$

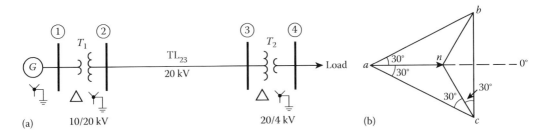

FIGURE J.7 System for Example J.7.

where

$$\mathbf{Z}_1 = \mathbf{Z}_{1,G} + \mathbf{Z}_{1,T_1} + \mathbf{Z}_{1,TL}$$

$$= j0.2 + j0.05 + (0.2 + j0.2)$$

$$= 0.2 + j0.45 \text{ pu}$$

and

$$\mathbf{Z}_2 = \mathbf{Z}_{2,G} + \mathbf{Z}_{2,T_1} + \mathbf{Z}_{2,TL}$$

$$= j0.1 + j0.05 + (0.2 + j0.2)$$

$$= 0.2 + j0.35 \text{ pu}$$

Therefore,

$$\mathbf{I}_{bf} = \sqrt{3}\mathbf{I}_{a1}\angle - 90°$$

$$= \sqrt{3}\,(3.571)\angle - 90°$$

$$= -6.186 \text{ pu}$$

and

$$\mathbf{I}_{bf} = \mathbf{I}_{a0} + a^2\mathbf{I}_{a1} + a\mathbf{I}_{a2}$$

$$= 0 + a^2\mathbf{I}_{a1} + a\mathbf{I}_{a2}$$

$$= (a^2 - a)\mathbf{I}_{a1}$$

$$= -j\sqrt{3}\,(1.118\angle - 63.4°)$$

$$\cong 1.94\angle 26.6° \text{ pu}$$

$$\cong (1.94\angle 26.6° \text{ pu})(577.35 \text{ A})$$

$$= 1120 \text{ A}$$

(b) The positive-sequence voltage at bus 2 is

$$\mathbf{V}_{a1}^{(2)} = 1.0\angle 0° - \mathbf{I}_{a1}\mathbf{Z}_1^{(2)}$$

$$= 1 - \frac{j0.25}{0.895\angle 63.4°}$$

$$= 0.75 - j0.121 \text{ pu}$$

$$= 0.76\angle - 9.2° \text{ pu}$$

so that

$$\mathbf{V}_{a2}^{(2)} = -\mathbf{Z}_2^{(2)} \times \mathbf{I}_{a2}$$

$$= \frac{j0.15}{0.895\angle 63.4°}$$

$$= 0.15 - j0.084$$

$$= 0.168\angle 26.6° \text{ pu}$$

and the faulted phase voltages are

$$\mathbf{V}_a^{(2)} = \mathbf{V}_{a0}^{(2)} + \mathbf{V}_{a1}^{(2)} + \mathbf{V}_{a2}^{(2)}$$

$$= 0 + 0.75 - j0.121 + 0.15 + j0.084$$

$$= 0.9 - j0.04 \text{ pu}$$

$$= 10.9 - j0.46 \text{ kV}$$

$$\mathbf{V}_b^{(2)} = \mathbf{V}_{a0}^{(2)} + a^2\mathbf{V}_{a1}^{(2)} + a\mathbf{V}_{a2}^{(2)}$$

$$= 0 + 0.76\angle -129.2° + 0.168\angle 46.6°$$

$$= -0.62 - j0.5 \text{ pu}$$

$$= -7.2 - j5.8 \text{ kV}$$

$$\mathbf{V}_c^{(2)} = \mathbf{V}_{a0}^{(2)} + a\mathbf{V}_{a1}^{(2)} + a^2\mathbf{V}_{a2}^{(2)}$$

$$= 0 + 0.76\angle 110.8° + 0.168\angle -93.4°$$

$$= -0.27 + j0.54 \text{ pu}$$

$$= -3.1 + j6.2 \text{ kV}$$

(c) The faulted line-to-line voltages are

$$\mathbf{V}_{ab} = \mathbf{V}_{an} - \mathbf{V}_{bn}$$

$$= 10.4 - j0.46 + 7.2 + j5.8$$

$$= 17.6 + j5.3 \text{ kV}$$

$$\mathbf{V}_{bc} = \mathbf{V}_{bn} - \mathbf{V}_{cn}$$

$$= -7.2 + j5.8 + 3.1 + j6.2$$

$$= -4.1 + j12 \text{ kV}$$

$$\mathbf{V}_{ca} = \mathbf{V}_{cn} - \mathbf{V}_{an}$$

$$= -3.1 + j6.2 - 10.4 + j0.46$$

$$= -13.5 + j6.7 \text{ kV}$$

(d) Generator line current is

$$\mathbf{I}_{a1} = -\mathbf{I}_{a2} = \frac{1.0\angle 0°}{\mathbf{Z}_1 + \mathbf{Z}_2}$$

$$= \frac{1.0\angle 0°}{0.4 + j0.80}$$

$$= \frac{1.0\angle 0°}{0.895\angle 63.4°}$$

$$= 1.12\angle -63.43° \text{ pu}$$

hence,

$$\mathbf{I}_{a1}^{(LV)} = 1.12\angle -93.4° \text{ pu}$$

$$\cong -j1.12 \text{ pu}$$

$$\mathbf{I}_{a2}^{(LV)} = -1.12\angle -33.4° \text{ pu}$$

$$\cong 0.935 - j0.615 \text{ pu}$$

Therefore,

$$\mathbf{I}_{a}^{(LV)} = -j1.12 - 0.935 - j0.615$$

$$= -0.935 - j0.5 \text{ pu}$$

$$= -1080 - j576 \text{ A}$$

$$\mathbf{I}_{b}^{(LV)} = 1.12\angle 146.6° - 1.21\angle 86.6°$$

$$= -0.935 + j0.615 - j1.12 \text{ pu}$$

$$= -0.935 - j0.5 \text{ pu}$$

$$= -1080 - j576 \text{ A}$$

$$\mathbf{I}_{c}^{(LV)} = 1.12\angle 26.6° - 1.21\angle -153.4°$$

$$= 1 + j0.5 + 1 + j0.5 \text{ pu}$$

$$= 2 + j1 \text{ pu}$$

$$= 2310 + j1155 \text{ A}$$

Note: Some of the calculations were done by slide rule, and thus, the answers are approximate.

Example J.8

Consider Figure J.8 and assume that the generator ratings are 2.40/4.16Y kV, 15 MW (3ϕ), 18.75 MVA (3ϕ), 80% PF, two poles, and 3600 rpm. Generator reactances are $X_1 = X_2 = 0.10$ pu and $X_0 = 0.05$ pu, all based on generator ratings. Note that the given value of X_1 is subtransient reactance X'', one of several different positive-sequence reactances of a synchronous machine. The subtransient reactance corresponds to the initial symmetrical fault current (the transient dc component not included) that occurs before demagnetizing armature magnetomotive force begins to weaken the net field excitation. If manufactured in accordance with US standards, the coils of a synchronous generator will withstand the mechanical forces that accompany a three-phase fault current, but not more. Assume that this generator is to supply a four-wire, wye-connected distribution. Therefore, the neutral grounding reactor X_n should have the smallest possible reactance. Consider both SLG and DLG faults. Assume the prefault positive-sequence internal voltage of phase a is 2500∠0° or 1.042 0° 1.042∠0° pu and determine the following:

(a) Specify X_n in ohms and in per units.
(b) Specify the minimum allowable momentary symmetrical current rating of the reactor in amperes.
(c) Find the initial symmetrical voltage across the reactor, $\mathbf{V}_n$, when a bolted SLG fault occurs on the OCB terminal in volts.

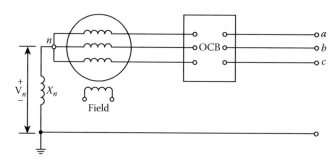

FIGURE J.8 System for Example J.8.

Solution

$$\mathbf{I}_{a(3\phi)} = \frac{\mathbf{V}_F}{\mathbf{Z}_1} = \frac{1.042\angle0°}{j0.1} = -j10.427 \text{ pu}$$

SLG fault

$$\left|\mathbf{I}_{a(\text{SLG})}\right| = 3\mathbf{I}_{a0} = 3\left(\frac{1.042\angle0°}{j(0.25+3X_n)}\right)$$

When $X_n = 0$,

$$\left|\mathbf{I}_{a(\text{SLG})}\right| = \left|3\left(\frac{1.042\angle0°}{j(0.25+3\times0)}\right)\right|$$

$$= \left|-j12.5040\,\text{pu}\right| = 12.5 \text{ pu}$$

DLG fault

$$\mathbf{V}_F - \mathbf{I}_{a1}\mathbf{Z}_1 = -\mathbf{I}_{a2}\mathbf{Z}_2 = \mathbf{I}_{a1}\mathbf{Z}_2 + \mathbf{I}_{a0}\mathbf{Z}_2$$

$$\mathbf{I}_{a0}(\mathbf{Z}_0 + 3\mathbf{Z}_n) = \mathbf{I}_{a1}\mathbf{Z}_2 + \mathbf{I}_{a0}\mathbf{Z}_2$$

Substituting values in these equations,

$$-\mathbf{I}_{a0}(j0.5+3\times jX_n) = j0.1\times\mathbf{I}_{a1} = j0.1\mathbf{I}_{a1} + j0.1\times\mathbf{I}_{a0}$$

$$-\mathbf{I}_{a0}(j0.05+3\times jX_n) = j0.1\mathbf{I}_{a1} + j0.1\mathbf{I}_{a0}$$

or

$$-j0.1\mathbf{I}_{a1} - j0.1\mathbf{I}_{a1} - j0.1\mathbf{I}_{a0} = -1.042\angle0°$$

$$-j0.05\mathbf{I}_{a0} - 3x_n\mathbf{I}_{a0} - j0.1\mathbf{I}_{a1} - j0.1\mathbf{I}_{a0} = 0$$

Since $1.042\angle0° = 1.042 + j0$, then

$$j0.2\mathbf{I}_{a1} - j0.1\mathbf{I}_{a0} = -1.042$$

$$j0.1\mathbf{I}_{a1} - j0.15\mathbf{I}_{a0} - j3X_n\times\mathbf{I}_{a0} = 0$$

By multiplying both equations by (-1), we get

$$j0.2\mathbf{I}_{a1} + j0.1\mathbf{I}_{a0} = 1.042$$

$$j0.1\mathbf{I}_{a1} + j(0.15-j3X_n)\times\mathbf{I}_{a0} = 0$$

After multiplying the last equation by (-2) and then adding it to the previous equation and then simplifying it,

$$-j(0.2+6X_n)\mathbf{I}_{a0} = 1.042$$

so that

$$\mathbf{I}_{a0} = \frac{1.042}{-j(0.2+6X_n)} \quad \text{or} \quad \mathbf{I}_{a0} = \frac{1.042}{j(0.2+6X_n)}$$

since $(1/-j) = j$. Thus,

$$\mathbf{I}_{a2} = \frac{j(0.05+3X_n)\mathbf{I}_{a0}}{j0.1}$$

$$= \frac{j(0.05+30X_n)\times 1.042}{0.2+6X_n}$$

Since $\mathbf{I}_{a1} + \mathbf{I}_{a2} + \mathbf{I}_{a0} = 0$, then $\mathbf{I}_{a1} = -\mathbf{I}_{a2} - \mathbf{I}_{a0}$. Thus,

$$\mathbf{I}_{a1} = \frac{j(0.05+30X_n)1.042}{0.2+6X_n} - j\frac{1.042}{0.2+6X_n}$$

$$\mathbf{I}_{a1} = \frac{-j(1.563+31.26X_n)}{0.2+6X_n}$$

Thus, $\mathbf{I}_{a(SLG)} = \mathbf{I}_{a0} + \mathbf{I}_{a1} + \mathbf{I}_{a2} = \mathbf{I}_{af} = 0$

$$\mathbf{I}_{b(SLG)} = \mathbf{I}_{a0} + a^2\mathbf{I}_{a1} + a\mathbf{I}_{a2}, \quad \text{and} \quad \text{since } \mathbf{I}_{a2} = -\mathbf{I}_{a1},$$

$$\mathbf{I}_{b(SLG)} = \mathbf{I}_{a0} + a^2\mathbf{I}_{a1} + a(-\mathbf{I}_{a1})$$

$$= \mathbf{I}_{a0} + \mathbf{I}_{a1}(a^2 - a)$$

Since $\mathbf{I}_{a0} = -(\mathbf{I}_{a1} + \mathbf{I}_{a2})$,

$$\mathbf{I}_{b(SLG)} = \mathbf{I}_{a0}(1-a) + \mathbf{I}_{a1}(a^2 - a)$$

$$= \frac{j1.042(1-a)}{0.2+6X_n} - \frac{j(1.563+31.26X_n)(a^2 - a)}{0.2+6X_n}$$

When $X_n = 0$,

$$\left|\mathbf{I}_{b(DLG)}\right| = \frac{j(1-a)1.042}{0.2} - \frac{j(a^2-a)1.563}{0.2}$$

$$= 11.9376 \, \text{pu}$$

Since $a = 1\angle 120°$ and $a^2 = 1\angle 240°$, then

$$\left|\mathbf{I}_{c(DLG)}\right| = \frac{j(1-a^2)1.042}{0.2} - \frac{j(a-a^2)1.563}{0.2}$$

$$= 11.9376 \, \text{pu}$$

(a) Since the SLG fault without grounding reactor is the most severe fault for the machine windings, the ground reactance X_n will have to be designed for the fault:

$$\left|\mathbf{I}_{a(\text{SLG})}\right| = \left|3\mathbf{I}_{a0}\right|$$

or

$$\frac{3 \times 1.042}{0.25 + 3X_n} = \frac{V_f}{X''}$$

$$\frac{3 \times 1.042}{0.25 + 3X_n} = \frac{1.042}{0.10}$$

or

$$X_n = 0.0167 \text{ pu}$$

or

$$X_n = 0.0167 \left(\frac{4.16^2}{18.75}\right) = 0.0154 \ \Omega$$

(b) Specify the minimum allowable momentary symmetrical current rating of the reactor in amperes:

$$\left|\mathbf{I}_{X_n(\text{SLG})}\right| = \left|\mathbf{I}_{a(\text{SLG})}\right|$$

$$= \frac{3 \times 1.042}{0.25 + 3 \times 0.0167}$$

$$= 10.42 \text{ pu}$$

and

$$\mathbf{I}_{X_n(\text{DLG})} = \mathbf{I}_{b(\text{DLG})} + \mathbf{I}_{c(\text{DLG})} = 3\mathbf{I}_{a0(\text{DLG})}$$

$$10.42 = \frac{3 \times 1.042}{0.2 + 6 \times 0.0167}$$

Therefore, the minimum allowable momentary symmetrical current rating of the reactor is 10.42 pu or

$$10.42 \left[\frac{18.75 \times 10^6}{\sqrt{3}\left(4.16 \times 10^3\right)}\right] = 27115.3387 \text{ A} \cong 27{,}000 \text{ A}$$

(c) Find the initial symmetrical voltage across the reactor V_n when a bolted fault occurs on the OCB terminal in volts:

$$V_n = -I_{af}Z_n = -\left(3I_{ao}\right)Z_n$$

$$= -\left(-j10.42\right)\left(j0.0167\right)$$

$$= -0.1737 \text{ pu} \quad \text{or} \quad -0.1737 \times 2.4 \text{ kV} = -416.8 \text{ V}$$

Example J.9

Consider the system shown in Figure J.9 and the following data:

> Generator G: $X_1 = X_2 = 0.10$ pu and $X_0 = 0.05$ pu based on its ratings.
> Motor: $X_1 = X_2 = 0.10$ pu and $X_0 = 0.05$ pu based on its ratings.
> Transformer T_1: $X_1 = X_2 = X_0 = 0.05$ pu based on its ratings.
> Transformer T_2: $X_1 = X_2 = X_0 = 0.10$ pu based on its ratings.
> Transmission line TL_{23}: $X_1 = X_2 = X_0 = 0.09$ pu based on 25 MVA.

Assume that bus 2 is faulted and determine the faulted phase currents.

(a) Determine the three-phase fault.
(b) Determine the line-to-ground fault involving phase a.
(c) Use the results of part (a) and calculate the line-to-neutral phase voltages at the fault point.

Solution

Based on the 25 MVA base
Generator: $X_1 = X_2 = j0.10$ pu and $X_0 = j0.5$ pu

Transformer T_1: $Z_1 = Z_2 = Z_0 = j0.05\left(\dfrac{25}{20}\right) = j0.0625$ pu

Line: $Z_1 = Z_2 = Z_0 = j0.09$ pu

Transformer T_2: $Z_1 = Z_2 = Z_0 = j0.10\left(\dfrac{25}{20}\right) = j0.125$ pu

Motor: $X_1 = X_2 = j0.10\left(\dfrac{25}{10}\right) = j0.25$ pu

$$X_0 = j0.05\left(\frac{25}{10}\right) = j0.125 \text{ pu}$$

(a) The positive-sequence Thévenin impedance at the fault point is

$$\mathbf{Z}_{1,th} = j\frac{(0.10+0.0625)(0.09+0.125+0.25)}{0.10+0.0625+0.09+0.125+0.25} = j0.1204 \text{ pu}$$

$$\mathbf{I}_{f(3\phi)} = \frac{\mathbf{V}_F}{\mathbf{Z}_{1,th}} = \frac{1.0}{j0.1204} = -j8.3044 \text{ pu}$$

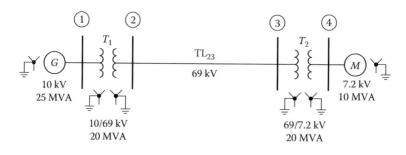

FIGURE J.9   System for Example J.9.

(b)

$$\mathbf{Z}_{0,th} = j\frac{(0.1125)(0.34)}{0.4525} = j0.0845 \ \text{pu}$$

$$\mathbf{Z}_{1,th} = \mathbf{Z}_{2,th} = j0.1204 \ \text{pu}$$

$$\mathbf{I}_{af} = \frac{3\mathbf{V}_F}{\mathbf{Z}_{1,th} + \mathbf{Z}_{2,th} + \mathbf{Z}_{0,th}}$$

$$= \frac{3(1.0\angle 0°)}{j0.1204 + j0.1204 + j0845}$$

$$= -j9.2214 \ \text{pu}$$

(c) Since the three-phase fault is a symmetrical one, at the fault point,

$$\mathbf{V}_a = \mathbf{V}_b = \mathbf{V}_c = 0$$

Example J.10

Consider the system given in Example J.9 and assume a line-to-line fault, involving phases b and c, at bus 2, and determine the faulted phase currents.

Solution

$$\mathbf{I}_{a1} = \frac{\mathbf{V}_F}{\mathbf{Z}_{1,th} + \mathbf{Z}_{2,th}}$$

$$= \frac{1.0\angle 0°}{j0.1204 + j0.1204}$$

$$= -j4.1522 \ \text{pu}$$

$$\mathbf{I}_{af} = 0$$

$$\mathbf{I}_{bf} = \sqrt{3}\mathbf{I}_{a1}\angle -90°$$

$$= \sqrt{3}(-j4.1522)(-j)$$

$$= -7.1918 \ \text{pu}$$

$$\mathbf{I}_{cf} = -\mathbf{I}_{bf} = 7.1918 \ \text{pu}$$

Example J.11

Consider the system shown in Figure J.11 and assume that the associated data are given in Table J.11 and are based on a 100 MVA base and referred to nominal system voltages.

   Assume that there is a three-phase fault at bus 6. Ignore the prefault currents and determine the following:

(a) Fault current in per units at faulted bus 6
(b) Fault current in per units in transmission line TL_{25}

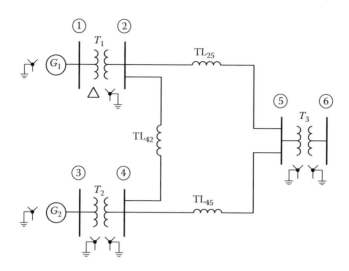

FIGURE J.11   System Example J.11.

TABLE J.11
Data for Example J.11

Network Component	X_1 (pu)	X_2 (pu)	X_3 (pu)
G_1	0.35	0.35	0.09
G_2	0.35	0.35	0.09
T_1	0.10	0.10	0.10
T_2	0.10	0.10	0.10
T_3	0.05	0.05	0.05
TL_{42}	0.45	0.45	1.80
TL_{25}	0.35	0.45	1.15
TL_{45}	0.35	0.35	1.15

Solution

Since $\mathbf{Z}_{1,th} = j0.45$ pu

(a)

$$\mathbf{I}_{f(3\phi)} = \frac{\mathbf{V}_F}{\mathbf{Z}_{1,th}}$$

$$= \frac{1.0\angle 0°}{j0.45}$$

$$= -j2.2222 \text{ pu}$$

(b)   The fault current in line TL_{25} is

$$\frac{\mathbf{I}_{f(3\phi)}}{2} = \frac{\mathbf{V}_F}{\mathbf{Z}_{1,th}} = \frac{1.0\angle 0°}{j0.45} = -j2.222 \text{ pu}$$

Example J.12

Use the results of Problem J.11 and calculate the line-to-neutral phase voltages at the faulted bus 6.

Solution

The three-phase fault is symmetrical. Thus,

$$\mathbf{V}_{a1} = \mathbf{V}_F - \mathbf{I}_{a1}\mathbf{Z}_1$$
$$= 1.0 - (j0.45)(-j2.222)$$
$$= 0$$

Since

$$\mathbf{V}_{a2} = \mathbf{V}_{a0} = 0$$

then

$$\mathbf{V}_{an} = \mathbf{V}_{a1} + \mathbf{V}_{a2} + \mathbf{V}_{a0} = 0$$

Therefore,

$$\mathbf{V}_{bn} = \mathbf{V}_{cn} = 0$$

Example J.13

Repeat Problem J.11 assuming a line-to-ground fault, with $\mathbf{Z}_f = 0$ pu, at bus 6.

Solution

(a) Since the fault is an SLG fault at bus 6,

$$\mathbf{Z}_{0,th} = j0.97744 \text{ pu}$$

$$\mathbf{Z}_{1,th} = \mathbf{Z}_{2,th} = j0.45 \text{ pu}$$

Thus,

$$\mathbf{I}_{a0} = \mathbf{I}_{a1} = \mathbf{I}_{a2} = \frac{\mathbf{V}_F}{\mathbf{Z}_{1,th} + \mathbf{Z}_{2,th} + \mathbf{Z}_{0,th}} = -j0.5326 \text{ pu}$$

$$\mathbf{I}_{a(\text{SLG})} = 3\mathbf{I}_{a0} = -j1.5979 \text{ pu}$$

(b) The sequence SLG fault currents in line TL_{25} are

$$\mathbf{I}'_{a1} = \mathbf{I}''_{a2} = \frac{\mathbf{I}_{a1}}{2} = \frac{-j0.5326}{2} = -j0.2663 \text{ pu}$$

$$\mathbf{I}'_{a0} = \mathbf{I}_{a0}\left(\frac{j1.8 + j1.15}{j1.15 + j1.15 + j1.8}\right)$$

$$= (-j0.5326 \text{ pu})\left(\frac{j2.95}{j4.1}\right)$$

$$= -j0.3832 \text{ pu}$$

Thus, the SLG fault current in line TL_{25} is

$$\mathbf{I}'_{a(\text{SLG})} = \mathbf{I}'_{a0} + \mathbf{I}'_{a1} + \mathbf{I}'_{a2}$$

$$= -j0.3832 - j0.2663 - j0.2663$$

$$= -j0.9159 \text{ pu}$$

Example J.14

Use results of Problem J.13 and calculate the line-to-neutral phase voltages at the following buses:

(a) Bus 6
(b) Bus 2

Solution

(a) At bus 6,

$$\mathbf{V}_{a1} = \mathbf{V}_F - \mathbf{I}_{a1}\mathbf{Z}_1 = 1 - (-j0.5326)(j0.45) = 0.7603 \text{ pu}$$

$$\mathbf{V}_{a2} = 0 - \mathbf{I}_{a2}\mathbf{Z}_2 = -(-j0.5326)(j0.45) = -0.2397 \text{ pu}$$

$$\mathbf{V}_{a0} = 0 - \mathbf{I}_{a0}\mathbf{Z}_0 = -(-j0.5326)(j0.9774) = -0.5206 \text{ pu}$$

so that

$$\mathbf{V}_{af} = \mathbf{V}_{a0} + \mathbf{V}_{a1} + \mathbf{V}_{a2} = -0.5206 + 0.7603 - 0.2397 = 0$$

$$\mathbf{V}_{bf} = \mathbf{V}_{a0} + a^2\mathbf{V}_{a1} + a\mathbf{V}_{a2}$$

$$= -0.5206 + (1\angle 240°)0.7603 + (1\angle 120°)(-0.2397)$$

$$= 1.1661\angle -132.0425° \text{ pu} \quad \text{or} \quad \cong 1.1661\angle 227.96°$$

$$\mathbf{V}_{cf} = \mathbf{V}_{a0} + a\mathbf{V}_{a1} + a^2\mathbf{V}_{a2}$$

$$= -0.5206 + (1\angle 120°)0.7603 + (1\angle 240°)(-0.2397)$$

$$= 1.1661\angle 132.0425° \text{ pu}$$

(b) *At bus 2*, it is left to the reader.

Example J.15

Repeat Problem J.11 assuming a line-to-line fault at bus 6.

Solution

(a) Since the fault at bus 6 is a line-to-line fault,

$$\mathbf{Z}_{1,th} = \mathbf{Z}_{2,th} = j0.45 \text{ pu}$$

$$\mathbf{I}_{a1} = \frac{\mathbf{V}_F}{\mathbf{Z}_{1,th} + \mathbf{Z}_{2,th}}$$

$$= \frac{1.0\angle 0°}{j0.45 + j0.45}$$

$$= -j1.1111 \text{ pu}$$

$$\mathbf{I}_{af} = 0$$

$$\mathbf{I}_{bf} = \sqrt{3}\mathbf{I}_{a1}\angle -90°$$

$$= \sqrt{3}(-j1.1111)(-j)$$

$$= -1.9245 \text{ pu}$$

$$\mathbf{I}_{cf} = -\mathbf{I}_{bf}$$

$$= 1.9245 \text{ pu}$$

(b) The L-L fault currents in line TL_{25} are

$$I'_{bf} = \frac{-1.9245}{2}$$

$$= -0.9623 \text{ pu}$$

$$I'_{cf} = \frac{-1.9245}{2}$$

$$= -0.9623 \text{ pu}$$

Example J.16

Repeat Problem J.11 assuming a DLG fault, with $\mathbf{Z}_f = 0$ and $\mathbf{Z}_g = 0$, at bus 6.

Solution

(a) Since the fault is a DLG fault,

$$I_{a1} = \frac{V_f}{\mathbf{Z}_1 + \dfrac{\mathbf{Z}_2 \times \mathbf{Z}_0}{\mathbf{Z}_2 + \mathbf{Z}_0}}$$

$$= \frac{1.0 \angle 90°}{j0.45 + \dfrac{(j0.977744)(j0.45)}{(j0.977744) + (j0.45)}}$$

$$= -j1.3190 \text{ pu}$$

$$\mathbf{V}_{a1} = \mathbf{V}_{a2} = \mathbf{V}_{a0} = \mathbf{V}_f - I_{a1}\mathbf{Z}_1$$

$$= 1.0 \angle 0° - (-j1.3190)(j0.45)$$

$$= 0.4064 \text{ pu}$$

$$I_{a2} = -\frac{\mathbf{V}_{a2}}{\mathbf{Z}_2} = -\frac{0.4064}{j0.45} = j0.9032 \text{ pu}$$

$$I_{a0} = -\frac{\mathbf{V}_{a0}}{\mathbf{Z}_0} = -\frac{0.4064}{j0.97744} = j0.4158 \text{ pu}$$

$$I_{af} = 0$$

$$I_{bf} = I_{a1}a^2 + I_{a2}a + I$$

$$= (-j1.3190)(1\angle -120°) + (j0.9032)(1\angle 120°) + j0.4158$$

$$= -1.9245 + j0.6237$$

$$\cong 2.0231 \angle 162.04° \text{ pu}$$

$$I_{cf} = I_{a1}a + I_{a2}a^2 + I_{a0}$$

$$= (-j1.3190)(1\angle 120°) + (j0.9032)(1\angle -120°) + j0.4158$$

$$= -1.9245 + j0.6237$$

$$\cong 2.0231 \angle 17.96° \text{ pu}$$

(b) Left to the reader.

Example J.17

Consider the system shown in Figure J.17 and data given in Table J.17. Assume there is a fault at bus 2. After drawing the corresponding sequence networks, reduce them to their Thévenin equivalents looking in at bus 2:

(a) Positive-sequence network
(b) Negative-sequence network
(c) Zero-sequence network

Solution

(a) For positive-sequence network,

$$
\begin{aligned}
\mathbf{Z}_{1,th} &= \frac{\left(\mathbf{Z}_{1,G_1} + \mathbf{Z}_{1,T_1} + \mathbf{Z}_{1,TL_{12}}\right)\left(\mathbf{Z}_{1,T_2} + \mathbf{Z}_{1,G_2}\right)}{\mathbf{Z}_{1,G_1} + \mathbf{Z}_{1,T_1} + \mathbf{Z}_{1,TL_{12}} + \mathbf{Z}_{1,T_2} + \mathbf{Z}_{1,G_2}} \\
&= \frac{j\left(0.2 + 0.2 + 0.6\right) \times j\left(0.15 + 0.3\right)}{j\left(0.2 + 0.2 + 0.6 + 0.15 + 0.3\right)} \\
&= j0.3103 \text{ pu}
\end{aligned}
$$

(b) For negative-sequence network,

$$
\begin{aligned}
\mathbf{Z}_{2,th} &= \frac{\left(\mathbf{Z}_{2,G_1} + \mathbf{Z}_{2,T_1} + \mathbf{Z}_{2,TL_{12}}\right)\left(\mathbf{Z}_{2,T_2} + \mathbf{Z}_{2,G_2}\right)}{\mathbf{Z}_{2,G_1} + \mathbf{Z}_{2,T_1} + \mathbf{Z}_{2,TL_{12}} + \mathbf{Z}_{2,T_2} + \mathbf{Z}_{2,G_2}} \\
&= \frac{j\left(0.15 + 0.2 + 0.6\right) \times j2}{j\left(0.15 + 0.2 + 0.6 + 0.15 + 0.2\right)} \\
&= j0.2558 \text{ pu}
\end{aligned}
$$

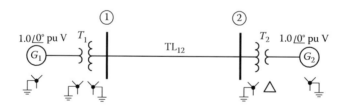

FIGURE J.17   System for Example J.17.

TABLE J.17
Table for Problem J.17

Network Component	MVA Base (pu)	X_1 (pu)	X_2 (pu)	X_0 (pu)
G_1	100	0.2	0.15	0.05
G_2	100	0.3	0.2	0.05
T_1	100	0.2	0.2	0.2
T_2	100	0.15	0.15	0.15
TL_{12}	100	0.6	0.6	0.9

(c) Foe zero-sequence network,

$$\mathbf{Z}_{0,th} = \frac{\left(\mathbf{Z}_{0,G_1} + \mathbf{Z}_{0,T_1} + \mathbf{Z}_{0,TL_{12}}\right)\left(\mathbf{Z}_{0,T_2}\right)}{\mathbf{Z}_{0,G_1} + \mathbf{Z}_{0,T_1} + \mathbf{Z}_{0,TL_{12}} + \mathbf{Z}_{0,T_2}}$$

$$= \frac{j\left(0.05 + 0.2 + 0.9\right) \times j\left(0.15\right)}{j\left(0.05 + 0.2 + 0.9 + 0.15\right)}$$

$$= j0.1327 \text{ pu}$$

Example J.18

Use the solution of Example J.17 and calculate the fault currents for the following faults and draw the corresponding interconnected sequence networks:

(a) SLG fault at bus 2 assuming faulted phase is phase a
(b) DLG fault at bus 2 involving phases b and c
(c) Three-phase fault at bus 2

Solution

(a) The SLG fault is at bus 2 and $\mathbf{Z}_f = 0$ and $\mathbf{Z}_g = 0$:

$$\mathbf{I}_{a0} = \mathbf{I}_{a1} = \mathbf{I}_{a2} = \frac{\mathbf{V}_F}{\mathbf{Z}_0 + \mathbf{Z}_1 + \mathbf{Z}_2}$$

$$= \frac{1.0\angle 0°}{j0.1327 + j0.3103 + j0.2558}$$

$$= -j1.4310 \text{ pu} = 1.4310\angle -90° \text{ pu}$$

$$\mathbf{I}_{af} = \mathbf{I}_{a0} + \mathbf{I}_{a1} + \mathbf{I}_{a2}$$

or

$$\mathbf{I}_{af} = 3\mathbf{I}_{a0} = 3\left(1.4031\angle -90°\right)$$

$$= 4.2931\angle -90° \text{ pu}$$

$$\mathbf{I}_{bf} = \mathbf{I}_{cf} = 0$$

(b) The DLG fault is at bus 2 involving phases b and c:
Since DLG fault, $\mathbf{I}_{af} = 0$

$$\mathbf{I}_{a1} = \frac{1.0\angle 0°}{\mathbf{Z}_1 + \dfrac{\mathbf{Z}_2 \times \mathbf{Z}_0}{\mathbf{Z}_2 + \mathbf{Z}_0}}$$

$$= \frac{1.0\angle 0°}{j0.3103 + \dfrac{\left(j0.2552\right) \times \left(j0.1327\right)}{\left(j0.2552\right) + \left(j0.1327\right)}}$$

$$= -j2.5146 \text{ pu} = 2.5146\angle -90° \text{ pu}$$

$$\mathbf{I}_{a0} = -\left(\frac{\mathbf{Z}_2}{\mathbf{Z}_0 + \mathbf{Z}_2}\right)\mathbf{I}_{a1}$$

$$= -\left(\frac{j0.2558}{j0.1327 + j0.2558}\right)(-j2.5146)$$

$$= 1.6557\angle 90° \text{ pu} \quad \text{or} \quad -1.6557\angle -90° \text{ pu}$$

$$\mathbf{I}_{a2} = -\left(\frac{\mathbf{Z}_0}{\mathbf{Z}_0 + \mathbf{Z}_2}\right)\mathbf{I}_{a1}$$

$$= -\left(\frac{j0.1327}{j0.1327 + j0.2558}\right)(-j2.5146)$$

$$= 0.8590\angle 90° \text{ pu} \quad \text{or} \quad -0.8590\angle -90° \text{ pu}$$

$$\mathbf{I}_{af} = 0$$

$$\mathbf{I}_{bf} = \mathbf{I}_{a0} + a^2\mathbf{I}_{a1} + a\mathbf{I}_{a2}$$

$$= 1.6557\angle 90° + (1\angle -120°)(2.5146\angle -90°) + (1\angle 120°)(0.8590\angle 90°)$$

$$= -2.9216 + j2.4835$$

$$= -2.8345\angle 139.034° \text{ pu}$$

$$\mathbf{I}_{cf} = \mathbf{I}_{a0} + a\mathbf{I}_{a1} + a^2\mathbf{I}_{a2}$$

$$= 1.6557\angle 90° + (1\angle 120°)(-j2.5146) + (1\angle -120°)(0.8590\angle 90°)$$

$$= 2.9216 + j2.4835$$

$$= 3.8345\angle 40.366° \text{ pu}$$

$$\mathbf{I}_{f(DLG)} = \mathbf{I}_{bf} + \mathbf{I}_{cf} = 3\mathbf{I}_{a0}$$

$$= 4.9671\angle 90° \text{ pu} \quad \text{or} \quad -4.9671\angle -90° \text{ pu}$$

(c) The three-phase fault is at bus 2:

$$\mathbf{I}_{a0} = \mathbf{I}_{a2} = 0$$

$$\mathbf{I}_{a1} = \frac{1.0\angle 0°}{\mathbf{Z}_1 + \mathbf{Z}_f}$$

$$= \frac{1.0\angle 0°}{\mathbf{Z}_1} \quad \text{since } \mathbf{Z}_f = 0$$

$$= \frac{1.0\angle 0°}{j0.3103}$$

$$= -j3.2227$$

$$= 3.2227\angle -90° \text{ pu}$$

$$\mathbf{I}_{af} = \mathbf{I}_{a1} = 3.2227\angle -90° \text{ pu}$$

$$\mathbf{I}_{bf} = a^2\mathbf{I}_{a1} = 3.2227\angle 150° \text{ pu}$$

$$\mathbf{I}_{cf} = a\mathbf{I}_{a1} = 3.2227\angle 30° \text{ pu}$$

Example J.19

Consider the system shown in Figure J.19 and data given in Table J.19. Assume that there is an SLG fault at bus 3. Determine the following:

(a) Thévenin equivalent positive-sequence impedance.
(b) Thévenin equivalent negative-sequence impedance.
(c) Thévenin equivalent zero-sequence impedance.
(d) Positive-, negative-, and zero-sequence currents.
(e) Phase currents in per units and amperes.
(f) Positive-, negative-, and zero-sequence voltages.
(g) Phase voltages in per units and kilovolts.
(h) Line-to-line voltages in per units and kilovolts.
(i) Draw a voltage phasor diagram using before-the-fault line-to-neutral and line-to-line voltage values.
(j) Draw a voltage phasor diagram using the resultant after-the-fault line-to-neutral and line-to-line voltage values.

Solution

(a)

$$\mathbf{Z}_{1,th} = j0.2097 \text{ pu}$$

(b)

$$\mathbf{Z}_{2,th} = j0.2097 \text{ pu}$$

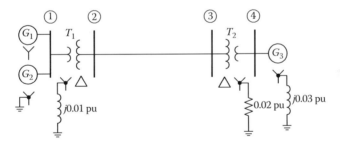

FIGURE J.19 System for Example J.19.

TABLE J.19
Table for Example J.19

Network Component	MVA Rating	Voltage Rating (kV)	X_1 (pu)	X_2 (pu)	X_0 (pu)
G_1	100	13.8	0.15	0.15	0.05
G_2	100	13.8	0.15	0.15	0.05
G_3	100	13.8	0.15	0.15	0.05
T_1	100	13.8/115	0.20	0.20	0.20
T_2	100	115/13.8	0.18	0.18	0.18
TL_{23}	100	115	0.30	0.30	0.90

(c)

$$\mathbf{Z}_{0,th} = 0$$

(d)

$$\mathbf{I}_{a0} = \mathbf{I}_{a1} = \mathbf{I}_{a2} = \frac{1.0\angle 0°}{0 + j0.2097 + j0.2097} = 2.3847\angle -90° \text{ pu}$$

(e)

$$\mathbf{I}_{af} = 3\mathbf{I}_{a0} = 3(2.3847\angle -90°) = 7.1531\angle -90° \text{ pu}$$

$$\mathbf{I}_{bf} = \mathbf{I}_{cf} = 0$$

$$I_B = \frac{S_B}{\sqrt{3}V_B} = \frac{100 \times 10^6}{\sqrt{3}(115 \times 10^3)} = 502.04 \text{ A}$$

$$\mathbf{I}_{af} = (7.1541\angle -90°)(502.04 \text{ A}) = 3591.67\angle -90° \text{ A}$$

(f)

$$\mathbf{V}_{a0} = \mathbf{I}_{a0}\mathbf{Z}_0 = 0$$

$$\mathbf{V}_{a0} = 1.0 - (2.3847\angle -90°)(j0.2097) = 0.5 \text{ pu}$$

$$\mathbf{V}_{a2} = -\mathbf{I}_{a2}\mathbf{Z}_2 = -(j0.2097)(2.3847\angle -90°) = -0.5 \text{ pu}$$

(g) $\mathbf{V}_{af} = \mathbf{V}_{a1} + \mathbf{V}_{a2} = 0$

$$\mathbf{V}_{bf} = a^2\mathbf{V}_{a1} + a\mathbf{V}_{a2}$$

$$= (1\angle 240°)(0.5) + (1\angle 120°)(0.5)$$

$$= 0.866\angle -90° \text{ pu}$$

$$\mathbf{V}_{cf} = a\mathbf{V}_{a1} + a^2\mathbf{V}_{a2}$$

$$= (1\angle 120°)(0.5) + (1\angle -120°)(0.5)$$

$$= 0.866\angle 90° \text{ pu}$$

$$\mathbf{V}_B = \frac{115}{\sqrt{3}} \text{ kV}$$

$$\mathbf{V}_a = 0$$

$$\mathbf{V}_b = (0.866\angle -90°)\left(\frac{115}{\sqrt{3}}\right) = 57.4983\angle -90° \text{ kV}$$

$$\mathbf{V}_c = (0.866\angle 90°)\left(\frac{115}{\sqrt{3}}\right) = 57.4983\angle 90° \text{ kV}$$

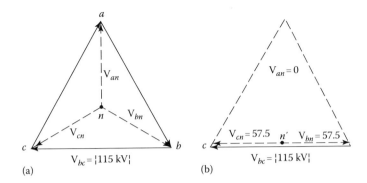

FIGURE J.20   The phasor diagrams for the line-to-neutral voltages and line-to-line voltages (a) before the fault and (b) after the fault.

(h)

$$\mathbf{V}_{ab} = \mathbf{V}_a - \mathbf{V}_b = 0 - 57.4983\angle{-90°} = -57.4983\angle{-90°} \text{ kV}$$

$$\mathbf{V}_{bc} = \mathbf{V}_b - \mathbf{V}_c = 57.4983\angle{-90°} - 57.4983\angle{90°} = 114.9966\angle{-90} \text{ kV}$$

$$\mathbf{V}_{ca} = \mathbf{V}_c - \mathbf{V}_a = 57.4983\angle{90°} - 0 = 57.4983\angle{90°} \text{ kV}$$

Or in per units,

$$\mathbf{V}_{ab} = \mathbf{V}_a - \mathbf{V}_b = -0.866\angle{-90°} \text{ pu}$$

$$\mathbf{V}_{bc} = \mathbf{V}_b - \mathbf{V}_c = 0.866\angle{-90°} - 0.866\angle{90°} = 1.732\angle{-90°} \text{ pu}$$

$$\mathbf{V}_{ca} = \mathbf{V}_c - \mathbf{V}_a = 0.866\angle{90°} \text{ pu}$$

(i) Figure J.20a shows the phasor diagram for the line-to-neutral voltage and line-to-line voltage values before the fault and after the fault.

(j) Figure J.20b shows the phasor diagram for the line-to-neutral voltage and line-to-line voltage values after the fault.

Appendix K: Additional Solved Examples of Shunt Faults Using MATLAB®

Example K.1

Solve Example J.1 given in Appendix J using MATLAB®.

```
%Consider the system shown in  Figure J.1 and the following data:
%Generator G1: 15 kV, 50 MVA, X1 = X2 = 0.10 pu and Xo = 0.05 pu based
on its own ratings.
%Synchronous motor M : 15 kV, 20 MVA, X1 = X2 = 0.20 pu and Xo = 0.07 pu
based on its own ratings.
%Transformer T1 : 15/115 kV, 30 MVA, X1 = X2 = Xo = 0.06 pu based on its
own ratings.
%Transformer T2: 115/15 kV, 25 MVA, X1 = X2 = Xo = 0.07 pu based on its
own ratings.
%Transmission line TL23: X1 = X2 = 0.03 pu and X0 = 0.10 pu based on its
own ratings.
%Assume a single line-to-ground fault at bus 4 and determine the fault
current in per units and amperes. Use 50 MVA as the%megavoltampere base
and assume that Zf is j0.l pu based on 50 MVA.
```

Solution

(a) MATLAB script for Example K.1

```
%
%Data
clear; clc;
format short g
Zb = 50 % System base
Zf = i*0.10 % Fault impedance
Vf = 1+i*0 %The voltage to ground of phase "a" at the fault point F
before the fault
%       occurred is Vf and it is usually selected as 1.0/_O pu.
Sb = 50e6 % 50MVA base
VLL = 115e3 %Voltage line to line

%Generator G1
G1b = 50
Z1G1 = i*0.10*(Zb/G1b)
Z2G1 = i*0.10*(Zb/G1b)
Z0G1 = i*0.05*(Zb/G1b)

%Generator G2
G2b = 20
Z1G2 = i*0.20*(Zb/G2b)
Z2G2 = i*0.20*(Zb/G2b)
Z0G2 = i*0.07*(Zb/G2b)
```

```
%Transformer T1
T1b = 30
Z1T1 = i*0.06*(Zb/T1b)
Z2T1 = i*0.06*(Zb/T1b)
Z0T1 = i*0.06*(Zb/T1b)

%Transformer T2
T2b = 25
Z1T2 = i*0.07*(Zb/T2b)
Z2T2 = i*0.07*(Zb/T2b)
Z0T2 = i*0.07*(Zb/T2b)

%Transmission line TL23
TL23b = 50
Z1TL23 = i*0.03*(Zb/TL23b)
Z2TL23 = i*0.03*(Zb/TL23b)
Z0TL23 = i*0.10*(Zb/TL23b)

%Z1 Thevenin
Z1Th = ((Z1G1+Z1T1+Z1TL23+Z1T2)*(Z1G2))/(Z1G1+Z1T1+Z1TL23+Z1T2+Z1G2)
%Z2 Thevenin
Z2Th = Z1Th
%Z0 Thevenin
Z0Th = ((Z0G1+Z0T1+Z0TL23+Z0T2)*(Z0G2))/(Z0G1+Z0T1+Z0TL23+Z0T2+Z0G2)

%Iaf = 3*Ia1 = 3*(Vf/Z1Th+Z2Th+Z0Th+3*Zf)

Ia1 = Vf/(Z1Th+Z2Th+Z0Th+3*Zf)
%the fault current for phase 'a' can be found as
Iaf_pu = 3*Ia1

IB_A = Sb/(sqrt(3)*VLL)

If_A = abs(Iaf_pu)*IB_A

disp('_____');
disp(' ');
disp(' ');
disp(' ');
disp(' #################### OR IN SUMMARY ##################');
disp(' ');
disp(' **** 1st Row G1; 2nd Row G2; 3rd Row T1; 4th Row T2; 5th Row
TL23 ****')
disp('        Z1           Z2           Z0 ');
disp(' ***********************************************************');
[Z1G1 Z2G1 Z0G1 ;Z1G2 Z2G2 Z0G2; Z1T1 Z2T1 Z0T1; Z1T2 Z2T2
Z0T2;Z1TL23 Z2TL23 Z0TL23]
disp('_____');
disp(' ');
disp(' ');
disp(' ');
disp('    Z1Th           Z2Th           Z0Th');
disp(' ***********************************************************');
[Z1Th Z2Th Z0Th]
disp('_____');
disp(' ');
disp(' ');
disp(' ');
disp('    Iaf_pu      IB_A           If_A ') ;
disp(' ***********************************************************');
[Iaf_pu IB_A If_A]
disp('_____');
```

```
disp(' ');
disp(' ');
disp(' ');
```

(b) MATLAB results for Example K.1

Zb =
   50

Zf =
      0 +   0.1i

Vf =
   1

Sb =
      50000000

VLL =
      115000

G1b =
   50

Z1G1 =
      0 +   0.1i

Z2G1 =
      0 +   0.1i

Z0G1 =
      0 + 0.05i

G2b =
   20

Z1G2 =
      0 +   0.5i

Z2G2 =
      0 +   0.5i

Z0G2 =
      0 + 0.175i

T1b =
   30

Z1T1 =
      0 +   0.1i

Z2T1 =
      0 +   0.1i

Z0T1 =
      0 +   0.1i

T2b =
   25

Z1T2 =
      0 + 0.14i

Z2T2 =
      0 + 0.14i

Z0T2 =
      0 + 0.14i

TL23b =
   50

Z1TL23 =
      0 + 0.03i

Z2TL23 =
        0 + 0.03i
Z0TL23 =
        0 +   0.1i
Z1Th =
        0 + 0.21264i
Z2Th =
        0 + 0.21264i
Z0Th =
        0 + 0.1208i
Ia1 =
        0 − 1.1819i
Iaf_pu =
        0 − 3.5457i
IB_A =
     192.45
If_A =
     890.06

############################   OR IN SUMMARY   ############################
************   1st Row G1; 2nd Row G2; 3rd Row T1; 4th Row T2; 5th Row TL23   ****************
            Z1   Z2   Z0
****
ans =
        0+   0.1i   0+   0.1i   0+   0.05i
        0+   0.5i   0+   0.5i   0+   0.175i
        0+   0.1i   0+   0.1i   0+   0.1i
        0+   0.14i   0+   0.14i   0+   0.14i
        0+   0.03i   0+   0.03i   0+   0.1i

        Z1Th   Z2Th   Z0Th
****
ans =
        0+ 0.21264i   0+ 0.21264i   0+ 0.1208i

        Iaf_pu   IB_A   If_A
****
ans =
        0−   3.5457i   192.45   682.37

Example K.2

Solve Example J.2 using MATLAB.

```
%Consider the system given in Example K.1 and assume that there is a
line-to-line fault at bus 3 involving phases b and c. Determine%the fault
currents for both phases in per units and amperes.
```

```
%Consider the system showing in Figure F.1 and the following data:
%Generator G1: 15 kV, 50 MVA, X1 = X2 = 0.10 pu and Xo = 0.05 pu based
on its own ratings.
%Generator G2: 15 kV, 20 MVA, X1 = X2 = 0.20 pu and Xo = 0.07 pu based
on its own ratings.
%Transformer T1: 15/115 kV, 30 MVA, X1 = X2 = Xo = 0.06 pu based on its
own ratings.
%Transformer T2: 115/15 kV, 25 MVA, X1 = X2 = Xo = 0.07 pu based on its
own ratings.
%Transmission line TL23: X1 = X2 = 0.03 pu and X0 = 0.10 pu based on its
own ratings.
%Assume a single line-to-ground fault at bus 4 and determine the fault
current in per units and amperes. Use 50 MVA as the%megavoltampere base
and assume that Zf is j0.1 pu based on 50 MVA.
```

Solution

(a) MATLAB script for Example K.2

```
%
clear; clc;
format short g
%Data
Zb = 50 % System base
Zf = i*0.10 % Fault impedance
Vf = 1+i*0 %The voltage to ground of phase "a" at the fault point F
before the fault
%       occurred is Vf and it is usually selected as 1.0/_0 pu.
Sb = 50e6 % 50MVA base
VLL = 115e3 %Voltage line to line

%Generator G1
G1b = 50
Z1G1 = i*0.10*(Zb/G1b)
Z2G1 = i*0.10*(Zb/G1b)
Z0G1 = i*0.05*(Zb/G1b)

%Generator G2
G2b = 20
Z1G2 = i*0.20*(Zb/G2b)
Z2G2 = i*0.20*(Zb/G2b)
Z0G2 = i*0.07*(Zb/G2b)

%Transformer T1
T1b = 30
Z1T1 = i*0.06*(Zb/T1b)
Z2T1 = i*0.06*(Zb/T1b)
Z0T1 = i*0.06*(Zb/T1b)

%Transformer T2
T2b = 25
Z1T2 = i*0.07*(Zb/T2b)
Z2T2 = i*0.07*(Zb/T2b)
Z0T2 = i*0.07*(Zb/T2b)

%Transmission line TL23
TL23b = 50
Z1TL23 = i*0.03*(Zb/TL23b)
Z2TL23 = i*0.03*(Zb/TL23b)
Z0TL23 = i*0.10*(Zb/TL23b)

%Z1 Thevenin
Z1Th = ((Z1G1+Z1T1+Z1TL23)*(Z1T2+Z1G2))/(Z1G1+Z1T1+Z1TL23+Z1T2+Z1G2)
%Z2 Thevenin
```

```
Z2Th = Z1Th
%Iaf = 3*Ia1 = 3*(Vf/Z1Th+Z2Th+Z0Th+3*Zf)

Ia1_pu = Vf/(Z1Th+Z2Th)
Ibf_pu = sqrt(3)*Ia1_pu*(-i)

IB_A = Sb/(sqrt(3)*VLL)

IBf_A = Ibf_pu*IB_A

Icf_pu = -Ibf_pu
Icf_A = -IBf_A

disp('_____');
disp(' ');
disp(' ');
disp(' ');
disp(' ################### OR IN SUMMARY ####################');
disp(' ');
disp(' **** 1st Row G1; 2nd Row G2; 3rd Row T1; 4th Row T2; 5th Row
TL23 ****')
disp('        Z1              Z2              Z0 ');
disp(' ****************************************************');
[Z1G1 Z2G1 Z0G1 ;Z1G2 Z2G2 Z0G2; Z1T1 Z2T1 Z0T1; Z1T2 Z2T2
Z0T2;Z1TL23 Z2TL23 Z0TL23]
disp('_____');
disp(' ');
disp(' ');
disp(' ');
disp('        Z1Th            Z2Th            Ia1_pu');
disp(' ****************************************************');
[Z1Th Z2Th Ia1_pu]
disp('_____');
disp(' ');
disp(' ');
disp(' ');
disp(' Ibf_pu IB_A   IBf_A Icf_pu Icf_A') ;
disp(' ****************************************************');
[Ibf_pu IB_A IBf_A Icf_pu Icf_A]
disp('_____');
disp(' ');
disp(' ');
disp(' ');
```

(b) MATLAB results for Example K.2

Zb =
    50
Zf =
        0 +   0.1i
Vf =
    1
Sb =
    50000000
VLL =
    115000

G1b =
 50
Z1G1 =
        0 +   0.1i
Z2G1 =
        0 +   0.1i
Z0G1 =
        0 + 0.05i
G2b =
 20
Z1G2 =
        0 +   0.5i
Z2G2 =
        0 +   0.5i
Z0G2 =
        0 + 0.175i
T1b =
 30
Z1T1 =
        0 +   0.1i
Z2T1 =
        0 +   0.1i
Z0T1 =
        0 +   0.1i
T2b =
 25
Z1T2 =
        0 + 0.14i
Z2T2 =
        0 + 0.14i
Z0T2 =
        0 + 0.14i
TL23b =
 50
Z1TL23 =
        0 + 0.03i
Z2TL23 =
        0 + 0.03i
Z0TL23 =
        0 +   0.1i
Z1Th =
        0 + 0.1692i
Z2Th =
        0 + 0.1692i
Ia1_pu =
        0 – 2.9552i
Ibf_pu =
   –5.1185

IB_A =
    251.02
IBf_A =
    −1284.9
Icf_pu =
    5.1185
Icf_A =
    1284.9

##########################   OR IN SUMMARY   ##########################
************** 1st Row G1; 2nd Row G2; 3rd Row T1; 4th Row T2; 5th Row TL23 **************
             Z1   Z2   Z0
****
ans =

0 +	0.1i	0 +	0.1i	0 +	0.05i
0 +	0.5i	0 +	0.5i	0 +	0.175i
0 +	0.1i	0 +	0.1i	0 +	0.1i
0 +	0.14i	0 +	0.14i	0 +	0.14i
0 +	0.03i	0 +	0.03i	0 +	0.1i

        Z1Th   Z2Th   Ia1_pu
****
ans =

    0 + 0.1692i   0 + 0.1692i   0 − 2.9552i

Ibf_pu IB_A IBf_A Icf_pu Icf_A
****
ans =
−5.1185 251.02 −1284.9 5.1185 1284.9

Example K.3

Solve Example J.3 using MATLAB.

```
%Consider the system given in Example J.3 and assume that there is a DLG
fault at bus 2, involving phases b and c. Assume that Zf is %j0.1 pu and
Zg is j0.2pu (where Zg is the neutral-to-ground impedance) both based on
50 VA. Consider the system showing in%Figure J.1 and the following data:
%Generator G1: 15 kV, 50 MVA, X1 = X2 = 0.10 pu and Xo = 0.05 pu based
on its own ratings.
%Generator G2: 15 kV, 20 MVA, X1 = X2 = 0.20 pu and Xo = 0.07 pu based
on its own ratings.
%Transformer T1: 15/115 kV, 30 MVA, X1 = X2 = Xo = 0.06 pu based on its
own ratings.
%Transformer T2: 115/15 kV, 25 MVA, X1 = X2 = Xo = 0.07 pu based on its
own ratings.
%Transmission line TL23: X1 = X2 = 0.03 pu and X0 = 0.10 pu based on its
own ratings.
%Assume a single line-to-ground fault at bus 4 and determine the fault
current in per units and amperes. Use 50 MVA as the%megavoltampere base
and assume that Zf is j0.1 pu based on 50 MVA.
```

Solution

(a) MATLAB script for Example K.3

```
%
clear; clc;
format short g
%Data
Zb = 50 % System base 50VA
Zf = i*0.10 % Fault impedance
Vf = 1+i*0 %The voltage to ground of phase "a" at the fault point F
before the fault
%       occurred is Vf and it is usually selected as 1.0/_0 pu.
Zg = i*0.20 % System base 50VA
Sb = 50e6 % 50MVA base
VLL = 115e3 %Voltage line to line

%Generator G1
G1b = 50
Z1G1 = i*0.10*(Zb/G1b)
Z2G1 = i*0.10*(Zb/G1b)
Z0G1 = i*0.05*(Zb/G1b)

%Generator G2
G2b = 20
Z1G2 = i*0.20*(Zb/G2b)
Z2G2 = i*0.20*(Zb/G2b)
Z0G2 = i*0.07*(Zb/G2b)

%Transformer T1
T1b = 30
Z1T1 = i*0.06*(Zb/T1b)
Z2T1 = i*0.06*(Zb/T1b)
Z0T1 = i*0.06*(Zb/T1b)

%Transformer T2
T2b = 25
Z1T2 = i*0.07*(Zb/T2b)
Z2T2 = i*0.07*(Zb/T2b)
Z0T2 = i*0.07*(Zb/T2b)

%Transmission line TL23
TL23b = 50
Z1TL23 = i*0.03*(Zb/TL23b)
Z2TL23 = i*0.03*(Zb/TL23b)
Z0TL23 = i*0.10*(Zb/TL23b)

%Z1 Thevenin
Z1Th = ((Z1G1+Z1T1)*(Z1TL23+Z1T2+Z1G2))/(Z1G1+Z1T1+Z1TL23+Z1T2+Z1G2)
%Z2 Thevenin
Z2Th = Z1Th
%Z0 Thevenin
Z0Th = ((Z0G1+Z0T1)*(Z0TL23+Z0T2+Z0G2))/(Z0G1+Z0T1+Z0TL23+Z0T2+Z0G2)
%Iaf = 3*Ia1 = 3*(Vf/Z1Th+Z2Th+Z0Th+3*Zf)
%
Ia1_pu = Vf/(Zf+Z1Th+(((Z2Th+Zf)*(Z0Th+Zf+3*Zg))/(Z2Th+Z0Th+2*Zf+3*Zg)))

Ia2_pu = -(((Z0Th+Zf+3*Zg)/(Z2Th+Z0Th+2*Zf+3*Zg)))*(Ia1_pu)

Ia0_pu = -(((Z2Th+Zf)/(Z2Th+Z0Th+2*Zf+3*Zg)))*(Ia1_pu)

IG = 3*Ia0_pu
```

```
IB_A = Sb/(sqrt(3)*VLL)
IB__A = abs(IG)*IB_A

a = -0.5+i*0.866
a2 = a^2

Ibf_pu = a^2*Ia1_pu+a*Ia2_pu+Ia0_pu

IBf_A = abs(Ibf_pu)*IB_A
%
Icf_pu = a*Ia1_pu+a^2*Ia2_pu+Ia0_pu

ICf_A = abs(Icf_pu)*IB_A

disp('                                                      ');
disp(' ');
disp(' ');
disp(' ');
disp(' #################### OR IN SUMMARY ####################');
disp(' ');
disp(' **** 1st Row G1; 2nd Row G2; 3rd Row T1; 4th Row T2; 5th Row
TL23 ****')
disp('        Z1              Z2              Z0 ');
disp(' ***********************************************************');
[Z1G1 Z2G1 Z0G1;Z1G2 Z2G2 Z0G2; Z1T1 Z2T1 Z0T1; Z1T2 Z2T2 Z0T2;
Z1TL23 Z2TL23 Z0TL23]
disp('                                                      ');
disp(' ');
disp(' ');
disp(' ');
disp('        Z1Th              Z2Th              Z0Th');
disp(' ***********************************************************');
[Z1Th Z2Th Z0Th]
disp('                                                      ');
disp(' ');
disp(' ');
disp(' ');

disp('        Ia1_pu              Ia2_pu              Ia0_pu ');
disp(' ***********************************************************');
[Ia1_pu Ia2_pu Ia0_pu]
disp('                                                      ');
disp(' ');
disp(' ');
disp(' ');

disp('        IG              IB_A              IB__A     ') ;
disp(' ***********************************************************');
[IG IB_A IB__A]
disp('                                                      ');
disp(' ');
disp(' ');
disp(' ');

disp('        Ibf_pu          IBf_A') ;
disp(' ***********************************************************');
[Ibf_pu IBf_A]
disp('                                                      ');
disp(' ');
disp(' ');
disp(' ');
```

```
disp('     Icf_pu     ICf_A') ;
disp(' *******************************************************');
[Icf_pu ICf_A]
disp('  _____  ');
disp(' ');
disp(' ');
disp(' ');
```

(b) MATLAB results for Example K.3

Zb =
  50
Zf =
        0 +   0.1i
Vf =
  1
Zg =
        0 +   0.2i
Sb =
  50000000

VLL =
  115000
G1b =
  50
Z1G1 =
        0 +   0.1i
Z2G1 =
        0 +   0.1i
Z0G1 =
        0 + 0.05i
G2b =
  20
Z1G2 =
        0 +   0.5i
Z2G2 =
        0 +   0.5i
Z0G2 =
        0 + 0.175i
T1b =
  30
Z1T1 =
        0 +   0.1i
Z2T1 =
        0 +   0.1i
Z0T1 =
        0 +   0.1i
T2b =
  25
Z1T2 =
        0 + 0.14i
Z2T2 =
        0 + 0.14i
```
```

Z0T2 =
          0 + 0.14i
TL23b =
     50
Z1TL23 =
          0 + 0.03i
Z2TL23 =
          0 + 0.03i
Z0TL23 =
          0 +   0.1i
Z1Th =
          0 + 0.15402i
Z2Th =
          0 + 0.15402i
Z0Th =
          0 + 0.11018i
Ia1_pu =
          0 − 2.2351i
Ia2_pu =
          0 + 1.7016i
Ia0_pu =
          0 + 0.53351i
IG =
          0 + 1.6005i
IB_A =
     251.02
IB__A =
     401.77
a =
          −0.5 + 0.866i
a2 =
          −0.49996 − 0.866i
Ibf_pu =
          −3.4091 + 0.80017i
IBf_A =
     879.02
Icf_pu =
          3.4091 + 0.80034i
ICf_A =
     879.03

_____

############################   OR IN SUMMARY   ############################
************ 1st Row G1; 2nd Row G2; 3rd Row T1; 4th Row T2; 5th Row TL23 ************
          Z1   Z2   Z0
****
ans =
     0+   0.1i   0+   0.1i   0+   0.05i
     0+   0.5i   0+   0.5i   0+   0.175i
     0+   0.1i   0+   0.1i   0+   0.1i

```
      0+      0.14i    0+      0.14i    0+      0.14i
      0+      0.03i    0+      0.03i    0+      0.1i
```

```
      Z1Th              Z2Th              Z0Th
******************************************************************************
ans =
      0+ 0.15402i     0+ 0.15402i     0+ 0.11018i
```

```
Ia1_pu          Ia2_pu          Ia0_pu
******************************************************************************
ans =
      0- 2.2351i      0+ 1.7016i      0+ 0.53351i
```

```
      IG              IB_A            IB__A
******************************************************************************
ans =
      0+ 1.6005i  251.02          401.77
```

```
      Ibf_pu   IBf_A
******************************************************************************
ans =
      -3.4091+ 0.80017i 879.02
```

```
      Icf_pu          ICf_A
******************************************************************************
ans =
      3.4091+ 0.80034i 879.03
```

Example K.4

Solve Example J.4 using MATLAB.

```
%Consider the system shown in Figure J.4 and assume that the generator
is loaded and running at the rated voltage with the circuit%breaker open
at bus 3. Assume that the reactance values of the generator are given as
Xd" = X1 = X2 = 0.14 pu and X0 = 0.08 pu%based on its ratings. The
transformer impedances are Z1 = Z2 = Z0 = j0.05 pu based on its ratings.
The transmission line TL23 has%Z1 = Z2 = j0.04pu and Z0 = j0.10 pu.
Assume that the fault point is located on bus 1. Select 25 MVA as the
megavoltampere base,%and 8.5 and 138 kV as the low-voltage and high-
voltage voltage bases, respectively,
%and determine the following:
      %(a) Subtransient fault current for three-phase fault in per units
           and amperes.
      %(b) Line-to-ground fault. [Also find the ratio of this line-to-
           ground fault current to the three-phase fault
           current found in part (a)].
      %(c) Line-to-line fault. (Also find the ratio of this line-to-line
           fault current to previously calculated three-
           phase fault current.)
      %(d) Double line-to-ground fault.
```

Solution

(a) MATLAB script for Example K.4

```
%
%Data
clear; clc;
format short g
Sb = 25 % System base 50VA
S = 25e6
Vf = 1+i*0 %The voltage to ground of phase "a" at the fault point F
before the fault
%        occurred is Vf and it is usually selected as 1.0/_0 pu.

VLL = 115e3 %Voltage line to line
%Generator G
Gb = 25
VLLG = 8.5e3
Z1G = i*0.14*(Sb/Gb)
Z2G = i*0.14*(Sb/Gb)
Z0G = i*0.08*(Sb/Gb)

% Part a L-G fault
%Iaf = 3*Ia0
Iaf_pu = 3*(Vf/(Z0G+Z1G+Z2G))

%If_LL = (sqrt(3)/2)*If_3phase
If_LG_pu = abs(Iaf_pu)
% See part "c" for If_3phase

%Part b L-L fault
% Ia0 = 0 ans Iaf = 0 therefore
Ia1_pu = Vf/(Z1G+Z2G)

Ibf_pu = sqrt(3)*Ia1_pu*(-i)
VLLG = 8.5e3
IB_A = S/(sqrt(3)*VLLG)
IBf_A = Ibf_pu*IB_A

Icf_pu = -Ibf_pu
Icf_A = -IBf_A

%If_LL = (sqrt(3)/2)*If_3phase
If_LL_pu = abs(Ibf_pu)
If_3phase = (2/sqrt(3))*If_LL_pu

If_LL_div_If_3phase = If_LL_pu/If_3phase
% Thus If_LL = 86.66% of If_3phase (check result to confirm)
%After finding If_3phase from If_Line-to-Line plug back into Part
"a" to find
%Line-to-Grnd/If3pase ratio

If_LG_div_If_3phase = If_LG_pu/If_3phase

%Part c DLG fault
I_a1_pu = Vf/((Z1G + ((Z2G*Z0G)/(Z2G+Z0G)))))
Va1 = Vf-I_a1_pu*Z1G

I_a2_pu = -Va1/Z2G
I_a0_pu = -Va1/Z0G
I_nf_pu = 3*I_a0_pu

a = -0.5+i*0.866
a2 = a^2
I_bf_pu = a^2*I_a1_pu+a*I_a2_pu+I_a0_pu
abs_I_bf_pu = abs(I_bf_pu)
```

```
I_cf_pu = a*I_a1_pu+a^2*I_a2_pu+I_a0_pu
abs_I_cf_pu = abs(I_cf_pu)

I_Bf_A = abs(I_bf_pu)*IB_A
I_Cf_A = abs(I_cf_pu)*IB_A

disp('  _____  ');
disp(' ');
disp(' ');
disp(' ');
disp(' #################### OR IN SUMMARY #####################');
disp(' ');
disp(' ########### RESULTS FOR LINE TO GROUND FAULT ############')
disp('       Z1G              Z2G              Z0G ');
disp(' ************************************************************');
[Z1G Z2G Z0G]
disp('  _____  ');
disp(' ');
disp(' ');
disp(' ');
disp('      Iaf_pu      If_LG_pu                ') ;
disp(' ************************************************************');
[Iaf_pu If_LG_pu]
disp('_____ ');
disp(' ');
disp(' ');
disp(' ');
disp(' If_3phase If_LG_div_If_3phase        ') ;
disp(' ************************************************************');
[If_3phase If_LG_div_If_3phase]
disp('  _____  ');
disp(' ');
disp(' ');
disp(' ');
disp(' ############# RESULTS FOR LINE TO LINE FAULT #############')

disp('    Ia1_pu    Ibf_pu          IB_A       IBf_A ') ;
disp(' ************************************************************');
[Ia1_pu Ibf_pu IB_A IBf_A]
disp('  _____  ');
disp(' ');
disp(' ');
disp(' ');
disp('   Icf_pu    Icf_A     If_LL_pu' ) ;
disp(' ************************************************************');
[Icf_pu Icf_A If_LL_pu]
disp('  _____  ');
disp(' ');
disp(' ');
disp(' ');
disp(' If_3phase If_LL_div_If_3phase             ' ) ;
disp(' ************************************************************');
[If_3phase If_LL_div_If_3phase]
disp('  _____  ');
disp(' ');
disp(' ');
disp(' ');
disp(' ########### RESULTS FOR DOUBLE LINE TO LINE FAULT ##########')
disp('   I_a1_pu    Va1          I_a2_pu          I_a0_pu ') ;
disp(' ************************************************************');
```

```
    [I_a1_pu Va1 I_a2_pu I_a0_pu ]
    disp(`_____');
    disp(' ');
    disp(' ');
    disp(' ');
    disp('    I_nf_pu          I_bf_pu      I_cf_pu      ' ) ;
    disp(' ***********************************************************');
    [I_nf_pu I_bf_pu I_cf_pu]
    disp(`_____');
    disp(' ');
    disp(' ');
    disp(' ');
    disp(' abs_I_bf_pu  I_Bf_A  abs_I_cf_pu  I_Cf_A   ' ) ;
    disp(' ***********************************************************');
    [abs_I_bf_pu I_Bf_A abs_I_cf_pu I_Cf_A]
    disp(`_____');
    disp(' ');
    disp(' ');
    disp(' ');
```

(b) MATLAB results for Example K.4

Sb =
   25
S =
   25000000
Vf =
   1
VLL =
   115000
Gb =
   25
VLLG =
   8500
Z1G =
       0 + 0.14i
Z2G =
       0 + 0.14i
Z0G =
       0 + 0.08i
Iaf_pu =
       0 − 8.3333i
If_LG_pu =
   8.3333
Ia1_pu =
       0 − 3.5714i
Ibf_pu =
   −6.1859
VLLG =
   8500
IB_A =
   1698.1
IBf_A =
   −10504

Icf_pu =
   6.1859
Icf_A =
   10504
If_LL_pu =
   6.1859
If_3phase =
   7.1429
If_LL_div_If_3phase =
   0.86603
If_LG_div_If_3phase =
   1.1667
I_a1_pu =
          0 − 5.2381i
Va1 =
   0.26667
I_a2_pu =
          0 + 1.9048i
I_a0_pu =
          0 + 3.3333i
I_nf_pu =
          0 +   10i
a =
          −0.5 + 0.866i
a2 =
          −0.49996 - 0.866i
I_bf_pu =
          −6.1857 + 4.9998i
abs_I_bf_pu =
   7.9537
I_cf_pu =
          6.1857 + 5.0001i
abs_I_cf_pu =
   7.9539
I_Bf_A =
   13506
I_Cf_A =
   13506

_____

######################   OR IN SUMMARY   ##########################
################   RESULTS FOR LINE TO GROUND FAULT   ################
          Z1G   Z2G   Z0G
****
ans =

          0+ 0.14i   0+ 0.14i   0+ 0.08i

_____

          Iaf_pu   If_LG_pu
****

ans =

          0– 8.3333i   8.3333

If_3phase If_LG_div_If_3phase
****
ans =

          7.1429   1.1667

################   RESULTS FOR LINE TO LINE FAULT   ################
          Ia1_pu   Ibf_pu   IB_A   IBf_A
****
ans =

          0– 3.5714i –6.1859   1698.1   –10504

          Icf_pu Icf_A If_LL_pu
****
ans =

          6.1859 10504 6.1859

If_3phase If_LL_div_If_3phase
****
ans =

          7.1429 0.86603

##############   RESULTS FOR DOUBLE LINE TO LINE FAULT   ##############
          I_al_pu   Va1   I_a2_pu   I_a0_pu
****
ans =

          0– 5.2381i 0.26667   0+ 1.9048i   0+ 3.3333i

          I_nf_pu   I_bf_pu   I_cf_pu
****
ans =

          0+ 10i –6.1857+ 4.9998i 6.1857+ 5.0001i

---

abs_I_bf_pu I_Bf_A abs_I_cf_pu I_Cf_A
****
ans =

          7.9537   13506   7.9539   13506

Example K.5

Solve Example J.5 using MATLAB.

```
%Consider the system shown in Figure J.5 and assume that the generator
is loaded and running at the rated voltage with the circuit%breaker open
at bus 3. Assume that the reactance values of the generator are given as
Xd" = X1 = X2 = 0.14 pu and X0 = 0.08 pu%based on its ratings. The
transformer impedances are Z1 = Z2 = Z0 = j0.05 pu based on its ratings.
The transmission line TL23 has%Z1 = Z2 = j0.04pu and Z0 = j0.10 pu.
```

Assume that the fault point is located on bus 1. Select 25 MVA as the megavoltampere base,%and 8.5 and 138 kV as the low-voltage and high-voltage voltage bases, respectively, and determine the following:

%(a) Subtransient fault current for three-phase fault in per units and amperes.

%(b) Line-to-ground fault. [Also find the ratio of this line-to-ground fault current to the three-phase fault current found in part (a)].

%(c) Line-to-line fault. (Also find the ratio of this line-to-line fault current to previously calculated three-phase fault current.)

%(d) Double line-to-ground fault.

Solution

(a) MATLAB script for Example K.5

```
%
%Data
clear; clc;
format short g
Sb = 25 % System base 50VA
S = 25e6
Vf = 1+i*0 %The voltage to ground of phase "a" at the fault point F
before the fault
%        occurred is Vf and it is usually selected as 1.0/_0 pu.

%
%Generator G
Gb = 25
VLLG = 8.5e3
Z1G = i*0.14*(Sb/Gb)
Z2G = i*0.14*(Sb/Gb)
Z0G = i*0.08*(Sb/Gb)

%Transformer T
Tb = 25
VLLT = 138e3
Z1T = i*0.05*(Sb/Tb)
Z2T = i*0.05*(Sb/Tb)
Z0T = i*0.05*(Sb/Tb)

% Part a L-G fault

Z1 = Z1G+Z1T
Z2 = Z2G+Z2T
Z0 = Z0T
%Iaf = 3*Ia0
Iaf_pu = 3*(Vf/(Z0+Z1+Z2))

IB_A = S/(sqrt(3)*VLLT)
Iaf_A = abs(Iaf_pu)*IB_A

%If_LL = (sqrt(3)/2)*If_3phase
If_LG_pu = abs(Iaf_pu)

%Part b L-L fault
%Assuming that the faulted phases are "b" and "c" Iaf = 0

Ia1_pu = Vf/(Z1+Z2)

Ibf_pu = sqrt(3)*Ia1_pu*(-i)
```

```
IB_A = S/(sqrt(3)*VLLT)
IBf_A = Ibf_pu*IB_A

Icf_pu = -Ibf_pu
Icf_A = -IBf_A

%If_LL = (sqrt(3)/2)*If_3phase
If_LL_pu = abs(Ibf_pu)
If_3phase = (2/sqrt(3))*If_LL_pu
If_LL_div_If_3phase = If_LL_pu/If_3phase

%After finding If_3phase from If_Line-to-Line plug back into Part
"a" to find
%Line-to-Grnd/If3pase ratio

If_LG_div_If_3phase = If_LG_pu/If_3phase
%Part c DLG fault
I_a1_pu = Vf/((Z1 + ((Z2*Z0)/(Z2+Z0)))))
Va1 = Vf-I_a1_pu*Z1

I_a2_pu = -Va1/Z2
I_a0_pu = -Va1/Z0
I_nf_pu = 3*I_a0_pu

a = -0.5+i*0.866
a2 = a^2
I_bf_pu = a^2*I_a1_pu+a*I_a2_pu+I_a0_pu
abs_I_bf_pu = abs(I_bf_pu)

I_cf_pu = a*I_a1_pu+a^2*I_a2_pu+I_a0_pu
abs_I_cf_pu = abs(I_cf_pu)

I_Bf_A = abs(I_bf_pu)*IB_A
I_Cf_A = abs(I_cf_pu)*IB_A

disp('_____');
disp(' ');
disp(' ');
disp(' ');
disp('#################  OR IN   SUMMARY #####################');
disp(' ');
disp('############ RESULTS FOR LINE TO GROUND FAULT ###########')
disp('**************    1st Row G; 2nd Row T    **************')
disp('     Z1              Z2            Z0 ');
disp(' *****************************************************');
[Z1G Z2G Z0G;Z1T Z2T Z0T]
disp('_____');
disp(' ');
disp(' ');
disp(' ');
disp('     Iaf_pu         IB_A            Iaf_A    If_LG_pu ');
disp('*****************************************************');
[Iaf_pu IB_A Iaf_A If_LG_pu]
disp('_____');
disp(' ');
disp(' ');
disp(' ');
```

```
disp(' If_3phase  If_LG_div_If_3phase          ') ;
disp('***********************************************');
[If_3phase If_LG_div_If_3phase]
disp('_____') ;
disp(' ');
disp(' ');
disp(' ');
disp('############## RESULTS FOR LINE TO LINE FAULT ############')
disp('    Ia1_pu    Ibf_pu       IB_A         IBf_A ') ;
disp('***********************************************');
[Ia1_pu Ibf_pu IB_A IBf_A]
disp('_____') ;
disp(' ');
disp(' ');
disp(' ');
disp('   Icf_pu  Icf_A  If_LL_pu' ) ;
disp('***********************************************');
[Icf_pu  Icf_A  If_LL_pu]
disp('_____') ;
disp(' ');
disp(' ');
disp(' ');
disp('If_3phase If_LL_div_If_3phase    ' ) ;
disp('***********************************************');
[If_3phase If_LL_div_If_3phase]
disp('_____') ;
disp(' ');
disp(' ');
disp(' ');
disp('########## RESULTS FOR DOUBLE LINE TO LINE FAULT ##########');
disp(' I_a1_pu       Va1          I_a2_pu      I_a0_pu ') ;
disp('***********************************************');
[I_a1_pu Va1 I_a2_pu I_a0_pu ]
disp('_____') ;
disp(' ');
disp(' ');
disp(' ');
disp(' I_nf_pu       I_bf_pu       I_cf_pu    ');
disp('***********************************************');
[I_nf_pu I_bf_pu I_cf_pu]
disp('_____') ;
disp(' ');
disp(' ');
disp(' ');
disp(' abs_I_bf_pu I_Bf_A abs_I_cf_pu I_Cf_A    ');
disp('***********************************************');
[abs_I_bf_pu I_Bf_A abs_I_cf_pu I_Cf_A]
disp('_____') ;
disp(' ');
disp(' ');
disp(' ');
```

(b) MATLAB results for Example K.5

    Sb =
       25
    S =
       25000000

Vf =
  1
Gb =
  25
VLLG =
  8500
Z1G =
    0 + 0.14i
Z2G =
    0 + 0.14i
Z0G =
    0 + 0.08i
Tb =
  25
VLLT =
  138000
Z1T =
    0 + 0.05i
Z2T =
    0 + 0.05i
Z0T =
    0 + 0.05i
Z1 =
    0 + 0.19i
Z2 =
    0 + 0.19i
Z0 =
    0 + 0.05i
Iaf_pu =
    0 – 6.9767i
IB_A =
  104.59
Iaf_A =
  729.71
If_LG_pu =
  6.9767
Ia1_pu =
    0 – 2.6316i
Ibf_pu =
  –4.558
IB_A =
  104.59
IBf_A =
  –476.74
Icf_pu =
  4.558
Icf_A =
  476.74
If_LL_pu =
  4.558

If_3phase =
   5.2632
If_LL_div_If_3phase =
   0.86603
If_LG_div_If_3phase =
   1.3256
I_a1_pu =
   0 −4.3557i
Va1 =
   0.17241
I_a2_pu =
        0 + 0.90744i
I_a0_pu =
        0 + 3.4483i
I_nf_pu =
        0 + 10.345i
a =
        −0.5 + 0.866i
a2 =
        −0.49996 − 0.866i
I_bf_pu =
        −4.5579 + 5.1722i
abs_I_bf_pu =
   6.8939
I_cf_pu =
        4.5579 + 5.1725i
abs_I_cf_pu =
   6.8941
I_Bf_A =
   721.05
I_Cf_A =
   721.07

############################   OR IN SUMMARY   ###########################
################## RESULTS FOR LINE TO GROUND FAULT ####################
***********************   1st Row G; 2nd Row T   ****************************
               Z1   Z2   Z0
****
ans =
        0+ 0.14i   0+ 0.14i   0+ 0.08i
        0+ 0.05i   0+ 0.05i   0+ 0.05i

   Iaf_pu   IB_A   Iaf_A   If_LG_pu
****
ans =
        0− 6.9767i   104.59   729.71   6.9767

If_3phase   If_LG_div_If_3phase
****

ans =
5.2632   1.3256

#################   RESULTS FOR LINE TO LINE FAULT   #################
Ia1_pu Ibf_pu   IB_A   IBf_A
****
ans =
0- 2.6316i   −4.558   104.59   −476.74

            Icf_pu Icf_A   If_LL_pu
****
ans =
            4.558 476.74   4.558

If_3phase If_LL_div_If_3phase
****
ans =
5.2632   0.86603

##############   RESULTS FOR DOUBLE LINE TO LINE FAULT   ##############
I_al_pu Va1   I_a2_pu   I_a0_pu
****
ans =
0- 4.3557i 0.17241   0+ 0.90744i   0+ 3.4483i

            I_nf_pu   I_bf_pu   I_cf_pu
****
ans =
            0+ 10.345i −4.5579+ 5.1722i 4.5579+ 5.1725i

---

abs_I_bf_pu   I_Bf_A   abs_I_cf_pu   I_Cf_A
****
ans =
6.8939   721.05   6.8941   721.07

Example K.6

Solve Example J.6 using MATLAB.

```
%Repeat J.5 assuming that the fault is located on bus 3
%Consider the system shown in Figure PJ.4 and assume that the%generator
is loaded and running at the rated voltage with the%circuit breaker open
at bus 3. Assume that the reactance values of the generator are given as
Xd" = X1 = X2 = 0.14 pu and X0 =%0.08 pu based on its ratings. The
transformer impedances are Z1 = Z2 = Z0 = j0.05 pu based on its ratings.
The transmission line%TL23 has Z1 = Z2 = j0.04pu and Z0 = j0.10 pu.
Assume that the fault point is located on bus 1. Select 25 MVA as
```

the%megavoltampere base, and 8.5 and 138 kV as the low-voltage and high-voltage voltage bases, respectively, and determine the%following:

%(a) Subtransient fault current for three-phase fault in per units and amperes.

%(b) Line-to-ground fault. [Also find the ratio of this line-to-ground fault current to the three-phase fault current found in part (a)].

%(c) Line-to-line fault. (Also find the ratio of this line-to-line fault current to previously calculated three-phase fault current.)

%(d) Double line-to-ground fault.

Solution

(a) MATLAB script for Example J.6

```
%
%Data
clear; clc;
format short g
Sb = 25 % System base 50VA
S = 25e6
Vf = 1+i*0 %The voltage to ground of phase "a" at the fault point
F before the fault
%        occurred is Vf and it is usually selected as 1.0/_O pu.

%Generator G
Gb = 25
VLLG = 8.5e3
Z1G = i*0.14*(Sb/Gb)
Z2G = i*0.14*(Sb/Gb)
Z0G = i*0.08*(Sb/Gb)

%Transformer T
Tb = 25
VLLT = 138e3
Z1T = i*0.05*(Sb/Tb)
Z2T = i*0.05*(Sb/Tb)
Z0T = i*0.05*(Sb/Tb)

%Transmission Line TL23
TL23b = 25
VLLT = 138e3
Z1TL = i*0.04*(Sb/Tb)
Z2TL = i*0.04*(Sb/Tb)
Z0TL = i*0.10*(Sb/Tb)
% Part a L-G fault

Z1 = Z1G+Z1T+Z1TL
Z2 = Z2G+Z2T+Z2TL
Z0 = Z0T+Z0TL
%Iaf = 3*Ia0
Iaf_pu = 3*(Vf/(Z0+Z1+Z2))

IB_A = S/(sqrt(3)*VLLT)
Iaf_A = abs(Iaf_pu)*IB_A
```

```
%If_LL = (sqrt(3)/2)*If_3phase

If_LG_pu = abs(Iaf_pu)
%Part b L-L fault
%Assuming that the faulted phases are "b" and "c" Iaf = 0

Ia1_pu = Vf/(Z1+Z2)

Ibf_pu = sqrt(3)*Ia1_pu*(-i)
IB_A = S/(sqrt(3)*VLLT)
IBf_A = Ibf_pu*IB_A

Icf_pu = -Ibf_pu
Icf_A = -IBf_A

%If_LL = (sqrt(3)/2)*If_3phase
If_LL_pu = abs(Ibf_pu)
If_3phase = (2/sqrt(3))*If_LL_pu

If_LL_div_If_3phase = If_LL_pu/If_3phase

%After finding If_3phase from If_Line-to-Line plug back into Part
"a" to find
%Line-to-Grnd/If3pase ratio

If_LG_div_If_3phase = If_LG_pu/If_3phase

%Part c DLG fault
I_a1_pu = Vf/((Z1 + ((Z2*Z0)/(Z2+Z0))))
Va1 = Vf-I_a1_pu*Z1

I_a2_pu = -Va1/Z2
I_a0_pu = -Va1/Z0
I_nf_pu = 3*I_a0_pu


a = -0.5+i*0.866
a2 = a^2
I_bf_pu = a^2*I_a1_pu+a*I_a2_pu+I_a0_pu
abs_I_bf_pu = abs(I_bf_pu)

I_cf_pu = a*I_a1_pu+a^2*I_a2_pu+I_a0_pu
abs_I_cf_pu = abs(I_cf_pu)

I_Bf_A = abs(I_bf_pu)*IB_A
I_Cf_A = abs(I_cf_pu)*IB_A


disp('_____');
disp(' ');
disp(' ');
disp(' ');
disp(' ##############      OR IN SUMMARY      ###############');
disp(' ');
```

```
disp(' ########### RESULTS FOR LINE TO GROUND FAULT ############')
disp(' *******1st Row G; 2nd Row T; 3rd Row TL23    ***********')
disp('     Z1              Z2              Z0 ');
disp('***************************************************************');
[Z1G Z2G Z0G;Z1T Z2T Z0T;Z1TL Z2TL Z0TL]
disp('_____');
disp(' ');
disp(' ');
disp(' ');
disp('    Iaf_pu        IB_A        Iaf_A        If_LG_pu ') ;
disp('***************************************************************');
[Iaf_pu IB_A Iaf_A If_LG_pu]
disp('_____');
disp(' ');
disp(' ');
disp(' ');
disp('If_3phase If_LG_div_If_3phase        ') ;
disp('***************************************************************');
[If_3phase If_LG_div_If_3phase]
disp('_____');
disp(' ');
disp(' ');
disp(' ');
disp('###########   RESULTS FOR LINE TO LINE FAULT   ############')
disp('    Ia1_pu       Ibf_pu       IB_A         IBf_A ') ;
disp('***************************************************************');
[Ia1_pu Ibf_pu IB_A IBf_A]
disp('_____');
disp(' ');
disp(' ');
disp(' ');
disp('Icf_pu Icf_A If_LL_pu' ) ;
disp('***************************************************************');
[Icf_pu Icf_A If_LL_pu]
disp('_____');
disp(' ');
disp(' ');
disp(' ');
disp('If_3phase If_LL_div_If_3phase     ' ) ;
disp('***************************************************************');
[If_3phase If_LL_div_If_3phase]
disp('_____');
disp(' ');
disp(' ');
```

```
disp(' ');
disp('#######  RESULTS FOR DOUBLE LINE TO LINE FAULT  ########')
disp(' I_a1_pu        Va1              I_a2_pu
I_a0_pu ');
disp('*******************************************************');
[I_a1_pu Va1 I_a2_pu I_a0_pu ]
disp('_____');
disp(' ');
disp(' ');
disp(' ');
disp(' I_nf_pu        I_bf_pu        I_cf_pu        ');
disp('*******************************************************');
[I_nf_pu I_bf_pu I_cf_pu]
disp('_____');
disp(' ');
disp(' ');
disp(' ');
disp('abs_I_bf_pu I_Bf_A abs_I_cf_pu I_Cf_A');
disp('*******************************************************');
[abs_I_bf_pu I_Bf_A abs_I_cf_pu I_Cf_A]
disp('_____');
disp(' ');
disp(' ');
disp(' ');
```

(b) MATLAB results for Problem K.6

Sb =
   25
S =
   25000000
Vf =
   1
Gb =
   25
VLLG =
   8500
Z1G =

        0 + 0.14i
Z2G =
        0 + 0.14i
Z0G =
        0 + 0.08i
Tb =
   25
VLLT =
   138000
Z1T =
        0 + 0.05i
Z2T =
        0 + 0.05i
Z0T =
        0 + 0.05i

TL23b =
  25
VLLT =
  138000
Z1TL =
          0 +   0.04i
Z2TL =
          0 +   0.04i
Z0TL =
          0 +   0.1i
Z1 =
          0 +   0.23i
Z2 =
          0 +   0.23i
Z0 =
          0 +   0.15i
Iaf_pu =
          0 −   4.918i
IB_A =
  104.59
Iaf_A =
  514.39
If_LG_pu =
  4.918
Ia1_pu =
          0 − 2.1739i
Ibf_pu =
  −3.7653
IB_A =
  104.59
IBf_A =
  −393.82
Icf_pu =
  3.7653
Icf_A =
  393.82
If_LL_pu =
  3.7653
If_3phase =
  4.3478
If_LL_div_If_3phase =
  0.86603
If_LG_div_If_3phase =
  1.1311
I_a1_pu =
          0 − 3.1173i
Va1 =
  0.28302
I_a2_pu =
          0 + 1.2305i

```
I_a0_pu =
        0 + 1.8868i
I_nf_pu =
        0 + 5.6604i
a =
        −0.5 + 0.866i
a2 =
        −0.49996 − 0.866i
I_bf_pu =
        −3.7652 + 2.8301i
abs_I_bf_pu =
    4.7102
I_cf_pu =
        3.7652 + 2.8302i
abs_I_cf_pu =
    4.7103
I_Bf_A =
    492.65
I_Cf_A =
    492.66
```

#############################   OR IN SUMMARY   ######################
################### RESULTS FOR LINE TO GROUND FAULT ##################
*********************   1st Row G; 2nd Row T; 3rd Row TL23   ******************

Z1		Z2	Z0

```
***************************************************************************
ans =
        0 + 0.14i    0 + 0.14i    0 + 0.08i
        0 + 0.05i    0 + 0.05i    0 + 0.05i
        0 + 0.04i    0 + 0.04i    0 + 0.1i
```

Iaf_pu   IB_A   Iaf_A   If_LG_pu
```
***************************************************************************
ans =
0−  4.918i    104.59              514.39              4.918
```

If_3phase   If_LG_div_If_3phase
```
***************************************************************************
ans =
    4.3478    1.1311
```

###################### RESULTS FOR LINE TO LINE FAULT ###################
Ial_pu   Ibf_pu   IB_A   IBf_A
```
***************************************************************************
ans =
    0−  2.1739i   −3.7653            104.59              −393.82
```

     Icf_pu   Icf_A   If_LL_pu
```
***************************************************************************
```

ans =
  3.7653 393.82 3.7653

If_3phase If_LL_div_If_3phase
****

ans =
  4.3478 0.86603

################# RESULTS FOR DOUBLE LINE TO LINE FAULT #################
I_a1_pu   Va1   I_a2_pu   I_a0_pu
****

ans =
  0− 3.1173i 0.28302   0+ 1.2305i   0+ 1.8868i

          I_nf_pu   I_bf_pu   I_cf_pu
****

ans =
          0+ 5.6604i   −3.7652+ 2.8301i   3.7652+ 2.8302i

---

abs_I_bf_pu I_Bf_A abs_I_cf_pu I_Cf_A
****

ans =
4.7102 492.65 4.7103 492.66

Example K.7

Solve Example J.7 using MATLAB.

```
%Consider the system shown in Figure J.7(a).  Assume that loads, line
capacitance, and transformer-magnetizing currents are%neglected and that
the following data is given based on 20 MVA and the line-to-line voltages
as shown in Figure J.7(a). Do not%neglect the resistance of the
transmission line TL23. The prefault positive-sequence voltage at bus 3
is Van = 1.0/_0 pu, as shown in%Figure J.7(b).

%Generator: X1 = 0.20 pu, X2 = 0.10 pu, Xo = 0.05 pu.
%Transformer T1 : X1 = X2 = 0.05 pu, Xo = X1 (looking into high-voltage
side).
%Transformer T2: X1 = X2 = 0.05 pu, X0 = inf. (looking into high-voltage
side).
%Transmission line: Z1 = Z2 = 0.2 + j0.2 pu, Zo = 0.6 + j0.6 pu.
%Assume that there is a bolted (i.e., with zero fault impedance) line-
to-line fault on phases b and c at bus 3 and determine the following:
    %(a) Fault current Ibf in per units and amperes.
    %(b) Phase voltages Va, Vb, and Vc at bus 2 in per units and
        kilovolts.
```

Solution

(a) MATLAB script for Example K.7
```
%
%Data
clear;
clc;
```

```
format short g
%data
S = 20 % System base 20 MVA
Sb = 20e6
VLL = 20e3
Vf = 1+i*0 %The voltage to ground of phase "a" at the fault point F
before the fault
%       occurred is Vf and it is usually selected as 1.0/_0 pu.


%Generator G
Gb = 20
VLLG = 10e3
Z1G = i*0.2*(S/Gb); Z2G = i*0.1*(S/Gb)
Z0G = i*0.05*(S/Gb)


%Transformer T1
T1b = 20
VLLT1 = 20e3
Z1T1 = i*0.05*(S/T1b)
Z2T1 = i*0.05*(S/T1b)
Z0T1 = i*0.05*(S/T1b)


%Transformer T2
T2b = 20
VLLT2 = 4e3
Z1T2 = i*0.05*(S/T2b)
Z2T2 = i*0.05*(S/T2b)
Z0T2 = i*Inf*(S/T2b)


%Transmission Line TL23
TLb = 20
VLLT = 20e3
Z1TL = 0.2+i*0.2
Z2TL = 0.2+i*0.2
Z0TL = 0.6+i*0.6

% Part (a) Fault current Ibf in per units and amperes.

Z1 = Z1G+Z1T1+Z1TL
Z2 = Z2G+Z2T1+Z2TL

Ia1_pu = Vf/(Z1+Z2)
abs_Ia1_pu = abs(Ia1_pu)
angle_Ia1_rad = angle(Ia1_pu)
angle_Ia1_deg = angle(Ia1_pu)*(180/pi)

%'a' in rectangular form
      a = (-0.5+i*0.866)    % polar: 1/_120
      a2 = (-0.5-i*0.866)   % polar: 1/_-120

a2 = a^2
Ibf_pu = (a^2-a)*Ia1_pu
abs_Ibf_pu = abs(Ibf_pu)
angle_Ibf_rad = angle(Ibf_pu)
angle_Ibf_deg = angle(Ibf_pu)*(180/pi) %Convert rad into degrees

IB_A = Sb/(sqrt(3)*VLL)
Ibf_A = abs(Ibf_pu)*IB_A
```

```
angle_Ibf_deg = angle_Ibf_deg+360 %Convert negative to positive
angle (+360)

% Part (b) Phase voltages Va, Vb, and Vc at bus 2 in per units and
kilovolts.
% The positive-sequence voltage at bus 2 is
Z1_2 = Z1G+Z1T1
Va1_2_pu = Vf-Z1_2*Ia1_pu
abs_Va1_2_pu = abs(Va1_2_pu)
angle_Va1_2_pu = angle(Va1_2_pu)
angle_Va1_2_deg_pu = angle_Va1_2_pu*(180/pi)

% The negative-sequence voltage at bus 2 is
Z2_2 = Z2G+Z2T1
Va2_2_pu = -Z2_2*Ia1_pu
abs_Va2_2_pu = abs(Va2_2_pu)
angle_Va2_2_rad_pu = angle(Va2_2_pu)
angle_Va2_2_deg_pu = angle(Va2_2_pu)*(180/pi)
angle_Va2_2_deg_pu = angle_Va2_2_deg_pu + 360

disp('_____');
disp(' ');
disp(' ');
disp(' ');
disp(' ###################    OR IN SUMMARY    ###############');
disp(' ');
disp(' ######### RESULTS FOR FAULT CURENT Ibf IN pu AND AMPERE
#########')
disp('********* 1st Row G; 2nd Row T1; 3rd Row T2; 4th Row TL23
*******')
disp('         Z1                    Z2          Z0 ');
disp('*******************************************************');
[Z1G Z2G Z0G;Z1T1 Z2T1 Z0T1;Z1T1 Z2T1 Z0T1; Z1TL Z2TL Z0TL]
disp('_____');
disp(' ');
disp(' ');
disp(' ');
disp('         Z1                    Z2                  ');
disp('*******************************************************');
[Z1 Z2]
disp('_____');
disp(' ');
disp(' ');
disp(' ');
disp(' Ia1_pu       abs_Ia1_pu         angle_Ia1_deg ');
disp('*******************************************************');
[Ia1_pu abs_Ia1_pu angle_Ia1_deg]
disp('_____');
disp(' ');
disp(' ');
disp(' ');
disp(' Ibf_pu       abs_Ibf_pu         angle_Ibf_deg ') ;
disp('*******************************************************');
[Ibf_pu abs_Ibf_pu angle_Ibf_deg]
disp('_____');
disp(' ');
disp(' ');
disp(' ');
disp(' IB_A   Ibf_A angle_Ibf_deg  ');
```

```
disp('*********************************************************');
[IB_A Ibf_A angle_Ibf_deg]
disp('_____');
disp(' ');
disp(' ');
disp(' ');
```

(b) MATLAB results for Example K.7

S =
    20
Sb =
    20000000
VLL =
    20000
Vf =
    1
Gb =
    20
VLLG =
    10000
Z2G =
        0 +   0.1i
Z0G =
        0 +   0.05i
T1b =
    20
VLLT1 =
    20000
Z1T1 =
        0 +   0.05i
Z2T1 =
        0 +   0.05i
Z0T1 =
        0 +   0.05i
T2b =
    20
VLLT2 =
    4000
Z1T2 =
        0 +   0.05i
Z2T2 =
        0 +   0.05i
Z0T2 =
        0 +   Infi
TLb =
    20
VLLT =
    20000
Z1TL =
        0.2 +   0.2i

Z2TL =
     0.2 +   0.2i

Z0TL =
     0.6 +   0.6i

Z1 =
     0.2 + 0.45i

Z2 =
     0.2 +   0.35i

Ia1_pu =
     0.5 −   1i

abs_Ia1_pu =

  1.118

angle_Ia1_rad =
  −1.1071

angle_Ia1_deg =
  −63.435

a =
     −0.5 +   0.866i

a2 =
     −0.5 −   0.866i

a2 =
     −0.49996 − 0.866i

Ibf_pu =
     −1.732 −   0.86604i

abs_Ibf_pu =
  1.9364

angle_Ibf_rad =
  −2.6779

angle_Ibf_deg =
  −153.43

IB_A =
  577.35

Ibf_A =
  1118

angle_Ibf_deg =
  206.57

Z1_2 =
  0 + 0.25i

Va1_2_pu =
     0.75 − 0.125i

abs_Va1_2_pu =

  0.76035

angle_Va1_2_pu =
  −0.16515

angle_Va1_2_deg_pu =
  −9.4623

Z2_2 =
        0 + 0.15i

Va2_2_pu =
        −0.15 − 0.075i

abs_Va2_2_pu =
   0.16771

angle_Va2_2_rad_pu =
   −2.6779

angle_Va2_2_deg_pu =
   −153.43

angle_Va2_2_deg_pu =
   206.57

###########################   OR IN SUMMARY   ###########################

############## RESULTS FOR FAULT CURENT Ibf IN pu AND AMPERES ############

******************* 1st Row G; 2nd Row T1; 3rd Row T2; 4th Row TL23 *****************
        Z1   Z2   Z0
****
ans =

0+	0.2i	0+	0.1i	0+	0.05i
0+	0.05i	0+	0.05i	0+	0.05i
0+	0.05i	0+	0.05i	0+	0.05i
0.2+	0.2i	0.2+	0.2i	0.6+	0.6i

          Z1   Z2
****
ans =

     0.2+ 0.45i   0.2+ 0.35i

    Ia1_pu   abs_Ia1_pu   angle_Ia1_deg
****
ans =

    0.5 −   1i   1.118   −63.435

    Ibf_pu   abs_Ibf_pu   angle_Ibf_deg
****
ans =

    −1.732   −0.86604i   1.9364   206.57

    IB_A   Ibf_A   angle_Ibf_deg
****
ans =

  577.35   1118   206.57

Example K.8

Solve Example J.8 using MATLAB.

Consider Figure PJ.8 and assume that the generator ratings are 2.40/4.16Y kV, 15 MW (3ϕ), 18.75 MVA (3ϕ), 80% power factor, two poles, 3600 rpm. Generator reactances are $X_1 = X_2 = 0.10$ pu and $X_0 = 0.05$ pu, all based on generator ratings. Note that the given value of X_1 is subtransient reactance ampere X'', one of several different positive-sequence reactances of a synchronous machine. The subtransient reactance corresponds to the initial symmetrical fault current (the transient dc component not included) that occurs before demagnetizing armature magnetomotive force begins to weaken the net field excitation. If manufactured in accordance with US standards, the coils of a synchronous generator will withstand the mechanical forces that accompany a three-phase fault current, but not more. Assume that this generator is to supply a four-wire, wye-connected distribution. Therefore, the neutral grounding reactor X_n should have the smallest possible reactance. Consider both SLG and DLG faults. Assume that the prefault positive-sequence internal voltage of phase a is 2500 ∠0° or 1.042 0° 1.042 ∠0° pu and determine the following:

(a) Specify X_n in ohms and in per units.
(b) Specify the minimum allowable momentary symmetrical current rating of the reactor in amperes.
(c) Find the initial symmetrical voltage across the reactor, V_n, when a bolted SLG fault occurs on the OCB terminal in volts.

Solution

(a) MATLAB script for Example K.8

```
%
%Data
clear; clc;
format short g
%data
% System base MVA

x0 = i*0.05;%pu
x1 = i*0.1; %pu
x2 = i*0.1; %pu all based on generator ratings

Vf = 1.042; %/1.042_0deg polar = 1.042 rectangular
Z1 = x1;
Z2 = x2;
```

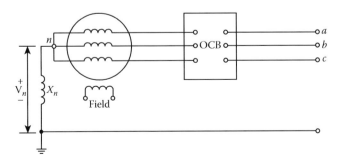

FIGURE PJ.8   System for Problem K.8.

```
%Part(a) Specify Xn, in ohms and in per units
Ia_3phase = Vf/Z1;
%SLG Fault:
Z = x0+x1+x2;
%For Xn = 0:
Xn = 0;
Ia0 = Vf/(Z+3*Xn);
Ia_SLG_abs = abs(3*Ia0); %pu

%DLG Fault
%Vf-Ia1*Z1 = -Ia2*Z2 = Ia1*Z2+Ia0*Z2-Ia0*(Z0+3*Zn)............(1)
%-Ia0(Z0+3Zn) = Ia1Z2+Ia0Z2.................................(2)
Ia0 = (i*1.042)/(0.2+6*Xn);%pu
Ia2 = (i*(0.05+3*Xn)*Ia0)/(i*0.1);%pu
Ia1 = -Ia2-Ia0; %pu
%'a' in rectangular form
        a = (-0.5+i*0.866);  % polar: 1/_120 deg
        a2 = (-0.5-i*0.866); % polar: 1/_-120 deg

Ib_DLG_abs = abs(Ia0*(1-a)+Ia1*(a^2-a)); %pu
Ic_DLG_abs = abs(Ia0*(1-a^2)+Ia1*(a-a^2)); %pu

%The grounding reactor Xn:

%Ia_LG_abs = abs(3*Ia0)

syms Vf Z_ q x2
%q = Xn;
%3*(Vf/(Z+3*q)) = Vf/x2
%Ia0 = Vf/(Z+3*Xn);
x0 = i*0.05;%pu
x1 = i*0.1; %pu
x2 = i*0.1; %pu all based on generator ratings
Z = x0+x1+x2;
Z_ = Z/i;
Vf = 1.042;
%3*(Vf/(Z+3*q)) = =Vf/x2
%Ia0 = Vf/(Z+3*Xn);
S = (3*Vf)/(Z_+3*q)-((Vf/(x2/i)));
q = solve(S,q);
%Xn in pu
Xn_pu = eval(q); %pu
%Xn in ohm
V_sec = 4.16E3; %V
B = 18.75E6; % VA base
Xn_ohm = Xn_pu*(V_sec^2/B); %ohm
```

(b) MATLAB results for Problem K.8

```
%Part (b) Specify the minimum allowable momentary symmetrical
current
%rating of the reactor in amperes.
IXn_DLG_pu = 3*(Vf/(Z_+3*Xn_pu)); %pu
IXn_DLG_A = IXn_DLG_pu*(B/(sqrt(3)*V_sec)); %pu
%Part (c) Find the initial symmetrical voltage across the reactor,
Vn, when a
%bolted SLG fault occurs on the oil circuit breaker (OCB) terminal
%in volts.
Zn = i*Xn_pu;
Vn_pu = -(-i*IXn_DLG_pu)*(Zn); %pu
V_pr = 2.4E3;
Vn_V = Vn_pu*V_pr;
```

```
        disp('_____');
        disp(' ');
        disp(' ');
        disp(' ');
        disp(' #################    OR IN SUMMARY    #############');
        disp(' ');
        disp(' Xn_pu   Xn_ohm        ');
        disp(' ************************************************************');
        [Xn_pu Xn_ohm]
        disp('_____');
        disp(' ');
        disp(' ');
        disp(' ');
        disp(' IXn_DLG_pu    IXn_DLG_A    ') ;
        disp(' ************************************************************');
        [IXn_DLG_pu    IXn_DLG_A]
        disp('_____');
        disp(' ');
        disp(' ');
        disp(' ');
        disp('Vn_pu            Vn_V     ') ;
        disp('************************************************************');
        [Vn_pu Vn_V]
        disp(' ');
        disp(' ');
        disp(' ');
```

Solutions

####################### OR IN SUMMARY ##########################

Xn_pu Xn_ohm

****

ans =
0.016667   0.015383

IXn_DLG_pu IXn_DLG_A

****

ans =
      10.42   27115

Vn_pu   Vn_V

****

ans =
 −0.17367 −416.8

Example K.9

Solve Example J.9 using MATLAB.

Consider the system shown in Figure PJ.9 and the following data:
Generator G: $X_1 = X_2 = 0.10$ pu and $X0 = 0.05$ pu based on its ratings.
Motor: $X_1 = X_2 = 0.10$ pu and $X_0 = 0.05$ pu based on its ratings.
Transformer T_1: $X_1 = X_2 = X_0 = 0.05$ pu based on its ratings.
Transformer T_2: $X_1 = X_2 = X_0 = 0.10$ pu based on its ratings.
Transmission line TL_{23}: $X_1 = X_2 = X_0 = 0.09$ pu based on 25 MVA.

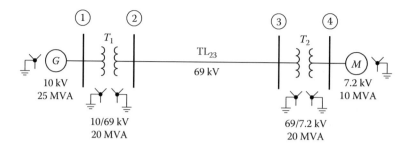

FIGURE PJ.9 System for Example K.9.

Assume that bus 2 is faulted and determine the faulted phase currents.

(a) Determine the three-phase fault.
(b) Determine the line-to-ground fault involving phase a.
(c) Use the results of part (a) and calculate the line-to-neutral phase voltages at the fault point.

Solution

(a) MATLAB script for Example K.9

```
%Data
clear; clc;
format short g
%data
%System base 25MVA
S = 25E6;% VA

%Generator:
X0 = i*0.05;%pu
X1 = i*0.1; %pu
X2 = i*0.1; %pu all based on 25MVA ratings

%Transformer T1:
T1_base = 20E6;%VA
Z0_1 = i*0.05;
Z1_1 = i*0.05;
Z2_1 = i*0.05;
Z0_T1 = i*0.05*(S/T1_base);
Z1_T1 = Z0_T1;
Z2_T1 = Z0_T1;

%Line
Z0_L = i*0.09;
Z1_L = i*0.09;
Z2_L = i*0.09;

%Transformer T2:
T2_base = 20E6;%MVA
Z0_2 = i*0.1;
Z1_2 = i*0.1;
Z2_2 = i*0.1;
Z0_T2 = i*0.1*(S/T2_base);
Z1_T2 = Z0_T2;
Z2_T2 = Z0_T2;
```

```
%Motor
M_base = 10E6;%MVA
X0_ = i*0.05;
X1_ = i*0.1;
X2_ = i*0.1;
X0_M = X0_*(S/M_base);
X1_M = X1_*(S/M_base);
X2_M = X1_M;


%Part(a)
Z1_Th = ((X1+Z1_T1)*(Z1_L+Z1_T2+X1_M))/
((X1+Z1_T1+Z1_L+Z1_T2+X1_M));%pu
Vf = 1.0;
If_3phase = Vf/Z1_Th; %pu


%Part(b)
Z0_Th = ((X0+Z0_T1)*(Z0_L+Z0_T2+X0_M))/
(X0+Z0_T1+Z0_L+Z0_T2+X0_M);%pu
Z2_Th = Z1_Th;
If = (3*Vf)/(Z0_Th+Z1_Th+Z2_Th);


%Part(c)
Va = 0;
Vb = Va;
Vc = Va;
disp('  _____  ');
disp(' ');
disp(' ');
disp(' ');
disp(' ############### OR IN SUMMARY    ###############');
disp(' ');
disp(' If_3phase      If            ');
disp(' ***********************************************************');
[If_3phase    If ]
disp('  _____  ');
disp(' ');
disp(' ');
disp(' ');
disp(' Va Vb Vc      ');
disp(' ***********************************************************');
[ Va Vb Vc]
```

Solutions

```
_____ _____
####################### OR IN SUMMARY      ####################
If_3phase      If
*************************************************************************
ans =
     0 - 8.3044i    0 - 9.2204i

_____
Va Vb Vc
*************************************************************************
ans =
0 0 0
```

Example K.10

Solve Example J.10 using MATLAB.

Consider the system given in Problem J.9 and assume a line-to-line fault, involving phases *b* and *c*, at bus 2, and determine the faulted phase currents.

Solution

(a)   MATLAB script for Example K.10

```
%Data
clear; clc;
format short g
%data
%System base 25MVA
S = 25E6;% VA

%Generator:
X0 = i*0.05;%pu
X1 = i*0.1; %pu
X2 = i*0.1; %pu all based on 25MVA ratings

%Transformer T1:
T1_base = 20E6;%VA
Z0_1 = i*0.05;
Z1_1 = i*0.05;
Z2_1 = i*0.05;
Z0_T1 = i*0.05*(S/T1_base);
Z1_T1 = Z0_T1;
Z2_T1 = Z0_T1;

%Line
Z0_L = i*0.09;
Z1_L = i*0.09;
Z2_L = i*0.09;

%Transformer T2:
T2_base = 20E6;%MVA
Z0_2 = i*0.1;
Z1_2 = i*0.1;
Z2_2 = i*0.1;
Z0_T2 = i*0.1*(S/T2_base);
Z1_T2 = Z0_T2;
Z2_T2 = Z0_T2;

%Motor
M_base = 10E6;%MVA
X0_ = i*0.05;
X1_ = i*0.1;
X2_ = i*0.1;
X0_M = X0_*(S/M_base);
X1_M = X1_*(S/M_base);
X2_M = X1_M;

%Part(a)
Z1_Th = ((X1+Z1_T1)*(Z1_L+Z1_T2+X1_M))/
((X1+Z1_T1+Z1_L+Z1_T2+X1_M));%pu
Vf = 1.0;
If_3phase = Vf/Z1_Th; %pu
```

```
%Part(b)
Z0_Th = ((X0+Z0_T1)*(Z0_L+Z0_T2+X0_M))/
(X0+Z0_T1+Z0_L+Z0_T2+X0_M);%pu
Z2_Th = Z1_Th;
If = (3*Vf)/(Z0_Th+Z1_Th+Z2_Th);%pu

%Part(c)
Va = 0;
Vb = Va;
Vc = Va;

%Assume L-L fault, involving phases b and c, at bus 2
Ia1 = Vf/(Z1_Th+Z2_Th); %pu
Iaf = 0 ;
Ibf = sqrt(3)*Ia1*(-i); %pu
Icf = -Ibf ;   %pu

disp('_____');
disp(' ');
disp(' ');
disp(' ');
disp('################## OR IN SUMMARY   #############');
disp(' ');
disp('Ia1 Iaf Ibf    Icf      ');
disp('***************************************************************');
[Ia1   Iaf Ibf Icf ]
disp('_____');
disp(' ');
disp(' ');
disp(' ');
```

Solutions

_____

########################### OR IN SUMMARY   ###########################

Ia1   Iaf   Ibf   Icf
****

ans =

0 − 4.1522i 0   −7.1918   7.1918

_____

Example K.11

Solve Example J.11 using MATLAB.

Consider the system shown in Figure PJ.11 and assume that the associated data are given in Table PJ.11 and are based on a 100 MVA base and referred to nominal system voltages.
  Assume that there is a three-phase fault at bus 6. Ignore the prefault currents and determine the following:

  (a) Fault current in per units at faulted bus 6
  (b) Fault current in per units in transmission line TL_{25}

Solution

(a) MATLAB script for Example K.11

```
%Data
clear; clc;
format short g
%data
%System base 100MVA
S = 100E6;% VA

%Generator 1:
X1_G1 = i*0.35;%pu
X2_G1 = i*0.35; %pu
X3_G1 = i*0.09; %pu all based on 100MVA ratings

%Generator 2:
X1_G2 = i*0.35;%pu
X2_G2 = i*0.35; %pu
X3_G2 = i*0.09; %pu all based on 100MVA ratings

%Transformer T1:
T1_base = 100E6;%VA
Z0_1 = i*0.1;
Z1_1 = i*0.1;
Z2_1 = i*0.1;
Z0_T1 = i*0.1*(S/T1_base);
Z1_T1 = Z0_T1;
Z2_T1 = Z0_T1;

%Transformer T2:
T2_base = 100E6;%VA
Z0_2 = i*0.1;
Z1_2 = i*0.1;
Z2_2 = i*0.1;
Z0_T2 = i*0.1*(S/T2_base);
Z1_T2 = Z0_T1;
Z2_T2 = Z0_T1;

%Transformer T3:
T3_base = 100E6;%VA
Z0_3 = i*0.05;
Z1_3 = i*0.05;
Z2_3 = i*0.05;
Z0_T3 = i*0.05*(S/T2_base);
Z1_T3 = Z0_T3;
Z2_T3 = Z0_T3;
```

TABLE PJ.11

Data for Problem J.11

Network Component	X_1 (pu)	X_2 (pu)	X_3 (pu)
G_1	0.35	0.35	0.09
G_2	0.35	0.35	0.09
T_1	0.10	0.10	0.10
T_2	0.10	0.10	0.10
T_3	0.05	0.05	0.05
TL_{42}	0.45	0.45	1.80
TL_{25}	0.35	0,45	1 15
TL_{45}	0.35	0.35	1.15

```
%Line TL42
Z0_TL42 = i*0.45;
Z1_TL42 = i*0.45;
Z2_TL42 = i*1.80;

%Line TL25
Z0_TL25 = i*0.35;
Z1_TL25 = i*0.45;
Z2_TL25 = i*1.15;
%Line TL45

Z0_TL45 = i*0.35;
Z1_TL45 = i*0.35;
Z2_TL45 = i*1.15;

%Part(a) from Example J.11
%Ia0 = Ia2 = 0
%Ia1 = Vf/(Z1+Zf)
Vf = 1.0;
Z1_Th = j*0.45;
If_3phase = Vf/Z1_Th; %pu

%Part(b) from Problem J.11
If_3phase_TL25 = (If_3phase)/(2);%pu
%The three phase fault is symmetrical therefore:
%Va1 = Vf-Ia1*Z1
Va1 = Vf-Z1_Th*If_3phase;
Va0 = Va1;
Va2 = Va1;
Van = Va1+Va2+Va0;
Vbn = Van;
Vcn = Van;

disp('_____');
disp(' ');
disp(' ');
disp(' ');
disp(' ############### OR IN SUMMARY      ###############');
disp(' ');
disp('Van Vbn Vcn                                    ');

disp('***************************************************************');
[ Van Vbn Vcn ]
disp('_____');
disp(' ');
disp(' ');
disp(' ');
```

Solutions

_____

####################   OR IN SUMMARY   ###############
Van Vbn Vcn
****

ans =

0 0 0

_____

Example K.12

Solve Example J.12 using MATLAB.

Use the results of Example J.11 and calculate the line-to-neutral phase voltages at the faulted bus 6.

Solution

(b) MATLAB script for Example K.12

```
%Data
clear; clc;
format short g
%data
%System base 100MVA
S = 100E6;% VA


%Generator 1:
X1_G1 = i*0.35;%pu
X2_G1 = i*0.35; %pu
X3_G1 = i*0.09; %pu all based on 100MVA ratings


%Generator 2:
X1_G2 = i*0.35;%pu
X2_G2 = i*0.35; %pu
X3_G2 = i*0.09; %pu all based on 100MVA ratings


%Transformer T1:
T1_base = 100E6;%VA
Z0_1 = i*0.1;
Z1_1 = i*0.1;
Z2_1 = i*0.1;
Z0_T1 = i*0.1*(S/T1_base);
Z1_T1 = Z0_T1;
Z2_T1 = Z0_T1;


%Transformer T2:
T2_base = 100E6;%VA
Z0_2 = i*0.1;
Z1_2 = i*0.1;
Z2_2 = i*0.1;
Z0_T2 = i*0.1*(S/T2_base);
Z1_T2 = Z0_T1;
Z2_T2 = Z0_T1;


%Transformer T3:
T3_base = 100E6;%VA
Z0_3 = i*0.05;
Z1_3 = i*0.05;
Z2_3 = i*0.05;
Z0_T3 = i*0.05*(S/T2_base);
Z1_T3 = Z0_T3;
Z2_T3 = Z0_T3;


%Line TL42
Z0_TL42 = i*0.45;
Z1_TL42 = i*0.45;
Z2_TL42 = i*1.80;
```

```
%Line TL25
Z0_TL25 = i*0.35;
Z1_TL25 = i*0.45;
Z2_TL25 = i*1.15;


%Line TL45
Z0_TL45 = i*0.35;
Z1_TL45 = i*0.35;
Z2_TL45 = i*1.15;


%Part(a) from Example J.11
%Ia0 = Ia2 = 0
%Ia1 = Vf/(Z1+Zf)
Vf = 1.0;
Z1_Th = j*0.45;
If_3phase = Vf/Z1_Th; %pu


%Part(b) from Problem J.11
If_3phase_TL25 = (If_3phase)/(2);%pu
%The three phase fault is symmetrical therefore:
%Va1 = Vf-Ia1*Z1
Va1 = Vf-Z1_Th*If_3phase;
Va0 = Va1;
Va2 = Va1;
Van = Va1+Va2+Va0;
Vbn = Van;
Vcn = Van;


disp('  _____ ');
disp(' ');
disp(' ');
disp(' ');
disp('############### OR IN SUMMARY ###############');
disp(' ');
disp('Van Vbn Vcn                                        ');
disp('***************************************************************');
[ Van Vbn Vcn ]
disp('_____ ');
disp(' ');
disp(' ');
disp(' ');
```

Solutions

############################ OR IN SUMMARY   ###########################
Van Vbn Vcn
****

ans =

0 0 0

Example K.13

Solve Example J.13 using MATLAB.

Repeat Example J.11 assuming a line-to-ground fault, with $\mathbf{Z}_f = 0$ pu, at bus 6.

Solution

(a) MATLAB script for Example K.13

```
%Data
clear; clc;
format short g
%data
%System base 100MVA
S = 100E6;% VA

%Generator 1:
X1_G1 = i*0.35;%pu
X2_G1 = i*0.35; %pu
X3_G1 = i*0.09; %pu all based on 100MVA ratings

%Generator 2:
X1_G2 = i*0.35;%pu
X2_G2 = i*0.35; %pu
X3_G2 = i*0.09; %pu all based on 100MVA ratings

%Transformer T1:
T1_base = 100E6;%VA
Z0_1 = i*0.1;
Z1_1 = i*0.1;
Z2_1 = i*0.1;
Z0_T1 = i*0.1*(S/T1_base);
Z1_T1 = Z0_T1;
Z2_T1 = Z0_T1;

%Transformer T2:
T2_base = 100E6;%VA
Z0_2 = i*0.1;
Z1_2 = i*0.1;
Z2_2 = i*0.1;
Z0_T2 = i*0.1*(S/T2_base);
Z1_T2 = Z0_T1;
Z2_T2 = Z0_T1;

%Transformer T3:
T3_base = 100E6;%VA
Z0_3 = i*0.05;
Z1_3 = i*0.05;
Z2_3 = i*0.05;
Z0_T3 = i*0.05*(S/T2_base);
Z1_T3 = Z0_T3;
Z2_T3 = Z0_T3;

%Line TL42
Z0_TL42 = i*0.45;
Z1_TL42 = i*0.45;
Z2_TL42 = i*1.80;

%Line TL25
Z0_TL25 = i*0.35;
```

```
Z1_TL25 = i*0.45;
Z2_TL25 = i*1.15;

%Line TL45
Z0_TL45 = i*0.35;
Z1_TL45 = i*0.35;
Z2_TL45 = i*1.15;

%Part(a)
Vf = 1.0;
Z0_Th = j*0.97744;
Z1_Th = j*0.45;
Z2_Th = j*0.45;
Ia1 = Vf/(Z1_Th+Z2_Th+Z0_Th);
Ia0 = Ia1;
Ia2 = Ia1;
Ia_SLG_pu = 3*Ia0;

%Part(b)
Ia1_TL25 = Ia1/2;
Ia2_TL25 = Ia1_TL25;
Ia2 = Ia1;
Ia0_TL25 = Ia0*((i*1.8+i*1.15)/(i*1.8+i*1.15+i*1.15));
Ia_SLG_TL25_pu = Ia1_TL25+Ia2_TL25+Ia0_TL25;

disp(' _____ ');
disp(' ');
disp(' ');
disp(' ');
disp(' ############  OR IN SUMMARY  ############');
disp(' ');
disp(' Ia_SLG_pu Ia_SLG_TL25_pu                        ');
disp(' ****************************************************************');
[       Ia_SLG_pu Ia_SLG_TL25_pu ]
disp(' _____ ');
disp(' ');
disp(' ');
disp(' ');
```

Solutions

_____

########################## OR IN SUMMARY ##########################
       Ia_SLG_pu   Ia_SLG_TL25_pu
****

ans =
        0 − 1.5979i   0 − 0.91588i

_____

Example K.14

Solve Example J.14 using MATLAB.

Use the results of Example J.13 and calculate the line-to-neutral phase voltages at the following buses:

(a) Bus 6
(b) Bus 2

Solution

(a)   MATLAB script for Example K.14

```
%Data
clear; clc;
format short g
%data
%System base 100MVA
S = 100E6;% VA

%Generator 1:
X1_G1 = i*0.35;%pu
X2_G1 = i*0.35; %pu
X3_G1 = i*0.09; %pu all based on 100MVA ratings

%Generator 2:
X1_G2 = i*0.35;%pu
X2_G2 = i*0.35; %pu
X3_G2 = i*0.09; %pu all based on 100MVA ratings

%Transformer T1:
T1_base = 100E6;%VA
Z0_1 = i*0.1;
Z1_1 = i*0.1;
Z2_1 = i*0.1;
Z0_T1 = i*0.1*(S/T1_base);
Z1_T1 = Z0_T1;
Z2_T1 = Z0_T1;

%Transformer T2:
T2_base = 100E6;%VA
Z0_2 = i*0.1;
Z1_2 = i*0.1;
Z2_2 = i*0.1;
Z0_T2 = i*0.1*(S/T2_base);
Z1_T2 = Z0_T1;
Z2_T2 = Z0_T1;

%Transformer T3:
T3_base = 100E6;%VA
Z0_3 = i*0.05;
Z1_3 = i*0.05;
Z2_3 = i*0.05;
Z0_T3 = i*0.05*(S/T2_base);
Z1_T3 = Z0_T3;
Z2_T3 = Z0_T3;

%Line TL42
Z0_TL42 = i*0.45;
Z1_TL42 = i*0.45;
Z2_TL42 = i*1.80;
%Line TL25
Z0_TL25 = i*0.35;
Z1_TL25 = i*0.45;
Z2_TL25 = i*1.15;

%Line TL45
Z0_TL45 = i*0.35;
Z1_TL45 = i*0.35;
Z2_TL45 = i*1.15;
```

```
%Part(a) from Example J.13
Vf = 1.0;
Z0_Th = j*0.97744;
Z1_Th = j*0.45;
Z2_Th = j*0.45;
Ia1 = Vf/(Z1_Th+Z2_Th+Z0_Th);
Ia0 = Ia1;
Ia2 = Ia1;
Ia_SLG_pu = 3*Ia0;

%Part(b) from Example J.13
Ia1_TL25 = Ia1/2;
Ia2_TL25 = Ia1_TL25;
Ia2 = Ia1;
Ia0_TL25 = Ia0*((i*1.8+i*1.15)/(i*1.8+i*1.15+i*1.15));
Ia_SLG_TL25_pu = Ia1_TL25+Ia2_TL25+Ia0_TL25;

%Part(a) at bus 6
Va1_pu = Vf-Ia1*Z1_Th;
Va2_pu = 0-Ia2*Z2_Th;
Va0_pu = 0-Ia0*Z0_Th;
Vaf_pu = Va1_pu+Va2_pu+Va0_pu;
[real, angle_rad, angle_deg] = cart2polar(Vaf_pu);

Vaf_pu_polar = [real angle_deg];
%'a' in rectangular form
        a = (-0.5+i*0.866);  % polar: 1/_120 deg
        a2 = (-0.5-i*0.866); % polar: 1/_-120 deg
Vbf_pu = Va0_pu+a^2*Va1_pu+a*Va2_pu;
[real, angle_rad, angle_deg] = cart2polar(Vbf_pu);
Vbf_pu_polar = [real angle_deg];
Vcf_pu = Va0_pu+a*Va1_pu+a^2*Va2_pu;
[real, angle_rad, angle_deg] = cart2polar(Vcf_pu);
Vcf_pu_polar = [real angle_deg];

disp('_____');
disp(' ');
disp(' ');
disp(' ');
disp(' ################## OR IN SUMMARY  ###############');
disp(' ');
disp(' Vaf_pu_polar Vbf_pu_polar   Vcf_pu_polar ');
disp(' ********************************************************');
[Vaf_pu_polar Vbf_pu_polar Vcf_pu_polar]
disp('_____');
disp(' ');
disp(' ');
disp(' ');
```

Solutions

_____

######################### OR IN SUMMARY   ########################
Vaf_pu_polar   Vbf_pu_polar   Vcf_pu_polar
****

ans =
0   0 1.1661 −132.04 1.1661 132.04

_____

Example K.15

Solve Example J.11 using MATLAB.

```
%Repeat Example J.11 assuming a line-to-line fault at bus 6.
```

Solution

(a) MATLAB script for Example K.15

```
%Data
clear; clc;
format short g
%data
%System base 100MVA
S = 100E6;% VA

%Generator 1:
X1_G1 = i*0.35;%pu
X2_G1 = i*0.35; %pu
X3_G1 = i*0.09; %pu all based on 100MVA ratings

%Generator 2:
X1_G2 = i*0.35;%pu
X2_G2 = i*0.35; %pu
X3_G2 = i*0.09; %pu all based on 100MVA ratings

%Transformer T1:
T1_base = 100E6;%VA
Z0_1 = i*0.1;
Z1_1 = i*0.1;
Z2_1 = i*0.1;
Z0_T1 = i*0.1*(S/T1_base);
Z1_T1 = Z0_T1;
Z2_T1 = Z0_T1;

%Transformer T2:
T2_base = 100E6;%VA
Z0_2 = i*0.1;
Z1_2 = i*0.1;
Z2_2 = i*0.1;
Z0_T2 = i*0.1*(S/T2_base);
Z1_T2 = Z0_T1;
Z2_T2 = Z0_T1;

%Transformer T3:
T3_base = 100E6;%VA
Z0_3 = i*0.05;
Z1_3 = i*0.05;
Z2_3 = i*0.05;
Z0_T3 = i*0.05*(S/T2_base);
Z1_T3 = Z0_T3;
Z2_T3 = Z0_T3;

%Line TL42
Z0_TL42 = i*0.45;
Z1_TL42 = i*0.45;
Z2_TL42 = i*1.80;

%Line TL25
Z0_TL25 = i*0.35;
```

```
        Z1_TL25 = i*0.45;
        Z2_TL25 = i*1.15;

        %Line TL45
        Z0_TL45 = i*0.35;
        Z1_TL45 = i*0.35;
        Z2_TL45 = i*1.15;

        %Part(a)
        %Ia0 = Ia2 = 0
        %Ia1 = -Ia2 = Vf/(Z1+Z2)
        Vf = 1.0;
        Z1_Th = j*0.45;
        Z2_Th = j*0.45;
        Ia1 = Vf/(Z1_Th+Z2_Th);
        Iaf = 0;
        Ibf = -i*sqrt(3)*(Vf/(Z2_Th+Z2_Th));
        Icf = -Ibf;

        %Part(b)
        Iaf_TL25_pu = 0;
        Ibf_TL25_pu = Ibf/2;
        Icf_TL25_pu = Icf/2;

        disp('_____');
        disp(' ');
        disp(' ');
        disp(' ');
        disp('############## OR IN SUMMARY ###############');
        disp(' ');
        disp('Iaf_pu Ibf_pu Icf_pu Iaf_TL25_pu Ibf_TL25_pu Icf_TL25_pu ');
        disp(' *********************************************************');
        [ Iaf Ibf Icf Iaf_TL25_pu Ibf_TL25_pu Icf_TL25_pu]
        disp('_____');
        disp(' ');
        disp(' ');
        disp(' ');
```

Solutions

################## IN SUMMARY ###############

Iaf_pu Ibf_pu Icf_pu Iaf_TL25_pu Ibf_TL25_pu Icf_TL25_pu

****

ans =

0 −1.9245 1.9245 0   −0.96225 0.96225

Example K.16

Solve Example J.11 using MATLAB.

```
%Repeat Example J.11 assuming a double line-to-ground fault, with
%Zf = 0 and Zg = 0, at bus 6.
```

Solution

(a) MATLAB script for Example K.16
```
      %Data
      clear; clc;
```

```
format short g
%data
%System base 100MVA
S = 100E6;% VA

%Generator 1:
X1_G1 = i*0.35;%pu
X2_G1 = i*0.35; %pu
X3_G1 = i*0.09; %pu all based on 100MVA ratings

%Generator 2:
X1_G2 = i*0.35;%pu
X2_G2 = i*0.35; %pu
X3_G2 = i*0.09; %pu all based on 100MVA ratings

%Transformer T1:
T1_base = 100E6;%VA
Z0_1 = i*0.1;
Z1_1 = i*0.1;
Z2_1 = i*0.1;
Z0_T1 = i*0.1*(S/T1_base);
Z1_T1 = Z0_T1;
Z2_T1 = Z0_T1;

%Transformer T2:
T2_base = 100E6;%VA
Z0_2 = i*0.1;
Z1_2 = i*0.1;
Z2_2 = i*0.1;
Z0_T2 = i*0.1*(S/T2_base);
Z1_T2 = Z0_T1;
Z2_T2 = Z0_T1;

%Transformer T3:
T3_base = 100E6;%VA
Z0_3 = i*0.05;
Z1_3 = i*0.05;
Z2_3 = i*0.05;
Z0_T3 = i*0.05*(S/T2_base);
Z1_T3 = Z0_T3;
Z2_T3 = Z0_T3;

%Line TL42
Z0_TL42 = i*0.45;
Z1_TL42 = i*0.45;
Z2_TL42 = i*1.80;

%Line TL25
Z0_TL25 = i*0.35;
Z1_TL25 = i*0.45;
Z2_TL25 = i*1.15;

%Line TL45
Z0_TL45 = i*0.35;
Z1_TL45 = i*0.35;
Z2_TL45 = i*1.15;

%Part(a)
%Ia0 = Ia2 = 0
%Ia1 = -Ia2 = Vf/(Z1+Z2)
```

```
Vf = 1.0;
Z1_Th = j*0.45;
Z0_Th = j*0.97744;
Z2_Th = j*0.45;
Ia1 = Vf/(Z1_Th+(Z2_Th*Z0_Th)/(Z2_Th+Z0_Th));

Va1 = Vf-Ia1*Z1_Th;
Va2 = Va1;
Va0 = Va1;
Ia2 = -Va2/Z2_Th;
Ia0 = -Va0/Z0_Th;
%'a' in rectangular form
        a = (-0.5+i*0.866);  % polar: 1/_120 deg
        a2 = (-0.5-i*0.866); % polar: 1/_-120 deg
Iaf = 0;
Ibf = a^2*Ia1+a*Ia2+Ia0;
[real, angle_rad, angle_deg] = cart2polar(Ibf);
Ibf = [real angle_deg];
Icf = a*Ia1+a^2*Ia2+Ia0;
[real, angle_rad, angle_deg] = cart2polar(Icf);
Icf = [real angle_deg];

disp('_____');
disp(' ');
disp(' ');
disp(' ');
disp(' ###############  OR IN SUMMARY   ##############');
disp(' ');
disp(' Iaf_pu Ibf_pu Icf_pu ');
disp('*******************************************************************');
[ Iaf Ibf Icf ]
disp('_____');
disp(' ');
disp(' ');
disp(' ');
```

Solutions

_____

#########################   OR IN SUMMARY   #####################
        Iaf_pu   Ibf_pu   Icf_pu
****

ans =

        0   2.023 162.04   2.023 17.959

_____

Example K.17

Solve Example J.17 using MATLAB.

```
%Consider the system shown in Figure PJ.17 and data given in Table
%PJ.17. Assume there is a fault at bus 2. After drawing the corresponding
%sequence networks, reduce them to their Thevenin equivalents
```

```
%looking in at bus 2.
  %(a) Positive-sequence network.
  %(b) Negative-sequence network.
  %(c) Zero-sequence network.

%TABLE PJ.17 Table for Example J.17
%Network Base      X1 X2 X0
%Component MVA (pu) (pu) (pu)
%G1          100    0.2   0.15  0.05
%G2          100    0.3   0.2   0.05
%T1          100    0.2   0.2   0.2
%T2          100    0.15  0.15  0.15
%TL12        100    0.6   0.6   0.9
```

Solution

(a) MATLAB script for Example K.17

```
%Data
clear; clc;
format short g
%data
%System base 100MVA
S = 100;% pu

%Generator 1:
Z1_G1 = i*0.20; %pu
Z2_G1 = i*0.15; %pu
Z0_G1 = i*0.05; %pu

%Generator 2:
Z1_G2 = i*0.30; %pu
Z2_G2 = i*0.20; %pu
Z0_G2 = i*0.05; %pu

%Transformer T1:
T1_base = 100; %pu
Z1_T1 = i*0.2; %pu
Z2_T1 = i*0.2; %pu
Z0_T1 = i*0.2; %pu

%Transformer T2:
T2_base = 100; %pu
Z1_T2 = i*0.15;%pu
Z2_T2 = i*0.15;%pu
Z0_T2 = i*0.15;%pu

%Line TL12
Z1_TL12 = i*0.60;%pu
Z2_TL12 = i*0.60;%pu
Z0_TL12 = i*0.90;%pu

%Part(a)
Z1_Th = ((Z1_G1+Z1_T1+Z1_TL12)*(Z1_T2+Z1_G2))/
(Z1_G1+Z1_T1+Z1_TL12+Z1_T2+Z1_G2);

%Part(b)
Z2_Th = ((Z2_G1+Z2_T1+Z2_TL12)*(Z2_T2+Z2_G2))/
(Z2_G1+Z2_T1+Z2_TL12+Z2_T2+Z2_G2);
```

```
%Part(c)
Z0_Th = ((Z0_G1+Z0_T1+Z0_TL12)*(Z0_T2))/(Z0_G1+Z0_T1+Z0_TL12+Z0_T2);
disp('_____');
disp(' ');
disp(' ');
disp(' ');
disp(' ###############  OR IN SUMMARY   ################');
disp(' ');
disp(' Z1_Th_pu       Z2_Th_pu            Z0_Th_pu       ');
disp(' *******************************************************');
[ Z1_Th Z2_Th Z0_Th]
disp('_____');
disp(' ');
disp(' ');
disp(' ');
```

Solutions

####################### OR IN SUMMARY #######################

Z1_Th_pu   Z2_Th_pu   Z0_Th_pu
****

ans =

0 + 0.31034i   0 + 0.25577i   0 + 0.13269i

Example K.18

Solve Example J.18 using MATLAB.

```
%Use the solution of Example J.18 and calculate the fault currents for
%the following faults and draw the corresponding interconnected sequence
%networks.
```

```
%(a) Single line-to-ground fault at bus 2 assuming faulted phase is%phase a.
%(b) Double line-to-ground fault at bus 2 involving phases b and c.
%(c) Three-phase fault at bus 2.
```

Solution

MATLAB script for Example K.18

```
%Data
clear; clc;
format short g
%data
%System base 100MVA
S = 100;% pu

%Generator 1:
Z1_G1 = i*0.20; %pu
```

```
Z2_G1 = i*0.15; %pu
Z0_G1 = i*0.05; %pu


%Generator 2:
Z1_G2 = i*0.30; %pu
Z2_G2 = i*0.20; %pu
Z0_G2 = i*0.05; %pu


%Transformer T1:
T1_base = 100; %pu
Z1_T1 = i*0.2; %pu
Z2_T1 = i*0.2; %pu
Z0_T1 = i*0.2; %pu


%Transformer T2:
T2_base = 100; %pu
Z1_T2 = i*0.15;%pu
Z2_T2 = i*0.15;%pu
Z0_T2 = i*0.15;%pu


%Line TL12
Z1_TL12 = i*0.60;%pu
Z2_TL12 = i*0.60;%pu
Z0_TL12 = i*0.90;%pu
Z1_Th = ((Z1_G1+Z1_T1+Z1_TL12)*(Z1_T2+Z1_G2))/
(Z1_G1+Z1_T1+Z1_TL12+Z1_T2+Z1_G2);
Z2_Th = ((Z2_G1+Z2_T1+Z2_TL12)*(Z2_T2+Z2_G2))/
(Z2_G1+Z2_T1+Z2_TL12+Z2_T2+Z2_G2);
Z0_Th = ((Z0_G1+Z0_T1+Z0_TL12)*(Z0_T2))/(Z0_G1+Z0_T1+Z0_TL12+Z0_T2);


%Part(a)
Vf = 1.0;
Ia1 = Vf/(Z1_Th+Z2_Th+Z0_Th);
Ia0 = Ia1;
Ia2 = Ia1;
Iaf_SLG_pu = 3*Ia0;
[real, angle_rad, angle_deg] = cart2polar(Iaf_SLG_pu);
Iaf_SLG_polar_pu = [real angle_deg];
Ibf_SLG_polar_pu = 0;
[real, angle_rad, angle_deg] = cart2polar(Ibf_SLG_polar_pu);
Ibf_SLG_polar_pu = [real angle_deg];
Icf_SLG_polar_pu = 0;
[real, angle_rad, angle_deg] = cart2polar(Icf_SLG_polar_pu);
Icf_SLG_polar_pu = [real angle_deg];


%Part(b)
Iaf_DLG_pu = 0;
[real, angle_rad, angle_deg] = cart2polar(Iaf_DLG_pu);
Iaf_DLG_polar_pu = [real angle_deg];
Ia1_DLG_pu = Vf/(Z1_Th+(Z2_Th*Z0_Th)/(Z2_Th+Z0_Th));
[real, angle_rad, angle_deg] = cart2polar(Ia1_DLG_pu);
Ia1_DLG_polar_pu = [real angle_deg];

Ia0_DLG_pu = -(Z2_Th/(Z0_Th+Z2_Th))*Ia1_DLG_pu;
[real, angle_rad, angle_deg] = cart2polar(Ia0_DLG_pu);
Ia0_DLG_polar_pu = [real angle_deg];
Ia2_DLG_pu = -(Z0_Th/(Z0_Th+Z2_Th))*Ia1_DLG_pu;
```

```
[real, angle_rad, angle_deg] = cart2polar(Ia2_DLG_pu);
Ia2_DLG_polar_pu = [real angle_deg];
%'a' in rectangular form
        a = (-0.5+i*0.866);  % polar: 1/_120
        a2 = (-0.5-i*0.866); % polar: 1/_-120


Ibf = Ia0_DLG_pu+a^2*Ia1_DLG_pu+a*Ia2_DLG_pu;
[real, angle_rad, angle_deg] = cart2polar(Ibf);
Ibf_DLG_polar_pu = [real angle_deg];

Icf = Ia0_DLG_pu+a*Ia1_DLG_pu+a^2*Ia2_DLG_pu;
[real, angle_rad, angle_deg] = cart2polar(Icf);
Icf_DLG_polar_pu = [real angle_deg];

%Part(c)
Ia0_3phase = 0;
Ia2_3phase = 0;
Ia1 = (Vf)/(Z1_Th);
[real, angle_rad, angle_deg] = cart2polar(Ia1);
Ia1_3phase_polar_pu = [real angle_deg];

Iaf = Ia1;
[real, angle_rad, angle_deg] = cart2polar(Iaf);
Iaf_3phase_polar_pu = [real angle_deg];

Ibf = a^2*Ia1;
[real, angle_rad, angle_deg] = cart2polar(Ibf);
Ibf_3phase_polar_pu = [real angle_deg];

Icf = a*Ia1;
[real, angle_rad, angle_deg] = cart2polar(Icf);
Icf_3phase_polar_pu = [real angle_deg];

disp('  _____  ');
disp(' ');
disp(' ');
disp(' ');
disp(' ################  OR IN SUMMARY  ################');
disp(' ');
disp('Iaf_SLG_polar_pu   Ibf_SLG_polar_pu   Icf_SLG_polar_pu   ');
disp(' ****************************************************************');
[     Iaf_SLG_polar_pu   Ibf_SLG_polar_pu   Icf_SLG_polar_pu]
disp('  _____  ');
disp(' ');
disp(' ');
disp(' ');
disp('Iaf_DLG_polar_pu   Ibf_DLG_polar_pu   Icf_DLG_polar_pu ');
disp('****************************************************************');
[     Iaf_DLG_polar_pu   Ibf_DLG_polar_pu   Icf_DLG_polar_pu]
disp('_____  ');
disp(' ');
disp(' ');
disp(' ');
disp('Iaf_3phase_polar_pu  Ibf_3phase_polar_pu  Icf_3phase_polar_pu ');
disp('****************************************************************');
[     Iaf_3phase_polar_pu  Ibf_3phase_polar_pu  Icf_3phase_polar_pu]
disp('_____  ');
disp(' ');
disp(' ');
disp(' ');
```

Solutions

############################ OR IN SUMMARY   ############################

Iaf_SLG_polar_pu   Ibf_SLG_polar_pu   Icf_SLG_polar_pu
****

ans =

  4.293 −90   0   0   0   0

Iaf_DLG_polar_pu   Ibf_DLG_polar_pu   Icf_DLG_polar_pu
****

ans =

0   0   3.834 139.63   3.8341 40.367

          Iaf_3phase_polar_pu   Ibf_3phase_polar_pu Icf_3phase_polar_pu
****

ans =

3.2222 −90 3.2221   150 3.2222 30.001

Example K.19

Solve Example J.19 using MATLAB.

```
%Consider the system shown in Figure PJ.19 and data given in Table PJ,19.
Assume that there is a SLG fault at bus 3. Determine the following:
 %(a)Thevenin equivalent positive-sequence impedance.
 %(b)Thevenin equivalent negative-sequence impedance.
 %(c)Thevenin equivalent zero-sequence impedance.
 %(d)Positive-, negative-, and zero-sequence currents.
 %(e)Phase currents in per units and amperes.
 %(f)Positive-, negative-, and zero-sequence voltages.
 %(g)Phase voltages in per units and kilovolts.
 %(h)Line-to-line voltages in per units and kilovolts.
 %(i)Draw a voltage phasor diagram using before-the-fault line-to-neutral
 % and line-to-line voltage values.
 %(j)Draw a voltage phasor diagram using the resultant after-the-fault
 %line-to-neutral and line-to-line voltage values.
```

TABLE PJ.19
Table for Example PJ.19

%Network %Component	Base MVA	Voltage (kV)	X1 (pu)	X2 (pu)	X0 (pu)
%G1	100	13.8	0.15	0.15	0.05
%G2	100	13.8	0.15	0.15	0.05
%G3	100	13.8	0.15	0.15	0.05
%T1	100	13.8/115	0.20	0.20	0.20
%T2	100	115/13.8	0.18	0.18	0.18
%TL12	100	115	0.30	0.30	0.90

Solution

(a) MATLAB script for Example K.19

```
%Data
clear; clc;
format short g
%data
%System base 100MVA
S = 100E6;% VA


%Generator 1:
X1_G1 = i*0.15; %pu
X2_G1 = i*0.15; %pu
X3_G1 = i*0.05; %pu all based on 100MVA ratings


%Generator 2:
X1_G2 = i*0.15; %pu
X2_G2 = i*0.15; %pu
X3_G2 = i*0.05; %pu all based on 100MVA ratings


%Generator 2:
X1_G3 = i*0.15; %pu
X2_G3 = i*0.15; %pu
X3_G3 = i*0.05; %pu all based on 100MVA ratings


%Transformer T1:
T1_base = 100E6;%VA
Z0_1 = i*0.20;
Z1_1 = i*0.20;
Z2_1 = i*0.20;
Z0_T1 = i*0.20*(S/T1_base);
Z1_T1 = Z0_T1;
Z2_T1 = Z0_T1;


%Transformer T2:
T2_base = 100E6;%VA
Z0_2 = i*0.18;
Z1_2 = i*0.18;
Z2_2 = i*0.18;
Z0_T2 = i*0.18*(S/T2_base);
Z1_T2 = Z0_T1;
Z2_T2 = Z0_T1;


%Line TL23
Z0_TL23 = i*0.30;
Z1_TL23 = i*0.30;
Z2_TL23 = i*0.90;


%Part(a)
Vf = 1.0;
Z1_Th = j*0.2097; %pu

%Part(b)
Z2_Th = j*0.2097; %pu

%Part(c)
Z0_Th = 0;      %pu
```

```
%Part(d)
Ia0 = Vf/(Z0_Th+Z1_Th+Z2_Th);
Ia1 = Ia0;
Ia2 = Ia0;
%polar to rectangular conversion using function:
%function [real, angle_rad, angle_deg] = cart2polar(x)
%real = abs(x);
%angle_rad = angle(x);
%angle_deg = angle_rad*180/pi;
[real, angle_rad, angle_deg] = cart2polar(Ia0);
Ia0_polar = [real angle_deg];
Ia1_polar = Ia0_polar;
Ia2_polar = Ia0_polar;

%Part(e)
Iaf_pu = 3*Ia0; %pu
[real, angle_rad, angle_deg] = cart2polar(Iaf_pu);
Iaf_pu_polar = [real angle_deg];
Ibf_pu = 0; %pu
[real, angle_rad, angle_deg] = cart2polar(Ibf_pu);
Ibf_pu_polar = [real angle_deg];
Icf_pu = 0; %pu
[real, angle_rad, angle_deg] = cart2polar(Icf_pu);
Icf_pu_polar = [real angle_deg];

Vbase = 115E3;
IB = S/(sqrt(3)*Vbase);
%Iaf in Amperes
Iaf_A = Iaf_pu*IB; % A
[real, angle_rad, angle_deg] = cart2polar(Iaf_A);
Iaf_A_polar = [real angle_deg];
Ibf_A_polar = 0; % A
[real, angle_rad, angle_deg] = cart2polar(Ibf_A_polar);
Ibf_A_polar = [real angle_deg];
Icf_A_polar = 0; % A
[real, angle_rad, angle_deg] = cart2polar(Icf_A_polar);
Icf_A_polar = [real angle_deg];

%Part(f)
Va0_pu = Ia0*Z0_Th;
Va1_pu = Vf-(Ia1*Z1_Th);
Va2_pu = -Ia2*Z2_Th;

%Part(g)
Vaf = Va1_pu+Va2_pu;
[real, angle_rad, angle_deg] = cart2polar(Vaf);
Vaf_pu_polar = [real angle_deg];
%'a' in rectangular form
        a = (-0.5+i*0.866);  % polar: 1/_120
        a2 = (-0.5-i*0.866); % polar: 1/_-120
Vbf = a^2*Va1_pu+a*Va2_pu;
[real, angle_rad, angle_deg] = cart2polar(Vbf);
Vbf_pu_polar = [real angle_deg];
Vcf = a*Va1_pu+a^2*Va2_pu;
[real, angle_rad, angle_deg] = cart2polar(Vcf);
Vcf_pu_polar = [real angle_deg];

%in kV
VBase = Vbase/sqrt(3);
```

```
Vaf_kV = Vaf*VBase;
[real, angle_rad, angle_deg] = cart2polar(Vaf_kV);
Vaf_kV_polar = [real angle_deg];
Vbf_kV = Vbf*VBase;
[real, angle_rad, angle_deg] = cart2polar(Vbf_kV);
Vbf_kV_polar = [real angle_deg];
Vcf_kV = Vcf*VBase;
[real, angle_rad, angle_deg] = cart2polar(Vcf_kV);
Vcf_kV_polar = [real angle_deg];

%Part(h)
%in kV
Vab_kV = Vaf_kV-Vbf_kV;
[real, angle_rad, angle_deg] = cart2polar(Vab_kV);
Vab_kV_polar = [real angle_deg];

Vbc_kV = Vbf_kV-Vcf_kV;
[real, angle_rad, angle_deg] = cart2polar(Vbc_kV);
Vbc_kV_polar = [real angle_deg];
Vca_kV = Vcf_kV-Vaf_kV;
[real, angle_rad, angle_deg] = cart2polar(Vca_kV);
Vca_kV_polar = [real angle_deg];

%in pu
Vab_pu = Vaf-Vbf;
[real, angle_rad, angle_deg] = cart2polar(Vab_pu);
Vab_pu_polar = [real angle_deg];

Vbc_pu = Vbf-Vcf;
[real, angle_rad, angle_deg] = cart2polar(Vbc_pu);
Vbc_pu_polar = [real angle_deg];

Vca_pu = Vcf-Vaf;
[real, angle_rad, angle_deg] = cart2polar(Vca_pu);
Vca_pu_polar = [real angle_deg];

disp('_____');
disp(' ');
disp(' ');
disp(' ');
disp(' ##########    OR IN SUMMARY    ##########');
disp(' ');
disp(' Z1_Th Z2_Th Z0_Th');
disp(' ****************************************************************');
[ Z1_Th Z2_Th Z0_Th ]
disp(' ');
disp(' ');
disp(' ');
disp(' Ia1_polar    Ia2_polar    Ia0_polar');
disp(' ****************************************************************');
[ Ia1_polar Ia2_polar Ia0_polar ]
disp('_____');
disp(' ');
disp(' ');
disp(' ');
disp(' Iaf_pu_polar  Ibf_pu_polar  Icf_pu_polar');
disp(' ****************************************************************');
[ Iaf_pu_polar Ibf_pu_polar Icf_pu_polar ]
disp(' ');
```

```
disp(' ');
disp(' ');
disp(' Iaf_A_polar    Ibf_A_polar    Icf_A_polar');
disp(' ***********************************************************');
[ Iaf_A_polar Ibf_A_polar Icf_A_polar ]
disp(' ');
disp(' ');
disp(' ');
disp(' Va1_pu         Va2_pu Va0_pu');
disp(' ***********************************************************');
[    Va1_pu Va2_pu Va0_pu]
disp(' ');
disp(' ');
disp(' ');
disp(' Vaf_pu_polar  Vbf_pu_polar   Vcf_pu_polar');
disp(' ***********************************************************');
[    Vaf_pu_polar Vbf_pu_polar Vcf_pu_polar]
disp(' ');
disp(' ');
disp(' ');
disp(' Vaf_kV_polar   Vbf_kV_polar   Vcf_kV_polar');
disp(' ***********************************************************');
[    Vaf_kV_polar Vbf_kV_polar Vcf_kV_polar]
disp(' ');
disp(' ');
disp(' ');
disp(' Vab_pu_polar   Vbc_pu_polar   Vca_pu_polar');
disp(' ***********************************************************');
[    Vab_pu_polar Vbc_pu_polar Vca_pu_polar]
disp(' ');
disp(' ');
disp(' ');
disp(' Vab_kV_polar   Vbc_kV_polar   Vca_kV_polar');
disp(' ***********************************************************');
[    Vab_kV_polar Vbc_kV_polar Vca_kV_polar]
```

Solutions

```
##############      IN SUMMARY    ###############

    Z1_Th      Z2_Th              Z0_Th
***************************************************************

ans =

    0 + 0.2097i   0 + 0.2097i        0
    Ia1_polar     Ia2_polar     Ia0_polar
***************************************************************

ans =

2.3844  -90    2.3844   -90    2.3844   -90
```

```
    Iaf_pu_polar          Ibf_pu_polar   Icf_pu_polar
***************************************************************

ans =

7.1531      -90      0        0        0        0
```

```
Iaf_A_polar                    Ibf_A_polar        Icf_A_polar
*********************************************************************


ans =

3591.2     -90     0          0          0        0
        Va1_pu    Va2_pu    Va0_pu
*********************************************************************


ans =

        0.5     -0.5     0
Vaf_pu_polar            Vbf_pu_polar        Vcf_pu_polar
*********************************************************************


ans =

5.5511e-017   0       0.866    -89.999   0.866    90.001
Vaf_kV_polar            Vbf_kV_polar        Vcf_kV_polar
*********************************************************************


ans =

3.6857e-012   0       57498    -89.999   57498    90.001
Vab_pu_polar            Vbc_pu_polar        Vca_pu_polar
*********************************************************************


ans =

0.866     90.001     1.732    -89.999   0.866    90.001
        Vab_kV_polar    Vbc_kV_polar        Vca_kV_polar
*********************************************************************


ans =

    57498 90.001 1.15e+005 -89.999 57498 90.001

%Part(a) Specify Xn, in ohms and in per units
Ia_3phase = Vf/Z1;

%SLG Fault:
Z = x0+x1+x2;
%For Xn = 0:
Xn = 0;
Ia0 = Vf/(Z+3*Xn);
Ia_SLG_abs = abs(3*Ia0); %pu

%DLG Fault
%Vf-Ia1*Z1 = -Ia2*Z2 = Ia1*Z2+Ia0*Z2-Ia0*(Z0+3*Zn)............(1)
%-Ia0(Z0+3Zn) = Ia1Z2+Ia0Z2..................................(2)

Ia0 = (i*1.042)/(0.2+6*Xn);%pu
Ia2 = (i*(0.05+3*Xn)*Ia0)/(i*0.1);%pu
Ia1 = -Ia2-Ia0; %pu

%'a' in rectangular form
        a = (-0.5+i*0.866);  % polar: 1/_120 deg
        a2 = (-0.5-i*0.866); % polar: 1/_-120 deg

Ib_DLG_abs = abs(Ia0*(1-a)+Ia1*(a^2-a)); %pu
```

```
Ic_DLG_abs = abs(Ia0*(1-a^2)+Ia1*(a-a^2)); %pu

%The grounding reactor Xn:
%Ia_LG_abs = abs(3*Ia0)

syms Vf Z_ q x2
%q = Xn;
%3*(Vf/(Z+3*q)) = Vf/x2
%Ia0 = Vf/(Z+3*Xn);

x0 = i*0.05;%pu
x1 = i*0.1; %pu
x2 = i*0.1; %pu all based on generator ratings
Z = x0+x1+x2;
Z_ = Z/i;
Vf = 1.042;
%3*(Vf/(Z+3*q)) = =Vf/x2
%Ia0 = Vf/(Z+3*Xn);
S = (3*Vf)/(Z_+3*q)-((Vf/(x2/i)));
q = solve(S,q);
%Xn in pu
Xn_pu = eval(q); %pu
%Xn in ohm
V_sec = 4.16E3; %V
B = 18.75E6; % VA base
Xn_ohm = Xn_pu*(V_sec^2/B); %ohm
```

Appendix L: Glossary for Transmission System Engineering Terminology

Some of the most commonly used terms, both in this book and in general usage, are defined on the following pages. Most of the definitions given in this glossary are based on Refs. [1–8].

AA: Abbreviation for all-aluminum conductors.

AAAC: Abbreviation for all-aluminum-alloy conductor. Aluminum alloy conductors have higher strength than those of the ordinary electric-conductor grade of aluminum.

ACAR: Abbreviation for aluminum conductor alloy-reinforced. It has a central core of higher-strength aluminum surrounded by layers of electric-conductor grade aluminum.

AC circuit breaker: A CB whose principal function is usually to interrupt short-circuit or fault currents.

Accuracy classification: The accuracy of an instrument transformer at specified burdens. The number used to indicate accuracy is the maximum allowable error of the transformer for specified burdens. For example, 0.2 accuracy class means the maximum error will not exceed 0.2% at rated burdens.

ACSR: An abbreviation for aluminum conductor, steel reinforced. It consists of a central core of steel strands surrounded by layers of aluminum strands.

Admittance: The ratio of the phasor equivalent of the steady-state sine-wave current to the phasor equivalent of the corresponding voltage.

Adverse weather: Weather conditions that cause an abnormally high rate of forced outages for exposed components during the periods such conditions persist, but which do not qualify as major storm disasters. Adverse weather conditions can be defined for a particular system by selecting the proper values and combinations of conditions reported by the weather bureau: thunderstorms, tornadoes, wind velocities, precipitation, temperature, etc.

Air blast transformer: A transformer cooled by forced circulation of air through its core and coils.

Air circuit breaker: A CB in which the interruption occurs in air.

Air switch: A switch in which the interruptions of the circuit occur in air.

Al: Symbol for aluminum.

Ampacity: Current rating in amperes, as of a conductor.

ANSI: Abbreviation for American National Standards Institute.

Apparent sag (at any point): The departure of the wire at the particular point in the span from the straight line between the two points of the span, at 60°F, with no wind loading.

Arc-back: A malfunctioning phenomenon in which a valve conducts in the reverse direction.

Arcing time of fuse: The time elapsing from the severance of the fuse link to the final interruption of the circuit under specified conditions.

Arc-over of insulator: A discharge of power current in the form of an arc following a surface discharge over an insulator.

Armored cable: A cable provided with a wrapping of metal, usually steel wires, primarily for the purpose of mechanical protection.

Askarel: A generic term for a group of nonflammable synthetic chlorinated hydrocarbons used as electrical insulating media. Askarels of various compositional types are used. Under arcing conditions, the gases produced, while consisting predominantly of noncombustible hydrogen chloride, can include varying amounts of combustible gases depending upon the askarel type. Because of environmental concerns, it is not used in new installations anymore.

Automatic reclosing: An intervention that is not manual. It probably requires specific interlocking such as a full or check synchronizing, voltage or switching device checks, or other safety or operating constrains. It can be high speed or delayed.

Automatic substations: Those in which switching operations are so controlled by relays that transformers or converting equipment are brought into or taken out of service as variations in load may require, and feeder CBs are closed and reclosed after being opened by overload relays.

Autotransformer: A transformer in which at least two windings have a common section.

Auxiliary relay: A relay that operates in response to the opening or closing of its operating circuit to assist another relay in the performance of its function.

AWG: Abbreviation for American wire gauge. It is also sometimes called the Brown and Sharpe wire gauge.

Base load: The minimum load over a given period of time.

Basic impulse insulation level: Reference levels expressed in impulse crest voltage with a standard wave not longer than 1.5×50 µs. The impulse waves are defined by a combination of two numbers. The first number is the time from the start of the wave to the instant crest value; the second number is the time from the start to the instant of half-crest value on the tail of the wave.

BIL: See *Basic impulse insulation level.*

Blocking: Preventing the relay from tripping due either to its own characteristic or to an additional relay.

Breakdown: Also termed puncture, denoting a disruptive discharge through insulation.

Breaker, primary feeder: A breaker located at the supply end of a primary feeder that opens on a primary-feeder fault if the fault current is of sufficient magnitude.

Breaker-and-a-half scheme: A scheme that provides the facilities of a double main bus at a reduction in equipment cost by using three CBs for each two circuits.

Burden: The loading imposed by the circuits of the relay on the energizing input power source or sources, that is, the relay burden is the power required to operate the relay.

Bus: A conductor or group of conductors that serves as a common connection for two or more circuits in a switchgear assembly.

Bus (or bus bar): An electrical connection of zero impedance joining several items such as lines and loads. *Bus* in a one-line diagram is essentially the same as that of a *node* in a circuit diagram. It is the term used for a main bar or conductor carrying an electric current to which many connections may be made. Buses are simply convenient means of connecting switches and other equipment into various arrangements. They can be in a variety of sizes and shapes. They can be made of rectangular bars, round solid bars, square tubes, open pairs, or even stranded cables. In substations, they are built above the head and supported by insulated metal structures. Bus materials, in general use, are aluminum and copper, with hard-drawn aluminum, especially in the tubular shape, the most widely used in HV and EHV open-type outdoor stations. Copper or aluminum tubing as well as special shapes is sometimes used for low-voltage distribution substation buses.

Bus, auxiliary: See *Transfer bus.*

Bus-tie circuit breaker: A CB that serves to connect buses or bus sections together.

Bus, transfer: A bus to which one circuit at a time can be transferred from the main bus.

Bushing: An insulating structure including a through conductor, or providing a passageway for such a conductor, with provision for mounting on a barrier, conductor or otherwise, for the purpose of insulating the conductor from the barrier and conducting from one side of the barrier to the other.

BVR: Abbreviation for bus voltage regulator or regulation.

BW: Abbreviation for bandwidth.

BX cable: A cable with galvanized interlocked steel spiral armor. It is known as ac cable and used in a damp or wet location in buildings at LV.

Cable: Either a standard conductor (single-conductor cable) or a combination of conductors insulated from one another (multiple-conductor cable).

Cable fault: A partial or total load failure in the insulation or continuity of the conductor.

Capability: The maximum load-carrying ability expressed in kilovolt-amperes or kilowatts of generating equipment or other electric apparatus under specified conditions for a given time interval.

Capability, net: The maximum generation expressed in kilowatt-hours per hour that a generating unit, station, power source, or system can be expected to supply under optimum operating conditions.

Capacitor bank: An assembly at one location of capacitors and all necessary accessories (switching equipment, protective equipment, controls, etc.) required for a complete operating installation.

Capacity: The rated load-carrying ability expressed in kilovolt-amperes or kilowatts of generating equipment or other electric apparatus.

Capacity factor: The ratio of the average load on a machine or equipment for the period of time considered to the capacity of the machine or equipment.

Characteristic quantity: The quantity or the value of which characterizes the operation of the relay.

Characteristics (of a relay in steady state): The locus of the pickup or reset when drawn on a graph.

Charge: The amount paid for a service rendered or facilities used or made available for use.

Chopped-wave insulation level: Determined by test using waves of the same shape to determine the BIL, with exception that the wave is chopped after about 3 μs.

CIGRÉ: It is the international conference of large HV electric systems. It is recognized as a permanent nongovernmental and nonprofit international association based in France. It focuses on issues related to the planning and operation of power systems, as well as the design, construction, maintenance, and disposal of HV equipment and plants.

Circuit breaker: A device that interrupts a circuit without injury to itself so that it can be reset and reused over again.

Circuit breaker mounting: Supporting structure for a CB.

Circuit, earth (ground) return: An electric circuit in which the earth serves to complete a path for current.

Circular mil: A unit of area equal to $i/4$ of a square mil (= 0.7854 square mil). The cross-sectional area of a circle in circular mils is therefore equal to the square of its diameter in mils. A circular inch is equal to 1 million circular mils. A mil is one one-thousandth of an inch. There are 1974 circular mils in a square millimeter. Abbreviated cmil.

CL: Abbreviation for current limiting (fuse).

cmil: Abbreviation for circular mil.

Commutation: The transfer of current from one valve to another in the same row.

Commutation margin angle (ζ): The time angle between the end of conduction and the reversal of the sign of the nonsinusoidal voltage across the outgoing valve of an inverter. Under normal operating conditions, the commutation margin angle is equal to the extinction advance angle.

Component: A piece of equipment, a line, a section of a line, or a group of items that is viewed as an entity.

Computer usage:
> **Off-line usage:** It includes research, routine calculations of the system performance, and data assimilations and retrieval.
> **Online usage:** It includes data logging and monitoring of the system state, including switching, safe interlocking, plant loading, postfault control, and load shedding.

Condenser: Also termed capacitor; a device whose primary purpose is to introduce capacitance into an electric circuit. The term condenser is deprecated.

Conductor: A substance that has free electrons or other charge carriers that permit charge flow when an electromotive force (emf) is applied across the substance.

Conductor tension, final unloaded: The longitudinal tension in a conductor after the conductor has been stretched by the application for an appreciable period, with subsequent release, of the loadings of ice and wind, at the temperature decrease assumed for the loading district in which the conductor is strung (or equivalent loading).

Congestion cost: The difference between the actual price of electricity at the point of usage and the lowest price on the grid.

Contactor: An electric power switch, which is not operated manually and designed for frequent operation.

Conventional RTU: Designated primarily for hardwired input/output (I/O) and has little or no capability to talk to downstream IEDs.

Converter: A machine, device, or system for changing ac power to dc power or vice versa.

Cress factor: A value that is displayed on many power quality monitoring instruments representing the ratio of the crest value of the measured waveform to the rms value of the waveform. For example, the cress factor of a sinusoidal wave is 1.414.

Critical flashover (CFO) voltage: The peak voltage for a 50% probability of flashover or disruptive discharge.

CT: Abbreviation for current transformer.

Cu: Symbol for copper.

Current transformer burdens: CT burdens are normally expressed in ohms impedance such as B-0.1, B-0.2, B-0.5, B-0.9, or B-1.8. Corresponding volt-ampere values are 2.5, 5.0, 12.5, 22.5, and 45.

Current transformer ratio: CT ratio is the ratio of primary to secondary current. For CT rated 200:5, the ratio is 200:5 or 40:1.

Current transformers: They are usually rated on the basis of 5 A secondary current and used to reduce primary current to usable levels for transformer-rated meters and to insulate and isolate meters from HV circuits.

Delay angle (α): The time, expressed in electrical degrees, by which the starting point of commutation is delayed. It cannot exceed 180°. It is also called *ignition angle* or *firing angle*.

Demand: The load at the receiving terminals averaged over a specified interval of time.

Demand factor: The ratio of the maximum coincident demand of a system, or part of a system, to the total connected load of the system, or part of the system, under consideration.

Demand, instantaneous: The load at any instant.

Demand, integrated: The demand integrated over a specified period.

Demand interval: The period of time during which the electric energy flow is integrated in determining demand.

Dependability (in protection): The certainty that a relay will respond correctly for all faults for which it is designed and applied to operate.

Dependability (in relays): The ability of a relay or relay system to provide correct operation when required.

Dependent time-delay relay: A time-delay relay in which the time delay varies with the value of the energizing quantity.

Depreciation: The component that represents an approximation of the value of the portion of plant consumed or *used up* in a given period by a utility.

Differential current relay: A fault-detecting relay that functions on a differential current of a given percentage or amount.

Directional (or directional overcurrent) relay: A relay that functions on a desired value of power flow in a given direction on a desired value of overcurrent with ac power flow in a given direction.

Disconnecting or isolating switch: A mechanical switching device used for changing the connections in a circuit or for isolating a circuit or equipment from the source of power.

Disconnector: A switch that is intended to open a circuit only after the load has been thrown off by other means. Manual switches designed for opening loaded circuits are usually installed in a circuit with disconnectors to provide a safe means for opening the circuit under load.

Displacement factor (DPF): The ratio of active power (watts) to apparent power (volt-amperes).

Distance relay: A relay that responds to input quantities as a function of the electrical circuit distance between the relay location and the point of faults.

Distribution center: A point of installation for automatic overload protective devices connected to buses where an electric supply is subdivided into feeders and/or branch circuits.

Distribution switchboard: A power switchboard used for the distribution of electric energy at the voltages common for such distribution within a building.

Distribution system: That portion of an electric system that delivers electric energy from transformation points in the transmission, or bulk power system, to the consumers.

Distribution transformer: A transformer for transferring electric energy from a primary distribution circuit to a secondary distribution circuit or consumer's service circuit; it is usually rated in the order of 5–500 kVA.

Diversity factor: The ratio of the sum of the individual maximum demands of the various subdivisions of a system to the maximum demand of the whole system.

Dropout or reset: A relay drops out when it moves from the energized position to the unenergized position.

Effectively grounded: Grounded by means of a ground connection of sufficiently low impedance that fault grounds that may occur cannot build up voltages dangerous to connected equipment.

EHV: Abbreviation for extra-high voltage.

Electric fields: They exist whenever voltage exists on a conductor. They are not dependent on the current.

Electric system loss: Total electric energy loss in the electric system. It consists of transmission, transformation, and distribution losses between sources of supply and points of delivery.

Electrical reserve: The capability in excess of that required to carry the system load.

Element: See *Unit*.

Emergency rating: Capability of installed equipment for a short time interval.

Energizing quantity: The electrical quantity, that is, current or voltage, either alone or in combination with other electrical quantities required for the function of the relay.

Energy: That which does work or is capable of doing work. As used by electric utilities, it is generally a reference to electric energy and is measured in kilowatt-hours.

Energy loss: The difference between energy input and output as a result of transfer of energy between two points.

Energy management system (EMS): A computer system that monitors, controls, and optimizes the transmission and generation facilities with advanced applications. A SCADA system is a subject of an EMS.

Equivalent commutating resistance (R_c): The ratio of drop of direct voltage to dc. However, it does not consume any power.

Express feeder: A feeder that serves the most distant networks and that must traverse the systems closest to the bulk power source.

Extinction (advance) angle (γ): The extinction angle of an inverter and is equal to $\pi - \gamma$ electrical degrees. It is defined as the time angle between the end of conduction and the reversal of the sign of the sinusoidal commutation voltage of the source.

Extinction angle (δ): The sum of the delay angle α and the overlap angle u of a rectifier and is expressed in degrees.

Extra-high voltage: A term applied to voltage levels higher than 230 kV. Abbreviated EHV.

Facilities charge: The amount paid by the customer as a lump sum or, periodically, as reimbursement for facilities furnished. The charge may include operation and maintenance as well as fixed costs.

Fault: It is a malfunctioning of the network, usually due to the short-circuiting of two or more conductors or live conductors connecting to earth.

Feeder: A set of conductors originating at a main distribution center and supplying one or more secondary distribution centers, one or more branch-circuit distribution centers, or any combination of these two types of load.

Feeder, multiple: Two or more feeders connected in parallel.

Feeder, tie: A feeder that connects two or more independent sources of power and has no tapped load between the terminals. The source of power may be a generating system, substation, or feeding point.

Fiber-optic cable: It is made up of varying number of either single or multimode fibers, with a strength member in the center of the cable and additional outer layers to provide support and protection against physical damage to the cable. Large amounts of data as high as gigabytes per second can be transmitted over the fiber. They have inherent immunity from electromagnetic interference and have high bandwidth. Two types are used by utilities: (1) optical power grid wire (OPGW) type and (2) all dielectric self-supporting (ADSS) type.

First-contingency outage: The outage of one primary feeder.

Fixed capacitor bank: A capacitor bank with fixed, not switchable, capacitors.

Flash: A term encompassing the entire electrical discharge from cloud to stricken object.

Flashover: An electrical discharge completed from an energized conductor to a grounded support. It may clear itself and trip a CB.

Flexible ac transmission systems (FACTS): They are the converter stations for ac transmission. It is an application of power electronics for control of the ac system to improve the power flow, operation, and control of the ac system.

Flicker: Impression of unsteadiness of visual sensation induced by a light stimulus whose luminance or spectral distribution fluctuates with time.

Forced interruption: It is an interruption caused by a forced outage.

Forced outage: It is an outage that results from emergency conditions directly associated with a component requiring that component to be taken out of service immediately, either automatically or as soon as switching operations can be performed, or an outage caused by improper operation of equipment or human error.

Frequency deviation: An increase or decrease in the power frequency. Its duration varies from few cycles to several hours.

Fuse: An overcurrent protective device with a circuit-opening fusible part that is heated and severed by the passage of overcurrent through it.

Fuse cutout: An assembly consisting of a fuse support and holder; it may also include a fuse link.

Gas-insulated transmission line (GIL): A system for the transmission of electricity at high power ratings over long distances. The GIL consists of three single-phase encapsulated aluminum tubes that can be directly buried into the ground, laid in a tunnel, or installed on steel structures at heights of 1–5 m aboveground.

Grip, conductor: A device designed to permit the pulling of conductor without splicing on fittings.

Ground: Also termed earth; a conductor connected between a circuit and the soil; an accidental ground occurs due to cable insulation faults, an insulator defect, etc.

Grounding: It is the connection of a conductor or frame of a device to the main body of the earth. Thus it must be done in a way to keep the resistance between the item and the earth under the limits. It is often that the burial of large assemblies of conducting rods in the earth and the use of connectors in large cross diameters are needed.

Ground protective relay: Relay that functions on the failure of insulation of a machine, transformer, or other apparatus to ground.

Ground wire: A conductor having grounding connections at intervals that is suspended usually above but not necessarily over the line conductor to provide a degree of protection against lightning discharges.

GTOs: It is gate turn-off thyristors.

Harmonic distortion: Periodic distortion of the sign wave.

Harmonic resonance: A condition in which the power system is resonating near one of the major harmonics being produced by nonlinear elements in the system, hence increasing the harmonic distortion.

Harmonics: Sinusoidal voltages or currents having frequencies that are integer multiples of the fundamental frequency at which the supply system is designed to operate.

Hazardous open circulating (in CTs): The operation of the CTs with the secondary winding open can result in an HV across the secondary terminals, which may be dangerous to the personnel or equipment. Therefore, the secondary terminals should always be short-circuited before a meter is removed from service.

High-speed relay: A relay that operates in less than a specified time. The specified time in present practice is 50 ms (i.e., 3 cycles on a 60 HZ system).

HV: Abbreviation for high voltage.

IED: See *Intelligent electronic device.*

IED integration: Integration of protection, control, and data acquisition functions into a minimal number of platforms to reduce capital and operating costs, reduce panel and control room space, and eliminate redundant equipment and data base.

Ignition angle (β): The delay angle of an inverter and is equal to π-α electrical degrees.

Impedance: The ratio of the phasor equivalent of a steady-state sine-wave voltage to the phasor equivalent of a steady-state sine-wave current.

Impedance relay: A relay that operates for all impedance values that are less than its setting, that is, for all points within the crosshatched circles.

Impulse ratio (flashover or puncture of insulation): It is the ratio of impulse peak voltage to the peak values of the 60 Hz voltage to cause flashover or puncture.

Impulsive transient: A sudden (nonpower) frequency change in the steady-state condition of the voltage or current that is unidirectional in polarity.

Incremental energy costs: The additional cost of producing or transmitting electric energy above some base cost.

Independent time-delay relay: A time-delay relay in which the time delay is independent of the energizing quantity.

Index of reliability: A ratio of cumulative customer minutes that service was available during a year to total customer minutes demanded; can be used by the utility for feeder reliability comparisons.

Infinite bus: A bus that represents a very large external system. It is considered that at such bus, voltage and frequency are constant. Typically, a large power system is considered as an infinite bus.

Installed reserve: The reserve capability installed on a system.

Instantaneous relay: A relay that operates and resets with no intentional time delay. Such relay operates as soon as secure decision is made. No intentional time delay is introduced to slow down the relay response.

Instrument transformer: A transformer that is used to produce safety for the operator and equipment from HV and to permit proper insulation levels and current-carrying capability in relays, meters, and other measurements.

Insulation coordination: It is the process of determining the proper insulation levels of various components in a power system and their arrangements. That is, it is the selection of an insulation structure that will withstand the voltage stresses to which the system or equipment will be subjected together with the proper surge arrester.

Intelligent electronic device: Any device incorporating one or more processors with the capability to receive or send data and control from or to an external source (e.g., electronic multifunction meters, digital relays, and controllers).

Integrated services digital network: It is a switched, end-to-end wide-area network designed to combine digital telephony and data transport services.

Interconnections: See *Tie lines.*

International Electrotechnical Commission (IEC): An international organization whose mission is to prepare and publish standards for all electrical, electronic, and related technologies.

Interruptible load: A load that can be interrupted as defined by contract.

Interruption: The loss of service to one or more consumers or other facilities and is the result of one or more component outages, depending on system configuration.

Interruption duration: The period from the initiation of an interruption to a consumer until service has been restored to that consumer.

Inverse time-delay relay: A dependent time-delay relay having an operating time that is an inverse function of the electrical characteristic quantity.

Inverse time-delay relay with definite minimum: A relay in which the time delay varies inversely with the characteristic quantity up to a certain value, after which the time delay becomes substantially independent.

Inverter: A converter for changing dc to ac.

Investment-related charges: Those certain charges incurred by a utility that are directly related to the capital investment of the utility.

ISO: Independent system operator.

Isokeraunic level: The average number of thunder-days per year at that locality (i.e., the average number of thunder will be heard during a 24 h period).

Isokeraunic map: A map showing mean annual days of thunderstorm activity within the continental United States.

Isolated ground: Originates at an isolated ground-type receptacle or equipment input terminal block and terminates at the point where neutral and ground are bonded at the power source. Its conductor is insulated from the metallic raceway and all ground points throughout its length.

kcmil: Abbreviation for thousand circular mils.

Keraunic level: See *Isokeraunic level.*

K factor: A factor used to quantify the load impact of electric arc furnaces on the power system.

Knee-point emf: That sinusoidal emf applied to the secondary terminals of a CT, which, when increased by 10%, causes the exciting current to increase by 50%.

Lag: Denotes that a given sine wave passes through its peak at a later time than a reference time wave.

Lambda: The incremental operating cost at the load center, commonly expressed in mils per kilowatt-hour.

Lightning arrestor: A device that reduces the voltage of a surge applied to its terminals and restores itself to its original operating condition.

Line: A component part of a system extending between adjacent stations or from a station to an adjacent interconnection point. A line may consist of one or more circuits.

Line loss: Energy loss on a transmission or distribution line.

Line, pilot: A lightweight line, normally synthetic fiber rope, or wire rope, used to pull heavier pulling lines that in turn are used to pull the conductor.

Line, pulling: A high-strength line, normally synthetic fiber rope, used to pull the conductor.

L-L: Abbreviation for line to line.

L-N: Abbreviation for line to neutral.

Load: May be used in a number of ways to indicate a device or collection of devices that consume electricity, or to indicate the power required from a given supply circuit, or the power or current being passed through a line or machine.

Load center: A point at which the load of a given area is assumed to be concentrated.

Load diversity: The difference between the sum of the maxima of two or more individual loads and the coincident or combined maximum load, usually measured in kilowatts over a specified period of time.

Load duration curve: A curve of loads, plotted in descending order of magnitude, against time intervals for a specified period.

Load factor: The ratio of the average load over a designated period of time to the peak load occurring in that period.

Load-interrupter switch: An interrupter switch designed to interrupt currents not in excess of the continuous-current rating of the switch.

Load, interruptible: A load that can be interrupted as defined by contract.

Load losses, transformer: Those losses that are incident to the carrying of a specified load. They include I^2R loss in the winding due to load and eddy currents, stray loss due to leakage fluxes in the windings, and the loss due to circulating currents in parallel windings.

Load management (also called demand-side management): It extends remote supervision and control to subtransmission and distribution circuits, including control of residential, commercial, and industrial loads.

Load tap changer: A selector switch device applied to power transformers to maintain a constant low-side or secondary voltage with a variable primary voltage supply or to hold a constant voltage out along the feeders on the low-voltage side for varying load conditions on the low-voltage side. Abbreviated LTC.

Load-tap-changing transformer: A transformer used to vary the voltage or phase angle or both of a regulated circuit in steps by means of a device that connects different taps of tapped winding(s) without interrupting the load.

Local backup: Those relays that do not suffer from the same difficulties as remote backup, but they are installed in the same substation and use some of the same elements as the primary protection.

Loss factor: The ratio of the average power loss to the peak load power loss during a specified period of time.

Low-side surges: The current surge that appears to be injected into the transformer secondary terminals upon a lighting strike to grounded conductors in the vicinity.

LTC: Abbreviation for load tap changer.

LV: Abbreviation for low voltage.

Magnetic fields: Such fields exist whenever current flows in a conductor. They are not voltage dependent.

Main bus: A bus that is normally used. It has a more elaborate system of instruments, relays, and so on associated with it.

Main distribution center: A distribution center supplied directly by mains.

Maintenance expenses: The expense required to keep the system or plant in proper operating repair.

Maximum demand: The largest of a particular type of demand occurring within a specified period.

Messenger cable: A galvanized steel or copperweld cable used in construction to support a suspended current-carrying cable.

Metal-clad switchgear, outdoor: A switchgear that can be mounted in suitable weatherproof enclosures for outdoor installations. The base units are the same for both indoor and outdoor applications. The weatherproof housing is constructed integrally with the basic structure and is not merely a steel enclosure. The basic structure, including the mounting details and withdrawal mechanisms for the CBs, bus compartments, transformer compartments, etc., is the same as that of indoor metal-clad switchgear. (Used in distribution systems.)

Minimum demand: The smallest of a particular type of demand occurring within a specified period.

Momentary interruption: An interruption of duration limited to the period required to restore service by automatic or supervisory controlled switching operations or by manual switching at locations where an operator is immediately available. Such switching operations are typically completed in a few minutes.

Monthly peak duration curve: A curve showing the total number of days within the month during which the net 60 min clock hour–integrated peak demand equals or exceeds the percent of monthly peak values shown.

MOV: It is the metal-oxide varistor that is built from zinc oxide disks connected in series and parallel arrangements to achieve the required protective level and energy requirement. It is similar to an HV surge arrester.

N.C.: Abbreviation for normally closed.

NESC: Abbreviation for National Electrical Safety Code.

Net system energy: Energy requirements of a system, including losses, defined as (1) net generation of the system, plus (2) energy received from others, less (3) energy delivered to other systems.

Network configurator: An application that determines the configuration of the power system based on telemetered breaker and switch statuses.

Network transmission system: A transmission system that has more than one simultaneous path of power flow to the load.

N.O.: Abbreviation for normally open.

Noise: An unwanted electrical signal with a less than 200 kHz superimposed upon the power system voltage or current inphase conductors or found on neutral conductors or signal lines. It is not a harmonic distortion or transient. It disturbs microcomputers and programmable controllers.

No-load current: The current demand of a transformer primary when no current demand is made on the secondary.

No-load loss: Energy losses in an electric facility when energized at rated voltage and frequency but not carrying load.

Nonlinear load: An electrical load that draws current discontinuously or whose impedances vary throughout the cycle of the input ac voltage waveform.

Normal rating: Capacity of installed equipment.

Normal weather: All weather not designated as adverse or major storm disaster.

Normally closed: Denotes the automatic closure of contacts in a relay when deenergized. Abbreviated N.C.

Normally open: Denotes the automatic opening of contacts in a relay when deenergized. Abbreviated N.O.

Notch: A switching (or other) disturbance of the normal power voltage waveform, lasting less than a half cycle, which is initially of opposite polarity than the waveform. It includes complete loss of voltage for up to a 0.5 cycle.

Notching: A periodic disturbance caused by normal operation of a power electronic device, when its current is commutated from one phase to another.

NSW: Abbreviation for nonswitched.

NX: Abbreviation for nonexpulsion (fuse).

Off-peak energy: Energy supplied during designated periods of relatively low system demands.

OH: Abbreviation for overhead.

On-peak energy: Energy supplied during designated periods of relatively high system demands.

Open systems: A computer system that embodies supplier-independent standards so that software can be applied on many different platforms and can interoperate with other applications on local and remote systems.

Operational data: Also called SCADA data; instantaneous values of power system analog and status points (e.g., volts, amps, MW, Mvar, CB status, and switch positions).

Operating expenses: The labor and material costs for operating the plant involved.

Oscillatory transient: A sudden and non-power-frequency change in the steady-state condition of voltage or current that includes both positive and negative polarity values.

Outage: It describes the state of a component when it is not available to perform its intended function due to some event *directly associated* with that component. An outage may or may not cause an interruption of service to consumers depending on system configuration.

Outage duration: The period from the initiation of an outage until the affected component or its replacement once again becomes available to perform its intended function.

Outage rate: For a particular classification of outage and type of component; the mean number of outages per-unit exposure time per component.

Overhead expenses: The costs that in addition to direct labor and material are incurred by all utilities.

Overlap angle (u): The time, expressed in degrees, during which the current is commutated between two rectifying elements. It is also called commutation time. In normal operation, it is less than 60° and is usually somewhere between 20° and 25° at full load.

Overload: Loading in excess of normal rating of equipment.

Overload protection: Interruption or reduction of current under conditions of excessive demand, provided by a protective device.

Overshoot time: The time during which stored operating energy dissipated after the characteristic quantity has been suddenly restored from a specified value to the value it had at the initial position of the relay.

Overvoltage: A voltage that has a value at least 10% above the nominal voltage for a period of time greater than 1 min.

Passive filter: A combination of inductors, capacitors, and resistors designed to eliminate one or more harmonics. The most common variety is simply an inductor in series with a shunt capacitor, which short-circuits the major distorting harmonic component from the system.

PE: An abbreviation used for polyethylene (cable insulation).

Peak current: The maximum value (crest value) of an ac.

Peak voltage: The maximum value (crest value) of an alternating voltage.

Peaking station: A generating station that is normally operated to provide power only during maximum load periods.

Peak-to-peak value: The value of an ac waveform from its positive peak to its negative peak. In the case of a sine wave, the peak-to-peak value is double the peak value.

Pedestal: A bottom support or base of a pillar, statue, etc.

Percent regulation: See *Percent voltage drop*.

Percent voltage drop: The ratio of VD in a circuit to voltage delivered by the circuit, multiplied by 100 to convert to percent.

Permanent forced outage: An outage whose cause is not immediately self-clearing but must be corrected by eliminating the hazard or by repairing or replacing the component before it can be returned to service. An example of a permanent forced outage is a lightning flashover that shatters an insulator, thereby disabling the component until repair or replacement can be made.

Permanent forced outage duration: The period from the initiation of the outage until the component is replaced or repaired.

Persistent forced outage: A component outage whose cause is not immediately self-clearing but must be corrected by eliminating the hazard or by repairing or replacing the affected component before it can be returned to service. An example of a persistent forced outage is a lightning flashover that shatters an insulator, thereby disabling the component until repair or replacement can be made.

Phase: The time of occurrence of the peak value of an ac waveform with respect to the time of occurrence of the peak value of a reference waveform.

Phase angle: An angular expression of phase difference.

Phase-angle measuring relay: A relay that functions at a predetermined phase angle between voltage and current.

Phase shift: The displacement in time of one voltage waveform relative to other voltage waveform(s).

Pickup: A relay is said to pick up when it moves from the unenergized position to the energized position (by closing its contacts).

Pilot channel: A means of interconnection between relaying points for the purpose of protection.

Planning, conceptual: A long range of guidelines for decision.

Planning, preliminary: A state of project decisions.

Polarity: The relative polarity of the primary and secondary windings of a CT is indicated by polarity marks, associated with one end of each winding. When current enters at the polarity end of the primary winding, a current in phase with it leaves the polarity end of the secondary winding.

Pole: A column of wood or steel, or some other material, supporting OH conductors, usually by means of arms or brackets.

Pole fixture: A structure installed in lieu of a single pole to increase the strength of a pole line or to provide better support for attachments than would be provided by a single pole. Examples are A fixtures and H fixtures.

Port: A communication pathway into or out of a computer or networked device such as a server. Well-known applications have standard port numbers.

Power: The rate (in kilowatts) of generating, transferring, or using energy.

Power, active: The product of the rms value of the voltage and the rms value of the inphase component of the current.

Power, apparent: The product of the rms value of the voltage and the rms value of the current.

Power factor: The ratio of active power to apparent power.

Power, instantaneous: The product of the instantaneous voltage multiplied by the instantaneous current.

Power line carrier (PLC): Systems operating on narrow channels between 30 and 50 kHz are frequently used for HV line protective relaying applications.

Power pool: A group of power systems operating as an interconnected system and pooling their resources.

Power, reactive: The product of the rms value of the voltage and the rms value of the quadrature component of the current.

Power system stability: The ability of an electric power system, for a given initial operating condition, to regain a state of operating equilibrium after being subjected to a physical disturbance.

Power transformer: A transformer that transfers electric energy in any part of the circuit between the generator and the distribution primary circuits.

Primary disconnecting devices: Self-coupling separable contacts provided to connect and disconnect the main circuits between the removable element and the housing.

Primary distribution feeder: A feeder operating at primary voltage supplying a distribution circuit.

Primary distribution mains: The conductors that feed from the center of distribution to direct primary loads or to transformers that feed secondary circuits.

Primary distribution network: A network consisting of primary distribution mains.

Primary distribution system: A system of ac distribution for supplying the primaries of distribution transformers from the generating station or substation distribution buses.

Primary distribution trunk line: A line acting as a main source of supply to a distribution system.

Primary feeder: That portion of the primary conductors between the substation or point of supply and the center of distribution.

Primary lateral: That portion of a primary distribution feeder that is supplied by a main feeder or other laterals and extends through the load area with connections to distribution transformers or primary loads.

Primary main feeder: The higher-capacity portion of a primary distribution feeder that acts as a main source of supply to primary laterals or directly connected distribution transformers and primary loads.

Primary network: A network supplying the primaries of transformers whose secondaries may be independent or connected to a secondary network.

Primary open-loop service: A service that consists of a single distribution transformer with dual primary switching, supplied from a single primary circuit that is arranged in an open-loop configuration.

Primary selective service: A service that consists of a single distribution transformer with primary throw-over switching, supplied by two independent primary circuits.

Primary transmission feeder: A feeder connected to a primary transmission circuit.

Primary unit substation: A unit substation in which the low-voltage section is rated above 1000 V.

Protective gear: The apparatus, including protective relays, transformers, and auxiliary equipment, for use in a protective system.

Protective relay: An electrical device whose function is to detect defective lines or apparatus or other power system conditions of an abnormal or dangerous nature and to initiate isolation of a part of an electrical system or to operate an alarm signal in the case of a fault or other abnormal condition.

Protective scheme: The coordinated arrangements for the protective of a power system.

Protective system: A combination of protective gears designed to secure, under predetermined conditions, usually abnormal, the disconnection of an element of a power system or to give an alarm signal or both.

Protective system usage: In protection system, it is used to compare relevant quantities and so replace slower, more conventional devices, based on the high-speed measurement of system parameters.

PT: Abbreviation for potential transformer.

pu: Abbreviation for per unit.

Puller, reel: A device designed to pull a conductor during stringing operations.

Pulse number (p): The number of pulsations (i.e., *cycles of ripple*) of the direct voltage per cycle of alternating voltage (e.g., pulse numbers for three-phase one-way and three-phase two-way rectifier bridges are 3 and 6, respectively).

Radial distribution system: A distribution system that has a single simultaneous path of power flow to the load.

Radial service: A service that consists of a single distribution transformer supplied by a single primary circuit.

Radial system, complete: A radial system that consists of a radial subtransmission circuit, a single substation, and a radial primary feeder with several distribution transformers each supplying radial secondaries; has the lowest degrees of service continuity.

Ratchet demand: The maximum past or present demands that are taken into account to establish billings for previous or subsequent periods.

Rate base: The net plant investment or valuation base specified by a regulatory authority upon which a utility is permitted to earn a specified rate of return.

Rated burden: It is the load that may be imposed on the transformer secondaries by associated meter coils, leads, and other connected devices without causing an error greater than the stated accuracy classification.

Rated continuous current: The maximum 60 Hz rms current that the breaker can carry continuously while it is in the closed position without overheating.

Rated impulse withstand voltage: The maximum crest voltage of a voltage pulse with standard rise and delay times that the breaker insulation can withstand.

Rated insulation class: It denotes the nominal (line-to-line) voltage of a circuit on which it should be used.

Rated interrupting MVA: For a three-phase CB, it is $\sqrt{3}$ times the rated maximum voltage in kV times the rated short-circuit current in kA. It is more common to work with current and voltage ratings than with MVA rating.

Rated interrupting time: The time in cycles on a 60 Hz basis from the instant the trip coil is energized to the instant the fault current is cleared.

Rated low-frequency withstanding voltage: The maximum 60 Hz rms line-to-line voltage that the CB can withstand without insulation damage.

Rated maximum voltage: Designated the maximum rms line-to-line operating voltage. The breaker should be used in systems with an operating voltage less than or equal to this rating.

Rated momentary current: The maximum rms asymmetrical current that the breaker can withstand while in the closed position without damage. Rated momentary current for standard breakers is 1.6 times the symmetrical interrupting capacity.

Rated short-circuit current: The maximum rms symmetrical current that the breaker can safely interrupt at rated maximum voltage.

Rated voltage range factor K: The range of voltage for which the symmetrical interrupting capability times the operating voltage is constant.

Ratio correction factor: The factor by which the marked ratio of a CT must be multiplied to obtain the true ratio.

Reach: A distance relay operates whenever the impedance seen by the relay is less than a prescribed value. This impedance or the corresponding distance is known as the reach of the relay.

Reactive power compensation: Shunt reactors, shunt capacitors, static var systems, and synchronous condensers are used to control voltage. SCs are used to reduce line impedance.

Reactor: An inductive reactor between the dc output of the converter and the load. It is used to smooth the ripple in the dc adequately, to reduce harmonic voltages and currents in the dc line, and to limit the magnitude of fault current. It is also called a *smoothing reactor.*

Recloser: A dual-timing device that can be set to operate quickly to prevent downline fuses from blowing.

Reclosing device: A control device that initiates the reclosing of a circuit after it has been opened by a protective relay.

Reclosing fuse: A combination of two or more fuse holders, fuse units, or fuse links mounted on a fuse support(s), mechanically or electrically interlocked, so that one fuse can be connected into the circuit at a time and the functioning of that fuse automatically connects the next fuse into the circuit, thereby permitting one or more service restorations without replacement of fuse links, refill units, or fuse units.

Reclosing relay: A programming relay whose function is to initiate the automatic reclosing of a CB.

Reclosure: The automatic closing of a circuit-interrupting device following automatic tripping. Reclosing may be programmed for any combination of instantaneous, time-delay, single-shot, multiple-shot, synchronism-check, deadline-live-bus, or dead-bus-live-line operation.

Recovery voltage: The voltage that occurs across the terminals of a pole of a circuit-interrupting device upon interruption of the current.

Rectifier: A converter for changing ac to dc.

Relays: A low-powered electrical device used to activate a high-powered electrical device. (In T & D systems, it is the job of relays to give the tripping commands to the right CBs.)

Remote access: Access to control systems or IED by a user whose operation terminal is not directly connected to the control systems or IED.

Remote backup: Those relays that are located in a separate location and are completely independent of the relays, transducers, batteries, and CBs that they are backing up.

Remote terminal unit (RTU): A hardware that telemeters system-wide data from various field locations (i.e., substations, generating plants to a central location). It includes the entire complement of devices, functional modules, and assemblies that are electrically interconnected to affect the remote station supervisory functions.

Required reserve: The system planned reserve capability needed to ensure a specified standard of service.

Resetting value: The maximum value of the energizing quantity that is insufficient to hold the relay contacts closed after operating.

Resistance: The real part of impedance.

Return on capital: The requirement that is necessary to pay for the cost of investment funds used by the utility.

Ripple: The ac component from dc power supply arising from sources within the power supply. It is expressed in peak, peak-to-peak, rms volts, or as percent rms. Since HVDC converters have large dc smoothing reactors, approximately 1 H, the resultant dc is constant (i.e., free from ripple). However, the direct voltage on the valve side of the smoothing reactor has ripple.

Ripple amplitude: The maximum value of the instantaneous difference between the average and instantaneous value of a pulsating unidirectional wave.

Risk: The probability that a particular threat will exploit a particular vulnerability of an equipment, plant, or system.

Risk management: Decisions to accept exposure or to reduce vulnerabilities by either mitigating the risks or applying cost-effective controls.

SA: Deployment of substation and feeder operating functions and applications ranging from SCADA and alarm processing to integrated volt/var control in order to optimize the management of capital assets and enhance operational and maintenance efficacies with minimal human intervention.

Sag: The distance measured vertically from a conductor to the straight line joining its two points of support. Unless otherwise stated, the sag referred to is the sag at the midpoint of the span.

Sag: A decrease to between 0.1 and 0.9 pu in rms voltage and current at the power frequency for a duration of 0.5 cycles to 1 min.

Sag, final unloaded: The sag of a conductor after it has been subjected for an appreciable period to the loading prescribed for the loading district in which it is situated, or equivalent loading, and the loading removed. Final unloaded sag includes the effect of inelastic deformation.

Sag, initial unloaded: The sag of a conductor prior to the application of any external load.

SAG of a conductor (at any point in a span): The distance measured vertically from the particular point in the conductor to a straight line between its two points of support.

Sag section: The section of line between snub structures. More than one sag section may be required to properly sag the actual length of conductor that has been strung.

Sag span: A span selected within a sag section and used as a control to determine the proper sag of the conductor, thus establishing the proper conductor level and tension. A minimum of two, but normally three, sag spans are required within a sag section to sag properly. In mountainous terrain or where span lengths vary radically, more than three sag spans could be required within a sag section.

SCADA: An abbreviation for supervisory control and data acquisition.

SCADA communication line: The communication link between the utility's control center and the RTU at the substation.

Scheduled interruption: An interruption caused by a scheduled outage.

Scheduled maintenance (generation): Capability that has been scheduled to be out of service for maintenance.

Scheduled outage: An outage that results when a component is deliberately taken out of service at a selected time, usually for purposes of construction, preventive maintenance, or repair. The key test to determine if an outage should be classified as forced or scheduled is as follows: if it is possible to defer the outage when such deferment is desirable, the outage is a scheduled outage; otherwise, the outage is a forced outage. Deferring an outage may be desirable, for example, to prevent overload of facilities or an interruption of service to consumers.

Scheduled outage duration: The period from the initiation of the outage until construction, preventive maintenance, or repair work is completed.

SCV: Abbreviation for steam-cured (cable insulation).

Seasonal diversity: Load diversity between two (or more) electric systems that occurs when their peak loads are in different seasons of the year.

Secondary current rating: The secondary current existing when the transformer is delivering rated kilovolt-amperes at rated secondary voltage.

Secondary disconnecting devices: Self-coupling separable contacts provided to connect and disconnect the auxiliary and control circuits between the removable element and the housing.

Secondary distributed network: A service consisting of a number of network transformer units at a number of locations in an urban load area connected to an extensive secondary cable grid system.

Secondary distribution feeder: A feeder operating at secondary voltage supplying a distribution circuit.

Secondary distribution mains: The conductors connected to the secondaries of distribution transformers from which consumers' services are supplied.

Secondary distribution network: A network consisting of secondary distribution mains.

Secondary fuse: A fuse used on the secondary-side circuits, restricted for use on a low-voltage secondary distribution system that connects the secondaries of distribution transformers to consumers' services.

Secondary mains: Those that operate at utilization voltage and serve as the local distribution main. In radial systems, secondary mains that supply general lighting and small power are usually separated from mains that supply three-phase power because of the dip in voltage caused by starting motors. This dip in voltage, if sufficiently large, causes an objectionable lamp flicker.

Secondary network: It consists of two or more network transformer units connected to a common secondary system and operating continuously in parallel.

Secondary network service: A service that consists of two or more network transformer units connected to a common secondary system and operating continuously in parallel.

Secondary system, banked: A system that consists of several transformers supplied from a single primary feeder, with the low-voltage terminals connected together through the secondary mains.

Secondary unit substation: A unit substation whose low-voltage section is rated 1000 V and below.

Secondary voltage regulation: A VD caused by the secondary system; it includes the drop in the transformer and in the secondary and service cables.

Second-contingency outage: The outage of a secondary primary feeder in addition to the first one.

Sectionalizer: A device that resembles an oil circuit recloser but lacks the interrupting capability.

Security: The measure that a relay will not operate incorrectly for any faults.

Security (in protection): The measure that a relay will not operate incorrectly for any fault.

Security (in relays): The ability of a relay or relaying system never to operate falsely.

Selector: See *Transfer switches.*

Sequence filters: Used in a three-phase systems to measure (and therefore to indicate the presence of) symmetrical components of current and voltage.

Service area: Territory in which a utility system is required or has the right to supply or make available electric service to ultimate consumers.

Service availability index: See *Index of reliability.*

Service drop: The OH conductors, through which electric service is supplied, between the last utility company pole and the point of their connection to the service facilities located at the building or other support used for the purpose.

Service entrance: All components between the point of termination of the OH service drop or underground service lateral and the building main disconnecting device, with the exception of the utility company's metering equipment.

Service entrance conductors: The conductors between the point of termination of the OH service drop or underground service lateral and the main disconnecting device in the building.

Service entrance equipment: Equipment located at the service entrance of a given building that provides overcurrent protection to the feeder and service conductors, provides a means of disconnecting the feeders from energized service conductors, and provides a means of measuring the energy used by the use of metering equipment.

Service lateral: The underground conductors, through which electric service is supplied, between the utility company's distribution facilities and the first point of their connection to the building or area service facilities located at the building or other support used for the purpose.

Setting: The actual value of the energizing or characteristic quantity of which the relay is designed to operate under given conditions.

SF6: Formula for sulfur hexafluoride (gas).

Shielding, effective: A shielding that has zero unprotective width.

Short-circuit selective relay: A relay that functions instantaneously on an excessive value of current.

Shunt capacitor bank: A large number of capacitor units connected in series and parallel arrangement to make up the required voltage and current ratings and connected between line and neutral or between line to line.

Skin effect: The phenomenon by which alternative current tends to flow in the outer layer of a conductor. It is a function of conductor size, frequency, and the relative resistance of the conductor material.

St: Abbreviation for steel.

Stability: The quality whereby a protective system remains in operative under all conditions other than those for which it is specifically designed to operate.

STATCOM: It is a static compensator. It provides variable lagging or leading reactive powers without using inductors or capacitors for var generation.

Static var system: It is a static var compensator that can also control mechanical switching of shunt capacitor banks or reactors.

Strand: One of the wires, or groups of wires, of any stranded conductor.

Stranded conductor: A conductor composed of a group of wires or of any combination of groups of wires. Usually, the wires are twisted together.

Strike distance: The distance that jumped an approaching flash to make contact.

Stroke: The high-current components in a flash. A single flash may contain several strokes.

Submarine cable: A cable designed for service underwater. It is usually a lead-covered cable with a steel armor applied between layers of jute.

Submersible transformer: A transformer so constructed as to be successfully operable when submerged in water under predetermined conditions of pressure and time.

Substation: An assemblage of equipment for purposes other than generation or utilization, through which electric energy in bulk is passed for the purpose of switching or modifying its characteristics. The term substation includes all stations classified as switching, collector bus, distribution, transmission, or bulk power substations.

Substation LAN: A communications network, typically high speed, and within the substation and extending into the switchyard.

Substation local area network (LAN): A technology that is used in a substation environment and facilitates interfacing to process-level equipment (IEDs and PLCs) while providing immunity and isolation to substation noise.

Substation voltage regulation: The regulation of the substation voltage by means of the voltage regulation equipment that can be LTC (load-tap-changing) mechanisms in the substation transformer, a separate regulator between the transformer and low-voltage bus, switched capacitors at the low-voltage bus, or separate regulators located in each individual feeder in the substation.

Subsynchronous: Electrical and mechanical quantities associated with frequencies below the synchronous frequency of a power system.

Subsynchronous oscillation: The exchange of energy between the electrical network and the mechanical spring-mass system of the turbine generator at subsynchronous frequencies.

Subsynchronous resonance: It is an electric power system condition where the electric power network exchanges energy with a turbine generator at one or more of the natural frequencies of the combined system below the synchronous frequency of the system.

Subtransmission: That part of the distribution system between bulk power source(s) (generating stations or power substations) and the distribution substation.

Supersynchronous: Electrical or mechanical quantities associated with frequencies above the synchronous frequency of a power system.

Supervisory control and data acquisition (SCADA): A computer system that performs data acquisition and remote control of a power system.

Supply security: Provision must be made to ensure continuity of supply to consumers even with certain items of plant out of action. Usually, two circuits in parallel are used and a system is said to be secure when continuity is assured. It is the prerequisite in design and operation.

Susceptance: The imaginary part of admittance.

Sustained interruption: The complete loss of voltage (<0.1 pu) on one or more phase conductors for a time greater than 1 min.

SVC: Static var compensator.

Swell: An increase to between 1.1 and 1.8 pu in rms voltage or current at the power frequency for durations from 0.5 cycle to 1 min.

Switch: A device for opening and closing or for changing connections in a circuit.

Switchboard: A large single panel, frame, or assembly of panels on which are mounted (on the face or back or both) switches, fuses, buses, and usually instruments.

Switched capacitor bank: A capacitor bank with switchable capacitors.

Switchgear: A general term covering switching or interrupting devices and their combination with associated control, instrumentation, metering, protective, and regulating devices; also assemblies of these devices with associated interconnections, accessories, and supporting structures.

Switching: Connecting or disconnecting parts of the system from each other. It is accomplished using breakers and/or switches.

Switching time: The period from the time a switching operation is required due to a forced outage until that switching operation is performed.

Switch, isolating: An auxiliary switch for isolating an electric circuit from its source of power; it is operated only after the circuit has been opened by other means.

System: A group of components connected together in some fashion to provide flow of power from one point or points to another point or points.

System interruption duration index: The ratio of the sum of all customer interruption durations per year to the number of customers served. It gives the number of minutes out per customer per year.

Systems: It is used to describe the complete electrical network, generators, loads, and prime movers.

TCR: It is a thyristor controlled reactor.

TCSC: It denotes thyristor-controlled series compensation. It provides fast control and variation of the impedance of the SC bank. It is part of the flexible system (FACTS).

Thyristor (SCR): A thyristor (silicon-controlled rectifier) is a semiconductor device with an anode, a cathode terminal, and a gate for the control of the firing.

Tie lines: The transmission lines between the electric power systems of separate utility companies.

Time delay: An intentional time delay is inserted between the relay decision time and the initiation of the trip action.

Time-delay relay: A relay having an intentional delaying device.

Total demand distortion (TDD): The ratio of the rms of the harmonic current to the rms value of the rated or maximum demand fundamental current, expressed as a percent.

Total harmonic distortion (THD): The ratio of the rms of the harmonic content to the rms value of the fundamental quantity, expressed as a percent of the fundamental.

Transfer bus: A bus used for the purpose of transferring a load.

Transfer switches: The switches that permit feeders or equipment to be connected to a bus.

Transformer ratio (TR): The total ratio of current and VTs. For 200:5 CT and 480:120 VT, $TR = 40 \times 4 = 160$.

Transient forced outage: A component outage whose cause is immediately self-clearing so that the affected component can be restored to service either automatically or as soon as a switch or a CB can be reclosed or a fuse replaced. An example of a transient forced outage is a lightning flashover that does not permanently disable the flashed component.

Traveler: A sheave complete with suspension arm or frame used separately or in groups and suspended from structures to permit the stringing of conductors.

Trip out: A flashover of a line that does not clear itself. It must be cleared by operation of a CB.

Triplen harmonics: A term frequency used to refer to the odd multiples of the third harmonic, which deserve special attention because of their natural tendency to be zero sequence.

True power factor (TPF): The ratio of the active power of the fundamental wave, in watts, to the apparent power of the fundamental wave, in rms volt-amperes (including the harmonic components).

TSC: It is a thyristor switched capacitor.

Ultrahigh speed: It is a term that is not included in the relay standards but is commonly considered to be in operation in 4 ms or less.

Underground distribution system: That portion of a primary or secondary distribution system that is constructed below the earth's surface. Transformers and equipment enclosures for such a system may be located either above or below the surface as long as the served and serving conductors are located underground.

Undervoltage: A voltage that has a value at least 10% below the nominal voltage for a period of time greater than 1 min.

Undervoltage relay: A relay that functions on a given value single-phase ac undervoltage.

Unit: A self-contained relay unit that in conjunction with one or more other relay units performs a complex relay function.

Unit substation: A substation consisting primarily of one or more transformers that are mechanically and electrically connected to and coordinated in design with one or more switchgear or motor control assemblies or combinations thereof.

Unreach: The tendency of the relay to restrain at impedances larger than its setting. That is, it is due to error in relay measurement resulting in wrong operation.

URD: Abbreviation for underground residential distribution.

Utilization factor: The ratio of the maximum demand of a system to the rated capacity of the system.

VD: Abbreviation for voltage drop.

VDIP: Abbreviation for voltage dip.

Voltage, base: A reference value that is a common denominator to the nominal voltage ratings of transmission and distribution lines, transmission and distribution equipment, and utilization equipment.

Voltage collapse: The process by which voltage instability leads to a very low–voltage profile in a significant part of the system.

Voltage dip: A voltage change resulting from a motor starting.

Voltage drop: The difference between the voltage at the transmitting and receiving ends of a feeder, main or service.

Voltage fluctuation: A series of voltage changes or a cyclical variation of the voltage envelope.

Voltage imbalance (or unbalance): The maximum deviation from the average of the three-phase voltages or currents divided by the average of the three-phase voltages or currents, expressed in percent.

Voltage interruption: Disappearance of the supply voltage on one or more phases. It can be momentary, temporary, or sustained.

Voltage magnification: The magnification of capacitor switching oscillatory transient voltage on the primary side by capacitors on the secondary side of a transformer.

Voltage, maximum: The greatest 5 min average or mean voltage.

Voltage, minimum: The least 5 min average or mean voltage.

Voltage, nominal: A nominal value assigned to a circuit or system of a given voltage class for the purpose of convenient designation.

Voltage, rated: The voltage at which operating and performance characteristics of equipment are referred.

Voltage regulation: The percent VD of a line with reference to the receiving-end voltage:

$$\%\text{Regulation} = \frac{\left|\overline{E}_s\right| - \left|\overline{E}_r\right|}{\left|\overline{E}_r\right|} \times 100$$

where

$\left|\overline{E}_s\right|$ is the magnitude of the sending-end voltage
$\left|\overline{E}_r\right|$ is the magnitude of the receiving-end voltage

Voltage regulator: An induction device having one or more windings in shunt with, and excited from, the primary circuit and having one or more windings in series between the primary circuit and the regulated circuit, all suitably adapted and arranged for the control of the voltage or of the phase angle or of both of the regulated circuit.

Voltage, service: Voltage measured at the terminals of the service entrance equipment.

Voltage spread: The difference between maximum and minimum voltages.

Voltage stability: The ability of a power system to maintain steady voltages at all buses in the system after being subjected to a disturbance from a given initial operational condition. It can be either fast (short term, with voltage collapse in the order of fractions of a few seconds) or slow (long term, with voltage collapse in minutes or hours).

Voltage stability problems: Manifested by low system voltage profiles, heavy reactive line flows, inadequate reactive support, and heavy-loaded power systems.

Voltage transformation: It is done by substation power transformers by raising or lowering the voltage.

Voltage transformer: The transformer that is connected across the points at which the voltage is to be measured.

Voltage transformer burdens: The VT burdens are normally expressed as volt-amperes at a designated PF. It may be a W, X, M, Y, or Z where W is 12.5 VA at 0.10 PF, X is 25 VA at 0.70 PF, M is 35 VA at 0.20 PF, Y is 75 VA at 0.85 PF, and Z is 200 VA at 0.85 PF. The complete expression for a CT accuracy classification might be 0.3 at B-0.1, B-0.2, and B-0.5, while the PT might be 0.3 at W, X, M, and Y.

Voltage transformer ratio: Also called the *VT ratio*. It is the ratio of primary to secondary voltage. For a VT rated 480:120, the ratio is 4:1, and for a VT rated 7200:120, it is 60:1.

Voltage, utilization: Voltage measured at the terminals of the machine or device.

VRR: Abbreviation for voltage-regulating relay.

Waveform distortion: A steady-state deviation from an ideal sine wave of power frequency principally characterized by the special content of the deviation.

Weatherability: The ability to operate in all weather conditions. For example, transformers are rated as indoor or outdoor, depending on their construction (including hardware).

Withstand voltage: The BIL that can be repeatedly applied to an equipment without any flashover, disruptive charge, puncture, or other electrical failure, under specified test conditions.

XLPE: Abbreviation for cross-linked polyethylene (cable insulation).

REFERENCES

1. IEEE Committee Report. Proposed definitions of terms for reporting and analyzing outages of electrical transmission and distribution facilities and interruptions, *IEEE Trans. Power Appar. Syst.* PAS-87 (5), May 1968, 1318–1323.
2. IEEE Committee Report. Guidelines for use in developing a specific underground distribution system design standard, *IEEE Trans. Power Appar. Syst.* PAS-97 (3), May/June 1978, 810–827.
3. *IEEE Standard Definitions in Power Operations Terminology*, IEEE Standard 346-1973, November 2, 1973.
4. *Proposed Standard Definitions of General Electrical and Electronics Terms*, IEEE Standard 270, 1966.
5. Pender, H. and Del Mar, W. A. *Electrical Engineers' Handbook—Electrical Power*, 4th edn., Wiley, New York, 1962.
6. *National Electrical Safety Code*, 1977 edn., ANSI C2, IEEE, New York, November 1977.
7. Fink, D. G. and Carroll, J. M., eds. *Standard Handbook for Electrical Engineers*, 10th edn., McGraw-Hill, New York, 1969.
8. *IEEE Standard Dictionary of Electrical and Electronics Terms*, IEEE, New York, 1972.

Index

For Product Safety Concerns and Information please contact our EU representative GPSR@taylorandfrancis.com Taylor & Francis Verlag GmbH, Kaufingerstraße 24, 80331 München, Germany

Printed and bound by CPI Group (UK) Ltd, Croydon, CR0 4YY

01/05/2025

01858608-0001